AF691957

Orthopaedic Basic Science

Foundations of Clinical Practice

FIFTH EDITION

Wolters Kluwer
Philadelphia • Baltimore • New York • London
Buenos Aires • Hong Kong • Sydney • Tokyo

AAOS
American Academy of Orthopaedic Surgeons

Orthopaedic Basic Science

Foundations of Clinical Practice

FIFTH EDITION

Edited by
ROY K. AARON, MD
Professor, Orthopedic Surgery
Professor, Molecular Pharmacology, Physiology, and Biotechnology
Warren Alpert Medical School of Brown University
Providence, Rhode Island

Wolters Kluwer
Philadelphia • Baltimore • New York • London
Buenos Aires • Hong Kong • Sydney • Tokyo

AAOS
American Academy of Orthopaedic Surgeons

AAOS
AMERICAN ACADEMY OF ORTHOPAEDIC SURGEONS

Board of Directors, 2019-2020

Kristy L. Weber, MD
President

Joseph A. Bosco, III, MD
1st Vice President

Daniel K. Guy, MD
2nd Vice President

Alan S. Hilibrand, MD, MBA
Treasurer

David A. Halsey, MD
Past President

Robert M. Orfaly, MD
Chair BOC

Thomas S. Muzzonigro, MD
Chair-Elect BOC

Wayne A. Johnson, MD
Secretary BOC

Dirk H. Alander, MD, MHA
Chair BOS

C. Craig Satterlee, MD
Chair-Elect BOS

Kevin D. Plancher, MD, MPH, MS
Secretary BOS

James J. Balaschak
Lay Member

Rachel Y. Goldstein, MD
Member at Large

James R. Ficke, MD
Member at Large

Elizabeth G. Matzkin, MD
Member at Large

Thomas W. Throckmorton, MD
Member at Large

Thomas E. Arend, Jr., Esq., CAE
Ex-Officio

Staff
American Academy of Orthopaedic Surgeons

Anna Salt Troise, MBA, *Chief Education Strategist*

Hans Koelsch, PhD, *Director, Publishing Partner Relationships*

Lisa Claxton Moore, *Senior Manager, Editorial*

Steven Kellert, *Senior Editor*

Wolters Kluwer Health

Brian Brown, *Director, Medical Practice*

Stacey Sebring, *Senior Development Editor*

Kerry McShane, *Senior Editorial Coordinator*

Erin Cantino, *Portfolio Marketing Manager*

David Saltzberg, *Production Project Manager*

Stephen Druding, *Design Coordinator*

Beth Welsh, *Senior Manufacturing Coordinator*

TNQ Technologies, *Prepress Vendor*

The material presented in the *Orthopaedic Basic Science, Fifth Edition* has been made available by the American Academy of Orthopaedic Surgeons for educational purposes only. This material is not intended to present the only, or necessarily best, methods or procedures for the medical situations discussed, but rather is intended to represent an approach, view, statement, or opinion of the author(s) or producer(s), which may be helpful to others who face similar situations. Some drugs or medical devices demonstrated in Academy courses or described in Academy print or electronic publications have not been cleared by the Food and Drug Administration (FDA) or have been cleared for specific uses only. The FDA has stated that it is the responsibility of the physician to determine the FDA clearance status of each drug or device he or she wishes to use in clinical practice. Furthermore, any statements about commercial products are solely the opinion(s) of the author(s) and do not represent an Academy endorsement or evaluation of these products. These statements may not be used in advertising or for any commercial purpose.

All rights reserved. No part of this publication may be reproduced, stored in a retrieval system, or transmitted, in any form, or by any means, electronic, mechanical, photocopying, recording, or otherwise, without prior written permission from the publisher.

ISBN 978-1-9751-4816-4

Library of Congress Control Number: Cataloging in Publication data available on request from publisher.

Printed in China

Published 2021 by the
American Academy of Orthopaedic Surgeons
9400 West Higgins Road
Rosemont, Illinois 60018

Copyright 2021 by the American Academy of Orthopaedic Surgeons

Bone and Joint Initiative USA

CCS1219

Acknowledgments

EDITORIAL BOARD
ORTHOPAEDIC BASIC SCIENCE 5

Editors

Roy K. Aaron, MD
Professor, Orthopedic Surgery
Professor, Molecular Pharmacology, Physiology, and Biotechnology
Warren Alpert Medical School of Brown University
Providence, Rhode Island

Section Reviewers

Kevin C. Baker, PhD *(Basic Disciplines in Orthopaedic Surgery)*
Director, Orthopaedic Research
Department of Orthopaedic Surgery
Beaumont Health
Royal Oak, Michigan

Joshua J. Jacobs, MD *(Basic Disciplines in Orthopaedic Surgery)*
William A. Hark, MD/Susanne G. Swift Professor and Chairman, Department of Orthopaedic Surgery
Vice Provost for Research
Rush University
Chicago, Illinois

Linda J. Sandell, PhD, C-IAYT *(Structure and Function of Musculoskeletal Tissues)*
Editor in Chief, Journal of Orthopaedic Research
Professor Emerita, Department of Orthopaedic Surgery
Washington University
St. Louis, Missouri

Robert H. Brophy, MD *(Pathophysiology and Orthopaedic Medicine)*
Professor
Department of Orthopaedic Surgery
Washington University School of Medicine
St. Louis, Missouri

Robert L. Sah, MD, ScD *(Repair and Regeneration)*
Professor
Department of Bioengineering
University of California, San Diego
La Jolla, California

Barbara D. Boyan, PhD *(Repair and Regeneration)*
Professor, Department of Biomedical Engineering
Alice T. and William H. Goodwin, Jr. Dean
College of Engineering
Virginia Commonwealth University
Richmond, Virginia

Kurt P. Spindler, MD *(Principles of Clinical Information)*
Vice-Chair of Research Orthopaedic and Rheumatology Professor, Orthopaedic Surgery
Cleveland Clinic
Cleveland, Ohio

Patricia D. Franklin, MD, MBA, MPH *(Principles of Clinical Information)*
Professor and Co-Director, Outcomes and Measurement Hub
Department of Medical Social Sciences
Northwestern University Feinberg School of Medicine
Chicago, Illinois

We want to thank Ms. Jennifer Racine-Avila for her editorial and graphics guidance and digital support. Her contributions to this edition were invaluable.

© 2021 American Academy of Orthopaedic Surgeons

Contributors

Roy K. Aaron, MD
Professor, Orthopedic Surgery
Professor, Molecular Pharmacology, Physiology, and Biotechnology
Warren Alpert Medical School of Brown University
Providence, Rhode Island

Kristen Allen, BS, RAC
Engagement Partner
Quality and Regulatory Affairs
Bruder Consulting & Venture Group
Franklin Lakes, New Jersey

Tamara Alliston, PhD
Professor
Department of Orthopaedic Surgery
University of California, San Francisco
San Francisco, California

Thomas P. Andriacchi, PhD
Professor (Emeritus)
Department of Mechanical Engineering
Stanford University
Stanford, California

Hiba K. Anis, MD
Research Fellow
Department of Orthopaedic Surgery
Cleveland Clinic Foundation
Cleveland, Ohio

Valentin Antoci Jr, MD, PhD
Director, Outpatient Adult Reconstruction
Assistant Professor of Orthopedic Surgery
Department of Orthopedic Surgery
Warren Alpert Medical School of Brown University
Providence, Rhode Island

Gerard A. Ateshian, PhD
Andrew Walz Professor of Mechanical Engineering
Professor of Biomedical Engineering
Department of Mechanical Engineering
Columbia University
New York, New York

Karsyn N. Bailey, BS
MD/PhD Candidate
UC Berkeley - UCSF Graduate Program in Bioengineering
University of California, San Francisco
San Francisco, California

Spencer Bailey, BS, MBA
Engagement Partner
Reimbursement and Health Economics
Bruder Consulting & Venture Group
Franklin Lakes, New Jersey

Keith D. Baldwin, MD, MSPT, MPH
Associate Professor
Department of Othopedic Surgery
University of Pennsylvania
Philadelphia, Pennsylvania

Alexander M. Ballatori, BS
Research Study Coordinator
Department of Orthopaedic Surgery
University of California, San Francisco
San Francisco, California

Joel A. Block, MD
The Willard L. Wood, MD Professor
Director, Division of Rheumatology
Rush Medical College
Rush University Medical Center
Chicago, Illinois

Barbara D. Boyan, PhD
Professor, Department of Biomedical Engineering
Alice T. and William H. Goodwin, Jr. Dean
College of Engineering
Virginia Commonwealth University
Richmond, Virginia

Brendan F. Boyce, MBChB
Professor
Department of Pathology and Laboratory Medicine
University of Rochester Medical Center
Rochester, New York

© 2021 American Academy of Orthopaedic Surgeons

Caroline Boyle, BA
Department of Sports Medicine
Hospital for Special Surgery
New York, New York

Kevin J. Bozic, MD, MBA
Professor and Chair
Department of Surgery and Perioperative Care
Dell Medical School at The University of Texas at Austin
Austin, Texas

Robert H. Brophy, MD
Professor, Department of Orthopaedic Surgery
Washington University School of Medicine
St. Louis, Missouri

Scott P. Bruder, MD, PhD
Founder and CEO
Bruder Consulting & Venture Group
Franklin Lakes, New Jersey

David B. Burr, PhD
Distinguished Professor Emeritus
Department of Anatomy, Cell Biology, and Physiology
Indiana University School of Medicine
Department of Biomedical Engineering
Indiana University-Purdue University, Indianapolis (IUPUI)
Indianapolis, Indiana

William A. Cantrell, BS
Medical Student, Orthopaedic Surgery
Department of Surgery
Cleveland Clinic
Cleveland, Ohio

Arthur L. Caplan, PhD
Drs. William F. and Virginia Connolly Mitty Professor of Bioethics
Department of Population Health
NYU School of Medicine
NYU Langone Health
New York, New York

Andrew K. Chan, MD
Resident Physician
Department of Neurological Surgery
University of California, San Francisco
San Francisco, California

Qian Chen, PhD
Michael G. Ehrlich, MD Professor of Orthopaedic Research
Department of Orthopaedics
Warren Alpert Medical School of Brown University
Rhode Island Hospital
Providence, Rhode Island

George J. Christ, PhD
Professor of Biomedical Engineering and Orthopaedic Surgery
Mary Muilenberg Stamp Professor of Orthopaedic Research
Director of Basic and Translational Research in Orthopaedic Surgery
Co-Director, Center for Advanced Biomanufacturing
Laboratory of Regenerative Therapeutics
University of Virginia, Virginia
Charlottesville, Virginia

Margaret E. Cooke, MD
Hand and Upper Extremity Surgery Fellow
Department of Orthopaedic Surgery
Hospital for Special Surgery
New York, New York

Alexus M. Cooper, BS
Research Fellow
Rothman Orthopaedic Institute
Thomas Jefferson University
Philadelphia, Pennsylvania

Matthew M. Counihan, MD
Orthopaedic Surgery Resident
Department of Orthopaedic Surgery
University of Pennsylvania
Philadelphia, Pennsylvania

Joseph O. Ehiorobo, MD
Research Fellow
Department of Orthopaedic Surgery
Northwell Health
New York, New York

Jennifer C. Erhart-Hledik, PhD
Instructor
Department of Orthopaedic Surgery
Stanford University
Stanford, California

Andrew R. Evans, MD, FACS
Assistant Professor of Orthopedic Surgery
Department of Orthopedic Surgery
Warren Alpert Medical School of Brown University
Providence, Rhode Island

Aaron J. Fields, PhD
Associate Professor
Department of Orthopaedic Surgery
University of California, San Francisco
San Francisco, California

© 2021 American Academy of Orthopaedic Surgeons

Jeffrey S. Fischgrund, MD
Professor and Chairman
Department of Orthopaedic Surgery
Oakland University, Willaim Beaumont School of Medicine
Royal Oak, Michigan

Patricia D. Franklin, MD, MBA, MPH
Professor and Co-Director, Outcomes and Measurement Hub
Department of Medical Social Sciences
Northwestern University Feinberg School of Medicine
Chicago, Illinois

Erica G. Gacasan, MS
Graduate Student
Department of Bioengineering
University of California, San Diego
La Jolla, California

Joel J. Gagnier, ND, MSc, PhD
Associate Professor
Department of Orthopaedic Surgery, Michigan Medicine
Department of Epidemiology, School of Public Health
University of Michigan
Ann Arbor, Michigan

Yun Gao, MD, PhD
Postdoctoral Research Associate
Department of Orthopaedic
Alpert Medical School of Brown University
Rhode Island Hospital
Providence, Rhode Island

Dioscaris R. Garcia, PhD
Assistant Professor
Department of Orthopaedics
Warren Alpert Medical School of Brown University
Providence, Rhode Island

Louis C. Gerstenfeld, PhD
Professor
Department of Orthopaedic Surgery
Boston University Medical Campus
Boston, Massachusetts

Austin P. Gillies, BA
Clinical Research Assistant
Division of Orthopaedic Surgery and Sports Medicine
Children's National Hospital
Washington, District of Columbia

Jillian L. Glasser, BA
Adult Reconstruction Research Fellow
Department of Orthopaedics
Warren Alpert Medical School of Brown University
Providence, Rhode Island

Stuart B. Goodman, MD, PhD, FRCSC, FACS, FBSE, FICORS
Robert L. and Mary Ellenburg Professor of Surgery
Professor, Department of Orthopaedic Surgery and Bioengineering
Stanford University Medical Center Outpatient Center
Redwood City, California

Karan Goswami, MD, MRCS
Research Fellow and PhD Candidate
Rothman Orthopaedic Institute
Thomas Jefferson University
Philadelphia, Pennsylvania

Roman A. Hayda, MD, Col (Ret.)
Associate Professor of Orthopedic Surgery
Department of Orthopedic Surgery
Warren Alpert Medical School of Brown University
Providence, Rhode Island

Michael Hausman, MD
Robert K. Lippmann Professor of Orthopaedic Surgery
Vice-Chairman, Department of Orthopaedic Surgery
Chief, Upper Extremity Surgery
Mount Sinai Health System
New York, New York

Jill Helms, DDS, PhD
Professor
Division of Plastic and Reconstructive Surgery
Department of Surgery
School of Medicine
Stanford University
Palo Alto, California

Patrick D.G. Henry, MD, FRSCS
Assistant Professor
Division of Orthopaedic Surgery, Sunnybrook Health Sciences Centre
University of Toronto
Toronto, Canada

Johnny Huard, PhD
Chief Scientific Officers
Steadman Philippon Research Institute
Director
Center for Regenerative Sports Medicine
Vail, Colorado

Clark T. Hung, PhD
Professor of Biomedical Engineering and Orthopedic Surgery
Department of Biomedical Engineering
Columbia University
New York, New York

© 2021 American Academy of Orthopaedic Surgeons

Jonathan E. Isaacs, MD
Herman M. & Vera H. Nachman Distinguished Research Professor
Professor and Chief, Division of Hand Surgery
Vice Chairman of Research and Education, Department of Orthopedic Surgery
VCU Medical Center
Hand and Wrist, Orthopedic Microsurgical Reconstruction
Richmond, Virginia

Jameel Iqbal, MD, PhD
Senior Faculty
Mount Sinai Bone Program
Icahn School of Medicine at Mount Sinai
New York, New York

Chathuraka T. Jayasuriya, PhD
Assistant Professor
Department of Orthopaedics
Warren Alpert Medical School of Brown University
Providence, Rhode Island

Derek R. Jenkins, MD
Assistant Professor
Department of Orthopaedic Surgery
Warren Alpert Medical School of Brown University
Providence, Rhode Island

Kenton Kaufman, PhD, PE
W. Hall Wendel Jr Musculoskeletal Research Professor
Professor of Biomedical Engineering
Departments of Orthopedic Surgery
Physiology and Biomedical Engineering
Mayo Clinic
Rochester, Minnesota

Oran D. Kennedy, PhD
Research Lecturer
Department of Anatomy and Regenerative Medicine
Royal College of Surgeons in Ireland
Dublin, Ireland

Jad G. Khalil, MD, FAOA
Assistant Professor of Orthopaedic Surgery
Oakland University William Beaumont Hospital
Royal Oak, Michigan

Se-Min Kim, MD
Assistant Professor
Mount Sinai Beth Israel
Icahn School of Medicine at Mount Sinai
New York, New York

Eiki Koyama, DDM, PhD
Associate Professor
Division of Orthopaedic Surgery
The Children's Hospital of Philadelphia
Philadelphia, Pennsylvania

Jeffrey K. Lange, MD
Instructor
Department of Orthopaedic Surgery
Harvard Medical School
Brigham and Women's Hospital
Boston, Massachusetts

Steve K. Lee, MD
Associate Professor of Orthopedic Surgery
Department of Orthopedic Surgery
Hospital for Special Surgery
Weill Medical College of Cornell University
New York, New York

Francis Y. Lee, MD, PhD
Department of Orthopedics and Rehabilitation
Department of Pathology
Yale University School of Medicine
New Haven, Connecticut

Zhijun Li, MD, PhD
Postdoctoral Researcher,
Division of Plastic and Reconstructive Surgery,
Department of Surgery,
School of Medicine,
Stanford University,
Palo Alto, California

Heng An Lin, MBBS, MMEd(Ortho), FRCSEd
Consultant Orthopaedic Surgeon
Department of Orthopaedic Surgery
Sengkang General Hospital Singapore Health Services
Singapore

Kenneth M. Lin, MD
Resident Physician
Department of Orthopaedic Surgery
Hospital for Special Surgery
New York, New York

Jeffrey C. Lotz, PhD
David S. Bradford, MD, Endowed Chair
Vice Chair for Research
Professor
Department of Orthopaedic Surgery
University of California, San Francisco
San Francisco, California

© 2021 American Academy of Orthopaedic Surgeons

Robert J. Majeska, PhD
Professor
Department of Biomedical Engineering
Grove School of Engineering
City College of New York
New York, New York

Anne-Marie Malfait, MD, PhD
Professor
Department of Internal Medicine
Rush University Medical Center
Chicago, Illinois

Niv Marom, MD
Department of Sports Medicine
Hospital for Special Surgery
New York, New York

Robert G. Marx, MD
Attending Orthopedic Surgeon
Professor of Orthopedic Surgery
Department of Sports Medicine
Hospital for Special Surgery
Weill Medical College of Cornell University
New York, New York

Robert L. Mauck, PhD
Mary Black Ralston Professor of Orthopaedic Surgery
Professor of Bioengineering
Department of Orthopaedic Surgery
University of Pennsylvania
Philadelphia, Pennsylvania

Courtney M. Mazur, BS
PhD Candidate
UC Berkeley - UCSF Graduate Program in Bioengineering
University of California, San Francisco
San Francisco, California

Michael J. McClure, PhD
Assistant Professor
Department of Biomedical Engineering
Virginia Commonwealth University
Richmond, Virginia

Jerry Menikoff, MD, JD
Director
Office for Human Research Protections
Department of Health & Human Services
Rockville, Maryland

Rachel E. Miller, PhD
Assistant Professor
Department of Internal Medicine
Rush University Medical Center
Chicago, Illinois

Michael A. Mont, MD
Chief of Joint Reconstruction, Vice President of Strategic Initiatives
Department of Orthopaedic Surgery
Northwell Health
New York, New York

Douglas C. Moore, MS
Clinical Assistant Professor
Associate Director, Bioengineering Laboratory
Department of Orthopaedic Surgery
Warren Alpert Medical School of Brown University
Providence, Rhode Island

Elise F. Morgan, PhD
Department of Mechanical Engineering
Boston University
Boston, Massachusetts

Saam Morshed, MD, PhD, MPH
Associate Professor
Departments of Orthopaedic Surgery, Epidemiology and Biostatistics
University of California, San Francisco
San Francisco, California

Maria New, MD
Professor
Department of Pediatrics
Icahn School of Medicine at Mount Sinai
New York, New York

Regis J. O'Keefe, MD, PhD
Fred C. Reynolds Professor and Chair
Department of Orthopaedic Surgery
Washington University
St. Louis, Missouri

Brett D. Owens, MD
Professor of Orthopaedics
Department of Orthopaedic Surgery
Warren Alpert Medical School of Brown University
Providence, Rhode Island

© 2021 American Academy of Orthopaedic Surgeons

Maurizio Pacifici, PhD
Professor and Director of Orthopaedic Research
Division of Orthopaedic Surgery
The Children's Hospital of Philadelphia
Philadelphia, Pennsylvania

Javad Parvizi, MD, FRCS
James Edwards Professor of Orthopaedic Surgery
Rothman Orthopaedic Institute
Thomas Jefferson University
Philadelphia, Pennsylvania

Joseph T. Patterson, MD
Clinical Instructor
Department of Orthopaedic Surgery and Sports Medicine
University of Washington
Seattle, Washington

Michael Pazianas, MD
Institute of Musculoskeletal Sciences
Oxford University
Oxford, England

Christian A. Pean, MD, MS
Resident Physician
Department of Orthopedic Surgery
NYU Langone Orthopedic Hospital
New York, New York

Vincent D. Pellegrini Jr, MD
Professor and Vice Chair for Education and Research
Department of Orthopaedics
Dartmouth-Hitchcock Medical Center
Geisel School of Medicine at Dartmouth
Lebanon, New Hampshire

James Petricek, MSE, MBA
Vice President
Bruder Consulting & Venture Group
Franklin Lakes, New Jersey

Marc J. Philippon, MD
Managing Partner
The Steadman Clinic
Co-Chairman of the Board
Steadman Philippon Research Institute
Vail, Colorado

Sameer K. Puri, MD
Assistant Professor, Hand and Upper Extremity Surgery
Department of Orthopaedic Surgery
Loyola University Medical Center
Stritch School of Medicine
Maywood, Illinois

Jennifer Racine-Avila, MBA
Program Manager, Clinical/Translational Research
Department of Orthopaedic Surgery
Warren Alpert Medical School of Brown University
Providence, Rhode Island

Muhammad Farooq Rai, PhD
Assistant Professor
Department of Orthopaedic Surgery
Washington University
St. Louis, Missouri

Sudheer K. Ravuri, PhD
Steadman Philippon Research Institute
Deputy Director
Center for Regenerative Sports Medicine
Vail, Colorado

Scott A. Rodeo, MD
Co-Chief Emeritus, Sports Medicine and Shoulder Service
Vice Chair of Orthopaedic Research
Co-Director, Orthopaedic Soft Tissue Research Program
Professor, Orthopaedic Surgery, Weill Medical College of Cornell University
Attending Orthopaedic Surgeon, The Hospital for Special Surgery
Head Team Physician, New York Giants Football
New York City, New York

James Ryaby, PhD
Chief Scientific Officer
Orthofix Inc.
Lewisville, Texas

Robert L. Sah, MD, ScD
Professor
Department of Bioengineering
University of California, San Diego
La Jolla, California

Mitchell B. Schaffler, PhD
CUNY Distinguished Professor and Wallace H. Coulter Professor
Department of Biomedical Engineering
Grove School of Engineering
City College of New York
New York, New York

David W. Shearer, MD, MPH
Assistant Professor in Residence
Department of Orthopaedic Surgery
University of California, San Francisco
San Francisco, California

© 2021 American Academy of Orthopaedic Surgeons

Anita Shukla, PhD
Assistant Professor of Engineering
School of Engineering, Center for Biomedical Engineering
Institute for Molecular and Nanoscale Innovation
Brown University
Providence, Rhode Island

Hamish Simpson, BM, BCh, DM(Oxon), MA(Cantab), FRCS(Eng & Ed)
Professor of Orthopaedics and Trauma
Department of Orthopaedic Surgery
University of Edinburgh
Edinburgh, Scotland, United Kingdom

Nipun Sodhi, MD
Resident
Department of Orthopaedic Surgery
Northwell Health
New York, New York

Louis J. Soslowsky, PhD
Fairhill Professor of Orthopaedic Surgery
Associate Dean for Research Integration
University of Pennsylvania
Philadelphia, Pennsylvania

Kurt P. Spindler, MD
Vice-Chair of Research Orthopaedic and Rheumatology, Professor
Orthopaedic Surgery
Cleveland Clinic
Cleveland, Ohio

Charit Taneja, MD
Resident Physician
Department of Medicine
Mount Sinai Beth Israel
Icahn School of Medicine at Mount Sinai
New York, New York

David J. Tennent, MD, MAJ MC
Department of Orthopedic Surgery
Keller Army Community Hospital
United States Military Academy
West Point, New York
Assistant Professor of Surgery
Uniformed Services University of the Health Sciences
School of Medicine
Bethesda, Maryland

Laura L. Tosi, MD
Associate Professor Pediatrics and Orthopaedics
Division of Orthopaedic Surgery and Sports Medicine
Children's National Hospital
The George Washington University
Washington, District of Columbia

John Twomey-Kozak, BS
Orthopaedic Research Assistant
Department of Orthopaedic Research
Warren Alpert Medical School of Brown University
Providence, Rhode Island

Hajime Utsunomiya, MD, PhD
Steadman Philippon Research Institute
Center for Regenerative Sports Medicine
Vail, Colorado

Emily A. Van Kouwenberg, MD
Assistant Professor of Surgery
Department of Surgery, Division of Plastic and Reconstructive Surgery
Rutgers Robert Wood Johnson Medical School
New Brunswick, New Jersey

Joseph M. Wallace, PhD
Associate Professor
Department of Biomedical Engineering
Indiana University-Purdue University, Indianapolis (IUPUI)
Indianapolis, Indiana

David Wasserstein, MD, MSc, MPH, FRCSC
Assistant Professor
Division of Orthopaedic Surgery, Sunnybrook Health Sciences Centre
University of Toronto
Toronto, Canada

Brad A. Webb, DO
Medical Education, Orthopedic Surgery
Grandview Hospital
Dayton, Ohio

Daniel Weltsch, MD
Department of Orthopedic Surgery
Tel Aviv University
Tel Aviv, Israel

Taylor J. Wiley, MD
University Orthopedics
East Providence, Rhode Island

© 2021 American Academy of Orthopaedic Surgeons

Rolanda A. Willacy, BA
Clinical Research Assistant
Division of Orthopaedic Surgery and Sports Medicine
Children's National Hospital
Washington, District of Columbia

Lianping Xing, PhD
Department of Pathology and Center for Musculoskeletal Research
University of Rochester Medical Center
Rochester, New York

Tony Yuen, PhD
Assistant Professor
Mount Sinai Bone Program
Icahn School of Medicine at Mount Sinai
New York, New York

Mone Zaidi, MD, PhD
Professor
Mount Sinai Bone Program
Icahn School of Medicine at Mount Sinai
New York, New York

Michael J. Zuscik, PhD
Mack Clayton Professor and Vice Chair of Research
Department of Orthopedics
Anschutz Medical Campus
University of Colorado
Aurora, Colorado

© 2021 American Academy of Orthopaedic Surgeons

Preface

This edition represents the scientific basis of orthopaedic surgery as of 2020. It is intended to inform clinical decision making by providing the basic sciences in a clinically relevant context.

The production of the fifth edition of *Orthopaedic Basic Science* was a substantial undertaking contributed to by each of the authors. The author list is comprised of senior scientists and clinicians, and rising stars, a healthy mixture that reflects well on both sustained personal commitments and expectations for the future.

This edition benefitted from an outstanding Editorial Advisory Board that provided important guidance on the inclusion of new subject matter and the revision of older material with a contemporary focus, as well as insightful reviews.

Reflecting the growth in orthopaedic scientific information, all the previously included chapters have been revised and many new chapters have been added. Molecular biology has been refocused to emphasize the role of epigenetics. Biomaterials, repair, and tissue engineering are also emphasized. The significance of articular crosstalk is presented together with new chapters on joint biology and osteoarthritis. Consideration of gender differences in preclinical and clinical studies recognizes the spectrum of biological responses and the presentation of metabolic bone diseases acknowledges the importance of secondary fracture prevention. A completely redone section on the generation of clinical information recognizes advances in methodology, the assessment of large databases and the growth of registries, and best-practice guidelines.

Two individuals from outside of the musculoskeletal community graciously made singular contributions. Arthur Caplan, the internationally recognized ethicist, provided a chapter on the ethics of clinical practice. Jerry Menikoff, Director of the Office of Human Research Protections at the Department of Health and Human Services, was extremely generous with his time and insights in contributing to the chapter on the ethics of clinical research in this, the year that the US Common Rule was, for the first time, revised.

That this is a fifth edition in a series recognizes that it is part of the ongoing development of the basic and clinical sciences. We are grateful to those who preceded us in revealing the nature of the musculoskeletal system upon which we could build. Isaac Newton famously paraphrased John of Salisbury, who wrote in 1159:

> "We are like dwarfs sitting on the shoulders of giants. We see more, and things that are more distant, than they did, not because our sight is superior or because we are taller than they, but because they raise us up, and by their great stature add to ours."

We are mindful that, during the writing of this book, we lost three of those giants, Henry Mankin, Michael Ehrlich, and Adele Boskey, all of whom were part of a generation that provided the framework for modern musculoskeletal science and clinical orthopaedics.

We must be mindful also that, as there were editions that preceded us, so will there be editions that succeed us. We can take pleasure in this continuum, and we can be grateful that we are part of the unfolding of science, while at the same time recognizing that, someday, there will be other volumes, other authors, and new knowledge. To those who are coming, I can recommend Louis Pasteur's words, "*Chance favors the prepared mind,*" and be optimistic that more secrets will be uncovered and that human health will be improved.

Roy Kenneth Aaron, MD
Providence, Rhode Island

Contents

Section 1

BASIC DISCIPLINES IN ORTHOPAEDIC SURGERY

Section Editors: Kevin C. Baker, PhD and Joshua J. Jacobs, MD

Section 2

STRUCTURE AND FUNCTION OF MUSCULOSKELETAL TISSUES

Section Editors: Linda J. Sandell, PhD, C-IAYT and Roy K. Aaron, MD

© 2021 American Academy of Orthopaedic Surgeons

© 2021 American Academy of Orthopaedic Surgeons

Section 5

PRINCIPLES OF CLINICAL INFORMATION

Section Editors: Kurt P. Spindler, MD and Patricia D. Franklin, MD, MBA, MPH

© 2021 American Academy of Orthopaedic Surgeons

1

BASIC DISCIPLINES IN ORTHOPAEDIC SURGERY

SECTION EDITORS

Kevin C. Baker, PhD
Joshua J. Jacobs, MD

1

Genetics, Gene Expression, and Epigenetics

Muhammad Farooq Rai, PhD
Regis J. O'Keefe, MD, PhD
Robert H. Brophy, MD

Keywords: *epigenetic modifications; epigenome; gene regulation; genome; transcriptome*

INTRODUCTION

Molecular genetics has improved the early detection of diseases through the identification of genetic markers. Epigenetics is a subdiscipline of genetics. Epigenetics refers to modifications independent of the nucleotide sequence that influence the folding of double helix DNA and regulate gene expression.

Genetics is now considered not merely a fundamental science but an applied science, applications of which are extending beyond gene mutations. Information on the coding and regulatory sequences facilitates the identification of disease-causing genes and gene variants. Some of these approaches employ gene expression strategies to measure the expression level as well as expression pattern of a transcript, a set of transcripts, or genome-wide transcripts in a disease. Both the magnitude and pattern of transcript expression provide further insight into dynamic differences in the genetic code and help measure even the smallest changes in the transcripts, thus facilitating the detection of transcript alterations associated with complex diseases such as osteoarthritis (OA). However, gene (transcript) expression changes are driven not only by the coding sequence of the genome (which makes up of 2% to 3% of human genome) but also by the large noncoding sequence (previously thought to be junk DNA) as well as epigenetic changes beyond the DNA sequence itself. For example, all cells in the human body contain the same DNA sequence, yet the function of each cell is different as changes in gene expression are mediated by other transcription-level changes commonly known as epigenetic modifications. Alterations in genes, gene expression, and epigenetic modifications may be a window into the early diagnosis of diseases and identification of patients at risk for developing a disease such as knee OA after meniscus or ligament injuries.

Genetic, transcriptomic, and epigenetic analyses generate a large number of big datasets. These datasets require sophisticated computational software and informational pipelines to maximize the extraction of useful information. This has revolutionized the field of computational biology, thus reshaping molecular genetics as a quantitative and computationally intensive science.

GENETICS

Every cell in the human body holds about 2 m of DNA, which contains the genetic information for every eukaryotic organism to sustain life. The entire genetic material in our body is termed as the genome. All nucleated cells contain chromosomes. Humans have altogether 46 chromosomes (23 pairs) stowed in the nucleus that contain DNA, which is composed of nucleic acid sequences that form genes. DNA is made up of a combination of four nucleotides: guanine (G), cytosine (C), adenine (A), and thymine (T) (**Figure 1**). Genes are a sequence or region of DNA that contains instructions for

Dr. Rai or an immediate family member serves as a board member, owner, officer, or committee member of the Orthopaedic Research Society; Dr. O'Keefe or an immediate family member has received royalties from Fate Therapeutics and serves as a board member, owner, officer, or committee member of the American Orthopaedic Association; and Dr. Brophy or an immediate family member serves as a board member, owner, officer, or committee member of the American Academy of Orthopaedic Surgeons, the American Orthopaedic Association, and the American Orthopaedic Society for Sports Medicine.

©Copyright 2021 American Academy of Orthopaedic Surgeons

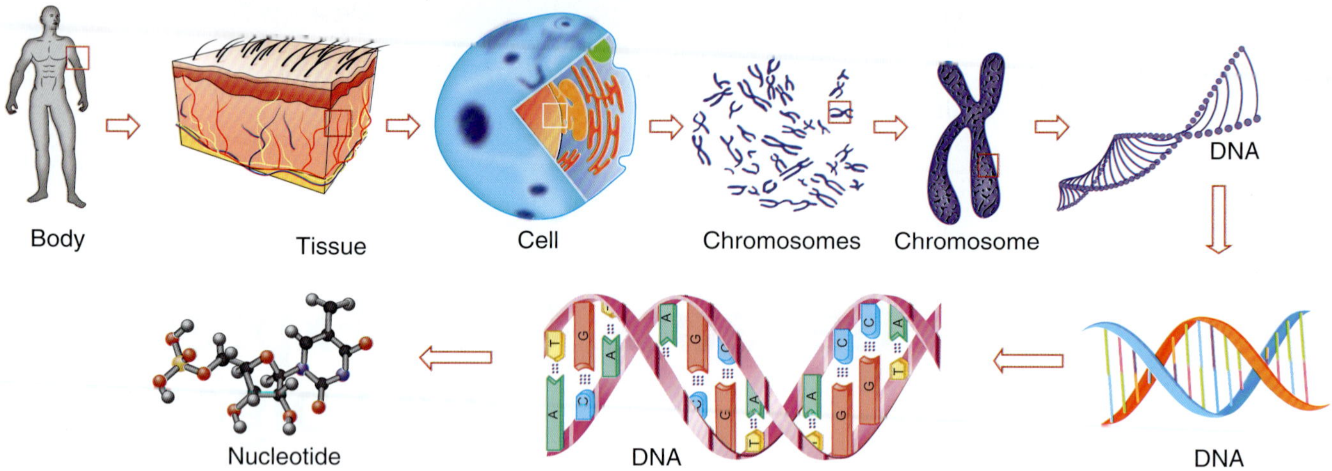

FIGURE 1 Illustration showing nucleotide making up DNA, which is stowed in chromosomes within the nucleus of cells that reside in every tissue of the body.

making functional molecules called proteins. Study of these genes (including other components such as enhancers and small ribonucleic acids or RNAs) is called genetics, which also encompasses other components such as heredity and genetic variation. Proteins alone or in complexes perform a variety of cellular functions. With the advancement of technology and discovery of new phenomena, the concept of a gene continues to be refined. For instance, regulatory regions of a gene may be far away from the coding regions, and coding regions may consist of several split exons (a segment of a DNA molecule containing information coding for peptides). The domain of genetics is broad and encompasses several conceptual frameworks that include but are not limited to genomics, transcriptomics, proteomics, heredity, evolutionary genetics, and genetic diseases (**Figure 2**).

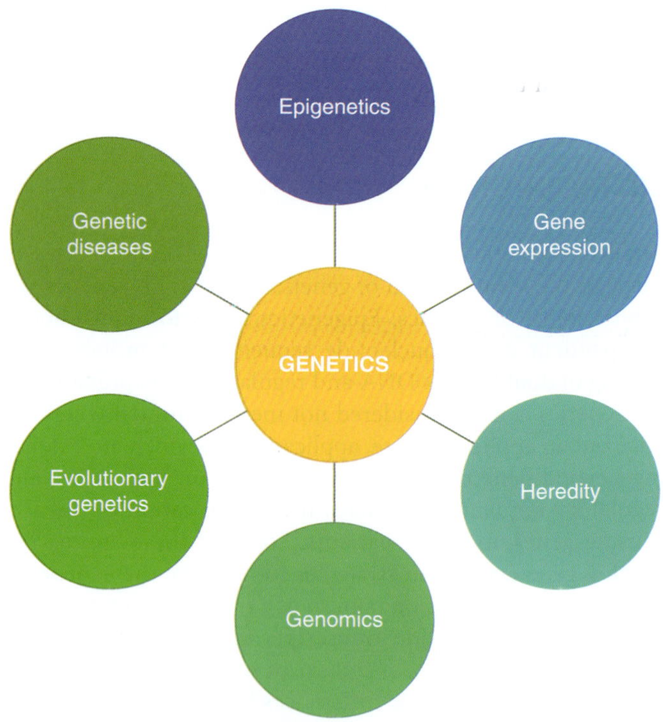

FIGURE 2 Illustration showing various domains of genetics.

GENOMICS AND DNA SEQUENCING

The genome is the complete set of DNA within a cell and the field of genomics deals with the genes and genetic information encoded in DNA. It also includes recombinant DNA technology, DNA sequencing methods, and bioinformatics to sequence, assemble, and analyze the function and structure of the genome. First-generation DNA sequencing is one of the most fundamental technologies developed in the 1970s to study genetics.[1] It uncovered the sequence of nucleotides in DNA fragments and has facilitated the study of the molecular sequences associated with multiple human diseases.[2] Despite being a groundbreaking technology, it certainly had many limitations and therefore efforts were directed to develop shotgun sequencing,[3,4] second-, third-, and next-generation sequencing technologies. These technologies enabled the sequencing of the genomes of many organisms through genome assembly and were used to sequence the complete human genome in 2003. The human genome is made up of 3 billion base pairs of DNA macromolecules of lengths varying from 33 to 250 million base pairs, distributed in the 23 paired chromosomes located in each human cell nucleus. Since its inception, the Human Genome Project has revolutionized the field of molecular medicine.

TRANSCRIPTOMICS

Following the sequencing of the human genome, efforts have been focused on the measurement of the expression of RNA transcripts. In an analogy to the genome, the term "transcriptome" was coined. The transcriptome is the sum of all of

©Copyright 2021 American Academy of Orthopaedic Surgeons

messenger RNA molecules in a cell or population of cells and contains the full information about all RNA transcribed by the genome in a specific tissue or cell type, at a certain developmental stage, and under explicit pathophysiological circumstances. For instance, we know that osteocytes are derived from osteoblast lineage cells that become progressively embedded in mineralized bone matrix in the adult skeleton.[5] These cells are morphologically, functionally, and genetically unique, due in part to the underlying expression of selective gene subsets that characterize the osteocyte phenotype. Although substantial changes in gene expression take place during osteoblast to osteocyte transition, the majority of the transcriptome remains qualitatively osteoblast-like.

Transcriptomics is the science that studies an organism's transcriptome and mechanism of expression. Overall, transcriptome analysis not only allows for the comprehension of the human genome at the transcript level but also provides a conceptual framework of gene structure and function, and gene expression regulation. Moreover, it may disclose the key alterations of biological processes triggering human diseases, thus offering novel tools useful not only for the comprehension of their underlying mechanisms but also for their molecular diagnosis and clinical therapy (see Gene Expression).

HEREDITY AND HERITABILITY

Heredity is the study of how traits are passed on from parents to progeny or how cells acquire the genetic information of parent cells. Heredity is a complex process that involves several steps such as segregation, assortment, and dominance. Through heredity, variations between individuals can accumulate and cause species to evolve by natural selection. Inherited traits are controlled by genes and the complete set of genes within an organism's genome is called its genotype. Genotype is part of the genetic makeup of the cells that determines, along with epigenetics and environmental factors (discussed later in this chapter), the phenotype of an individual. Phenotype refers to observable characteristics or traits, such as form and structure, developmental processes, and numerous biochemical and physiological properties. The distinction between genotype and phenotype is commonly experienced when studying family patterns for different hereditary diseases. As we know, humans and most mammals are diploid (containing two complete sets of chromosomes); thus, there can be more than one allele (one of a number of alternative forms of the same gene or same genetic locus) for any given gene. These alleles can be the same (homozygous) or different (heterozygous), depending on the individual. With a dominant allele, the offspring is guaranteed to inherit the trait in question irrespective of the second allele.

An organism's genotype can be uncovered by a process called genotyping, which uses a variety of biological methods such as polymerase chain reaction (PCR), DNA fragment analysis, nucleic acid hybridization, restriction fragment length polymorphism, microarrays, and other high-throughput techniques such as RNA sequencing. Phenotypic traits can be monogenic (due to one gene) or polygenic (attributable to two or more genes). Polygenic traits can be measured by heritability estimates.

Genetic heritability is the estimation of the degree of variation in a phenotypic trait in a population that is the result of genetic variation between individuals in that population. This type of heritability is termed as broad-sense heritability and is denoted by H^2. In medical context, H^2 can be construed as a measure of the proportion of the variance in liability to a disease or trait caused by additive and nonadditive genetic effects.[6] H^2 ranges from 0 to 1.0, with higher numbers implying that the genetic component of a trait or disease is more dominant than environmental factors.

Recently, a substantial genetic component has been recognized for many common musculoskeletal diseases such as OA of the hip, knee, and hand; rheumatoid arthritis (RA); ankylosing spondylitis; and others. Heritability estimates that determine the genetic contribution have been measured for a number of musculoskeletal diseases, for example, tendinopathy (0.40),[7] rotator cuff tear (0.82),[8] primary hip (0.60),[9] and knee OA (0.42).[10]

GENE MUTATIONS

A quantitative trait locus (QTL) is a region of DNA associated with a particular phenotypic trait. It varies in degree and can be attributed to polygenic effects, that is, the product of two or more genes, and their environment. QTLs are often found on different chromosomes. The number of QTLs explaining variation in a phenotypic trait indicates the genetic architecture of a trait. It may indicate that a disease is controlled by many genes of small effect, or by a few genes of large effect. QTLs are mapped by identifying which molecular markers correlate with an observed trait. The molecular marker usually consists of a single nucleotide polymorphism (SNP) and refers to a variation in a single nucleotide that occurs at a specific position in the genome. For instance, the C nucleotide may appear in a majority of individuals, but in some individuals, the position is occupied by an A. This means that there is a SNP at this specific position, and the two possible nucleotide variations—C or A—are called alleles for this position. Such SNP variation is present to a certain degree within a population and results from gene mutations that potentially impact gene function and expression of disease phenotypes.

SNPs underlie differences in our susceptibility to a wide range of diseases. For instance, a single-base mutation in the type II procollagen gene (COL2A1) is associated with susceptibility to OA. Not all SNPs are the same. Some SNPs fall within the coding sequence (a sequence that encodes a protein) of a gene, some in noncoding region (a sequence that does not encode a protein) of a gene, and yet others in the intergenic region (a sequence located between genes). SNPs within a coding sequence do not always result in a change in the amino acid sequence of the protein and can be divided into

©Copyright 2021 American Academy of Orthopaedic Surgeons

two types: synonymous and nonsynonymous. Synonymous SNPs do not affect the protein sequence, whereas nonsynonymous SNPs change the amino acid sequence of a protein. SNPs that are not in protein-coding regions may still affect gene splicing, transcription factor binding, messenger RNA degradation, or the sequence of noncoding RNA. Gene expression affected by this type of SNP is referred to as an eSNP (expression SNP). Besides SNPs, there also exist several other forms of genetic variations such as copy number variations (CNVs). A CNV is a type of structural change (deletions, insertions, duplications, and complex multisite variants) in the genome in which the sections of genome (a DNA segment of 1 kb or large) are repeated in the form of gain or loss of segments of genomic DNA relative to a reference sequence.[11] CNVs are as important a component of genomic diversity as SNPs. Although SNPs are variations at the level of single nucleotide and account for less than 1% of human genome, CNVs affect regions >1 kb and cover roughly 35% of genome.[12]

GENETIC LINKAGE ANALYSIS

Genetic linkage is a powerful tool for successfully detecting chromosomal locations for causative genes in monogenic diseases and can be used to identify patients with familial risk factors. As genetic mutations causing Mendelian disease are rare in the general population, linkage of a chromosomal locus with disease is evident when genetic markers at or near that locus are co-segregated with disease phenotype within families. Although genetic linkage could map monogenic diseases and localize areas of disease risk, its application in polygenic diseases such as OA and osteoporosis has not been as successful,[13] partly due to the requirement of a large number of families with many affected generations. With the advent of whole-genome sequencing, linkage analysis is again emerging as an important and powerful analytical tool for the identification of disease-causing genes through SNPs generated by the whole-genome sequencing.[14]

GENOME-WIDE ASSOCIATION STUDIES

The limitations associated with genetic linkage analysis for complex (polygenic) diseases can be overcome with linkage disequilibrium mapping to perform large-scale genome-wide association studies (GWAS). A major advantage is that this approach does not require families but instead could use unrelated cases and controls.

Plausible associations between common genetic variants (SNPs) and traits (ie, specific disease phenotypes) are screened by GWAS. GWAS offer an unbiased approach to identify new candidate genes for human diseases that can be confirmed by further candidate gene expression and functional studies. A number of large-scale GWAS have identified a number of OA-associated gene variants with generally small effect sizes (**Table 1**).

UNDERSTANDING THE FUNCTION OF A GENE

Gene targeting provides a valuable resource to alter a specified gene in order to discern its biological function. Remarkable genetic similarity between mice and humans allows for study of the function of single genes in mice. The mouse is a powerful experimental model, not only because many disease phenotypes can be induced, but also because DNA sequences of genes of interest can be introduced into the germline genome randomly or into a specific locus by recombination.[15] A common application of gene targeting is to generate gene knockout mice. Gene knockout mice can be produced as an animal model for a number of human diseases, offering a biological context in which pharmacological and gene therapies can be developed and tested.[16] The number of genes that have been knocked out in mice is expanding. In 2007, it was estimated that at least 11,000 gene knockouts have been conducted.[17] The Knockout Mouse Phenotyping Program, in partnership with International Mouse Phenotyping Consortium, now aims to generate 20,000 “knocked out mice” genes with disrupted genes throughout 90% of the mouse genome. Some relevant terms are defined in **Table 2**.

TOOLS FOR GENE KNOCKOUT AND GENOME EDITING

A variety of different approaches have been used to inhibit specific gene expression in mammalian systems. A knockout of a gene or an insertion of a gene to the mouse genome may involve many steps such as specific gene ablation by homologous recombination in embryonic stem cells, introducing mutation(s) into a targeted gene, suppression of gene function (using, eg, antisense DNA or RNA that hybridizes to a protein-coding single-stranded mRNA and blocks its translation into protein), and gene editing. A number of techniques can be used, many of which are becoming obsolete with the development of novel and crisp classes of nucleases such as zinc finger nucleases (ZFNs), transcription activator–like effector nucleases (TALENs), and clustered regularly interspaced palindromic repeats (CRISPR)/CRISPR-associated protein 9 (Cas9) system (**Figure 3**) in achieving targeted genome modifications.[18] An overview of these systems is provided in **Table 3**.

CLINICAL SIGNIFICANCE OF GENETIC STUDIES IN THE MUSCULOSKELETAL SYSTEM

Genetics and genomics not only provide useful tools for better understanding of the diseases through the identification of measurable gene variants to identify individuals at (higher) risk of developing a disease but also help screen clinically relevant treatment options to prevent, halt, or

©Copyright 2021 American Academy of Orthopaedic Surgeons

TABLE 1 Significant SNPs Associated With Hip, Knee, and Hand OA

Gene	SNP	Locus	Joint	OR	P value	Cases	Controls	References
CHADL	rs532464664	22q13.2	Hip	7.71	5×10^{-18}	4,657	207,514	62
CAMK2B	rs3757837	7p13	Hip	1.27	8×10^{-10}	11,277	67,473	63
NACA2	rs17610181	17q23	Hip	1.12	8×10^{-6}	11,277	67,473	63
RPL35AP, LOC102723442	rs6094710	20q13	Hip	1.28	2×10^{-10}	11,277	67,473	63
NPM1P14, LSMEM1	rs5009270	7q31	Hip	1.1	3×10^{-6}	11,277	67,473	63
A2BP1	rs716508	16p13.3	Hand	NR	1.81×10^{-5}	2,277	NR	64
BTNL2, LOC101929163,	rs10947262	Chr. 6	Knee	1.32	6.73×10^{-8}	960	3,396	65
HLA-DQB1, rs7775228	rs7775228	Chr. 6	Knee	1.34	2.43×10^{-8}	960	3,396	65
ALDH1A2	rs3204689	15q22	Hand	1.46	1.1×10^{-11}	623	69,153	66
DUS4L	rs4730250	7q22	Knee	1.15	9.2×10^{-9}	2,371	35,909	67
DOT1L	rs12982744	19p13.3	Hip	NR	1×10^{-11}	3,717	10,013	68
GNL3	rs11177	Chr. 3	Hip	1.09	5.13×10^{-9}	7,473	42,938	69
FTO	rs8044769	Chr. 16	Hip	1.07	3.56×10^{-06}	7,473	42,938	69
PACERR, PLA2G4A	rs4140564	1q25	Knee	1.59	3×10^{-6}	387	255	69
PARD3B	rs1207421	2q33	Knee	1.46	6×10^{-6}	387	255	70
COG5	rs3815148	7q22	Knee/hand	1.14	8×10^{-8}	14,938	39,000	71
TGFA	rs3771501	Chr. 2	Hip/knee/hand	0.94	1.66×10^{-8}	10,083	12,658	72
DYNC1I1	rs1352413	Chr. 7	Knee	1.39	6×10^{-6}	3,898	3,168	73
FRMD4A	rs7079380	Chr. 10	Knee	1.25	6×10^{-6}	3,898	3,168	73
NOD1	rs6963954	Chr. 7	Knee	1.41	5×10^{-6}	3,898	3,168	73
MCF2L	rs11842874	13q34	Knee	1.17	2×10^{-8}	3,177	4,894	74
DOT1L	rs11880992	Chr. 19	Hip	NR	3×10^{-16}	8,649	>57,000	75
TGFA	rs2862851	Chr. 2	Hip	NR	5×10^{-11}	8,649	>57,000	75
RUNX2	rs12206662	Chr. 6	Hip	NR	1×10^{-9}	8,649	>57,000	75
SMAD3	rs12901071	NR	Knee/hip	1.08	3.12×10^{-10}	23,425	236,814	76
GLIS3	rs10116772	Chr. 9	Knee/hip	1.03	4×10^{-8}	5,414	9,939	77

Chr. = chromosome, NR = not reported, OR = odds ratio

reverse disease progression. Genomic studies have provided important insights into the biologic mechanisms underlying differences in susceptibility or resistance of an individual to musculoskeletal diseases such as RA, OA, and systemic lupus erythematosus. It has been estimated that 39% to 78% cases of OA can be attributed to genetics.[19] Genetics also plays a crucial role in drug development. For example, pharmacogenomics involves genetic variants that impact expression of genes affecting drug pharmacodynamics such as absorption, distribution, action, metabolism, and toxicity of a drug. The term pharmacogenomics is often used interchangeably with the term pharmacogenetics. Pharmacogenetics refers to inherited genetic differences in drug metabolic pathways. It also pertains to other pharmacological principles such as enzymes, messengers, and receptors, which can affect individual responses to drugs, in terms of both therapeutic benefits and adverse effects.

©Copyright 2021 American Academy of Orthopaedic Surgeons

TABLE 2 Definitions of Some Gene Knockout Strategies

Terms	Definition
Transgenic	Refers to any mouse whose genome contains an inserted piece of DNA, originating from the mouse genome or from the genome of another species, and the term includes the standard transgenic mouse as well as a knock in or knockout mouse
Knockout (global)	A genetically modified mouse in which researchers have inactivated, or "knocked out," an existing gene by replacing it or disrupting it with an artificial piece of DNA
Knock-in	A knock-in refers to a genetic engineering method that involves the one-for-one substitution of DNA sequence information in a genetic locus or the insertion of sequence information not found within the locus.
Tissue-specific knockout	An animal model in which a gene of interest is "floxed" and thus inactivated in specific cell types in a specific tissue. The most commonly used technique is the Cre-lox recombination system. This whole system is inducible, so a chemical can be added to knock genes out. This is often also referred to as "conditional" knockout as a specific genes can be eliminated at a specific time as needed.

GENE EXPRESSION

The process by which information from a gene is used in the synthesis of a functional gene product is called gene expression. Gene expression products are generally proteins but can be functional RNA. The gene expression process is complex in nature and involves a number of important steps (**Figure 4**).

TRANSCRIPTION

Transcription is the first step in the gene expression process initiated by an enzyme called RNA polymerase that catalyzes the initiation and elongation of RNA chains from the DNA template. Because both DNA and RNA are nucleic acids in nature, they employ base pairs of nucleotides as complementary semantics. Specifically, RNA polymerase reads and binds to a particular sequence of the DNA (the promoter) terminating into a complementary, antiparallel messenger RNA strand known as messenger RNA (mRNA). The transcription is a very complex process and involves a number of additional intermediate steps such as polyadenylation, capping, and splicing in a mechanism called posttranscriptional modification. In this mechanism, which is tightly regulated in the cell, chemical alternations take place in mRNA. Such alterations are crucial for the correct translation of genome because the initial precursor mRNA produced by transcription is often comprised of both exons (coding sequences) and introns (noncoding sequences). Although the capping and polyadenylation facilitate the transport of the mRNA to a ribosome, (alternative) splicing removes the introns and links the exons directly, thus allowing a single gene to code for multiple related or unrelated proteins. Chemical alternations in mRNA result in a functional RNA molecule that contains information essential for building a polypeptide during the process of translation.

TRANSLATION

In translation, the mRNA transcript is decoded in a ribosome that assembles around the target mRNA to produce the first codon (triplets of nucleotides). Then transfer RNA (tRNA) transfers an amino acid to the tRNA corresponding to the next codon, thus creating an amino acid chain or polypeptides. This process is terminated when one of the termination or stop codons signals the release of a completed polypeptide chain. The ribosome that initially assembled around the target mRNA disengages from the mRNA and the ribosomal subunits dissociate, ready to start the cycle again. The resulting peptides undergo numerous posttranslational modification steps before performing their functional role.

POSTTRANSLATIONAL MODIFICATIONS

Proteins generated in previous step are not able to perform their dedicated function unless they undergo some posttranslational modifications. A posttranslational modification refers

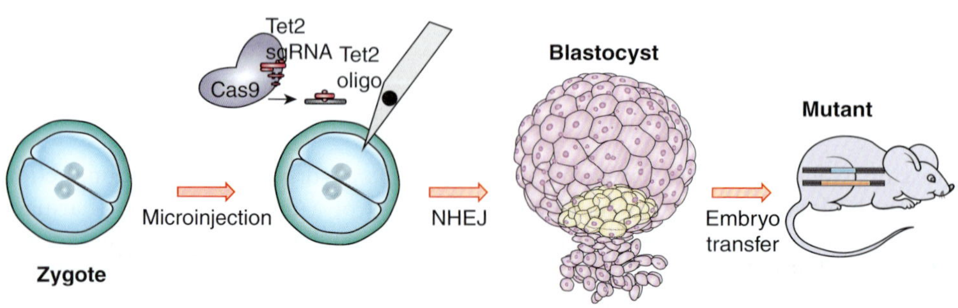

FIGURE 3 Illustration showing generation of mutant mouse. To create a mutant mouse, a guide RNA with the desired sequence is inserted into an isolated (single cell) mouse zygote using microinjection. Then, nonhomologous end-joining, to repair double-strand breaks in DNA, occurs naturally within some cells within a blastocyst. A blastocyst is transferred to a pseudo-pregnant female mouse, replacing the gene of interest with the designed transgene.

©Copyright 2021 American Academy of Orthopaedic Surgeons

TABLE 3 Genome Editing Tools

Method	Alias	Principle	Pros	Cons	Year	References
Zinc finger nucleases	*ZFNs*	Comprise nonspecific artificial restriction enzymes generated by fusing a zinc finger DNA-binding domain to a DNA-binding domain	Target any genomic sequence; reasonable specificity; fewer off-target mutations	Laborious (takes months); expensive; intermediate efficiency; target only one site at a time; difficult to multiplex	1996	78
Transcription activator–like effector nucleases	*TALENs*	Transcription activator–like effector nucleases are restriction enzymes that can be engineered to cut specific sequences of DNA.	Acceptable efficiency; good specificity; easy design (take weeks); target any genomic sequence	Laborious and time consuming; low efficiency; target only one site at a time; sensitive to target DNA methylation; difficult to multiplex	2010	79
Clustered regularly interspaced short palindromic repeat	*CRISPR*	*CRISPR-Cas9* enables editing parts of the genome by removing, adding, or altering sections of the DNA sequence.	Simple; easy design (takes days); high efficiency; targets multiple sites simultaneously; easy multiplex	More potential for off-target effects; limited target selection	2012	80

to the covalent modification of proteins following their biosynthesis to increase the functional diversity of the proteome. One example of such modifications is phosphorylation. In this process, a phosphoryl group is attached to a protein that in turn activates or deactivates the protein, thereby regulating its function. Other examples include methylation, glycosylation, acetylation, and ubiquitination, all of which influence almost all aspects of normal cell biology and pathogenesis.

Regulation of Gene Expression

Regulation of gene expression is an intricate, yet complex and variable, phenomenon that occurs during transcription and translation processes. Any step of gene expression can be modulated, from transcriptional initiation, to RNA processing, and to the posttranslational modification of a protein (**Figure 5**). The intricate regulatory framework controls or regulates genes and their interaction with each other. This process not only provides the cell control over structure and function but is also a fundamental process for differentiation, morphogenesis, and adaptability of cells and organism. Both differentiation and morphogenesis processes may lead to generation of different cell types with different gene expression patterns essentially originating from the same initial genome sequence.

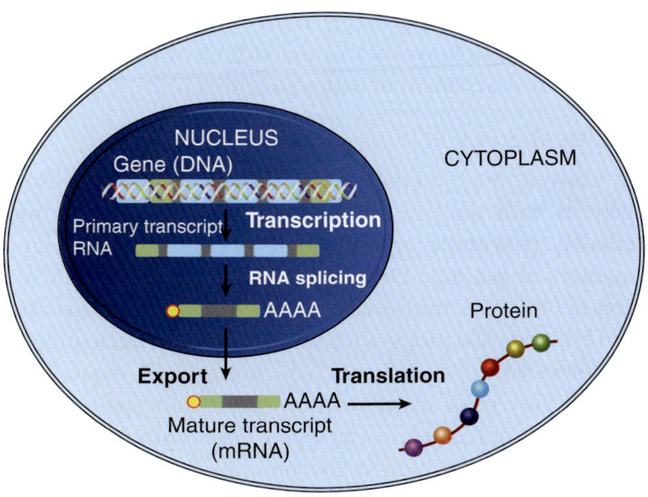

FIGURE 4 Illustration showing gene expression process.

Gene regulation may also serve as a substrate for evolutionary change, because control of the timing, location, and amount of gene expression can exert a profound effect on gene function. Gene expression regulation involves a variety of mechanisms that are used by cells to increase or decrease the production of specific gene products (protein or RNA). There have been a number of studies that study the impact of genetics on gene expression to get more insights into a disease process.[20] Likewise, epigenetics also plays a significant role in modulating gene expression as reviewed elsewhere.[21] Examples of gene expression regulation include processes that trigger developmental pathways, responses to stimuli, or physiological adaptations to alterations in diet.

Gene Expression Pattern

Gene expression can virtually be measured in any cell or tissue of the body. Most tissues, particularly in the musculoskeletal system, are quiescent unless injured or diseased, so their expression remains undetectable or low. However, in response to an injury or stimulus, the expression of certain genes is

©Copyright 2021 American Academy of Orthopaedic Surgeons

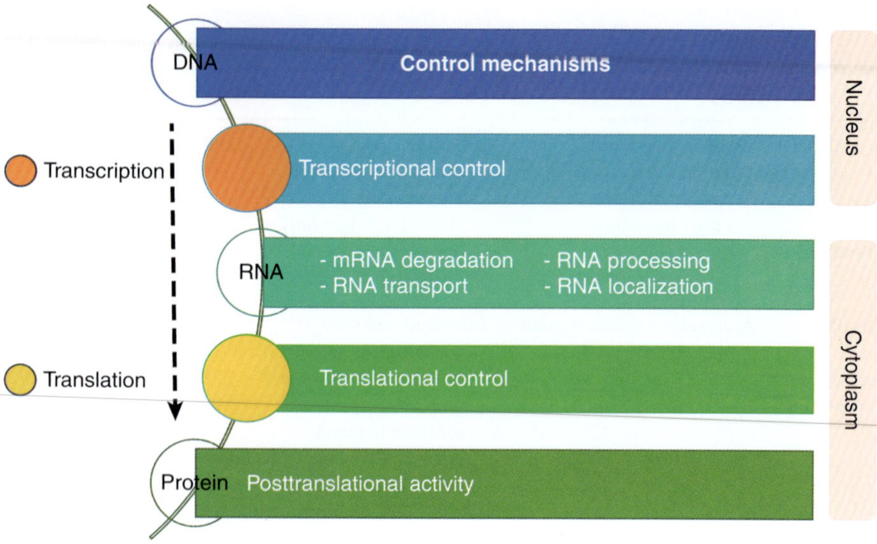

FIGURE 5 Illustration showing regulation of gene expression at transcriptional and translational levels along with posttranslational activity.

elevated. This is called positive gene regulation or gene upregulation. Upregulation of a gene or a set of genes may result in the elevation of protein expression for which these genes are encoded. In addition, upregulation of gene expression can also occur when a cell is deficient in some sort of surface receptor. Increased receptor protein is synthesized and transported to the cell membrane, thus bringing back the sensitivity of the cell to a normal homeostatic level. The other alteration of gene expression occurs when a gene or a set of genes decrease their expression following a stimulus. This phenomenon also results in suppression of expression of the corresponding protein(s). Downregulation of gene expression may also result from overstimulation of cells (eg, by a drug) in which case the expression of the receptor is decreased, thus blocking the continued effect of the drug on a target cell.

Early gene expression studies in musculoskeletal medicine have primarily been descriptive. A number of studies have looked at how patient and injury factors relate to gene expression in the meniscus,[22] articular cartilage,[23-25] and anterior cruciate ligament[26] from the knee. Other studies have looked at gene expression in rotator cuff tears[27] and intervertebral disks.[28]

Transcription Factors and Cell Signaling

Transcription factors or sequence-specific DNA binding factors are proteins, which regulate rate of transcription as well as spatiotemporal expression pattern of genes. Gene regulation and expression is a multifaceted phenomenon and is mediated by transcription factors alone or in combination with proteins. For instance, activator transcription factors stimulate transcription of genes and repressor transcription factors suppress gene transcription (mainly by blocking RNA polymerases). Furthermore, groups of transcription factor binding sites called enhancers and silencers can turn an adjacent gene on and off, respectively, in specific cells and tissues. Transcription factors regulate gene expression through epigenetic mechanisms such as histone modifications. Activation and deactivation of transcription factors is also mediated through signal sensing domains, for example, ligand binding and phosphorylation. Receptor activation caused by a ligand binding to a receptor is coupled with the cell's response to the ligand. Ligand binding influences the location of transcription factors within a cell and affects the activity of transcription factors and their ability to bind with DNA. To bind to DNA and to be activated, transcription factors undergo phosphorylation and interact with other transcription factors. Cell signaling, a process in which cells respond to stimuli, also modulates the activity of various transcription factors.

Analysis of Differentially Expressed Genes

Scientists have always been interested in measuring the transcriptional response of the genome to different stimuli such as injury and disease. There are a number of tools that measure such responses, and many of the traditional methods, such as northern blotting, are no longer commonly used. Gene expression, specifically mRNA expression, is measured on RNA samples extracted directly from tissues or from cells isolated from tissues. Interestingly, RNA often needs to be reverse transcribed to first synthesize the strand of complementary DNA before assessment of expression level.

Amplification by PCR

The conventional methods to measure the expression of a gene is with the use of PCR, which is based on primer-mediated enzymatic amplification of specific gene target sequences in genomic DNA. This results[29] in the exponential increase (100,000s times) of target DNA copies. In this assay, an enzyme is used along with some deoxyribonucleotide triphosphates (dNTPs). Primers, which are DNA sequences of 20 to 25 base pairs in length that specifically span a region of the transcript, bind to unzipped DNA through variation of temperatures resulting in the generation of large numbers of copies of the targeted DNA segment. These signals can be analyzed semiquantitatively by running on agarose gels or

 ©Copyright 2021 American Academy of Orthopaedic Surgeons

quantitatively by addition of fluorescent dyes (eg, Sybr green) during amplification steps.

Fluorescent In Situ Hybridization

Fluorescent in situ hybridization (FISH) allows the detection of individual mRNAs at single cell resolution. This method allows absolute quantitative measurement of mRNA expression. Moreover, it also allows examination of many aspects of mRNA metabolism such as mRNA localization and degradation.

Microarrays

Microarrays detect gene expression change of a multitude of genes simultaneously.[30,31] These arrays, unlike, PCR or equivalent, do not have a priori information of candidate genes and instead scan the changes in the entire transcriptome. Microarrays are thus discovery-oriented tools and are useful in the generation of marker panels to aid in future diagnostic studies. Microarrays employ a hybridization strategy and detect the signals of genes that are converted into numerical values. Microarrays have a number of shortcomings such as cross-hybridization artifacts, poor quantification of genes that are either very low or very high in expression, and limited access to rare gene isoforms.[32,33]

RNA Sequencing

RNA sequencing (RNA-seq) is a revolutionary tool for transcriptome profiling and has clear advantages over hybridization-based assays such as microarray.[32,33] This technique utilizes next-generation sequencing to unravel the amount of RNA in biological samples.[34] This technology has the power to analyze the continuously changing cellular transcriptome, thus facilitating the examination of alternative gene splicing (splice variants), gene fusion, and posttranscriptional modifications as well as temporal gene expression within a tissue/cell and differential expression between different tissues/cells.[35] Although microarrays generally identify mRNAs and some specific microRNAs, RNA-seq can examine all of the RNA in the cells, as well as a number of RNA populations such as total RNA, mRNA, small RNA, miRNA, lncRNA, and tRNAs. Another application of RNA-seq is its ability to determine exon-intron boundaries. This is an important application since sequencing reads harboring an exon-intron boundary indicate a biological process of junction alteration and, possibly, altered splicing.[36]

Single Cell RNA-seq

Although both microarrays and RNA-seq provide phenotype of a disease based on global gene expression, cutting edge single cell RNA-seq (scRNA-seq) technology defines cell phenotypes within a diseased tissue based on gene expression profile, for example, as in the case of OA.[37] In contrast to bulk RNA-seq that uses RNA from mixed population of thousands of pooled cells, scRNA-seq measures gene expression in hundreds of individual cells, thus unmasking previously undetectable cellular properties.[38] Furthermore, only scRNA-seq has the capability to show the genotype and phenotype differentiation branch points when a large population of progenitor cells are examined.

PROTEOMICS

Proteomics is the study of proteome (totality of protein products of encoded genome) and deals with questions such as how do proteins interact and how is information encoded in a protein. Proteomics has enabled the identification of ever-increasing numbers of proteins. Proteomics is an interdisciplinary domain that has benefitted greatly from the genetic information of the Human Genome Project. It covers the exploration of proteomes from the overall level of protein composition, structure, and activity.

There are a number of techniques that can quantitate or semiquantitate the expression of proteins in biological samples to compare, for example, samples from healthy and diseased individuals. Qualitative assessment of proteins as in the case of general proteomics only provides a list of proteins present in a sample. In contrast, quantitative proteomics enables researcher to identify the amount of any given protein in a biological sample. Quantification of proteins is possible by many methods including spectrophotometry, two-dimensional gel electrophoreses, and, more reliably, by mass spectrometry.

Mass spectrometry ionizes chemical species and sorts the ions based on their mass-to-charge ratio to identify and quantify molecules in a biological sample. The development of high-throughput and quantitative mass spectrometry proteomics has significantly improved our understanding of the structure, function, modification, and dynamics of proteins.

METABOLOMICS

For biological phenotyping, genomics, transcriptomics, proteomics, and epigenomics study, respectively, DNA, RNA, protein, and epigenome, whereas metabolomics is the study of metabolites (**Figure 6**). Metabolites are small chemical entities that are the intermediate end-product of metabolism.[39] In addition to their involvement in growth and nutrition, metabolites play a number of important roles, such as fuel sources, structural elements, cell signaling, and catalytic activity of enzymes. Because metabolites serve as direct signatures of biochemical activity and provide functional readouts of cellular state, their assessment (phenotyping) has become a powerful tool in clinical diagnostics. Targeted metabolomic studies are designed to selectively extract information regarding a group of related metabolites from the complex mixture of biomolecules in a hypothesis-driven manner.[40] In contrast, untargeted metabolomics is more global in scope and is discovery oriented.[39]

©Copyright 2021 American Academy of Orthopaedic Surgeons

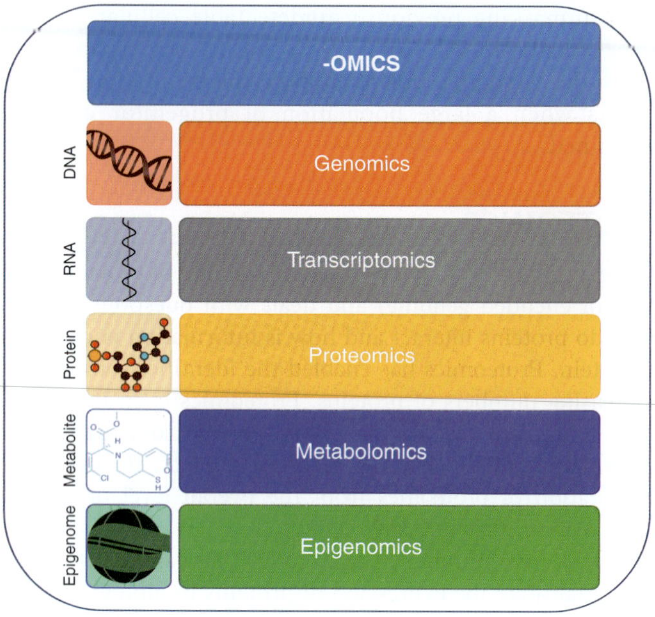

FIGURE 6 Illustration showing an overview of various -omics technologies with their respective molecule.

BIG DATA SETS, GENE ONTOLOGY, AND PATHWAY ANALYSIS

Microarrays, RNA-seq, and scRNA-seq platforms not only yield an unbiased assessment of gene expression signatures from the entire genome but also enable us to explore signaling pathways and biological and molecular processes based on the expression pattern of hundreds and thousands of genes. These platforms yield large datasets and form the basis for large databases. These databases are publicly available on specific servers. The purpose is to give access to other scientists to compare their own data as well as draw additional conclusions from the same data by looking at different aspects of the original data. For example, a recent study on meniscus gene expression has used previously published datasets to focus on new genes.[41]

A commonly used platform for submission of large transcriptomic data is the NIH-supported Gene Expression Omnibus (GEO, https://www.ncbi.nlm.nih.gov/geo/), for proteomics is Proteomics DB (https://www.proteomicsdb.org/), and for epigenome is Roadmap Epigenomics Project (http://www.roadmapepigenomics.org/).

Several other specific databases also exist for miRNAs, proteomics, and metabolomics datasets. The miRNA datasets are deposited to miRNA database called miRBase (http://www.mirbase.org/). The PRIDE (PRoteomics IDEntifications) database is a centralized, standards compliant, public data repository for proteomics data (https://www.ebi.ac.uk/pride/archive/). Metabolomics datasets are deposited to a designated repository called MetaboLights (https://www.ebi.ac.uk/metabolights/index) that contains metabolomics experiments and derived information. A number of working groups are in the process of developing Big Data Knowledge Portals to integrate all human datasets and databases.

Most of genes in our genome work in concert with other genes, therefore necessitating the need to look at them collectively. For this purpose, a number of bioinformatics resources have been developed. The purpose of these resources is to interpret genes in the context of biological process that a gene or a group of genes are collectively involved in. The Database for Annotation, Visualization and Integrated Discovery (DAVID, https://david.ncifcrf.gov), Ingenuity pathways analysis (https://analysis.ingenuity.com), PANTHER (http://www.pantherdb.org), and GeneGo MetaCore (https://portal.genego.com) are all examples of bioinformatics tools being used to interpret gene interaction. In addition, a gene ontology consortium has been established that consists of biological databases from over 100 species (geneontology.org). The main objective of this consortium is to generate and maintain a structured, precisely defined, controlled vocabulary of biological process for the description of the roles of genes.

EPIGENETICS

Epigenetic modification brings about dynamic changes in gene expression, which was originally thought to be a nongenetic transgenerational inheritance. We now know that epigenetic signatures are also inherited. The current definition of epigenetics, however, is a change in gene expression between cell divisions and generations, without changes in the underlying DNA sequence.

Unlike genetic defects, epigenetic defects are potentially reversible and are therefore more amenable to corrective therapeutic reversal. This realization has driven the rapid emergence and expansion of epigenetic drug discovery, and drug-targeting epigenetic enzymes are in the clinic for the treatment of human disorders, especially for clinical management of hematological malignancies and neurological disorders.[42,43] However, treatments with epi-drugs still need to overcome the challenge of avoiding off-target effects. Epigenetic target discovery in musculoskeletal disorders is expected to mirror the efforts directed toward epigenetic drug development in the field of cancer. Early musculoskeletal epigenetics has primarily been in the area of orthopedic oncology.

Some of the main types of epigenetic mechanisms include DNA methylation and demethylation, histone modifications (acetylation and deacetylation), microRNAs, and long noncoding RNAs.

DNA METHYLATION AND DEMETHYLATION

DNA methylation is a phenomenon by which a methyl group is added directly to a cytosine residue. Methylation can change the activity of a DNA segment without changing the sequence.

©Copyright 2021 American Academy of Orthopaedic Surgeons

Cytosine residue exists in a cytosine guanine sequence or CpG sequence. Many CpG sites make up the CpG Island where cytosines are methylated. When located in a gene promoter, the methylation of CpG sites typically correlates negatively with gene expression and acts to repress gene transcription. DNA methylation generally affects the transcription of genes in two ways. First, the methylation of DNA itself may physically impede the binding of transcriptional proteins to the gene. Second, methylated DNA may be bound by proteins known as methyl-CpG-binding domain proteins. These proteins then recruit additional proteins to the locus, such as histone deacetylases and other chromatin remodeling proteins that can modify histones, thereby forming compact, inactive chromatin, termed heterochromatin.

In mammals, DNA methylation is catalyzed by DNA methyl transferases (DNMTs), which are encoded by DNMT1, DNMT3A, and DNMT3B.[44,45] Interestingly, little is known about variation in the methylation status of epigenetic regulators, although there is now a great interest and focus on the expression pattern of DNMT3B. For instance, Dnmt3b has recently has been shown to have a critical role in regulating chondrogenic differentiation and participate in the pathogenesis of impaired fracture repair and other chondrogenesis-associated disorders.[46]

DNA methylation process is reversible, contrary to what was thought initially, since a methyl group in a nucleotide can generally be replaced by a hydrogen atom in a process called DNA demethylation. We now know that ten-eleven translocation proteins (TETs) are capable of modifying methylcytosine and erase DNA methylation.[47] Although DNA methylation culminates in gene silencing, demethylation on a gene promoter is associated with transcriptional activation and gene expression. Both of these processes are important in epigenetic studies and play a significant role in mediating gene expression changes.

HISTONE MODIFICATIONS

Cells package their DNA together with proteins called histones. This DNA and protein complex is known as chromatin. DNA is wrapped around histone proteins forming repeated units called nucleosomes that look like beads on a string. Chromatin also functions to preclude DNA strands from becoming tangled, reinforcing the DNA during cell division and preventing DNA damage. The core of one nucleosome is composed of DNA wrapped around a histone octamer that consists of two copies of the major types of histones called H2A, H2B, H3, and H4. This organized DNA protein complex allows the cells to regulate what genes are expressed and when. Although all the cells in our body contain the same DNA sequence, they have different structures and functions. The reason is that different cells only use or express certain genes. Within each cell, the DNA and histones can be tagged by tiny chemicals that modify gene expression. These chemical tags cause some genes to be turned on and some genes turned off. For example, bone cells will have genes turned on that a bone cell requires and will turn off genes that tendon cells require. Similarly, tendon cells will have genes for bones turned off and genes the tendons require turned on. These modifications are known as epigenetic modifications (**Figure 7**). There are two major types of histone modifications, namely histone acetylation and deacetylation.

In histone acetylation, an acetyl or methyl group can be directly added onto histone tails to modify gene expression. For example, histone3k9 (H3K9) acylation correlates with transcription activation and H3K27 trimethylation with transcription repression. Genome-wide patterns of DNA and histone modifications, or cellular epigenome, are established during early development and are maintained during cell differentiation. In disease states, these patterns are altered and disrupted. In contrast, histone deacetylation,

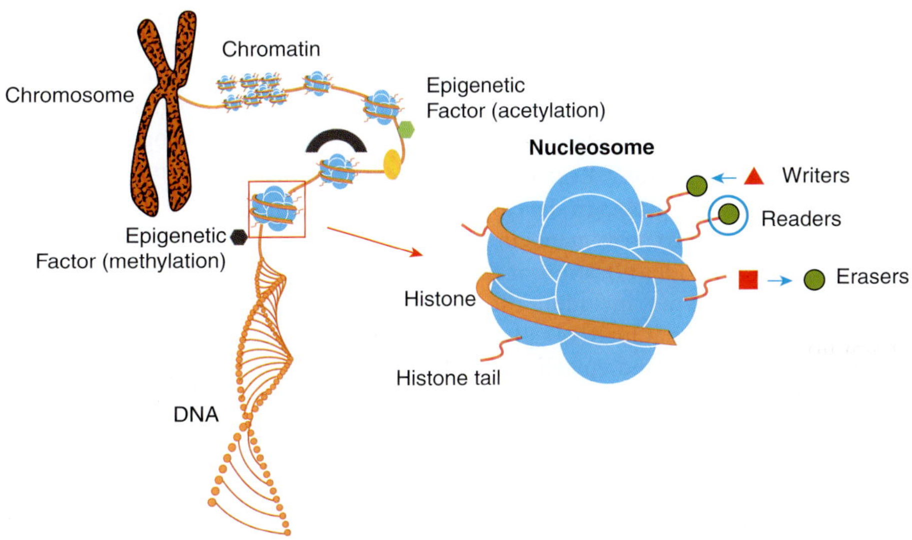

FIGURE 7 Illustration showing epigenetic mechanism.

©Copyright 2021 American Academy of Orthopaedic Surgeons

in which an acetyl molecule is replaced by another molecule, is associated with transcriptional deactivation. This process is achieved by the activity of a class of enzymes called histone deacetylases. Both histone acetylation and deacetylation are important processes in epigenetics and are essential parts of gene regulation.

MICRORNAS

MicroRNAs are small (only 20 to 23 nucleotides) noncoding single-stranded RNAs that are processed from longer transcripts. Although they are too short to code for a protein, they play an important role in cells. Initially it was thought that microRNAs fine-tune gene expression post-transcriptionally by binding to complementary sequences in the coding or 3' untranslated region of target mRNAs targets via mRNA degradation and/or translational repression.[48] However, current knowledge stemming from mechanistic studies and from specific microRNA knockout mice suggests that the biogenesis and function of miRNAs are related to the molecular mechanisms of various clinical diseases, and that they can potentially regulate every aspect of cellular activity such as differentiation and development, metabolism, proliferation, apoptotic cell death, viral infection, and tumorigenesis.[48,49]

LONG NONCODING RNAS

The rapid development of new-generation sequencing technology has deepened the understanding of genome and functional products such as RNAs and proteins. RNA sequencing studies in mammals have revealed that about 85% of the DNA sequences have RNA products over 200 nucleotides in length called long noncoding RNAs (lncRNA). They do not encode proteins and lack >100 amino acid open reading frame (a translatable segment of reading sequence). Today, we understand that lncRNAs play key roles in epigenetic regulation and gene expression, genetic imprinting, histone modification, and chromatin dynamics.[50] LncRNAs are thought to encompass nearly 30,000 different transcripts in humans; hence lncRNA transcripts account for the major part of the noncoding transcriptome. There are many specialized lncRNA databases, which are organized and centralized through RNAcentral.[51] Recently, a significant role has been identified for lncRNAs in developing and maintaining cellular phenotypes. Improvements in sequencing technologies have led to the identification of thousands of lncRNAs across diverse cell types, including the cells within cartilage and bone. It is clear that lncRNAs play critical roles in regulating gene expression and epigenetic modifications.[52,53] For example, they can function as epigenetic regulators in the nucleus via chromatin modulation to control gene transcription, or in the cytoplasm, where they can function as scaffolds for protein-binding partners or modulate the activity of other coding and noncoding RNAs.

ROLE OF EPIGENETICS IN DEVELOPMENT, INFLAMMATION, INJURY, AND OA

Although genetics looks at the sequence of the genetic code, epigenetics is the study of the other factors that influence how and when a gene is expressed. Epigenetic modifications result in altered gene expression and are associated with various disease conditions, including inflammation and aging.[54] Because both environmental stimuli and aging are important risk factors for OA, aberrant epigenetic modifications are likely to impact the disease pathogenesis. For instance, the incremental influence of risk factors that elicit epigenetic responses (DNA methylation and histone modifications) in chondrocytes may cause aberrant gene expression from a variety of molecules, disrupting cartilage homeostasis and contributing to cartilage degradation.[55] Epigenetics is a molecular link between environmental factors and diseases development.[56,57] Thus epigenetics can be affected by a number of intrinsic and extrinsic factors such as diet, lifestyle, aging, exercise, injury, smoking, diabetes, and disease.[58]

EPIGENOMICS

Epigenomics is the study of the complete set of epigenetic modifications on the genetic material of a cell, known as the epigenome. Epigenomics is performed to characterize epigenetic changes in the cell at the genome-wide level to make inferences about epigenetic modifications, which might not otherwise be possible through analysis of a specific locus. Epigenomic activities can be detected by a number of assays, and a Roadmap Epigenomics project has been developed that provides 111 reference epigenomes of various cell lines, primary cells, and tissues.[59] Each reference epigenome comprises about five histone marks and is often complemented with DNA methylation, chromatin accessibility, and transcriptomic data.[60]

SIMILARITIES AND DIFFERENCES BETWEEN GENETICS AND EPIGENETICS

It seems suitable here to describe the fact that although epigenetics is a subspecialty of genetics, both study genes. The changes of the entities studied in both genetics and epigenetics are inheritable and are involved in the control of the formation and functions of a particular organism. Despite these similarities, there are a number of differences between the two as summarized in **Table 4**.

CLINICAL SIGNIFICANCE OF EPIGENETIC STUDIES IN MUSCULOSKELETAL FIELD

The impact of DNA methylation on human disease is known for many decades. Cancer was the first human disease that was linked to DNA methylation. A large body of literature supports the involvement of epigenetic dysregulation in cancer,

©Copyright 2021 American Academy of Orthopaedic Surgeons

TABLE 4 Differences Between Genetics and Epigenetics

Parameter	Genetics	Epigenetics
Inventor	Gregor Mendel	Conrad Waddington
Year	1865	1942
Definition	Study of genes, genetic variation, and heredity	Study of the alterations in inheritable traits in gene expression that involves no change in the underlying DNA sequence
Focus	Structure, function, alteration, and interaction of genes	Modification of gene expression
Domains	Genomics, transcriptomics, proteomics, heredity, evolutionary genetics, genetic diseases	Gene regulation and interaction of gene/protein with environment
Gene level	Combination of alleles	DNA methylation and acylation
Phenotypic traits	Develop with the inheritance of genetic information in the form of genes	Occurs due to external factors such as environmental and behavioral patterns

but only a handful of studies have been conducted to determine the relationship between epigenetic changes and musculoskeletal problems (reviewed in Ref. 61), although research in this area is emerging.

SUMMARY

Understanding the genetic underpinning of a disease is of paramount interest for better diagnosis and treatment of a disease. Although a great deal of data are generated through animal models, the rapid technological development of single-cell RNA sequencing and genome editing tools have made it feasible to perform functional genetic studies directly in human cells. An area with great potential for further study is the 97% to 98% of the human genome that is noncoding. These rapid advancements in basic science are just beginning to be translated into clinically relevant information and applications for musculoskeletal medicine.

REFERENCES

1. Maxam AM, Gilbert W: A new method for sequencing DNA. *Proc Natl Acad Sci USA* 1977;74(2):560-564.
2. Sanger F, Coulson AR: A rapid method for determining sequences in DNA by primed synthesis with DNA polymerase. *J Mol Biol* 1975;94(3):441-448.
3. Staden R: A strategy of DNA sequencing employing computer programs. *Nucleic Acids Res* 1979;6(7):2601-2610.
4. Gardner RC, Howarth AJ, Hahn P, Brown-Luedi M, Shepherd RJ, Messing J: The complete nucleotide sequence of an infectious clone of cauliflower mosaic virus by M13mp7 shotgun sequencing. *Nucleic Acids Res* 1981;9(12):2871-2888.
5. Dallas SL, Bonewald LF: Dynamics of the transition from osteoblast to osteocyte. *Ann N Y Acad Sci* 2010;1192:437-443.
6. Falconer DS: The inheritance of liability to diseases with variable age of onset, with particular reference to diabetes mellitus. *Ann Hum Genet* 1967;31(1):1-20.
7. Hakim AJ, Cherkas LF, Spector TD, MacGregor AJ: Genetic associations between frozen shoulder and tennis elbow: A female twin study. *Rheumatology* 2003;42(6):739-742.
8. Gumina S, Arceri V, Fagnani C, et al: Subacromial space width: Does overuse or genetics play a greater role in determining it? An MRI study on elderly twins. *J Bone Joint Surg Am* 2015;97(20):1647-1652.
9. MacGregor AJ, Antoniades L, Matson M, Andrew T, Spector TD: The genetic contribution to radiographic hip osteoarthritis in women: Results of a classic twin study. *Arthritis Rheum* 2000;43(11):2410-2416.
10. Felson DT, Couropmitree NN, Chaisson CE, et al: Evidence for a Mendelian gene in a segregation analysis of generalized radiographic osteoarthritis: The Framingham Study. *Arthritis Rheum* 1998;41(6):1064-1071.
11. Redon R, Ishikawa S, Fitch KR, et al: Global variation in copy number in the human genome. *Nature* 2006;444(7118):444-454.
12. Zhang F, Gu W, Hurles ME, Lupski JR: Copy number variation in human health, disease, and evolution. *Annu Rev Genomics Hum Genet* 2009;10:451-481.
13. Pulst SM: Genetic linkage analysis. *Arch Neurol* 1999;56(6):667-672.
14. Ott J, Wang J, Leal SM: Genetic linkage analysis in the age of whole-genome sequencing. *Nat Rev Genet* 2015;16(5):275-284.
15. Bouabe H, Okkenhaug K: Gene targeting in mice: A review. *Methods Mol Biol* 2013;1064:315-336.
16. Hall B, Limaye A, Kulkarni AB: Overview: Generation of gene knockout mice. *Curr Protoc Cell Biol* 2009;44(1):19.12.1-19.12.17.
17. Vogel G: Nobel Prizes. A knockout award in medicine. *Science* 2007;318(5848):178-179.
18. Govindan G, Ramalingam S: Programmable site-specific nucleases for targeted genome engineering in higher eukaryotes. *J Cell Physiol* 2016;231(11):2380-2392.
19. Sandell LJ: Etiology of osteoarthritis: Genetics and synovial joint development. *Nat Rev Rheumatol* 2012;8(2):77-89.
20. Emilsson V, Thorleifsson G, Zhang B, et al: Genetics of gene expression and its effect on disease. *Nature* 2008;452(7186):423-428.
21. Gibney ER, Nolan CM: Epigenetics and gene expression. *Heredity* 2010;105(1):4-13.
22. Brophy RH, Zhang B, Cai L, Wright RW, Sandell LJ, Rai MF: Transcriptome comparison of meniscus from patients with and without osteoarthritis. *Osteoarthr Cartil* 2018;26(3):422-432.
23. Ajekigbe B, Cheung K, Xu Y, et al: Identification of long non-coding RNAs expressed in knee and hip osteoarthritic cartilage. *Osteoarthr Cartil* 2019;27(4):694-702.
24. Rai MF, Sandell LJ, Barrack TN, et al: A microarray study of articular cartilage in relation to obesity and severity of knee osteoarthritis. *Cartilage* 2018:1947603518796122.

©Copyright 2021 American Academy of Orthopaedic Surgeons

25. Rai MF, Sandell LJ, Zhang B, Wright RW, Brophy RH: RNA microarray analysis of macroscopically normal articular cartilage from knees undergoing partial medial meniscectomy: Potential prediction of the risk for developing osteoarthritis. *PLoS One* 2016;11(5):e0155373.
26. Brophy RH, Rothermich MA, Tycksen ED, Cai L, Rai MF: Presence of meniscus tear alters gene expression profile of anterior cruciate ligament tears. *J Orthop Res* 2018;36(10):2612-2621.
27. Ren YM, Duan YH, Sun YB, Yang T, Tian MQ: Bioinformatics analysis of differentially expressed genes in rotator cuff tear patients using microarray data. *J Orthop Surg Res* 2018;13(1):284.
28. Wan ZY, Song F, Sun Z, et al: Aberrantly expressed long noncoding RNAs in human intervertebral disc degeneration: A microarray related study. *Arthritis Res Ther* 2014;16(5):465.
29. Saiki RK, Scharf S, Faloona F, et al: Enzymatic amplification of beta-globin genomic sequences and restriction site analysis for diagnosis of sickle cell anemia. *Science* 1985;230(4732):1350-1354.
30. Schena M, Shalon D, Davis RW, Brown PO: Quantitative monitoring of gene expression patterns with a complementary DNA microarray. *Science* 1995;270(5235):467-470.
31. Schena M, Shalon D, Heller R, Chai A, Brown PO, Davis RW: Parallel human genome analysis: Microarray-based expression monitoring of 1000 genes. *Proc Natl Acad Sci USA* 1996;93(20):10614-10619.
32. Rai MF, Tycksen ED, Sandell LJ, Brophy RH: Advantages of RNA-seq compared to RNA microarrays for transcriptome profiling of anterior cruciate ligament tears. *J Orthop Res* 2018;36(1):484-497.
33. Wang Z, Gerstein M, Snyder M: RNA-seq: A revolutionary tool for transcriptomics. *Nat Rev Genet* 2009;10(1):57-63.
34. Brenner S, Johnson M, Bridgham J, et al: Gene expression analysis by massively parallel signature sequencing (MPSS) on microbead arrays. *Nat Biotechnol* 2000;18(6):630-634.
35. Maher CA, Kumar-Sinha C, Cao X, et al: Transcriptome sequencing to detect gene fusions in cancer. *Nature* 2009;458(7234):97-101.
36. Mudvari P, Movassagh M, Kowsari K, et al: SNPlice: Variants that modulate intron retention from RNA-sequencing data. *Bioinformatics* 2015;31(8):1191-1198.
37. Ji Q, Zheng Y, Zhang G, et al: Single-cell RNA-seq analysis reveals the progression of human osteoarthritis. *Ann Rheum Dis* 2019;78(1):100-110.
38. Kanter I, Kalisky T: Single cell transcriptomics: Methods and applications. *Front Oncol* 2015;5:53.
39. Patti GJ, Yanes O, Siuzdak G: Innovation: Metabolomics. The apogee of the omics trilogy. *Nat Rev Mol Cell Biol* 2012;13(4):263-269.
40. Dudley E, Yousef M, Wang Y, Griffiths WJ: Targeted metabolomics and mass spectrometry. *Adv Protein Chem Struct Biol* 2010;80:45-83.
41. Huang P, Gu J, Wu J, et al: Microarray analysis of the molecular mechanisms associated with age and body mass index in human meniscal injury. *Mol Med Rep* 2019;19(1):93-102.
42. de Lera AR, Ganesan A: Epigenetic polypharmacology: From combination therapy to multitargeted drugs. *Clin Epigenetics* 2016;8:105.
43. Delgado-Morales R, Agis-Balboa RC, Esteller M, Berdasco M: Epigenetic mechanisms during ageing and neurogenesis as novel therapeutic avenues in human brain disorders. *Clin Epigenetics* 2017;9:67.
44. Rajendran G, Shanmuganandam K, Bendre A, Muzumdar D, Goel A, Shiras A: Epigenetic regulation of DNA methyltransferases: DNMT1 and DNMT3B in gliomas. *J Neuro Oncol* 2011;104(2):483-494.
45. Uysal F, Ozturk S, Akkoyunlu G: DNMT1, DNMT3A and DNMT3B proteins are differently expressed in mouse oocytes and early embryos. *J Mol Histol* 2017;48(5-6):417-426.
46. Wang C, Abu-Amer Y, O'Keefe RJ, Shen J: Loss of Dnmt3b in chondrocytes leads to delayed endochondral ossification and fracture repair. *J Bone Miner Res* 2018;33(2):283-297.
47. Rasmussen KD, Helin K: Role of TET enzymes in DNA methylation, development, and cancer. *Genes Dev* 2016;30(7):733-750.
48. Huang Y, Shen XJ, Zou Q, Wang SP, Tang SM, Zhang GZ: Biological functions of microRNAs: A review. *J Physiol Biochem* 2011;67(1):129-139.
49. McAlinden A, Im GI: MicroRNAs in orthopaedic research: Disease associations, potential therapeutic applications, and perspectives. *J Orthop Res* 2018;36(1):33-51.
50. Wang C, Wang L, Ding Y, et al: LncRNA structural characteristics in epigenetic regulation. *Int J Mol Sci* 2017;18(12):1-11.
51. Bateman A, Agrawal S, Birney E, et al: RNAcentral: A vision for an international database of RNA sequences. *RNA* 2011;17(11):1941-1946.
52. Huynh NP, Anderson BA, Guilak F, McAlinden A: Emerging roles for long noncoding RNAs in skeletal biology and disease. *Connect Tissue Res* 2017;58(1):116-141.
53. Cao J: The functional role of long non-coding RNAs and epigenetics. *Biol Proced Online* 2014;16:11.
54. Shen J, Abu-Amer Y, O'Keefe RJ, McAlinden A: Inflammation and epigenetic regulation in osteoarthritis. *Connect Tissue Res* 2017;58(1):49-63.
55. Zhang M, Wang J: Epigenetics and osteoarthritis. *Genes Dis* 2015;2(1):69-75.
56. Skinner MK, Manikkam M, Guerrero-Bosagna C: Epigenetic transgenerational actions of environmental factors in disease etiology. *Trends Endocrinol Metab* 2010;21(4):214-222.
57. Ling C, Groop L: Epigenetics: A molecular link between environmental factors and type 2 diabetes. *Diabetes* 2009;58(12):2718-2725.
58. Torano EG, Garcia MG, Fernandez-Morera JL, Nino-Garcia P, Fernandez AF: The impact of external factors on the epigenome: In Utero and over Lifetime. *BioMed Res Int* 2016;2016:2568635.
59. Roadmap Epigenomics C, Kundaje A, Meuleman W, et al: Integrative analysis of 111 reference human epigenomes. *Nature* 2015;518(7539):317-330.
60. Klein HU, De Jager PL: How do we measure the epigenome(s)? *Mult Scler* 2018;24(4):446-448.
61. Oppermann U: Why is epigenetics important in understanding the pathogenesis of inflammatory musculoskeletal diseases? *Arthritis Res Ther* 2013;15(2):209.
62. Styrkarsdottir U, Helgason H, Sigurdsson A, et al: Whole-genome sequencing identifies rare genotypes in COMP and CHADL associated with high risk of hip osteoarthritis. *Nat Genet* 2017;49(5):801-805.
63. Evangelou E, Kerkhof HJ, Styrkarsdottir U, et al: A meta-analysis of genome-wide association studies identifies novel variants associated with osteoarthritis of the hip. *Ann Rheum Dis* 2014;73(12):2130-2136.
64. Zhai G, van Meurs JB, Livshits G, et al: A genome-wide association study suggests that a locus within the ataxin 2 binding protein 1 gene is associated with hand osteoarthritis: The Treat-OA consortium. *J Med Genet* 2009;46(9):614-616.
65. Nakajima M, Takahashi A, Kou I, et al: New sequence variants in HLA class II/III region associated with susceptibility to knee osteoarthritis identified by genome-wide association study. *PLoS One* 2010;5(3):e9723.
66. Styrkarsdottir U, Thorleifsson G, Helgadottir HT, et al: Severe osteoarthritis of the hand associates with common variants within the ALDH1A2 gene and with rare variants at 1p31. *Nat Genet* 2014;46(5):498-502.
67. Evangelou E, Valdes AM, Kerkhof HJ, et al: Meta-analysis of genome-wide association studies confirms a susceptibility locus for knee osteoarthritis on chromosome 7q22. *Ann Rheum Dis* 2011;70(2):349-355.
68. Castano Betancourt MC, Cailotto F, Kerkhof HJ, et al: Genome-wide association and functional studies identify the DOT1L gene to be involved in cartilage thickness and hip osteoarthritis. *Proc Natl Acad Sci USA* 2012;109(21):8218-8223.
69. arc OC, arc OC, Zeggini E, et al: Identification of new susceptibility loci for osteoarthritis (arcOGEN): A genome-wide association study. *Lancet* 2012;380(9844):815-823.
70. Valdes AM, Loughlin J, Timms KM, et al: Genome-wide association scan identifies a prostaglandin-endoperoxide synthase 2 variant involved in risk of knee osteoarthritis. *Am J Hum Genet* 2008;82(6):1231-1240.
71. Kerkhof HJ, Lories RJ, Meulenbelt I, et al: A genome-wide association study identifies an osteoarthritis susceptibility locus on chromosome 7q22. *Arthritis Rheum* 2010;62(2):499-510.

©Copyright 2021 American Academy of Orthopaedic Surgeons

72. Zengini E, Hatzikotoulas K, Tachmazidou I, et al: Genome-wide analyses using UK Biobank data provide insights into the genetic architecture of osteoarthritis. *Nat Genet* 2018;50(4):549-558.
73. Yau MS, Yerges-Armstrong LM, Liu Y, et al: Genome-wide association study of radiographic knee osteoarthritis in North American Caucasians. *Arthritis Rheumatol* 2017;69(2):343-351.
74. Day-Williams AG, Southam L, Panoutsopoulou K, et al: A variant in MCF2L is associated with osteoarthritis. *Am J Hum Genet* 2011;89(3):446-450.
75. Castano-Betancourt MC, Evans DS, Ramos YF, et al: Novel genetic variants for cartilage thickness and hip osteoarthritis. *PLoS Genet* 2016;12(10):e1006260.
76. Hackinger S, Trajanoska K, Styrkarsdottir U, et al: Evaluation of shared genetic aetiology between osteoarthritis and bone mineral density identifies SMAD3 as a novel osteoarthritis risk locus. *Hum Mol Genet* 2017;26(19):3850-3858.
77. Casalone E, Tachmazidou I, Zengini E, et al: A novel variant in GLIS3 is associated with osteoarthritis. *Ann Rheum Dis* 2018;77(4):620-623.
78. Ainley WM, Sastry-Dent L, Welter ME, et al: Trait stacking via targeted genome editing. *Plant Biotechnol J* 2013;11(9):1126-1134.
79. Boch J, Scholze H, Schornack S, et al: Breaking the code of DNA binding specificity of TAL-type III effectors. *Science* 2009;326(5959):1509-1512.
80. Jinek M, Chylinski K, Fonfara I, Hauer M, Doudna JA, Charpentier E: A programmable dual-RNA-guided DNA endonuclease in adaptive bacterial immunity. *Science* 2012;337(6096):816-821.

©Copyright 2021 American Academy of Orthopaedic Surgeons

2

Cell Biology, Cell Differentiation, and Stem Cells of the Skeletal System

Michael J. Zuscik, PhD
Lianping Xing, PhD
Brendan F. Boyce, MBChB
Francis Y. Lee, MD, PhD

Keywords: *chondrocyte; mesenchymal stem cell; osteoblast; osteoclast; osteocyte*

INTRODUCTION

The skeleton and the bones that comprise it are formed during embryonic development through two distinct processes: endochondral and intramembranous ossification. These processes involve the commitment and differentiation of cells arising from both the mesenchymal and hematopoietic lineages, and a coordinated interaction of these cells, particularly chondrocytes, osteoblasts (OBs), osteocytes, and osteoclasts (OCs) (**Figure 1**), is required to regulate cartilage and bone formation and resorption (**Figure 2**). These coordinated interactions support development, growth, repair, and homeostasis of skeletal tissues. When they are disrupted, skeletal diseases manifest themselves.

Dr. Zuscik or an immediate family member serves as an unpaid consultant to Solarea BIO. Dr. Lee or an immediate family member has stock or stock options held in L&J BIO and has received research or institutional support from Musculoskeletal Transplant Foundation, National Institutes of Health (NIAMS & NICHD), and OREF. Neither of the following authors nor any immediate family member has received anything of value from or has stock or stock options held in a commercial company or institution related directly or indirectly to the subject of this chapter: Dr. Xing and Dr. Boyce.

Long bones of the appendicular skeleton are primarily formed by the process of endochondral ossification initiated in limb buds arising from the lateral plate mesoderm that comprises the trunk of an embryo. The buds are the epicenter of the formation of cartilage templates (cartilage anlagen), which provide a structural scaffold for the formation of each skeletal element leading up to fully formed and anatomically correct bones (**Figure 3**). Chondroblasts, the cells that produce the cartilaginous matrix of the anlagen, arise from mesenchymal stem cells (MSCs). In addition to chondro-lineage cells, MSCs are pluripotent cells possessing the ability to differentiate into numerous other musculoskeletal cell lineages including OBs, fibroblasts, adipocytes, striated muscle, and endothelial cells.[1] Chondroblasts in the central parts of the anlagen differentiate from early chondroprogenitors into hypertrophic chondrocytes, and the matrix around the hypertrophic chondrocytes calcifies to create the first mineralized tissues.[1] Some of these chondroprogenitors positioned near the proximal and distal ends of bones where joints will form differentiate into articular chondrocytes. Blood vessels grow into the calcified cartilage, followed by matrix degrading enzymes, including various metalloproteinases, which served to remove the mineralized cartilage at the midshaft of the developing bone. Parallel to this, the hypertrophic chondrocytes in the remodeling anlagen undergo apoptosis. As calcified cartilage is removed and chondrocytes die off, OBs that have mainly differentiated from MSCs in the limb bud and precursors circulating in the blood[2] replace it with new bone organized into rod- and plate-shaped structures called trabeculae. Some OBs residing on the new trabeculae or on the endosteal (ie, inside) surface of the shaft of the

©Copyright 2021 American Academy of Orthopaedic Surgeons

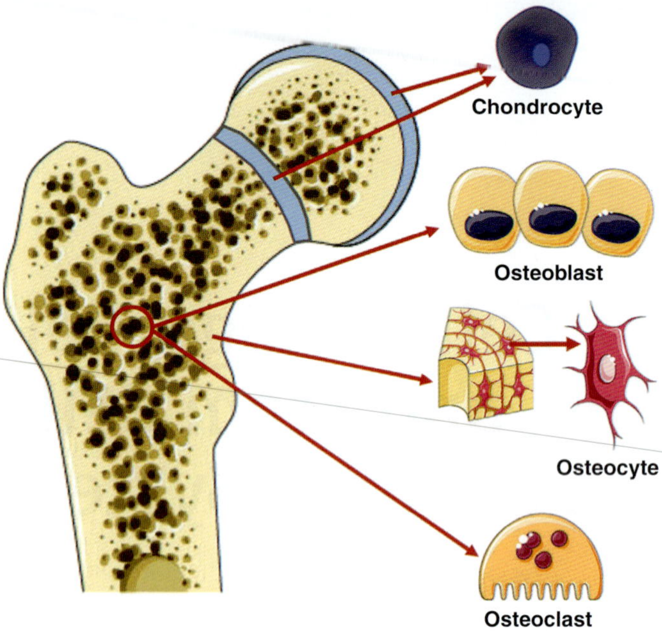

FIGURE 1 Graphical images of the main skeletal cell types and where they reside. A femoral head is shown with the rough locations identified for the four key cells described in this chapter: chondrocytes, osteoblasts, osteocytes, and osteoclasts.

long bone will encase themselves in unmineralized collagen-proteoglycan matrix known as osteoid that can bind calcium.[3] The binding of calcium to osteoid results in hardening of the matrix, encasement of OBs, and their terminal differentiation into osteocytes. Osteocytes have numerous functions within and outside of bone, most important being their role as load sensors that translate mechanical stresses in bones into cellular signals that control bone remodeling/homeostasis to maximize bone strength in response to load-bearing requirements.[4]

Growth of long bones perpendicular to their long axis (ie, radial growth) as well as the formation and expansion of flat bones such as the calvarial plates in the skull is supported by the process of intramembranous ossification. This process involves the direct conversion of mesenchymal tissue into bone and the differentiation of MSCs into OBs.[5] Although this process does not involve a cartilage precursor, as in endochondral ossification, OBs participating in intramembranous bone formation can also encase themselves in mineralized osteoid and terminally differentiate into osteocytes.

A portion of new bone must be removed to accommodate the formation of bone marrow cavities during skeletal development and the removal of bone throughout life in a tight balance with OBs to support remodeling and homeostasis. The process of bone resorption in these contexts is supported by OCs, which resorb matrix on bone surfaces to create trenches that are subsequently filled with new bone produced by OBs (**Figure 2**). The OCs that perform this work arise from myeloid lineage hematopoietic cells that also give rise to macrophages.[6] OCs are multinucleated cells formed by cytoplasmic fusion of these hematopoietic precursors in response to cues from various cytokines and growth factors.

With all of these in mind, this chapter will focus on describing the main cells that contribute to skeletal system development, growth, and maintenance: chondrocytes, OBs, osteocytes, and OCs (**Figure 1**). This is not to suggest that other cell types are not involved or critical to the skeletal system, but these groups of cells are the dominant players in bone and cartilage biology. The central factors and signaling pathways that regulate progenitor cell differentiation to these key lineages will also be presented as foundational information to establish the mechanisms underlying how these cells create and maintain the skeleton by carrying out the key functions that are specific to their differentiated phenotypes.

CHONDROCYTES

CHONDROCYTE DIFFERENTIATION

Chondrocytes undergo differentiation along two major distinct pathways. During endochondral ossification, cells undergo maturation, hypertrophy, and apoptosis, ultimately supporting matrix calcification. This pathway is used in the physes (ie, growth plates) of growing adolescent vertebrates and is recapitulated in bone repair following fracture. The second pathway of chondrocyte differentiation takes place in hyaline cartilage. In this context, cells are relatively quiescent, carrying out structural or load-bearing functions in the articular cartilages of joints. In either case, chondrogenesis is required to initiate differentiation of chondrocyte progenitors toward their fate in these related but functionally distinct tissues.

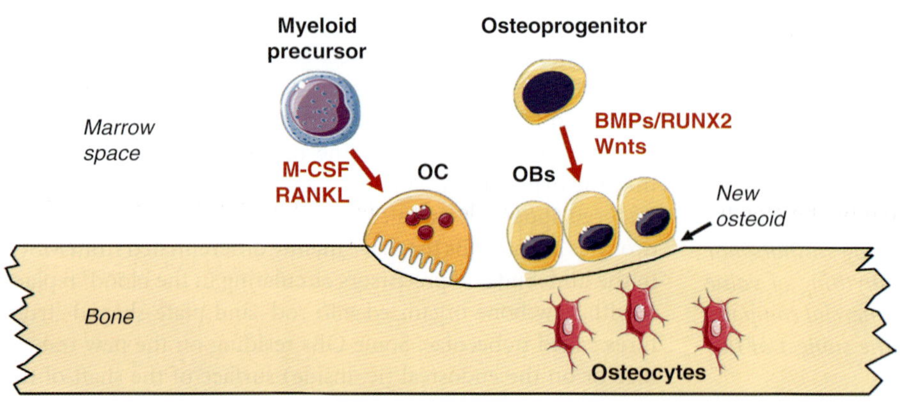

FIGURE 2 Illustrated model of osteoclast-Osteoblast (OC-OB) coupling during bone turnover. Active OCs excavate trenches in bony tissue, followed by OBs, which lay down new mineral at sites that have been resorbed. Key factors that drive myeloid precursor differentiation into OCs and osteoprogenitors into OBs are depicted.

©Copyright 2021 American Academy of Orthopaedic Surgeons

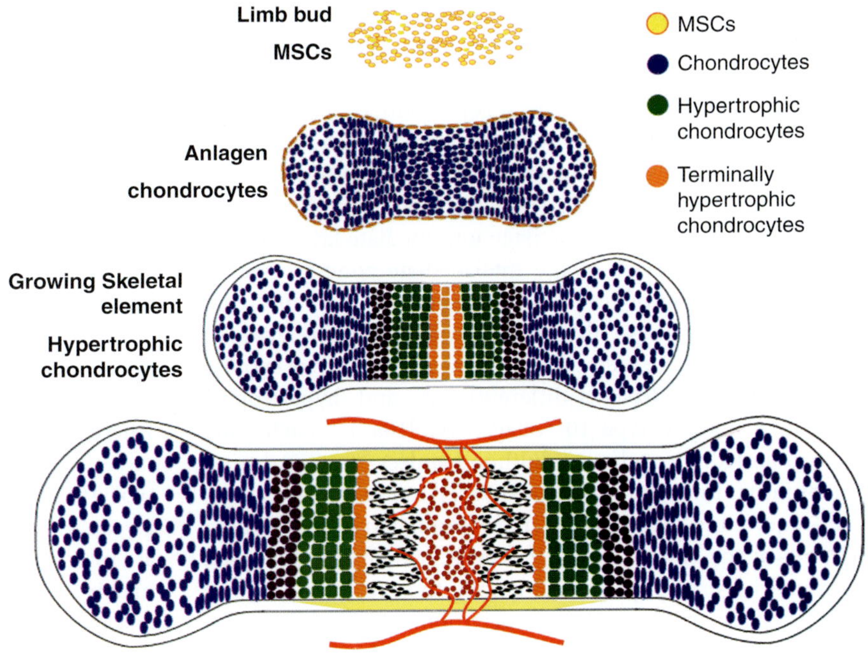

FIGURE 3 Illustrated summary of endochondral ossification. Each stage of endochondral ossification is depicted from mesenchymal stem cell (MSC) condensations in the limb bud through to the development of a mineralizing skeletal element with chondrocytes spanning the spectrum of differentiation from pre-hypertrophic to terminally differentiated cells. Colors denote cell differentiation stage. Blood supply is depicted in red.

Differentiation of Chondrocytes During Endochondral Ossification

In skeletal development, chondrogenesis begins with the aggregation and condensation of loose mesenchymal tissue to form anlagen comprised of cells that actively express various extracellular matrix and cell adhesion molecules, including aggrecan and the IIa splice variant of the type 2 collagen α1 chain.[7] The appropriate temporal and spatial secretion of extracellular matrix and the associated steps of chondrocyte differentiation rely on the action of various morphogens/growth factors, their cognate receptors and the downstream signaling pathways, and transcription factors. The earliest events in the mesenchyme that participate in anlagen formation are initially driven by the morphogen Sonic Hedgehog (Shh) via its transmembrane receptors Patched 1 and 2 (Ptc1,2), leading to recruitment of another transmembrane protein Smoothened (Smo) and activation of Gli transcription factors.[8] Activation of this signaling system leads to the induction of various targets including the master transcriptional regulator of chondrogenesis, Sox9,[9] and NK3 homeobox 2 (Nkx3-2), another transcription factor necessary to maintain Sox9 expression in condensing cells.[10]

Once signals downstream of Shh initiate Sox9 upregulation in early development, its tight regulation by a series of other signaling pathways sets the pace for appropriate progression of chondrogenesis. Deceleration of chondroprogenitor entry into the chondrocyte lineage is in part facilitated by the Notch receptor family which comprises four different single-pass transmembrane receptors consisting of extracellular, transmembrane, and intracellular domains that determine cell fate. Notch receptor activation by its agonist ligands Delta-like 1, 3 and 4 (Dll1, 3 and 4) and Jagged 1 and 2 (Jag1 and 2) inhibits Sox9 via the Notch-activated transcription factor, RBP-Jκ, and the downstream activation of various other transcriptional regulators including HES1 and HES5. Chondrogenesis ensues only following reduced signaling on the Notch pathway (ie, reduced transcriptional repression of Sox9 by RBP-Jκ).[11] Once this Notch repression is overcome, several key pathways strongly drive Sox9 upregulation, expansion of chondrogenesis, and entry into the chondrocyte hypertrophic program. These include fibroblast growth factors (FGFs),[12] hypoxic conditions, and the concomitant upregulation of hypoxia-inducible factor 1α (HIF-1α),[13] and transforming growth factor-β (TGFβ).[14] Bone morphogenic proteins (BMPs), members of the TGFβ superfamily, also possess potent chondrogenic activity. Consistent with this, blockade of BMP signaling by overexpressing the soluble decoy receptor Noggin, which competes away BMPs from their cognate receptors, inhibits cartilage formation.[15] Overall, these signaling pathways work in concert with each other to modulate MSC/progenitor cell commitment to the chondrocyte lineage. These events are critical to the expansion and conversion of anlagen into mineralized skeletal elements (**Figure 3**).

Differentiation of Chondrocytes in Hyaline Cartilage

Articular cartilage development begins during embryogenesis at sites of synovial joint formation through a sequential series of steps that include patterning of the joint site, interzone formation, cavitation, and morphogenesis.[16] Articular chondrocytes are formed from interzone cells and, unlike chondrocytes participating in endochondral ossification in the epiphyseal plate which are removed completely following adolescent growth, these chondrocytes persist. The tissue left behind

©Copyright 2021 American Academy of Orthopaedic Surgeons

postnatally and in adulthood is articular cartilage, which is maintained as four distinct cellular zones from the surface to the underlying bone: superficial, intermediate, radial, and calcified cartilage. The superficial zone consists of one to two cell layers of flattened chondrocytes expressing Proteoglycan 4 (Prg4) (also known as superficial zone protein or lubricin), Sox9, type 2 collagen Col2a1(IIb), aggrecan (Acan), tenascin C (Tnc) and low levels of cartilage intermediate layer protein (Cilp).[16] Chondrocytes of the intermediate zone are round and express many of the same molecules as the superficial zone except for Prg4, although they have higher levels of Cilp. Radial and calcified cartilage zone chondrocytes express markers of chondrocyte differentiation and hypertrophy, including, notably, type 10 collagen (Col10a1).[16] Each zone is maintained throughout adulthood unless stress-inducing injury, inflammation, or genetic defects lead to loss of the signals required to maintain the appropriate matrix homeostatic activity of the chondrocytes and prevent their inappropriate terminal hypertrophy. Central among these cytokine signals that suppress inappropriate hypertrophic differentiation is the TGF-β/Smad signaling pathway.[17] When this pathway and others that decelerate or prevent chondrocyte hypertrophy are disrupted or impaired, chondrocytes become hypertrophic, increasing their expression of matrix degrading enzymes such as matrix metalloproteinase (MMP)-9 and MMP-13 and members of the A Disintegrin And Metalloprotease with Thrombospondin Motifs (ADAMTS) family.[18] Coupled with enzyme-driven progressive loss of biomechanically appropriate articular cartilage matrix is the terminal maturation of chondrocytes, which make Col10a1 and ultimately apoptose. These matrix and cellular changes lead to degenerative diseases such as osteoarthritis.[18]

CHONDROCYTE FUNCTION

Chondrocytes can be grown and studied in culture, with numerous 2-D and 3-D culturing conditions that support the chondro-differentiated phenotype. Isolation of chondrocytes can be accomplished by the digestion of cartilage with collagenase or combinations of enzymes including collagenase, hyaluronidase, and trypsin. Chondrocytes in monolayer culture tend to dedifferentiate into type 1 collagen-expressing fibroblast-like cells and lose their ability to express Col2a1 and other matrix components such as proteoglycans.[18] When cultured in a suspension culture or in a three-dimensional gel made of collagen, agar, or alginate, the cells will maintain their chondrocytic phenotype,[19] emphasizing the importance of cell-matrix interactions in controlling gene expression, chondrocyte differentiation, and maintaining the chondrocyte phenotype.

The predominant matrix protein in cartilage is type II collagen, which is composed of a single chain forming a triple helix.[20] Like type I collagen, it is secreted as triple helical pro-protein, which is cleaved extracellularly by proteinases.[21] The other major organic component of the matrix is proteoglycan, which includes several proteins containing covalently bound glycosaminoglycan side chains.[22] The major proteoglycan is aggrecan, which consists of a protein core and chondroitin sulfate and keratan sulfate side chains. The proteoglycans confer many of the unique mechanical properties of cartilage, including its ability to absorb repetitive compressive mechanical loads without damage. Aggrecan molecules form aggregates with hyaluronic acid and a link glycoprotein. In addition, cartilage contains small proteoglycans, such as decorin and biglycan. In addition to type II collagen and aggrecan, there are a series of minor collagens that also contribute to the chondrocytic phenotype. These include type VI, IX, X, and XI collagens.[20] Type VI collagen is a pericellular matrix protein, whereas type IX is a collagen molecule with a proteoglycan moiety. Type IX collagen molecules coat the outer surface of type II collagen fibrils and interact with the matrix proteoglycan via proteoglycan moieties. This is thought to serve as an interconnection between the collagen and proteoglycan matrix. Type XI collagen is localized within the type II fibrils and may regulate the diameters of fibrils.

Several chondrocyte phenotypic markers are specific to the differentiation pathway of the chondrocyte. For instance, type X collagen is only expressed by hypertrophic chondrocytes and is a specific marker for this phenotype.[18,22] In addition, these cells express high levels of alkaline phosphatase, in contrast to the minimal expression observed in chondrocytes that are not committed to maturation. Chondrocytes committed to the endochondral calcification pathway also express and respond to several growth factors, including several BMPs[21] and the cell signaling protein Indian hedgehog (IHH),[23] which promote chondrocyte maturation, and parathyroid hormone-related protein (PTHrp)[24] which inhibits it via inhibition of RUNX2 by cyclic AMP response element binding protein (CREBP). Differential expression of these genes in articular and epiphyseal plate chondrocytes demonstrates the critical role of regulatory gene products that may operate as determinants of chondrocytic phenotypes. **Figure 4** summarizes the key signaling, matrix and phenotypic genes expressed, and chondrocyte functional activities at each stage of chondrocyte differentiation, and **Table 1** compiles information about the key pathways that impact chondrocyte differentiation and function.

OSTEOBLASTS

OB DIFFERENTIATION

OB formation from MSCs, which occurs in endochondral ossification and intramembranous bone formation, is a two-step process involving (1) lineage commitment of MSCs to osteogenic precursors followed by (2) differentiation of pre-OBs and their maturation into OBs. Several critical signaling pathways and transcription factors are involved. Key regulators include the BMPs and their signaling pathways, the

 ©Copyright 2021 American Academy of Orthopaedic Surgeons

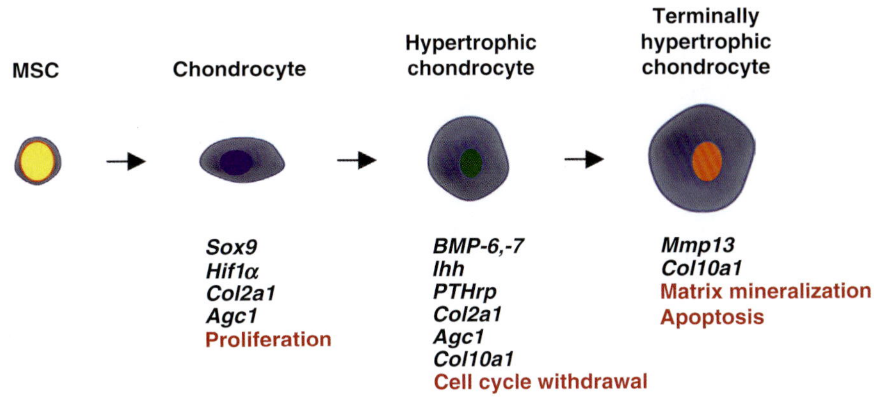

FIGURE 4 Pictorial representation of Chondrocyte differentiation. The key stages of chondrocyte differentiation from mesenchymal stem cells (MSCs) into terminally hypertrophic chondrocytes are depicted. Listed for each differentiation stage are the central factors, phenotypic genes, and important cellular activities.

transcription factor RUNX2, the Wingless (Wnt)-β-catenin signaling pathway, and the Notch pathway. A broad literature documents the central roles of each of these factors and signaling cascades; these concepts are summarized below and in **Table 1**, and their net effects in OB differentiation are summarized in **Figure 5**.

1. *The BMP signaling pathway.* BMP signaling involves as many as 20 agonist ligands which are members of the TGFβ superfamily of growth factors. BMPs bind to their cognate transmembrane serine-threonine kinase receptors to activate canonical Smad1,5,8-dependent and noncanonical p38 mitogen-activated protein kinase (p38 MAPK) signaling.[25] When the Smad molecules are activated, they serve as transcription factors that can directly target gene expression. Comparatively, active p38 MAPK serves as a signal transducer that induces various transcription factors to become active. Overall, stimulation of these signaling cascades results in expression of RUNX2, an essential transcription factor for OB differentiation[26] and development of a mineralized skeleton.[27] It should be noted that BMPs often have redundant roles in OB development. For example, although BMP2, BMP4, and BMP7 all regulate limb development, single knockout mice for individual family members have normal limb development and appropriate skeletal mineralization.[28]
2. *RUNX2: A master regulator of bone formation.* Downstream of the BMP signaling pathways, RUNX2 plays essential roles in bone formation by transactivating many genes required for OB differentiation and skeletal mineralization. RUNX2 is initially expressed in mesenchymal condensations during anlagen formation, well before the appearance of chondroblasts or OBs at the very earliest stages of endochondral ossification.[26] Its levels are tightly controlled by multiple processes, including transcriptional regulation and protein modifications including phosphorylation and ubiquitination. It is essential for vascular invasion of the calcified hypertrophic cartilage in anlagen by directly regulating the vascular endothelial growth factor A (VEGF-A) gene, a master regulator of vasculogenesis in nascent (ie, anlagen) or healing tissue fields.[29] Access to blood supply under these conditions is a critical requirement for OBs to form, become anabolic, and mineralize the matrix.
   Recently it has been understood that OB differentiation is tightly associated with increased energy demand involving glucose metabolism and protein synthesis, both of which are regulated by factors that drive OB differentiation. Glucose enters OBs through the glucose transporter (Glut1) whose expression in pre-OBs requires RUNX2. Crosstalk between Glut1 and RUNX2 determines the onset of OB differentiation and the extent of bone formation,[30] linking cellular metabolic activity with RUNX2 in progenitor cell commitment to the OB fate.
3. *The Wnt-β-catenin signaling pathway.* The Wnt-β-catenin signaling family consists of a large number of secreted glycoproteins, which function by either paracrine or autocrine mechanisms. Under conditions where the pathway is not active, the transcriptional regulator β-catenin is bound to a complex of proteins that target it for proteasomal degradation, thus blocking signaling. When Wnt ligands bind to the 7-transmembrane domain-spanning Frizzled (Fzd) receptor and LRP5/6 co-receptors, the complex that is binding β-catenin dissociates and β-catenin escapes the proteasome and is free to translocate to the nucleus to function as a transcription factor. Reduced signaling on this pathway via deletion of LRP co-receptor genes leads to a delay in OB differentiation that skeletally manifests as reduced bone mineral density and smaller bones in the axial skeleton.[31] Conversely, mice expressing a mutant Lrp5 (G171V) allele have more OBs and increased bone mass.[32] Finally, *Lrp6–/–* mice are perinatal lethal due to developmental abnormalities, including truncations of the axial skeleton, limb defects, and loss of the paraxial mesoderm.[33] Consistent with this, OB-specific Lrp6 deletion leads to significantly reduced bone mass, fewer OBs, and lower bone formation rates.[34]
4. *Notch signaling.* Notch receptor family members influence OB fate following activation by five different agonistic ligands mentioned previously (Dll1, 3, and 4 and Jag1 and 2). As in chondrocytes, upon agonist binding, the

©Copyright 2021 American Academy of Orthopaedic Surgeons

TABLE 1 Summary of the Main Signaling Pathway Networks and Their Effects in Chondro- and Osteo-Lineage Cells

Pathway	Factor(s)	Receptor Signaling Molecule(s)	Cell Effect(s)
Hedgehog	Shh Ihh	Ptc1, 2 and Smo receptors Gli transcription factors	***Chondrocytes:*** Activation of Sox9 and Nkx3-2 Chondrogenesis Induces hypertrophy
Notch	Dll1, 3, and 4 Jag1 and 2	Notch1 and 2 receptors γ-Secretase and NICD RBP-jκ transcription factor	***Chondrocytes:*** Activation of Hes1 and 5 Inhibits chondrogenesis ***OBs:*** Activation of Hes1 and Hey-like Inhibits differentiation
TGFβ (canonical)	TGFβ	Nine TGFβ receptor subunits Smad2, 3 transcription factors	***Chondrocytes:*** Activation of Sox9 Chondrogenesis Inhibits hypertrophy ***OBs:*** Progenitor Proliferation Osteoblast Lineage Commitment
BMP (canonical)	BMP	Four BMP receptor subunits Smad1, 5, 8 transcription factors	***Chondrocytes:*** Activation of Sox9 and RUNX2 Chondrogenesis Induces hypertrophy ***OBs:*** Activation of RUNX2 Induces differentiation
PTHrP	PTHrP, PTH	PTH1R CREBP transcription factor	***Chondrocytes:*** Inhibits RUNX2 Inhibits hypertrophy ***OBs:*** Induces deposition of bone matrix
Wnt-β-catenin	19 different Wnt ligands	FZD receptor, LRP coreceptors β-Catenin transcription factor	***OBs:*** Activates RUNX2 Induces differentiation

Notch intracellular domain (NICD) of activated receptors is cleaved by the γ-secretase enzyme and translocates to the nucleus where it regulates expression of target genes, including the transcription factors Hes1 and Hey-like, both of which act to suppress osteo-lineage commitment.[35] Genetically modified mice with depletion of Notch[36] or γ-secretase[37] in the limb mesenchyme or OB precursors have markedly increased bone mass in adolescence followed by severe osteopenia as they age as a result of precocious OB differentiation. This led to the general concept that Notch signaling acts normally to maintain a pool of mesenchymal progenitors and inhibit OB precursor differentiation.[38]

OB FUNCTION

OBs have several phenotypic characteristics that are required for confirmation of lineage commitment and support the physiochemical regulatory steps that lead to bone formation. The key extracellular steps contributing to nucleation of mineral crystal and production of mineralized tissue are described elsewhere in this compendium. This chapter, on the other hand, describes the biological and physiologic aspects of OB function that support matrix mineralization.

OBs produce and secrete structural proteins such as collagen and regulatory proteins including numerous growth factors,[39] all of which are critical in the ultimate production of mineralized matrix. The study of OBs has been facilitated by the development of methods for isolating them from intact bone tissue, usually by collagenase digestions of rodent calvarial or long bone specimens, or human trabecular bone specimens. Osteoblastic cells are also derived from tumors or immortalization by viral transformations. Commonly used cell lines include ROS 17.28 (rat), UMR106 (rat), SAOS2 (human), MG63 (human), and MC3T3 (murine).[40] The most abundant extracellular matrix produced by OBs is known as osteoid, which comprises an unmineralized type I collagen-proteoglycan matrix that biochemically facilitates binding of calcium and phosphate.[3] When this matrix is mineralized with crystalline hydroxyapatite, the matrix becomes what is macroscopically appreciated to be bone tissue. The major matrix protein synthesized by osteoblastic cells, which comprises more than 90% of the organic matrix of bone, is type I collagen. Type I collagen is synthesized and secreted as a triple helix with two α1 and one α2 chains (genes designated as COLIA1 and COLIA2).[41] The amino-terminal and carboxy-terminal propeptides are cleaved extracellularly, and the collagen molecules spontaneously self-assemble into collagen microfibrils and fibrils with a quarter-staggered arrangement of the individual molecules. The C-propeptide is cleaved by the proteolytic activity of BMP-1, a member of the BMP family that lacks osteoinductive capacity but has some homology to the other members.[42] The C-propeptide and N-propeptide fragments can be detected in serum; these fragments are indicative of bone formation rates.[43] Bone matrix also contains small amounts of type III and type V collagens. The collagen fibrils are laid down parallel to the surface of the OB and spontaneously nucleate hydroxyapatite crystals that initially form

©Copyright 2021 American Academy of Orthopaedic Surgeons

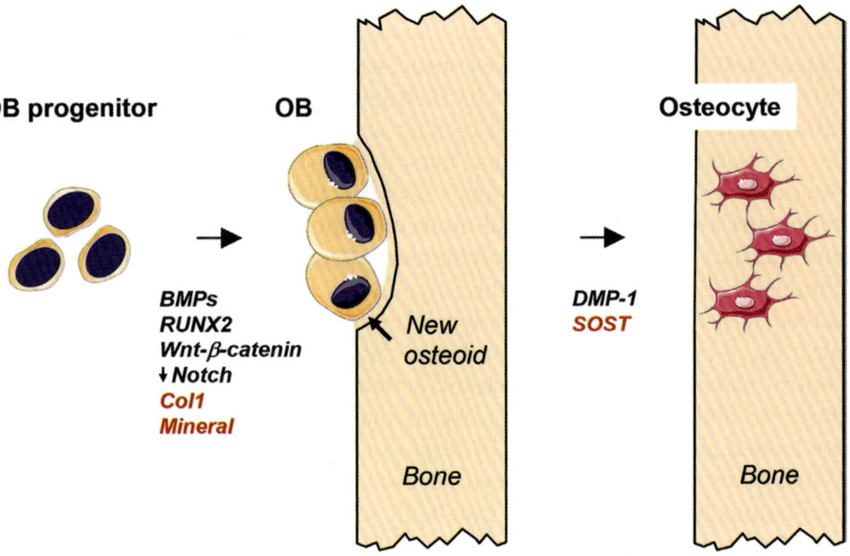

FIGURE 5 Pictorial representation of osteoblast (OB) differentiation. The stages of OB differentiation, starting from osteoprogenitor cells, leading to mature OBs producing osteoid, and culminating in the encasement of the most mature cells in bone matrix as osteocytes, are illustrated. The central regulators of each differentiation step are listed.

between the quarter-staggered collagen molecules.[44] With a periodicity related to the bone formation rate, the orientation of the fibrils changes 90° to the preceding layer, resulting in a plywood-like layered structure that maximizes the tensile strength of the material.[44]

The carboxyglutamic acid–containing glycoprotein, osteocalcin, along with two other glycoproteins, osteopontin and osteonectin, are the next most abundant extracellular matrix protein constituents produced by OBs.[45] Osteonectin may function to enhance the binding of hydroxyapatite crystals to the collagen matrix as mineralization proceeds.[46] Osteocalcin is thought to facilitate recruitment of OCs to bone surfaces for bone resorption along with playing a role in glucose metabolism in OBs,[47] and osteopontin is thought to modulate immune and inflammatory responses and possibly enhance OB survival by inhibiting apoptosis.[48] Bone matrix also contains a sialoprotein and small amounts of several other glycoproteins and phosphoproteins of uncertain function.[45]

Overall, the extracellular matrix structural proteins produced by OBs are one set of phenotypic parameters that define the lineage. During OB differentiation, there are several shifts in protein synthesis: (1) from a mixture of type III and type I collagen to predominantly type I collagen; (2) from low to high levels of alkaline phosphatase; (3) from versican to fibronectin expression; and (4) from expression of an attachment protein called thrombospondin to expression of the bone glycoproteins, osteonectin, osteocalcin, osteopontin, and sialoprotein.[22] These phenotypic shifts during differentiation are indicative of the differentiated state of OBs, serving as a powerful tool to stage the progression of differentiation. Bone matrix also contains several regulatory proteins deposited by OBs. These include growth factors such as TGF-β, IGF-I and IGF-II, FGFs, PDGF, and BMPs.[22] Although present quantitatively in minute amounts, these proteins are extremely important in regulating bone remodeling and in conferring osteoinductive capacity to bone.

In terms of endocrine regulation of bone, OBs display responsiveness of various hormones and vitamins in addition to the local paracrine signaling molecules mentioned above. OBs respond to PTH because of their expression of the PTH receptor (PTH1R) and exhibit intracellular signaling responses to receptor activation that can be important in endocrine regulation of circulating calcium levels, and under specific conditions, increased deposition of bone matrix.[24] OBs also express the vitamin D receptor and consequently have vitamin D responsiveness that supports enhanced mineral matrix deposition.[49] It is for these reasons that frontline approaches to deal with bone loss, particularly in osteoporosis, involve calcium and vitamin D supplementation,[50] or in severe bone loss situations, treatment with PTH analogs (ie, teriparatide or the new PTH-related protein derivative, abaloparatide).[51,52] Glucocorticoids have complex effects on bone, stimulating differentiation of pre-OBs in culture through a BMP-6–mediated pathway, while inhibiting OB proliferation and decreasing bone formation, resorption, and net mass when given systemically in vivo.[53]

OSTEOCYTES

OSTEOCYTE DIFFERENTIATION

A subset of OBs undergo a further terminal differentiation step and become osteocytes encased in secreted matrix.[22] OBs fated to undergo this transition encase themselves in osteoid that ultimately mineralizes to completely surround the cell in bone (**Figures 1**, **2**, and **5**). In addition to vitamin D and the impact of the surrounding matrix,[54] dentin matrix protein-1 (DMP-1) is important in driving osteocyte maturation, with its genetic deletion resulting in immature osteocytes, osteomalacia, and rickets.[55] Similarly, inactivation of the transcription factor Osterix in early OBs leads to defects in osteocyte maturation and a parallel loss of bone mass.[56]

©Copyright 2021 American Academy of Orthopaedic Surgeons

OSTEOCYTE FUNCTION

Osteocytes have numerous cell processes that extend throughout the bone matrix in channels known as canaliculi; these processes are often in contact with the cell processes of other osteocytes.[22] It has been demonstrated that osteocytes express cell-cell channels (gap junctions) called connexins, through which small molecules, including second messengers, can pass,[57] implying that osteocytes are in communication with one another. A putative function of osteocyte-osteocyte communication within the larger organization of bone is in sensing and modulating signals that control osteoblastic and osteoclastic activity, enabling the observed ability of bone to increase its mass in areas that are loaded and decrease mass in response to unloading.[58] When bones are loaded, osteocytes sense loading-induced oscillations in fluid flow in the canaliculi and perceive tensile strains during normal activities, facilitating paracrine signaling events that modulate bone homeostasis in this context.[4] For example, sclerostin, a Wnt ligand decoy receptor encoded by the SOST gene, is secreted by osteocytes in response to loading,[59] serving as a negative regulator of osteoblastic bone formation by reducing Wnt-β-catenin canonical signaling in OBs.

OSTEOCLASTS

OC DIFFERENTIATION

OCs are multinucleated cells formed by cytoplasmic fusion of committed precursors derived from the myeloid lineage of hematopoietic cells that also gives rise to macrophages.[6] Differentiation of OC progenitor cells requires their expression of cytokine receptors and numerous transcription factors and signaling molecules that regulate osteoclastogenesis. Macrophage-colony stimulating factor (M-CSF) and RANKL are the two most important cytokines required for OC formation under basal and pathologic conditions,[6] but co-stimulatory signaling through other receptors also mediates osteoclastogenesis, particularly in response to inflammation.[60] Other pro-osteoclastogenic cytokines are IL-1, granulocyte M-CSF, IL-6, and prostaglandin E2.[61] Anti-osteoclastogenic cytokines are IFN-β, IFN-γ, and IL-4, and these suppress RANKL-induced osteoclastogenesis.[61] Also inhibiting OC differentiation is osteoprotegerin (OPG), a decoy receptor for RANKL that reduces RANKL action in precursor populations and stalls OC differentiation.[62] OPG can function at any step along the path to activation of multinucleated OCs. These factors ultimately interact to modulate differentiation through the formation of preosteoclasts, to multinucleated OCs (ie, fused polykaryons) to actively resorbing mature OCs (**Figure 6**).

OC FUNCTION

OCs attach to bone surfaces through a specific cell attachment receptor called an integrin. This OC-specific integrin is known as $\alpha_v\beta3$, or the vitronectin receptor.[62] Several bone matrix proteins, including type I collagen, fibronectin, and osteopontin, contain the attachment arginine-glycine-aspartate (RGD) sequences.[63] After attachment to a bone surface, the integrins activate focal adhesion kinases, including c-src, which is a regulatory kinase that contributes to the induction of OC polarization. Polarization involves formation of an extensive series of microscopic invaginations of the plasma membrane surface against the bone matrix surface. These invaginations are referred to as the ruffled border, which is a structure that serves to markedly increase the surface area of membrane next to the bone. A plasma membrane proton pump moves to the ruffled border and pumps protons from the cytosol into the sealed space between the OC and the bone. This acidifies the bone surface, resulting in dissolution of the hydroxyapatite mineral phase of the bone.[63]

Lysosomes move to the ruffled border and discharge their contents of lysosomal enzymes into the resorption region. These enzymes include acid-activated hydrolases such as cathepsin, which degrades the collagen in the matrix. Furthermore, OCs express an isoform of carbonic anhydrase (CAII), which generates intracellular protons for the acidification process. OCs also express matrix metalloproteinase (gelatinase B, or MMP) and a specific phosphatase, tartrate resistant acid phosphatase (TRAP), but the functions of these enzymes remain unclear.[63] TRAP and other lysosomal enzymes are deposited on the resorption surface and remain

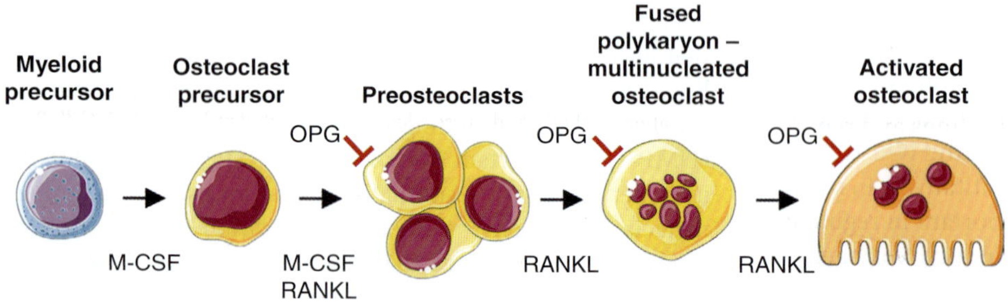

FIGURE 6 Pictorial representation of osteoclast (OC) differentiation. The stages of OC differentiation, starting from myeloid precursors and progressing to multinuclear OCs (fused polykaryon) and active OCs, are summarized. The central regulators of each differentiation step are also included.

©Copyright 2021 American Academy of Orthopaedic Surgeons

there even after the OC has moved away. Many of these enzymes contain glycosylations, which permit these enzymes to bind to receptors such as the IFGII/mannose-6-phosphate receptor.[63] This receptor is expressed by OBs, and when stimulated, it causes anabolic effects and stimulates matrix synthesis. Theoretically, the residue of glycosylated enzymes on the resorption surface may function to target OBs to this location and initiate bone formation, thus representing part of the site-directing coupling mechanism between bone formation and resorption (**Figure 2**). OCs contain a calcium receptor that may be involved in the induction of pseudopodia to enable OCs to become motile and creep along the bone surface as they excavate the matrix. When the pseudopodia lift up from the bone surface and move to reattach, the high concentration of inorganic calcium and phosphate ions that have accumulated from bone matrix resorption becomes discharged into the extracellular space. Some of the matrix and mineral may be removed by endocytosis and transport across the OC, but this is controversial. OCs have a finite lifetime and are active in bone resorption for an estimated 2 weeks, after which they undergo apoptosis.[20]

Several key hormones and local factors control OC function. Systemically, PTH stimulates bone resorption.[24] However, only OBs and not OCs express the PTH receptor. Therefore, the stimulation of resorption by PTH is mediated through indirect signaling from OBs to OCs.[24] One of these signals may be IL-6, a stimulator of OC formation and resorptive activity. Similar to IL-1, TNF-α is an extremely potent stimulator of OC progenitor proliferation, fusion, and activation of osteoclastic bone resorption. TNF-α, IL-1, and IL-6 are produced by many inflammatory processes and are collectively known as proinflammatory cytokines.[64] These factors are critical to many important clinical disorders and have been implicated in pathologic bone resorption in metastatic and primary bone tumors, infection, prosthetic loosening, nonunion of fractures, osteoporosis, and periarticular bone loss in inflammatory arthropathies.

As mentioned, OCs are short-lived cells, and when apoptosis is initiated, they die predominantly in the central and deeper parts of resorption lacunae as new OCs form at the cutting edges of the lacunae by addition of new mononuclear cells.[6] The same cytokines that induce osteoclastogenesis (ie, RANKL, M-CSF, TNF, IL-1, and VEGF-A) also prevent their apoptosis.[6] Withdrawal of these cytokines from OC cultures leads to rapid induction of apoptosis. OCs have long been considered to be merely bone-degrading cells whose formation and functions were under the control of osteoblastic, stromal, and immune cells in the marrow. However, OCs and their precursors interact with, and positively and negatively regulate, the formation and functions of these and other cell types, and they can behave as immune cells.[65] These findings and reports of OCs having regulatory roles in autoimmune and inflammatory diseases affecting the skeleton spawned the field of osteoimmunology,[60] which has at its core an immunomodulatory role for the OC that goes beyond its classic role as a bone resorbing cell.

SUMMARY

This chapter has aimed to provide a concise summary of cell biology in the context of the central cell types that participate in the biology that plays out in the bony skeleton. MSCs and populations of progenitor cells, chondrocytes, OBs, osteocytes, and OCs each have a unique role to play in development, growth and homeostasis of bone and cartilage, and the key regulators of these cell types are described to set the stage for understanding how dysregulation of these regulatory pathways leads to disease. Many of the signaling molecules and transcription factors mentioned here will be important in subsequent chapters where the molecular basis of skeletal control and disease progression is more deeply discussed.

REFERENCES

1. Karsenty G, Kronenberg HM, Settembre C: Genetic control of bone formation. *Annu Rev Cell Dev Biol* 2009;25:629-648.
2. Undale A, Srinivasan B, Drake M, et al: Circulating osteogenic cells: Characterization and relationship to rates of bone loss in postmenopausal women. *Bone* 2010;47:83-92.
3. Anderson HC: Mechanism of mineral formation in bone. *Lab Invest* 1989;60:320-330.
4. Bonewald LF: The role of the osteocyte in bone and Nonbone disease. *Endocrinol Metab Clin North Am* 2017;46:1-18.
5. Percival CJ, Richtsmeier JT: Angiogenesis and intramembranous osteogenesis. *Dev Dyn* 2013;242:909-922.
6. Boyce BF: Advances in osteoclast biology reveal potential new drug targets and new roles for osteoclasts. *J Bone Miner Res* 2013;28:711-722.
7. Samsa WE, Zhou X, Zhou G: Signaling pathways regulating cartilage growth plate formation and activity. *Semin Cell Dev Biol* 2017;62:3-15.
8. Wilson CW, Chuang PT: Mechanism and evolution of cytosolic Hedgehog signal transduction. *Development* 2010;137:2079-2094.
9. Monsoro-Burq AH: Sclerotome development and morphogenesis: When experimental embryology meets genetics. *Int J Dev Biol* 2005;49:301-308.
10. Zeng L, Kempf H, Murtaugh LC, Sato ME, Lassar AB: Shh establishes an Nkx3.2/Sox9 autoregulatory loop that is maintained by BMP signals to induce somitic chondrogenesis. *Genes Dev* 2002;16:1990-2005.
11. Rutkowski TP, Kohn A, Sharma D, et al: HES factors regulate specific aspects of chondrogenesis and chondrocyte hypertrophy during cartilage development. *J Cell Sci* 2016;129:2145-2155.
12. ten Berge D, Brugmann SA, Helms JA, Nusse R: Wnt and FGF signals interact to coordinate growth with cell fate specification during limb development. *Development* 2008;135:3247-3257.
13. Provot S, Zinyk D, Gunes Y, et al: Hif-1alpha regulates differentiation of limb bud mesenchyme and joint development. *J Cell Biol* 2007;177:451-464.
14. Karamboulas K, Dranse HJ, Underhill TM: Regulation of BMP-dependent chondrogenesis in early limb mesenchyme by TGFbeta signals. *J Cell Sci* 2010;123:2068-2076.
15. Rosen V: BMP and BMP inhibitors in bone. *Ann N Y Acad Sci* 2006;1068:19-25.

©Copyright 2021 American Academy of Orthopaedic Surgeons

16. Las Heras F, Gahunia HK, Pritzker KP: Articular cartilage development: A molecular perspective. *Orthop Clin N Am* 2012;43:155-171, v.

17. Yang X, Chen L, Xu X, et al: TGF-beta/Smad3 signals repress chondrocyte hypertrophic differentiation and are required for maintaining articular cartilage. *J Cell Biol* 2001;153:35-46.

18. Buckwalter JA, Mankin HJ, Grodzinsky AJ: Articular cartilage and osteoarthritis. *Instr Course Lect* 2005;54:465-480.

19. Schulze-Tanzil G: Activation and dedifferentiation of chondrocytes: Implications in cartilage injury and repair. *Ann Anat* 2009;191:325-338.

20. Bilezikian JP, Raisz LG, Rodan GA. *Principles of Bone Biology*. San Diego, CA: Academic Press; 1996.

21. Karsenty G: Transcriptional control of skeletogenesis. *Annu Rev Genomics Hum Genet* 2008;9:183-196.

22. Buckwalter JA, Ehrlich MG, Sandell LJ, Trippel SB. *Skeletal Growth and Development: Clinical Issues and Basic Science Advances*. Rosemont, IL: American Academy of Orthopaedic Surgeons; 1998.

23. Maeda Y, Nakamura E, Nguyen MT, et al: Indian Hedgehog produced by postnatal chondrocytes is essential for maintaining a growth plate and trabecular bone. *Proc Natl Acad Sci USA* 2007;104:6382-6387.

24. Kronenberg HM: PTHrP and skeletal development. *Ann N Y Acad Sci* 2006;1068:1-13.

25. Sanchez-Duffhues G, Hiepen C, Knaus P, Ten Dijke P: Bone morphogenetic protein signaling in bone homeostasis. *Bone* 2015;80:43-59.

26. Vimalraj S, Arumugam B, Miranda PJ, Selvamurugan N: Runx2: Structure, function, and phosphorylation in osteoblast differentiation. *Int J Biol Macromol* 2015;78:202-208.

27. Komori T: Runx2, a multifunctional transcription factor in skeletal development. *J Cell Biochem* 2002;87:1-8.

28. Kamiya N, Mishina Y: New insights on the roles of BMP signaling in bone-A review of recent mouse genetic studies. *Biofactors* 2011;37:75-82.

29. Zelzer E, Glotzer DJ, Hartmann C, et al: Tissue specific regulation of VEGF expression during bone development requires Cbfa1/Runx2. *Mech Dev* 2001;106:97-106.

30. Wei J, Shimazu J, Makinistoglu MP, et al: Glucose uptake and Runx2 synergize to orchestrate osteoblast differentiation and bone formation. *Cell* 2015;161:1576-1591.

31. Zhao L, Shim JW, Dodge TR, Robling AG, Yokota H: Inactivation of Lrp5 in osteocytes reduces young's modulus and responsiveness to the mechanical loading. *Bone* 2013;54:35-43.

32. Frey JL, Li Z, Ellis JM, et al: Wnt-Lrp5 signaling regulates fatty acid metabolism in the osteoblast. *Mol Cell Biol* 2015;35:1979-1991.

33. Williams BO, Insogna KL: Where Wnts went: The exploding field of Lrp5 and Lrp6 signaling in bone. *J Bone Miner Res* 2009;24:171-178.

34. Li C, Xing Q, Yu B, et al: Disruption of LRP6 in osteoblasts blunts the bone anabolic activity of PTH. *J Bone Miner Res* 2013;28:2094-2108.

35. Zanotti S, Canalis E: Notch and the skeleton. *Mol Cell Biol* 2010;30:886-896.

36. Engin F, Yao Z, Yang T, et al: Dimorphic effects of Notch signaling in bone homeostasis. *Nat Med* 2008;14:299-305.

37. Hilton MJ, Tu X, Wu X, et al: Notch signaling maintains bone marrow mesenchymal progenitors by suppressing osteoblast differentiation. *NatMed* 2008;14:306-314.

38. Zanotti S, Smerdel-Ramoya A, Stadmeyer L, et al: Notch inhibits osteoblast differentiation and causes osteopenia. *Endocrinology* 2008;149:3890-3899.

39. DiGirolamo DJ, Clemens TL, Kousteni S: The skeleton as an endocrine organ. *Nat Rev Rheumatol* 2012;8:674-683.

40. Kartsogiannis V, Ng KW: Cell lines and primary cell cultures in the study of bone cell biology. *Mol Cell Endocrinol* 2004;228:79-102.

41. Nagler-Anderson C, Bober LA, Robinson ME, Siskind GW, Thorbecke GJ: Suppression of type II collagen-induced arthritis by intragastric administration of soluble type II collagen. *Proc Natl Acad Sci USA* 1986;83:7443-7446.

42. Hoffmann A, Gross G: BMP signaling pathways in cartilage and bone formation. *Crit RevEukaryot Gene Expr* 2001;11:23-45.

43. Viguet-Carrin S, Garnero P, Delmas PD: The role of collagen in bone strength. *Osteoporos Int* 2006;17:319-336.

44. Katz EP, Wachtel E, Yamauchi M, Mechanic GL: The structure of mineralized collagen fibrils. *Connect Tissue Res* 1989;21:149-154; discussion 155-148.

45. Young MF, Kerr JM, Ibaraki K, Heegaard AM, Robey PG: Structure, expression, and regulation of the major noncollagenous matrix proteins of bone. *Clin Orthop Relat Res* 1992:275-294.

46. Fujisawa R, Wada Y, Nodasaka Y, Kuboki Y: Acidic amino acid-rich sequences as binding sites of osteonectin to hydroxyapatite crystals. *Biochim Biophys Acta* 1996;1292:53-60.

47. Mizokami A, Kawakubo-Yasukochi T, Hirata M: Osteocalcin and its endocrine functions. *Biochem Pharmacol* 2017;132:1-8.

48. Denhardt DT, Noda M: Osteopontin expression and function: Role in bone remodeling. *J Cell Biochem* 1998;72 Suppl 30-31:92-102.

49. Owen TA, Aronow MS, Barone LM, et al: Pleiotropic effects of vitamin D on osteoblast gene expression are related to the proliferative and differentiated state of the bone cell phenotype: Dependency upon basal levels of gene expression, duration of exposure, and bone matrix competency in normal rat osteoblast cultures. *Endocrinology* 1991;128:1496-1504.

50. Sunyecz JA: The use of calcium and vitamin D in the management of osteoporosis. *Ther Clin Risk Manag* 2008;4:827-836.

51. Bazaldua OV, Bruder J: Teriparatide (Forteo) for osteoporosis. *Am Fam Physician* 2004;69:1983-1984.

52. Boyce EG, Mai Y, Pham C: Abaloparatide: Review of a next-generation parathyroid hormone agonist. *Ann Pharmacother* 2018;52:462-472.

53. Cooper MS, Hewison M, Stewart PM: Glucocorticoid activity, inactivity and the osteoblast. *J Endocrinol* 1999;163:159-164.

54. Turner AG, Hanrath MA, Morris HA, Atkins GJ, Anderson PH: The local production of 1,25(OH)2D3 promotes osteoblast and osteocyte maturation. *J Steroid Biochem Mol Biol* 2014;144 Pt A:114-118.

55. Feng JQ, Ward LM, Liu S, et al: Loss of DMP1 causes rickets and osteomalacia and identifies a role for osteocytes in mineral metabolism. *Nat Genet* 2006;38:1310-1315.

56. Sinha KM, Zhou X: Genetic and molecular control of osterix in skeletal formation. *J Cell Biochem* 2013;114:975-984.

57. Kogianni G, Noble BS: The biology of osteocytes. *Curr Osteoporos Rep* 2007;5:81-86.

58. Uda Y, Azab E, Sun N, Shi C, Pajevic PD: Osteocyte mechanobiology. *Curr Osteoporos Rep* 2017;15:318-325.

59. Galea GL, Lanyon LE, Price JS: Sclerostin's role in bone's adaptive response to mechanical loading. *Bone* 2017;96:38-44.

60. Takayanagi H: Osteoimmunology in 2014: Two-faced immunology-from osteogenesis to bone resorption. *Nat Rev Rheumatol* 2015;11:74-76.

61. Lee SK, Lorenzo J: Cytokines regulating osteoclast formation and function. *Curr Opin Rheumatol* 2006;18:411-418.

62. Boyce BF, Xing L: Functions of RANKL/RANK/OPG in bone modeling and remodeling. *Arch Biochem Biophys* 2008;473:139-146.

63. Teitelbaum SL: Bone resorption by osteoclasts. *Science* 2000;289:1504-1508.

64. Borish LC, Steinke JW: 2. Cytokines and chemokines. *J Allergy Clin Immunol* 2003;111:S460-S475.

65. Boyce BF, Yao Z, Xing L: Osteoclasts have multiple roles in bone in addition to bone resorption. *Crit Rev Eukaryot Gene Expr* 2009;19:171-180.

©Copyright 2021 American Academy of Orthopaedic Surgeons

Biology and Mechanics of the Skeletal Extracellular Matrix

Zhijun Li, MD, PhD
Jill Helms, DDS, PhD

Keywords: *aged; bone; cartilage; stem cell*

INTRODUCTION TO THE SKELETAL EXTRACELLULAR MATRIX

The extracellular matrix is defined as the organic substance found between most eukaryotic cells and has three general functions. The first purpose is the most obvious: the extracellular matrix of the skeleton serves a structural role, in that it acts both as a substrate for cells and as a shape-maintaining scaffold for the body in response to gravity and other physical loads. A second function of the extracellular matrix is as a storage site for growth factors and cytokines. Some growth factors adhere to the matrix until released by action of matrix metalloproteinases and other enzymes, thereby making it an active participant in establishing morphogen gradients during development[1] and tissue repair.[2] A third function of the extracellular matrix is in communication: via molecules that span the membrane, cells attached to the matrix can sense and respond to changes in their environment.

Turnover rates in the extracellular matrix vary widely depending on anatomic location and the age of the animal. In general, cartilage extracellular matrix remains relatively stable throughout life with very slow rates of remodeling, except when degenerative changes are triggered by trauma or aging (reviewed in Ref. 3). This low remodeling rate is reflected in a minimal mitotic activity by cells in the articular cartilage,[4] and instead, the primary mode by which the size of the articular cartilage is increased is via matrix deposition.[5]

Neither of the following authors nor any immediate family member has received anything of value from or has stock or stock options held in a commercial company or institution related directly or indirectly to the subject of this chapter: Dr. Li and Dr. Helms.

Bone extracellular matrix, in contrast, undergoes nearly continual remodeling. Bone regularly sustains microdamage that, if not repaired, can accumulate and lead to fractures,[6] and osteocytes embedded in this bone extracellular matrix play an active role in orchestrating the action of osteoblasts and osteoclasts that remodel this microdamage (reviewed in Ref. 7). One molecular pathway that is particularly important in this regard is regulating by Wnt signaling. Osteocytes express Sclerostin, an inhibitor of the Wnt pathway,[8] and Sclerostin in turn acts as an inhibitor of bone formation.[9] In response to anabolic stimuli in the environment, Wnt signaling is activated, Sclerostin expression in osteocytes is downregulated, and osteoblasts are activated.[10] Through such mechanisms linking a physical stimulus with a molecular pathway, osteocytes can coordinate resorptive and formative actions that maintain the structural integrity of bone.

COLLAGEN COMPOSITION OF THE SKELETAL EXTRACELLULAR MATRICES

BONE EXTRACELLULAR MATRIX

Bone extracellular matrix is composed of an organic matrix, osteoid, that is strengthened by deposits of calcium phosphate. Approximately 95% of the osteoid matrix is composed of type I collagen, a fibrillar protein arranged in a triple helical pattern that gives the matrix high tensile strength. Type I collagen is comprised of heterotrimeric molecules, for example, two α1 (I) chains and one α2(I) chain,[11] and this structural heterogeneity is important. A case in point: in the disease state of osteogenesis imperfecta (OI), bones are exceedingly brittle.[12] The basis for these brittle bones appears to lie in the fact that OA bones are comprised of collagen that, instead of a heterotrimeric structure of two α1 (I) chains and one α2(I) chain, is a homotrimer molecule.[13]

©Copyright 2021 American Academy of Orthopaedic Surgeons

Homotrimeric isoforms of type I collagen are also found in fetal tissues, fibrosing conditions, and in cancers.[14] Precisely why a homotrimeric form of collagen has such a profound effect on skeletal fragility is not entirely clear, but structural studies of the molecule suggest that compared with heterotrimeric collagen, homotrimeric collagens form kinks, which in turn affect intermolecular cross-linking and ultimately affect the mechanical strength of the bone.[13]

The remaining 5% of the organic matrix of osteoid is composed of proteoglycans and other noncollagenous proteins. Proteoglycans act as a space-filling material. Because these molecules can absorb and release water, a proteoglycan-rich extracellular matrix can withstand substantial compressive forces without collapsing. The combination of a collagen- and proteoglycan-rich extracellular matrix is therefore ideally suited to the load-bearing function of the skeleton.

CARTILAGE EXTRACELLULAR MATRIX

Cartilage extracellular matrix differs substantially from bone extracellular matrix. Cartilage extracellular matrix is secreted by chondroblasts, and although it has a similar collagen content (~90% in bone versus ~90% to 95% in cartilage), cartilage has a much higher water content (~30% in bone and ~80% in cartilage) and a much higher concentration of proteoglycans (less than 1% in bone and ~15% in cartilage). Cartilage extracellular matrix also contains chondroitin sulfate, a sulfated glycosaminoglycan that provides resistance to compression.

In contrast to bone that is composed of type I collagen, cartilage is primarily composed of type II collagen that is formed from three identical α1 (II) chains. Mutations in the Col2A1 gene are responsible for a range of collagenopathies from a chondrogenesis type II (OMIM 200610), Stickler syndrome (OMIM 108300), to Legg-Calve-Perthes disease (OMIM 150600) and osteoarthritis with mild chondrodysplasia (OMIM 604864). The Col2A1 gene mutations responsible for these syndromes include point, missense, deletion, and insertion mutations, as well as complex rearrangements and frameshift mutations. Precisely how these mutations affect the structure of the collagen type II molecule is not fully understood, but current theories suggest that the mutations cause helical instability and inappropriate folding of the molecule.[15]

In the cartilage extracellular matrix, collagen fibrils are interspersed with densely packed proteoglycans, and this arrangement is key to the biomechanical function of the tissue. For example, when one of these components, for example, the proteoglycan aggrecan, is degraded, the result is a change in the biomechanical stability of cartilage. In the case of aggrecan, its degradation can lead to a decrease in the load-bearing capacity of cartilage, which can then progress to osteoarthritis (OA; reviewed in Ref. 16; see also OMIM 165800). In addition, mutations in type II collagen, cartilage oligomeric matrix protein (COMP), and the matrilins, which enhance collagen type II and aggrecan expression, are also associated with OA.[17]

THE SKELETAL EXTRACELLULAR MATRIX AS A BIOLOGICAL REPOSITORY

THE SKELETAL EXTRACELLULAR MATRIX AS A CALCIUM STORE

The skeleton contains 99% of the body's calcium, and this mineral is essential for a variety of physiological processes including vascular contraction, vasodilation, muscle functions, nerve transmission, intracellular signaling, and hormonal secretion. Calcium is stored in the skeleton as hydroxyapatite, which is released from the skeletal extracellular matrix in response to parathyroid hormone (PTH). PTH, in turn, is triggered when the concentration of Ca^{2+} drops in the blood. PTH has two major mechanisms for promoting the absorption of calcium: directly, by increasing Ca^{2+} reabsorption by the kidneys, and indirectly, by stimulating vitamin D activity (**Figure 1**). Another hormone, calcitonin, is produced by the parafollicular cells in the thyroid gland. Calcitonin also regulates levels of calcium in the blood, opposing the action of PTH and, in doing so, reduces osteoclast activity and decreases bone resorption. The functions of PTH and calcitonin are presented in detail elsewhere in this book; here, our focus will remain on the function of the extracellular matrix as an enzymatically accessible repository for growth factors.

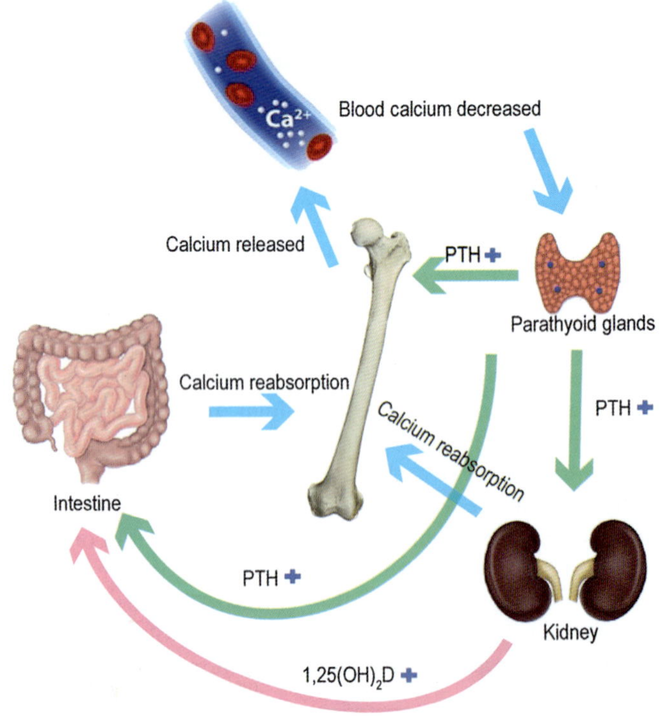

FIGURE 1 Illustration demonstrating that the skeletal extracellular matrix is a biological calcium store. Parathyroid glands produce parathyroid hormone that (PTH) controls body calcium level through bone, intestine and kidneys.

 ©Copyright 2021 American Academy of Orthopaedic Surgeons

THE SKELETAL EXTRACELLULAR MATRIX AS A GROWTH FACTOR STORE

Growth factors including fibroblast growth factors (FGFs), vascular endothelial growth factors (VEGFs), transforming growth factors (TGFs) bone morphogenetic proteins (BMPs), and Wnts can all bind to components of proteoglycans that are part of the skeletal extracellular matrix. This binding affinity between various growth factors and heparan sulfates has led to the idea that the extracellular matrix acts as a reservoir for growth factors, maybe even playing a role in establishing gradients of the growth factors that are necessary for developmental patterning.[1]

The release of growth factors from the extracellular matrix is governed in part by matrix metalloproteinases (MMPs), which places these molecules in an important position for regulating cell-extracellular matrix signaling during development, repair, and some disease states including cancer. It should also be noted that some growth factors use heparan sulfate as a cofactor in binding to their receptors, which then implicates the extracellular matrix as an active mediator of morphogenetic signaling.

ESTABLISHING THE SHAPE OF THE SKELETAL EXTRACELLULAR MATRIX

The ancient homeobox-containing Hox gene family was first identified because of its role in shaping the fruit fly body axis; this same family of transcription factors is now known to shape the structural framework of the skeleton. From ancient marine animals to today's man, Hox genes provide cells with a zip code of sorts, by which their position and ultimately their fate as skeletal cells are specified.

In the developing embryo, Hox genes are expressed in skeletal elements derived from the mesoderm, for example, the axial and appendicular skeletons. Hox genes are notably absent from the head and facial skeletons, which are derived from neural crest. This Hox-free status in neural crest cells is associated with remarkable plasticity and stem-like characteristics in this population.[18]

This Hox code also exists in the postnatal skeleton and during tissue repair.[19] Current understanding of the postnatal function of the Hox code is still being developed, but the fact that Hox genes are expressed in the stem/progenitor cells of the periosteum,[20] where they are involved in maintaining the multipotency of this progenitor population.[20]

ESTABLISHING THE CHONDROGENIC AND OSTEOGENIC LINEAGES

Once the molecular pattern of the skeleton is established, cells differentiate into chondrocytes and osteoblasts and produce the characteristic cartilaginous and bone extracellular matrices of the skeleton. How this decision is made is beginning to be understood as at least part of the answer lies in the balance of two transcription factors. Sox9 is a Sry-related transcription factor involved in the regulation of cartilage-specific genes. Runt-related transcription factor Runx2 (also known as Cbfa1) regulates the expression of genes such as ollagen type I and Osteocalcin and is required for both bone and cartilage formation.

Our current understanding is that the levels of Sox9 relative to Runx2 dictate whether cells adopt a chondrogenic or an osteogenic lineage. In brief, when Sox9 levels are elevated and Runx2 levels are low then cells adopt a chondrogenic fate; conversely, when Runx2 levels are high and Sox9 levels are low, cells adopt an osteogenic fate (**Figure 2**). By this mechanism, cells commit to a chondrogenic or osteogenic fate and produce the extracellular matrix unique to their fate.

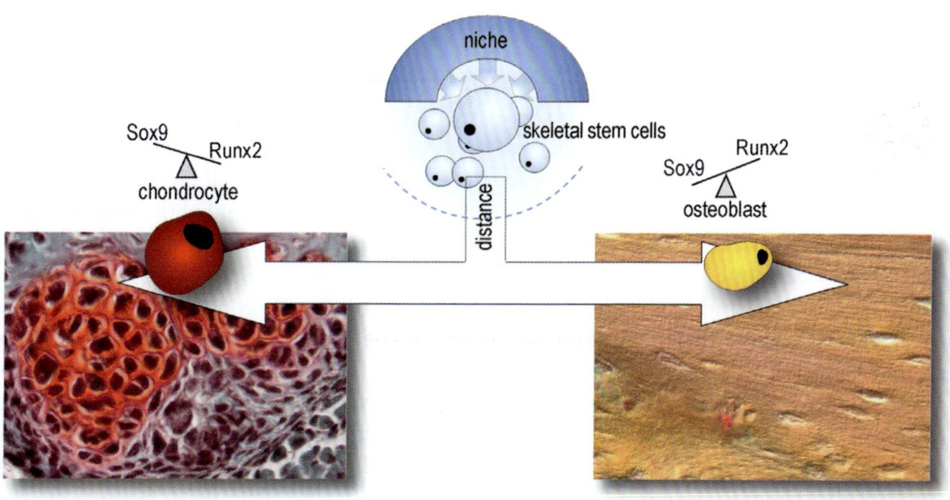

FIGURE 2 Illustration demonstrating that when the Sox9 expressing levels are high and Runx2 levels are low, then the skeletal stem cells adopt a chondrogenic fate. Conversely, when Runx2 levels are high and Sox9 levels are low, skeletal stem cells adopt an osteogenic fate.

©Copyright 2021 American Academy of Orthopaedic Surgeons

MECHANICAL SIGNALS SHAPE THE SKELETAL EXTRACELLULAR MATRIX

Around 400 million years ago, as animals transitioned from an aquatic to a terrestrial environment, the skeleton was placed under dramatically different physical demands. As a consequence, the weight of the skeletal extracellular matrix decreased and its flexibility increased. How did the skeleton get lighter without losing its strength? One evolved mechanism was to reduce the overall thickness of the extracellular matrix. Hollow bones are a generalized theropod condition and, compared with solid or virtually solid bones of the same diameter, are both lighter and stronger in bending.[21] The trabecular portion of the skeleton is lightweight and rapidly remodeled, and although it may appear to be randomly oriented, it is not. In fact, bone trabeculae remodel according to patterns of tension and compression.

As mentioned previously, one of the important functions of the extracellular matrix is communication and perhaps the best understood of the molecules responsible for this function are the integrins. As the extracellular matrix changes its stiffness, stem cells respond by altering their fate. For example, stem cells grown on a soft substrate, which replicates the elasticity of brain tissue, adopt a neuronal phenotype whereas cells grown on a stiff substrate, which mimics bone tissue, assume an osteoblast phenotype.[22] These data exemplify the intimate relationship that exists between the behavior of a cell and the extracellular matrix to which it is attached.

How do cells perceive the stiffness of the extracellular matrix? Integrins are prime candidates because they span the cell membrane, connecting the cytoskeleton to the extracellular matrix. In some biological systems, integrins are converted to a high affinity state in response to a mechanical force, but precisely how physical stimuli are transduced into biological responses via integrins remains poorly understood. Equally puzzling is how integrin-mediated responses are then integrated across multiple cell types and ultimately synchronized into a coordinated tissue-level response in a living organism.[23]

ORGANIZATION OF THE EXTRACELLULAR MATRIX INTO CORTICAL AND CANCELLOUS BONE

Morphologically, there are two organized forms of bone extracellular matrix: cortical (compact) and cancellous (trabecular) bone. In cortical bone, densely packed collagen fibrils form concentric lamellae, and the fibrils in adjacent lamellae run in perpendicular planes. Cancellous bone, on the other hand, has a more loosely organized, porous matrix.

A variety of classification schemes have been proposed that are loosely based on the proportion of compact cortical bone relative to spongy trabecular bone. For example, one clinical classification scheme[24] describes "type I" bone to be the least vascular and most homogenous; "type II" is a combination of cortical bone with a marrow cavity; "type III" is predominantly composed of trabecular bone; and "type IV" is described as having a very thin cortex and low-density trabeculae.

These different types of bone have biological significance. First, compared with type I bone, type III bone has significantly more proliferating cells in the periosteum.[25,26] Second, compare to type I bone, type III bone exhibits significantly more remodeling activity.[25] For example, some estimates suggest that in adult humans, 25% of trabecular bone volume is renewed each year, compared with only ~2% to 3% of cortical bone. A third biological difference is that type III bone had significantly more Wnt stem/osteoprogenitor cells, and significantly higher expression of Wnt target genes, than type I bone.[25]

These biological data have direct implications for clinical bone repair: In bones with greater regenerative potential (eg, type III bones), osteoprogenitor cells are more abundant, proliferate more readily, and deposit a collagen matrix sooner that begins to mineralize faster.[25] The presence of a mineralizing matrix stiffens the injury environment, which in turn lowers tissue strain, which then favors bone formation. This positive feedback loop exists in type III bone and ultimately manifests as faster healing. In type I bone, there is a notably lower rate of cell proliferation that is coupled with minimal collagen deposition; slower mineralization means that interfacial tissues fail to stiffen, and strains remain high; this high-strain environment favors the formation of fibrous tissue.[27]

ORGANIZATION OF THE EXTRACELLULAR MATRIX INTO HYALINE CARTILAGE

Hyaline cartilage covers the subchondral bone of most joint surfaces and is described as having a glassy appearance. The structure of hyaline cartilage allows for the near-frictionless movement of articulating joints while simultaneously absorbing the compressive forces generated by weight bearing (**Figure 3**). At a molecular level, the primary organic matrix of hyaline cartilage is comprised of collagen types II and IX. These collagens differ from collagen type I (found in bone) primarily because type II collagen is a homotrimer with a chain composition of $[\alpha1(II)]_3$.[11]

Hyaline cartilage has a layered arrangement. The most superficial layer is the thinnest and is in direct contact with synovial fluid of the joint. Underneath is a transitional zone comprised of chondrocytes embedded in their extracellular matrix. Collagen fibers in this zone are randomly arranged, and proteoglycan content is higher than in the superficial zone. Beneath the transition zone is the radial zone where cell density is lower, and viability is maintained by diffusion rather than vascularization. The calcified cartilage zone is deepest and is in contact with the underlying (subchondral) bone. Chondrocytes in this region synthesize type X collagen and were once thought to be metabolically inactive; this has since been disproven.

©Copyright 2021 American Academy of Orthopaedic Surgeons

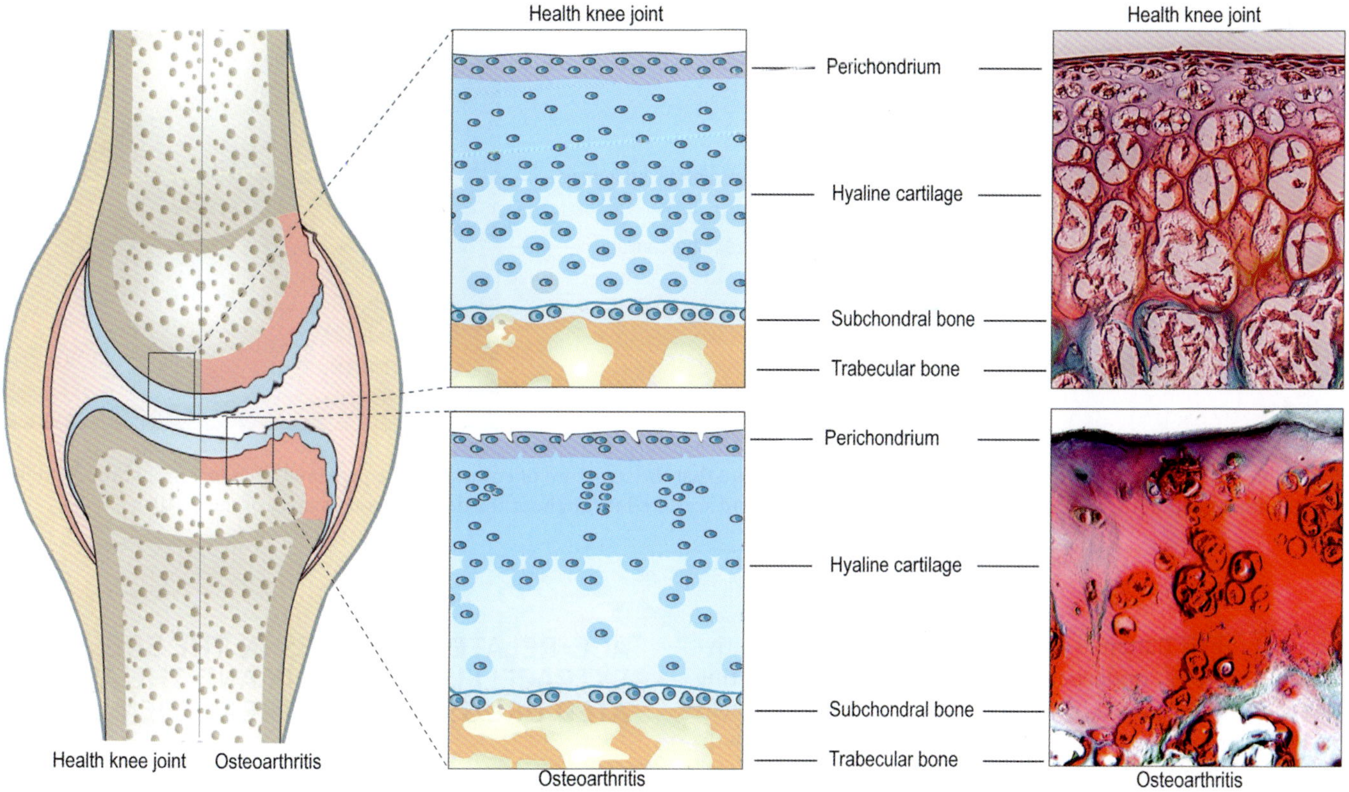

FIGURE 3 Schematics and Safranin O stained images show both healthy and osteoarthritic articular cartilage of the knee joint in a mouse model. Osteoarthritis (OA) is characterized by the loss of cartilage extracellular matrix and remodeling of subchondral bone.

Hyaline cartilage does not regenerate following injury. When hyaline cartilage is damaged, chondrocytes are the only cell type present and they must both degrade as well as synthesize the new hyaline cartilage extracellular matrix. The metabolic activity of these chondrocytes is under the control of anabolic and catabolic growth factors that include—but are not limited to—insulinlike growth factor, TGF-β, and components of the Wnt pathway. An increase in catabolic signaling induces the expression of matrix metalloproteinases and other enzymes that degrade the cartilage extracellular matrix. Chronic injury of the hyaline cartilage often leads to osteoarthritis.[28]

ORGANIZATION OF THE EXTRACELLULAR MATRIX INTO FIBROCARTILAGE

Fibrocartilage is typically found in the ventral part of the ribs (ie, costal cartilages), the nose, the larynx, the trachea, the intervertebral disks, menisci, and the triangular fibrocartilage complex of the wrist. Fibrocartilage is also referred to as white fibrocartilage, and its extracellular matrix is dominated by a dense, regular network of collagen fiber bundles that are arranged parallel to each other in several layers. Adjacent layers have these collagen bundles oriented in different directions, which produces an extracellular matrix with moderate elasticity (**Figure 4**). In its most typical form, fibrocartilage is predominantly composed of types I and II collagen; the relative proportions of these collagens can vary. For example, the knee joint menisci contains more type I collagen than type II, whereas the anulus fibrosus of the spine contains roughly equal quantities of collagen types I and II.[29] Osteophytic fibrocartilage, on the other hand, lacks type I collagen completely (**Figure 5**).

Fibrocartilage can undergo limited repair. For example, the meniscus is composed of fibrocartilage; the outer layer is vascularized; and this "red zone" of the meniscus can undergo repair. In contrast, the inner "white zone" is not vascularized, and when it is injured, healing is typically insufficient. The triangular fibrocartilage complex of the wrist is also composed of fibrocartilage, and in this case of ligament-to-bone repair, healing is typically inadequate. The basis for this limited healing potential is currently unknown.

ORGANIZATION OF THE EXTRACELLULAR MATRIX INTO EPIPHYSEAL PLATE CARTILAGE

Epiphyseal plate cartilage has a layered arrangement. Similar to articular cartilage, the zone closest to the primary ossification center is comprised of "resting" chondrocytes, so-called

©Copyright 2021 American Academy of Orthopaedic Surgeons

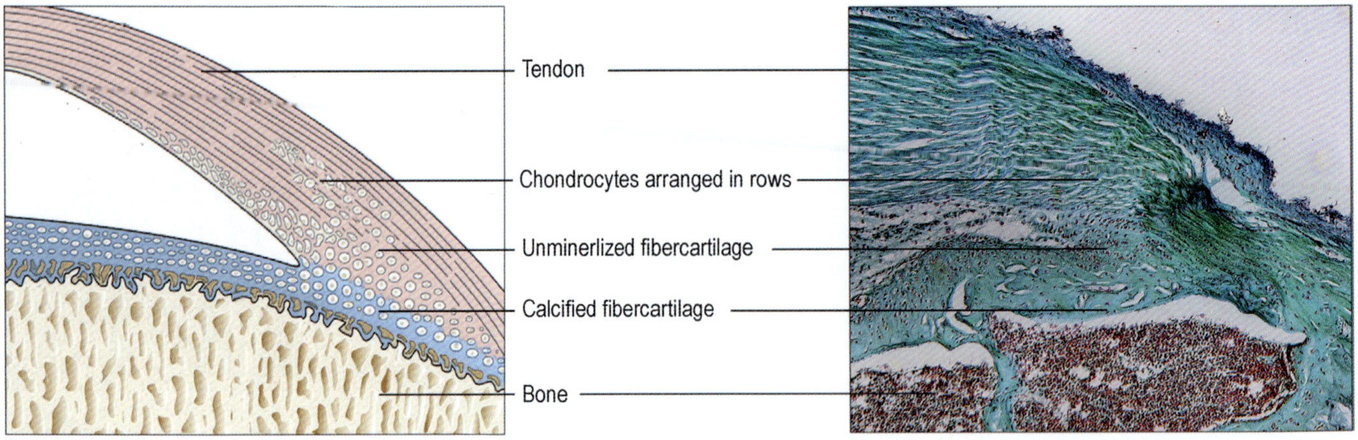

FIGURE 4 Schematic and Safranin O stained images demonstrate that the structure of enthesis at the proximal tibia in a mouse model. Fibers from tendon attach to the periosteum; chondrocytes are small and scattered throughout the dense fibrous matrix of the cartilage.

because of their flattened appearance and low mitotic activity. Immediately underneath this zone are proliferating chondrocytes, arranged in columns. These proliferating cells are the source of new cells that lead to long bone growth. The next layer is composed of prehypertrophic chondrocytes followed by hypertrophic chondrocytes. Hypertrophic chondrocytes are so named because the volume of their cytoplasm is significantly greater than that in other chondrocytes in the epiphyseal plate. Hypertrophic chondrocytes are also embedded in a calcified extracellular matrix. For many years, hypertrophy was considered the terminal state of chondrocyte differentiation because below this layer is trabecular bone. New studies, however, provide evidence that hypertrophic chondrocytes can transdifferentiate into osteoblasts that contribute to this new bone at the growing ends of appendicular skeletal elements.[30]

AGE-RELATED CHANGES IN THE SKELETAL EXTRACELLULAR MATRIX AND THE ASSOCIATED DRUGS USED TO TREAT THEM

The extracellular matrix of the skeleton changes with age, and one of the most obvious alterations is the loss of mass and volume (**Figure 6**). Low bone mass diseases including osteopenia/osteoporosis are characterized by a decrease in bone volume and bone mineral density, making the skeleton more fragile and therefore prone to fracture.

A decline in bone quantity is often equated with a decrease in bone quality, but this relationship is not so straightforward. For example, two individuals with the same bone mineral density may have dramatically different fracture risk profiles, if, for example, one individual is aged and the other is young.[31] New data indicate that the age-related increase in fracture

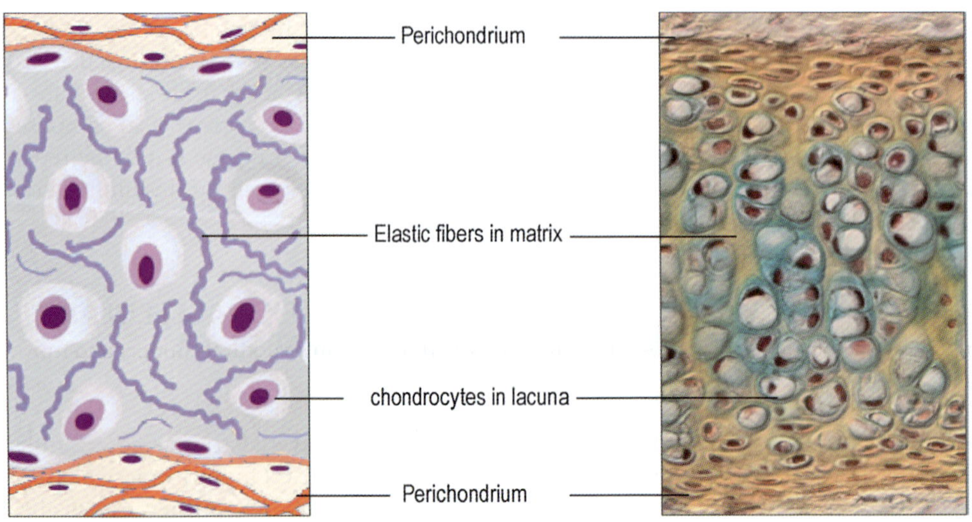

FIGURE 5 Schematic and pentachrome-stained image of mouse's ear section demonstrate that elastic cartilage contains elastic fibers comprising the extracellular matrix. These fibers form bundles that appear yellow in a pentachrome stained tissue. Chondrocytes lie between the fibers.

 ©Copyright 2021 American Academy of Orthopaedic Surgeons

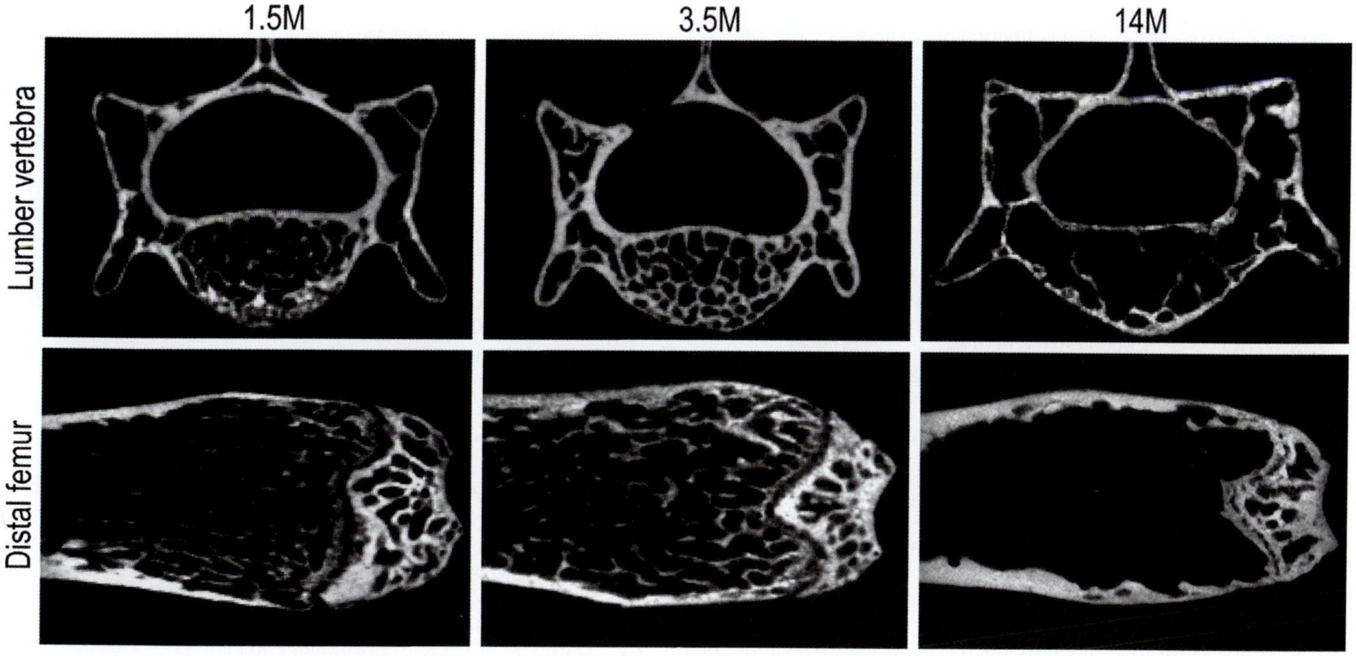

FIGURE 6 Two-dimensional reconstruction of μCT imaging performed on 1.5-month (**A**), 3.5-month (**B**), and 14-month-old mice (**C**) in the lumbar spine and the distal femur. Bone loss in the axial, appendicular skeletons that occurs as a consequence of age in these animals is analogous to that reported in human populations.

risk is more likely attributable to a decline in remodeling and repair functions.[32] As we age, our ability to repair microdamaged bone diminishes, and this weakens the skeletal extracellular matrix, making it more prone to failure.

Drugs that target this remodeling activity, that is, bisphosphonates (BPs) and receptor activator of nuclear factor kappa-B ligand (RANKL) inhibitors, result in bone accrual over time, but can also lead to accumulated microdamage.[33] Although the absolute risk is small, there is nonetheless a high prevalence of atypical femoral fractures in patients who are long-term BP users.[34] For example, in a 2014 report published by the American Society for Bone and Mineral Research, the assigned task force noted that there is a significant positive association between the use of BPs and the prevalence of atypical femur fractures (AFFs). The task force specifically stated, "Although the relative risk of patients with AFFs taking BPs is high, the absolute risk of AFFs in patients on BPs is low, ranging from 3.2 to 50 cases per 100,000 person-years."[35]

To address this shortcoming of BPs, other drugs have been developed. For example, another drug that blocks bone resorption is denosumab, a human monoclonal antibody that binds RANKL, preventing RANKL from activating RANK, its receptor on the osteoclast surface. With reduced RANK–RANKL binding, osteoclast formation, function, and survival are inhibited, and bone resorption decreases.[36]

The N-terminal portion of recombinant human PTH consisting of the 34-amino acid peptide hPTH(1-34), for example, teriparatide is a bone anabolic agent intended for use in the treatment of postmenopausal osteoporosis. The physiological role of PTH on skeletal homeostasis is complex and likely involves roles in bone remodeling as well as bone formation; consequently, the pharmacologic mechanism of teriparatide is not entirely clear. In general, the synthetic version of hPTH(1-34), Forteo, regulates calcium metabolism, and clinical use demonstrates its ability to promote bone formation rather than inhibit bone resorption as BPs do.

Another new drug in development that acts as an anabolic agent to stimulate bone accrual via activation of the Wnt pathway is the anti-Sclerostin antibody, for example, romosozumab. Wnt proteins are potent pro-osteogenic signals[37,38] that activate bone-forming, osteoblastic[39] pathways and repress bone-resorbing osteoclastic[40] pathways. Data accrued from a wide array of nonclinical studies definitively validate Wnt pathway agonists as bone-forming agents.[41] Wnt signaling declines with age,[41,42] and in the approach taken here, inhibiting the Wnt inhibitor, Sclerostin is thought to elevate Wnt signaling levels.[43] Early clinical trial results have shown promising results, although there are also reported side effects that may curtail their use.[44]

THE SKELETON AS A STEM CELL NICHE

Aside from its classic functions in structural support and movement, the skeleton acts as a stem cell niche for hematopoiesis and osteogenesis. In tissues that turn over rapidly, adult stem cells tend to be mitotically active; in tissues that have minimal turnover, stem cell pools tend to be quiescent. In both cases, these stem cell pools rapidly expand in response to injury.[45]

©Copyright 2021 American Academy of Orthopaedic Surgeons

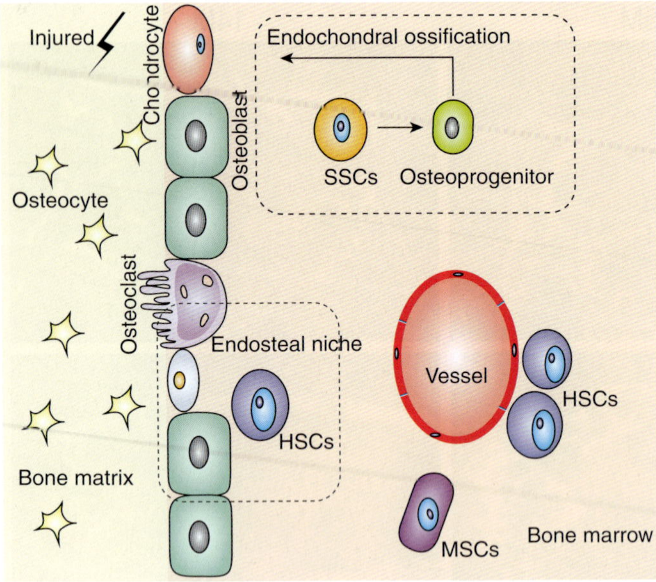

FIGURE 7 Illustration demonstrating that hematopoietic stem cells (HSCs) reside close to osteoblasts on the endosteal surface of the bone marrow, or adjacent to endothelial cells. Skeletal stem cells (SSCs) are also located in the bone marrow cavity, lining the trabeculae and in this location give rise to chondrocytes and osteoblasts. MSC = mesenchymal stem cell.

The bone marrow cavity is one such stem cell niche. Hematopoietic stem cells often reside adjacent to osteoblasts lining the endosteal surface of the bone in the marrow cavity. This physical proximity has suggested that the two cell types interact, and data supporting this conclusion have come from studies showing that osteoblasts produce hematopoietic stem cell–activating proteins. Skeletal stem cells also exist in the bone marrow cavity, and at least in some in vitro assays, these cells can give rise to cartilage and bone through a process akin to endochondral ossification.[46] The periosteum is another source of skeletal stem cells,[47] which give rise to new bone via intramembranous ossification. This pool of stem cells exhibits plasticity, in that they can also give rise to cartilage in the event of an injury (**Figure 7**). Given the location of these two skeletal stem cell populations, it is tempting to speculate that diseases which diminish their niches would necessarily diminish the stem cell pool. Indeed, this appears to be the case in diseases such as osteopetrosis and osteoporosis.[48]

REFERENCES

1. Brown NH: Extracellular matrix in development: Insights from mechanisms conserved between invertebrates and vertebrates. *Cold Spring Harb Perspect Biol* 2011;3(12).
2. Checa S, Rausch MK, Petersen A, Kuhl E, Duda GN: The emergence of extracellular matrix mechanics and cell traction forces as important regulators of cellular self-organization. *Biomech Model Mechanobiol* 2015;14(1):1-13.
3. Asanbaeva A, Masuda K, Thonar EJ, Klisch SM, Sah RL: Cartilage growth and remodeling: Modulation of balance between proteoglycan and collagen network in vitro with beta-aminopropionitrile. *Osteoarthr Cartil* 2008;16(1):1-11.
4. Kavanagh E, Abiri M, Bland YS, Ashhurst DE: Division and death of cells in developing synovial joints and long bones. *Cell Biol Int* 2002;26(8):679-688.
5. Williamson AK, Chen AC, Masuda K, Thonar EJ, Sah RL: Tensile mechanical properties of bovine articular cartilage: Variations with growth and relationships to collagen network components. *J Orthop Res* 2003;21(5):872-880.
6. Donahue SW, Sharkey NA, Modanlou KA, Sequeira LN, Martin RB: Bone strain and microcracks at stress fracture sites in human metatarsals. *Bone* 2000;27(6):827-833.
7. Bonewald LF: The amazing osteocyte. *J Bone Miner Res* 2011;26(2):229-238.
8. Delgado-Calle J, Sato AY, Bellido T: Role and mechanism of action of sclerostin in bone. *Bone* 2017;96:29-37.
9. van Bezooijen RL, Roelen BA, Visser A, et al: Sclerostin is an osteocyte-expressed negative regulator of bone formation, but not a classical BMP antagonist. *J Exp Med* 2004;199(6):805-814.
10. Babij P, Zhao W, Small C, et al: High bone mass in mice expressing a mutant LRP5 gene. *J Bone Miner Res* 2003;18(6):960-974.
11. Shoulders MD, Raines RT: Collagen structure and stability. *Annu Rev Biochem* 2009;78:929-958.
12. Tournis S, Dede AD: Osteogenesis imperfecta – a clinical update. *Metabolism* 2018;80:27-37.
13. Chang SW, Shefelbine SJ, Buehler MJ: Structural and mechanical differences between collagen homo- and heterotrimers: Relevance for the molecular origin of brittle bone disease. *Biophys J* 2012;102(3):640-648.
14. Sharma U, Carrique L, Vadon-Le Goff S, et al: Structural basis of homo- and heterotrimerization of collagen I. *Nat Commun* 2017;8:14671.
15. Barat-Houari M, Sarrabay G, Gatinois V, et al: Mutation update for COL2A1 gene variants associated with type II collagenopathies. *Hum Mutat* 2016;37(1):7-15.
16. Heinegard D, Saxne T: The role of the cartilage matrix in osteoarthritis. *Nat Rev Rheumatol* 2011;7(1):50-56.
17. Muttigi MS, Han I, Park HK, Park H, Lee SH: Matrilin-3 role in cartilage development and osteoarthritis. *Int J Mol Sci* 2016;17(4):590.
18. Le Douarin NM, Creuzet S, Couly G, Dupin E: Neural crest cell plasticity and its limits. *Development* 2004;131(19):4637-4650.
19. Leucht P, Kim J-B, Amasha RR, Girod SA, Helms JA: Embryonic origin and Hox status determine progenitor cell fate during adult bone regeneration. *Development* 2008;135(17):2845-2854.
20. Bradaschia-Correa V, Leclerc K, Josephson AM, et al: Hox gene expression determines cell fate of adult periosteal stem/progenitor cells. *Sci Rep* 2019;9(1):5043.
21. Currey JD: The many adaptations of bone. *J Biomech* 2003;36(10):1487-1495.
22. Engler AJ, Sen S, Sweeney HL, Discher DE: Matrix elasticity directs stem cell lineage specification. *Cell* 2006;126(4):677-689.
23. Leucht P, Kim JB, Currey JA, Brunski J, Helms JA: FAK-mediated mechanotransduction in skeletal regeneration. *PLoS One* 2007;2:e390.
24. Misch CE: Bone classification, training keys to implant success. *Dent Today* 1989;8(4):39-44.
25. Li J, Yin X, Huang L, et al: Relationships among bone quality, implant osseointegration, and Wnt signaling. *J Dent Res* 2017;96(7):822-831.
26. Mouraret S, Von Kaeppler E, Bardet C, et al: The potential for vertical bone regeneration via maxillary periosteal elevation. *J Clin Periodontol* 2014;41(12):1170-1177.
27. Carter D, Beaupré G. *Skeletal Function and Form: Mechanobiology of Skeletal Development, Aging, and Regeneration*. Cambridge, New York, Cambridge University Press, 2001.
28. Boehme KA, Rolauffs B: Onset and progression of human osteoarthritis-can growth factors, inflammatory cytokines, or differential miRNA expression concomitantly induce proliferation, ECM degradation, and inflammation in articular cartilage? *Int J Mol Sci* 2018;19(8):2282.

 ©Copyright 2021 American Academy of Orthopaedic Surgeons

29. Eyre DR, Matsui Y, Wu JJ: Collagen polymorphisms of the intervertebral disc. *Biochem Soc Trans* 2002;30(pt 6):844-848.
30. Zhou BO, Yue R, Murphy MM, Peyer JG, Morrison SJ: Leptin-receptor-expressing mesenchymal stromal cells represent the main source of bone formed by adult bone marrow. *Cell Stem Cell* 2014;15(2):154-168.
31. Fonseca H, Moreira-Goncalves D, Coriolano HJ, Duarte JA: Bone quality: The determinants of bone strength and fragility. *Sports Med* 2014;44(1):37-53.
32. Gibon E, Lu L, Goodman SB: Aging, inflammation, stem cells, and bone healing. *Stem Cell Res Ther* 2016;7:44.
33. Allen MR, Burr DB: Bisphosphonate effects on bone turnover, microdamage, and mechanical properties: What we think we know and what we know that we don't know. *Bone* 2011;49(1):56-65.
34. Stevenson JC: Bisphosphonates and atypical femoral shaft fractures. *N Engl J Med* 2011;365(4):377; author reply.
35. Shane E, Burr D, Abrahamsen B, et al: Atypical subtrochanteric and diaphyseal femoral fractures: Second report of a task force of the American Society for Bone and Mineral Research. *J Bone Miner Res* 2014;29(1):1-23.
36. Baron R, Ferrari S, Russell RG: Denosumab and bisphosphonates: Different mechanisms of action and effects. *Bone* 2011;48(4):677-692.
37. Chen J, Lan Y, Baek JA, Gao Y, Jiang R: Wnt/beta-catenin signaling plays an essential role in activation of odontogenic mesenchyme during early tooth development. *Dev Biol* 2009;334(1):174-185.
38. Leucht P, Helms JA: Wnt signaling: An emerging target for bone regeneration. *J Am Acad Orthop Surg* 2015;23(1):67-68.
39. Chen J, Tu X, Esen E, et al: WNT7B promotes bone formation in part through mTORC1. *PLoS Genet* 2014;10(1):e1004145.
40. Weivoda MM, Ruan M, Hachfeld CM, et al: Wnt signaling inhibits osteoclast differentiation by activating canonical and noncanonical cAMP/PKA pathways. *J Bone Miner Res* 2016;31(1):65-75.
41. Roforth MM, Fujita K, McGregor UI, et al: Effects of age on bone mRNA levels of sclerostin and other genes relevant to bone metabolism in humans. *Bone* 2014;59:1-6.
42. Almeida M: Aging mechanisms in bone. *Bonekey Rep* 2012;1:102.
43. Costa AG, Bilezikian JP: Sclerostin: Therapeutic horizons based upon its actions. *Curr Osteoporos Rep* 2012;10(1):64-72.
44. Saag KG, Petersen J, Brandi ML, et al: Romosozumab or Alendronate for fracture prevention in women with osteoporosis. *N Engl J Med* 2017;377(15):1417-1427.
45. Whyte JL, Smith AA, Helms JA: Wnt signaling and injury repair. *Cold Spring Harb Perspect Biol* 2012;4(8):a008078.
46. Chan CK, Chen CC, Luppen CA, et al: Endochondral ossification is required for haematopoietic stem-cell niche formation. *Nature* 2009;457(7228):490-494.
47. Zhang J, Niu C, Ye L, et al: Identification of the haematopoietic stem cell niche and control of the niche size. *Nature* 2003;425(6960):836-841.
48. Arioka M, Zhang X, Li Z, et al: Osteoporotic changes in the periodontium impair alveolar bone healing. *J Dent Res* 2019;98(4):450-458. 22034518818456.

©Copyright 2021 American Academy of Orthopaedic Surgeons

4

Biomechanics of the Skeletal System

Kenton Kaufman, PhD, PE

Keywords: *biomechanics; euler angles; helical axis; instant center of rotation; joint-articulating surface motion; kinematics; kinetics; screw axis*

INTRODUCTION

Mechanics is a branch of physics that is concerned with motion and deformation of bodies that are acted upon by mechanical forces. Mechanics is one of the oldest physical sciences, dating back to Aristotle (384-322 B.C.), who conducted and organized analytical analysis of animal movement. Leonardo daVinci (1452-1519) investigated the mechanics of the human body, and his detailed anatomic sketches represent the birth of anatomy as a discipline and of mechanics as a science governing human motion. Although daVinci wrote extensively on body mechanics, the man generally credited to be the father of modern biomechanics is Giovanni Alfonso Borelli (1608-1679). His book *De Motu Animalium* provided a quantitative graphical solution to a musculoskeletal biomechanics problem.

Engineering mechanics is the applied mechanics branch of the physical sciences. Biomechanics is the application of engineering mechanics to study the structure and function of the musculoskeletal system. Biomechanical principles are used to understand the mechanical influence on biological systems. Forces that load joints are generated by muscles and transmitted by tendons. Bones withstand these forces. Developments in the field of orthopaedic biomechanics have improved our understanding of normal and pathological movement, neuromuscular control, and mechanics of growth and form. Knowledge of biomechanical principles has improved fracture repair and joint reconstruction. It has provided the basis for the design and manufacture of implants and orthotic devices and has enhanced rehabilitation therapy practices. Biomechanics has also been used to improve human performance and reduce workplace injuries. Basic biomechanics relies heavily on Newtonian mechanics. These laws were introduced by Sir Isaac Newton and form the basis for analyses. The general field of dynamics consists of two major areas: kinematics and kinetics. The purpose of this chapter is to give a brief overview of biomechanics and its application to the musculoskeletal system.

Dr. Kaufman has received research or institutional support from American Orthotic and Prosthetic Association.

KINEMATICS

Kinematics is the subdivision of mechanics that deals with the description of motion without regard to the forces causing this motion. Kinematics describes motion in terms of displacement, velocity, and acceleration in space. To study kinematics in an organized manner, it is common to classify the motion as translational, rotational, or general. Translational motion occurs when a straight line drawn between two points on the body remains in the same direction during the motion. Translational motion can be either rectilinear (if the paths are straight lines) or curvilinear (if the paths are curved lines) (**Figure 1**). Rotational motion occurs when the points on the body move in a circular path about a central line known as the axis of rotation, which lies perpendicular to the plane of motion (**Figure 2**). The third class of motion is called general motion, or displacement, which occurs if a body undergoes both translational and rotational motion simultaneously.

Degrees of freedom (DOF) is a term that describes the ability of an object to move in space. The number of DOF of a system is the number of independent modes of motion that must be specified to define the location and orientation of the object. Rigid body motion in three-dimensional space without any constraint has six DOF: three in rotation and three in translation. This means that there are three coordinates

©Copyright 2021 American Academy of Orthopaedic Surgeons

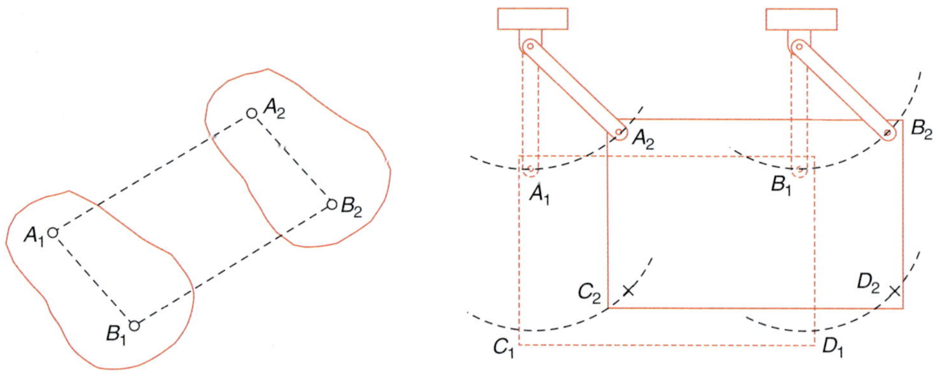

FIGURE 1 Examples of bodies undergoing translation. All points on the body move in a parallel fashion.

needed to locate a reference point on the body and three angles with respect to a set of reference axes are needed to specify its orientation. In reality, all anatomic joints have six DOF that consist of three rotational and three translations. However, if the motion of the joint is limited by anatomic constraints, the number of DOF is reduced. In this case, the combination of the number of DOF and the number of constraints in general three-dimensional space is six.

There are a number of simple mechanisms that are used for describing joint motion. A joint with one DOF is called a hinge joint (**Figure 3**). Examples of a hinge joint are the interphalangeal joints of the hand and foot. A joint with two DOF is called a universal joint. An example is the MCP joint of the hand (**Figure 4**). A joint with three DOF in rotation is called a ball joint. The hip joint is an example of a ball joint which is able to rotate about three planes, that is, flexion/extension, abduction/adduction, and internal/external rotation (**Figure 5**).

Given the wide range of possible types of motion, care must be taken in describing or interpreting the biomechanics of human movement. The type of movement (linear or angular), the reference frame, as well as the dimensions of the moment (DOF) must be defined. The motion of a body may be grouped into three general categories: planar motion, rotational three-dimensional motion, and generalized six DOF joint motion.

PLANAR MOTION

Planar motion is the simplest but most common model used to represent an anatomical joint moving about a single axis embedded in a fixed segment, that is, a single DOF. In this case, points on the limb describe a circular path around a fixed center of rotation. The limb undergoes simple angular motion. The center of rotation is the point that has zero velocity relative to all points of the body that are rotating around it. This point is said to be the instant center of rotation (ICR). Two methods can be used to locate the ICR. In the first method, the velocities of two points on the moving segment are required. Points A and B undergo an angular displacement in space as shown by the two velocity vectors (**Figure 6**). It is easy to find the location of the ICR, which does not necessarily lie on the body in question. Draw lines perpendicular to each of the velocity vectors. A velocity vector has no component perpendicular to itself, and therefore, velocity is

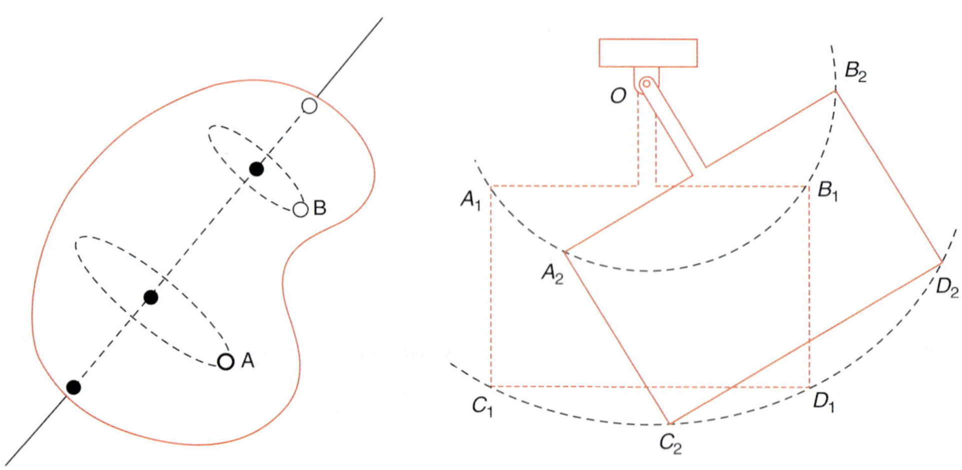

FIGURE 2 Examples of bodies undergoing rotation. All points on the body move in circular fashion around an axis of rotation.

©Copyright 2021 American Academy of Orthopaedic Surgeons

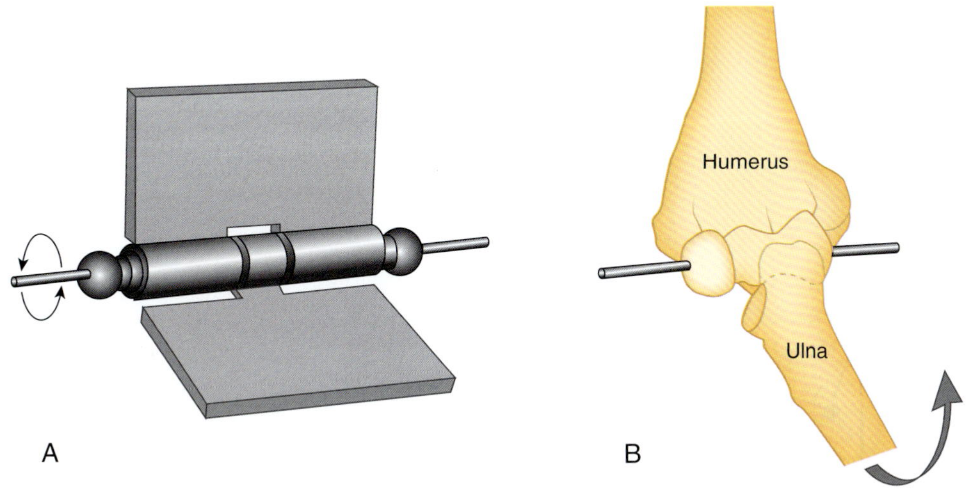

FIGURE 3 A hinge joint allows rotation of one rigid body with respect to another rigid body about a common axis. A hinge joint has one degree of freedom. The elbow can be considered a hinge joint.

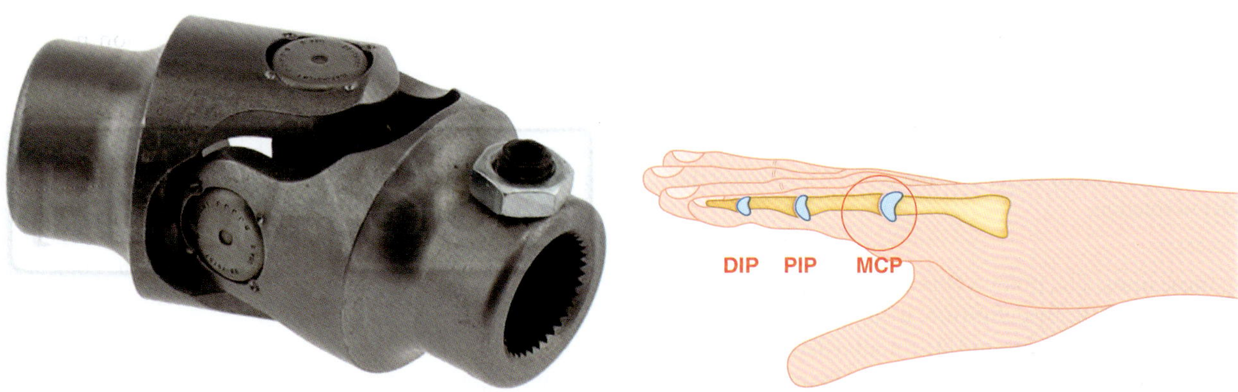

FIGURE 4 A universal joint consists of a pair of hinges located close together, oriented at 90° to each other, connected by a cross shaft. A universal joint has two degrees of freedom (ie, rotation around two axes). The MCP can be considered a universal joint. DIP = distal interphalangeal; MCP = metacarpophalangeal; PIP = proximal interphalangeal.

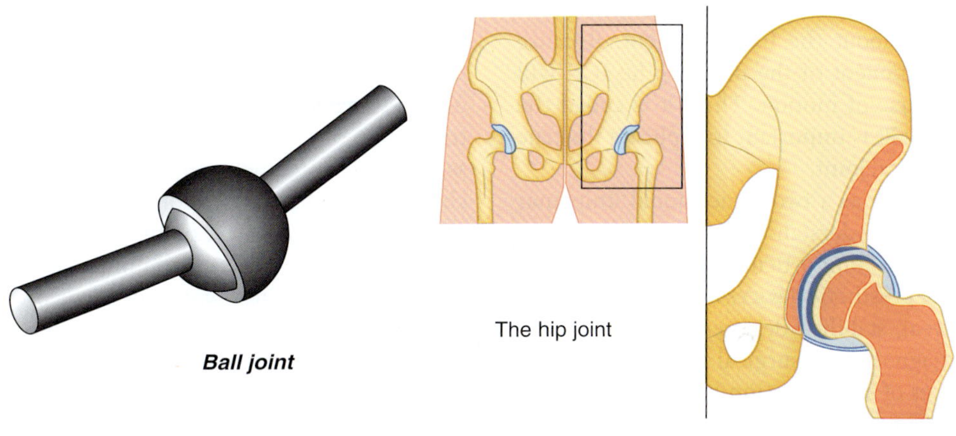

FIGURE 5 A ball-and-socket joint has a ball shaped surface of one rigid body fitting into a cup shaped depression of a second rigid body. A ball and socket joint has three degrees of freedom (ie, rotation about three orthogonal axes). The hip joint is a ball-and-socket joint.

©Copyright 2021 American Academy of Orthopaedic Surgeons

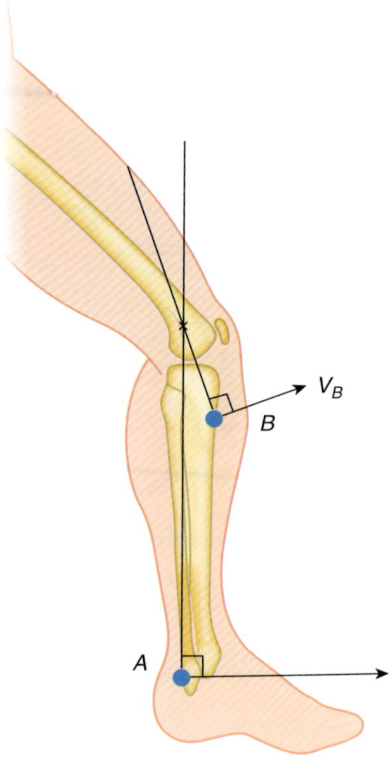

FIGURE 6 Illustration of the method to determine the instant center of rotation of the knee using the velocities at two points *A* and *B*. The perpendiculars to the velocity vector at points A and B intersect at the instant center of rotation.

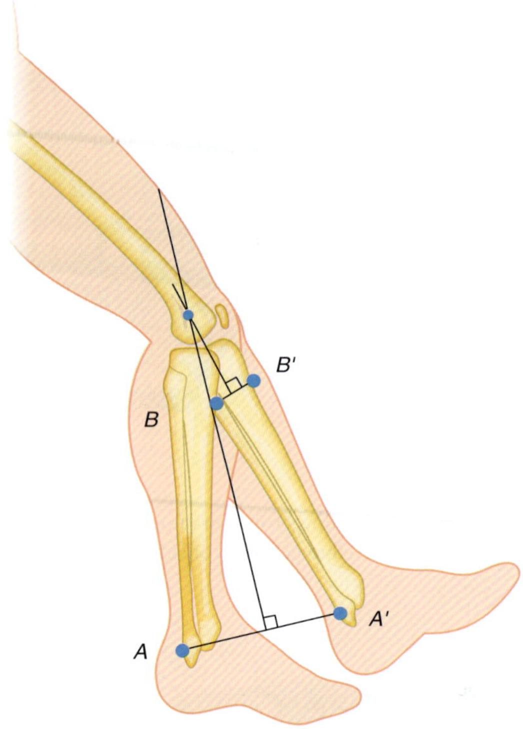

FIGURE 7 Illustration of the method to determine the instant center of rotation using Reuleaux method. The points *A* and *B* are displaced to *A′* and *B′*, respectively, during rotation of the moving segment. Straight connecting lines are drawn between *A* and *A′*, and between *B* and *B′*. Perpendicular bisectors of these two displacement lines are drawn at a point halfway between *A*-*A′* and *B*-*B′*. The point at which the perpendicular bisectors intersect is the instant center of rotation.

zero along these lines. The point where the two perpendicular lines intersect is the ICR. By definition, it has zero velocity relative to the points rotating around it. An alternative method for approximating the ICR was described by Franz Reuleaux in 1876. In this method, the instant location of two points on the moving segment are identified from two consecutive positions within a short period of time and the intersection of the bisectors of the line joining the same points at the two positions define the ICR (**Figure 7**). For a true hinged motion, the ICR will be a fixed point throughout the movement. In general planar motion, the moving limb segment can have both translation and rotation about the fixed segment. Because of the translational component of the motion, the ICR will change through the course of motion. Thus, it is called the ICR. Knowledge of the ICR is important to replicate the true kinematics of an anatomical joint.

Representation of a joint as a two dimensional uniplanar "hinge" joint is useful for understand joint articulating surface motion. Knowledge of joint articulating surface motion is essential for design of prosthetic devices to restore function, assessment of joint wear, stability, degeneration, and determination of proper diagnosis and surgical treatment of joint disease. Various degrees of simplification have been used for kinematic modeling of joints. A hinged joint is the simplest and most common used to simulate an anatomical joint in planar motion about a single axis embedded in the fixed segment. Experimental methods have been developed for determination of the ICR for planar motion. ICR is defined as the point of zero velocity. For a true hinged motion, the ICR will be a fixed point throughout the movement. Otherwise, the loci of the ICR will vary. The center of curvature has also been used to define joint anatomy. The center of curvature is defined as a geometric center of coordinates of the articulating surface.

For more general planar motion of an articulating surface, the term "sliding," "rolling," and "spinning" are commonly used (**Figure 8**). Sliding (gliding) motion is defined as the pure translation of a moving segment against the surface of a fixed segment. The contact point of the moving segment does not change while the contact point of the fixed segment has a constantly changing contact point. In this case, assuming that the wear couple is comprised of similar materials (eg, cartilage on cartilage), the greatest wear will occur on the contact point of the moving segment. If the surface of the fixed segment is flat, the ICR is located at infinity. Otherwise, it is located at the center of curvature of the fixed surface. Spinning motion (rotation) is the exact opposite of sliding motion. In this case, the moving segment rotates and the contact point on the fixed surface does not change. The ICR is located at the center of curvature

©Copyright 2021 American Academy of Orthopaedic Surgeons

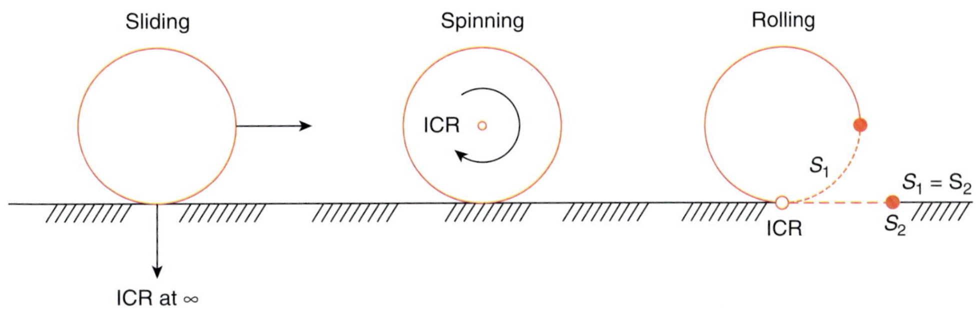

FIGURE 8 Illustration of the three types of joint articulating surface motion used to describe general planar motion: sliding, spinning and rolling. ICR = instant center of rotation.

of the spinning body that is undergoing pure rotation. For spinning motion, the greatest wear occurs on the contact point of the fixed surface. Rolling motion occurs between moving and fixed segments where the contact points of each surface are constantly changing and the arc lengths of contact are equal on each segment. The ICR is located at the contact point. In this case, the wear is minimal. Most planar motion of anatomic joints can be described by using any two of these three basic descriptions. An illustrious example can be given for the knee joint (**Figure 9**). In the case of spinning, knee flexion can occur while the contact on the tibial plateau remains in a single point (**Figures 9** and **10**, A). For sliding, the knee remains in a fully extended position while the location of the contact point moves posterior due entirely to translation. For rolling, as the knee flexes, the contact location on the tibial plateau moves posterior in a linear fashion (**Figures 9** and **10**, B). Normal knee motion is a combination of both rolling and sliding. As the knee flexes, the tibiofemoral contact point moves posterior due to rolling but slides forward to maintain contact with the tibial plateau (**Figures 9** and **10**, C). From this illustration, it becomes obvious that a unicentric hinge axis for the knee will not adequately represent knee kinematics of the articulating surface. Due to this requirement, the polycentric knee was designed to more truly replicate knee kinematics (**Figure 9**).

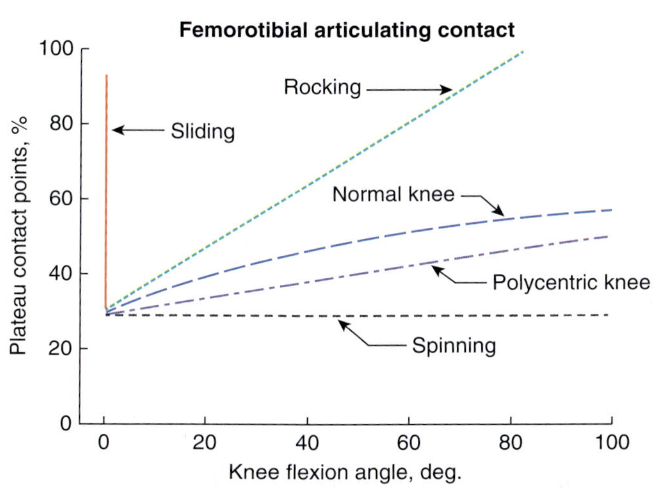

FIGURE 9 Femorotibial articulation surface motion patterns. Knee flexion is shown on the horizontal axis and the location of the tibiofibular articular contact is shown on the vertical axis with 0% indicating the most anterior part of the tibial plateau and 100% indication the most posterior part of the tibial plateau.

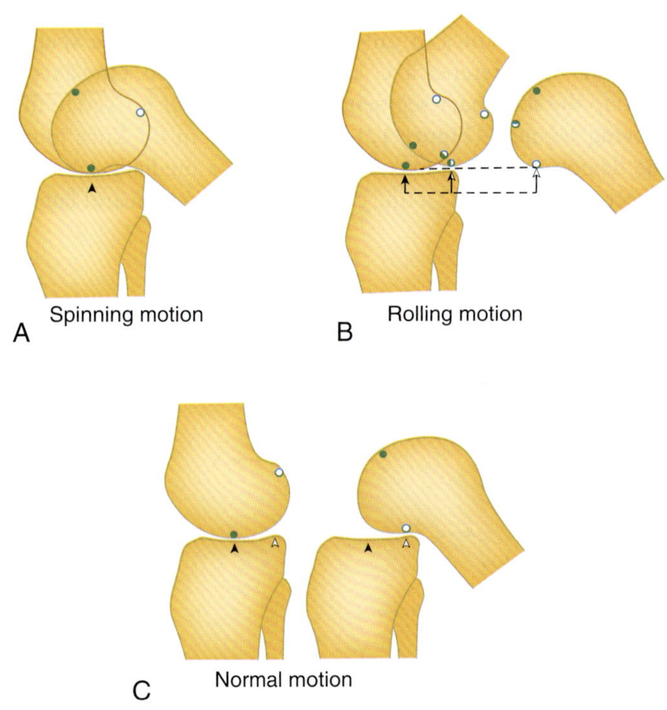

FIGURE 10 Illustration of types of knee motion. **A**, Spinning motion. The femur flexes while the contact stays in one point on the tibial plateau. For this type of motion, the metaphysis of the femur would engage on the posterior rim of the tibial plateau at ~130° of flexion, thereby limiting knee flexion. **B**, Rolling motion. For this type of motion, the femur would roll off the tibial plateau at ~45° flexion. If a knee was designed with only rolling motion, it would be necessary to increase the depth of the tibial plateau. This would result in more weight and humans would become immobile. **C**, Normal motion is a combination of rolling and sliding. The femur rolls back and slides forward to maintain contact on the tibial plateau.

©Copyright 2021 American Academy of Orthopaedic Surgeons

ROTATIONAL THREE-DIMENSIONAL MOTION

Very commonly, when describing an anatomical joint, only the rotational motions are considered. A spherical or ball-and-socket joint is commonly used to represent a joint that allows three DOF and rotation. Three angles are required to specify the relative position between the moving and fixed segments. For finite spatial rotation, the sequence of rotation is extremely important and must be specified for a unique description of joint motion. For the same amount of rotation, different final orientations will result from different sequences of rotation (**Figure 11**). This phenomenon was first noticed by Boston surgeon Codman in 1935 and is referred to as Codman's paradox. This behavior demonstrates the rotation is not a vector. The order of rotation cannot be interchanged. Rotation around the Z-axis plus rotation around the X-axis does not equal rotation around the X-axis plus rotation around the Z-axis. Stated another way, rigid body motion is sequence dependent. However, with proper selection and definition of the axes of rotation between two bony segments, it is possible to construct consistent rotation definitions.

The concept of Eulerian angles has been adopted in orthopaedic biomechanics to unify the definition of finite spatial rotation. The reference axes are carefully selected. One axis is fixed to the stationary segment and another axis is fixed to the moving segment (**Figure 12**). For example, in the knee joint, the flexion-extension axis occurs around a medially-laterally directed axis defining a line connecting the medial and lateral femoral condyles. The axial rotation axis is measured about an axis defined by the line along the shaft of the tibia. The third axis, also defined as the floating axis, is orthogonal to the other two axes and defines abduction-adduction.

GENERALIZED SIX DEGREES OF FREEDOM MOTION

For general unconstrained movement in 3D space, three translations and three rotations are required to completely describe the joint motion. In this situation, displacement of the moving segment may take place along any one of an infinite number of paths. It is convenient to describe the displacement in terms of the simplest motion that can produce it. The most commonly used analytical method for description of six DOF displacement of a rigid body is the screw displacement axis or helical axis. The motion of the moving segment from one position to another can be defined in terms of a simultaneous rotation (phi) around and a translation (t) along a unique axis called a screw displacement axis which is fixed in the fixed segment (**Figure 13**). Four additional parameters are required to completely describe the displacement of the moving body (**Figure 14**). These additional parameters are the inclination and location of the screw displacement axis. The screw displacement axis is a true vector quantity. Its magnitude can be decomposed along any coordinate axes used for the analysis. However, the amount of finite screw rotation is not a vector quantity and the decomposition of it must be carefully interpreted because of the noncommutative nature of the finite rotation.

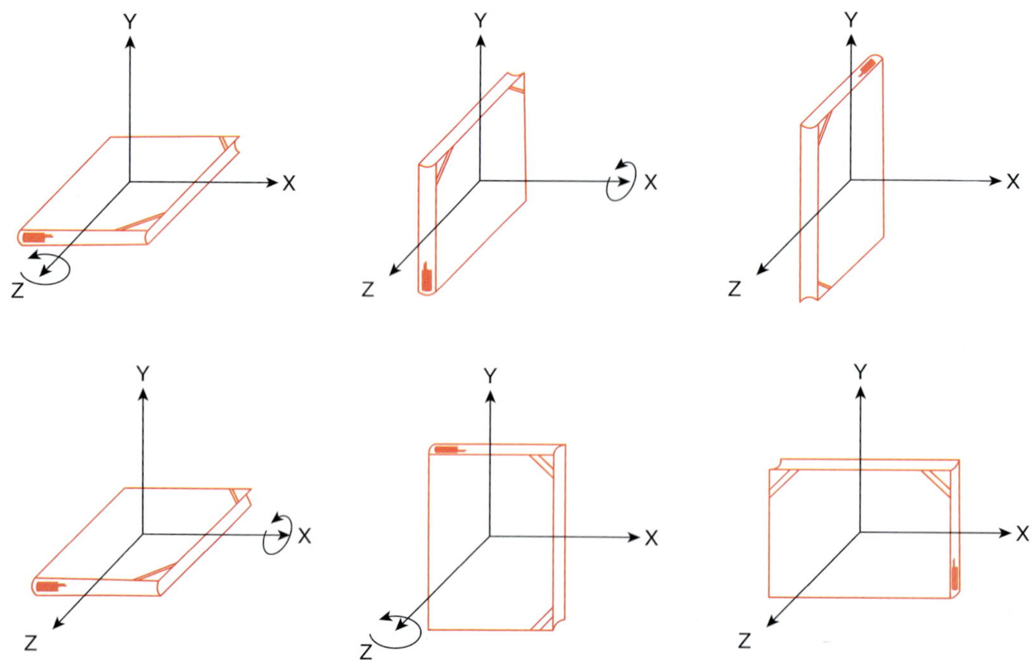

FIGURE 11 Pictorial illustration of how the sequence of rigid body motion affects the final orientation of the rigid body. In the top sequence, rotation occurs around the Z-axis and then the X-axis. In the bottom sequence, rotation first occurs around the X-axis and then the Z-axis. For the same amount of rotation, different final orientation result from the different sequences of rotation.

©Copyright 2021 American Academy of Orthopaedic Surgeons

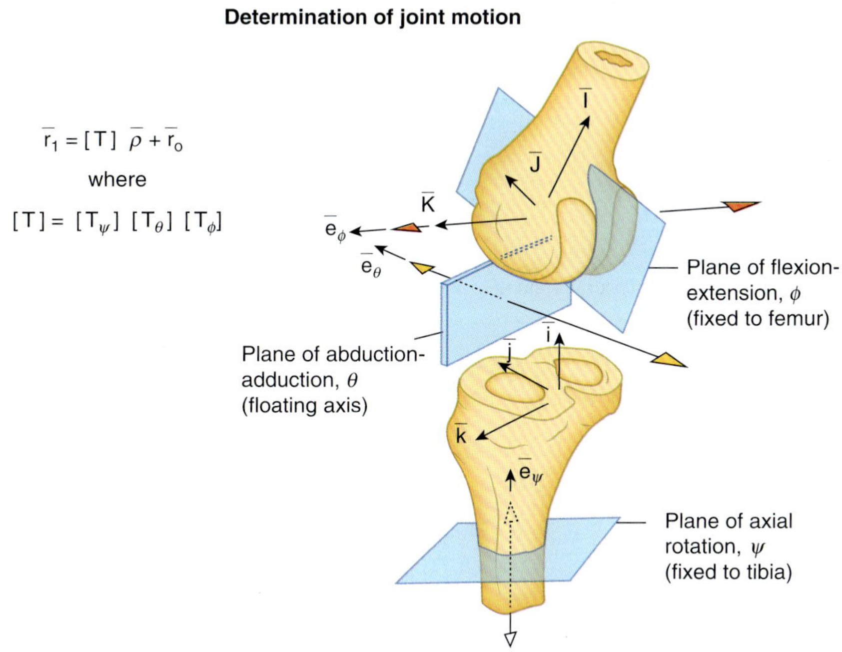

FIGURE 12 Description of knee joint motion using the Eulerian angle system. The axis fixed to the distal femur defines the flexion-extension motion, ϕ. The axis fixed to the proximal tibia along its anatomic axis defines internal-external rotation, ψ. The floating axis is orthogonal to the other two axes and is used to measure abduction-adduction, θ. (Redrawn with permission from Mayo Clinic.)

There are several advantages of using the screw displacement axis. First, the orientation of the screw axis is invariant regardless of the reference coordinate system used. Second, the gimbal lock situation can be avoided. Gimbal lock occurs when the orientation cannot be uniquely described using Eulerian angles. In this situation, that is, shoulder joint motion, the axial rotation axis of the moving segment (humerus) coincides with the flexion axis of the fixed segment (trunk). Third, the screw displacement axis can be composed into orthogonal axes which may be better suited for decomposing other vectorial entities such as force and moment vectors.

KINETICS

Kinetics is the study of the relationship between the rigid body motion and the forces causing the motion. When unbalanced forces or moments are acting on a rigid body, it is under a nonequilibrium or dynamic condition resulting in motion. A rigid body is defined as one whose deformation in the application of a set of forces may be considered negligible. Understanding the kinetics of human movement produces a fundamental understanding of the musculoskeletal system. Before one can begin to analyze the forces during human movement, some basic definitions are necessary and some basic assumptions must be made.

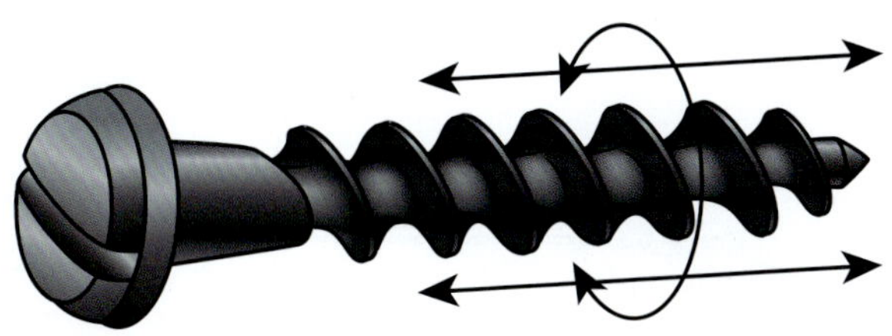

FIGURE 13 The screw axis or helical axis describes a straight line about which a rigid body rotates and translates as it moves through space.

DEFINITIONS

The key quantities in kinetics are *force*, *moment*, and *torque*. A force represents the interaction between two bodies. According to Newton's Second Law, force is any action that tends to change the state of rest or state of motion of a body to which it is applied. Forces can be contact forces (when bodies touch each other) or field forces (such as gravitational, electric, or magnetic forces where the bodies are separated by a distance). Forces are represented by *vectors*, which are composed of four components: magnitude, direction, sense, and point of application. Force vectors may be resolved into component forces along specified, usually perpendicular, coordinate axes. Conversely, component forces can be summed using vectorial addition.

A moment represents the turning, twisting, or rotational effect of a force. An off-axis force, applied at a distance from an actual or potential axis of rotation of an object, tends to cause angular displacement. It is defined as the product of the force and the perpendicular distance between the line of action of the force and the axis of rotation of the motion that the force produces (**Figure 15**). Its magnitude is the force times the perpendicular distance to the axis of rotation. The moment arm is the shortest distance from the force action line to the actual or pivotal point of the system, regardless of the state of motion. The direction of the moment is along the axis of rotation (or potential rotation) and is perpendicular to the plane in which the force is applied. Skeletal motion is the result of

©Copyright 2021 American Academy of Orthopaedic Surgeons

$$\bar{r}p_2 = [T]\,\bar{r}p_1 + \bar{d}$$

also

$$\bar{r}p_2 = \bar{r}p_1 + t\bar{\rho} + \Delta\bar{r}$$

where

$$\Delta\bar{r} = (I - \cos\Phi)\,(\bar{\rho} \times (\bar{\rho} \times \bar{r})) + \sin\Phi\,(\bar{\rho} \times \bar{r})$$

$$\bar{r} = \bar{r}p_1 - \bar{s}$$

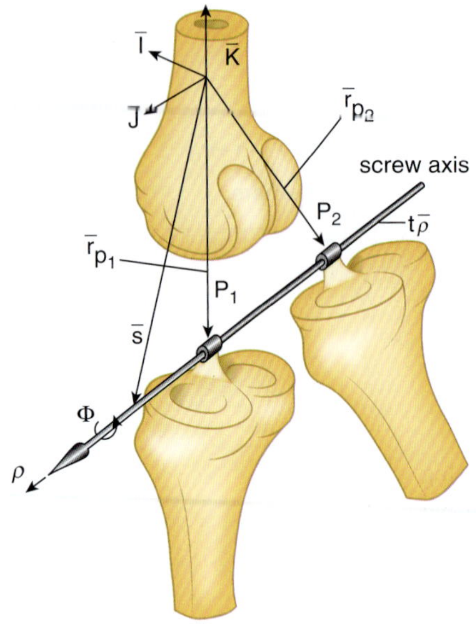

FIGURE 14 The screw displacement axis can be used to describe general spatial motion. The tibia moves from position 1 to position 2 by rotation about the screw axis by an amount ϕ and by translating along the screw axis, ρ, by an amount τ.

the moments applied by muscles that cross the joints on which they act. A moment of force about an axis measures the tendency of the force to impart rotational motion about a fixed axis. A moment is a vector quantity with (1) a magnitude given by the product of the force times lever arm distance from the force to the rotation axis and (2) direction defined by the "right-hand rule" (**Figure 15**). To apply the right-hand rule, one curls the fingers of the right hand in the direction that the force would rotate the object and then the thumb points in the direction of the positive moment.

A torque is a special type of moment that results when a pair of forces has equal magnitude, parallel lines of action, and opposite sense act on a body (**Figure 16**). The magnitude of the torque is the product of the applied force (*F*) and the perpendicular distance (*D*) between the two forces that is, $F \times D$. The resultant force is zero because the two forces are equal and opposite each other.

EXTERNAL AND INTERNAL FORCES

Kinetics can be used to analyze forces affecting the musculoskeletal system. These forces can be classified as either external or internal forces. External forces represent the action of objects contacting the body, gravitational forces, or forces due to body inertia. Internal forces are the body's response to external forces. Internal forces consist of muscles, ligament, and joint contact forces. In general, the limb segments are assumed to be

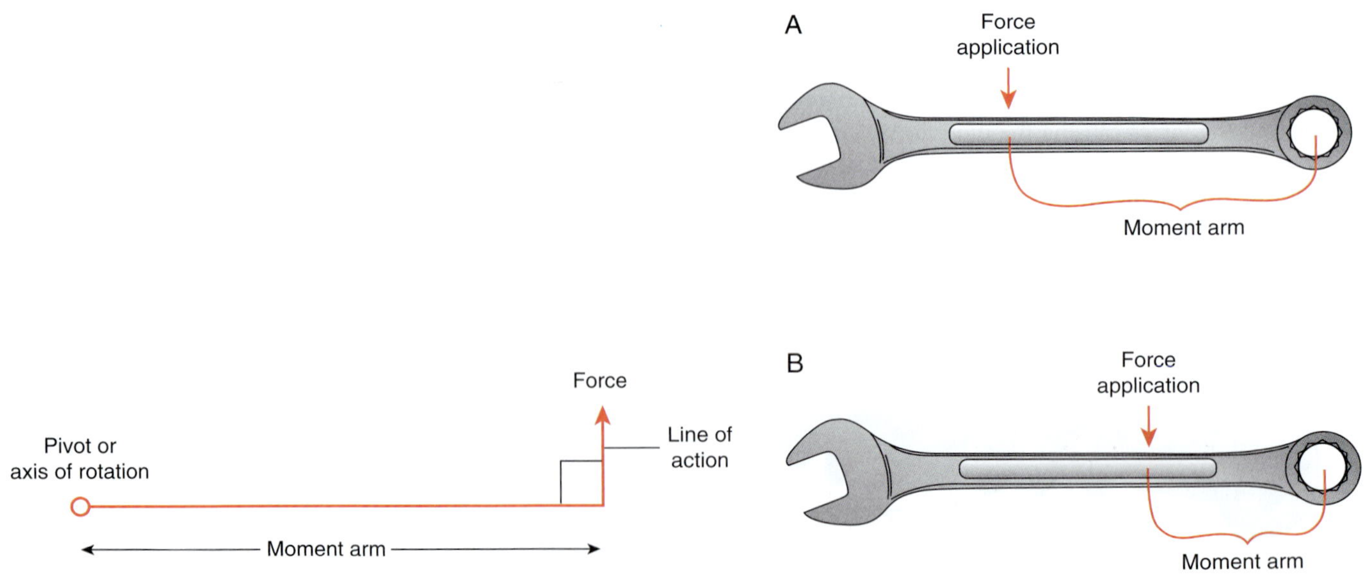

FIGURE 15 Example of how a moment is created by a force acting at a perpendicular distance from an axis of rotation. The moment magnitude can be modified by changing the amount of force or the point of application of the force.

©Copyright 2021 American Academy of Orthopaedic Surgeons

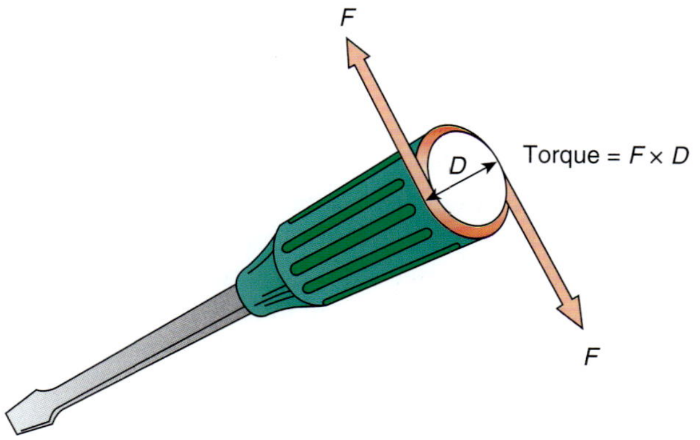

FIGURE 16 Example of how a torque is generated to rotate a screw driver. A torque is a pair of equal, parallel, and opposite forces acting on a body and separated by an equal distance from one another.

rigid which simplifies analysis because it is assumed that the structure does not deform under load. Furthermore, joints are assumed to be frictionless hinges because the articular surface has a very low coefficient of friction. For example, during gait at a particular instant in time, the ground reaction force passes behind the knee joint center. This creates an external flexion moment which tends to flex the knee. The internal response is an internal extension moment due to contraction of the quadriceps muscle to balance the external demand (**Figure 17**).

The technique used to solve kinetic problems is called free-body analysis. The following examples will explain the approach and teach you how to use it. After you work through the examples, you will be able to perform a simplified analysis on your own. This will add precision to your clinical estimates of potentially damaging forces.

COMPOSITION AND RESOLUTION OF FORCES

While solving kinetic problems in biomechanics, we must take into account all the forces that are acting on the body of interest. When two or more forces are acting in the same plane and at the same point, we often wish to show their combined effect as a single force. Any set of coplanar concurrent forces may be replaced by a single force having the same effect as that of the given forces. This single force, obtained by combining the given forces, is called the resultant force. Vectors may be combined by addition and subtraction. Consider the rotator cuff where three muscles, the infraspinatus, supraspinatus, and subscapularis pull on the humerus. Determine the resultant force of these muscles and its resultant direction (**Figure 18**). To solve this problem, the horizontal and vertical components of each muscle must be determined. The infraspinatus acts with the magnitude of 75 N at an angle of 70° from the horizontal. The vertical component of the infraspinatus is

$$F_y = 75\sin\theta = 75(\sin 70°) = 75(0.9397) = 70.5\,\text{N}$$

and horizontal component is

$$F_x = -75\cos\theta = -75(\cos 70°) = -75(0.3420) = -25.7\,\text{N}$$

The negative sign indicates that the horizontal component act in the negative X-direction.

The supraspinatus acts with a magnitude of 100 N in the vertical direction only. Thus,

$$F_y = 100\,\text{N and } F_x = 0\,\text{N}$$

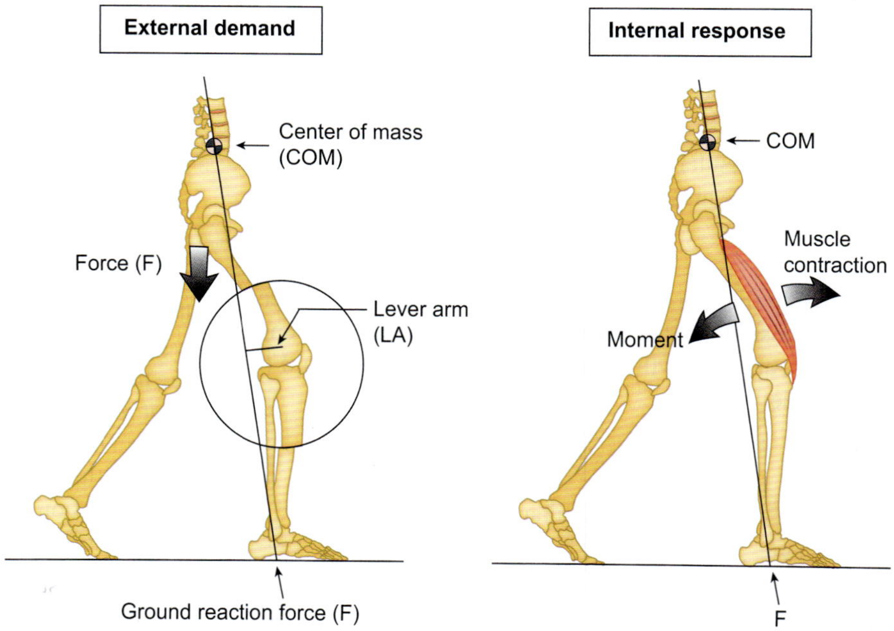

FIGURE 17 Illustration of how external forces generated during walking are balanced by internal forces. During gait the external forces generated by the ground reaction force, gravity, and inertial are balanced by internal forces generated by muscles, ligaments, and joint articulating surface contact. The ground reaction force passes behind the knee joint center creating an external moment which causes the knee to flex. The external demand is balanced by the internal response of the muscles. In this point during the gait cycle, the quadriceps contract to generate an internal knee extensor moment.

©Copyright 2021 American Academy of Orthopaedic Surgeons

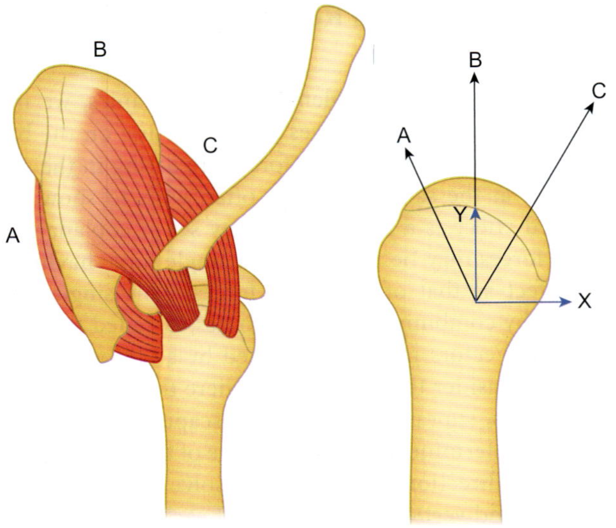

FIGURE 18 Illustration of the concurrent force system of the shoulder. The infraspinatus, A, is contracting with a force of 75 N at an angle of 70° from the horizontal. The supraspinatus, B, is contracting with a force of 100 N in the vertical direction. The subscapularis, C, is contracting with a force of 100 N at an angle of 60° from the horizontal. A Cartesian coordinate system, ie, X-Y axes shown in blue, is used to resolve each force into components along the X-axis and the Y-axis.

The subscapularis has a magnitude of 100 N and a direction of 60° from the horizontal. So the vertical component for the subscapularis is

$$F_y = 100 \sin\theta = 100 \sin 60° = 100(0.866) = 86.6\,\text{N}$$

The horizontal component of the subscapularis is

$$F_x = 100 \cos\theta = 100 \cos 60° = 100(0.5) = 50\,\text{N}$$

The Y component of the resultant effect of the three muscles is obtained by summing the effects of each muscle in the Y-direction. The Greek letter sigma (Σ) is used to indicate summation. In this notation, the resultant y component (R_y) is

$$R_y = \Sigma F_y = 70.5 + 100 + 86.6 = 257.1\,\text{N}$$

Similarly, the resultant component (R_x) is the sum of the x values for the three muscles

$$R_x = \Sigma F_x = -25.7 + 0 + 50 = 24.3\,\text{N}$$

Identifying the horizontal and vertical force components makes it possible to determine the resultant vector. A triangle is formed, and the Pythagorean Theorem is used to find the hypotenuse.

$$R = \sqrt[2]{R_x^{\,2} + R_y^{\,2}} = \sqrt{24.3^2 + 257.1^2} = 258.1\,\text{N}$$

The line of action, θ, of the resultant is

$$\theta = \tan^{-1} R_y / R_x = \tan^{-1}(257/24.3) = 84.6°$$

from the positive X-direction.

Thus the composite muscle pull is 258 N pulling at an angle of 84.6° from the horizontal. This example demonstrates that the combined effort of several forces acting on a single bone can be determined by finding the force resultant.

In the previous example, all forces were concurrent, that is, acting at a single point. Thus, there was no net rotational effect or rotational moment of these forces. Now let us solve a problem where the forces are no longer concurrent and the object needs to maintain rotational equilibrium. The laws of equilibrium require that for a body or structure to be in equilibrium, two conditions must be satisfied:

$$\Sigma \mathbf{F} = 0, \text{ and}$$

$$\Sigma \mathbf{M} = 0$$

If all the force and moment vectors acting on a body or structure are resolved into their components along the three axes, X, Y, and Z of a three-dimensional coordinate system, then it is possible to set up mathematical expressions describing the equilibrium conditions for translation and rotation. Representing the forces and moment components by F_x, F_y and F_z and M_x, M_y and M_z respectively, the six equilibrium equations in three dimensional space are:

Force equilibrium equations

$$\Sigma F_x = 0, \quad \Sigma F_y = 0, \quad \Sigma F_z = 0$$

Moment equilibrium equations

$$\Sigma M_x = 0, \quad \Sigma M_y = 0, \quad \Sigma M_z = 0$$

These six equations are required since a rigid body in 3D space has six DOF.

If we simplify to a planar problem, that is, 2D space, then we have two translations and one rotation that must be maintained for equilibrium. The condition for translational equilibrium can be written

$$\Sigma F_x = 0, \text{ and } \Sigma F_y = 0$$

For the body to be in rotational equilibrium, the sum of moments about a point must equal to zero,

$$\Sigma M_z = 0$$

These equations are referred to as planar equilibrium equations. Consider a person in single limb stance (**Figure 19**). The person weighs 120 lbs, so the ground reaction force is 120 lbs. The weight of the lower leg is 18 lbs, or 15% of total body weight of 120 lbs. The hip abductor force acts at 60° above the horizontal and the joint reaction force is unknown. As the joint reaction force is unknown, we put an unknown reaction force in the positive X-direction, R_x, and an unknown reaction force in the positive Y-direction, R_y. After solving the equilibrium equations, if we have a negative value, it simply means that the force direction we assumed is incorrect and the force is acting in the opposite direction. We have three unknown forces, R_x, R_y and F_{abd}. We also have three equations. As there

©Copyright 2021 American Academy of Orthopaedic Surgeons

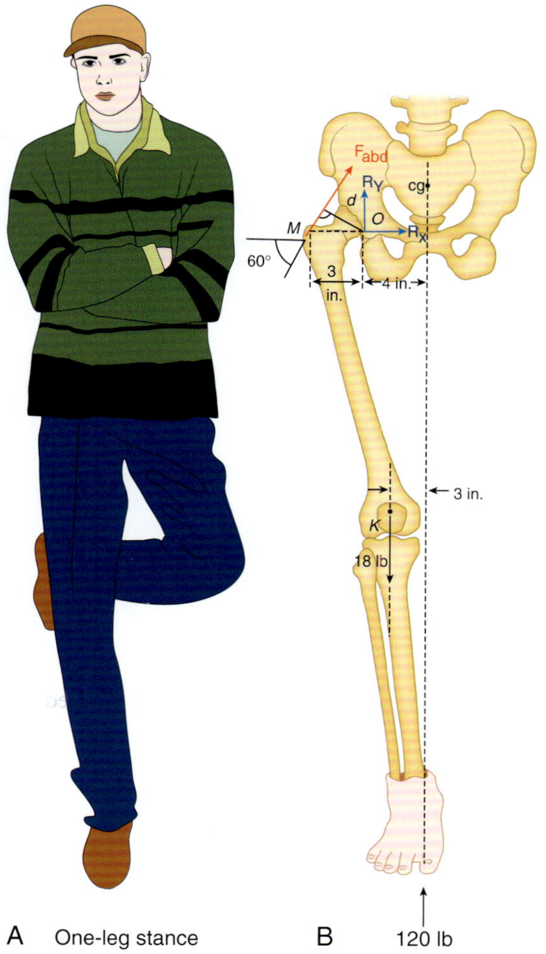

FIGURE 19 Illustration of a general force system. **A**, A person is standing in single-limb stance. The person weighs 120 lbs. The weight of the right lower extremity is 18 lbs. **B**, A free-body diagram is created to solve for the hip abductor force and the joint reaction force. The hip abductor contracts at an angle of 60° from the horizontal. The dimensions are shown in the illustration.

are three unknowns and three equations, there is a determinant solution for this problem. First let us satisfy the moment equilibrium equation. By summing moments about the hip center, the unknown forces R_x and R_y have no lever arm and do not enter into the moment equation. Thus, the moment equation is

$$\Sigma M_z = (120 \text{ lbs} \times 4\text{in}) - (18 \text{ lbs} \times 3\text{in}) - F_{abd}(\sin 60°)(3\text{in})$$

Solving this equation, F_{abd} = 178 lbs.
Next satisfying the equation for translational equilibrium in the X-direction (horizontal),

$$\Sigma F_x = 0 = R_x + F_{abd}(\cos 60°)$$

Solving this equation, R_x = −89 lbs. Thus, we assumed the incorrect direction for the resultant force in the X-direction.

Next, assessing translational equilibrium in the Y-direction (vertical),

$$\Sigma F_y = 0 = 120 - 18 + R_y + F_{abd}(\sin 60°)$$

Solving, R_y = −256 lbs. Once again, the force is negative, so the assumed direction for the joint reaction force was incorrect.

Now, solving for the resultant joint reaction force,

$$R = \sqrt[2]{R_x^2 + R_y^2} = \sqrt[2]{(-89)^2 + (-256)^2} = 271 \text{lbs}$$

The direction of the joint reaction force can be solved relative to the horizontal

$$\theta = \tan^{-1}(R_y / R_x) = \tan^{-1}(-256/-89) = 71°$$

You will note that due to the small lever arm of the hip abductor force, the joint reaction force is larger than the muscle force but the resultant direction is close to that of the muscle force and only modified slightly by the vertical direction of the ground reaction force.

To summarize, when an object is known to be at rest, the equations of equilibrium may be applied. A free-body diagram needs to be created that shows all forces acting. These forces must be represented as vectors, showing their direction (with letters being assigned to them to represent their magnitudes). All forces pertinent to the problem must be included. The steps to solve the equilibrium problem are as follows:

1. Create a free-body diagram that includes the unknown forces
2. Choose coordinate axes
3. Substitute the forces into the equations of motion, (ie, $\Sigma F = 0$, $\Sigma M = 0$)
4. Solve the equations of equilibrium to obtain the unknown forces

SUMMARY

Knowledge of biomechanics of the musculoskeletal system is essential for an orthopaedic surgeon. These basic concepts will help an orthopaedic surgeon understand the mechanical basis of the musculoskeletal system function, facilitate their diagnosis and treatment, evaluate and improve treatment procedures, and understand biomechanical research findings. The rudimentary concepts presented in this chapter provide a foundation for understanding why a patient may complain about instability following joint replacement, why a patient's bone broke, how to repair such a fracture, or why a certain repair technique did not succeed. As a patient who has received orthopaedic care, I was pleased to know that the orthopaedic surgeon caring for me had received training in biomechanics.

©Copyright 2021 American Academy of Orthopaedic Surgeons

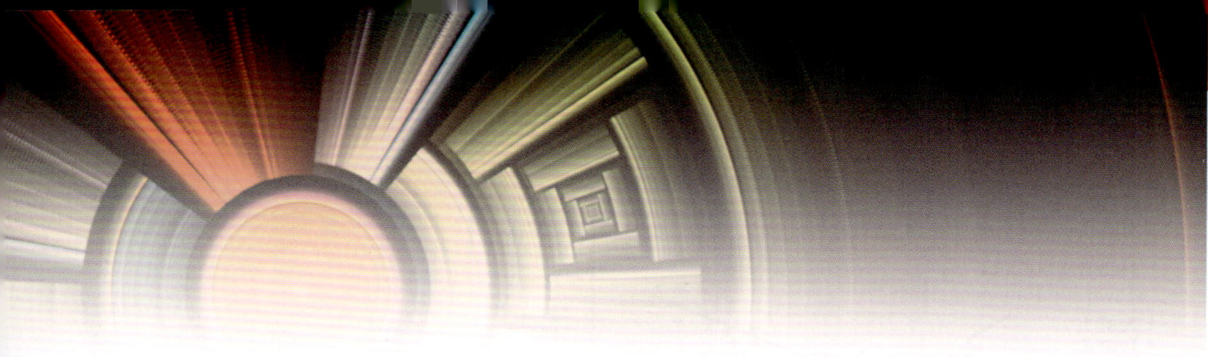

5

Gait and Gait Disturbances

Thomas P. Andriacchi, PhD
Jennifer C. Erhart-Hledik, PhD

Keywords: *Clinical applications of gait analysis; gait disturbances; gait measures*

INTRODUCTION

The purpose of this chapter is to highlight new evidence that shows specific elements of gait can be used to assess functional health, the state of many pathological conditions, and the risk of progression of pathological conditions and provide objective assessment of treatment outcome. This information is particularly important for orthopedic practice because one of the primary goals of orthopedic treatment is restoration of function.

The field of gait analysis continues to evolve producing clinically relevant new information. Section 2 provides definitions and methods for interpreting gait measures that can be considered signals for both musculoskeletal pathology as well as tissue adaptation. Section 3 illustrates how musculoskeletal pathology provides a signaling pathway for gait disturbances that reflect the underlying pathology. Conversely, Section 4 will illustrate how specific features of gait mechanics can stimulate a signaling pathway where tissue structure and biology adapt to gait mechanics. Both signaling pathways suggest there are interactions between the elements of gait mechanics, biology, and structure that offer new opportunities to address the multifaceted complexity of musculoskeletal pathology.

Dr. Erhart-Hledik or an immediate family member serves as a paid consultant to or is an employee of HingeHealth and Moximed. Neither Dr. Andriacchi nor any immediate family member has received anything of value from or has stock or stock options held in a commercial company or institution related directly or indirectly to the subject of this chapter.

GAIT MEASURES DEFINITION AND INTERPRETATION

Time-distance measures offer an assessment of the overall pattern of gait that can provide an objective test for gait disturbances associated with pathology and assess treatment outcomes. These measures are among the easiest gait measures to capture[1] and are usually quantified by walking speed (average speed of forward progression in meters/second), stride length (distance between ipsilateral heel strikes in meters), and cadence (steps per unit time in step count/minute). In some cases, stride length can be normalized to height or lower extremity length to allow for comparisons among individuals with differences in statures.

It is important to note that time-distance measures are interrelated with strong associations between metrics such as stride length and walking speed. For example, a healthy subject has a shorter stride length when walking slower, and stride length linearly increases with walking speed (**Figure 1**). The fact that gait metrics like stride length are dependent on walking speed is critical to the clinical application of gait analysis because patients with gait disturbances often walk slower than healthy subjects (**Figure 1**). Thus, gait metric comparisons between healthy subjects and patients should account for the influence of walking speed.[2]

The fact that gait measures are reproducible is another important consideration in the clinical application of gait analysis as illustrated in **Figure 1**. A healthy subject tested on two occasions will have the same relationship between stride length and walking speed. The reproducibility of gait mechanics for healthy subjects is governed by minimizing metabolic energy consumption[3,4] that permits walking efficiently for long distances. Thus, any changes in the stride length-walking speed relationship would suggest a change in the health status of the subject. The clinical application of time-distance measures will be discussed further in the Clinical Applications section.

©Copyright 2021 American Academy of Orthopaedic Surgeons

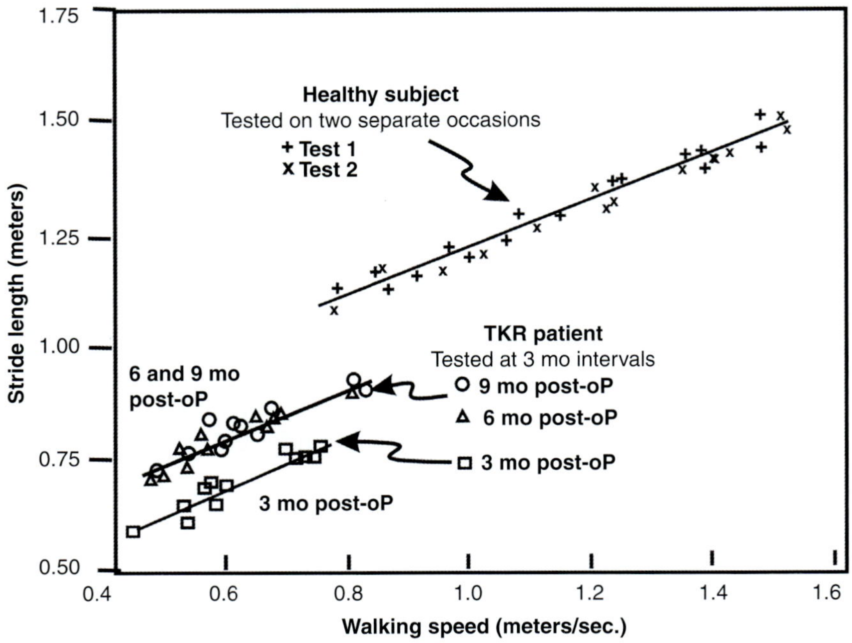

FIGURE 1 Graph showing that the relationship between stride length and walking speed can be used to objectively assess the change in ambulatory function following total knee replacement (TKR). The reproducibility of gait for a healthy subject is illustrated for the healthy subject tested on two separate occasions. Note: The speed dependence of most gait parameters makes it important to account for differences in walking speed when comparing gait between subjects. (Data from Andriacchi TP, Ogle JA, Galante JO: Walking speed as a basis for normal and abnormal gait measurements. *J Biomech* 1977;10:261-268.)

Kinematics measures during gait provide more specific information than time-distance measures which can be related to the motion of individual joints. Joint kinematics is normally described in terms of relative angles between adjacent limb segments. In practice, human gait[5] is often described in terms of the sagittal plane motion (eg, flexion-extension at the hip and knee as well as dorsiflexion-plantar flexion at the ankle). The patterns of flexion-extension motion are reproducible among the normal population. As illustrated for healthy gait (**Figure 2**): hip motion smoothly cycles from a peak flexion at heel strike (~20°) to peak extension prior to toe off to reaching a peak in flexion during swing phase; knee motion cycles from extension at heel strike, to local maximum flexion (~20°) during midstance phase (load response), toward extension in late stance (terminal extension) and flexes again prior to swing phase where the knee flexes to approximately 60°; ankle motion cycles from plantar flexion in early stance phase to dorsiflexion in late stance phase and reverses to plantar flexion during swing phase returning to a neutral position prior to heel strike. The smooth patterns of motions illustrated in **Figure 2** are consistent with walking with an energy-efficient gait that allows walking long distances with minimal fatigue. In addition, these motion patterns allow for some of the impact load to be absorbed by soft tissues and reduce impact directly on the joint surfaces. For example, knee flexion during midstance (**Figure 2**), commonly called load response, allows for some of the downward load in early stance to be absorbed through the extensor mechanism rather than through the cartilage at the knee.

The smooth patterns of motion during healthy gait can substantially change with musculoskeletal pathology because gait patterns will be reprogrammed to adapt to conditions such as pain, instability, or disruption of normal muscle activation. As such, gait disturbances typically can cause untimely fatigue during walking as the pattern of gait is no longer programmed to optimize energy consumption but rather to adapt to the specific nature of the pathological condition.

Kinetic measurements provide clinically important measures that can be related to the loading on the musculoskeletal system. Commonly, musculoskeletal loading during gait is described in terms of forces and moments. As will be illustrated in this chapter, gait analysis can provide a useful tool to noninvasively measure joint loading (forces and moments at the joints) during ambulation. At present, these kinetic measures have been primarily the domain of the research laboratory and have not migrated to routine clinical practice or thinking, yet an understanding of joint loading during gait can provide a deeper comprehension of the treatment of musculoskeletal injury and disease.

Given the clinical importance of understanding the nature of joint loading during gait, it is useful to explore some of the methods and assumptions used when capturing and interpreting kinetic measures. The fact that forces and moments are abstract constructs that cannot be seen often presents a barrier to clinical interpretation. Understanding a few general concepts (illustrated for the knee in **Figure 3**) will help facilitate clinical interpretation of kinetic measures. Most clinical gait studies are conducted noninvasively with external sensors. As such, direct gait loading measured in the laboratory is described as "external loading". These external loading measures during walking include the external ground reaction and inertial forces/moments (due to mass, inertia, velocity, and acceleration) that act on each limb segment (**Figure 3**, A and D). These forces and moments can be resolved to the joint center[6] and are described as external measures.

©Copyright 2021 American Academy of Orthopaedic Surgeons

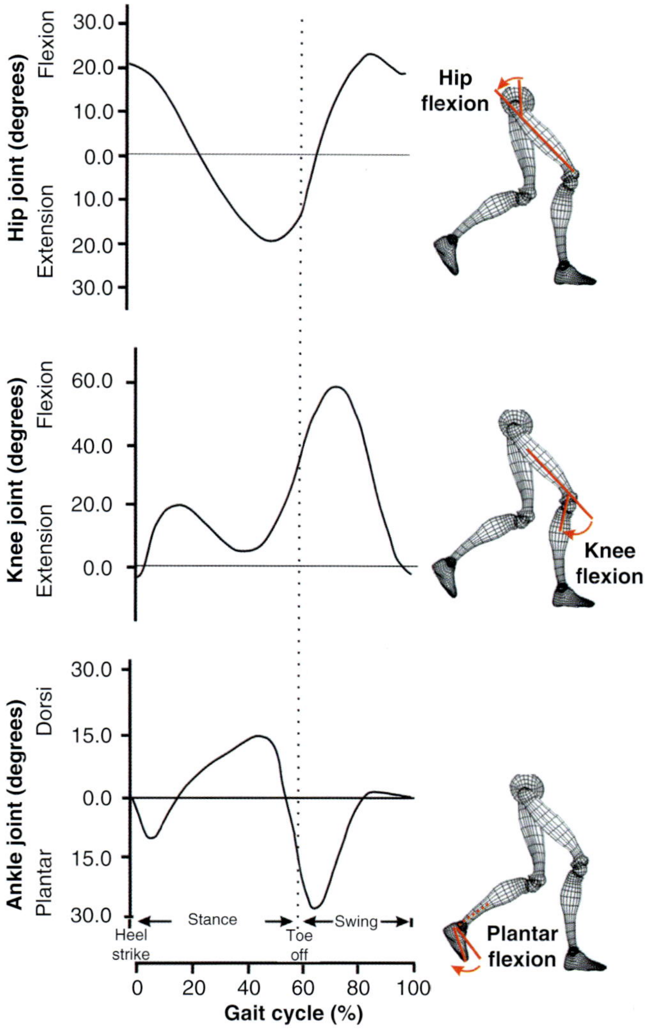

FIGURE 2 An illustration of the typical cyclic patterns of motion in the sagittal plane during healthy walking. The smooth transitions from flexion to extension allow for energy-efficient gait. The amplitude of the motion will change with walking speed, but the patterns remain the same. (Data from Chehab EF, Andriacchi TP, Favre J: Speed, age, sex, and body mass index provide a rigorous basis for comparing the kinematic and kinetic profiles of the lower extremity during walking. *J Biomech* 2017;58:11-20.)

Clinical interpretation of the external measurement requires relating the external loads to internal loads[7] generated by muscles and joint contact forces (**Figure 3**, B and E). For the knee joint example (**Figure 3**, A), the external flexion moment is important because this moment must be balanced by a force generated by the quadriceps muscle (**Figure 3**, B), and patterns of the flexion-extension moment can be interpreted as reflecting quadriceps function during walking. Again, using the knee example, the external adduction moment can be related to the internal joint reaction forces on the medial and lateral compartment of the knee and provides a basis for understanding why there are greater forces on the medial compartment of the knee relative to the lateral compartment.[7]

The moment magnitudes are dependent on walking speed, and comparisons between moment magnitudes should also account for walking speed. The moment magnitude is also dependent on weight and height (which influences lever arms, or the distance over which the force acts on the joint); thus, moments are often normalized by expressing the moment as a percentage of body weight X height to allow comparison between subjects of different stature. Finally, the interpretation of the external moment should include the possibility that the internal moment balance can be due to the summation of both antagonistic and synergistic muscle forces. For example, an external moment tending to flex the knee would be balanced by a "net" (extensors minus flexors) internal moment tending to extend the knee. In spite of the numerous factors that could influence the moment, these patterns are quite repeatable for healthy gait.[8] The repeatability of these patterns is important because changes from these patterns can be used to identify gait disturbances that are associated with specific pathology. Some examples are given in the Clinical Applications section later in this chapter.

Reproducibility of gait measures is in general critical to the clinical application of gait. Specifically, gait patterns are governed by criteria that act at the interface between physics and human physiology in a manner that the mechanics of healthy gait are ruled by a tendency to optimize metabolic energy consumption. For example, self-selected walking speed (mechanical metric) for healthy subjects is directly associated with optimizing energy expenditure.[3,4] As such, healthy gait patterns at self-selected speeds reflect the tendency to optimize the capacity to walk with minimal energy consumption and provide a basis for explaining why healthy gait patterns are highly repeatable.

A pathological condition that causes pain or instability or affects muscle activation or strength will cause the body to reprogram gait patterns based on the pathological condition. For example, a limp due to pain reflects a reprogramming of the pattern of locomotion (gait disturbance) that is governed by the pathological condition rather than optimizing energy consumption. Evidence[2,5] that specific gait disturbances are also reproducible and can be related to the pathological condition when controlled for speed provides a basis for using gait to assess musculoskeletal pathology.

Another important consideration in utilizing gait measures is that the gait-testing modality should not encumber natural patterns of locomotion to avoid masking the nature of any adaptive gait disturbances that reflect adaptations to the underlying pathology. Many orthopedic conditions such as osteoarthritis are influenced by cyclic loading associated with the repeated patterns of movement during natural gait. Even testing methods such as walking on a treadmill can create gait changes relative to natural overground walking[9] (eg, significant changes in muscle activation and joint moments) that can mask the true nature of a clinically relevant adaptive gait pattern. Thus, capturing the unencumbered characteristics of gait is important for evaluating musculoskeletal pathology.

©Copyright 2021 American Academy of Orthopaedic Surgeons

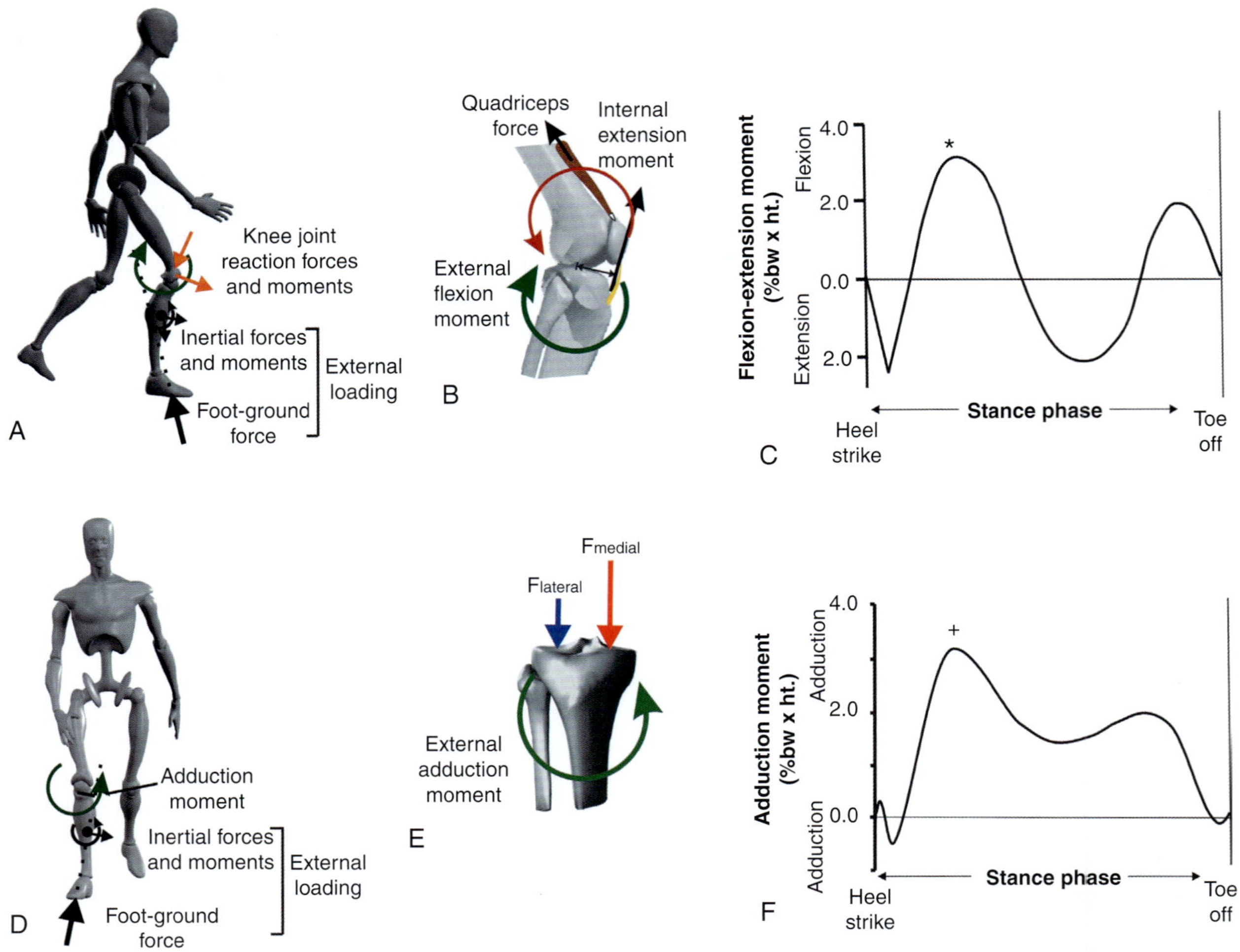

FIGURE 3 Illustrations demonstrate the following. Sagittal plane: **A**, External forces produce a flexion moment at the knee. **B**, Internal forces generated by the quadriceps muscle have been related to the external flexion moment. **C**, Reductions in the first peak (*) of the flexion moment have been related to reduced quadriceps function. Frontal plane: **D**, External forces produce an adduction moment at the knee. **E**, The internal force distribution produces a higher medial force (F_{medial}) than lateral ($F_{lateral}$) related to the adduction moment. **F**, An increase in the first peak (+) of the adduction moment has been related to increase in F_{medial}.

Finally, it should be noted that the methods and principles summarized above for the knee can be applied to the hip and ankle where additional detail can be found in the literature.[6,8]

CLINICAL APPLICATIONS OF GAIT ANALYSIS

Certain types of musculoskeletal pathology provide signals to the locomotor system to modify patterns of locomotion (a gait disturbance) that reflect the presence and nature of the pathological condition. Gait disturbances can be positive (mitigate pathology) or negative (intensify pathology) depending on the individual patient's capacity to respond to the pathological signaling.

Objective assessment of patients with total knee replacement (TKR) can be quite variable using common clinical methods based on patient-reported outcomes. However, it has been shown that objective assessment of functional improvement following TKR can be achieved using relatively inexpensive and efficient time-distance measures. The analysis was based on the fact that time-distance measures are highly reproducible (**Figure 1**) for healthy subjects and provides a useful basis for detecting general disturbances in gait patterns. Treatments, therefore, can be evaluated by testing changes in these measures over time. Given the walking speed dependency of gait measures, it is useful to test these measures as a function of walking speed by asking a subject to walk at their comfortable normal speed, slower than normal, and faster than normal. The resulting data will present a spread of measures over a range of walking speeds. The stride length-walking speed relationship (**Figure 1**) is linear over a range of speeds, and this relationship can be useful for making comparison to healthy subjects as well as comparing changes in patient gait patterns following treatment.

A study[2] of patients at 3, 6, and 9 months following TKR surgery was conducted to test the length of time it took for

 ©Copyright 2021 American Academy of Orthopaedic Surgeons

a patient to recover stable gait following surgery (**Figure 1**) relative to healthy gait patterns. TKR patients and healthy subjects were tested for differences in stride length over a range of speeds to address the walking speed influence. The results showed that the TKR patient walked slower than a healthy subject. Further, the TKR patient had a stride length-walking speed relationship that was different from healthy subjects at the three time points following surgery, and the patient did not return to normal gait at 9 months past surgery (**Figure 1**). However, the results did demonstrate that the gait of the TKR subject changed toward normal between 3 and 6 months past surgery but did not change between 6 and 9 months past surgery, suggesting that gait changes following TKR stabilize at 6 months past surgery.

The above example illustrates that time-distance measurements can be useful for objective assessment of treatment outcome. Given that patient-reported outcomes alone can vary substantially among patients, the potential to have a simple metric that can objectively assess functional outcome could be important in evaluating the efficacy of procedures such as TKR. In addition, these measures can be obtained using simple sensors without the need of a full gait laboratory. Although useful, these measures cannot give the specific cause of the gait disturbance.

Hip osteoarthritis (OA) and femoral acetabular impingement (FAI) have common kinematic gait disturbances that provide insight into the pathomechanics of these conditions as well as a basis for evaluating treatment outcomes. Patients with hip OA were studied[10] to test for gait characteristics that could be associated with motion of the hip during walking. Specifically, hip flexion-extension motion was studied in patients with unilateral OA of the hip and compared with a group of healthy subjects with a similar demographic distribution. The patients who had hip OA had a consistent gait disturbance that was characterized by a decreased dynamic range of motion of the hip and with a disturbance in the normal smooth pattern of hip flexion during gait. The disturbance was characterized by a hesitation or reversal in the direction of the sagittal plane motion as the hip extended in midstance (**Figure 4**). This reversal was documented in 74% of the OA patients and was evident in only 5% of the healthy subjects.[10] The gait adaptations in patients who had hip OA were related to pain and limitations in passive motion. Many of the features of the adaptations were subtle and not detectable through visual observation alone. As such, the nature of the gait disturbance illustrated in **Figure 4** provides an objective marker of the state of OA at the hip.

Interestingly, FAI patients were found to have a similar pattern of hip motion during gait to patients with hip OA.[11] The presence of these reversals in FAI patients reinforces the idea of FAI being a precursor to hip OA. This observation is important because FAI was thought to be a risk factor for developing hip OA. Thus, an objective functional marker for the risk of hip OA was needed as clinical outcome measures are generally subjective or not conducted under actual activities of daily living.

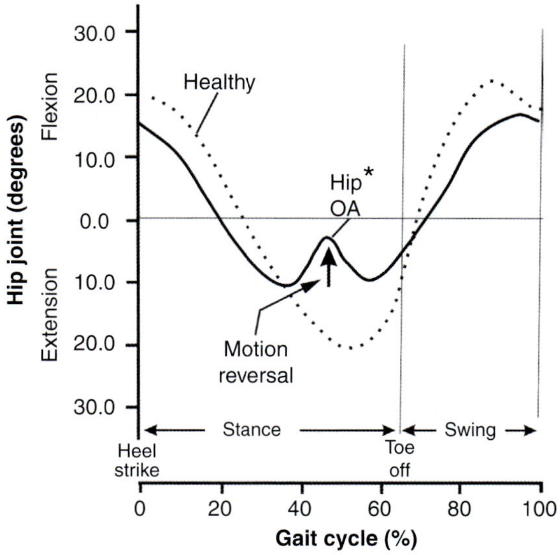

FIGURE 4 Graph illustrating patients with unilateral hip osteoarthritis (OA) had a change in hip motion that was characterized by a reversal (reduced extension) as the hip was moving from flexion to extension at midstance. *Interestingly, patients with femoral acetabular impingement (FAI) had a similar pattern of hip motion to the patients with hip OA. (Data from Hurwitz DE, Hulet CH, Andriacchi TP, et al: Gait compensations in patients with osteoarthritis of the hip and their relationship to pain and passive hip motion. *J Orthop Res* 1997;15:629-635 and Rylander JH, Shu B, Andriacchi TP, et al: Preoperative and postoperative sagittal plane hip kinematics in patients with femoroacetabular impingement during level walking. *Am J Sports Med* 2011;39 Suppl:36S-42S.)

The above observations were used in a subsequent study[12] to evaluate the outcome of treatment for FAI. Specifically, the study[12] demonstrated that the pattern of hip flexion-extension motion during walking returned to normal after arthroscopic surgery was performed to treat FAI. These findings suggest that walking mechanics can provide a useful objective measure to quantitatively assess the outcome of surgical intervention for FAI. The patterns of changes in motion with FAI provide insight into the functional pathologic abnormalities of the disease. The observed reduced hip flexion-extension motion preoperatively may be the result of an adaptive response to pain emanating from labral tears and chondral defects and/or mechanical abutment of the abnormal bony morphology commonly located on the anterior region of the hip joint. The results help establish motion capture as a potential method for quantitatively assessing the outcome in FAI surgical interventions.

Gait kinematic changes with aging have been used to assess the risk of developing knee OA with age.[13] Specifically, the angle of knee flexion at heel strike (the beginning of stance phase) is typically near zero or in slight extension (**Figure 5**) in a younger (29±4 years) population. In contrast, a healthy older (59±9 years) population showed a higher knee flexion at heel strike that was similar to patients with mild knee OA.

©Copyright 2021 American Academy of Orthopaedic Surgeons

Interestingly, patients with more severe knee OA had an even higher knee flexion angle at heel strike (**Figure 5**). Given the fact that aging is the highest risk factor for knee OA, these data (**Figure 5**) suggest an association between the angle of knee flexion at heel strike and the development of knee OA. As such, one could assume that increasing knee flexion at heel strike during gait is a marker of the risk for developing knee OA.

The assumption regarding the potential that changes in kinematics during gait can signal the risk of developing knee OA is important to consider because the field needs early markers sensitive to the risk for knee OA progression. Current imaging and biological markers have not been shown to have enough sensitivity to provide a rigorous basis for evaluating new interventions for OA leaving radiographic evidence as the gold standard. However, clinical trials with radiographic metrics as an outcome measure require large populations and long follow-up periods to evaluate the efficacy of new OA interventions. Thus, clinical trials of new OA interventions are very expensive, and at present, there is a paucity of disease-modifying interventions for OA. Thus, there is a critical need for new efficient methods to assess the state of OA as well as the risk of rapid progression from a mild to severe and disabling state.

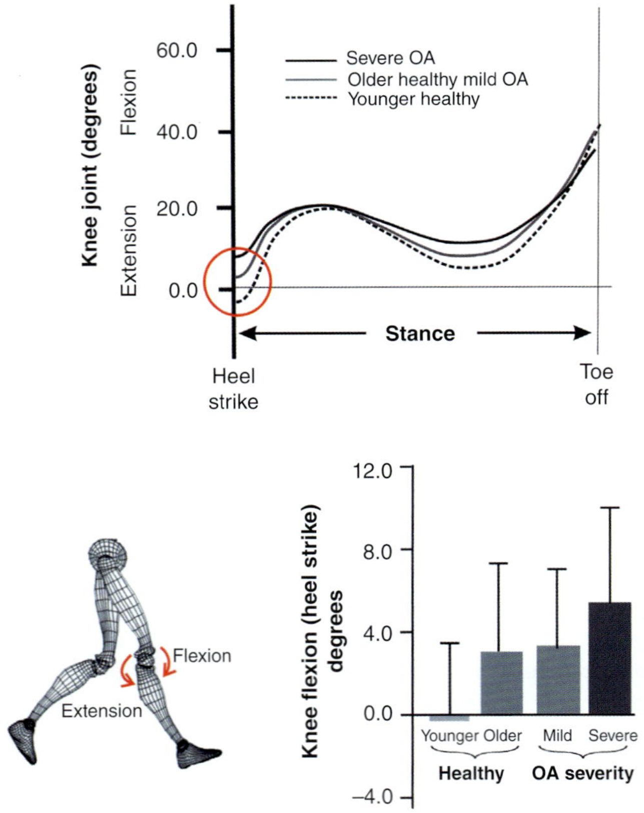

FIGURE 5 Graphs demonstrating the knee flexion at heel strike is greater in older healthy subjects in a manner similar to patterns seen in patients with mild knee osteoarthritis (OA). Knee flexion was greater in patients with more severe knee OA. (Data from Favre J, Erhart-Hledik JC, Andriacchi TP: Age-related differences in sagittal-plane knee function at heel-strike of walking are increased in osteoarthritic patients. *Osteoarthritis Cartilage* 2014;22:464-471.)

Quadriceps inhibition associated with anterior cruciate ligament (ACL) injury was among the first gait disturbances identified in patients with ACL-deficient knees.[14] One of the key findings reported[14] was that patients had a reduction in the magnitude of the moment that tended to flex the knee during walking (**Figure 3**, C) in early stance. As noted above (**Figure 3**, B), the external flexion moment is balanced internally by net quadriceps contraction, and the gait pattern was described as a "quadriceps avoidance" suggesting an avoidance or reduction in quadriceps muscle activation. One cause for this gait disturbance was suggested to be the tendency of quadriceps contraction to produce an anterior pull on the tibia at lower flexion angles (20° or less) in the early stance phase of gait. Thus, in the absence of an ACL, a patient adopting a gait pattern that reduces quadriceps contraction can mitigate the anterior pull on the tibia. This adaptation represents a neuromuscular change to the loss of a functioning ACL that would be difficult to detect without quantitative gait analysis. Yet the nature of this adaptation is clinically important because it helps to explain rapid quadriceps atrophy[15] after injury. There have been a number of subsequent studies[16,17] reporting the loss of quadriceps function following ACL injury.

The functional role of ACL graft orientation has been shown[18] to substantially influence the peak external knee flexion moment (net quadriceps moment) during walking (**Figure 3**, C) in patients following ACL reconstruction (ACLR). Patients tested in the gait laboratory were given an MRI to quantify the three-dimensional orientation of the ACL graft. The results indicated that when the ACL graft placement deviated from an anatomical location to a more vertical coronal orientation, patients reduced their net quadriceps usage during walking to a pattern consistent with ACL-deficient patients described above. It is important to note that the reconstructed knees were stable based on clinical testing, and it was the gait test that identified the functional change associated with a nonanatomical placement of the ACL graft. The sensitivity of quadriceps function to graft placement could help explain the reported variability in the knee flexion moment[19-21] after ACLR based on intersurgeon preferences for graft placement.

The finding that quadriceps function is reduced during gait when grafts are placed in a nonanatomical position is clinically important if one considers the risk of developing knee OA in an ACLR population. As will be discussed later in this chapter, the loss of quadriceps function is one of the critical gait disturbances frequently seen in patients with knee OA. Given the importance of quadriceps function for maintaining a healthy knee,[22,23] this gait study[18] provided important insight into the role of ACL graft placement in mitigating the risk of developing premature knee OA.

The association between knee OA progression and the adduction moment during gait was first identified in a

©Copyright 2021 American Academy of Orthopaedic Surgeons

longitudinal study[24] of patients with medial compartment knee OA treated with a high tibial osteotomy (HTO) to correct varus alignment. Patients were tested before surgery, 1 year after surgery, and 3 years after surgery. The results indicated that patients with a lower preoperative peak magnitude of the external knee adduction moment (indicated by plus sign on **Figure 3**, F) had significantly better postoperative clinical results than patients with a higher adduction moment. The high adduction moment and low adduction moment groups were indistinguishable based on preoperative knee score, initial varus deformity, immediate postoperative correction, age, and weight. These results suggest a low adduction moment mitigates the rate of OA progression in patients with medial knee OA. The underlying scientific basis for the relationship between medial compartment knee OA and the adduction moment was supported in an analysis[7] between the external moments and the internal contact force (**Figure 3**, E) which shows that a high adduction moment can be associated with a higher medial compartment force. Thus, the adduction moment provides a noninvasive surrogate for assessing internal loading on the medial compartment during walking that is useful for assessing knee OA.

Clinical applications of the knee adduction moment as a surrogate measure for medial compartment load have been used to enhance our understanding of etiologies of OA. For example, the knee adduction moment has been shown to influence treatment outcome[24] and disease progression[25] in patients with medial compartment knee OA. Thus, a high adduction moment can be considered an effective marker for risk of progression of knee OA as well as a target for intervention for patients with early knee OA or at risk for developing knee OA.

Several load-modifying interventions have been designed to lower the adduction moment during walking. Bracing has been shown to reduce the adduction moment at the knee, yet long-term studies of load-shifting brace treatments reported that compliance declined over time due to bulk and inconvenience, poor fit, leg swelling, and skin irritation.[26] Lateral wedges have also been shown[27] to reduce the adduction moment, yet discomfort has limited clinical use of lateral wedges.[28,29] Gait retraining has also been shown to reduce the adduction moment[30]; however, optimal strategies for clinical implementation have yet to be determined. Some issues with bracing/lateral wedges and certain gait retraining methods is that they either force the limb into a static position or result in extreme movements which can impede normal adaptations of the neuromuscular systems in a manner that can be uncomfortable and diminish compliance.

An alternative to the lateral wedge was introduced with a variable-stiffness shoe that was shown to reduce the adduction moment and pain.[31] The variable-stiffness shoe does not force the limb into a set static position, and this primary difference as compared with a brace or fixed lateral wedge provides some insight into different methods to reduce the adduction moment. The variable-stiffness shoe produces a dynamic stimulus during walking that results in a reduction in the lever arm of the adduction moment.[32] The dynamic stimulus is believed to activate the neuromuscular system during walking in a manner that shifts the center of mass laterally to reduce the adduction moment. Thus, the adduction moment reduction with the variable-stiffness shoe is controlled by the neuromuscular response of the patient, whereas a wedge or brace holds the limb in a fixed position. The clinical importance of the above observations is the capacity of the neuromuscular system to adapt to external stimuli in the form of interventions to modify gait.

The flexion moment is important to understanding knee OA because there is evidence[33] that the flexion moment as well as the adduction moment at baseline can influence cartilage changes 5 years later in patients with medial knee OA as assessed by MRI. Thus, evaluating any intervention for reducing the adduction moment should also test for changes in the flexion moment because both the flexion and adduction moment contribute to the loading at the knee joint. Again, as shown in **Figure 3**, C, the flexion moment can be considered a surrogate for the quadriceps function. Patients with knee OA have been shown[34] to have quadriceps deficits like that described above in patients with ACL injury. However, the quadriceps deficit in patients with knee OA appears to be related to pain.

In examining the role of the flexion moment relative to knee OA, it is useful to consider the contribution of the flexion and adduction moments components to the magnitude of the total moment at the knee during walking. The total moment (**Figure 6**, A) is the vector magnitude determined from the flexion, adduction, and rotation components of the total moment vector, and more detail can be found in the literature.[34] The rotation moment is very small and can be considered negligible relative to the adduction and flexion moment components. As such, this discussion will focus on the contributions of the flexion and adduction moments to the total moment. It can be seen by comparing flexion and adduction moment curves (**Figure 3**, C and F) to the total moment curve (**Figure 6**, A) that all three curves reach a peak at nearly the same time in early stance phase.

An analysis of the relative contributions of the adduction and flexion moments to the total moment in patients with medial knee OA provides unique insight into the pathomechanics of the disease. Specifically, patients with knee OA were studied over a period of 5 years.[34] Interestingly, the total moment remained constant over the 5-year period, but the relative contributions of the flexion and adduction moments substantially changed (**Figure 6**, B). As knee OA advanced over 5 years, there was a transition in gait to reduce the flexion moment and increase the adduction moment. This increase in the contribution of the adduction moment to the total moment is consistent with evidence that shows patients with more severe knee OA have a higher adduction moment.[35] The changing role of the flexion and adduction moments reflects different aspects of knee OA. The adduction moment increase

©Copyright 2021 American Academy of Orthopaedic Surgeons

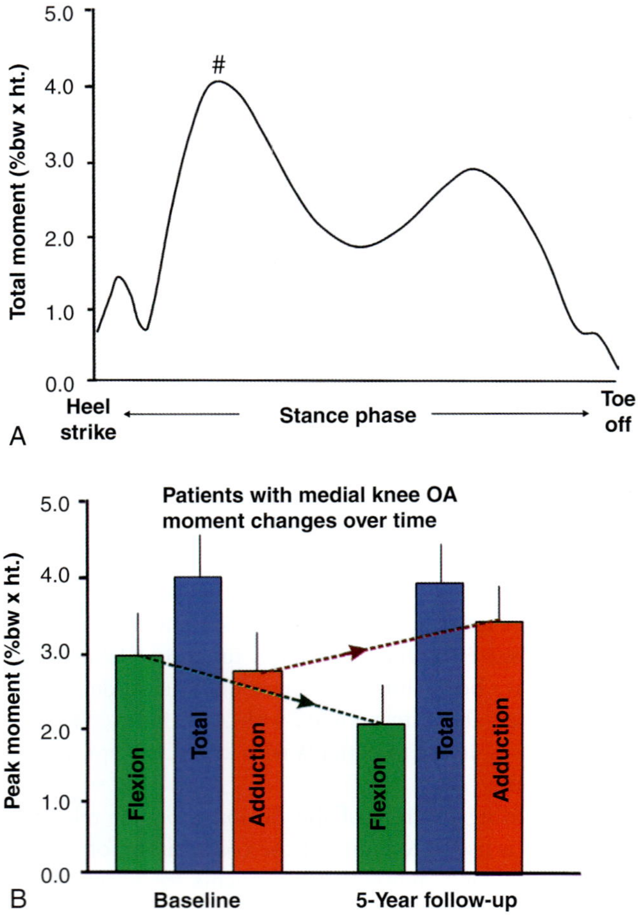

FIGURE 6 **A**, An illustration of the typical pattern of total joint moment that is calculated based primarily on the flexion and adduction moments (**Figure 3**) during walking. Note: The peak of the total moment (#) occurs early in stance near the instance of the peak of the flexion (**Figure 3**, C) and adduction moments (**Figure 3**, F). **B**, A bar graph demonstrating that at baseline, the peaks of the flexion moment (green) and adduction moment (red) are statistically the same. However, at the 5-year follow-up the peak flexion moment decreases while the peak adduction moment increases.

with OA severity appears to reflect structural changes in varus alignment likely due cartilage thinning in the medial compartment. A reduced flexion moment as the disease progresses likely reflects increased pain with more severe OA. The relationship between the flexion moment and pain is important because the flexion moment shows the potential as an objective marker of pain.

Evidence of the flexion moment as a marker of pain has been shown[36,37] in placebo-controlled studies of patients with knee OA. Specifically, in these studies, pain was modified through controlled administration of analgesic or anti-inflammatory medications and was related to a change in the magnitude of the flexion moment. Similarly, pain created in healthy subjects through injection of isotonic saline[38] was also associated with a reduction in the magnitude of the flexion moment. Thus, it appears that reducing the flexion moment is a common adaptation to pain. Given the fact that the flexion moment is balanced by net quadriceps contraction, the reduced quadriceps strength[39] reported with advancing stages of knee OA is consistent with an ambulatory adaptation to pain. In general, muscle function is altered as the severity of the disease becomes worse. Rehabilitation programs achieving quadriceps strengthening have been shown to reduce pain and disability in subjects with knee OA.[39]

SUMMARY OF CLINICAL APPLICATIONS

The clinical examples presented in this section demonstrate that gait disturbances appear as adaptations to a specific musculoskeletal pathology. The stimulus for the gait disturbance frequently comes from pain, muscle weakness, neuromuscular changes, or instability. The fact that gait disturbances can vary among patients is very important because differences in the patient adaptation can provide an objective marker for treatment planning or evaluation. Thus, the pathological condition acts as a signal for patients to adopt patterns of locomotion to accommodate biological or structural changes associated with specific clinical changes. Conversely, specific characteristics of gait mechanics can provide signals that influence biological and structural changes.

GAIT MECHANICS SIGNAL TISSUE ADAPTATION

Gait mechanics provide a signal[40] at the macroscale that can produce a response at the microscale (cellular level) that is reflected in structural and biological changes. The following section provides evidence that tissue adapts to signals that result from gait mechanics, and understanding these signals are fundamental to understanding the principles that underlie the clinical findings described above.

Evidence that cartilage morphology adapts to the adduction moment signal has important implications to help explain the mechanism underlying the clinical relationship between the adduction moment and progression of medial knee OA. Identifying the mechanism becomes clearer when examining a study[41] that showed healthy subjects with a higher adduction moment also had thicker cartilage in the medial knee compartment relative to the lateral compartment. Specifically, the ratio of the medial-to-lateral cartilage thickness positively correlated (**Figure 7**) with the adduction moment. Thus, the shift in the cartilage ratio toward the medial compartment is explained by the fact that the shift in the force distribution to the medial compartment is related to the adduction moment (**Figure 3**). The fact that healthy cartilage is thicker in regions that sustain higher cyclic loads during gait suggests a positive tissue adaptation to load.

The positive adaptation of healthy cartilage to loading at first might seem to contradict studies in patients with knee OA, where clinical function declines with increasing load.

©Copyright 2021 American Academy of Orthopaedic Surgeons

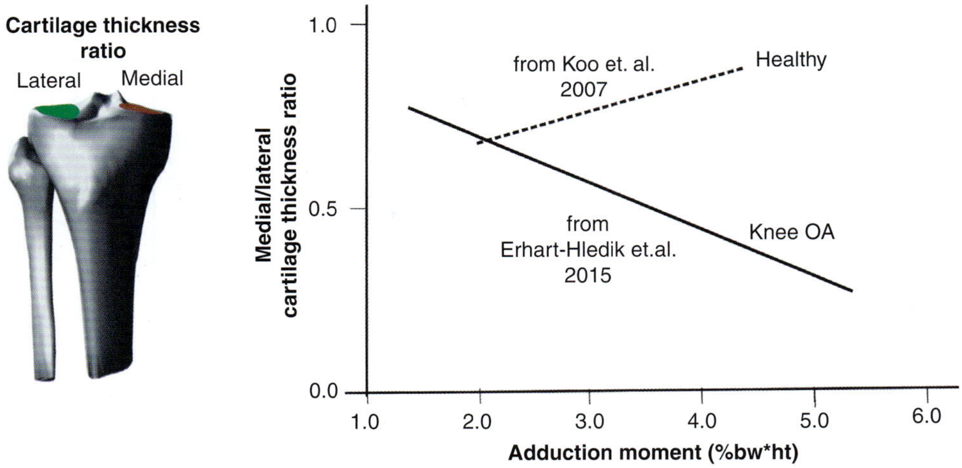

FIGURE 7 Illustration demonstrating that the ratio of medial-to-lateral cartilage thickness increases with the higher adduction moment in healthy subjects (dashed line) and decreases with higher adduction moment in patients with knee OA (solid line). These observations support the role of the adduction moment in the progression of medial knee OA.

However, probing deeper, the mechanosensitivity of cartilage (ie, cellular response to mechanical stimuli) helps explain this paradox. In general, cartilage health is maintained by a balance between synthesis and degradation that reflects a homeostasis modulated by mechanical loading[42] during gait. However, it appears that this homeostasis is not maintained in patients with knee OA, as it has been shown[43] that there is a negative relationship (**Figure 7**) between the adduction moment and the medial-to-lateral thickness ratio in patients with medial compartment knee OA. Thus, as the adduction moment increases, cartilage is thinner in these patients. This change in load sensitivity is likely related to a common finding that the chondrocyte is metabolically more active in OA cartilage reflecting a loss of normal homeostasis. This metabolic activity is accelerated with mechanical stimuli and can lead to further tissue degradation. As such, cartilage becomes thinner with increasing load in cartilage with knee OA.

Evidence that cartilage morphology adapts to a kinematics change during walking is relevant to understanding the risk of developing premature knee OA following ACL injury as well as understanding the increased risk of developing knee OA with aging. There is evidence that the variation in the thickness of healthy knee cartilage is related to the same kinematic measures (knee flexion at heel strike) found in subjects at risk for OA and increased in subjects with more severe knee OA. Specifically, it has been shown[44,45] that in healthy subjects the location of the thickest cartilage on the medial femoral condyle is associated with the knee flexion angle at heel strike (**Figure 8**). This is the same location in the gait cycle that has been shown to change as risk and severity of knee OA advances (**Figure 5**, A).

The clinical relevance of knee kinematics can be explained by examining the causes for the relationship between knee flexion at heel strike and cartilage thickness. At heel strike (**Figure 8**, A), the location of tibial-femoral contact is associated with the angle of knee flexion, and contact location changes as the knee flexes (**Figure 8**, B). The fact that individual variations in the location of the thickest cartilage (**Figure 8**, B) are related to knee kinematics during walking in healthy subjects suggests that regional cartilage adapts to local variations in loading during walking. Thus, local homeostasis of cartilage cells is conditioned by the cyclic walking loads that occur in a specific location. This conditioning of cartilage to its local mechanical environment provides a basis for explaining why patients with conditions (eg, aging and ACL injury) associated with kinematic changes at the knee (**Figure 5**) are at greater risk for developing knee OA. These observations suggest that if a condition develops resulting in a kinematic change at the knee which changes the location of the tibial-femoral loading during walking and that region cannot adapt to the local change in load, then the cartilage will progress on a degenerative pathway leading to knee OA.[46]

The biological response to gait mechanics helps to consolidate the interaction of mechanical and structural components that suggest analysis of musculoskeletal pathology should be treated as system.[42] Interpretation of conditions such as OA should include a comprehensive view that integrates mechanics, structure, and biology. For example, there are several studies[47-49] that showed that mechanical loading during walking can stimulate changes in serum concentration of cartilage oligomeric matrix protein (COMP), a marker of cartilage matrix turnover. Specifically, serum concentrations of COMP were taken at rest and after a mechanical stimulus in the form of a 30-minute walk (**Figure 9**). The serum concentrations of COMP were found to change after the mechanical stimulus relative to the resting levels, and the changes were found to differ between younger and older healthy subjects.[48] In a subsequent analysis of patients with knee OA,[47] it was found that the change in serum COMP concentration of the healthy older population was the same as patients with knee OA. Interestingly, the results were similar to the differences in knee flexion that occur with aging and disease severity with knee OA, suggesting the interactions between biology and gait mechanics.

The direct clinical significance of the biological response to a mechanical stimulus was identified in a study[49] that showed the change in serum COMP concentration levels

©Copyright 2021 American Academy of Orthopaedic Surgeons

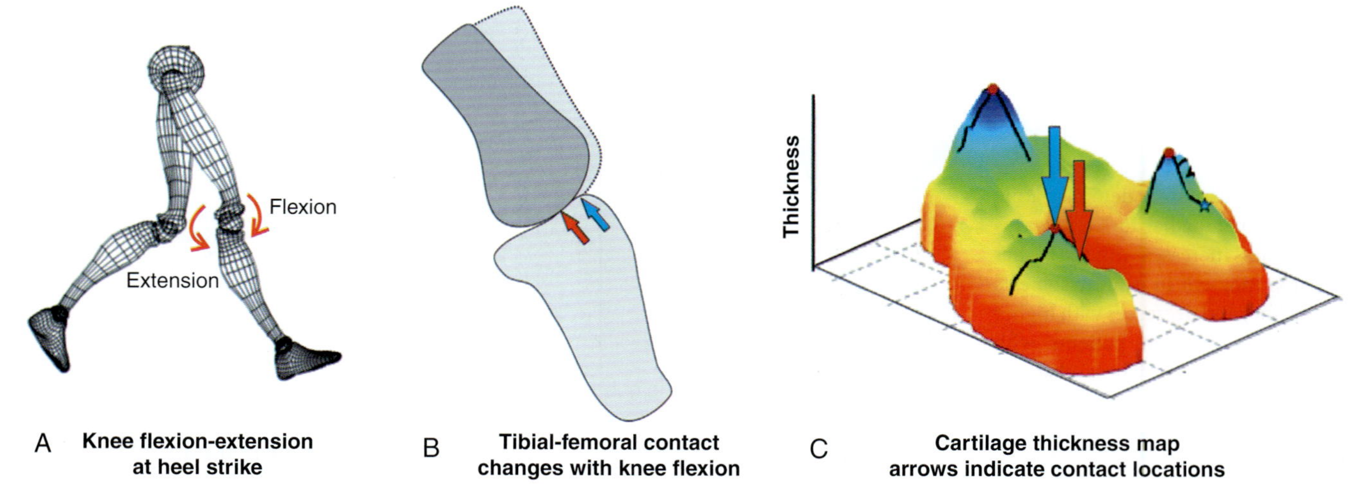

FIGURE 8 Illustration demonstrating that the angle of knee flexion-extension at heel strike (**A**) influences the location of tibial-femoral contact (**B**) and helps explain why the location of the thickest cartilage on the medial femoral condyle (**C**) is correlated to the knee flexion angle at heel strike. Aging and progressive knee OA associated with increased knee flexion at heel strike (**Figure 5**) can shift loading away from the thickest cartilage to regions that cannot adapt to the change in load and thus can initiate or accelerate a degenerative pathway. (Data from Scanlan SF, Favre J, Andriacchi TP: The relationship between peak knee extension at heel-strike of walking and the location of thickest femoral cartilage in ACL reconstructed and healthy contralateral knees. *J Biomech* 2013;46:849-854 and Koo S, Rylander JH, Andriacchi TP: Knee joint kinematics during walking influences the spatial cartilage thickness distribution in the knee. *J Biomech* 2011;44:1405-1409.)

following the mechanical stimulus (30-minute walk) at baseline was correlated with cartilage thickness changes derived from MRI at 5-year follow-up in knee OA patients. Clinically, the finding of this study is important because it provides a potential test method for the early detection of patients at risk for developing cartilage changes associated with OA progression. Introducing the mechanical stimulus appears to enhance the sensitivity of the biomarker response. As noted in the study of HTO patients,[24] the individual variations in the nature of a patient's adaptation to a particular condition can influence the risk of advancing disease. Thus, integrating a gait stimulus with a biological response provides a tool similar to a cardiac stress test in the form of an OA stress test.

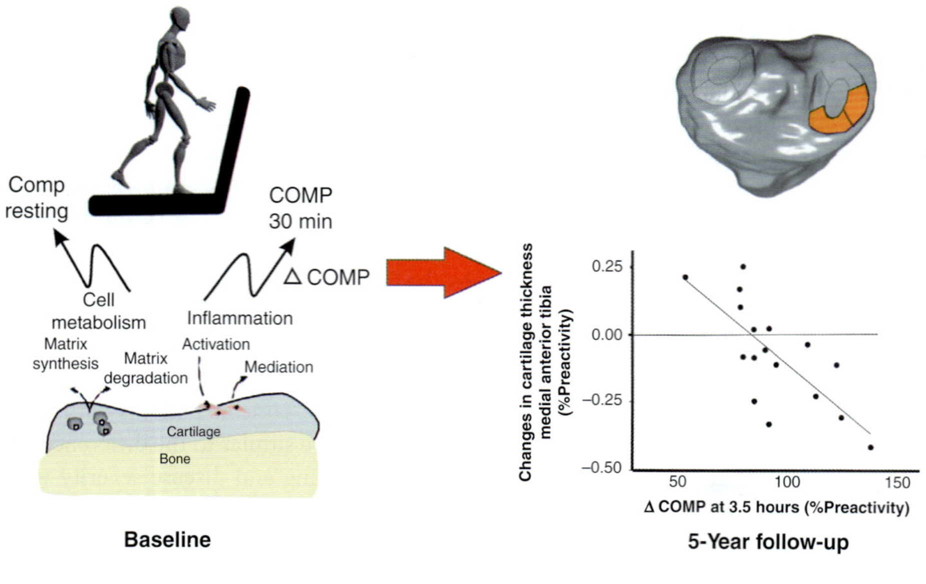

FIGURE 9 Illustration demonstrating that mechanical loading during a 30-minute walk can stimulate changes in serum concentrations of cartilage oligomeric matrix protein (COMP), a marker of cartilage matrix turnover. The change in serum COMP concentration levels following the mechanical stimulus (30-minute walk) at a baseline test was correlated with cartilage thickness changes derived from MRI at 5-year follow-up in knee OA patients. (Data from Erhart-Hledik JC, Favre J, Asay JL, et al: A relationship between mechanically-induced changes in serum cartilage oligomeric matrix protein (COMP) and changes in cartilage thickness after 5 years. *Osteoarthritis Cartilage* 2012;20:1309-1315.)

©Copyright 2021 American Academy of Orthopaedic Surgeons

SUMMARY

This chapter has presented a broad range of observations that apply to the clinical application of gait analysis. The observations show that measures obtained during gait provide signals reflecting adaptations to stimuli such as pain, instability, and muscle weakness and provide a basis for assessing disease state. Importantly, not all subjects adopt the same type of gait in response to an injury or disease, and the difference in the nature of the change in gait can explain why some subjects at risk do not develop progressive changes. For example, about 50% of patients with ACL injury[50] develop premature knee OA, and it possible that the nature of gait patterns of these patients mitigates the risk. Conversely, it has been shown that tissue (structure and biology) can adapt to the cyclic loads that occur during walking. This observation is also clinically important because it provides a basis for understanding why certain gait disturbances can lead to degenerative changes by shifting load to areas not conditioned to the new change in loading. Finally, our understanding of gait mechanics has evolved to seamlessly integrate gait with the structural and biological elements that influence musculoskeletal health and pathology in a manner that will continue to expand applications of gait analysis to address unsolved clinical problems.

KEY TAKEAWAY POINTS

- External measures obtained with gait analysis can reflect internal tissue response indicating the state of functional health.
- Gait measures are reproducible for healthy gait due to locomotor programming tuned to minimize energy expenditure during walking.
- Gait disturbances are also reproducible and reflect a reprogramming to adapt to specific pathological conditions.
- Patients adopt different specific patterns of ambulation in response to injury or disease, and the nature of the adaptation can influence clinical outcome.
- Gait mechanics interact with biomarkers and structural changes.
- Gait mechanics are fundamental to understanding disease, injury, and treatment outcomes that are addressed by numerous orthopedic procedures.
- Gait analysis methods should avoid introducing unnatural external stimuli that could mask the nature of the adaptation to pathological conditions.

REFERENCES

1. Grieve DW, Gear RJ: The relationships between length of stride, step frequency, time of swing and speed of walking for children and adults. *Ergonomics* 1966;9:379-399.
2. Andriacchi TP, Ogle JA, Galante JO: Walking speed as a basis for normal and abnormal gait measurements. *J Biomech* 1977;10:261-268.
3. Waters RL, Mulroy S: The energy expenditure of normal and pathologic gait. *Gait Posture* 1999;9:207-231.
4. Inman VT, Ralston HJ, Todd F, et al: *Human Walking*. Baltimore: Williams & Wilkins, 1981, xi, p 154.
5. Murray MP, Gore DR, Clarkson BH: Walking patterns of patients with unilateral hip pain due to osteo-arthritis and avascular necrosis. *J Bone Joint Surg Am* 1971;53:259-274.
6. Andriacchi TPJT, Hurwitz DE, Nataraja RN: Musculoskeletal dynamics, locomotion, and clinical applications, in Mow VC, Huiskes R, eds: *Basic Orthopaedic Biomechanics and Mechano-Biology*, ed 3. Philadelphia, PA: Lippincott Williams & Wilkins, 2005, pp 91-122.
7. Schipplein OD, Andriacchi TP: Interaction between active and passive knee stabilizers during level walking. *J Orthop Res* 1991;9:113-119.
8. Chehab EF, Andriacchi TP, Favre J: Speed, age, sex, and body mass index provide a rigorous basis for comparing the kinematic and kinetic profiles of the lower extremity during walking. *J Biomech* 2017;58:11-20.
9. Lee SJ, Hidler J: Biomechanics of overground vs. treadmill walking in healthy individuals. *J Appl Physiol (1985)* 2008;104:747-755.
10. Hurwitz DE, Hulet CH, Andriacchi TP, et al: Gait compensations in patients with osteoarthritis of the hip and their relationship to pain and passive hip motion. *J Orthop Res* 1997;15:629-635.
11. Rylander JH, Shu B, Andriacchi TP, et al: Preoperative and postoperative sagittal plane hip kinematics in patients with femoroacetabular impingement during level walking. *Am J Sports Med* 2011;39 suppl:36S-42S.
12. Rylander J, Shu B, Favre J, et al: Functional testing provides unique insights into the pathomechanics of femoroacetabular impingement and an objective basis for evaluating treatment outcome. *J Orthop Res* 2013;31:1461-1468.
13. Favre J, Erhart-Hledik JC, Andriacchi TP: Age-related differences in sagittal-plane knee function at heel-strike of walking are increased in osteoarthritic patients. *Osteoarthritis Cartilage* 2014;22:464-471.
14. Berchuck M, Andriacchi TP, Bach BR, et al: Gait adaptations by patients who have a deficient anterior cruciate ligament. *J Bone Joint Surg Am* 1990;72:871-877.
15. Thomas AC, Wojtys EM, Brandon C, et al: Muscle atrophy contributes to quadriceps weakness after anterior cruciate ligament reconstruction. *J Sci Med Sport* 2016;19:7-11.
16. Zabala ME, Favre J, Scanlan SF, et al: Three-dimensional knee moments of ACL reconstructed and control subjects during gait, stair ascent, and stair descent. *J Biomech* 2013;46:515-520.
17. Erhart-Hledik JC, Chu CR, Asay JL, et al: Gait mechanics 2 years after anterior cruciate ligament reconstruction are associated with longer-term changes in patient-reported outcomes. *J Orthop Res* 2017;35:634-640.
18. Scanlan SF, Blazek K, Chaudhari AM, et al: Graft orientation influences the knee flexion moment during walking in patients with anterior cruciate ligament reconstruction. *Am J Sports Med* 2009;37:2173-2178.
19. Webster KE, Wittwer JE, O'Brien J, et al: Gait patterns after anterior cruciate ligament reconstruction are related to graft type. *Am J Sports Med* 2005;33:247-254.
20. DeVita P, Hortobagyi T, Barrier J: Gait biomechanics are not normal after anterior cruciate ligament reconstruction and accelerated rehabilitation. *Med Sci Sports Exerc* 1998;30:1481-1488.
21. Bulgheroni P, Bulgheroni MV, Andrini L, et al: Gait patterns after anterior cruciate ligament reconstruction. *Knee Surg Sports Traumatol Arthrosc* 1997;5:14-21.

©Copyright 2021 American Academy of Orthopaedic Surgeons

22. Shelbourne KD, Gray T: Minimum 10-year results after anterior cruciate ligament reconstruction: how the loss of normal knee motion compounds other factors related to the development of osteoarthritis after surgery. *Am J Sports Med* 2009;37:471-480.

23. Lewek M, Rudolph K, Axe M, et al: The effect of insufficient quadriceps strength on gait after anterior cruciate ligament reconstruction. *Clin Biomech (Bristol, Avon)* 2002;17:56-63.

24. Prodromos CC, Andriacchi TP, Galante JO: A relationship between gait and clinical changes following high tibial osteotomy. *J Bone Joint Surg Am* 1985;67:1188-1194.

25. Miyazaki T: Dynamic load at baseline can predict radiographic disease progression in medial compartment knee osteoarthritis. *Annals of the Rheumatic Diseases* 2002;61:617-622.

26. Brouwer RW, van Raaij TM, Verhaar JA, et al: Brace treatment for osteoarthritis of the knee: a prospective randomized multi-centre trial. *Osteoarthritis Cartilage* 2006;14:777-783.

27. Fisher DS, Dyrby CO, Mundermann A, et al: In healthy subjects without knee osteoarthritis, the peak knee adduction moment influences the acute effect of shoe interventions designed to reduce medial compartment knee load. *J Orthop Res* 2007;25:540-546.

28. Kakihana W, Akai M, Nakazawa K, et al: Inconsistent knee varus moment reduction caused by a lateral wedge in knee osteoarthritis. *Am J Phys Med Rehabil* 2007;86:446-454.

29. Kerrigan DC, Lelas JL, Goggins J, et al: Effectiveness of a lateral-wedge insole on knee varus torque in patients with knee osteoarthritis. *Arch Phys Med Rehabil* 2002;83:889-893.

30. Eddo O, Lindsey B, Caswell SV, et al: Current evidence of gait modification with real-time biofeedback to alter kinetic, temporospatial, and function-related outcomes: A review. *Int J Kinesiology and Sports Sci* 2017;5(3):35.

31. Erhart JC, Mundermann A, Elspas B, et al: A variable-stiffness shoe lowers the knee adduction moment in subjects with symptoms of medial compartment knee osteoarthritis. *J Biomech* 2008;41:2720-2725.

32. Jenkyn TR, Erhart JC, Andriacchi TP: An analysis of the mechanisms for reducing the knee adduction moment during walking using a variable stiffness shoe in subjects with knee osteoarthritis. *J Biomech* 2011;44:1271-1276.

33. Chehab EF, Favre J, Erhart-Hledik JC, et al: Baseline knee adduction and flexion moments during walking are both associated with 5 year cartilage changes in patients with medial knee osteoarthritis. *Osteoarthritis Cartilage* 2014. 22:1833-1839.

34. Asay JL, Erhart-Hledik JC, Andriacchi TP: Changes in the total knee joint moment in patients with medial compartment knee osteoarthritis over 5 years. *J Orthop Res*.2018;36(9):2373-2379.

35. Mundermann A, Dyrby CO, Hurwitz DE, et al: Potential strategies to reduce medial compartment loading in patients with knee osteoarthritis of varying severity: reduced walking speed. *Arthritis Rheum* 2004;50:1172-1178.

36. Hurwitz DE, Ryals AR, Block JA, et al: Knee pain and joint loading in subjects with osteoarthritis of the knee. *J Orthop Res* 2000;18:572-579.

37. Boyer KA, Angst MS, Asay J, et al: Sensitivity of gait parameters to the effects of anti-inflammatory and opioid treatments in knee osteoarthritis patients. *J Orthop Res* 2012;30:1118-1124.

38. Henriksen M, Graven-Nielsen T, Aaboe J, et al: Gait changes in patients with knee osteoarthritis are replicated by experimental knee pain. *Arthritis Care Res (Hoboken)* 2010;62:501-509.

39. Anwer S, Alghadir A: Effect of isometric quadriceps exercise on muscle strength, pain, and function in patients with knee osteoarthritis: a randomized controlled study. *J Phys Ther Sci* 2014;26:745-748.

40. Andriacchi TP, Favre J: The nature of in vivo mechanical signals that influence cartilage health and progression to knee osteoarthritis. *Curr Rheumatol Rep* 2014;16:463.

41. Koo S, Andriacchi TP: A comparison of the influence of global functional loads vs. local contact anatomy on articular cartilage thickness at the knee. *J Biomech* 2007;40:2961-2966.

42. Andriacchi TP, Favre J, Erhart-Hledik JC, et al: A systems view of risk factors for knee osteoarthritis reveals insights into the pathogenesis of the disease. *Ann Biomed Eng* 2015;43:376-387.

43. Erhart-Hledik JC, Favre J, Andriacchi TP: New insight in the relationship between regional patterns of knee cartilage thickness, osteoarthritis disease severity, and gait mechanics. *J Biomech* 2015;48:3868-3875.

44. Scanlan SF, Favre J, Andriacchi TP: The relationship between peak knee extension at heel-strike of walking and the location of thickest femoral cartilage in ACL reconstructed and healthy contralateral knees. *J Biomech* 2013;46:849-854.

45. Koo S, Rylander JH, Andriacchi TP: Knee joint kinematics during walking influences the spatial cartilage thickness distribution in the knee. *J Biomech* 2011;44:1405-1409.

46. Andriacchi TP, Koo S, Scanlan SF: Gait mechanics influence healthy cartilage morphology and osteoarthritis of the knee. *J Bone Joint Surg Am* 2009;91(suppl 1):95-101.

47. Mundermann A, King KB, Smith RL, et al: Change in serum COMP concentration due to ambulatory load is not related to knee OA status. *J Orthop Res* 2009;27:1408-1413.

48. Mundermann A, Dyrby CO, Andriacchi TP, et al: Serum concentration of cartilage oligomeric matrix protein (COMP) is sensitive to physiological cyclic loading in healthy adults. *Osteoarthritis Cartilage* 2005;13:34-38.

49. Erhart-Hledik JC, Favre J, Asay JL, et al: A relationship between mechanically-induced changes in serum cartilage oligomeric matrix protein (COMP) and changes in cartilage thickness after 5 years. *Osteoarthritis Cartilage* 2012;20:1309-1315.

50. Lohmander LS, Ostenberg A, Englund M, et al: High prevalence of knee osteoarthritis, pain, and functional limitations in female soccer players twelve years after anterior cruciate ligament injury. *Arthritis Rheum* 2004;50:3145-3152.

©Copyright 2021 American Academy of Orthopaedic Surgeons

6

Biomaterials in Orthopaedic Practice

Derek R. Jenkins, MD
Douglas C. Moore, MS

Keywords: *biomaterials; engineering; preclinical*

INTRODUCTION

Biomaterials are composed of synthetic and natural substances used in orthopaedic implants and devices applied in biological systems. The field of biomaterials represents a convergence of biology, chemistry, physics, engineering, and medicine and is relatively young, at less than 100 years old, but has come in recent years to significantly impact healthcare and the economy.[1-4] Biomaterials are used in trauma surgery in plates, screws, and intramedullary rods, and as prostheses in joint replacement surgeries, but also as sutures, adhesives, and drug-eluting devices. The main classes of synthetic biomaterials are metals, polymers, ceramics, and composites. As the world population ages and standard of living improves, it can be expected that the field of biomaterials will become more and more prominent in the practice of orthopaedics, and so it is paramount as responsible surgeons that we have a fundamental understanding of basic principles to guide us in our ethical and effective employment of these technological foundations of our practice.

Neither of the following authors nor any immediate family member has received anything of value from or has stock or stock options held in a commercial company or institution related directly or indirectly to the subject of this chapter: Dr. Moore and Dr. Jenkins.

BIOCOMPATIBILITY

Interactions between a biomaterial and the host biological system will lead to success or failure of the material. Failure can be due to the biomaterial's local or systemic adverse effect on the biological system or due to the biological system's adverse effect or degradation of the biomaterial. Biocompatibility is a term used to describe the functional integration of the biomaterial into the host biological system.[5] Biocompatibility is affected by chemistry of the biomaterial, leachables, shape, mechanics, and design. Some of the early work on the materials used in orthopaedics was done in concert with dentistry, including poly methyl methacrylate, cobalt-chromium-molybdenum and titanium alloys. A biomaterial can be inert, interactive, or viable. Inert biomaterials are bulk materials having little or no adverse biologic response. Interactive biomaterials are passive materials designed to elicit a specific biologic response such as bony ingrowth. Viable biomaterials integrate or attract cells and are subsequently remodeled or resorbed. It is important to note that a biomaterial may be inert in bulk form but can elicit a local adverse effect if corrosion occurs in the host biological environment, or if mechanical wear produces particulates of a certain size and concentration. It is also important to recognize that there is often a change over time in the interaction of host to biomaterial, and biomaterial to host, and this biocompatibility is a dynamic relationship.[6,7]

At the cellular level, biocompatibility is influenced by the toxic effects of leachates, microbiologic or endotoxin contamination, mechanical interaction at the implant-tissue interface, and direct cell-biomaterial interactions. The vast majority of

This chapter is adapted from Mann KA, Allen MJ: Biomaterials in Orthopaedic Practice, in O'Keefe RJ, Jacobs JJ, Chu CR, Einhorn TA, eds: *Orthopaedic Basic Science*, ed 4. Rosemont, IL, American Academy of Orthopaedic Surgeons, 2013, pp 69-85.

©Copyright 2021 American Academy of Orthopaedic Surgeons

TABLE 1 Most Common Orthopaedic Biomaterials

Material	Primary Use(s)
Metals	
Ti alloy (Ti-6%/Al-4%V)	Plates, screws, TJA components (nonbearing surfaces)
Co-Cr-Mo alloy	TJA components
Stainless Steel	TJA components, screws, plates, cabling
Tantalum	TJA components, bone substitute augments
Zr-Nb alloys	TJA bearing surfaces, when oxidized
Polymers	
Poly methyl methacrylate (PMMA)	Bone cement
Ultra-high-molecular-weight polyethylene (UHMWPE)	Low-friction inserts for bearing surfaces in TKA
Ceramics	
Alumina (Al_2O_3)	Bearing surface TJA components
Zirconia (ZrO_2)	Bearing surface TJA components
Hydroxyapatite	Bioactive coatings
Calcium phosphate	Bone defect augmentation

TJA = total joint arthroplasty, TKA = total knee arthroplasty
Reproduced from Ratner BD, Hoffman AS, Schoen FJ, Lemons JE, eds: *Biomaterials Science: An Introduction to Materials in Medicine*. ed 3. Amsterdam, Elsevier/Academic Press, 2013. Table. II.5.6.1

orthopaedic implants are fabricated from a short list of metals, polymers, and ceramics (**Table 1**). All are well characterized and most have decades of successful use.

MECHANICAL BEHAVIOR OF ORTHOPAEDIC BIOMATERIALS

Electromagnetic interactions hold atoms together in ascending order of strength of bonding through van der Waals forces, hydrogen bonding, metallic forces, covalent interactions, and ionic forces. Materials are formed when these forces combine atoms or covalently bound atoms (molecules). How the atoms or molecules are organized and bound will determine their mechanical properties. Atoms are about the scale of 0.2 nm in diameter, molecules range from 1 to 100 nm, and molecules are organized into much larger structures. Structural units at the surface of a material are acted upon by different forces than those inside the material bulk and as such have a surface energy which leads to reactivity and unique properties.

Most orthopaedic implants are used in load-bearing applications, to replace damaged or diseased tissue (eg, joint replacement), or to provide structural support during healing (eg, internal fixation). As such, they must have *structural properties* appropriate for their intended applications. They must be sufficiently strong and have sufficient fatigue resistance to withstand any applied loads, and it is important that their stiffness is tuned to positively influence healing. Compliant implants stimulate bone formation through load sharing and, in the case of fracture fixation, controlled micromotion. Implant structural properties are determined via modeling (eg, finite element analysis), or laboratory testing. There are numerous ASTM standards for implant testing. Testing of unique configurations is routinely reported in the literature.

Implant structural properties are a function of (1) component geometry and (2) the mechanical properties of the material(s) used for fabrication. Component geometry is determined during design, within the anatomic and functional constraints of the application. The mechanical properties of materials are a function of their internal structure—specifically, the atoms and molecules they contain, and how the atoms and molecules are organized at the crystalline and microstructural levels. Material properties are determined empirically; they cannot be predicted analytically.

It is also important to distinguish between the concepts of bulk and surface properties of biomaterials as both are important to the success or failure of the material. Mechanical bulk properties dictate a material's ability to carry loads over multiple cycles over time without deformation or failure. Surface properties of biomaterials will determine interactions between the material and its host environment.

BULK MATERIAL PROPERTIES

Bulk material properties depend on the types of atoms and molecules it contains and also their arrangement, called *microstructure*. Microstructure concerns very small scales of the order 10^{-4} to 10^{-9} m. Bulk properties that depend on the type or composition of the material and not on microstructure are called *intrinsic properties* and include density and heat capacity. Bulk properties that depend on the microstructure of the material are called *extrinsic properties* and include yield strength and stiffness.

LOAD, STRESS, AND STRAIN

When a force or *load* is applied to an object, it can translate (move), rotate, and deform. To quantify material properties and make comparisons between different materials, it is important to standardize the shape and size of materials to be tested. Specifically, to discuss the concepts of stress and strain, we prepare a sample such that the cross section perpendicular to the applied force is the same, such as a cylinder or rectangular prism, and apply a force perpendicular to a pair of opposite faces of this material.

STANDARD BIOMECHANICAL TESTING OF MATERIALS[8-10]

The most widely used tests to characterize material properties are monotonic tensile tests. Monotonic tests provide information about a material's ability to withstand a single maximum applied load. In these tests, force is measured as material specimens are elongated until they break. The specimens are carefully machined to precise diameters and lengths, and the data

©Copyright 2021 American Academy of Orthopaedic Surgeons

are reported in terms of applied force per unit cross-sectional area, or *stress* ($\sigma = F/A_0$), and deformation per unit length, or *strain* ($\varepsilon = (L_f - L_0)/L_0$) (**Figure 1**). Stress-strain plots are important graphical representations of a material's inherent mechanical properties.

Elastic Behavior

Typical stress-strain plots include an initial linear region where stress increases proportionally with strain, followed by a nonlinear region that continues to the point of failure (**Figure 1**). The linear region reflects the fact that at low strains many materials behave elastically, recovering completely when the load is removed. The constant of proportionality, or slope, of the linear elastic region is defined as the *modulus of elasticity*, E ($E = \sigma/\varepsilon$). The modulus of elasticity reflects the stiffness of a material. Materials with a relatively high modulus of elasticity deform less under load than those with a low modulus of elasticity.[11-14]

Materials used as load-bearing implants should have elastic properties similar to the tissue to which they are adjacent. This would prevent differential motion at the interface between dissimilarly elastic materials, which could lead to loosening and failure. It follows then that titanium alloys are particularly good materials for total hip stems, and that poly methyl methacrylate is a useful intermediary between the more stiff cobalt-chromium–bearing surfaces and the adjacent host bone.

Plastic Behavior and Failure

The elastic limit, or *yield point*, marks the transition from elastic to plastic behavior. At the yield point the internal structure of the material begins to rearrange irreversibly, resulting in a permanent residual strain that is not lost on unloading. Closely related to the yield point is the *yield strength*, which is defined as the stress that results in plastic deformation of the material. Beyond the yield point molecular rearrangement results in a generalized decrease in the cross-sectional area along the length of the specimen. Ultimately, the plastic deformation localizes to a small region of the specimen that constricts ("necks") preferentially on the way to failure, and stress decreases with increasing strain. *Tensile strength* reflects the maximum stress a material can withstand before failing, and *breaking strength* is the stress when the material finally breaks catastrophically.

Other important mechanical properties that are reflected in stress-strain curves are *ductility* and *toughness*. Ductility is a material's ability to withstand plastic strain before fracture. Ductility may be reported as elongation at failure, $(L_f - L_0)/L_0$, or reduction in cross-sectional area $(A_0 - A_f)/A_0$ of the necked region. In general, metals and polymers are ductile because they exhibit significant plastic deformation before failure. Ceramics, on the other hand, are brittle because they fracture with little, if any, plastic deformation. Toughness is a measure of the amount of energy required to break a material. Toughness is determined by integrating the area under the load-displacement curve. *Resilience* is the elastic energy stored in a unit volume of stressed material. It represents the area under the stress-strain curve extending from zero strain to the strain at which the yield point is reached. *Hardness* is determined by deformation on a material surface caused by a small indenter tip under a constant load over a certain period of time. Hardness is measured on a relative scale and increases as the relative deformation decreases.

Fatigue

The stresses a material can withstand under cyclic loading are much less than the yield or ultimate strengths determined via monotonic tensile testing. This is important because implants

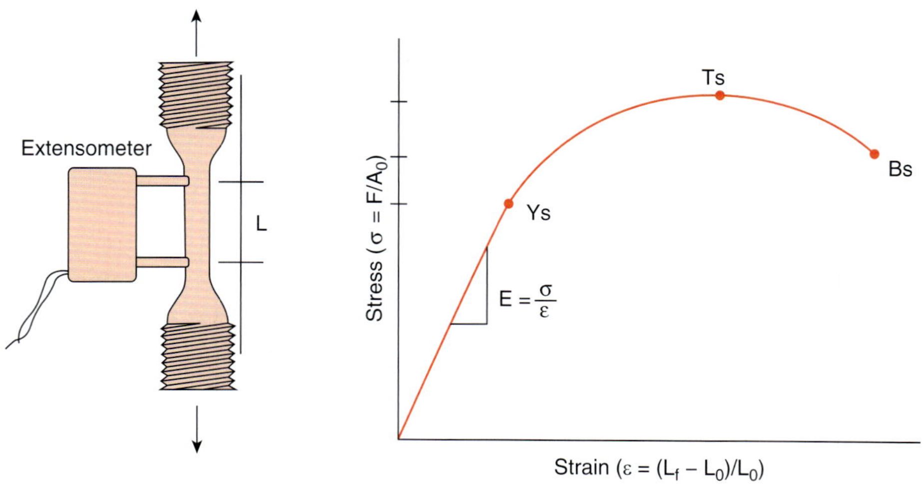

FIGURE 1 Schematic of tensile test. Samples machined to precise diameters and lengths (L_0) are loaded to failure in tension and the data are reported in terms of applied force per unit cross-sectional area, or *stress* ($\sigma = F/A_0$), and deformation per unit length, or *strain* ($\varepsilon = (L_f - L_0)/L_0$). Typical stress-strain plots include an initial linear region where stress increases proportionally with strain. The slope of the linear elastic region is defined as the *modulus of elasticity*, E ($E = \sigma/\varepsilon$). The *yield strength* (YS) reflects the stress that results in plastic deformation of the material. The *tensile strength* (TS) is the maximum stress the material can withstand before failing, and the *breaking strength* (BS) is the stress when the material finally fails catastrophically.

©Copyright 2021 American Academy of Orthopaedic Surgeons

routinely experience cyclic loading, especially weight-bearing implants in the lower extremity and spine. *Fracture toughness* measures the ability of a material to resist crack propagation. Fatigue failure occurs by crack propagation, driven by locally high stresses at the crack tip with each loading cycle. The cracks usually start at surface irregularities where bending or torsion leads to high tensile stresses, and catastrophic failure occurs when the cross-sectional area is reduced below the ability to carry the applied load. In general, the number of cycles to failure is inversely proportional to the applied stress.

The ability of a material to withstand fatigue is determined by cyclically loading specimens to different levels of maximum stress (S) and recording the number of cycles to failure (N). Plotted logarithmically, S-N has an inverse sigmoid shape (**Figure 2**). Specimens fail quickly when the cyclic stress is between the tensile strength and yield strength (*low cycle fatigue*), and after increasingly more cycles as the stress is reduced below the yield strength (*high cycle fatigue*). In many materials there is a lower limit of cyclic stress that will cause fatigue failure. The stress corresponding to this lower limit is called the *endurance limit*, or *fatigue limit*.

The rate of the applied strain also affects mechanical properties. Over a long period of time, a constantly applied stress below yield strength can cause deformation called *creep*.

Isotropy and Anisotropy

Materials are classified as being isotropic or anisotropic depending on whether their mechanical properties are directionally dependent. Isotropic materials have the same material properties in all directions, whereas in anisotropic materials, material properties vary by the direction of loading. In their raw forms, the metals, plastics, and ceramics used in orthopaedic implants are isotropic. However, in practice many are anisotropic. Anisotropy can be introduced into implant materials during manufacturing (eg, forging of metals, or extrusion of UHMWE). Allografts are anisotropic, a reflection of their complex hierarchically organized structure.

Failure Criteria

Most orthopaedic implants are designed using computers and analyzed numerically (ie, finite element analysis, FEA) before being fabricated, tested, and placed into service. Material properties obtained from laboratory tests are used as model inputs, and anticipated loads are used as boundary conditions. FEA models return predicted implant stresses during use. Because implants need to maintain their shape during use and withstand repeated loading, design stresses are held below the yield stress and endurance limit, depending on the application.

Biomaterials and implant standards are set by ASTM Committee F04 on Medical and Surgical Materials and Devices. Material standards describe the chemical, mechanical, and metallurgical properties of the raw materials used in fabrication, while device standards define requirements for implant performance in specified laboratory testing conditions.

SURFACE PROPERTIES

Atoms and molecules at the surface of a biomaterial have important particular properties to consider as they will be the interface between material and host. An important question in biocompatibility is how the material influences the response of the host cells and extracellular matrix. Material properties, surface geometry, and local chemistry will all affect host response and incorporation or alternatively failure of the material. Prevention of contamination of a surface is also a concern when we are aiming for a specific host response, whether that be from a biological (bacterial for instance) or chemical (oxidation) process. Contamination or alteration of a material can occur because of contact with packaging, exposure to sterilization methods, from the environment, and from the host.

Properties of surfaces of importance to biomaterials include roughness, morphology, wettability, surface mobility, chemical composition, electrical charge, crystallinity, and modulus.

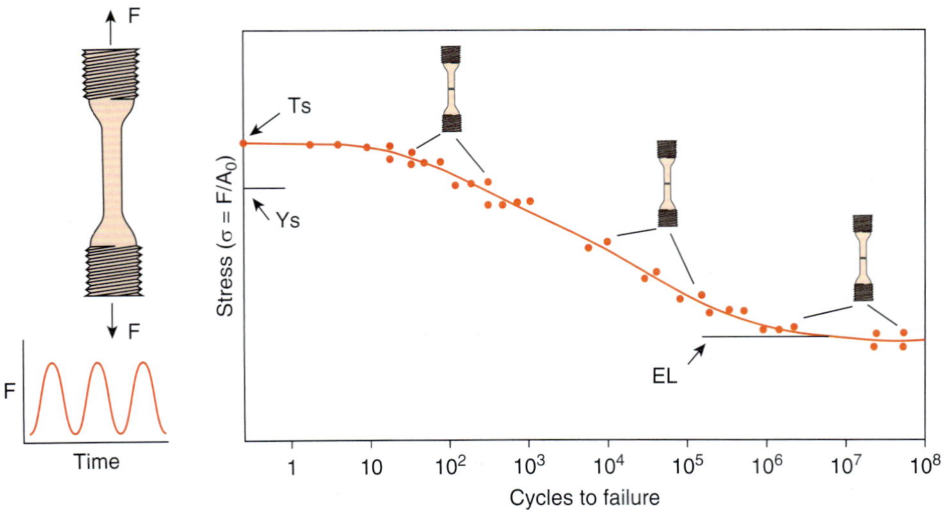

FIGURE 2 Schematic of fatigue test. Carefully machined specimens are cyclically loaded to different levels of maximum *stress* ($\sigma = F/A_0$) and the number of cycles to failure (N) is recorded. Specimens fail quickly when the cyclic stress is high, and after more cycles when the cyclic stress is low. In many materials there is a lower limit of cyclic stress that will cause fatigue failure. This lower limit is called the endurance limit (EL), or fatigue limit. TS = *tensile strength* (TS), YS = *yield strength* (YS).

©Copyright 2021 American Academy of Orthopaedic Surgeons

Tests to evaluate material surfaces include scanning electron microscopy to test morphology and electron spectroscopy to determine chemical analysis.

WEAR AND CORROSION

Wear is defined as the removal of surface material by mechanical motion. Wear is caused by friction, motion, and loading of an interface between materials. Lubrication mechanisms act to reduce friction and wear. There are three main types of wear: abrasive, adhesive, and third-body wear. Abrasive wear occurs when a rougher, harder surface moves against a softer surface, generating particulate debris from the softer surface. Adhesive wear results between two moving objects in contact whereby a thin layer of material is transferred from one surface to another. Wear occurs in the material which donates the film. Third-body wear results when an additional particle is present between the two main bearing surfaces, leading to friction and loss of material at the contact surface.

Corrosion occurs between metal surfaces as a combination of mechanical and chemical reactions.[15] Galvanic corrosion occurs at the interface of two dissimilar metals creating an electric potential. Fretting occurs because of micromotion at the interface of two metals, disrupting the passivation layer. Crevice corrosion involves the development of microscopic cracks, which creates a microenvironment that disrupts the passivation layer. Pitting corrosion occurs because of small surface defects in the passivation layer. Intergranular corrosion occurs at the interface of grain boundaries where carbides may be present.[16,17]

METALS

GENERAL STRUCTURE OF ORTHOPAEDIC METALS AND ALLOYS

Metal alloys are the most frequently used biomaterials in orthopaedic surgery, because of their high strength and load-bearing capacity. Alloys are metals in which additional elements are admixed with a base metal. The quantities of the alloying elements are tightly controlled to optimize material properties and biocompatibility. Mixing is performed by melting the combined elements together under controlled conditions.

At the atomic level, solid metals form densely packed crystalline lattices in which individual atoms are bonded together by the shared cloud, or sea, of delocalized free valence electrons. The most common lattice packing arrangements in metals are body-centered cubic (BCC), face-centered cubic (FCC), and hexagonal close-packed (HCP) (**Figure 3**).

At the microscopic level, metals are composed of small crystals, called grains. As molten metal is cooled, individual, randomly oriented grains nucleate and grow until they encounter neighboring grains. Depending on the solubility of the alloying elements, neighboring grains may have different elemental compositions and different crystal structures, or *phases*. The interfaces between adjacent grains are called grain boundaries. The material properties of metals are determined by their atomic and microscopic structures. Metallic bonding confers strength and hardness, as well as malleability and ductility. The microstructure (crystalline structure and grain size) influences most mechanical properties. In general, stiffness, yield strength, tensile strength, and fatigue strength all increase with decreasing grain size.

Implant alloys are initially manufactured as raw castings (ingots). Most implants are processed to near-final implant form by casting or forging, and then finished by machining (**Figure 4**). Casting involves remelting the alloy, pouring it into a mold, and cooling it under controlled conditions. During forging, a solid blank (cast ingot, bar, or rod) is heated until it is malleable and then it is shaped to final form by compression in a progressive series of dies. Hot forging results in metal that is stronger than cast or machined metal parts. Other, less common fabrication methods include powdered metallurgy, where powdered alloy is fused by sintering in heated dies, computer-controlled machining, or mechanical forming by rolling, drawing, or extrusion. The choice of fabrication method depends on the shape and complexity of the implant, characteristics of the alloy being used, intended use of the implant, and cost.

Manufacturing processes influence implant structural properties by altering the microstructure of the alloy. During casting, the rate of cooling can be used to control grain size, to a degree, because grain growth is a function of time and temperature. More rapid cooling yields a finer grain size, whereas slower cooling yields larger grains. During forging, the individual grains are distorted in the direction of the metal flow or plastic deformation, conforming to the shape of the implant as it is progressively shaped. The microstructural changes associated with forging increase tensile strength, yield strength, fatigue strength, and ductility. Final profile shaping is done via numerically controlled machining and/or abrasive grinding.

Once an implant is fabricated, heat treatment may be used to alter the mechanical properties of the alloy. The forming of implants can introduce residual stresses and work hardening. These can be relieved by *annealing*, which involves heating the part above the recrystallization temperature for a set period of time, followed by cooling at a controlled rate. Annealing increases ductility and reduces hardness. Raw castings typically contain internal voids and microporosity, which reduce fatigue resistance. Casting quality can be improved by a process called *hot isostatic pressing*, which involves simultaneous heating and pressurization with an inert gas in a high-pressure containment vessel. Hot isostatic pressing consolidates the casting by solid state diffusion.[18]

After bulk processing, several techniques are used for surface finishing. Nitriding and ion implantation are used to harden the load-bearing surface of stainless steel and titanium implants to increase wear resistance. Nitriding involves the exposure to a nitrogen-rich gas (eg, ammonia) at elevated temperatures.[19,20]

©Copyright 2021 American Academy of Orthopaedic Surgeons

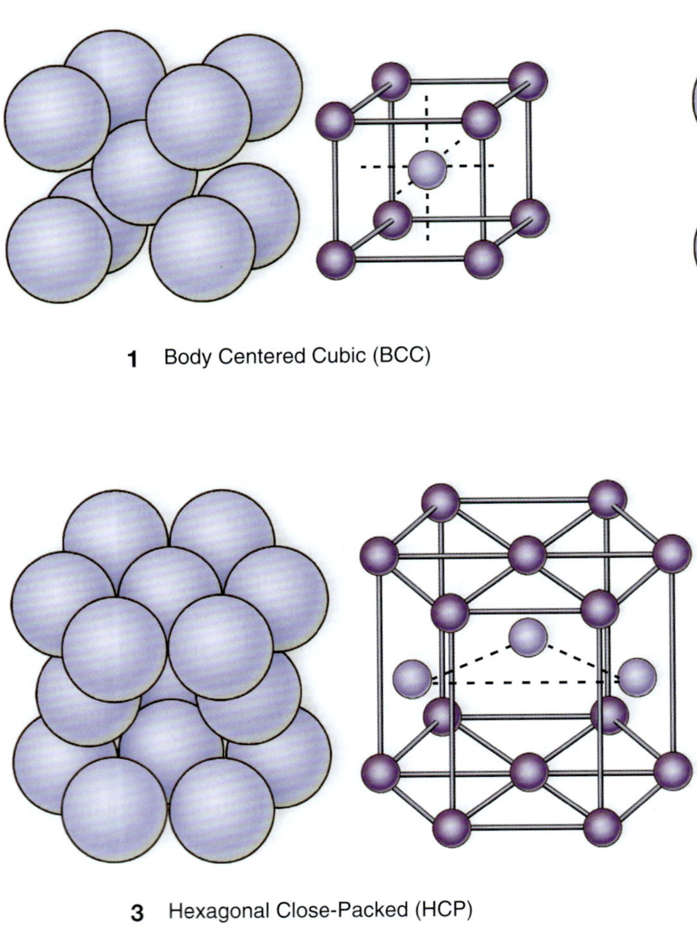

FIGURE 3 Illustration showing three most common crystal structures found in orthopaedic alloys: (**A**) body-centered cubic (BCC), (**B**) face-centered cubic (FCC), and (**C**) hexagonal close-packed (HCP). (Redrawn with permission from Gibbs K. The Structure of Solids. School Physics. http://www.schoolphysics.org/age16-19/properties%20of%20matter/elasticity/text/Structure_of_solids/index.html. Accessed August 13, 2019.)

The dissociated nitrogen diffuses into the surface of the part and bonds with the base metals to yield thin layers or iron or titanium nitride. Grind lines, scratches, and pits are removed by polishing with engineered abrasives. Articulating surfaces are buffed to a final mirror-like finish by a rotating cloth wheel that is impregnated with fine abrasive compounds.

The alloys used in orthopaedic implants spontaneously form metal oxide films in their surfaces that protect the underlying metal from further oxidative damage. However, these films are thin and may be porous. Accordingly, all metallic implants are passivated by acid treatment to form a thicker, more mechanically robust oxide layer.

STAINLESS STEEL

Stainless steel is the most commonly used orthopaedic implant metal and has the advantage of being relatively resistant to corrosion. Similar to traditional carbon steels, stainless steels are alloys of iron and carbon, but differ in that they contain significant amounts of chromium (17% to 20%), nickel (10% to 17%), and molybdenum (2% to 4%) as well as smaller amounts of manganese, sulfur, silicon, and phosphorus (2% to 8%). The carbon content of medical-grade stainless steel is usually low. Most stainless steels used in orthopaedics have an FCC microstructure. Common alloys include 316 L and 316LVM (L refers to low carbon content, and VM refers to vacuum melt). Annealed stainless steel and 30% cold worked stainless steel (ASTM F138 and F139) are the two manufactured forms of forged stainless steel most commonly used in orthopaedics. Processing of these stainless steels usually involves a passivation step with acid treatment to produce a surface oxide layer. Stainless steel is commonly used in fracture plates, pins, screws, cables, and wires.

COBALT-CHROMIUM ALLOYS

Cobalt-chromium (Co-Cr) is a commonly used metal in arthroplasty surgery, specifically cobalt-chromium-molybdenum (Co-Cr-Mo). Co-Cr has low ductility and is difficult to machine, but it is relatively cost-effective and easy

 ©Copyright 2021 American Academy of Orthopaedic Surgeons

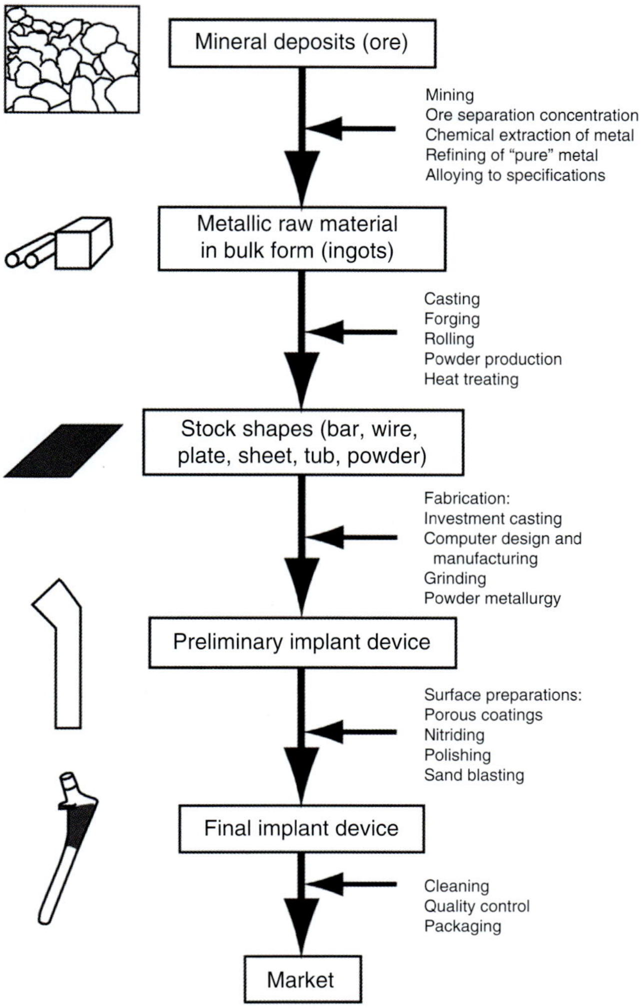

FIGURE 4 Schematic diagram depicting stages in processing of metal alloys into orthopaedic implants. (Adapted with permission from Ratner BD, Hoffman AS, Schoen FJ, Lemons JE, eds: *Biomaterials Science: An Introduction to Materials in Medicine*, ed 2. San Diego, CA, Academic Press, 2004, p 138.)

to manufacture into a complex shape using investment casting. Porosity can be reduced by hot isostatic pressing. Warm or hot forging of Co-Cr-Mo billets results in a wrought product (ASTM F799) with greater fatigue strength, yield strength, and ultimate tensile strength than the cast alloy. Co-Cr alloys are well suited for use as an ingrowth or ongrowth surfaces and had historically significant use in the PCA and AML hip arthroplasty stems, but the material's stiffness (high elastic modulus) led to end of stem pain and stress shielding issues.[21] The wear properties of Co-Cr alloys are superior to those of stainless steel or titanium alloys and therefore are commonly used in the manufacture of modular femoral heads.

TITANIUM AND TITANIUM ALLOYS

Titanium and titanium alloys have reduced elastic modulus (100 to 110 GPa) compared with Co-Cr alloys (200 to 220 GPa) as well as excellent biocompatibility and increased resistance to corrosion. Both commercially pure (CP) titanium and titanium alloys are available for use in orthopaedic applications. The most commonly used titanium alloy in orthopaedics combines titanium with 6% aluminum and 4% vanadium and is abbreviated as Ti6Al4V. The excellent biocompatibility of titanium and its alloys is largely due to the rapid formation of a stable surface oxide layer because of passivation. CP titanium is used as a porous bone ingrowth or ongrowth surface which can be deposited by plasma spray.[22,23] The surface finish produced by plasma spray is rough, which facilitates an initial press fit and eventual osseointegration as bone grows onto the microasperities. Three-dimensional porous forms of CP titanium are approved by the FDA for use as porous metal bone substitutes and bone ingrowth implant coatings. The wear properties of Ti6Al4V are inferior to those of Co-Cr alloys. Because of this, titanium and titanium alloys are not commonly used as bearings but are commonly used as hip arthroplasty stems and sockets and tibial components in total knee implants. Oftentimes titanium alloy hip stems are coupled with cobalt-chromium femoral heads using a modular taper junction, which can lead to corrosion at the interfaces due to mechanically assisted crevice corrosion. Bead forms of Ti6Al4V can be sintered onto other metals to form a bone ingrowth fixation surface. Beta-titanium alloys were developed to produce a less stiff hip stem, in an effort to improve rates of ingrowth, and decrease end of stem pain, which had been reported with the use of stiffer hip stem designs. One such of these beta-titanium alloys is TMZF (Ti-12Mo-6Zr-2Fe), a proprietary Stryker product introduced in 2002, which has shown successful bone ingrowth, but also some concerning reports of failure at the stem trunnion–head bore interface.

ZIRCONIUM-NIOBIUM ALLOYS

Zirconium-Niobium Alloys (Zr-Nb) have been developed for use in arthroplasty bearing surfaces. Although the base metal is relatively soft compared with other metals used in the production of orthopaedic implants, processing of the Zr-Nb by oxidation in high-temperature air transforms the surface to a stable, durable, low-friction oxide ceramic. Processing Zr-2.5Nb alloy in this way produces the Smith & Nephew product Oxinium with a nominally 5-micrometer-thick oxide surface. This material has very low reported rates of fracture and trunnion-related femoral head failure; however, failure has been reported because of other mechanisms, such as when surface oxidation is damaged and the underlying softer alloy is exposed to articular wear.

TANTALUM

Tantalum is a rare earth element that has a modulus of elasticity that closely approximates bone. It is biocompatible, forming surface oxides as a barrier to corrosion. Tantalum is most often used as a three-dimensional porous bone substitute and ingrowth surface for primary and revision arthroplasties.[24]

©Copyright 2021 American Academy of Orthopaedic Surgeons

POLYMERS

Polymers are the largest class of materials used in medicine in general and consist of repeating patterns of atomic units. Polymer molecules have high molecular weight and can be organized into different structures which will affect their function. Common morphologies of polymers include a linear chain, which can be modified to include sequences of different polymers. Branched structures also exist, where a central polymer chain has smaller side chains extending from it. More complex structures are also possible whereby cross-links between chains are formed to make a network polymer.

Polymers exhibit areas of random organization of chains called "amorphous regions" and areas of more organized chains called "crystalline regions." Crystalline regions stiffen and reinforce the bulk material. Adjacent polymer chains are bound by relatively weak attractive forces such as dipole-dipole interactions, hydrogen bonding, and London forces. Cross-linking, crystallinity, and copolymerization affect the physical behavior of polymers.

POLY METHYL METHACRYLATE BONE CEMENT

Poly methyl methacrylate (PMMA) bone cement is a room-temperature polymerizing material that is mixed at the time of use to produce a viscous liquid which can be worked and molded before hardening into a solid after a period of time to cure. PMMA bone cement is used as a grout to secure arthroplasty components to bone, stabilize fractures of the spine, and fill defects in bone.[25,26] Commercial PMMA bone cement is available for use in the operating room as powder and liquid components which are mixed at the time of use. The powder consists of beads of PMMA or methyl methacrylate-styrene copolymer; barium sulfate or zirconium dioxide as a radiopacifier; and benzoyl peroxide as a chemical initiator. The liquid component is primarily methyl methacrylate monomer and N,N dimethyl-p-toluidine, which accelerates the polymerization process when the liquid and powder are mixed. Also included in the liquid component is hydroquinone which acts as a stabilizer and prevents premature polymerization from heat or light during storage.

The polymerization of PMMA cement is an exothermic reaction whereby double carbon bonds of the methyl methacrylate monomer are broken so they can bond to the rapidly elongating polymer chain. This process can increase the temperature of the cement to more than 100°C, which is hot enough to potentially burn a patient or tissues.[27] Heat produced varies with mass of cement and ability of adjacent materials to dissipate the heat. Because the cement mantle used in joint replacement is typically thin and adjacent structures act as a heat sink, temperatures would rarely be high enough for thermal necrosis. However, when used to fill cavitary defects such as those left from tumor excision, the mass of cement may be large enough to produce temperatures sufficient to cause adjacent cell damage, which may have the benefit of reduction of any residual tumor cells remaining in the cavity.

Handling characteristics of PMMA bone cement vary with time from mix and across manufacturer's products. Viscosity is a measure of resistance to shear stress. Low-viscosity cements flow easily after mixing and high-viscosity cements are much more doughy. The working curve of a bone cement illustrates how its handling characteristics (viscosity) change over time and with temperature. Cements polymerize more quickly if they are mixed at a higher temperature or at higher humidity. The surgical art of the application of cement involves its use at an optimal viscosity to interlock well with trabecular bone.[28] Polymerization decreases cement volume by about 7% as it sets into a solid from a liquid, which can introduce defects into a cement mantle and potentially create an area of weakness.[29,30] Mixing cement in a vacuum removes entrapped air before use and so can decrease porosity of the final product, which decreases defects which may be a nidus for fracture propagation.[31] Fracturing of cement may be most likely to occur at sharp corners of an implant, pores in the cement mantle, or irregularities at the cement-bone interface. PMMA strength is weaker in tension (25 to 45 MPa) than in compression (85 to 110 MPa), and it has a fatigue strength of approximately 10 MPa.

PMMA bone cements can be modified according to their intended use.[32,33] Cements used in vertebral augmentation are prepared with increased radiopacifier to improve visualization, and reaction chemistry is modified to increase working time to allow injection into the spine. As an example, Simplex P (Stryker Orthopaedics) bone cement used in hip and knee arthroplasty has a working time of 3 minutes at 22°C, whereas KyphX (Medtronic Spine LLC) has a working time of 8 minutes.

ULTRA-HIGH-MOLECULAR-WEIGHT POLYETHYLENE

Ultra-high-molecular-weight polyethylene (UHMWPE) is commonly used in the bearings of total joint arthroplasties coupled with cobalt-chromium or ceramic. Sir John Charnley first used UHMWPE in the bearing of his low-friction hip arthroplasty[34] and it continues to be used though modified over the years since its first use to improve longevity and decrease wear.[35] UHMWPE has a low sliding friction, high material toughness, and high resistance to wear and is biologically inert in bulk form.[36-39]

UHMWPE is composed of very long chains of polyethylene ([C2H4]n) with degree of polymerization (n) between 71,000 (molecular weight of 2 million g/mol) and 214,000 (molecular weight of 6 million g/mol).[40] In comparison, high-density polyethylene (HDPE) has a molecular weight of about 500,000 g/mol. Mechanical properties of impact strength and wear resistance are dramatically improved with the extension of molecular chain length from HDPE to UHMWPE.

©Copyright 2021 American Academy of Orthopaedic Surgeons

UHMWPE is a linear, nonbranching polymer which consists of crystalline and amorphous phases. The crystalline phase is formed by repeated folding of the polymer chain upon itself to create highly oriented layers. The amorphous phase consists of tangled, randomly oriented chain segments. UHMWPE with higher crystallinity is generally superior in characteristics of use as it will have increased yield strength and resistance to fatigue crack propagation.[41]

Processing, sterilization, and packaging affect the two phases of UHMWPE which, in turn, affect material properties and mechanical performance.[42] UHMWPE is processed into the final implant part through multiple steps. This begins with resin powder which is formed into larger rods, sheets, or a molded shape by pressure applied with heat. Ram bar extrusion of the resin powder through a heated die can produce a rod, compression molding by heated platens can produce sheets of material, and direct compression molding can produce a nearly completed part. Rods and sheets are further machined into final dimensions of the implant to specific tolerances.

Sterilization and cross-linking of UHMWPE can affect its longevity and mechanical properties.[43-45] It was found in the 1980s and 1990s that sterilization by exposure to gamma radiation in air led to a decrease in mechanical properties and effective life of the material. The high-energy radiation in air altered the structure of the UHMWPE to produce free radicals which became active in the process of oxidative degradation and led to failure.[46-49] Since that time, manufacturers have altered their sterilization process such that it occurs in an inert gas or vacuum rather than air to decrease oxidation and chain scission after the production of free radicals.[50] Packaging has also been improved to prevent oxidative degradation and increase shelf life of implants. Exposure to high-energy gamma radiation did have the positive effect of forming chain cross-linkages, which improved mechanical properties of the material. To further decrease the concentration of reactive free radicals after irradiation, the additional processing improvements of annealing and remelting were introduced to allow unpaired electrons to find a mate and form a bond and prevent chain scission. Annealing is a process whereby irradiated UHMWPE is heated to just below its melt temperature, and remelting is a process whereby irradiated UHMWPE is heated above the melt temperature. Annealing slightly increases crystallinity, but is not as effective in quenching free radicals and preventing future oxidative damage. Remelting decreases crystallinity but more effectively quenches free radicals.

Wear rates of highly cross-linked UHMWPE acetabular components treated with annealing or remelting (first generation) have been shown to be superior to conventional polyethylenes, with radiographic femoral head penetration rates below the threshold of osteolysis (0.1 mm per year).[51-55] A second-generation of highly cross-linked UHMWPE has been developed to reduce free radicals further and improve mechanical properties, with process modifications including sequential annealing, and addition of antioxidants such as vitamin E.[56]

RESORBABLE POLYMERS

Resorbable polymers are made to degrade in vivo over time, which is particularly useful for devices that are only needed for a short period of time. This property is particularly useful for sutures and suture anchors which may only be needed during the initial healing process. After healing, the strength of the fixation would transition to biologic tissue and the polymer would degrade to prevent any untoward consequence such as becoming a source of pain or a surface for adherence of bacteria, leading to a local infection. The most commonly used resorbable copolymers are polyglycolic acid, polylactic acid, and derivatives. Both of these substances degrade by hydrolysis over time to their monomers. Mechanical properties and degradative times vary depending on the formulation and range from 2 to 7 GPa elastic modulus and 1 to 24 months resorption time.[57]

CERAMICS

Ceramics consist of a complex organized structure of metallic and nonmetallic elements held together with ionic and covalent bonds. In orthopaedics, ceramics such as alumina (dense aluminum oxide) and zirconia (zirconium oxide) are used in the manufacture of bearings used in hip replacements, and ceramics such as hydroxyapatite are used as surface coatings to promote fixation of implants to bone. Ceramics are hard substances that have excellent compressive strength. They have a high melting point and are nonductile (brittle). Most ceramics have a grain microstructure which can be made to vary with processing to alter mechanical properties.

Dense inert ceramic implants such as femoral heads are manufactured by molding a mixture of fine powder and water with a binder into a desired shape. The mold is heated which burns off the binder and evaporates the water, and further sintered at high temperature (about 1,600°C) to fuse the particles together. The strength of dense inert ceramics varies inversely with grain size and porosity. Thin-film bioactive ceramics such as a hydroxyapatite coating are produced by plasma spray or solution deposition. In the process of plasma spray, powdered ceramic is heated in gas plasma and then a mist of molten ceramic is then sprayed onto another material such as a titanium alloy hip arthroplasty stem. An advantage of plasma spray is that it can be uniformly applied to complex shaped parts.

INERT CERAMICS

Alumina has excellent biocompatibility and a very low coefficient of friction when coupled with UHMWPE in a bearing.[58] Alumina has a high wettability, and so lubrication is improved and friction decreased. These properties make alumina an ideal material for the manufacture of femoral heads. Fracture

©Copyright 2021 American Academy of Orthopaedic Surgeons

toughness was a concern for early iterations of alumina ceramic femoral heads, but improvements in manufacture of the heads and the trunnions of stems have decreased catastrophic failures.[59] Alumina can also be mated with alumina in hip prosthetic bearings with a potentially extremely low wear rate. However, sound production from the articulation (squeaking) likely due to variations in component position and loss of fluid film lubrication can be bothersome to patients.[60-62]

Zirconia can be used to produce femoral heads for hip replacements with potential advantages over alumina as being stronger and denser and more highly polished, though fracture toughness is also a concern.[63-65] Newer formulations of mixed alumina and zirconia have had excellent results. Zirconia-toughened alumina (Biolox Delta) has been shown to have greater strength and fracture toughness than either alumina or zirconia alone.[66]

BIOACTIVE CERAMICS

Bioactive ceramics are biocompatible, inducing osseointegration and extremely strong bonding to bone. Calcium phosphate-based coatings such as hydroxyapatite and beta-tricalcium phosphate are the most widely used in orthopaedic applications, most often in noncemented total hip arthroplasty. Hydroxyapatite (Ca10[PO4]6[OH]2) is the main inorganic component of naturally occurring bone.[67] Initially used in dentistry, hydroxyapatite has been adapted for wide use in orthopaedic applications.[67,68] Over time, the bioactive ceramic coating is absorbed and replaced with new bone over a course of weeks to years, depending on the formulation and processing of the coating.[69-71]

COMPOSITES

Composite materials are composed of two or more separate substances. The term composite as it applies to biomaterials usually refers to a material consisting of constituents in the nano to macro size range, each having a distinct interface separating them. Usually these composites include one or more discontinuous phases embedded in a continuous phase. Because the discontinuous phase is usually harder and stronger than the continuous phase, it is called the reinforcing material, and the continuous phase is called the matrix. Reinforcement materials and phases can be varied depending on the desired performance and application, optimizing hardness, strength, toughness, or bioactivity. Properties of the composite depend on the properties of the constituent materials, their distribution, and interface and interphase interactions between them. A hydroxyapatite coating on a titanium alloy hip stem can add a bioactive ingrowth phase to the device conferring desired bioactivity to the implant. Fused monoblock acetabular components consisting of a porous tantalum ingrowth shell welded to a polyethylene bearing are another example of a composite biomaterial implant. Other composite designs for implants have been conceived and produced with less optimal results, including carbon fiber–reinforced polyethylenes briefly used in total knee arthroplasty bearing surfaces which were subject to early failure due to less desirable mechanical properties than standard polyethylenes in use at the time.

CLINICAL ENGINEERING CASE STUDY: HIP STEM TRUNNION CORROSION AND FAILURE

The morse taper was invented by Stephen A. Morse in 1864 as a way to join large machine parts during the industrial revolution in southern Massachusetts. The design involves mating together a truncated cone called a trunnion into a conical cavity called a bore. The taper of these parts is machined to produce an interference fit. In the 1980s the morse taper was adapted for use in orthopaedics in the manufacture of hip stems to allow modularity because most hip stems at the time were a one-unit stem and head (monoblock). Modular heads are useful to the surgeon for many reasons. For example, the transition from cemented to press fit stems results in more variation in final stem position so that intraoperative modification of neck length and offset is necessary to produce optimal hip mechanics and stability. Modular head neck junctions have since become the standard in hip replacement implants, though this has also introduced another level of complexity in the hip replacement biomaterial system. The femoral head is manufactured with a bore and is impacted onto the trunnion on the hip stem to obtain mechanical locking of the parts due to frictional forces generated by the interference fit. The security of the interference fit depends on the contact length, taper angle, surface finish, material properties of the head and the stem, the diameter of the femoral head, impaction force, and presence of contaminants at the taper junction.

CASE STUDY

A 62-year-old male patient with history of bilateral THA at an outside institution presents to a tertiary referral hospital without a preceding traumatic event, limp, weakness, or chronic pain with sudden inability to bear weight on the right lower extremity. He reports hearing some "clicking" in his hip in the preceding week. Radiographs revealed intraprosthetic dissociation of his right noncemented total hip replacement (**Figure 5**, A). Record retrieval from index surgeries showed bilateral TMZF hip stems. Infection screening tests were of low suspicion and so patient was brought to the operating room for hip stem revision and the implant was sent to laboratory for analysis (**Figure 5**, B). A metal-filled pseudotumor was found and débrided at the time of surgery.

 ©Copyright 2021 American Academy of Orthopaedic Surgeons

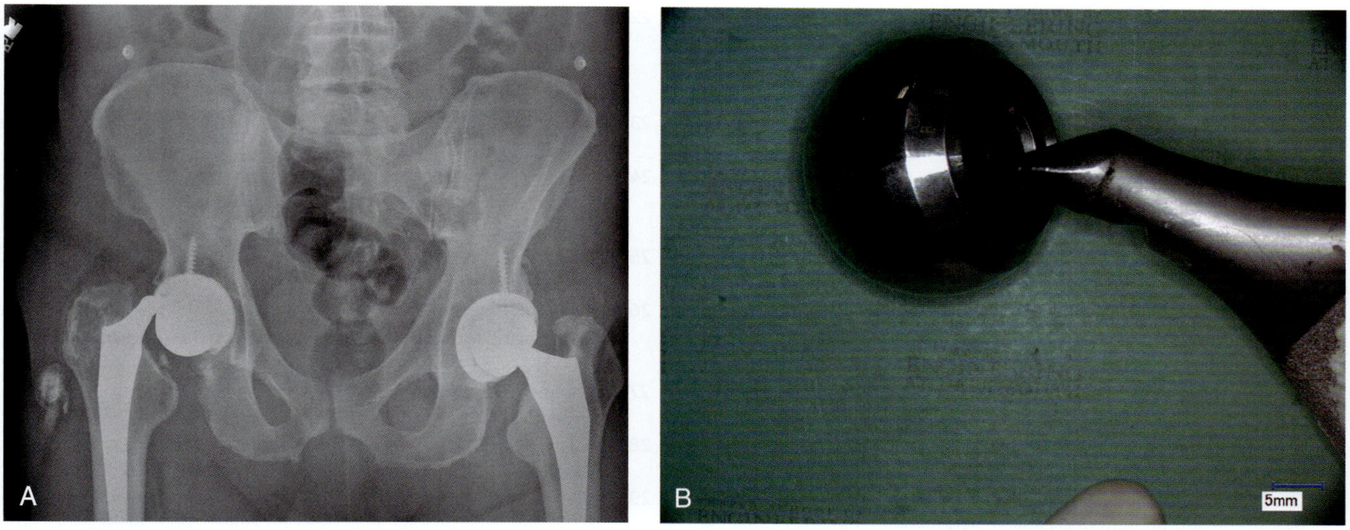

FIGURE 5 **A**, AP radiograph showing right noncemented total hip replacement with intraprosthetic dissociation. **B**, Photograph of gross retrieval hip stem specimen demonstrating a catastrophic gross trunnion failure.

Geometries of hip stem tapers vary significantly between manufacturers and implant design, with different lengths, taper angles, contact areas, and surface finishes. Most hip stems are produced from titanium alloys, the most common being Ti6Al4V alloys. A less stiff novel titanium alloy, Ti-12Mo-6Zr-2Fe was developed in the the early 2000s by a manufacturer with the potential benefit of more closely reproducing the modulus of elasticity of cortical bone. Although ingrowth rates of this stem were satisfactory, there have been cases reported of catastrophic trunnion failure such as illustrated in the above case study. In addition, the trunnion geometry of this implant is shorter and of smaller diameter compared with other trunnion designs. The manufacturer in 2016 issued a recall of a certain proportion of their Co-Cr 36 and larger diameter heads with higher neck lengths (+4 and above) reporting a potential manufacturing irregularity with the bores.[72]

This biomaterial system failure illustrates many of the important preclinical topics reviewed in this chapter. The material of the hip stem involved in failure was less stiff (lower young's modulus) compared with standard titanium alloy stems and the stiff Co-Cr heads, and the surface interface of the taper failed because of fretting and corrosion.[73,74] This process of trunnion failure is described as being mostly due to what has been termed mechanically assisted crevice corrosion.[75] In this case of gross trunnion failure, abrasive wear after the interference fit had been compromised led to loss of material from the trunnion and dissociation at the head-neck junction. Failures such as shown above have been reported less commonly with smaller diameter heads and ceramic heads. This particular stem design was replaced with an updated version in 2012 which is made from a Ti6Al4V alloy.

SUMMARY

The orthopaedic surgeon employs a wide armamentarium of surgical instruments, devices, and implants. The production of these requires the processing and manufacturing of biomaterials including metals, polymers, and ceramics. Material composition, structure, and manufacture will determine the mechanical properties of the material and its biocompatibility. The field of orthopaedic biomaterials is continually changing, and even those materials which have been used for years are being modified and updated to optimize their performance. As new materials and iterations of more familiar materials are produced, it is the responsibility of the surgeon to determine the potential risk and benefit of incorporating new technologies into patient care.

Our case study illustrates how materials engineering–related issues can impact orthopaedic practice; it is important for the orthopaedic surgeon to have an understanding of these disciplines to provide the best care to our patients. As we make our myriad of daily clinical decisions in practice regarding the implants we use and how we couple them together, we need to rely on our understanding of the properties of these materials and their potential interactions over time to guide our judgment. Thoughtful decisions guided by engineering and surgical principles will help us as surgeons toward our goal of the best long-term outcomes for our patients.

©Copyright 2021 American Academy of Orthopaedic Surgeons

REFERENCES

1. Von Recum A, Jacobi JE, eds: *Handbook of Biomaterials Evaluation: Scientific, Technical, and Clinical Testing of Implant Materials*, ed 2. Philadelphia, PA, Taylor & Francis, 1999.
2. Buckwalter JA, Einhorn TA, O'Keefe RJ, American Academy of Orthopaedic Surgeons: *Orthopaedic Basic Science: Foundations of Clinical Practice.* Rosemont, IL, American Academy of Orthopaedic Surgeons, 2007.
3. Ratner BD, Hoffman AS, Schoen FJ, Lemons JE, eds: *Biomaterials Science: An Introduction to Materials in Medicine*, ed 3. Amsterdam, Elsevier/Academic Press, 2013.
4. Skinner: *Current Diagnosis and Treatment in Orthopedics.* Appleton & Lange, 1999.
5. O'Keefe RJ, Jacobs JJ, Chu CR, Einhorn TA: *Orthopaedic Basic Science: Foundations of Clinical Practice.* Rosemont, IL, American Academy of Orthopaedic Surgeons, 2013.
6. Gibon E, Amanatullah DF, Loi F, et al: The biological response to orthopaedic implants for joint replacement: Part I: Metals. *J Biomed Mater Res B Appl Biomater* 2017;105(7):2162-2173.
7. Gibon E, Córdova LA, Lu L, et al: The biological response to orthopedic implants for joint replacement. II: Polyethylene, ceramics, PMMA, and the foreign body reaction. *J Biomed Mater Res B Appl Biomater* 2017;105(6):1685-1691.
8. Mow VC, Huiskes R, eds: *Basic Orthopaedic Biomechanics & Mechano-Biology*, ed 3. Philadelphia, Lippincott, Williams & Wilkins, 2005.
9. Murphy W, Black J, Hastings GW: *Handbook of Biomaterial Properties.* New York, Springer-Verlag,2016.
10. Ong KL, Lovald S, Black J: *Orthopaedic Biomaterials in Research and Practice.* CRC Press, 2014.
11. Bartel DL, Davy DT, Keaveny TM: *Orthopaedic Biomechanics: Mechanics and Design in Musculoskeletal Systems.* Upper Saddle River, NJ, Pearson/Prentice Hall, 2006.
12. Lewis G: Properties of acrylic bone cement: State of the art review. *J Biomed Mater Res* 1997;38(2):155-182.
13. Lewis G: Percutaneous vertebroplasty and kyphoplasty for the stand-alone augmentation of osteoporosis-induced vertebral compression fractures: Present status and future directions. *J Biomed Mater Res Part B Appl Biomater* 2007;81(2):371-386.
14. Lewis G: Properties of antibiotic-loaded acrylic bone cements for use in cemented arthroplasties: A state-of-the-art review. *J Biomed Mater Res Part B Appl Biomater* 2009;89(2):558-574.
15. Jacobs JJ, Gilbert JL, Urban RM: Corrosion of metal orthopaedic implants. *J Bone Joint Surg Am* 1998;80(2):268-282.
16. Weiser MC, Lavernia CJ: Trunnionosis in total hip arthroplasty: *J Bone Jt. Surg* 2017;99(17):1489-1501.
17. Wright TM, Goodman SB, American Academy of Orthopaedic Surgeons , eds: *Implant Wear in Total Joint Replacement: Clinical and Biologic Issues, Material and Design Considerations: Symposium, Oakbrook, Illinois, October 2000.* ed 1. Rosemont, IL, American Academy of Orthopaedic Surgeons, 2001.
18. Rostoker W, Chao EY, Galante JO: Defects in failed stems of hip prostheses. *J Biomed Mater Res* 1978;12(5):635-651.
19. McKellop HA, Röstlund TV: The wear behavior of ion-implanted Ti-6A1-4V against UHMW polyethylene. *J Biomed Mater Res* 1990;24(11):1413-1425.
20. Gil FJ, Canedo R, Padrós A, Sada E: Enhanced wear resistance of ball-and-socket joints of dental implants by means of titanium gaseous nitriding. *J Biomater Appl* 2002;17(1):31-43.
21. Brown TE, Larson B, Shen F, Moskal JT: Thigh pain after cementless total hip arthroplasty: Evaluation and management. *J Am Acad Orthop Surg* 2002;10(6):385-392.
22. Simmons CA, Valiquette N, Pilliar RM: Osseointegration of sintered porous-surfaced and plasma spray-coated implants: An animal model study of early postimplantation healing response and mechanical stability. *J Biomed Mater Res* 1999;47(2):127-138.
23. Pohler OE: Unalloyed titanium for implants in bone surgery. *Injury* 2000;31 suppl 4:7-13.
24. Bobyn JD, Stackpool GJ, Hacking SA, Tanzer M, Krygier JJ: Characteristics of bone ingrowth and interface mechanics of a new porous tantalum biomaterial. *J Bone Joint Surg Br* 1999;81(5):907-914.
25. Kuehn K-D, Ege W, Gopp U: Acrylic bone cements: Mechanical and physical properties. *Orthop Clin North Am* 2005;36(1):29-39, v-vi.
26. Webb JCJ, Spencer RF: The role of polymethylmethacrylate bone cement in modern orthopaedic surgery. *J Bone Joint Surg Br* 2007;89(7):851-857.
27. Reckling FW, Dillon WL: The bone-cement interface temperature during total joint replacement. *J Bone Joint Surg Am* 1977;59(1):80-82.
28. Ranawat CS: *Total-Condylar Knee Arthroplasty: Technique, Results, and Complications.* New York, NY, Springer New York, 1985.
29. Gilbert JL, Hasenwinkel JM, Wixson RL, Lautenschlager EP: A theoretical and experimental analysis of polymerization shrinkage of bone cement: A potential major source of porosity. *J Biomed Mater Res* 2000;52(1):210-218.
30. Messick KJ, Miller MA, Damron LA, Race A, Clarke MT, Mann KA: Vacuum-mixing cement does not decrease overall porosity in cemented femoral stems: An in vitro laboratory investigation. *J Bone Joint Surg Br* 2007;89(8):1115-1121.
31. Herberts P, Malchau H: Long-term registration has improved the quality of hip replacement: A review of the Swedish THR register comparing 160,000 cases. *Acta Orthop Scand* 2000;71(2):111-121.
32. Engesaeter LB, Lie SA, Espehaug B, Furnes O, Vollset SE, Havelin LI: Antibiotic prophylaxis in total hip arthroplasty: Effects of antibiotic prophylaxis systemically and in bone cement on the revision rate of 22,170 primary hip replacements followed 0-14 years in the Norwegian arthroplasty register. *Acta Orthop Scand* 2003;74(6):644-651.
33. Kane RJ, Yue W, Mason JJ, Roeder RK: Improved fatigue life of acrylic bone cements reinforced with zirconia fibers. *J Mech Behav Biomed Mater* 2010;3(7):504-511.
34. Charnley J: *Low Friction Arthroplasty of the Hip: Theory and Practice.* Berlin, Springer, 1979.
35. Wroblewski BM, Siney PD, Fleming PA: *Charnley Low-Frictional Torque Arthroplasty of the Hip Practice and Results.* Switzerland, Springer International Publishing, 2016.
36. Kurtz SM, Kurtz SM: *UHMWPE Biomaterials Handbook: Ultra High Molecular Weight Polyethylene in Total Joint Replacement and Medical Devices.* Amsterdam; Boston, Elsevier/Academic Press, 2009.
37. Kurtz SM, Medel FJ, MacDonald DW, Parvizi J, Kraay MJ, Rimnac CM: Reasons for revision of first-generation highly cross-linked polyethylenes. *J Arthroplasty* 2010;25(6 suppl):67-74.
38. Kurtz SM, Gawel HA, Patel JD: History and systematic review of wear and osteolysis outcomes for first-generation highly crosslinked polyethylene. *Clin Orthop Relat Res* 2011;469(8):2262-2277.
39. Lachiewicz PF, Soileau ES, Martell JM: Wear and osteolysis of highly crosslinked polyethylene at 10 to 14 Years: The effect of femoral head size. *Clin Orthop Relat Res* 2016;474(2):365-371.
40. Sobieraj MC, Rimnac CM: Ultra high molecular weight polyethylene: Mechanics, morphology, and clinical behavior. *J Mech Behav Biomed Mater* 2009;2(5):433-443.
41. Baker DA, Bellare A, Pruitt L: The effects of degree of crosslinking on the fatigue crack initiation and propagation resistance of orthopedic-grade polyethylene. *J Biomed Mater Res A* 2003;66(1):146-154.
42. Berry DJ, Currier BH, Mayor MB, Collier JP: Gamma-irradiation sterilization in an inert environment: A partial solution. *Clin Orthop Relat Res* 2012;470(7):1805-1813.

©Copyright 2021 American Academy of Orthopaedic Surgeons

43. Reinitz SD, Currier BH, Levine RA, Van Citters DW: Crosslink density, oxidation and chain scission in retrieved, highly cross-linked UHMWPE tibial bearings. *Biomaterials* 2014;35(15):4436-4440.
44. Reinitz SD, Currier BH, Van Citters DW, Levine RA, Collier JP: Oxidation and other property changes of retrieved sequentially annealed UHMWPE acetabular and tibial bearings. *J Biomed Mater Res Part B Appl Biomater* 2015;103(3):578-586.
45. Reinitz SD, Currier BH, Levine RAC, Collier JP, Van Citters DW: Oxidation and other property changes of a remelted highly crosslinked UHMWPE in retrieved tibial bearings. *J Biomed Mater Res Part B Appl Biomater* 2017;105(1):39-45.
46. Currier BH, Van Citters DW, Currier JH, Collier JP: In vivo oxidation in remelted highly cross-linked retrievals. *J Bone Joint Surg Am* 2010;92(14):2409-2418.
47. Currier BH, Van Citters DW, Currier JH, Carlson EM, Tibbo ME, Collier JP: In vivo oxidation in retrieved highly crosslinked tibial inserts. *J Biomed Mater Res Part B Appl Biomater* 2013;101(3):441-448.
48. Currier BH, Currier JH, Franklin KJ, Mayor MB, Reinitz SD, Van Citters DW: Comparison of wear and oxidation in retrieved conventional and highly cross-linked UHMWPE tibial inserts. *J Arthroplasty* 2015;30(12):2349-2353.
49. Tower SS, Currier JH, Currier BH, Lyford KA, Van Citters DW, Mayor MB: Rim cracking of the cross-linked longevity polyethylene acetabular liner after total hip arthroplasty. *J Bone Joint Surg Am* 2007;89(10):2212-2217.
50. Dumbleton JH, D'Antonio JA, Manley MT, Capello WN, Wang A: The basis for a second-generation highly cross-linked UHMWPE. *Clin Orthop Relat Res* 2006;453:265-271.
51. Bragdon CR, Doerner M, Martell J, et al: The 2012 John Charnley Award: Clinical multicenter studies of the wear performance of highly crosslinked remelted polyethylene in THA. *Clin Orthop Relat Res* 2013;471(2):393-402.
52. Bragdon CR, Martell JM, Greene ME, et al: Comparison of femoral head penetration using RSA and the Martell method. *Clin Orthop Relat Res* 2006;448:52-57.
53. Sochart DH: Relationship of acetabular wear to osteolysis and loosening in total hip arthroplasty. *Clin Orthop Relat Res* 1999;363:135-150.
54. Jacobs CA, Christensen CP, Greenwald AS, McKellop H: Clinical performance of highly cross-linked polyethylenes in total hip arthroplasty. *J Bone Joint Surg Am* 2007;89(12):2779-2786.
55. Brown TS, Van Citters DW, Berry DJ, Abdel MP: The use of highly crosslinked polyethylene in total knee arthroplasty. *Bone Joint Lett J* 2017;99-B(8):996-1002.
56. Currier BH, Currier JH, Holdcroft LA, Van Citters DW: Effectiveness of anti-oxidant polyethylene: What early retrievals can tell us. *J Biomed Mater Res Part B Appl Biomater* 2018;106(1):353-359.
57. Middleton JC, Tipton AJ: Synthetic biodegradable polymers as orthopedic devices. *Biomaterials* 2000;21(23):2335-2346.
58. Urban JA, Garvin KL, Boese CK, et al: Ceramic-on-polyethylene bearing surfaces in total hip arthroplasty. Seventeen to twenty-one-year results. *J Bone Joint Surg Am* 2001;83-A(11):1688-1694.
59. Huet R, Sakona A, Kurtz SM: Strength and reliability of alumina ceramic femoral heads: Review of design, testing, and retrieval analysis. *J Mech Behav Biomed Mater* 2011;4(3):476-483.
60. Hamadouche M, Boutin P, Daussange J, Bolander ME, Sedel L: Alumina-on-alumina total hip arthroplasty: A minimum 18.5-year follow-up study. *J Bone Joint Surg Am* 2002;84-A(1):69-77.
61. Willmann G: Ceramic femoral head retrieval data. *Clin Orthop Relat Res* 2000;379:22-28.
62. Chevillotte C, Trousdale RT, Chen Q, Guyen O, An K-N: The 2009 Frank Stinchfield Award: "Hip squeaking": A biomechanical study of ceramic-on-ceramic bearing surfaces. *Clin Orthop Relat Res* 2010;468(2):345-350.
63. Kumar P, Oka M, Ikeuchi K, et al: Low wear rate of UHMWPE against zirconia ceramic (Y-PSZ) in comparison to alumina ceramic and SUS 316L alloy. *J Biomed Mater Res* 1991;25(7):813-828.
64. Clarke IC, Manaka M, Green DD, et al: Current status of zirconia used in total hip implants. *J Bone Joint Surg Am* 2003;85-A(suppl 4):73-84.
65. Derbyshire B, Fisher J, Dowson D, Hardaker C, Brummitt K: Comparative study of the wear of UHMWPE with zirconia ceramic and stainless steel femoral heads in artificial hip joints. *Med Eng Phys* 1994;16(3):229-236.
66. Heyse TJ, Elpers ME, Nawabi DH, Wright TM, Haas SB: Oxidized zirconium versus cobalt-chromium in TKA: Profilometry of retrieved femoral components. *Clin Orthop Relat Res* 2014;472(1):277-283.
67. Cook SD, Thomas KA, Kay JF, Jarcho M: Hydroxyapatite-coated titanium for orthopedic implant applications. *Clin Orthop Relat Res* 1988;(232):225-243.
68. Sun L, Berndt CC, Khor KA, Cheang HN, Gross KA: Surface characteristics and dissolution behavior of plasma-sprayed hydroxyapatite coating. *J Biomed Mater Res* 2002;62(2):228-236.
69. Søballe K, Overgaard S, Hansen ES, Brokstedt-Rasmussen H, Lind M, Bünger C: A review of ceramic coatings for implant fixation. *J Long Term Eff Med Implants* 1999;9(1-2):131-151.
70. Ban S, Maruno S, Arimoto N, Harada A, Hasegawa J: Effect of electrochemically deposited apatite coating on bonding of bone to the HA-G-Ti composite and titanium. *J Biomed Mater Res* 1997;36(1):9-15.
71. Spivak JM, Ricci JL, Blumenthal NC, Alexander H: A new canine model to evaluate the biological response of intramedullary bone to implant materials and surfaces. *J Biomed Mater Res* 1990;24(9):1121-1149.
72. Morlock MM, Dickinson EC, Günther K-P, Bünte D, Polster V: Head taper corrosion causing head bottoming out and consecutive gross stem taper failure in total hip arthroplasty. *J Arthroplast* 2018;33(11):3581-3590.
73. Kao Y-YJ, Koch CN, Wright TM, et al: Affect fretting of the femoral stem trunnion in total hip arthroplasty. *J Arthroplast.* 2016;31(9 suppl):254-258.
74. Martin AJ, Jenkins DR, Van Citters DW: Role of corrosion in taper failure and head disassociation in total hip arthroplasty of a single design. *J Orthop Res* 2018;36(11):2996-3003.
75. Cooper HJ, Della Valle CJ, Berger RA, et al: Corrosion at the head-neck taper as a cause for adverse local tissue reactions after total hip arthroplasty. *J Bone Joint Surg Am* 2012;94(18):1655-1661.

©Copyright 2021 American Academy of Orthopaedic Surgeons

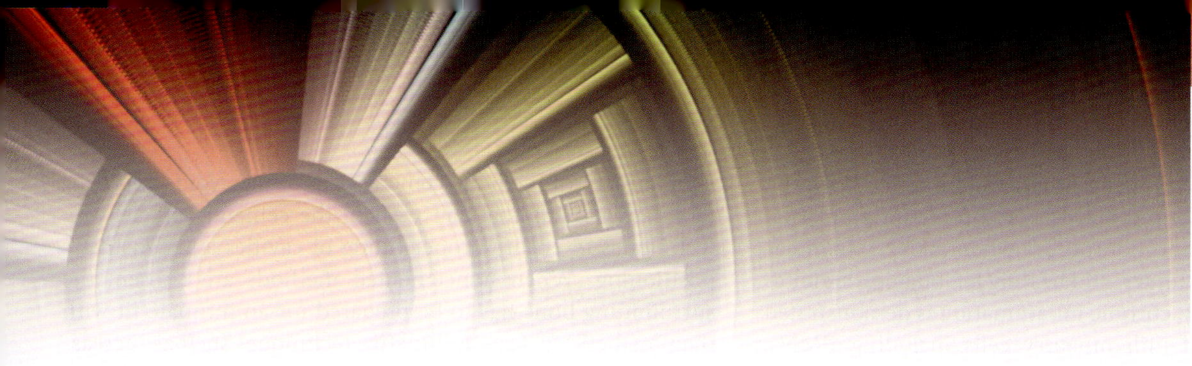

7

The Biologic Response to Orthopaedic Implants

Stuart B. Goodman, MD, PhD, FRCSC, FACS, FBSE, FICORS

Keywords: *biocompatibility; biomaterials; joint replacement; orthopaedic implants; osseointegration*

INTRODUCTION

Orthopaedic implants are commonly used as internal and external fixation devices for fracture repair, for stabilization/correction of spine fractures and deformities, for joint replacement procedures, and for other reconstructive purposes. Orthopaedic implants are usually made of materials and substances that normally do not reside in the body (eg, metallic, artificial polymeric, and ceramic devices) or are biologically based and manufactured or manipulated (such as hyaluronic acid for injection or musculoskeletal allografts). These materials may be permanent in nature, or biodegradable. This chapter will focus on the biological response to orthopaedic implants that are intended to remain permanently in the body or degrade slowly. Other chapters will review biologically based autograft and allograft implants and related materials.

Permanent orthopaedic biomaterials must demonstrate several fundamental properties to be successful for patient care. First, orthopaedic implants must accomplish their intended clinical function in exemplary fashion, that is to say they must be efficacious. Second, orthopaedic implants must be safe, and not lead to any major or minor local or systemic adverse effects in the majority of patients. Finally, for the benefit of society, these implants must be cost-effective.

A related topic is the concept of biocompatibility. Professor David Williams defines the term as follows: "Biocompatibility refers to the ability of a biomaterial to perform its desired function with respect to a medical therapy, without eliciting any undesirable local or systemic effects in the recipient or beneficiary of that therapy, but generating the most appropriate beneficial cellular or tissue response in that specific situation, and optimizing the clinically relevant performance of that therapy."[1] These key concepts: safety, efficacy, and biocompatibility of orthopaedic implants must be considered on a backdrop of acute inflammation that accompanies all surgical procedures during which an implant is placed.

ORTHOPAEDIC IMPLANTS AND INFLAMMATION—GENERAL PRINCIPLES

Whenever a surgical procedure is performed (whether an implant is used or not), the inflammatory cascade of events is initiated.[2-4] The surgical insult leads to local tissue destruction and the liberation of factors such as the pro-inflammatory cytokines (tumor necrosis factor [TNF], interleukin 1, and others), chemotactic cytokines or chemokines (interleukin-8, macrophage chemotactic protein, macrophage inflammatory protein, and others), nitric oxide and peroxide metabolites, and other substances that initiate local tissue necrosis and the migration of leukocytes both locally and systemically. This acute inflammatory response is universal and is orchestrated by polymorphonuclear leukocytes (PMNs) and macrophages. The local hematoma becomes rich in these inflammatory factors and cells, which continue the inflammatory cascade. Acute inflammation usually resolves to reconstitute relatively

Dr. Goodman or an immediate family member serves as a paid consultant to or is an employee of DePuy, A Johnson & Johnson Company, Integra, Pluristem, and Wishbone Medical; serves as an unpaid consultant to Accelalox and Biomimedica; has stock or stock options held in Accelalox, Arquos, and Biomimedica; and serves as a board member, owner, officer, or committee member of the Association of Residency Coordinators in Orthopaedic Surgery.

©Copyright 2021 American Academy of Orthopaedic Surgeons

normal tissue architectural and functional integrity; however, if this does not occur, either fibrosis or chronic inflammation follows.[3] The latter condition occurs when active inflammation, continued tissue injury, and healing are ongoing simultaneously. Histologically, chronic inflammation is demonstrated by the persistence of inflammatory cells including PMNs, macrophages, foreign-body giant cells, lymphocytes, and plasma cells, in conjunction with continued fibrosis and angiogenesis. This scenario may persist or resolve. Granulomatous inflammation is a unique type of chronic inflammation, in which activated macrophages play a prominent role histologically, assuming a squamous or epithelioid appearance. This may result from microorganisms (some bacteria, parasites, fungi), organic and inorganic particulate material, etc. Granulomatous inflammation may be divided into two types: (1) the foreign body granuloma, which is nonantigen based and therefore nonspecific and contains few lymphocytes, and (2) the immune granuloma, which is antigen based and contains higher numbers of lymphocytes.[4] These terms are extremely important when one considers the biological response to different materials and their byproducts. For example, sufficient numbers of polyethylene and poly methyl methacrylate (PMMA) particles elicit a foreign body granuloma, whereas in specific patients, byproducts of cobalt-chromium prostheses may induce an immune granuloma, often accompanied by more widespread tissue necrosis.

BIOLOGIC RESPONSE TO IMPLANTS USED IN AND AROUND BONE

BIOLOGIC RESPONSE TO IMPLANTS FOR JOINT REPLACEMENT

Joint replacement, particularly of the hip and knee, and to a lesser degree of the shoulder, elbow, finger joints, ankle, and feet, is a commonly performed surgical procedure worldwide. According to the July 2018 issue of *Orthopedic Network News* by Mendenhall and Associates, in the United States alone, there were 625,600 hip replacements and 966,900 knee replacements performed in 2017.[5] These operations are among the most cost-effective surgeries, improving pain, function, and psychosocial well-being. Long-term survivorship of these operations has been over 90% or higher at 15 years of follow-up for good prosthetic designs.[6,7]

The goal of joint replacement is to perform the surgical procedure meticulously in an appropriately selected patient to optimize long-term function and prosthetic fixation. Typically, there are two general methods for fixation of joint replacements to the skeleton. Joint replacements can be fixed to bone with poly methyl methacrylate (PMMA), which functions as a grout; alternatively, stable fixation to the surrounding bone can be accomplished using noncemented technique. When PMMA is used, state-of-the-art techniques are used including careful cleaning and drying of the bone, manipulation and containment of the bone cement to minimize voids and contaminating fluids that can weaken the cement, and delivery techniques to ensure proper filling of cavities and prosthetic positioning. When noncemented methods are chosen, the surrounding bone has to be prepared for an intimate fit with the prosthetic surface. Adjunctive techniques such as increasing the roughness of the prosthetic surface; porous or bioactive coatings; and screws, pegs, and other mechanical methods of fixation are also commonly used.

CEMENTED METAL-ON-POLYETHYLENE IMPLANTS

Sir John Charnley and others have documented the characteristics of the interface between well-fixed cemented implants and bone from postmortem human retrievals.[8-11] Charnley reported that the interface displayed cellular damage (loss of the definition of fat and hematopoietic cells) in a 500 μm radius from the cement several weeks after the surgical procedure, due to chemical, thermal, and mechanical trauma. This interface developed into a fibrous or fibrocartilaginous zone containing circular PMMA bead impressions in some areas; elsewhere, PMMA beads directly abutted bony trabecula and cortical bone. In some localized areas, the original necrotic bone subsequently underwent regeneration, with or without an intervening layer of fibrous tissue or fibrocartilage; this layer then underwent metaplasia to mature cancellous or lamellar bone over many months to years. A foreign-body giant cell reaction was rarely seen at the interface of well-fixed cemented femoral hip components. Harris' group found close bone-cement apposition and little evidence of fibrous tissue at the interface surrounding well-fixed femoral implants up to 17 years postoperatively.[10] Similar to Charnley's observations, they found that a secondary, circumferential, trabecular "neocortex" formed around the cement; this neocortex communicated with the internally expanded natural cortex via radial spicules of bone. However, Fornasier found evidence of an evolving foreign body response even when the cemented femoral implants at autopsy were not loose.[11] The presence of macrophages and foreign-body giant cells in the tissues correlated with the time after surgery, the thickness of the periprosthetic membrane, and the density of polyethylene particles. Cemented acetabular components demonstrated a progressive centripetally developing foreign body reaction to polyethylene and cement wear particles.[12] The linear osteolytic areas continued to grow with the generation of increasing amounts of wear particles and even ballooned into the bony supporting foundation until the prosthesis became mechanically loose.

NONCEMENTED METAL-ON-POLYETHYLENE IMPLANTS

When noncemented implants are used, the bone is prepared to achieve stable fixation to minimize micromotion and facilitate bone ongrowth or ingrowth without an intermediary grouting material (**Figure 1**). This goal is achieved by proper sizing of the implant and "machining" the bone for an intimate fit with

©Copyright 2021 American Academy of Orthopaedic Surgeons

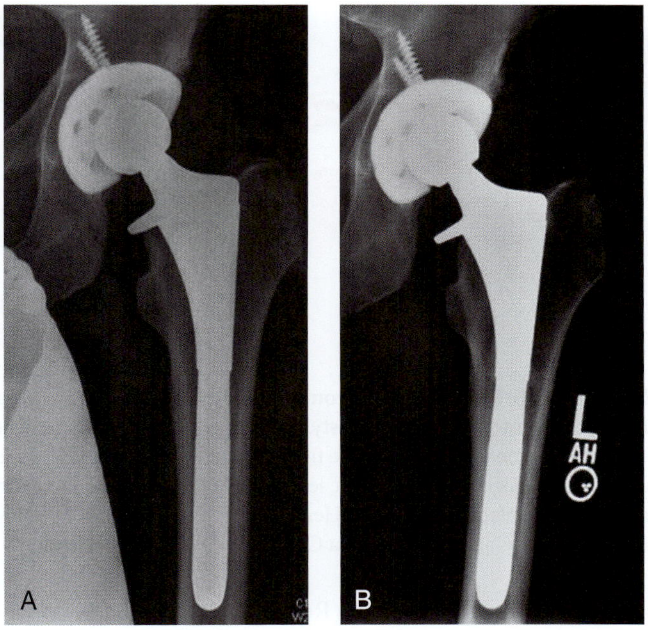

FIGURE 1 AP radiograph of osseointegrated noncemented total hip replacement. **A**, 6 weeks post noncemented total hip replacement. **B**, 5 years post total hip replacement. Note the rounding off of the calcar femorale underneath the collar of the femoral implant. The pertrochanteric area is less radiodense than previously. There are also "spot welds" at the termination of the porous coating at the midlevel of the femoral implant.

the prosthesis. Surface roughening, porous coating, and bioactive coating of the implant surface (eg, with hydroxyapatite) are adjunctive methods to achieve this goal. The aim is to induce prosthetic osseointegration, a stable physical and biofunctional incorporation of the implant within bone.[13] Interfacial micromotion beyond approximately 50 μm will lead to fibrous tissue formation, rather than bone. More conventional porous coatings (such as metallic beads and wires) and newer highly porous roughened cancellous-like metallic surfaces (such as porous tantalum or titanium) have demonstrated great success in facilitating osseointegration.[14-16] For porous coatings, a pore size of approximately 100 to 400 μm is optimal.[15]

The biological stages of bone ingrowth into stable porous coated implants parallel those of primary fracture healing. The initial hematoma that forms at the interface after noncemented prosthesis implantation is composed of localized areas of tissue necrosis, pro- and anti-inflammatory factors, and cells that consolidate into an amorphous gel. Mesenchymal stem cells migrate into the hematoma and, in the appropriate stable environment, begin to form immature woven bone via intramembranous ossification over several weeks to months. This bone undergoes remodeling to more mature cancellous and cortical bone over subsequent months to years. However, in an unstable environment with excessive micromotion, a large gap or poor vascularity, fibrous tissue, fibrocartilage, and a synovial lining layer form, and bone ingrowth is minimal. Infection will also produce a chronic inflammatory membranous interface that inhibits bone formation.

Much information concerning the interface between stable noncemented implants and bone can be learned from examining well-functioning implants retrieved at autopsy, rather than from specimens gathered at revision surgery. The latter implants are usually revised because of clinical failure due to chronic dislocation, unexplained pain, excessive wear or implant breakage, etc.[17] Clinically successful noncemented implants that have been retrieved at autopsy minimize these confounding variables.[18,19] The amount of bone within pores or adjacent to the metal surface has varied widely.[17-19] The location and orientation of fibrous tissue and bone around porous coated implants is determined by numerous factors including the material and design of the prosthesis, the location and extent of porous coating, the size of the pores, the addition of screws, the intimacy of the fit of the prosthesis with bone, and other variables.[18] Bone ingrowth is greater in titanium alloy stems where the porous coating ends, adjacent to screws, and in locations of compressive load where there is an intimate prosthetic fit.[18] Bone ingrowth is less around smooth as opposed to roughened surfaces, and in areas of localized infection or excessive motion. In such locations, fibrous tissue or an inflammatory membrane forms and may be associated with absorption of the adjacent bone. Unfilled screw holes containing fibrous tissue can provide a conduit for the migration of particles into the underlying cancellous bone. Bone ingrowth/ongrowth provides a more robust interface, preventing polyethylene particle migration compared with smooth implants.[20] Hydroxyapatite coatings can facilitate bone ongrowth, and preventing particle migration. However, at least one study reported a higher incidence of loosening when hydroxyapatite coatings are used to facilitate acetabular cup fixation.[21]

Recently, highly porous, corrosion-resistant metallic coatings and devices made out of tantalum, titanium, and other materials have been introduced to mimic the structure of cancellous bone.[16,22,23] These new materials are manufactured with a higher coefficient of friction, encouraging the adhesion and proliferation of osteoprogenitor cells and other mesenchymal tissues. These materials are particularly useful in the reconstruction of areas of bone deficiency and act as a scaffold for bone formation. Porous metallic implants are often used as a substitute for the use of bulk allografts.

Loose Metal-on-Polyethylene Implants

Loose cemented implants demonstrate radiolucent lines at the bone-cement and/or cement-prosthesis interface, and the implants often migrate from their original positions (**Figure 2**). These implants are surrounded by a fibro-inflammatory membrane up to several millimeters in thickness and contain particulate debris (**Figures 3** and **4**). The cellular components of this chronic inflammatory and foreign body reaction include fibroblasts, macrophages, giant cells, and vascular structures, but only scant numbers of lymphocytes and PMNs (**Figure 5**). If interfacial motion

©Copyright 2021 American Academy of Orthopaedic Surgeons

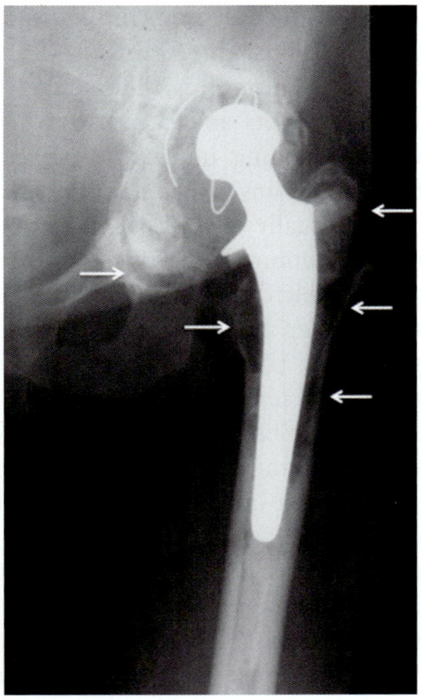

FIGURE 2 **AP radiograph of a loose cemented total hip replacement with osteolysis.** This failed hip replacement demonstrates loosening with osteolysis (arrows) of the acetabular and femoral components secondary to cement debris.

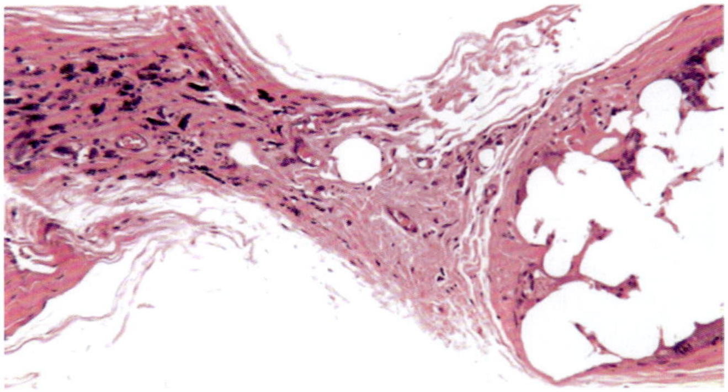

FIGURE 4 **Histologic section from the bone-cement interface of a revised cemented hip arthroplasty.** The large white circular cement "ghosts" are seen to the right of the figure, surrounded by fibrous tissue and scattered macrophages. To the left of the figure, macrophages have phagocytosed black metal debris. Hematoxylin and Eosin stain (magnification ×40). (Courtesy of Patricia Campbell, PhD, Los Angeles, CA.)

occurs, a synovial-like surface layer develops adjacent to the cement.[24,25] Large "cement lakes" in the retrieved tissue contain the remnants of PMMA (when used). Shards of polyethylene particles, which are birefringent under polarized light and stain positively with Oil Red O are seen in the interstitium and within mono- and multinucleated macrophages (**Figure 5**). These particles are often needle-like and may be up to a 1 mm or longer, but most the particulate debris are in the range of 0.3 to 5 μm in length. There is much heterogeneity throughout different locations of the tissue histologically, varying from highly oriented fibrous tissue to granulomatous inflammation, dependent on the concentration of polyethylene particles. High concentrations of osteoclasts line the membrane where bone resorption occurs; this coincides with the scalloped appearance seen around the cement mantle radiographically. Interestingly, evidence of active new bone formation is a predominant finding in the implant bone bed

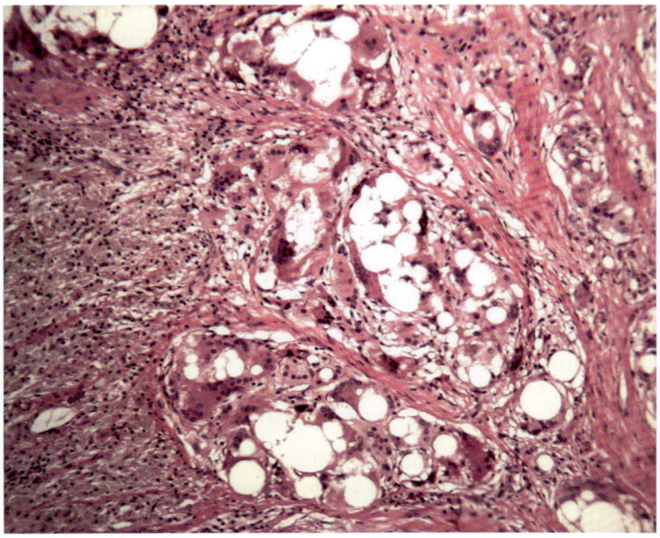

FIGURE 3 **Histologic section of a granulomatous reaction to cement debris.** Section from the bone-cement interface of a revised hip replacement demonstrates cement wear particles (larger and small round white cement "ghosts"), surrounded by a nonspecific granulomatous reaction composed of mono- and multinucleated macrophages and fibrous tissue. Hematoxylin and Eosin stain (magnification ×40). (Courtesy of Patricia Campbell, PhD, Los Angeles, CA.)

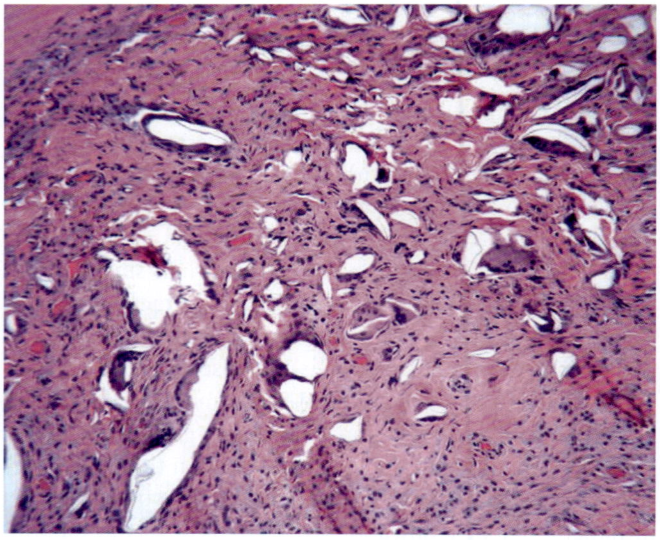

FIGURE 5 **Histologic section showing the biological reaction to polyethylene wear debris.** Large white shards of polyethylene are surrounded by macrophages and foreign-body giant cells. Hematoxylin and Eosin stain (magnification ×40). (Courtesy of Patricia Campbell, PhD, Los Angeles, CA.)

©Copyright 2021 American Academy of Orthopaedic Surgeons

histologically.[26] Loose noncemented implants display a similar histological finding, except that the fibrous tissue layer is usually thinner and contains macrophages and giant cells with phagocytosed polyethylene particles.

Osteolysis

Particle-associated periprosthetic bone loss is simply designated "osteolysis," although this term is also used in other contexts when discussing more rapid bone loss associated with aggressive tumors, infections, sustained localized pressure, and other causes. In joint replacement, osteolysis refers to a radiographic phenomenon in which progressive linear, scalloped, or larger areas of bone loss are noted in conjunction with excessive wear debris (**Figures 2** and **6**). The wear debris and inflammatory fluid from chronic synovitis are pumped around the prosthesis, insinuating into the cancellous bone by waves of high pressure generated during episodic loading of the limb. Thus, the debris can be located at a great distance from where it was generated. Wear particles have been found in the local lymph nodes, in other reticuloendothelial organs such as the liver and spleen.

Osteolysis is a phenomenon in which bone degradation is accelerated and bone formation is depressed by the production of and biological reaction to excessive wear particles. In some cases, an aggressive granulomatous lesion develops; this consists of a rapidly progressive radiographic lucent area containing well-organized connective tissue, sheets of macrophages, and fibrocystic reactive zones in a highly vascularized stroma. Aggressive granulomatosis may be due to "uncoupling of the normal sequence of monocyte-macrophage-mediated clearance of foreign material and tissue debris that is normally followed by fibroblast-mediated synthesis and remodeling of the extracellular matrix."[27]

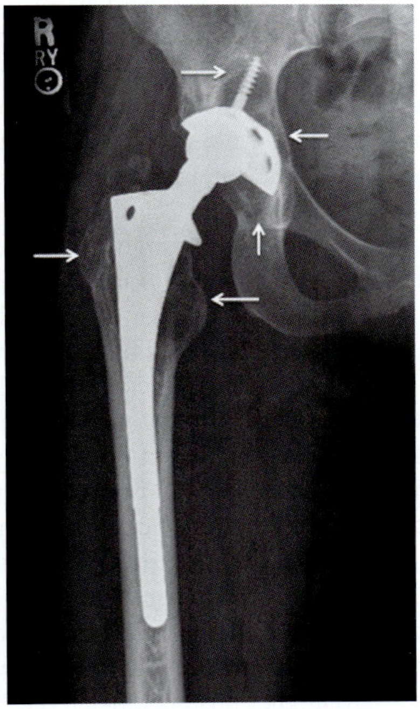

FIGURE 6 AP radiograph of a noncemented hip replacement with osteolysis due to polyethylene wear debris. This well-fixed noncemented total hip replacement demonstrates eccentric positioning of the femoral head in the acetabulum due to polyethylene wear. Note the severe polyethylene particle-associated periprosthetic osteolysis (arrows).

In vitro, in vivo, and human retrieval studies have demonstrated an association between wear particles from joint replacements and periprosthetic osteolysis.[28] Substances including prostaglandins (especially PGE2), cytokines (such as TNFa, interleukins 1 beta, 6, 8, and others), chemokines (primarily macrophage chemotactic and inhibitory proteins), nitric oxide and peroxide metabolic intermediates, and other factors are liberated by particle-activated cells that initiate the inflammatory cascade.[29] This results in the degradation of bone and suppression of bone lineage cells, leading to radiographic osteolysis. Other factors may be contributory including fluid flow–induced mechanical pressure, other mechanical factors, previous low grade infection, etc.[30]

TNFa, interleukin-1b, and many other pro- and anti-inflammatory cytokines and substances are regulated primarily by the transcription factor NFkB. This transcription factor has great relevance to periprosthetic osteolysis associated with wear particles. RANK (receptor activator of NFkB) activates the transcription factor NFkB and is a membrane bound receptor on the surface of osteoclasts. Osteoblasts, stromal cells, and other activated cells in the inflammatory process release RANK receptor ligand (RANKL), a member of the TNF superfamily. RANKL interacts with RANK located on osteoclasts, and the cytokine macrophage colony stimulating factor (GM-CSF) to upregulate the differentiation and maturation of tissue macrophages into osteoclasts. The soluble decoy protein receptor antagonist osteoprotegerin (OPG) inhibits RANKL and is part of the homeostatic mechanism controlling bone mass. Studies have demonstrated an imbalance in the RANKL:GM-CSF:OPG axis in vitro, and in vivo experiments with wear particle challenge and in cases of periprosthetic osteolysis.[31]

Although biological treatments for osteolysis have not yet reached the clinical arena, strategies to treat wear particle–associated dysregulatory processes leading to enhanced bone destruction and depressed bone formation are being addressed using in vitro and in vivo models. For example, our group has embarked on three biological strategies to address the particle-induced chronic inflammation and osteolysis: (1) by curtailing macrophage migration to particles using local delivery of a recombinant protein called 7ND, that functions as a mutant monocyte chemoattractant protein-1 (MCP-1/CCL2); (2) by modulating local macrophage function by polarizing them from a pro-inflammatory to an anti-inflammatory phenotype using local delivery of interleukin-4 (IL-4) via direct cytokine infusion or controlled release scaffolds, or by delivery of mesenchymal stem cells that overexpress IL-4; (3) by interfering with NFkB, the key pro-inflammatory transcription factor.[32-36] All of these strategies have been successful in vitro and in small animals. Further research using larger animals to demonstrate efficacy and safety profiles of these treatments is planned.

©Copyright 2021 American Academy of Orthopaedic Surgeons

Alternative Bearings

Wear and periprosthetic osteolysis has stimulated research into alternative bearing surfaces with improved wear characteristics. These new articulations include primarily newer polyethylenes, ceramic-on-ceramic, and metal-on-metal bearings. Conventional polyethylenes were originally sterilized with gamma irradiation in air and were usually stored in air containing packaging on the shelf until used. This caused oxidative degradation of the polyethylene and suboptimal wear characteristics when implanted in vivo. More recently, the more highly cross-linked polyethylenes that are heated at or above the melting temperature and/or annealed have shown improved wear characteristics in vitro and in vivo up to 10 to 15 years postoperatively. Moreover, the particle burden is less, although the particles are slightly smaller in size.[37] However, the very small number of particles generated more than compensates for the potential for increased particle-associated inflammation. Newer polyethylenes that are doped with the free radical scavenger vitamin D, or repetitively melted and annealed, may show even more promise.[38]

Ceramic-on-ceramic bearings are more popular in Europe and the Far East compared with America. Although the wear particles generated are few in number secondary to extremely low volumetric wear of this bearing couple, their biologic potential is similar to polyethylene.[37,39] Most of the particles generated are in the nanometer size range, although damaged surfaces can generate particles of a larger size. Issues related to particle generation include surface damage during initial placement or loss of the lubricating layer, striped wear, suboptimal placement of the components with impingement or edge loading, chipping, and catastrophic fracture.

Metal-on-metal (MOM) bearing surfaces have been used for over four decades, first as the McKee Farrar and Ring prostheses in Great Britain, and more recently worldwide, as the materials, tribological characteristics, and design of implants were improved. In addition, the resurgence of resurfacing arthroplasty of the hip (mostly in North America, Northern Europe, and Australia) encouraged a reconsideration of MOM bearing surfaces. Normally, wear with MOM bearings is particularly low because of the smaller clearance of the components that generates thin fluid film lubrication and the self-polishing nature of this articulation.[37,40] Implants manufactured with higher carbon alloys have demonstrated better wear characteristics compared with those with lower carbon alloys.[37,40] Although some MOM implants have functioned very well, new issues have arisen that have been a cause of great concern.

Metallic debris has been found in the periprosthetic tissues of metal-on-polyethylene joint replacements. This debris may be generated in large amounts in specific situations (eg, from corroding interfaces or particles, impingement, or when the femoral head wears completely through the polyethylene liner and articulates with the metal shell). However in MOM arthroplasty, the debris is produced in greater quantity and the particles are very small, in the order of 10 to 50 nm and have a large surface area.[37,40] Furthermore, ions of cobalt (Co) and chromium (Cr) are produced and can be found in the surrounding and remote tissues, blood, and urine. Although high levels of ions are associated with specific types of cancer in animal models, to date there is no evidence of this in humans.[37]

Retrieval and revision specimens from MOM prostheses demonstrate different histological findings compared with metal-on-polyethylene implants. Macrophage-laden particles are far less pervasive in MOM specimens. Professor Willert and colleagues in Germany brought to our attention a subset of 19 patients with pristine looking radiographs postoperatively, who had early recurrence of their preoperative pain, poor function, and a joint effusion associated with a second-generation MOM articulation.[41] Five of the 19 hips subsequently developed radiolucent lines and another 7 hips developed osteolysis, before revision. At surgery, the hip components were well fixed in nine patients; "the characteristic histological features were diffuse and perivascular infiltrates of T and B lymphocytes and plasma cells, high endothelial venules, massive fibrin exudation, accumulation of macrophages with drop-like inclusions, and infiltrates of eosinophilic granulocytes and necrosis."[41] The authors also found that the MOM retrievals showed pronounced ulceration superficial to the areas demonstrating peri-lymphocytic vascular infiltration.[42] The lymphocytic infiltration was more pronounced in specimens from MOM cases with prosthesis loosening compared with autopsy specimens or those undergoing arthrotomy. The above findings suggested that degradation products from MOM implants may be associated with an allergic hypersensitivity reaction, confirmed by a positive lymphocyte transformation test in 10/16 patients (62%) in a subsequent report.[43]

The debris produced by metal-on-polyethylene bearings is primarily polymeric and evokes a nonspecific, nonantigenic chronic inflammatory and foreign body reaction (a nonspecific granulomatous reaction). However, metal-on-metal articulations produce metallic byproducts that are soluble and can complex with serum proteins to form haptens, and subsequently, a hypersensitivity reaction mediated by the adaptive immune system involving T and B lymphocytes (immune granuloma). The most common metallic sensitizers include nickel, cobalt, and chromium. Rarely, metals such as titanium, vanadium, and tantalum function in this capacity. This allergic reaction is classified as a type IV delayed hypersensitivity immune reaction. Corrosion byproducts including $CrPO_4$ may also develop from MOM bearing surfaces, and other nonarticulating locations (eg, the femoral head and trunnion). These byproducts can elicit an immune response and act as agents promoting third body wear. In addition, patients with a MOM bearing surface have higher postoperative levels of cobalt and chromium ions in their blood, serum, erythrocytes, and urine, compared with preoperative values and others with a metal-on-polyethylene bearing.

Pseudotumor formation is a unique adverse reaction that has been described regarding MOM bearing implants.

©Copyright 2021 American Academy of Orthopaedic Surgeons

Pseudotumors are composed of large granulomatous masses of inflammatory cells (macrophages, T lymphocytes, plasma cells), fibrous tissue, and widespread tissue necrosis in conjunction with with MOM bearings[44,45] (**Figure 7**). The etiology appears to be both a cytotoxic response and delayed hypersensitivity reaction to cobalt-chromium particles and their byproducts. These masses may be asymptomatic at first, but often become symptomatic with time, and can cause a mass effect on the surrounding neurovascular structures, muscle, and bone. Risk factors for this reaction appear to be younger women with small sized components, hip dysplasia, malposition, edge loading, and impingement of the components.[46] Particularly worrisome is the high complication and poor outcome of revision of these cases. Surgical débridement demonstrates more widespread necrosis of soft tissue and bone than was originally suspected, often compromising subsequent function. The consensus appears to be that cases with pseudotumor formation should be revised early to a non-MOM bearing surface to avoid long-term tissue necrosis and functional loss.

Recently systematic reviews and meta-analyses reported higher early and intermediate revision rates for metal-on-metal primary resurfacing and total hip arthroplasties, compared with metal- or ceramic-on-conventional polyethylene primary total hip arthroplasties.[47,48] Given the fact that the newer highly cross-linked polyethylenes are even more durable than conventional polyethylenes, the utility of metal-on-metal articulations is questionable at this time.[49] Although many surgeons have changed from a cobalt-chromium to a ceramic femoral head articulating with highly cross-linked polyethylene, there is very limited evidence supporting this approach, other than the theoretical avoidance of "trunnionosis."

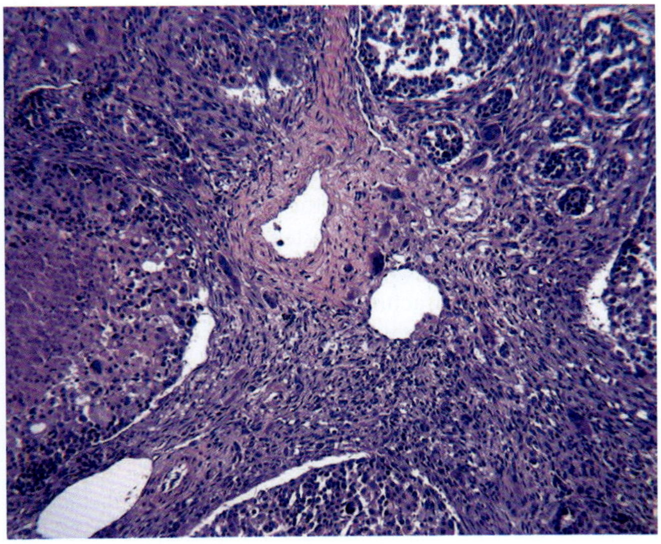

FIGURE 7 Histologic section of a metal-induced granulomatous reaction. Section from the tissue interface of a revised metal-on-metal implant demonstrating widespread infiltration of macrophages and lymphocytes in response to metal debris, in a fibrous stroma background. To the left of the photomicrograph, there are areas of tissue necrosis. Hematoxylin and Eosin stain (magnification ×40). (Courtesy of Patricia Campbell, PhD, Los Angeles, CA.)

Stress-Induced Bone Remodeling

In addition to affecting the biological environment, orthopaedic implants placed within bone profoundly affect the mechanical environment. Noncemented femoral implants were originally made of cobalt-chromium alloy, a material that is very stiff compared with both cortical and cancellous bone. As load was transmitted through the intramedullary stem from proximally to distally, bypassing the proximal femur, remodeling of the proximal femur over time according to biomechanical principles known as Wolff's law took place. The resulting radiographic findings, termed "stress shielding" or "adverse bone remodeling," showed marked atrophy of the proximal metaphysis of the femur and hypertrophy of the femur adjacent to the distal end of the implant, especially at the end of the porous coating (**Figure 1**). Larger stem sizes had a more profound effect.[50] Although these radiological events have not been associated with clinical failure of the femoral implant, the rapid disappearance of bone over time on follow-up radiographs can be daunting and might compromise the available bone stock if revision surgery should be necessary in the future. To mitigate these adverse bone remodeling changes, modern femoral implants have been designed to provide better proximal metaphyseal fit and fill (and therefore more metaphyseal loading), and many have special features such as a tapered design that does not engage the cortex distally, metal cutouts along the length of the stem, or a compressible double pronged distal end. Another approach has been to use materials that have a lower modulus of elasticity and are therefore less stiff than conventional stems, for example, titanium alloys or composite materials.[51]

Originally, porous coating was placed over the full length of the femoral implant to enhance mechanical fixation primarily by gaining a better initial "scratch fit," and a more extensive surface for bone ingrowth. Fully porous coated stems were thought to be another contributing factor to stress shielding.[52] To date, there is general agreement that large diameter longer stems made of stiffer materials result in more stress shielding than shorter stems of a smaller diameter.

Carcinogenesis

The potential for carcinogenesis due to the presence of orthopaedic implants is a particularly germane subject, given the fact that millions of implants are placed each year worldwide for joint replacement, fracture fixation, spine fusion, and other reconstructive procedures. Furthermore, joint replacements and other implants are currently being performed in younger patients who may have the device in situ for many decades. There is also controversy as to whether fixation devices such as intramedullary rods, plates, screws, wires, spinal implants, etc. should be excised when their presence is no longer needed. These devices prevent normal loading of the adjacent bone and release byproducts that may have biological sequela.

©Copyright 2021 American Academy of Orthopaedic Surgeons

As discussed above, most orthopaedic polymers and ceramics have few biological effects in bulk form. The particulates of these materials stimulate a nonspecific chronic inflammatory and foreign body reaction. In other organ systems subjected to chronic inflammatory processes, cellular metaplasia may occur; however, this does seem to be the case when discussing orthopaedic implants made of polymers and ceramics. Metallic implants present a slightly different scenario because the byproducts of corrosion and other processes can result in the formation of metallic-protein complexes that can function as antigenic haptens. Prolonged high levels of metallic ions and complexes containing cobalt, chrome, and nickel in rodents have been associated with sarcoma and lymphoma formation. Stainless steel fixation devices have been associated with sarcomas in dogs and cats. These concerns have stimulated controversy in the use of metal-on-metal bearing surfaces in younger patients, whose blood and tissues may potentially exhibit elevated metal ion levels for many decades.

Perhaps the most recent and comprehensive examination of cancer and metallic implants has come from Visuri's group.[53] They reviewed a total of 46 cases of malignant tumor formation at the site of total hip replacements reported in the Western literature between 1974 and 2003. These cases included 41 sarcomas, 4 lymphomas, and 1 epidermoid carcinoma. Thirty-one of the tumors were soft-tissue carcinomas, whereas 10 were located in bones. The most common soft-tissue sarcoma was the malignant fibrous histiocytoma in 20 of the 31 cases. The mean period of latency from the first operation was 6 years (range, 0.5 to 20 years). Predisposing factors included secondary osteoarthritis, previous local complications, chronic infection, and known preconditions for cancer such as irradiation. The sarcomas were highly aggressive, with 77% of patients dying within 1 year of diagnosis. The authors concluded that particle-associated chronic inflammation did not appear to be a risk factor for the development of cancer, given the large numbers of joint replacements performed each year worldwide. However, cancers associated with joint replacements and other metallic fixation devices are probably underreported.

When discussing the risk of cancer around orthopaedic implants with patients, the health care team should remember that the latency for most cancers in general is many years, if not decades. Although no direct association between metal implants and cancer has been established to date, long-term follow-up and continued epidemiologic studies are warranted.

BIOLOGIC RESPONSE TO IMPLANTS USED FOR FRACTURE FIXATION

The biological and biomechanical principles, and the materials used in the treatment of fractures are common with those in adult reconstructive surgery and joint replacement. Fracture fixation devices including intramedullary rods, plates, screws, wires, and other implants are generally manufactured from metal alloys such as stainless steel, cobalt-chromium, titanium alloy, other metallic and nonmetallic alloys and composites, and biodegradable polymeric devices. The biology and biomechanics of intramedullary nailing have been known for many years and have recently been reviewed.[54] Important factors that impact the local and systemic effects of intramedullary implants include the general condition of the patient, specific biomechanics and vascular supply of the bone involved, the type of fracture and injury characteristics, whether the canal is reamed, the type of reamer used, the design and material composition of the nail, whether it is locked with screws, and subsequent loading protocols during rehabilitation. Intramedullary reaming is superimposed on the injury to the affected bone and destroys the endosteal blood supply and the medullary contents. Reaming negatively affects cortical blood flow but increases blood flow to the surrounding muscle and soft tissues.[54] Endosteal blood supply appears to normalize within about 12 weeks in large animals. Reaming also facilitates the local deposition of marrow contents, and pro- and anti-inflammatory factors that promote osteogenesis. Whether reaming has an effect on the local rate of infection of open fractures is controversial, but at least one human study does not support this contention. Intramedullary reaming has the potential to embolize marrow contents into the systemic circulation and may affect the immune system both locally and systemically. Marrow embolization is dependent on the design of the reamer and the intramedullary pressures generated during the procedure. New directions include the use of new materials and bioactive coating of the nail to inhibit infection or promote fracture healing.

The use of plates and screws for fracture fixation, especially for peri-articular fractures, has a long successful history. Traditionally, the use of full contact plates and screws placed by wide surgical exposures has led to adverse bone remodeling, because of local alteration of the biomechanical environment and interference with local blood supply. More recently, screws and plates made of newer alloys and designs have demonstrated less corrosive byproducts and more limited contact with the underlying bone, minimizing local compressive forces exerted by the plate on the bone. Technical advances include preservation of the periosteum, and less invasive indirect reduction and bridging osteosynthesis (instead of reduction of every single fracture fragment) to better preserve the surrounding soft tissue and blood supply.[55]

Böstman's group in Finland has played a seminal role in defining the biocompatibility of bioabsorbable bone fixation devices.[56,57] They report a series of 2,528 fractures and other disorders in which pins, rods, bolts, and screws were used for fixation. These devices were made of polyglycolic acid or polylactic acid. These implants were generally used around the ankle, foot, and elbow. Clinically significant foreign body reactions to the breakdown products of these polymers were seen in 4.3% of cases and manifested as a painful erythematous fluctuating papule or discharging sinus. Fifty-seven percent of these cases exhibited localized osteolytic lesions at the site of the internal fixation device. The risk of this adverse reaction was dependent on the type of polymer implanted.

©Copyright 2021 American Academy of Orthopaedic Surgeons

Polyglycolic acid implants were associated with a 5.3% incidence of significant foreign body reaction, whereas only one case (0.2%) of polylactic acid implants demonstrated this reaction. Polyglycolic acid implants exhibited this reaction earlier (2 to 3 months) than polylactic acid (4.3 years). Polylactic acid is hydrophobic and has a known longer degradation time than polyglycolic acid. The presence of quinone dye additive exacerbated the inflammatory reaction. Screws and serrated bolts showed a greater propensity for this reaction compared with pins and rods, probably because of the former's increased surface area. Poorly vascularized areas were particularly susceptible. The lesions were débrided in all cases of significant reaction. Histological specimens showed a nonspecific inflammatory foreign body mono- and multinucleated cell reaction to extracellular polymeric debris, approximately 25 μm in size. Important factors to consider include the molecular weight of the polymer, the thermal history, crystallinity, porosity, and presence of residual impurities and additives, as well as the methods of fabrication and sterilization. Newer polymers are being developed that may mitigate these adverse reactions.

IMAGING OF THE BONE-IMPLANT INTERFACE

The bone-implant interface has traditionally been assessed using standard radiographs in at least two perpendicular planes. Further oblique views may be necessary if the anatomic details of interest are masked by the implant. With joint replacements, the classic radiographic determinants of implant loosening include migration of the implant within bone, progressive circumferential lucent lines, fracture of the cement mantle supporting the prosthesis, or fracture of the implant. With fracture fixations devices, implant failure is usually identified by fracture or migration of the implant with/without continued fracture nonunion, or progressive halos around screws or pins which signify loss of mechanical fixation or ongoing infection. The use of CT scans can further delineate the relationship between implant and surrounding bone using multiple thinner radiographic sections, compared with plain radiographs.[58] However, CT exposes the patient to ionizing radiation and is subject to beam hardening artifact due to the metallic implants.[58] For these reasons, recently, magnetic resonance imaging protocols have been developed that include algorithms to suppress metal artifact.[58-60] This avoids the use of ionizing radiation and can yield important information concerning the bone and surrounding soft tissues including the prosthetic interface. Specifically, this technique can identify areas of bone edema, synovitis associated with infection, wear particle disease or other causes, fluid collections, sinus tracts, probable implant loosening, etc.[58] Other techniques for investigation of implants and bones such as ultrasonography, tomosynthesis, nuclear imaging, and positron emission tomography (PET) scans are used rarely, and for specific indications, for example, ultrasonography as an initial screening tool for the presence of masses or fluid collections, nuclear imaging for difficult cases of suspected infection.

SURFACE MODIFICATION OF IMPLANTS

Implant surfaces can be modified physically and/or chemically to enhance osseointegration, prevent implant loosening, or provide delivery for molecules to enter the surrounding tissues.[61-64] Reviews of this subject with respect to prophylaxis and treatment of infection are provided in another chapter in this text and elsewhere.[62,63,65]

The surface of implants, especially metals, can be intentionally altered with regard to their topography, chemistry, oxidation, and hydrophilicity to optimize protein absorption, and key aspects related to cell attachment, function, and signaling pathways.[66,67] Techniques such as etching, blasting, plasma spraying, attaching porous coatings of various types, and nanopatterning of the surface to alter the surface topography and roughness are all being explored. Many of these technologies have been adapted from the dental field. Precise reproducibility of complex topographical features is difficult to achieve on a batch-to-batch basis, which limits the translational application of in vitro and in vivo experimental studies. However, with the advent of 3D printing technologies, composite surface modifications may now be easier to achieve. Chemical modification of metallic surfaces can be accomplished by physicochemical adsorption, covalent bonding of molecules, or by the use of carriers; however, physical methods also change the surface chemistry to a greater or lesser degree.[66] Specific coatings can be added to functionalize the prosthesis for enhanced osteogenesis and prevention of infection; however, the criteria which must be fulfilled are daunting.[68] Inorganic coatings such as calcium phosphates, including hydroxyapatite, and diphosphonates have been successful in vitro and in vivo, but have not achieved extensive clinical translation to humans because of questionable efficacy.[69] Other molecules have been added to calcium phosphate coatings including fluoride, strontium, zinc, and silver, to enhance osteogenesis and mitigate infection.

Biomolecular coatings can incorporate extracellular matrix proteins (such as collagen-mimetic peptides, chondroitin sulfate, and silk), short peptides such as Arg-Gly-Asp (RGD), growth factors (such as BMP-2), cellular chemotactic proteins (such as SDF-1), DNA molecules, and others to further functionalize the implant interface.[61,63] These coatings are still in the preclinical stage and will have significant challenges in completing the complex regulatory pathways involved in combination products.

Another innovation pertains to coating technologies associated with absorbable magnesium strontium alloys used for fracture fixation. These alloys enhance osteogenesis but are rapidly degraded in vivo. However, calcium phosphate microarc oxidation coating appeared to optimize corrosion resistance and cellular response when cultured with MC3T3-E1 preosteoblasts in vitro.[70]

©Copyright 2021 American Academy of Orthopaedic Surgeons

SUMMARY

Implants have revolutionized the treatment of traumatic injuries and orthopaedic reconstructive procedures worldwide. These devices are tightly regulated in the United States by the FDA, in Canada by the Medical Devices Bureau of Health Canada, in the UK by Medicines and Healthcare Products Regulatory Agency, in the European Union by the Ministry of Health in each member state (although European Union certification is designated by the CE mark), and by other regulatory bodies in other countries around the world. These devices generally undergo exhaustive preclinical and clinical studies before use in the United States.[71] A comprehensive system is also in place for reporting of device-associated adverse events by the hospital and physician. It should be emphasized that most current devices have changed the lives of millions of patients for the better, in ways that could not have been imagined. Internal fixation of fractures, hip and knee replacement, correction of spinal deformity, etc. are but a few examples of how our society has benefited from the use of orthopaedic implants to decrease pain, disability, functional loss, and deformity. However, with these benefits, there is risk, including perioperative complications, long-term adverse reactions, and even failure of the device.

Most implants placed within the body function well in the intermediate to long term and obtain a homeostatic level of biocompatibility with the surrounding tissues and systemic organ systems. However, some implants continue to liberate byproducts that are a function of continued use, mechanical loading protocols, exposure to biological fluids, biodegradability, and other factors. Thus constant vigilance for continued normal function of the implant and prompt adverse event reporting are crucial to the success of these devices in the long term. In this respect, orthopaedic device registries can play an important role. One other point relates to off-label use of orthopaedic devices. This practice is very common by orthopaedic surgeons and related specialties. The surgeon should use medical devices in an off-label manner judiciously, according to their best knowledge and educated good medical judgment.[72] The patient's best interests are placed above all else. Further improvements and newer orthopaedic devices for expanded indications will continue to improve the quality of life for our patients.

REFERENCES

1. Williams DF: On the mechanisms of biocompatibility. *Biomaterials* 2008;29(20):2941-2953.
2. Anderson JA: *Inflammation, Wound Healing, and the Foreign-Body Response*. San Diego, CA, USA, Elsevier, 2004.
3. Kumar V, Cotran RS, Robbins SL: *Robbins Basic Pathology*, ed 7. Philadelphia, Saunders, 2002.
4. Majno G, Joris I: *Cells Tissues and Disease: Principles of General Pathology*. Malden, MA, USA, Blackwell Science, 1996.
5. Mendenhall S: 2018 hip and knee implant review. *Orthopedic Network News* July 2018:1-23.
6. Vessely MB, Whaley AL, Harmsen WS, Schleck CD, Berry DJ: The Chitranjan Ranawat Award: Long-term survivorship and failure modes of 1000 cemented condylar total knee arthroplasties. *Clin Orthop Relat Res* 2006;452:28-34.
7. Callaghan JJ, Albright JC, Goetz DD, Olejniczak JP, Johnston RC: Charnley total hip arthroplasty with cement. Minimum twenty-five-year follow-up. *J Bone Joint Surg Am* 2000;82(4):487-497.
8. Charnley J. *Low Friction Arthroplasty of the Hip*. New York, Springer-Verlag, 1979.
9. Charnley J: The reaction of bone to self-curing acrylic cement. A long-term histological study in man. *J Bone Joint Surg Br* 1970;52(2):340-353.
10. Maloney WJ, Jasty M, Burke DW, et al: Biomechanical and histologic investigation of cemented total hip arthroplasties. A study of autopsy-retrieved femurs after in vivo cycling. *Clin Orthop Relat Res* 1989;(249):129-140.
11. Fornasier V, Wright J, Seligman J: The histomorphologic and morphometric study of asymptomatic hip arthroplasty. A postmortem study. *Clin Orthop Relat Res* 1991;(271):272-282.
12. Schmalzried TP, Kwong LM, Jasty M, et al: The mechanism of loosening of cemented acetabular components in total hip arthroplasty. Analysis of specimens retrieved at autopsy. *Clin Orthop Relat Res* 1992;(274):60-78.
13. Albrektsson T, Albrektsson B: Osseointegration of bone implants. A review of an alternative mode of fixation. *Acta Orthop Scand* 1987;58(5):567-577.
14. Galante J. *Bone Ingrowth in Porous Materials*. Park Ridge, American Academy of Orthopaedic Surgeons, 1985.
15. Bobyn JD, Pilliar RM, Cameron HU, Weatherly GC: The optimum pore size for the fixation of porous-surfaced metal implants by the ingrowth of bone. *Clin Orthop Relat Res* 1980;(150):263-270.
16. Patil N, Lee K, Goodman SB: Porous tantalum in hip and knee reconstructive surgery. *J Biomed Mater Res B Appl Biomater* 2009;89(1):242-251.
17. Cook SD, Thomas KA, Haddad RJ Jr: Histologic analysis of retrieved human porous-coated total joint components. *Clin Orthop Relat Res* 1988;(234):90-101.
18. Hirakawa K, Jacobs JJ, Urban R, Saito T: Mechanisms of failure of total hip replacements: Lessons learned from retrieval studies. *Clin Orthop Relat Res* 2004;(420):10-17.
19. Engh CA, Zettl-Schaffer KF, Kukita Y, Sweet D, Jasty M, Bragdon C: Histological and radiographic assessment of well functioning porous-coated acetabular components. A human postmortem retrieval study. *J Bone Joint Surg Am* 1993;75(6):814-824.
20. Bobyn JD, Jacobs JJ, Tanzer M, et al: The susceptibility of smooth implant surfaces to periimplant fibrosis and migration of polyethylene wear debris. *Clin Orthop Relat Res* 1995;(311):21-39.
21. Stilling M, Rahbek O, Soballe K: Inferior survival of hydroxyapatite versus titanium-coated cups at 15 years. *Clin Orthop Relat Res* 2009;467(11):2872-2879.
22. Issack PS: Use of porous tantalum for acetabular reconstruction in revision hip arthroplasty. *J Bone Joint Surg Am* 2013;95(21):1981-1987.
23. Migaud H, Common H, Girard J, Huten D, Putman S: Acetabular reconstruction using porous metallic material in complex revision total hip arthroplasty: A systematic review. *Orthop Traumatol Surg Res* 2019;105(1S):S53-S61. PMID:30138711.
24. Goldring SR, Schiller AL, Roelke M, Rourke CM, O'Neil DA, Harris WH: The synovial-like membrane at the bone-cement interface in loose total hip replacements and its proposed role in bone lysis. *J Bone Joint Surg Am* 1983;65(5):575-584.
25. Goodman SB, Chin RC, Chiou SS, Schurman DJ, Woolson ST, Masada MP: A clinical-pathologic-biochemical study of the membrane surrounding loosened and nonloosened total hip arthroplasties. *Clin Orthop Relat Res* 1989;(244):182-187.

©Copyright 2021 American Academy of Orthopaedic Surgeons

26. Kadoya Y, Revell PA, al-Saffar N, Kobayashi A, Scott G, Freeman MA: bone formation and bone resorption in failed total joint arthroplasties: Histomorphometric analysis with histochemical and immunohistochemical technique. *J Orthop Res* 1996;14(3):473-482.
27. Santavirta S, Konttinen YT, Bergroth V, Eskola A, Tallroth K, Lindholm TS: Aggressive granulomatous lesions associated with hip arthroplasty. Immunopathological studies. *J Bone Joint Surg Am* 1990;72(2):252-258.
28. Bostrom M, O'Keefe R: What experimental approaches (eg, in vivo, in vitro, tissue retrieval) are effective in investigating the biologic effects of particles? *J Am Acad Orthop Surg* 2008;16 suppl 1:S63-S67.
29. Tuan RS, Lee FY, Y TK, Wilkinson JM, Smith RL: What are the local and systemic biologic reactions and mediators to wear debris, and what host factors determine or modulate the biologic response to wear particles? *J Am Acad Orthop Surg* 2008;16 suppl 1:S42-S48.
30. Greenfield EM, Bechtold J: What other biologic and mechanical factors might contribute to osteolysis? *J Am Acad Orthop Surg* 2008;16 suppl 1:S56-S62.
31. Schwarz EM: What potential biologic treatments are available for osteolysis? *J Am Acad Orthop Surg* 2008;16 suppl 1:S72-S75.
32. Lin T, Pajarinen J, Nabeshima A, et al: Orthopaedic wear particle-induced bone loss and exogenous macrophage infiltration is mitigated by local infusion of NF-kappaB decoy oligodeoxynucleotide. *J Biomed Mater Res A* 2017;105(11):3169-3175.
33. Lin T, Pajarinen J, Nabeshima A, et al: Establishment of NF-kappaB sensing and interleukin-4 secreting mesenchymal stromal cells as an "on-demand" drug delivery system to modulate inflammation. *Cytotherapy* 2017;19(9):1025-1034.
34. Nabeshima A, Pajarinen J, Lin TH, et al: Mutant CCL2 protein coating mitigates wear particle-induced bone loss in a murine continuous polyethylene infusion model. *Biomaterials* 2017;117:1-9.
35. Sato T, Pajarinen J, Behn A, et al: The effect of local IL-4 delivery or CCL2 blockade on implant fixation and bone structural properties in a mouse model of wear particle induced osteolysis. *J Biomed Mater Res A* 2016;104(9):2255-2262.
36. Goodman SB, Gibon E, Pajarinen J, et al: Novel biological strategies for treatment of wear particle-induced periprosthetic osteolysis of orthopaedic implants for joint replacement. *J R Soc Interface* 2014;11(93):20130962.
37. Campbell P, Shen FW, McKellop H: Biologic and tribologic considerations of alternative bearing surfaces. *Clin Orthop Relat Res* 2004;(418):98-111.
38. Jarrett BT, Cofske J, Rosenberg AE, Oral E, Muratoglu O, Malchau H: In vivo biological response to vitamin e and vitamin-e-doped polyethylene. *J Bone Joint Surg Am* 2010;92(16):2672-2681.
39. D'Antonio JA, Sutton K: Ceramic materials as bearing surfaces for total hip arthroplasty. *J Am Acad Orthop Surg* 2009;17(2):63-68.
40. Jacobs JJ, Urban RM, Hallab NJ, Skipor AK, Fischer A, Wimmer MA: Metal-on-metal bearing surfaces. *J Am Acad Orthop Surg* 2009;17(2):69-76.
41. Willert HG, Buchhorn GH, Fayyazi A, et al: Metal-on-metal bearings and hypersensitivity in patients with artificial hip joints. A clinical and histomorphological study. *J Bone Joint Surg Am* 2005;87(1):28-36.
42. Davies AP, Willert HG, Campbell PA, Learmonth ID, Case CP: An unusual lymphocytic perivascular infiltration in tissues around contemporary metal-on-metal joint replacements. *J Bone Joint Surg Am* 2005;87(1):18-27.
43. Thomas P, Braathen LR, Dorig M, et al: Increased metal allergy in patients with failed metal-on-metal hip arthroplasty and peri-implant T-lymphocytic inflammation. *Allergy* 2009;64(8):1157-1165.
44. Mahendra G, Pandit H, Kliskey K, Murray D, Gill HS, Athanasou N: Necrotic and inflammatory changes in metal-on-metal resurfacing hip arthroplasties. *Acta Orthop* 2009;80(6):653-659.
45. Pandit H, Glyn-Jones S, McLardy-Smith P, et al: Pseudotumours associated with metal-on-metal hip resurfacings. *J Bone Joint Surg Br* 2008;90(7):847-851.
46. Glyn-Jones S, Pandit H, Kwon YM, Doll H, Gill HS, Murray DW: Risk factors for inflammatory pseudotumour formation following hip resurfacing. *J Bone Joint Surg Br* 2009;91(12):1566-1574.
47. Clarke A, Pulikottil-Jacob R, Grove A, et al: Total hip replacement and surface replacement for the treatment of pain and disability resulting from end-stage arthritis of the hip (review of technology appraisal guidance 2 and 44): Systematic review and economic evaluation. *Health Technol Assess* 2015;19(10):1-668, vii-viii.
48. Lopez-Lopez JA, Humphriss RL, Beswick AD, et al: Choice of implant combinations in total hip replacement: Systematic review and network meta-analysis. *BMJ* 2017;359:j4651.
49. Cafri G, Paxton EW, Love R, Bini SA, Kurtz SM: Is there a difference in revision risk between metal and ceramic heads on highly crosslinked polyethylene liners? *Clin Orthop Relat Res* 2017;475(5):1349-1355.
50. Engh CA, Bobyn JD: The influence of stem size and extent of porous coating on femoral bone resorption after primary cementless hip arthroplasty. *Clin Orthop Relat Res* 1988;(231):7-28.
51. Hartzband MA, Glassman AH, Goldberg VM, et al: Survivorship of a low-stiffness extensively porous-coated femoral stem at 10 years. *Clin Orthop Relat Res* 2010;468(2):433-440.
52. McAuley JP, Sychterz CJ, Engh CA Sr: Influence of porous coating level on proximal femoral remodeling. A postmortem analysis. *Clin Orthop Relat Res* 2000;(371):146-153.
53. Visuri T, Pulkkinen P, Paavolainen P: Malignant tumors at the site of total hip prosthesis. Analytic review of 46 cases. *J Arthroplasty* 2006;21(3):311-323.
54. Bong MR, Kummer FJ, Koval KJ, Egol KA: Intramedullary nailing of the lower extremity: Biomechanics and biology. *J Am Acad Orthop Surg* 2007;15(2):97-106.
55. Wagner M: General principles for the clinical use of the LCP. *Injury* 2003;34 suppl 2:B31-B42.
56. Bostman O, Pihlajamaki H: Clinical biocompatibility of biodegradable orthopaedic implants for internal fixation: A review. *Biomaterials* 2000;21(24):2615-2621.
57. Bostman OM, Pihlajamaki HK: Adverse tissue reactions to bioabsorbable fixation devices. *Clin Orthop Relat Res* 2000;(371):216-227.
58. Koff MF, Burge AJ, Koch KM, Potter HG: Imaging near orthopedic hardware. *J Magn Reson Imaging* 2017;46(1):24-39.
59. Jungmann PM, Agten CA, Pfirrmann CW, Sutter R: Advances in MRI around metal. *J Magn Reson Imaging* 2017;46(4):972-991.
60. Choi SJ, Koch KM, Hargreaves BA, Stevens KJ, Gold GE: Metal artifact reduction with MAVRIC SL at 3-T MRI in patients with hip arthroplasty. *AJR Am J Roentgenol* 2015;204(1):140-147.
61. Goodman SB, Yao Z, Keeney M, Yang F: The future of biologic coatings for orthopaedic implants. *Biomaterials* 2013;34(13):3174-3183.
62. Raphel J, Holodniy M, Goodman SB, Heilshorn SC: Multifunctional coatings to simultaneously promote osseointegration and prevent infection of orthopaedic implants. *Biomaterials* 2016;84:301-314.
63. Zhang BG, Myers DE, Wallace GG, Brandt M, Choong PF: Bioactive coatings for orthopaedic implants-recent trends in development of implant coatings. *Int J Mol Sci* 2014;15(7):11878-11921.
64. Orapiriyakul W, Young PS, Damiati L, Tsimbouri PM: Antibacterial surface modification of titanium implants in orthopaedics. *J Tissue Eng* 2018;9:2041731418789838.
65. Kargupta R, Bok S, Darr CM, et al: Coatings and surface modifications imparting antimicrobial activity to orthopedic implants. *Wiley Interdiscip Rev Nanomed Nanobiotechnol* 2014;6(5):475-495.
66. Damiati L, Eales MG, Nobbs AH, et al: Impact of surface topography and coating on osteogenesis and bacterial attachment on titanium implsnts. *J Tissue Eng* 2018;9:2041731418790694.
67. Boyan BD, Lotz EM, Schwartz Z: (*) roughness and hydrophilicity as osteogenic biomimetic surface properties. *Tissue Eng Part A* 2017;23(23-24):1479-1489.
68. Tobin EJ: Recent coating developments for combination devices in orthopedic and dental applications: A literature review. *Adv Drug Deliv Rev* 2017;112:88-100.

©Copyright 2021 American Academy of Orthopaedic Surgeons

69. Surmenev RA, Surmeneva MA, Ivanova AA: Significance of calcium phosphate coatings for the enhancement of new bone osteogenesis–a review. *Acta Biomater* 2014;10(2):557-579.

70. Shangguan Y, Sun L, Wan P, et al: Comparison study of different coatings on degradation performance and cell response of Mg-Sr alloy. *Mater Sci Eng C Mater Biol Appl* 2016;69:95-107.

71. Kirkpatrick JS, Stevens T: The FDA process for the evaluation and approval of orthopaedic devices. *J Am Acad Orthop Surg* 2008;16(5):260-267.

72. Buch B: FDA medical device approval: Things you didn't learn in medical school or residency. *Am J Orthop (Belle Mead NJ)* 2007;36(8):407-412.

©Copyright 2021 American Academy of Orthopaedic Surgeons

8

Osteolysis and Implant Loosening

Valentin Antoci Jr, MD, PhD
Dioscaris R. Garcia, PhD
Jillian L. Glasser, BA
Anita Shukla, PhD

Keywords: *implant; osteolysis; particle disease; polyethylene; wear*

INTRODUCTION

Modern trends in total joint arthroplasty indicate a sharp increase in demand with the inclusion of younger and more active patients. Implant survival curves suggest increased implant durability and previously described wear patterns are less relevant.[1] The introduction of highly cross-linked polyethylene two decades ago has resulted in less particulate wear and decreased osteolysis. Nevertheless, aseptic loosening is still the prevalent cause of implant failure, significantly outpacing the rates of periprosthetic infection, instability, and mechanical breakage.[2] Persistent development and changes in implant surface design and biocompatibility have had a relatively small impact on outcomes. The original Charnley hip has shown 85% survival at 25 years, which is very impressive considering the use of small diameter heads, cement, and early generation polyethylene formulations.[3] Early data on modern polyethylene show no penetration on radiographs at 10 years, suggesting very limited wear.[4] Does that suggest that implant wear, osteolysis, and loosening are problems of the past? To answer that question, the current chapter will focus on the biology of osteolysis, cellular interactions, molecular signaling cascades, and potential therapies for osteolysis and associated bone loss.

Dr. Garcia or an immediate family member serves as an unpaid consultant to BI Medical, LLC. Dr. Shukla or an immediate family member has received research or institutional support from Takeda. Neither of the following authors nor any immediate family member has received anything of value from or has stock or stock options held in a commercial company or institution related directly or indirectly to the subject of this chapter: Dr. Antoci and Dr. Glasser.

PARTICULATE WEAR PATTERNS

Even though implants are generally designed to be relatively inert, our bodies interact with them at the cellular and molecular levels. A foreign-body reaction is mediated by a cascade that results from (1) associated injury, (2) local hematoma, (3) recruitment of host inflammatory cells, (4) acute to chronic inflammation, and (5) fibrosis or granuloma formation. Foreign-body reactions can originate at the time of implant insertion through immediate tissue damage, or later due to wear particles and debris. Wear may be defined as loss of material volume with generation of material particles resulting from motion between two opposed surfaces.[5] In the case of joint replacement implants, such wear occurs at the bearing surface, where most motion takes place, or at the implant-bone interface. The inflammation produced locally leads to bone loss termed *osteolysis.* The initial loss of bone support around the implant leads to increased mechanical strains and micromotion. Cyclical micromotion then acts as a pump with subsequent pressurization that carries particles to other areas of the interfaces and can produce massive and extensive osteolysis.

The original design of total hip arthroplasty involved a polytetrafluorethylene (Teflon) bearing surface, and Charnley documented a very high failure rate of 95% between 1959 and 1962, mostly from osteolysis and implant loosening. Nevertheless, the process of osteolysis was not recognized as a biologic event until both Willert and Harris separately

©Copyright 2021 American Academy of Orthopaedic Surgeons

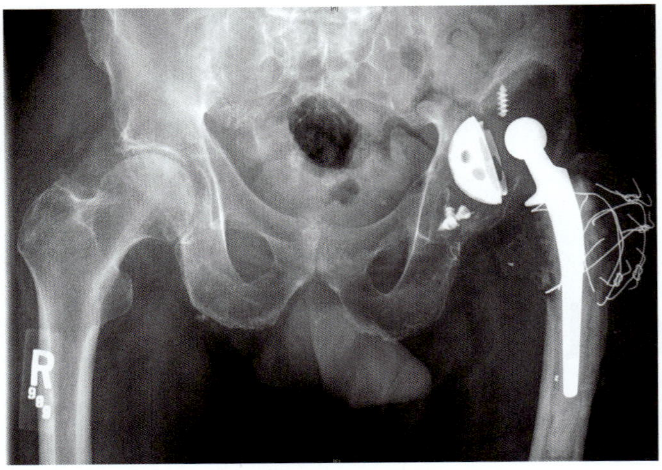

FIGURE 1 AP radiograph of total hip arthroplasty with extensive osteolysis throughout, bone loss, and loosening of components.

described the lysis derived from macrophages around loose implants, which was later mistakenly termed "cement disease" by Jones and Hungerford in 1987.[6] The so called "cement disease" was thought to be the product of cement particles produced around a total implant from abnormal motion and poor cement technique.[7] Methyl methacrylate, a monomer of acrylic resin, has revolutionized total joint arthroplasty by allowing early fixation of implants into bone. Nevertheless, loosening at the implant-cement interface or cement-bone interfaces allowed for generation of small debris that initiated the inflammatory cascade and led to extensive osteolysis. In severe cases of "cement disease," the entirety of the proximal femur and pelvic columns can show resorption and associated bone loss (**Figure 1**). The severity of the problem and the hypothesis that it was related to the cement itself led to the design of noncemented total hip arthroplasty in the 1980s, only to see the persistence of osteolysis. Osteolysis remains a major mechanism of failure in total joint arthroplasty, now reported around 21.8% in revision hip arthroplasty[8] compared with around 40% several decades ago.[9]

Osteolysis and concomitant loosening of implants can result from a variety of causes in both cemented and noncemented implants. The term "cement disease" has been replaced by "particle disease" through better understanding of the mechanical and physiological processes associated with orthopaedic implants. The typical response to particles can be split into three specific phases. In response to debris, a chronic activation of the immune system takes place through both cellular and cytokine responses. An increased number of macrophages, fibroblasts, and osteoclasts then disrupts the periprosthetic bone environment causing tissue breakdown. Finally, this process disrupts bone regeneration and remodeling by direct cytotoxic effect on mesenchymal osteoprogenitor cells.

Wear debris are constantly produced at joint bearing surfaces, modular interfaces, and other implant-implant or implant-bone interfaces. The particle size, composition, and shape are dependent on the material, with a wide range of particles identified. The accumulation of particles at the bone-implant interface stimulates the recruitment of immune cells, which interact with the particulate debris through direct surface antibodies or phagocytosis by macrophages or lymphocytes. Particles in the 0.2 to 10 μm range involve a macrophage driven response, while smaller metal particles in the nanometer range can elicit a lymphocyte response.[10] Ultimately, particle volume and rate of accumulation leads to a nonspecific immune response with an expansive foreign body reaction and chronic inflammation that mimics chronic infection. Furthermore, in vitro studies have documented a linear increase in transcriptional activity and cytokine responses to particulate volume. A threshold effect has been proposed for wear rate and associated osteolysis, for example, wear rates above 0.1 mm per year are at significant risk of osteolysis.[11]

MATERIAL PROPERTIES

Different materials provide for different particulate debris characteristics, including size, composition, and shape, that influence the interactions with the local cellular environment. Polyethylene is the most common source for particle matter around bearings. Polyethylene is a commonly used plastic dating back to 1898 when Hans von Pechmann prepared it serendipitously from diazomethane.[12] The manufacturing process directly affects the material characteristics including shaping by machining or compression molding, irradiation, and thermal processing, as well as end point sterilization and packaging. Conventional polyethylene was sterilized by gamma radiation in air which led to oxidative damage and increased wear and particle production contributing to long-term osteolysis. Contemporary orthopaedic devices take advantage of ultra-high–molecular-weight polyethylene (UHMWPE) which contains extremely long chains of two to six million monomer units. UHMWPE increases cross-linking which improves wear resistance at a cost of decreased mechanical properties and increased free radical formation. In the latest generation polyethylene, advances in radiation and annealing techniques as well as adjuvants such as vitamin E reduce free radicals and improve mechanical and fatigue properties. This does not mean that UHMWPE is less likely to produce osteolysis.

Understanding failure mechanisms is further complicated by the different mechanical environments encountered at various interfaces. The polyethylene wear particles are different in the knee compared with the hip. Failed total knee arthroplasties have large-size debris, which are associated with polyethylene delamination, pitting, and fatigue wear less likely to produce a large macrophage response (**Figure 2**). The prevalence of osteolysis after total knee arthroplasty ranges from 5% to 20% at 15 years. The knee differs from the hip due to the complex geometry and less congruent surfaces that produce multiaxial movement including sliding, rolling, and rotation. In contrast, the hip is largely exposed to cyclical motion that

©Copyright 2021 American Academy of Orthopaedic Surgeons

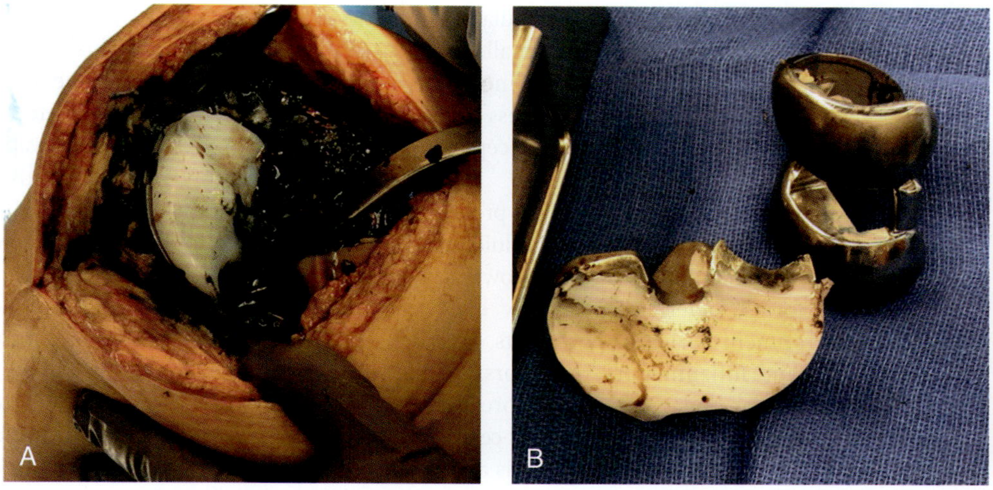

FIGURE 2 Photographs showing polyethylene wear and backside wear. **A**, Polyethylene wear due to postfracture delamination. **B**, Backside wear including extensive synovitis with polyethylene and metal particle debris.

leads to wear mainly through adhesion and abrasion mechanisms. Backside wear is not common at the hip, while it remains an important failure mechanism at the knee.

To address the debris problems of polyethylene, alternative bearing surfaces have been proposed including the use of ceramic and metal. Ceramic bearings have the lowest wear rates of any bearing combination, with less than 0.5 to 2.5 µm per year. However, ceramic-on-ceramic bearings have a much smaller window of error in component position, with early designs showing increased squeaking and breakage. Unfortunately, breakage of a ceramic bearing leads to disastrous particulate debris formation that produces extensive osteolysis, with revisions showing poor results due to the persistent particulate presence, third body wear, and continued osteolysis. A broken ceramic liner has to be replaced with another ceramic liner, as other materials such as polyethylene are softer and fail rapidly in response to ceramic debris. Alternatively, ceramic on polyethylene bearings have similar results to metal on polyethylene, even though possible decreased wear in the range of less than 150 µm has been reported. The low wear would suggest ceramic-on-polyethylene to be an ideal bearing, but subsequent possible damage to the ceramic head can lead to increased abrasive wear. Specifically, ceramic heads can show stripe wear as well as lead pencil-like wear, which increase surface roughness but also predispose the head to fracture in overweight or higher activity patients.

Metal-on-metal bearings produce smaller particles and lower wear rates compared with bearings that include polyethylene. An annual linear wear rate of less than 5 µm per year has been reported. The lower wear rates as well as improved material properties allowed for larger heads, increased stability, and theoretically a more forgiving surface. Interestingly, some small head metal-on-metal bearings had acceptable results with long-term follow-up of over 20 years. Unfortunately, some large head metal-on-metal bearings that followed had a high rate of failure due to significant adverse reactions both around the implant as well as the systemic toxicity of plasma metal levels.[13] The one aspect not accounted for was the significantly higher particulate presence. The metal particles are very small, in the range of 50 nm, but their numbers are up to 500 times higher compared with metal on polyethylene bearings. This significant volume of particulate matter leads to aggressive recruitment of the immune system and development of aseptic lymphocyte-dominated vasculitis-associated lesions (ALVAL) and pseudotumors.[14] This response is significantly different than the macrophage-driven response in polyethylene particle wear. The response to metal particles can be massive, involving extensive tissue necrosis, macrophagic response with phagocytosed metallic debris, granulomas, progressive perivascular lymphocytic infiltrate and ALVAL, lymphoid neogenesis, and large invasive fluid collections. Just like ceramic bearings, the component position is an important factor in bearing surface performance, with overabducted cups showing higher serum ion levels. Cases of adjacent tissue invasion have been widely described, including damage to nearby vascular and nervous planes. Ultimately, the high rate of failure in registries across the world lead to a quick response and recall of some designs, with most patients either now revised or remaining asymptomatic. The problem of metal interfaces has persisted, with fretting corrosion wear now described with modular implants at dual taper neck junctions and trunnions.[15]

THE BIOLOGY OF OSTEOLYSIS

Osteolysis is the process of bone loss triggered by implant material degradation, polyethylene, metal, or ceramic, that leads to immune system recruitment and local infiltration of macrophages and lymphocytes, subsequent chronic inflammatory reaction, and dissemination of particulate debris that expands the inflammatory process and ultimately leads to prosthesis loosening.[10] Willert et al[16] have speculated that a constant equilibrium is required between the amount of debris produced and the mechanisms responsible for removing the debris. Both biologic and mechanical factors have been implicated in the progression of osteolysis. For example, particles in

©Copyright 2021 American Academy of Orthopaedic Surgeons

the 0.3 to 1.0 μm are the most common stimulators of mononuclear phagocytes in vivo, while particles smaller than 0.3 μm are typically eliminated from the joint by pinocytosis rather than phagocytosis.[17] Pinocytosis is a much less inflammatory process that typically does not involve receptor-mediated responses.

The early stages of osteolysis mimic the process of healing with increased circulation and elevated fluid levels in the affected tissues. As the fluid expands, a growing, synovial-like membrane forms, determining a new effective joint space. This environment is rich in fibroblasts, macrophages, endothelial cells, and inflammatory mediators. Unlike healing though, the cellular and inflammatory processes do not subside but increase with the progression to cellular infiltration and bone loss through osteoclastogenesis and osteolysis. Simple models of polyethylene-induced osteolysis in mouse calvaria show extensive pitting and loss of bone surface similar to the periprosthetic environment (**Figure 3**). The normal regenerative process is disrupted and histological slices show extensive damage to the microarchitecture of bone and presence of immune cells and osteoclasts.

Osteoclasts are multinucleated giant cells derived from the monocytic/macrophage cell line and differentiated to function in bone resorption and remodeling. The osteoclast precursor is a circulatory cell that is activated upon physical contact with specific mesenchymal cells such as osteoblasts or marrow stromal cells. Stromal cells modulate resorption and bone deposition by direct inhibition of receptor activator of nuclear factor kappa B ligand (RANKL) by osteoprotegerin (OPG) which competes with receptor activator of nuclear factor kappa B (RANK) as a soluble decoy receptor. Mice overexpressing OPG develop osteopetrosis. In cases of material debris, the fibroblast-like cells present in the synovial membrane secrete RANKL in response to increase presence of inflammatory mediators such as prostaglandin E_2 (PGE_2). The binding of RANKL to RANK activates key transcription factors responsible for osteoclast differentiation. This family of transcription factors consists of several family members that form heterodimers and are typically found bound to an inhibitory (I-κB) protein. Stimulation by RANKL leads to activation of upstream I-κB kinases (IKKs), which phosphorylate I-κB leading to its dissociation from the nuclear factor kappa B (NF-κB) complex. NF-κB is then translocated to the nucleus where in induces specific gene transcription essential for osteoclast differentiation.

While osteoclasts are the ultimate destructive force behind osteolysis, the innate immune system is the primary player involved in the response to particulate debris. The cellular response is not limited to macrophages and lymphocytes, but also involves a vast interplay among osteoblasts and mesenchymal cells, osteoclasts, and fibroblasts. A wide array of proinflammatory cytokines such as tumor necrosis factor alpha (TNF-α), interleukins 1 and 6 (IL-1 and IL-6), PGE_2, and matrix metalloproteinases are evident in the response and support the nonspecific nature of the process. This macrophagic and cytokine response is associated with the osteolytic process, compared with loose implants without osteolysis that show mainly fibrous tissue. The release of cytokines is dose dependent and is also a function of particle size, concentration, and surface area. The inflammatory activation is not limited to phagocytosis; direct particle/cell interactions are adequate to activate osteoclastogenic signaling pathways. As such, T lymphocytes are not uncommon and may constitute up to 10% of cells at the interface of loose implants. As in the case of metallosis, the lymphocytes may have a modulatory effect on the local responses to polyethylene or cement particles. The specific function of the adaptive immune system in the response to polyethylene and cement particles is not well defined.

The mechanism underlying particle induction of cellular responses and osteolysis is not well understood, with research at times contradictory.[18] The primary response relies

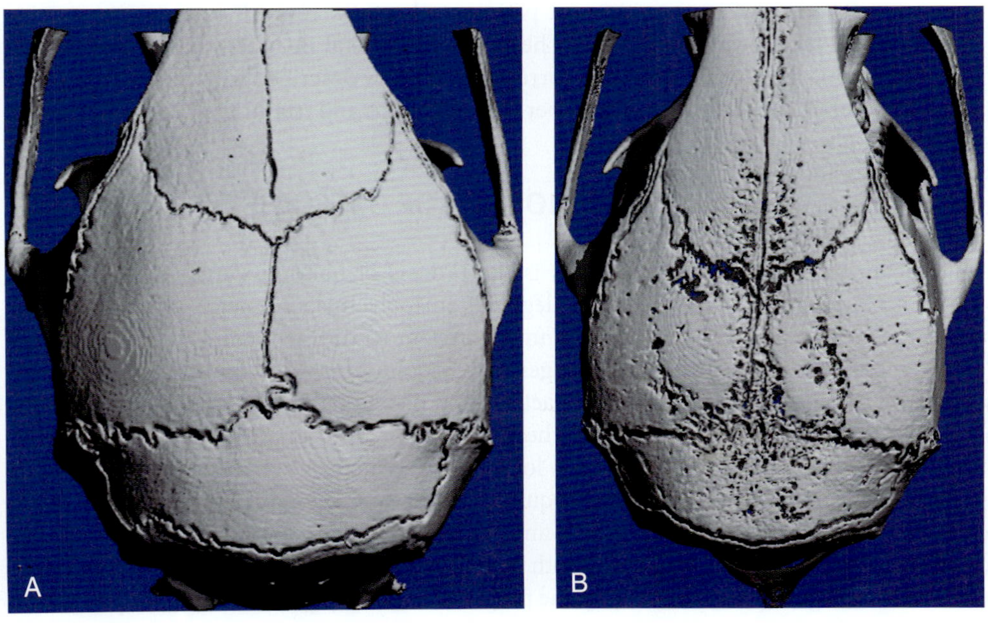

FIGURE 3 Models of polyethylene-induced osteolysis using mouse calvaria show extensive bone destruction, pitting, and bone loss in response to polyethylene particles packed in the subperiosteal space. **A**, Normal calvaria. **B**, Calvaria with osteolysis.

©Copyright 2021 American Academy of Orthopaedic Surgeons

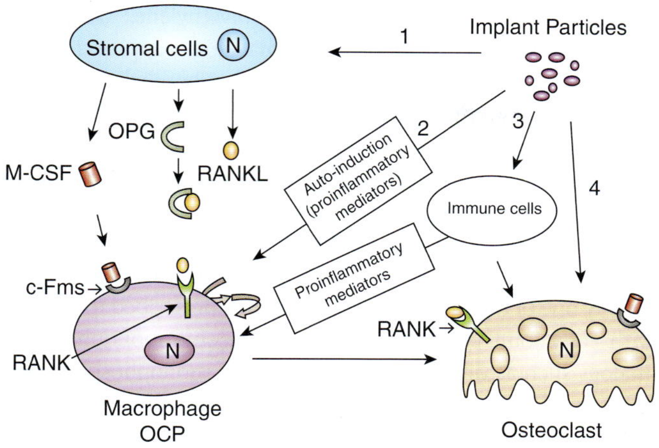

FIGURE 4 Diagram shows how implant particles induce osteoclast differentiation through direct stimulation of stromal cells, activation of immune cells and cytokine cascades, as well as by direct signaling to macrophages and osteoclasts. c-FMS = colony-stimulating factor 1 receptor, M-CSF = macrophage colony-stimulating factor, OCP = osteoclast precursor, OPG = osteoprotegerin, RANK = receptor activator of nuclear factor kappa B, RANKL = receptor activator of nuclear factor kappa B ligand.

on phagocytosis of small particles by macrophages (**Figure 4**). Within 48 hours of exposure to debris, the macrophages increase in size from about 10 to 20 μm to 40 to 50 μm and release proinflammatory markers such as TNF-α, monocyte chemotactic protein-1 (MCP1), and macrophage inflammatory protein-1 alpha (MIP1α). MCP1 accelerates the response by recruiting further monocytes and osteoclasts which all derive from the same lineage. The classic macrophage activation pathway is mainly enhanced by T-helper 1 cells and their specific cytokine groups, especially interferon-gamma, leading to IL-1, and TNF-α production by the macrophages. The main alternative macrophage activation pathway, which consists of a broad spectrum of responses, is mainly regulated by T-helper 2 cytokines, mainly IL-4 and IL-13. This pathway activation leads to the secretion of different cytokines by the macrophages, including PGE_2, as well as to the stimulation of variant detrimental cellular reactions, such as the NF-κB apoptotic pathway and the mitogen-activated protein kinases, an intracellular stress and inflammatory signal transduction trail. Other pathways are also hypothesized, even though limited in vitro modeling exists to reproduce in vivo osteolytic processes.

Histopathologically, the periprosthetic tissue is a fibrous granulomatous tissue composed of a complex amalgam of cellular infiltration and particulate debris (**Figure 5**). The cellular component of this tissue includes histiocytes, macrophages, foreign-body giant cells, fibroblasts, osteoblasts, osteoclasts, synovial cells, endothelial cells, and less commonly lymphocytes. All these cell types actively interact with each other, where for example, fibroblasts trigger the formation of foreign body giant cells, and osteoblasts contribute to the differentiation and maturation of osteoclasts. Studies have shown that fibroblasts release osteolytic enzymes in response to debris exposure, especially stromelysin and collagenase in the presence of titanium particles. Lymphocytes likely play a mediator type role. A few studies suggest that endotoxin, a bacterial protein, becomes concentrated on the surface of particles and induces an inflammatory reaction in immune cells. Immunoglobulin complexes with polyethylene can fix complement, which could then attract inflammatory cells to the polyethylene surface. Nevertheless, the few T lymphocytes found in retrieved periprosthetic tissues were not activated, as the interleukin-2 receptor (IL-2R), interleukin-2 (IL-2), interferon gamma, and TNF-β) were not expressed. Whether T lymphocytes are innocent bystanders or active participants in the reaction to loose implants containing polymers is still unresolved.[10]

Ultimately macrophage pathways are stimulated by implant particles either directly or indirectly through cytokine pathways. TNF-α and RANKL play critical roles in upregulating

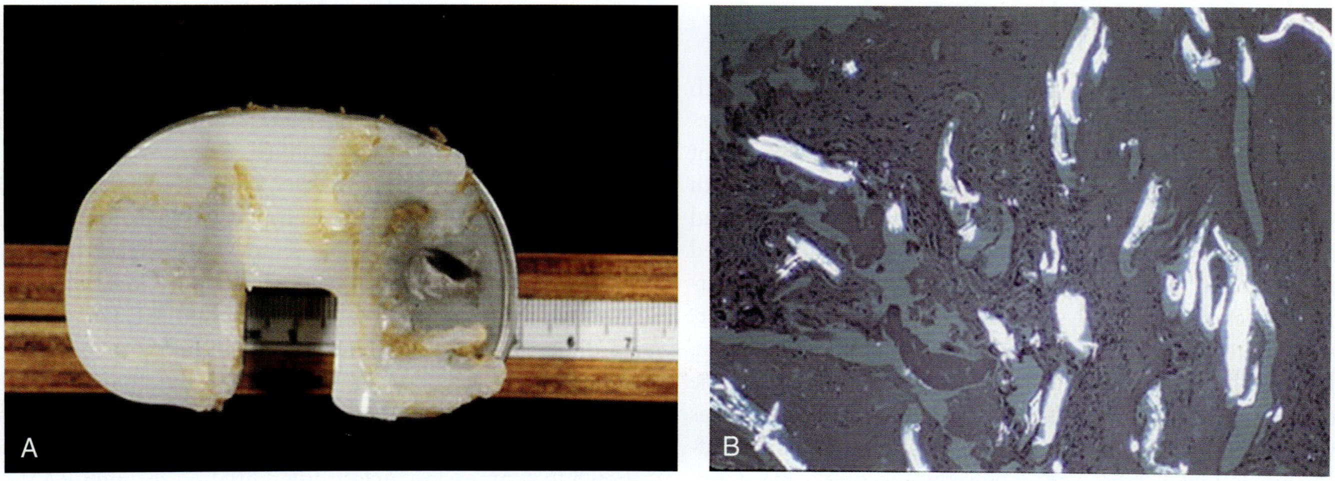

FIGURE 5 Polyethylene wear from tibial insert wear (**A**) causing extensive synovitis with particulate debris and an amalgamation of cells seen under polarized light (**B**). This is a consequence of loss of bulk polyethylene from the tibial plateau. (Courtesy of Roy Aaron, MD.)

©Copyright 2021 American Academy of Orthopaedic Surgeons

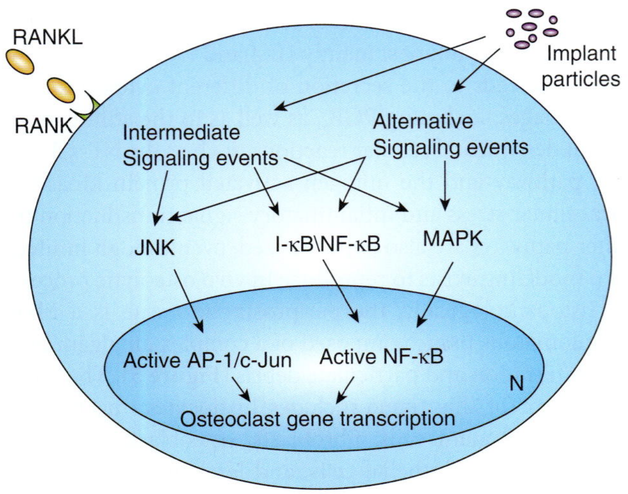

FIGURE 6 Diagram showing that osteoclast stimulation and differentiation is usually mediated through RANKL pathways. Nevertheless, implant particles can stimulate osteoclast activation directly through JNK, NF-κB, and MAPK pathways. AP-1 = activator protein-1, I-κB = inhibitory kappa B, JNK = Jun N-terminal kinase, MAPK = mitogen-activated protein kinase, NF-κB = nuclear factor kappa B, RANK = receptor activator of nuclear factor kappa B, RANKL = receptor activator of nuclear factor kappa B ligand.

the osteolytic process. In TNF-α or RANKL knockouts, cement particles fail to stimulate osteolysis. This is not unexpected as both TNF-α and RANKL are important in osteoclast differentiation and activation. Furthermore, downstream signaling by wear particles overlaps the RANKL pathways with activation of kinases and recruitment of molecules essential for osteoclastogenesis. Many of the pathways are being defined, including the tyrosine kinase c-src, mitogen-activated protein kinases, and the NF-κB cascade (**Figure 6**). Even though it would appear that the kinase/NF-κB pathway is secondary, blockage of this pathway inhibits the process of osteolysis.

POTENTIAL THERAPIES FOR OSTEOLYSIS

The process of osteolysis is initiated by particulate debris which triggers an inflammatory cascade with increased fluid and dissemination of the debris throughout an "effective total joint space." This is followed by the recruitment of macrophages with subsequent TNF-α- and RANKL-mediated differentiation and activation of osteoclasts. The continued research and improved understanding of the pathways involved in the response to particulate debris and osteolysis provide targets of possible interventions to decrease or terminate the foreign-body reaction, thus possibly preserving the implant or at least minimizing the associated soft-tissue destruction and bone loss. Research has resulted in improved implant materials, with second- and third-generation highly cross-linked polyethylene producing a significantly smaller volume of debris. Despite that, such particles can actually produce as much as 100-fold higher inflammatory response compared with conventional polyethylene.[17] To address these inflammatory reactions, pharmacologic approaches can target each step of the cascade including possibly chelating debris, inhibiting the proinflammatory cytokine cascade, limiting macrophage or lymphocyte modulation, inhibiting osteoclastogenesis, or altering the balance between osteoclast and osteoblast activity by increasing new bone formation.

Considering the role of cytokines and inflammation, anti-inflammatory agents may play a role in inhibiting osteolysis and is usually one of the first lines of medications prescribed to patients with early joint pain. Active cyclic adenosine monophosphate analogs such as dibutyryl cyclic adenosine monophosphate and PGE_1 and PGE_2 enhance IL-6 production but inhibit TNF-α. In contrast to expectations, indomethacin has been shown to actually potentiate cytokine production with a multifold increase in TNF-α function. These effects are paradoxical and underline the complex interactions, autoregulation, and overlapping pathways involved in osteolysis. Downregulation of one cytokine pathway may potentiate others.

Attempting to target more end-stage elements, MCP-1 mutant proteins have been delivered with a biodegradable layer-by-layer coating on femoral implants with good results. Similarly, targeting Src-homology region 2-containing protein tyrosine phosphatase 2 (SHP-2) has been shown to inhibit osteoclast formation in knockout mice, while specific targeting using oral SHP099 (an allosteric inhibitor of SHP-2) allowed focused targeting of osteoclast in osteolytic clinical scenarios. Since the actual bone resorption is largely produced by osteoclast function, this step of the process is an ideal target to inhibit osteolysis and the associated bone destruction. We have previously proposed implant delivery mechanisms that are capable of unloading therapeutic doses of SHP099 in the local bone environment, showing significant inhibition of osteoclasts and thus potentially inhibiting osteolysis. Such surfaces can theoretically be used in revision cases or high osteolytic pathology to curtail the destructive biology and promote bone formation and healing. At the same time though, the osteoclast resorptive activity is tightly coupled with osteoblast bone deposition, and inhibiting the osteoclastic pathway alone may result in disastrous consequence for skeletal remodeling and healing. This has not been observed in vivo,[19] with knockout mice showing normal osteoblast biology. Nevertheless, the pathways are complex and not fully understood, with specific indications for available drugs still being identified.

The local and systemic toxicity associated with metallosis has triggered research focused on particle chelation, antioxidative properties, and possible removal of material from the local environment. Cobalt and chromium chelation using N-acetylcysteine, edetate calcium disodium (EDTA), sodium 2,3-dimercaptopropane sulfonate, and dimercaprol have been reported.[20] N-acetylcysteine (NAC) is a glutathione precursor which acts as the most abundant endogenous antioxidant with vast interactions across the body. Glutathione has been shown to suppress osteoclast differentiation through RANKL signaling.[21] Cao et al[22] have shown increased bone volume and decreased osteoclast differentiation in mice supplemented

 ©Copyright 2021 American Academy of Orthopaedic Surgeons

with NAC. Fang et al[23] have pretreated tissues with NAC before exposure to poly methyl methacrylate and have shown inhibition of osteoclastogenesis and suppression of particle-induced osteolysis. Nevertheless, paradoxical effects have been documented in the case of NAC and glutathione too. Fujita et al[21] have shown that glutathione facilitates nuclear localization of the nuclear factor of activated T cells c1. In their experiments, NAC stimulated osteoclast formation and a fivefold increase in osteolytic volume. These observations fit the overarching theme of multiple competitive pathways playing critical roles in osteolysis with the science limited and lacking complete understanding. Interestingly though, NAC has several thiol groups that may provide chelating sites for metals. Giampreti et al[20] report on the clinical use of NAC to reduce systemic cobalt levels from approximately 16 to 20 mcg/L to less than 7 mcg/L, with increased excretion and decreased local presence. Nevertheless, a rebound effect was noted, hypothesized to be related to redistribution of metal ions and possible renal impairment.

Other current medications have been shown to have unexpected effects on bone. Statins are widely used for lowering serum cholesterol and potentially reducing the risk of cardiovascular events. Interestingly, several studies have shown the potential anti-inflammatory and antioxidative effects of statins. In a nationwide population-based case-control study of 4,698 patients after total hip arthroplasty, Thillemann et al[24] report an adjusted relative risk of revision of 0.34 with the use of statins. It is important to note though that the reduced risk was due to multiple causes including infection, aseptic loosening, and miscellaneous causes. Still, Lubbeke et al[25] document a 0.38 adjusted risk ratio of femoral osteolysis with the use of statins, supporting that a significant factor in the benefit of statin is possibly the effect on osteolysis pathways. Nevertheless, the data are still limited and does not provide support for using statins in healthy patients after total hip arthroplasty.

Bisphosphonates have been used specifically to balance the interplay between bone deposition and bone loss such as in osteoporosis and Paget disease. This family of pharmacologic agents attach to hydroxyapatite binding sites, targeting osteoclasts by inhibiting their ability to form the ruffled border, adhere to bone surfaces, and produce the protons necessary for continued bone resorption. Bisphosphonates also reduce osteoclast progenitor development and recruitment by promoting osteoclast apoptosis. At the same time, bisphosphonates prevent osteocyte and osteoblast apoptosis thus potentially increasing bone deposition. Several animal models demonstrate the inhibitory effect of bisphosphonates on particle-induced bone resorption by both inhibiting osteolysis in response to alendronate and reversing bone loss by disodium pamidronate. Several other studies support the beneficial effects of bisphosphonates on increased periprosthetic bone mass. A clinical study showed that parenteral (intramuscular) administration of neridronate, every fortnight for the first three months then every month for the remaining period of 1-year follow-up, reduced pain, improved function, and halted the roentgenographic evolution of periprosthetic osteolysis, as well as amplified periprosthetic bone mineral density as confirmed by dual-energy x-ray absorptiometry measurements.[18]

SUMMARY

Osteolysis and implant loosening are complex processes of significant clinical relevance that costs our health care system billions of dollars every year. Even though the goal of this work was to focus on the preclinical aspects of osteolysis, a complete understanding of patient presentations, imaging, diagnosis, and both medical as well as surgical treatment is important.

- Osteolysis is a largely innate immune system–mediated process that responds to a local irritant such as particulate debris by recruiting macrophages and monocytes which trigger a cytokine cascade leading to inflammation, fluid mobilization, and ultimately osteoclast recruitment and differentiation.
- The immune system response is dependent on particle size, volume, composition, and shape. Polyethylene or cement particles of sizes 0.2 to 10 μm are phagocytosed by macrophages while metal particles in the 50 nm range typically produce an ALVAL reaction.
- A proinflammatory cascade is modulated by TNF-α, MCP1, and PGE_2, which ultimately leads to osteoclast differentiation through a RANKL/OPG interplay.
- Targeting particle production and inflammatory cascades with statins and antioxidants such as ascorbic acid and N-acetylcysteine, or osteoclast differentiation by blocking RANKL, TNF-α, and MCP1, or osteoclast function through use of bisphosphonates are potential venues for future pharmacologic control of this damaging process

REFERENCES

1. Paxton EW, Cafri G, Nemes S, et al: An international comparison of THA patients, implants, techniques, and survivorship in Sweden, Australia, and the United States. *Acta Orthop* 2019;93:1-8.
2. Vijayvargiya M, Shetty V, Makwana K, Suri HS: Mid-term results of an uncemented tapered femoral stem and various factors affecting survivorship. *J Clin Orthop Trauma* 2019;10:368-373.
3. Caton J, Prudhon JL: Over 25 years survival after Charnley's total hip arthroplasty. *Int Orthop* 2011;35:185-188.
4. Baxter RM, MacDonald DW, Kurtz SM, Steinbeck MJ: Characteristics of highly cross-linked polyethylene wear debris in vivo. *J Biomed Mater Res Part B Appl Biomater* 2013;101:467-475.
5. Bauer TW, Schils J: The pathology of total joint arthroplasty. *Skeletal Radiol* 1999;28:483-497.

©Copyright 2021 American Academy of Orthopaedic Surgeons

6. Harris WH: Osteolysis and particle disease in hip replacement. A review. *Acta Orthop Scand* 1994;65:113-123.
7. Jones LC, Hungerford DS: Cement disease. *Clin Orthop Relat Res* 1987:192-206.
8. Haynes JA, Stambough JB, Sassoon AA, Johnson SR, Clohisy JC, Nunley RM: Contemporary surgical indications and referral trends in revision total hip arthroplasty: A 10-year review. *J Arthroplasty* 2016;31:622-625.
9. Morscher EW: Failures and successes in total hip replacement–why good ideas may not work. *Scand J Surg* 2003;92:113-120.
10. Goodman SB: Wear particles, periprosthetic osteolysis and the immune system. *Biomaterials* 2007;28:5044-5048.
11. Dumbleton JH, Manley MT, Edidin AA: A literature review of the association between wear rate and osteolysis in total hip arthroplasty. *J Arthroplast* 2002;17:649-661.
12. Chakrabarty G, Vashishtha M, Leeder D: Polyethylene in knee arthroplasty: A review. *J Clin Orthop Trauma* 2015;6:108-112.
13. Mabilleau G, Kwon Y-M, Pandit H, Murray DW, Sabokbar A: Metal-on-metal hip resurfacing arthroplasty: A review of periprosthetic biological reactions. *Acta Orthop* 2008;79:734-747.
14. Natu S, Sidaginamale RP, Gandhi J, Langton DJ, Nargol AVF: Adverse reactions to metal debris: Histopathological features of periprosthetic soft tissue reactions seen in association with failed metal on metal hip arthroplasties. *J Clin Pathol* 2012;65(5):409-418.
15. Vierra BM, Blumenthal SR, Amanatullah DF: Modularity in total hip arthroplasty: Benefits, risks, mechanisms, diagnosis, and management. *Orthopedics* 2017;40:355-366.
16. Willert HG, Semlitsch M: Reactions of the articular capsule to wear products of artificial joint prostheses. *J Biomed Mater Res* 1977;11:157-164.
17. Sukur E, Akman YE, Ozturkmen Y, Kucukdurmaz F: Particle disease: A current review of the biological mechanisms in periprosthetic osteolysis after hip arthroplasty. *Open Orthop J* 2016;10:241-251.
18. Bitar D, Parvizi J: Biological response to prosthetic debris. *World J Orthop* 2015;6:172-189.
19. Zhou Y, Mohan A, Moore DC, et al: SHP2 regulates osteoclastogenesis by promoting preosteoclast fusion. *Faseb J* 2015;29:1635-1645.
20. Giampreti A, Lonati D, Ragghianti B, et al: N-acetyl-cysteine as effective and safe chelating agent in metal-on-metal hip-implanted patients: Two cases. *Case Rep Orthop* 2016;2016, Article ID: 8682737, 7pp.
21. Fujita H, Ochi M, Ono M, et al: Glutathione accelerates osteoclast differentiation and inflammatory bone destruction. *Free Radic Res* 2019;53:226-236.
22. Cao JJ, Picklo MJ: N-acetylcysteine supplementation decreases osteoclast differentiation and increases bone mass in mice fed a high-fat diet. *J Nutr* 2014;144:289-296.
23. Fang Q, Wang H, Zhu S, Zhu Q: N-acetyl-L-cysteine inhibits wear particle-induced prosthesis loosening. *J Surg Res* 2011;168:e163-e172.
24. Thillemann TM, Pedersen AB, Mehnert F, Johnsen SP, Søballe K: The risk of revision after primary total hip arthroplasty among statin users: A nationwide population-based nested case-control study. *J Bone Joint Surg Am* 2010;92:1063-1072.
25. Lübbeke A, Garavaglia G, Rothman KJ, et al: Statins may reduce femoral osteolysis in patients with total hip arthroplasty. *J Orthop Res* 2013;31:814-820.

 ©Copyright 2021 American Academy of Orthopaedic Surgeons

2

STRUCTURE AND FUNCTION OF MUSCULOSKELETAL TISSUES

SECTION EDITORS

Linda J. Sandell, PhD, C-IAYT
Roy K. Aaron, MD

9

The Development, Growth, and Morphogenesis of the Skeleton

Maurizio Pacifici, PhD
Eiki Koyama, DDM, PhD

Keywords: *growth plate; joint formation; morphogenesis; pediatric skeletal disorders; skeletal development*

INTRODUCTION

The skeleton can be thought of as the ultimate morphogenetic machine determining the overall shape, size, organization, and features of the body. Paleontologists and biological anthropologists have long used bone fragments to envision and reconstruct the anatomic features of distant human ancestors, down to the level of facial composition and expression.[1] Thus, the formation, sculpting, and growth of the skeletal elements must be regarded as a feat of development, structure, organization, and evolution.[2] Biomedical research over recent decades has provided many important data and insights into mechanisms by which the skeletal tissues form and grow during fetal and postnatal life, how they develop their organization and structure, and how the major skeletal cell types (chondrocytes, osteoblasts, osteocytes, and osteoclasts) acquire their diversified and essential phenotypic functions.[3-8] Most skeletal elements, including the long bones, ribs, vertebrae, cranial base, vertebrae, and pelvis, are formed through endochondral ossification. During this process, mesenchymal cells differentiate into chondrocytes that produce and assemble the initial cartilaginous skeletal primordia and templates at prescribed sites and times, which serve as the blueprint for the corresponding ossified elements in the adult skeleton. The chondrocytes become organized into growth plates that represent the major engine of skeletal expansion and elongation. In the growth plates, the chondrocytes proliferate, accumulate large amounts of extracellular matrix, and undergo hypertrophy. The hypertrophic chondrocytes mineralize their matrix and provide the mineralized scaffold onto which osteoprogenitor cells differentiate and produce endochondral bone tissue.[6] The remaining skeletal elements including the calvaria, mandible, and a portion of the clavicle form through intramembranous ossification.[9] Ectomesenchymal cells differentiate directly into bone cells during this process.

Though distinct in many respects, the endochondral and intramembranous processes are more intimately connected than might be apparent. The first bone tissue to form in a developing long bone is intramembranous and is called the bone collar because it surrounds the incipient diaphysis. Likewise, the mandible forms in intimate association with the Meckel cartilage. The mandibular condyle, which articulates with the glenoid fossa to form the temporomandibular joint, is entirely endochondral. Research has also revealed that cells similar to chondrocytes are transiently present during the early stages of calvaria bone formation.[10]

In sum, cartilage and bone form and work in concert at multiple places and times during prenatal and postnatal life to bring about skeletogenesis and skeletal growth and morphogenesis. This chapter describes the key steps in the formation of the craniofacial, axial, and appendicular skeleton and discusses recent data on mechanisms regulating the behavior and function of skeletal progenitor and differentiated cells and the growth of skeletal elements. It also describes salient examples

Neither of the following authors nor any immediate family member has received anything of value from or has stock or stock options held in a commercial company or institution related directly or indirectly to the subject of this chapter: Dr. Pacifici and Dr. Koyama.

©Copyright 2021 American Academy of Orthopaedic Surgeons

of defects in such basic growth and developmental mechanisms that lead to congenital and acquired skeletal conditions in children and adults.

CRANIOFACIAL DEVELOPMENT AND GROWTH

The progenitor cells responsible for formation of the craniofacial skeletal elements originate embryonically from the ectodermal neural crest, the unsegmented paraxial mesoderm, and the most cephalic somites.[11,12] Between the first and second month of gestation, the progenitors migrate from their points of origin, proliferate, and assemble to form cell condensations at appropriate sites, producing initially over 100 distinct skeletogenic centers in the prospective skull.[12] Over increasing gestation time, consolidation and fusion amongst these skeletal primordial centers elicit formation of 45 skeletal elements by birth. Postnatal processes bring about a final reduction in number and the assembly of the mature 22 bones in the adult skull.

The different skull skeletal elements brought about by the above processes arise via an intramembranous or endochondral ossification process. The intramembranous elements (also called dermal bones) include the frontal and parietal cranial vault bones, the squama of the occipital and temporal bones, the zygomatic bone, the maxilla, and the mandible (**Figure 1**). The endochondral elements include the occipital bone, the cranial base, the mandibular condyle, the auditory ossicles, and the nasal bones (**Figure 1**). An alternative and common classification of skull skeletal elements takes into account their function rather than origin. Thus, the neurocranium includes the elements that surround and protect the brain—cranial vault and cranial base—and the sensory organs. The viscerocranium includes the elements of the face and pharyngeal arches.

Three-dimensional growth of the intramembranous elements continues through the remaining months of gestation and into early childhood. The process occurs mostly by apposition, during which progenitor cells differentiate into osteoblasts and are apposed onto the preexisting bone tissue. The progenitor cells responsible for appositional growth of the cranial vault elements are part of the fibrous connective and mesenchymal tissue masses called sutures and are connected at the fontanelles located at the corners where the elements meet (**Figure 1**). Progenitor cell function and differentiation in the sutures are controlled by various mechanisms. Chief among these mechanisms is action by members of the fibroblast growth factor (FGF) and hedgehog families of signaling proteins that may also be important in dictating progenitor cell function during skull fracture repair.[13,14] Growth and expansion of the cranial vault are closely coordinated with growth and expansion of the brain. The posterior and anterolateral fontanelles close during the first 3 months after birth; the other fontanelles remain open and close at approximately the age of 2 years. Defects and discoordination of these processes can have serious pathological consequences (see below).

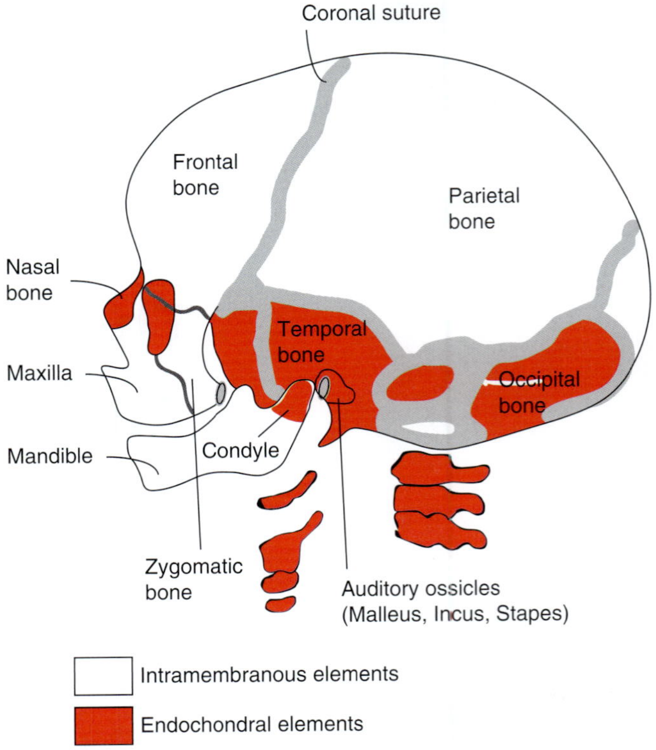

FIGURE 1 Schematic of craniofacial bones and their developmental nature. The intramembranous elements include the frontal and parietal cranial vault bones, the zygomatic bone, the maxilla, the mandible, and the squama of the occipital and temporal bones. The endochondral elements include the occipital and temporal bones, the mandibular condyle, the auditory ossicles, the nasal bones, and other cranial base elements.

The growth plates are responsible for enlargement and elongation of the craniofacial endochondral elements. Because the growth plates can be oriented in different directions and vary in size, they support and regulate skeletal elongation and ossification in distinct spatiotemporal directions and can fine-tune morphogenesis in three dimensions. One example is the exquisite shape and organization of the sella turcica of the sphenoid bone, which accommodates the pituitary gland. A special group of growth plates is present in the cranial base that is composed of the ethmoid, sphenoid, and occipital bones and other elements. These growth plates are called synchondroses, are active during fetal and early postnatal life, and are named according to their anatomical location: intrasphenoidal, spheno-occipital, and intraoccipital synchondroses (**Figure 2**, A and B). Each synchondrosis consists of two opposing, mirror-image growth plates that share a central reserve chondrocyte zone, display two proliferative, two prehypertrophic, and two hypertrophic zones, and sustain bidirectional growth along the naso-occipital axis (**Figure 2**, C and D). Despite their unique dual structure, the synchondrosis growth plates are regulated by most of the mechanisms that control the activity of single growth

 ©Copyright 2021 American Academy of Orthopaedic Surgeons

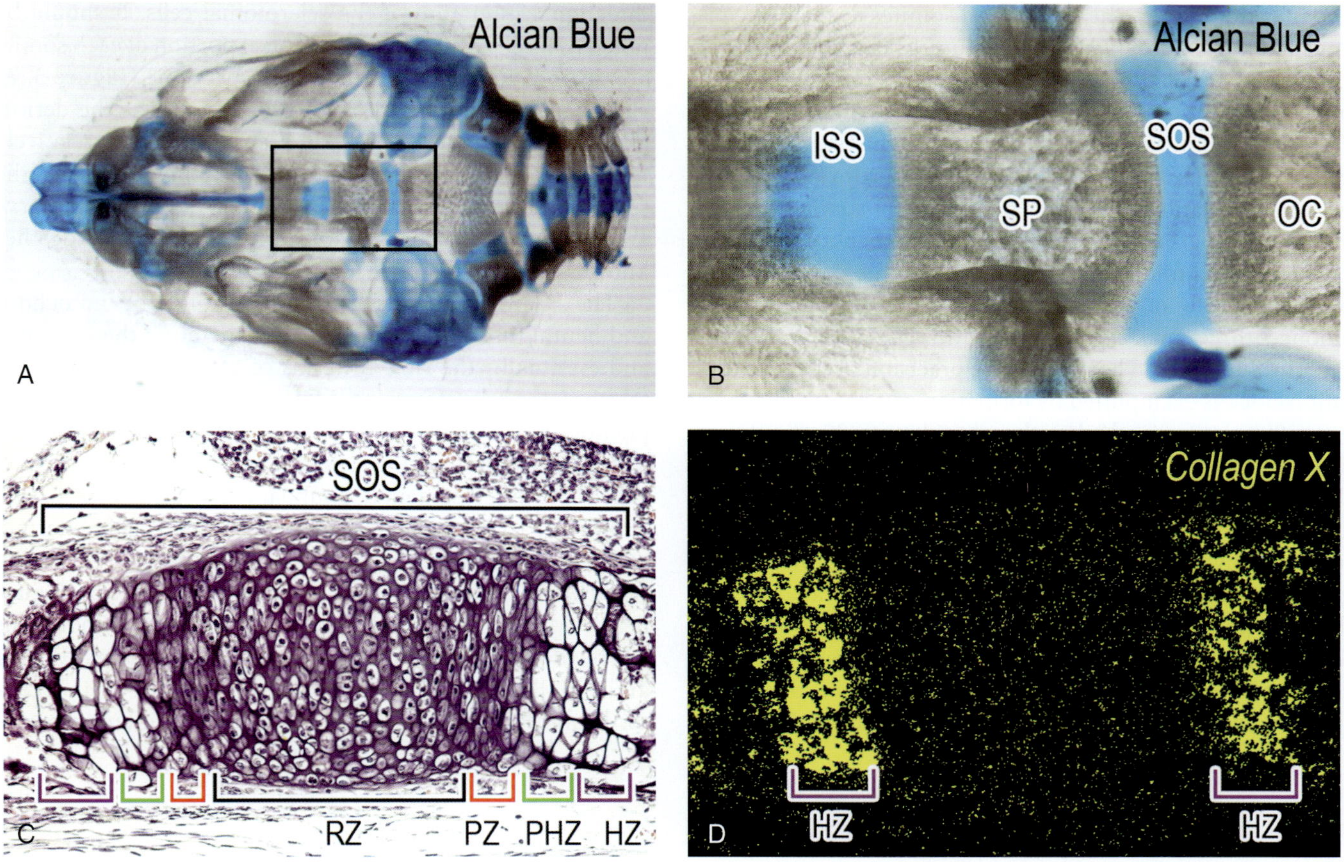

FIGURE 2 Whole mount and histological analyses of neonatal mouse skull. **A**, Bird-eye view of an alcian blue-stained specimen reveals the cartilaginous portions of the skull, including the cranial base synchondroses (box) and the nasal bones (on the left). **B**, High-magnification picture of the boxed area in (**A**) showing the intrasphenoid synchondrosis (ISS), the spheno-occipital synchondrosis (SOS), and the occipital (OC) and sphenoid (SP) bones. **C**, The pictures show the histological organization of the SOS dual growth plate with a central shared resting zone (RZ) that is flanked by two proliferative (PZ), prehypertrophic (PHZ), and hypertrophic (HZ) zones. **D**, The hypertrophic zones exhibit typical and very high *collagen X* gene expression revealed by in situ hybridization.

plates in all other locations in the developing and growing skeleton.[15,16] Under normal circumstances, the intraoccipital synchondrosis closes at the age of 1 to 3 years, while the spheno-occipital synchondrosis closes at puberty.

Clinically, defects in suture growth function and/or timing of closure can cause craniosynostoses that affect cranial base elongation and growth coordination and often have severe pathologic repercussions on brain development. Most craniosynostosis cases are due to gain-of-function mutations in the FGF receptor genes *FGFR1, FGFR2,* or *FGFR3* that alter the fine physiologic balance between proliferation and differentiation of progenitor cells, cause excessive bone differentiation, and provoke dysfunction and premature closure of the sutures.[17,18] Craniosynostoses affecting specifically the coronal suture are seen in patients with mutations in the transcription factor TWIST or the membrane-bound protein EPHRIN-B1. One side of the coronal suture arises from neural crest progenitors and the opposite side arises from mesodermal cells, and the boundary appears to be particularly sensitive to those mutations.[19] Defects in synchondrosis growth plate function and elongation rates can cause hypoplasia of the cranial base, as seen in Apert and Crouzon syndromes, and can have negative repercussions on overall skull growth, structure and organization.[20] Holoprosencephaly is a devastating condition caused by loss-of-function mutations in genes encoding Sonic hedgehog (*SHH*) or its receptor *PATCHED1*.[21] Hedgehog signaling is mediated by primary cilia on the surface of most cell types, and human syndromes affecting the craniofacial skeleton and other organs, such as Meckel-Gruber syndrome, are caused by malfunction of primary cilia-associated proteins.[22]

SOMITOGENESIS AND AXIAL SKELETON DEVELOPMENT

Beginning at approximately the third week of gestation, mesodermal cells flanking the neural tube and notochord (collectively called paraxial mesoderm) begin to locally condense, undergo a mesenchymal-to-epithelial transition

©Copyright 2021 American Academy of Orthopaedic Surgeons

(MET), and produce the first pair of somites near the incipient anatomical border between the future head and the trunk (**Figure 3**, A, left panel).[23] Additional pairs of somites form by the same process at very regular, short intervals along the cranial-to-sacral axis, a process known as the "segmentation clock." Somitogenesis is completed in approximately 1 week with the formation of more than 40 pairs of somites located all along the left and right sides of the notochord and neural tube. Rhythmic formation of each somite pair is driven by rapid cycles of activity by—and molecular integration among—three major signaling pathways: Notch, Wnt/β-catenin, and FGF.[24] The remarkable precision of the segmentation clock is exemplified by formation of a new somite pair every 90 minutes in chick embryos and every 20 minutes in zebrafish embryos.[25] Soon thereafter, the cells constituting the ventral portion of each somite pair (collectively known as the sclerotome) undergo an inverse process of epithelial-to-mesenchymal transition (EMT) and migrate toward and gather around the notochord, which remains located immediately below the neural tube (**Figure 3**, A, middle panel). Sonic hedgehog secreted by both the notochord and the adjacent ventral portion of the neural tube creates a concentration gradient in its surroundings and is responsible for such directional migration of the sclerotomal cells. It should be noted that cells constituting the dorsal portion of each somite are distinct and represent the dermomyotome (**Figure 3**, A, right panel) that will give rise to such tissues as the dermis and skeletal muscles in the trunk and limbs. The relatively few cells sandwiched between the dermomyotome and the sclerotome become marked by *scleraxis* expression, serve as progenitors for axial tendon formation and are together known as the syndetome (**Figure 3**, A, right panel).[26]

The sclerotomal cells gathering around the notochord and neural tube are responsible for generating the vertebrae and eventually, the ribs. In terms of vertebral developmental steps, the sclerotomal cells from each somite first become phenotypically subdivided into a larger cranial portion and a smaller caudal portion, and the border between them is called the intersegmental boundary or von Ebner fissure (**Figure 3**, B). Cranial cells from one somite pair intermix and condense with the caudal cells from the preceding somite pair and together, will produce each vertebra (**Figure 3**, B). Mixing and condensation of these subpopulations are regulated by expression of the ephrin receptors EPHA4 and EPHB3 in cranial cells and expression of their receptor ligand EPHRIN-B1 in caudal cells.[27] The intersegmental

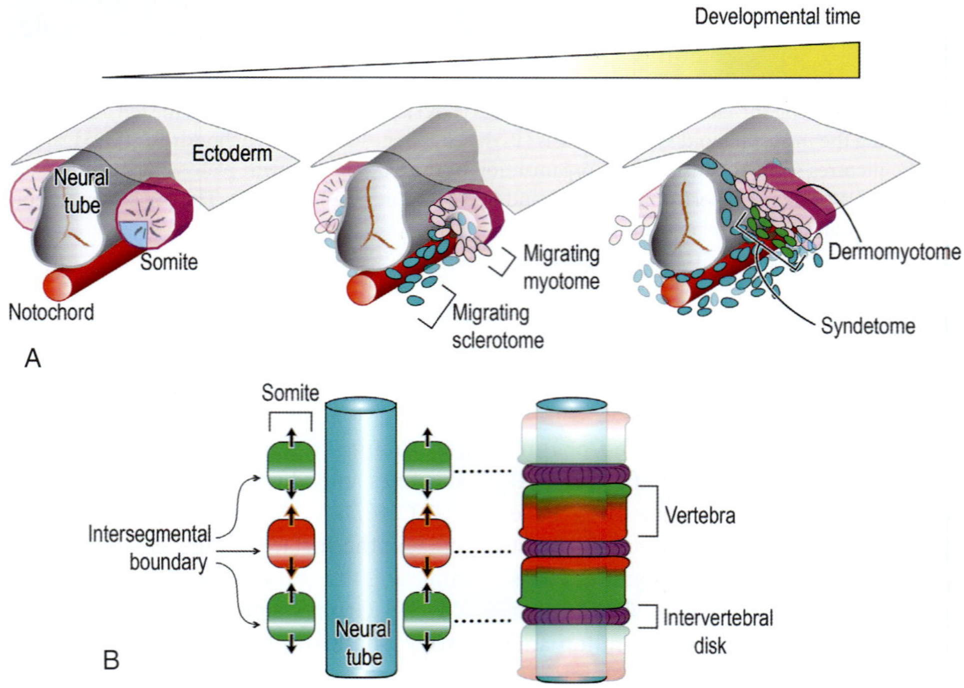

FIGURE 3 Schematics showing the formation of somites and the fate and roles of their cells. **A**, Somites initially form on each side of the neural tube (left panel). Following epithelial-to-mesenchymal transition, the sclerotomal cells migrate toward and surround the notochord and neural tube (middle and right panels). The more dorsal somatic cells give rise to the dermomyotome contributing to dermis and muscle development, while the intervening syndetome cells will generate axial skeleton ligaments. **B**, The schematic on the left shows somite pairs flanking the neural tube in which each somite is separated into cranial and caudal portions (in green and red colors) by an intervening intersegmental boundary. The schematic on the right shows that each vertebra is generated by the intermixing of cranial cells from one somite pair with caudal cells from the preceding somite pair. The location of the intersegmental boundary dictates where the intervertebral disks form and where peripheral nerves leave the neural tube.

 ©Copyright 2021 American Academy of Orthopaedic Surgeons

boundary within each somite represents the location where the intervertebral disk forms (**Figure 3**, B) and where the spinal nerves leave the spinal cord to innervate their diverse peripheral targets. To produce each vertebra, the condensed sclerotomal cells first undergo chondrogenesis and produce three-dimensionally complex cartilaginous templates corresponding to the distinct structure and portions of each vertebra, including the vertebral body, neural arches around the future vertebral foramen, and transverse processes. The notochordal cells trapped within the developing vertebral body undergo involution and disappear. The newly formed chondrocytes become organized into distinct growth plates, undergo hypertrophy and endochondral ossification, and produce the definitive bony vertebrae that surround the spinal cord. Spared from these maturation and hypertrophic processes are the chondrocytes located at the cranial and caudal vertebral ends that remain cartilaginous and produce the end plates articulating with the intervertebral disks (see below). As pointed out above, more than 40 somite pairs form initially.[23] However, the initial sclerotomes from the four occipital somites and the first cervical sclerotome aggregate to produce parachordal cartilages which fuse at midline and produce the occipital bone of the skull. In addition, many pairs of sacral somitic sclerotomes fuse to produce the sacrum and the coccyx, eventually leading to the establishment of the definitive 24 vertebrae. As these developmental and growth processes proceed, the spine acquires its typical species-specific curvature, as required for its normal biomechanical function and movement.[28] Very little is known of the mechanisms that regulate the spatiotemporal acquisition of normal spine curvature.

The intervertebral disks are critical for spine movement and shock absorption function. Each disk is composed of a centrally located nucleus pulposus and a surrounding anulus fibrosus (**Figure 4**, A). These two components have distinct embryologic origin. The progenitor cells producing the anulus fibrosus are those sclerotome cells located along the intersegmental boundary that do not participate in vertebra formation. The cells are still gathered around the notochord, but undergo differentiation into fibrocartilaginous cells that produce and deposit a matrix rich in collagens I and II endowed with stiffness and tensile strength, all needed for proper biomechanical function by the annulus. Instead, the progenitor cells responsible for nucleus pulposus formation are notochord cells, specifically those that become surrounded by intersegmental sclerotome cells.[29] Unlike the ephemeral notochord cells within each developing vertebral body, these notochord cells persist, differentiate into chondrocyte-like cells, and produce and accumulate a large amount of cartilaginous extracellular matrix. This matrix is rich in aggrecan and other proteoglycans but poor in collagen; it attracts a large quantity of water and ions and establishes a high osmotic pressure, which is believed to be essential for establishing the functional springiness and resilience of the disk. The intervertebral disk (anulus fibrosus plus nucleus pulposus) and flanking vertebral end plates together make up the joints of the spine, which, similar to synovial joints in the limbs, are characterized by local production of lubricating molecules such as lubricin (proteoglycan 4) that sustain movement and functional longevity and minimize mechanical friction (**Figure 4**, B and C).

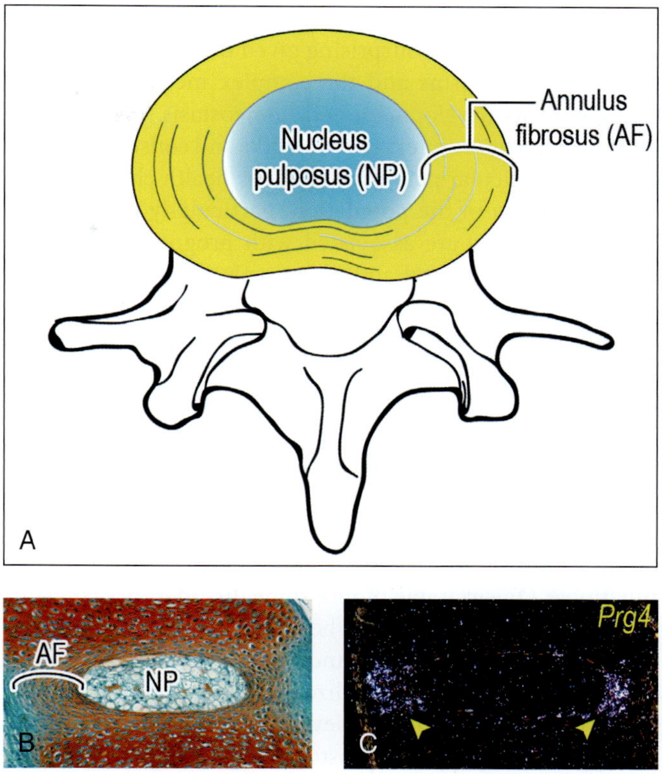

FIGURE 4 Structure and organization of an intervertebral disk and expression of joint lubricants. **A**, The schematic depicts the nucleus pulposus (NP, in blue) and anulus fibrosus (AF, in yellow) constituting the intervertebral disk that overlay the vertebral body connected to arches surrounding the spinal canal. **B**, Histological image showing the natural appearance of the NP and AF in the mouse spine, with adjacent end plate cartilage on both sides. **C**, Contiguous histological section processed for in situ hybridization showing that Prg4/lubricin is expressed all along the boundary between NP and AF.

With regard to the ribs, their development initiates at approximately the fifth week of embryogenesis with formation of small protrusions of lateral sclerotome-derived mesenchymal cells along the arches of all developing vertebrae. Only those in the thoracic region continue to grow and with time, curve ventrally to provide appropriate directionality to the mature ribs. The elongating thoracic ribs reach the developing sternum by embryonic day 45. Five additional lumbar ribs form that, however, are short, do not articulate with the sternum, and are called false ribs. All ribs are endochondral elements; they develop and elongate through the activities of a single growth plate that progressively shifts in relative position from dorsal toward ventral over time. The most ventral tip of the true ribs maintains a cartilaginous character to provide articulation with the sternum.

©Copyright 2021 American Academy of Orthopaedic Surgeons

Clinically, a number of common and rare disorders affect the axial skeleton, not surprising given the many demanding functions it performs and the complex mechanisms regulating both its development and homeostasis. For example, degeneration of the intervertebral disks and consequent back, neck, and radicular pain remain major health challenges for a large fraction of the population, particularly the elderly.[30] These conditions are associated with progressive derangement of disk structural and phenotypic integrity, including loss of extracellular proteoglycan matrix and water, thinning and stiffening of the tissues, and, ultimately, loss of functional resilience. Major pathogenic mechanisms include death of notochord-derived nucleus pulposus cells by apoptosis; increased levels of proinflammatory cytokines and immune cell infiltration; and ectopic appearance of microvessels and nerve fibers.[31] Current therapeutic attempts include stem cell therapies with notochord-like progenitors, surgical implantation of bioengineered disks, and antagonism of cytokine function.[32] One example of rare spine disorders are congenital forms of scoliosis that can be very pernicious, encompass several phenotypic patterns, and are difficult to treat.[33] Their pathogenesis includes generalized abnormalities in fetal vertebral segmentation and rib development as seen in patients with spondylothoracic dysostosis; regional abnormalities affecting a portion of the spine, such as cervical defects in Klippel-Feil patients; and local abnormalities affecting one or two vertebrae. Identification of siblings with congenital scoliosis has led to identification of possible causative mutations in genes that, interestingly, regulate the somatic segmentation clock and include such Notch signaling pathway components as *DLL3*, *HES7*, and *LUNATIC FRINGE*.[24]

LIMB PATTERNING AND ONSET OF SKELETOGENESIS

At approximately 3 weeks of embryogenesis, small protrusions known as limb buds begin to form along the incipient trunk at prescribed locations and represent the first overt sign of forelimb (arm) and hindlimb (leg) development. The limb buds are composed of an ectodermal tissue layer and are filled with mesenchymal cells. The latter originate from the lateral mesoderm, the somitic dermomyotome, and the neural crest,[12] and this triple origin reflects their distinct developmental fates and contributions over time. Thus, lateral mesoderm cells will produce all the limb skeletal elements, connective tissues, and ligaments; the somitic cells will produce all the limb skeletal muscles and endothelial cells; and the neural crest cells will produce melanocytes and Schwann cells. Once the limb buds appear, their further outgrowth progresses rapidly and is propelled and oriented by three key signaling centers acting along the proximal-distal, posterior-anterior, and dorsal-ventral axes of symmetry[34,35] (**Figure 5**, A and B). The apical ectodermal ridge (AER) is located at the very tip of the limb bud and regulates outgrowth and patterning along the proximal-to-distal axis (**Figure 5**, A). The AER cells produce FGF4, FGF8, FGF9, and FGF17, which diffuse and stimulate proliferation of the adjacent mesenchymal cells (collectively known as the progress zone), resulting in limb outgrowth. Experimentally, limb elongation stops if the ectodermal ridge is removed, but it can resume with application of exogenous recombinant FGFs. The zone of polarizing activity (ZPA) regulates patterning along the posterior-anterior axis. The ZPA consists of mesenchymal cells specifically located at the posterior margin of each limb bud that produce sonic hedgehog (**Figure 5**, B). SHH diffuses away from the cells, forms a concentration gradient along the posterior-to-anterior axis, and regulates patterning and skeletal element identity. For example, the high posterior concentration of SHH favors small finger formation, and the low anterior concentration of SHH favors thumb/big toe development. If the ZPA is

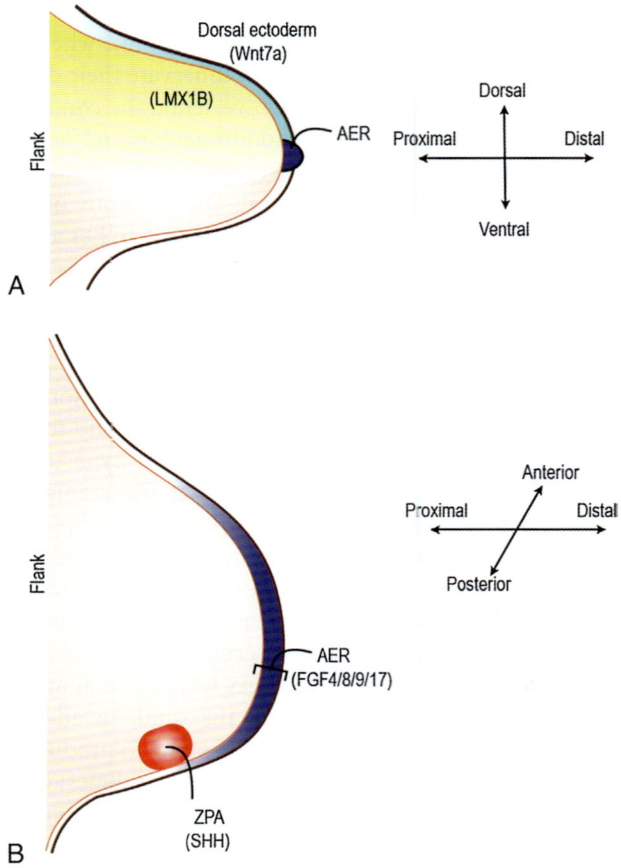

FIGURE 5 Schematics showing location of the major signaling centers in the limb bud. **A**, Transverse representation of a stereotypic limb bud. The apical ectodermal ridge (AER) at the distal tip directs development along the proximo-distal axis, while the dorsal ectoderm dictates development along the dorsal-ventral axis. **B**, Sagittal representation of the limb bud showing that the AER occupies a long equatorial portion of the limb bud and produces several fibroblast growth factors (FGFs) dictating cell proliferation in the progress zone and limb but outgrowth. The zone of polarizing activity (ZPA) is restricted to the posterior margin of the limb bud, produces Sonic Hedgehog (SHH), and regulates development along the posterior-anterior axis via a SHH-based gradient.

©Copyright 2021 American Academy of Orthopaedic Surgeons

microsurgically removed, the posterior-anterior axis of symmetry is completely disrupted. On the other hand, if an additional ZPA from a donor embryo is implanted into the anterior margin of a host limb bud (so that the host limb has two ZPAs and, thus, two opposite sources of SHH), two sets of limb skeletal elements form over time and are oriented in a mirror-image fashion along the posterior-to-anterior axis. Lastly, cells present in the dorsal ectoderm regulate limb patterning and skeletal growth along the dorsal-to-ventral axis and express factors such as wingless-type family member 7A (WNT7A) and homeobox protein LMX1B. When the dorsal ectoderm is microsurgically removed and transplanted to the ventral side, the dorsal-ventral axis is reversed 180° (eg, foot pads form on the dorsal side). A similar axis inversion is seen in transgenic *Wnt7a*-null mice. WNT7A function is mediated by LMX1B. Mice that are mutant for *Lmx1b* in the limbs lack dorsal structures; they also have defects along the posterior-anterior axis because *Lmx1b* regulates *Shh* expression in the ZPA.[36]

The AER, the ZPA, and the dorsal ectoderm interact and work in concert over time to regulate the emergence of mesenchymal preskeletal cell condensations within the core region of the limb bud, each condensation corresponding to a specific future skeletal element. The identity and character of the condensations—and the exact skeletal element to which each will give rise to—are under the regulatory jurisdiction of *HOX* genes (**Figure 6**). As revealed in mouse studies, *HOX10* paralogous genes dictate humerus and femur development (in the "stylopod" region of the limb), *HOX11* paralogous genes dictate development of radius and ulna and tibia and fibula (in the "zeugopod" region), and *HOX12* and *HOX13* genes regulate development of wrist, ankle, and digit skeletal elements (in the "autopod" region)[37,38] (**Figure 6**, A and B). For example, when all the six *HOX11* paralogous genes are concurrently ablated in mice, formation and growth of radius and ulna in the forelimb and tibia and fibula in the hindlimb are drastically reduced; however, the remaining elements in the stylopod and autopod remain normal[38,39] (**Figure 6**, C). The HOX genes likely influence formation and character of all other tissues and structures specific for each portion of the limb, including skeletal muscles and ligaments. To give rise to their respective specified skeletal elements, the mesenchymal cells within each condensation undergo chondrogenic cell differentiation and produce and assemble the initial cartilaginous template and backbone of each element. Chondrogenic differentiation requires positive action by transcription factors SOX5, SOX6, and SOX9 (the so-called SOX trio), bone morphogenetic proteins (BMPs), protein kinase A, and Hif1α[5,7,40] (**Figure 7**, A) and the concurrent reduction of inhibitory effectors and pathways including Wnt/beta-catenin, Notch and retinoid signaling.[41,42] The cartilaginous primordia become appreciable in the proximal region of the limb at about the fifth week of embryogenesis and in the distal region at about the sixth and seventh weeks.

In addition to the generation of new cells for growth, the normal development of the limb requires the elimination

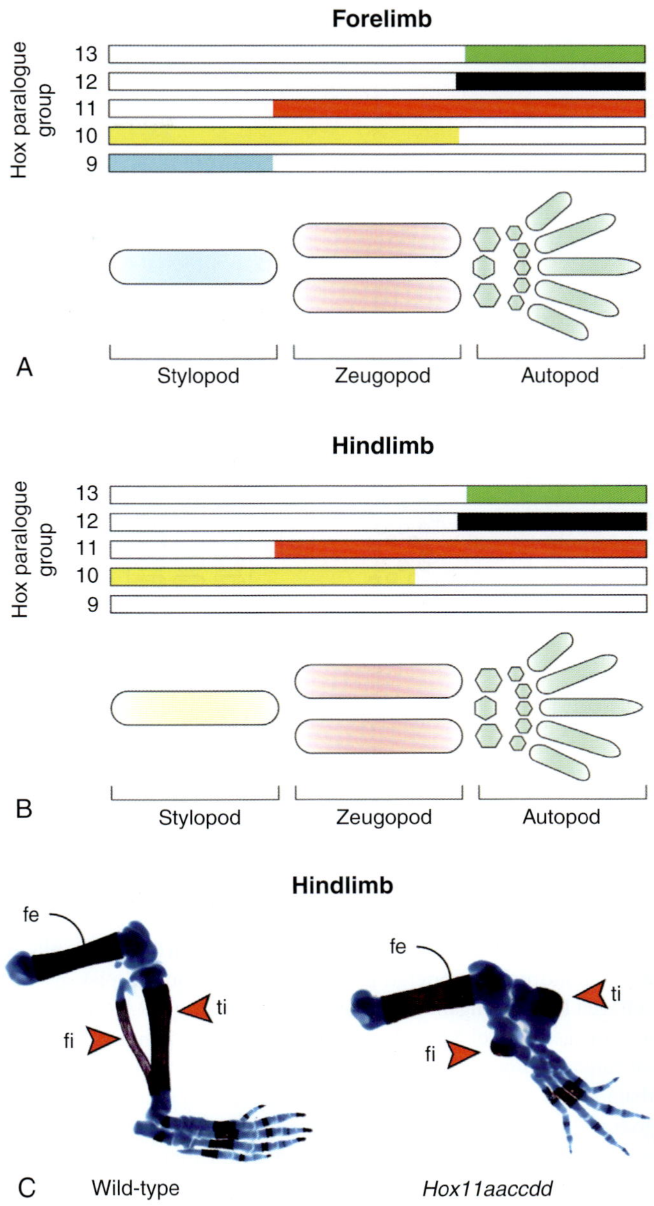

FIGURE 6 HOX gene expression patterns and regulation of limb skeletal element identity. **A** and **B**, Schematics of the gene expression domains of *HOX9* to *HOX13* paralogue genes depicted in different solid colors within the horizontal bars and juxtaposed to schematics of forelimb and hindlimb stylopods, zeugopods, and autopods. As an example, *HOX12* and *HOX13* genes are largely expressed in the autopod region, explaining why mutations in those genes cause various hand and foot skeletal defects in patients. **C**, Neonatal mouse hindlimb skeletons stained with alcian blue to reveal cartilage and alizarin red to reveal bone. Specimen on the left is from a normal wild-type mouse and shows normal skeletal elements including femur (fe), tibia (ti) and fibula (fi). Specimen on the right is from a companion mouse in which both alleles of *HOX11* paralogous genes (*Hoxa11*, *Hoxc11* and *Hoxd11*) were deleted. Because *HOX11* genes are mostly expressed in the zeugopod normally (see **A** and **B**), their complete deletion caused a severe reduction of tibia and fibula development, while femur and foot skeletal elements were unaffected.

©Copyright 2021 American Academy of Orthopaedic Surgeons

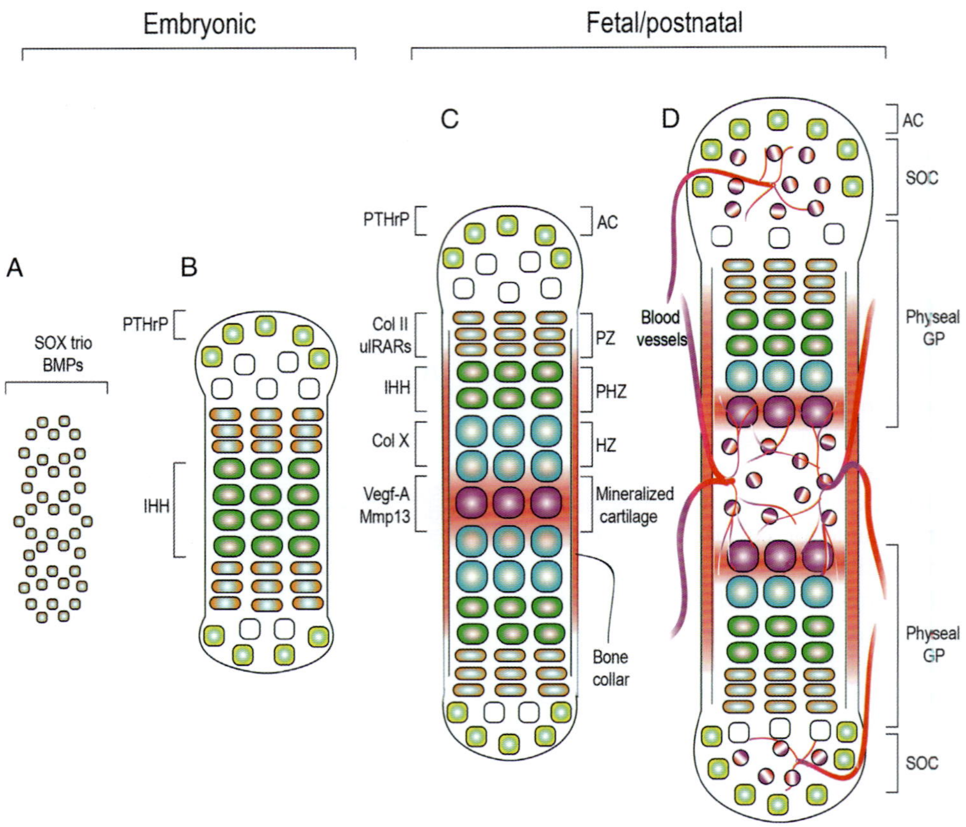

FIGURE 7 Schematic diagrams showing long bone inception, development, and growth. **A**, At early embryonic stages, condensed mesenchymal cells undergo chondrogenesis under SOX trio and BMP regulation and produce cartilaginous primordia. **B**, Soon after, the chondrocytes organize incipient growth plate zones in which IHH-expressing chondrocytes occupy the entire diaphyseal region and are flanked on both sides by flat proliferating cells and primitive periarticular/articular cells expressing PTHrP, establishing the IHH-PTHrP loop. **C**, With time, the long bone chondrocytes undergo further maturation and display all the typical growth plate zones, including a proliferative zone (PZ) expressing collagen II and unliganded retinoic acid receptors (ulRARs); a prehypertrophic zone (PHZ) expressing IHH; a hypertrophic zone (HZ) expressing collagen X (Col X); and a mineralizing zone expressing VEGF-A and MMP13. IHH diffusing into perichondrium triggers formation of the intramembranous bone collar around the incipient diaphysis. The most epiphyseal chondrocytes differentiate into permanent chondrocytes that assemble articular cartilage (AC) and sustain joint function. **D**, Later in fetal life and continuing postnatally, the diaphyseal region undergoes endochondral ossification following blood vessel invasion and formation of bone and marrow. Eventually, the epiphyses undergo ossification as well with formation of secondary ossification centers (SOC) and leading to the definition of the physeal growth plate (GP).

of certain populations of cells by programmed cell death (apoptosis). An important example of this mechanism can be seen in the autopod during the sixth and seventh weeks of embryogenesis, when the interdigit tissues are progressively eliminated to free the developing fingers and toes (the digit rays). Interdigit cell death depends on the concerted action of retinoic acid signaling, BMP family members, metalloproteinases, and HOXD13.[43-45] Increases or decreases in these regulators are known to lead to excessive or suboptimal cell death. Interdigit cell death is evolutionary and developmentally controlled; it does not occur in animals such as ducks in which the interdigit tissues are retained and are used to facilitate propulsion in water.

Clinically, aberrations in above mechanisms during early limb developmental stages can cause a number of pediatric pathologies. For instance, excessive signaling and action by SHH-dependent mechanisms in the ZPA are likely to be responsible for the formation of extra digits in patients with polydactyly.[46] Synpolydactyly and brachydactyly types D and E have been linked to mutations in *HOXD13*, while mutations in *HOXA13* have been documented in patients with hand-foot-genital syndrome.[47,48] Syndactyly is also observed in patients with Pfeiffer, Apert, or Jackson-Weiss syndromes who bear gain-of-function mutations in *FGFR2*.[49] It is believed that the resulting constitutive FGF signaling by mutant FGFR2 counters local BMP signaling, elicits survival of interdigit tissues, and results in webbing and syndactyly. Patients with Fuhrmann syndrome bear loss-of-function mutations in *WNT7A*, have defects in dorsal-ventral limb axis specification, and exhibit hypoplastic/aplastic nails and dorsal ectopic palms.[50]

©Copyright 2021 American Academy of Orthopaedic Surgeons

GROWTH PLATE ASSEMBLY AND ACTIVITY AND INDUCTION OF BONE FORMATION

Once the mesenchymal cells within each limb bud condensation undergo chondrogenesis and assemble the corresponding cartilaginous long bone primordia between approximately by the fourth to fifth week of embryogenesis (**Figure** 7, A), the chondrocytes organize themselves into a growth plate-like structure (**Figure** 7, B). Those occupying the entire diaphyseal region of each primordium begin to mature, enlarge into prehypertrophic chondrocytes, and turn on the expression of Indian hedgehog (IHH)[51,52] (**Figure** 7, B). The IHH-expressing chondrocytes interact with incipient most epiphyseal periarticular chondrocytes and induce them to express parathyroid hormone–related protein (PTHrP). The resulting IHH-PTHrP loop stimulates mitotic activity in underlying chondrocytes together with cyclin-D1 and SOX9, thus establishing proliferative zones and sustaining the initial elongation of the still cartilaginous long bone primordia. Shortly thereafter, the most diaphyseal chondrocytes further mature and develop into hypertrophic collagen X–producing cells. Formation of hypertrophic chondrocytes requires the action of RUNT-related transcription factors RUNX2 and RUNX3, FOXA2 and FOXA3, and MEF2C, a member of the myocyte enhancer factor-2; is promoted by Wnt/β-catenin and retinoid signaling; and is aided by effectors including WNT5A and NOTCH.[5,53-55] Thereafter, the hypertrophic chondrocytes reach their terminal stage of development, at which they change their phenotype (see below) and mineralize their matrix (**Figure** 7, C). The latter is an essential step because only mineralized matrix can serve as a suitable substrate for endochondral ossification that will follow. Mineralization involves the deposition and accumulation of hydroxyapatite crystals and is closely and topographically controlled by the hypertrophic chondrocytes by production and release of matrix vesicles.[56] The vesicles bud from the surface of the cells and already contain small preformed hydroxyapatite-rich crystals in their interior, in addition to calcium channels and alkaline phosphatase. The channels are thought to facilitate ingress of calcium and further growth of the crystals, that puncture the membrane, spread onto the surrounding matrix, and self-propagate in the presence of adequate levels of calcium, inorganic phosphate, and alkaline phosphatase. A number of mechanisms exist that are needed to restrict, limit, and delimit mineralization in terms of topography and extent, including pyrophosphate, osteopontin, matrix extracellular phosphoglycoprotein (MEPE), and matrix GLA protein (MGP). Excessive mineralization at ectopic sites such as aorta and connective tissues can occur after treatment with MGP inhibitors such as warfarin or in mice lacking *Mgp*.[57] By the end of this sequence of events, the fetal long bone elements contain a zone of terminally differentiated mineralizing hypertrophic chondrocytes occupying the diaphysis that are flanked on each side by zones of hypertrophic, prehypertrophic, and proliferating chondrocytes oriented toward the opposing epiphyses (**Figure** 7, C). The most epiphyseal cells will give rise to articular chondrocytes.

In addition to the IHH-PTHrP loop, there are other mechanisms that control and fine-tune the overall rates of chondrocyte proliferation, maturation, and hypertrophy. Prominent among these mechanisms are the FGF receptors and their ligands.[53] *FGFR3* is expressed in the proliferative zone, while *FGFR1* is expressed in the hypertrophic zone. Based on the phenotype of mice lacking *Fgfr3* and in patients with activating *FGFR3* mutations (see below), FGFR3 is known to serve as an important negative regulator of chondrocyte proliferation and hypertrophy. FGFR1 appears to exert similar, but lesser, roles. Ligands for these receptors are FGF9 and FGF18 that are produced by the surrounding perichondrium and are thought to diffuse into the chondrocyte zones, engage their receptors and elicit signaling via the STAT1 and MAPK pathways in coordination with the moderating action of C-type natriuretic peptide (CNP) and cyclic GMP. An additional and well-characterized moderator of chondrocyte maturation and hypertrophy is histone deacetylase 4 (HDAC4).[58] This protein is mostly expressed by prehypertrophic chondrocytes and represses production and activity of RUNX2 and MEF2 members, limiting the rates of hypertrophy. Another moderating mechanism is signaling by epidermal growth factor (EGF) receptor and ligands such as EGF and transforming growth factor-α (TGF-α). These components are all expressed in the prehypertrophic and hypertrophic zones and act to dampen the transition from hypertrophic to terminally differentiated mineralizing chondrocytes.[59] Lastly, additional regulators of growth plate functioning are the nuclear retinoic acid receptors (RARs). Data show that RARα and RARγ are dynamically expressed in the growth plate and operate as unliganded transcriptional repressors; their compound ablation markedly deranges growth plate function and skeletal elongation, indicating that they normally regulate overall growth rates.[55]

The first bone tissue that forms at the above embryonic stages of long bone development is intramembranous, and its formation is triggered by IHH produced by prehypertrophic chondrocytes. IHH diffuses into the adjacent perichondrium and induces resident progenitor mesenchymal cells to activate expression of osteogenic master genes—RUNX2 and Osterix (OSX)—and to directly differentiate into osteoblasts with the aid of WNT/β-catenin, BMP, and FGF signaling, resulting in formation of the so-called bone collar[51,60,61] (**Figure** 7, C). In the meantime, the hypertrophic and mineralizing chondrocytes begin to produce factors that are needed for endochondral ossification while concurrently turning off collagen X expression. Those factors include (i) vascular endothelial growth factor A (VEGF-A) and RANKL that facilitate invasion

2: Structure and Function of Musculoskeletal Tissues

©Copyright 2021 American Academy of Orthopaedic Surgeons

of mineralized cartilage by vascular, osteoprogenitor and osteoclastogenic cells from surrounding periosteal tissues; and matrix metalloproteases (MMPs) such as MMP9 and MMP13, which promote matrix breakdown, tissue remodeling and angiogenesis.[62-64] The concerted action by these and other factors and the differentiation of progenitors into their respective cell types elicit the replacement of mineralized hypertrophic cartilage with endochondral bone, vascular elements, and marrow (primary spongiosa) (**Figure** 7, D). Osteogenic cell differentiation is regulated by all the mechanisms described above that are involved in intramembranous bone collar formation, including RUNX2, OSX and WNT/β-catenin signaling, and osteoblasts proceed over time to further develop into osteocytes. It should be noted that the bone collar serves as the initial manifestation of cortical bone formation, a process that then continues over time by a mechanism of appositional growth by progenitors residing in periosteum and dependent on the unique action of BMP2.[65]

Genetic cell lineage tracing-tracking studies in mice have provided the experimental evidence for the sequence of cellular events leading to the above processes of osteogenesis. In particular, data do show that perichondrial/periosteal progenitors are responsible for bone collar formation and constitute the main cellular source for formation of cortical bone, whereas progenitor cells associated with invading blood vessels represent the main contingent for formation of endochondral bone in primary spongiosa trabecular bone.[62] These data agree with the long held idea that most hypertrophic mineralizing chondrocytes undergo apoptosis, are eliminated, and do not become bone cells themselves.[66] However, morphological studies had originally indicated that, occasionally, some hypertrophic chondrocytes survive and are incorporated into bone tissue.[67] Recent studies using genetic cell tracing with *Col10-CreER/LacZ* mice have found that an appreciable number of reporter-expressing hypertrophic chondrocytes survive and develop into osteoblasts and osteocytes within the primary spongiosa.[68] Thus, the exact roles and contributions of surviving hypertrophic chondrocytes versus osteoprogenitor cells in overall bone formation are issues that are still to be fully clarified.[69]

SECONDARY OSSIFICATION CENTER FORMATION AND PHYSEAL PLATE DEFINITION, ACTIVITY, AND CLOSURE

Toward the end of embryogenesis and early postnatal life, the cartilaginous epiphyseal portions of the long bone elements undergo endochondral ossification, eventually resulting in the formation of a secondary ossification center (SOC) (**Figure** 7, D). Thus, chondrocytes located in the deepest, central portion of the epiphysis begin to enlarge and mature into prehypertrophic and hypertrophic chondrocytes. Concurrently, blood vessels and connective tissue cells originating in surrounding tissues penetrate the epiphyses from very specific locations—forming cartilage canals—and reach the central core.[70] The arrival of blood vessels allows the chondrocyte maturation process to be completed with the generation of endochondral bone that spreads radially within the epiphysis at nearly 360°. Endochondral ossification in the SOC obeys all the major mechanisms that regulate primary ossification in the diaphysis, including RUNX2/OSX, metalloproteases, and Wnt/β-catenin and EGFR signaling.[71,72] One notable difference is that while angiogenic and osteoprogenitor cells invaded mineralized hypertrophic cartilage during primary ossification in the diaphysis, the cells need to invade nonhypertrophic and unmineralized cartilage during the early phases of SOC formation. Most long bones have two SOCs, although the metacarpals and metatarsals have only one. Spared from maturation, hypertrophy, and ossification are the most epiphyseal articular chondrocytes abutting the synovial cavity that retain a permanent phenotype, assemble articular cartilage, and sustain joint function throughout life (see below).

The formation of the SOCs thus leads to the definition of the growth plate as the classic postnatal "physeal plate" flanked by bone on both sides. Most long bones have two growth plates each located toward the epiphyseal end. Interestingly, the growth plates have distinct rates of activity and contribution to elongation even within the same skeletal elements, as seen in the proximal and distal growth plates in the radius and ulna.[73] It is likely that these divergent rates of postnatal growth activity are due to intrinsic mechanisms normally operating in growth plate—including the IHH-PTHrP loop and FGFR-FGF signaling—as well as to systemic factors. The most prominent among the latter are growth hormone, liver-derived insulinlike growth factor–1, thyroid hormone (TH), and vitamin D. For example, the TH receptors TRα1, TRα2, and TRβ1 are expressed in the growth plate—particularly in the proliferative and prehypertrophic zones—and interact with the IHH-PTHrP loop to regulate the overall rates of chondrocyte proliferation and maturation.[74] It has also been observed that TH action influences the columnar and zonal organization of growth plate chondrocytes and, hence, their functioning. Indeed, TH deficiencies can lead to short stature, disorganization of the growth plate, and delays in endochondral ossification as also mouse studies suggest.[75]

It should be noted that chondrocyte hypertrophy is the main propeller of overall skeletal growth and elongation, with chondrocyte proliferation and cartilaginous matrix accumulation acting as additional but not major contributors.[76] Notably, skeletal growth and long bone elongation are not continuous, but are most prominent at night. This recumbency pattern suggests that the growth plates can pause in their activity and that intrinsic and systemic circadian mechanisms and circuits play major roles in their

 ©Copyright 2021 American Academy of Orthopaedic Surgeons

discontinuous activity and skeletal growth rates.[77] This is in keeping with the fact that biomechanical loading and compression forces across the growth plate are known to reduce growth (the Heuter-Volkmann law), while increases in tensile forces can stimulate growth (the Delpech law). Thus, the relatively prominent growth during recumbency is likely to reflect a relaxation of compression. Under normal circumstances, the growth plates continue to operate under the influence of all of the above complex local and systemic factors and pathways through the end of puberty, when skeletal growth is complete and the growth plates close under the influence of mechanisms including estrogen, which acts through its receptors ERα and ERβ.[78]

GROWTH PLATE PATHOLOGIES

Given the multitude of mechanisms regulating the development and functioning of growth plates prenatally and postnatally, it is not surprising that growth plate function can be deranged in multiple manners, leading to a broad spectrum of skeletal dysplasias and other pathologies.[79] One example is achondroplasia that is the most common form of dwarfism in humans. The disease is caused by autosomal dominant mutations in *FGFR3* that stabilize the receptor, favor receptor dimerization, and enhance its tyrosine kinase activity.[80] Given that FGFR3 normally acts to limit and reduce chondrocyte proliferation, the constitutive activity of its mutant form in achondroplasia results in severe suppression of chondrocyte proliferation, precocious chondrocyte hypertrophy, and growth stoppage. Short limbs and dwarfism also are seen in Jansen-type metaphyseal chondrodysplasia caused by activating mutations in the PTH/PTHrP receptor 1 (*PTHR1*), which are found to cause a severe retardation of chondrocyte maturation, chondrocyte hypertrophy, and matrix mineralization and are associated with hypercalcemia. Nutritional rickets is caused by a vitamin D deficiency that disturbs calcium and phosphate homeostasis and causes low serum phosphate levels.[81] In turn, these changes lead to substandard growth plate and bone mineralization and culminate with broadening and weakening of the hypertrophic zone and osteomalacia, with collateral pathologies including hypocalcemic seizures and heart failure. Because phosphate has a role in apoptosis of hypertrophic chondrocytes, it is likely that the broadening of the hypertrophic zone is caused by inhibition of apoptosis, while osteomalacia would be caused by defective mineralization of preexisting bone during remodeling. Hypophosphatasia, a related condition, is caused by missense mutations in the tissue-nonspecific alkaline phosphatase gene (*ALPL*).[82] Its clinical expression ranges from prenatal death with severe hypomineralization to an adult propensity to fracture, probably related to the severity of the mutation and loss of function. Mutations in *IHH* that reduce its bioactivity are associated with brachydactyly type A1 and other skeletal growth deficiencies, reflecting the broadly relevant roles of *IHH* in skeletal development and growth plate function.[83] Hereditary multiple exostoses (also known as multiple osteochondroma) is a pediatric disorder characterized by osteochondroma formation next to the growth plate, causing major health problems that include skeletal growth retardation, deformities, and chronic pain.[84] HME is caused by mutations in *EXT1* or *EXT2* that are responsible for heparan sulfate (HS) synthesis.[85] The resulting HS deficiency leads to ectopic distribution and action by HS-binding signaling proteins—most prominently BMPs—in perichondrium, triggering ectopic chondrogenesis and osteogenesis and, in turn, osteochondroma development. Ectopic BMP signaling has been shown to be an effective therapeutic target for HME.[86]

JOINT FORMATION, ORGANIZATION, AND VULNERABILITIES

The skeletal elements articulate with one another by means of three main types of joints. Synarthroses are fibrous joints that connect neighboring bones but allow little or no movement; examples are the joints between the cranial bones. Amphiarthroses are fibrocartilaginous joints that allow some movement; important examples are the intervertebral joints (disks), the costochondral joints, and the pubic symphysis. Diarthroses are joints that allow full and largely free movement of the skeletal elements, and a prominent example are the limb synovial joints. These joints are isolated from the surrounding environment and tissues by the synovial capsule that encloses a synovial cavity filled with fluid and lubricants, including hyaluronan, lubricin, and phospholipids. Most current information on joint development is related to the formation of limb synovial joints,[87-91] and thus, the focus here is on these joints.

The onset of limb joint formation becomes histologically apparent during embryonic life with the emergence of the so-called mesenchymal "interzone" at each prescribed joint location, first proximally and then distally (**Figure 8**, A and B). The interzone at the elbow and knee locations forms at approximately the fifth week of gestation, and the interzones between phalangeal elements appear at approximately the sixth week. The interzone is composed of flat, tightly packed mesenchymal cells that initially define and delineate the anatomic boundary between the adjacent cartilaginous long bone primordia. Several signaling molecules and pathways converge on the interzone cells to establish their mesenchymal character at these early stages of joint formation, including GDF5, WNT9A and WNT4, the BMP signaling inhibitor Noggin, the hedgehog signaling modulator HIP-1, members of the nuclear retinoic acid receptor family, and members

©Copyright 2021 American Academy of Orthopaedic Surgeons

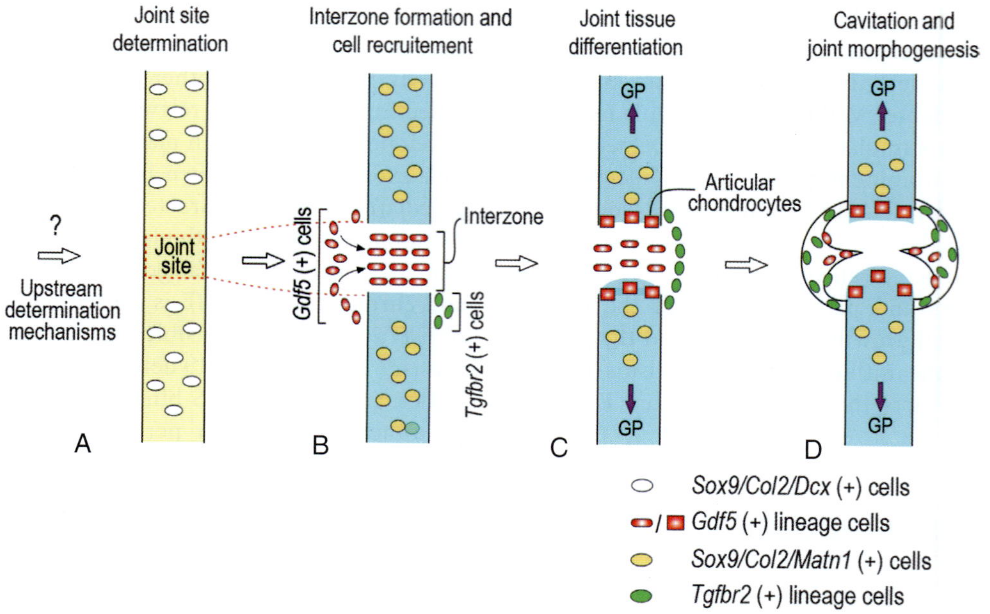

FIGURE 8 Schematic depicting the major phases of synovial joint development. **A**, At early embryonic stages, the limb skeletal primordia are composed of condensed cells descendants of progenitors expressing *Sox9*, *Col2*, and *Dcx* (*Sox9/Col2/Dcx+* lineage cells) with no overt sign of joint formation. Anatomical location of the future joint is determined by as yet obscure upstream site determination mechanisms. **B**, Soon after, the condensed cells undergo chondrogenesis and give rise to the cartilaginous primordia (in blue), while the joint site becomes occupied by flat-shaped and compacted interzone cells expressing *Gdf5* (*Gdf5+* lineage cells). Progenitors near the joint site are distinguished by *Tgfbr2* expression (*Tgfbr2+* lineage cells in green). **C**, With time, the chondrocytes in the shaft (*Sox9/Col2/Matn1+* lineage cells) become organized in growth plates (GP), while the interzone *Gdf5+* progenitors plus additional neighboring flanking cells give rise to most if not all differentiated joint tissues, including articular chondrocytes (in red). **D**, Eventually, the incipient joints undergo cavitation and morphogenesis, creating a synovial cavity filled with lubricants and a capsule insulating the joint from the body environment. Cell lineage tracing suggest that the *Gdf5+* flanking cells and the *Tgfbr2+* cells would together give rise primarily to capsule and synovial lining.

of the TGF-β family. With further time, the incipient joints become more distinct with the differentiation of typical tissues including articular cartilage, and joint cavitation and morphogenesis and capsule formation become apparent (**Figure 8**, C and D).

Decades ago, classic experiments showed that microsurgical removal of the interzone in early embryos causes joint ablation and fusion, demonstrating that the interzone is not merely a transient mesenchymal boundary but is needed for joint formation. Subsequent genetic cell lineage tracing using *GDF5Cre/reporter* mouse embryos revealed that the *GDF5*-expressing interzone cells (*GDF5+*) give rise to most if not all joint tissues over developmental time, including articular cartilage, intrajoint ligaments, synovial lining, and inner capsule[92] (**Figure 9**). These experiments demonstrated that interzone cells represent a specialized subset of limb mesenchymal progenitor cells that are endowed with the unique capacity to produce joint tissues. What still remains unclear is how the interzone cells enter specific differentiation paths and lineages to produce the diverse joint tissues. Recent studies have suggested that the initial interzone cells present from the very onset of joint formation give rise to centrally located tissues including articular cartilage and intrajoint ligaments, while additional surrounding *GDF5+* cells and *Tgfbr2+* cells are recruited and would mainly contribute to capsule and synovial lining formation (**Figure 8**, C and D). These possibilities need to be further tested. In addition, it remains essentially a mystery how articular chondrocytes differentiate from interzone cells and retain a stable cartilage phenotype lasting through life, thus avoiding the maturation and hypertrophy and the ephemeral character of growth plate chondrocytes. Equally unclear is exactly how during postnatal life articular cartilage acquires its functional thickness and multizone organization that are required for its functional biomechanical properties.

Clinically, synovial joints are affected by a number of pathologies. Osteoarthritis is a most common condition affecting the majority of people older than 65 years and involves the progressive structural and phenotypic deterioration of articular cartilage and loss of joint function. There is also a pediatric condition, osteochondritis dissecans (OCD), that affects juvenile patients—and females in particular—and is characterized by segmental loss of articular cartilage. These and other joint conditions are particularly challenging because articular cartilage has very poor intrinsic repair and regenerative capacity, possibly due to

©Copyright 2021 American Academy of Orthopaedic Surgeons

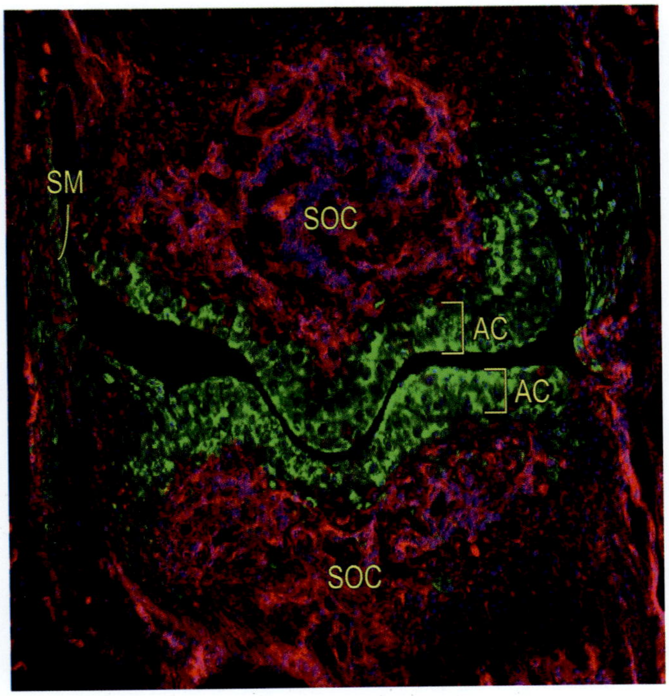

FIGURE 9 Genetic cell tracing analysis of joint development. This fluorescent image shows a metatarsal joint in a P14 transgenic *Gdf5Cre/R26-mTmG* mouse in which *Gdf5+* lineage cells produce green fluorescent protein (GFP), while all the other surrounding cells and issues produce red fluorescent protein (RFP). The data clearly show that the *Gdf5+* cells are restricted to, and produce only, joint tissues including articular cartilage (AC) and synovial membrane (SM). SOC = secondary ossification center. (These data were part of studies conducted by Dr. Rebekah S. Decker, a former postdoctoral researcher in the authors' laboratories.)

its normal lack of a blood supply and despite the presence of progenitor cells in its superficial lubricant-producing zone.[88] Thus, major efforts have long been directed to testing combinations of marrow- or fat-derived progenitor stem cells with bioengineering tools to heal and/or regenerate damaged articular cartilage. Most often, however, the repair tissue displays a cartilaginous character early on after therapeutic intervention, but it does not maintain it over time and eventually acquires a fibrous phenotype, with poor biomechanical characteristics and poor functional resilience.[93] While there are many possible reasons as to why these therapeutic strategies continue to be substandard and ineffective, the current lack of in-depth knowledge about articular cartilage developmental biology is not helping either. We can thus hope that major advances in the latter area will allow the creation of novel future therapies that combine principles and mechanisms of developmental biology with progenitor cells and bioengineering tools to re-create and reestablish a functional articular cartilage tissue in affected patients, young and older alike.

SUMMARY

This synopsis of skeletal development and growth in the skull, trunk, and limbs summarizes the remarkable features of these processes as well as their sheer complexity. The work of many biomedical and clinical research groups over past years has provided much information and insights on the cellular, biochemical, molecular, and biomechanical regulation of normal skeletal development, growth, and morphogenesis, and the resulting information has clarified the pathogenic basis of several skeletal diseases. However, much remains to be discovered. Undoubtedly, such concerted efforts will continue to broaden and deepen basic information on skeletal development, will yield new insights into pathogenesis, and will in turn lead to new diagnostic strategies and therapeutic tools to treat congenital and acquired skeletal disorders.

REFERENCES

1. Trinkaus E: Neandertal faces were not long; modern human faces are short. *Proc Natl Acad Sci USA* 2003;100:8142-8145.
2. Hall BK: *Bones and Cartilage. Developmental and Evolutionary Skeletal Biology*. San Diego, Elsevier Academic Press, 2005.
3. Dallas SL, Prideaux M, Bonewald LF: The osteocyte: An endocrine cell... and more. *Endocrine Rev* 2013;34:658-690.
4. Feng X, Teitelbaum SL: Osteoclasts: New insights. *Bone Res* 2013;29:11-26.
5. Kozhemyakina E, Lassar AB, Zelzer E: A pathway to bone: Signaling molecules and transcription factors involved in chondrocyte development and maturation. *Development* 2015;142:817-831.
6. Kronenberg HM: Developmental regulation of the growth plate. *Nature* 2003;423:332-336.
7. Lefebvre V, Bhattaram P: Vertebrate skeletogenesis. *Curr Top Dev Biol* 2010;90:291-317.
8. Long F: Building strong bones: Molecular regulation of the osteoblast lineage. *Nat Rev Mol Cell Biol* 2012;13:27-38.
9. Helms JA, Schneider RA: Cranial skeletal biology. *Science* 2003;423:326-331.
10. Nah H-D, Pacifici M, Gerstenfeld LC, Adams SL, Kirsch T: A transient chondrogenic phase in intramembranous pathway during normal skeletal development. *J Bone Min Res* 2000;15:522-533.
11. Couly GF, Coltey PM, Le Douarin NM: The triple origin of skull in higher vertebrate: A study in quail-chick chimeras. *Development* 1993;117:409-429.
12. Schoenwolf GC, Bleyl SB, Brauer PR, Francis-West PH: *Origin of skull*, in *Larsen's Human Embryology*, ed 5. Philadelphia, Churchill Livingstone Elsevier, 2015, pp 431-440.
13. Ornitz DM, Marie PJ: FGF signaling pathways in endochondral and intramembranous bone development and human genetic disease. *Genes Dev* 2002;16:1446-1465.
14. Zhao H, Feng JQ, Ho T-V, Grimes W, Urata M, Chai Y: The suture provides a niche for mesenchymal stem cells of craniofacial bones. *Nat Cell Biol* 2015;17:386-398.
15. Koyama E, Young B, Nagayama M, et al: Conditional Kif3a ablation causes abnormal hedgehog signaling topography, growth plate dysfunction, and excessive bone and cartilage formation during mouse skeletogenesis. *Development* 2007;134:2159-2169.

©Copyright 2021 American Academy of Orthopaedic Surgeons

16. Shum L, Kane AA, Nuckolls GH: BMP4 promotes chondrocyte proliferation and hypertrophy in the endochondral cranial base. *Int J Dev Biol* 2003;47:423-431.
17. Marie PJ, Coffin JD, Hurley MM: FGF and FGFR signaling in chondrodysplasia and craniosynostosis. *J Cell Biochem* 2005;96:888-896.
18. Johnson D, Wilkie AO: Craniosynostosis. *Eur J Hum Genet* 2011;19:369-376.
19. Zafeiriou DI, Pavidou EL, Vargiami E: Diverse clinical and genetic aspects of craniofrontonasal syndrome. *Pediatr Neurol* 2011;44:83-87.
20. Wilkie AOM: Craniosynostosis: Genes and mechanisms. *Hum Mol Genet* 1997;6:1647-1656.
21. Roessier E, Belloni E, Gaudenz K, et al: Mutations in the human Sonic hedgehog gene cause holoprosencephaly. *Nature Genet* 1996;14:357-360.
22. Hildebrandt F, Benzing T, Katsanis N: Ciliopathies. *N Engl J Med* 2011;364:1533-1543.
23. Schoenwolf GC, Bleyl SB, Brauer PR, Francis-West PH: *Development of the musculoskeletal system*, in *Larsen's Human Embryology*, ed 5. Philadelphia, Churchill Livingstone Elsevier, 2015, pp 172-196.
24. Pourquie O: Vertebrate segmentation: From cyclic gene networks to scoliosis. *Cell* 2011;145:650-663.
25. Aulehla A, Johnson RL: Dynamic expression of lunatic fringe suggests a link between notch signaling and an autonomous cellular oscillator driving somite segmentation. *Dev Biol* 1999;207:49-61.
26. Brent AE, Schweitzer R, Tabin CJ: A somitic compartment of tendon progenitors. *Cell* 2003;113:235-248.
27. Durbin L, Brennan C, Shiomi K, et al: Eph signaling is required for segmentation and differentiation of the somites. *Genes Dev* 1998;12:3096-3109.
28. Burwell RG, James NJ, Johnson F, Webb JK, Wilson YG: Standardised trunk asymmetry scores. A study of back contour of health school children. *J Bone Joint Surg Br* 1983;65:452-463.
29. Choi KS, Cohn MJ, Harfe BD: Identification of nucleus pulposus precursor cells and notochord remnants in the mouse: Implications for disk degeneration and chordoma formation. *Dev Dyn* 2008;237:3953-3958.
30. Walker BF: The prevalence of low back pain: A systematic review of the literature from 1966 to 1998. *J Spinal Disord* 2000;13:205-217.
31. Risbud MV, Shapiro IM: Role of cytokines in intervertebral disc degeneration: Pain and disc content. *Nature Rev Rheumatol* 2014;10:44-56.
32. Shapiro IM, Risbud MV: *The Intervertebral Disc: Molecular and Structural Studies of the Disc in Health and Disease*. Vienna, Springer Verlag GMBH, 2016.
33. Janicki JA, Alman B: Scoliosis: Review of diagnosis and treatment. *Paediatr Child Health* 2007;12:771-776.
34. Towers M, Tickle C: Growing models of vertebrate limb development. *Development* 2009;136:179-190.
35. Zeller R, Lopez-Rios J, Zuniga A: Vertebrate limb bud development: Moving towards integrative analysis of organogenesis. *Nature Rev Genet* 2009;10:845-858.
36. Yang Y, Niswander L: Interactions between the signaling molecules Wnt7a and Shh during vertebrate limb development: Dorsal signals regulate anteroposterior patterning. *Cell* 1995;80:939-947.
37. Koyama E, Yasuda T, Wellik DM, Pacifici M: Hox11 paralogous genes are required for formation of wrist and ankle joints and articular surface organization. *Ann NY Acad Sci* 2010;1192:307-316.
38. Wellik DM, Capecchi MR: Hox10 and Hox11 genes are required to globally pattern the mammalian skeleton. *Science* 2003;301:363-367.
39. Koyama E, Yasuda T, Minugh-Purvis N, et al: Hox11 genes establish synovial joint organization and phylogenetic characteristics in developing mouse zeugopod skeletal elements. *Development* 2010;137:3795-3800.
40. Hojo H, McMahon AP, Ohba S: An emerging regulatory landscape for skeletal development. *Trends Genet* 2016;32:774-787.
41. Day TF, Guo X, Garrett-Beal L, Yang Y: Wnt/β-catenin signaling in mesenchymal progenitors controls osteoblast and chondrocyte differentiation during vertebrate skeletogenesis. *Dev Cell* 2005;8:739-750.
42. Weston AD, Chandraratna RAS, Torchia J, Underhill TM: Requirement for RAR-mediated gene repression in skeletal progenitor differentiation. *J Cell Biol* 2002;158:39-51.
43. Schoenwolf GC, Bleyl SB, Brauer PR, Francis-West PH: *Development of the limbs*, in *Larsen's Human Embryology*. Philadelphia, Churchill Livingstone Elsevier, 2015, pp 501-523.
44. Weston AD, Hoffman LM, Underhill TM: Revisiting the role of retinoid signaling in skeletal development. *Birth Defects Res C Embryo Today* 2003;69:156-173.
45. Zou H, Niswander L: Requirement of BMP signaling in interdigital apoptosis and scale formation. *Science* 1996;272:738-741.
46. Lettice LA, Heaney SJH, Purdie LA, et al: A long-range Shh enhancer regulates expression in the developing limb and fin and is associated with preaxial polydactyly. *Hum Mol Genet* 2003;12:1725-1735.
47. Johnson D, Kan S-H, Oldridge M, et al: Missense mutations in the homeodomain of HOXD13 are associated with brachydatyly types D and E. *Am J Hum Genet* 2003;72:984-997.
48. Mortlock DP, Innis JW: Mutation in HOXA13 in hand-foot-genital syndrome. *Nat Genet* 1997;15:179-180.
49. Slaney SF, Oldridge M, Hurst JA, et al: Differential effects of FGFR2 mutations on syndactyly and cleft palate in Apert syndrome. *Am J Hum Genet* 1996;58:923-932.
50. Woods CG, Stricker S, Seemann P, et al: Mutations in WNT7A cause a range of limb malformations, including Fuhrmann syndrome and Al-Awadi/Raas-Rothschild/Schinzel phocomelia syndrome. *Am J Hum Genet* 2006;79:402-408.
51. Koyama E, Leatherman JL, Noji S, Pacifici M: Early chick limb cartilaginous elements possess polarizing activity and express *Hedgehog*-related morphogenetic factors. *Dev Dynam* 1996;207(3):344-354.
52. Vortkamp A, Lee K, Lanske B, Segre GV, Kronenberg HM, Tabin CJ: Regulation of rate of cartilage differentiation by Indian hedgehog and PTH-related protein. *Science* 1996;273:613-622.
53. Long F, Ornitz DM: Development of the endochondral skeleton. *Cold Spring Harb Perspect Biol* 2013;5:a008334.
54. Pacifici M: Retinoid roles and action in skeletal development and growth provide the rationale for an ongoing heterotopic ossification prevention trial. *Bone* 2018;109:267-275.
55. Williams JA, Kondo N, Okabe T, et al: Retinoic acid receptors are required for skeletal growth, matrix homeostasis and growth plate function in postnatal mouse. *Dev Biol* 2009;328:315-327.
56. Anderson HC, Garimella R, Tague SE: The role of matrix vesicles in growth plate development and mineralization. *Front Biosci* 2005;10:822-837.
57. Luo G, Ducy P, McKee MD, et al: Spontaneous calcification of arteries and cartilage in mice lacking matrix GLA protein. *Nature* 1997;386:78-81.
58. Kozhemyakina E, Cohen T, Yao T-P, Lassar AB: Parathyroid hormone-related peptide represses chondrocyte hypertrophy through a protein phosphatase 2A/histone deacetylase4/MEF2 pathway. *Mol Cell Biol* 2009;29:5751-5762.
59. Zhang X, Siclari VA, Lan S, et al: The critical role of the epidermal growth factor receptor in endochondral ossification. *J Bone Min Res* 2011;26:2622-2633.
60. Hojo H, Ohba S, Taniguchi K, et al: Hedgehog-Gli activators direct osteo-chondrogenic function in bone morphogenetic protein toward osteogenesis in the perichondrium. *J Biol Chem* 2013;288:9924-9932.
61. St-Jacques B, Hammerschmidt M, McMahon AP: Indian hedgehog signaling regulates proliferation and differentiation of chondrocytes and is essential for bone formation. *Genes Dev* 1999;13:2076-2086.
62. Maes C, Kobayashi T, Selig MK, et al: Osteoblast precursors, but not mature osteoblasts, move into developing and fractured bones along with invading blood vessels. *Dev Cell* 2010;19:329-344.
63. Page-McCaw A, Ewald AJ, Werb Z: Matrix metalloproteases and the regulation of tissue remodeling. *Nature Rev Mol Cell Biol* 2007;8:221-233.

©Copyright 2021 American Academy of Orthopaedic Surgeons

64. Zelzer E, McLean W, Ng YS, et al: Skeletal defects in VEGF(120/120) mice reveal multiple roles of VEGF in skeletogenesis. *Development* 2002;129:1893-1904.
65. Salazar VS, Gamer LW, Rosen V: BMP signaling in skeletal development, disease and repair. *Nat Rev Endocrinol* 2016;12:203-221.
66. Gibson GJ: Active role of chondrocyte apoptosis in endochondral ossification. *Microsc Res Tech* 1998;43:191-204.
67. Roach HI, Erenpreisa J, Aigner T: Osteogenic differentiation of hypertrophic chondrocytes involves asymmetric cell divisions and apoptosis. *J Cell Biol* 1995;131:483-494.
68. Yang L, Tsang KY, Tang HC, Chan D, Cheah KSE: Hypertrophic chondrocytes can become osteoblasts and osteocytes in endochondral bone formation. *Proc Natl Acad Sci USA* 2014;111:12097-12102.
69. Samsa WE, Zhou X, Zhou G: Signaling pathways regulating cartilage growth plate formation and activity. *Sem Cell Dev Biol* 2017;62:3-15.
70. Blumer MJ, Longato S, Richter E, Perez MT, Konakci KZ, Fritsch H: The role of cartilage canals in endochondral and perichondral bone formation: Are there similarities between these two processes? *J Anat* 2005;206:359-372.
71. Dao DY, Jonason JH, Zhang Y, et al: Cartilage-specific β-catenin signaling regulates chondrocyte maturation, generation of ossification centers, and perichondrial bone formation during skeletal development. *J Bone Min Res* 2012;27:1680-1694.
72. Zhang X, Zhu J, Li Y, et al: Epidermal growth factor receptor (EGFR) signaling regulates epiphyseal cartilage development through β-catenin-dependent and -independent pathways. *J Biol Chem* 2013;288:32229-32240.
73. Wilsman NJ, Farnum CE, Green EM, Lieferman EM, Clayton MK: Cell cycle analysis of proliferative zone chondrocytes in growth plates elongating at different rates. *J Orthop Res* 1996;14:562-572.
74. Robson H, Siebler T, Stevens DA, Shalet SM, Williams GH: Thyroid hormone acts directly on the growth plate chondrocytes to promote hypertrophic differentiation and inhibit clonal expansion and cell proliferation. *Endocrinology* 2000;141:3887-3897.
75. Gouveia CHA, Miranda-Rodrigues M, Martins GM, Neofiti-Papi B: Thyroid hormone and skeletal development. *Vitam Horm* 2018;106:383-472.
76. Breur GJ, VanEnkevort BA, Farnum CE, Wilsman NJ: Linear relationship between the volume of hypertrophic chondrocytes and the rate of longitudinal bone growth in growth plates. *J Ortho Res* 1991;9:348-359.
77. Noonan KJ, Farnum CE, Leifeman EM, Lampl M, Markel M, Wilsman NJ: Growing pains: Are they due to increased growth during recumbency as documented in a lamb model? *J Pediatr Orthop* 2004;24:726-731.
78. Weise M, De Levi S, Barnes KM, Gafni RI, Abad V, Baron J: Effects of estrogen on growth plate senescence and epiphyseal fusion. *Proc Natl Acad Sci USA* 2001;98:6871-6876.
79. Zelzer E, Olsen BR: The genetic basis of skeletal diseases. *Nature* 2003;423:343-348.
80. Ornitz DM, Legeai-Mallet L: Achondroplasia: Development, pathogenesis, and therapy. *Dev Dyn* 2017;246:291-309.
81. Pettifor JM: Nutrional rickes: Pathogenesis and prevention. *Pediatr Endocrinol Rev* 2013;10:347-353.
82. Whyte MP: Hypophosphatasia, In Glorieux FH, Jueppner H, Pettifor J, eds: *Pediatric Bone: Biology and Diseases*, ed 3. San Diego, CA, Academic Press, 2012, pp 771-794.
83. Gao B, Guo J, She C, et al: Mutations in IHH, encoding Indian hedgehog, cause brachydactyly type A-1. *Nature Genet* 2001;28:386-388.
84. Pacifici M: Hereditary mutliple exostoses: New insights into pathogenesis, clinical complications, and potential treatments. *Curr Osteoporos Rep* 2017;15:142-152.
85. Huegel J, Sgariglia F, Enomoto-Iwamoto M, Koyama E, Dormans JP, Pacifici M: Heparan sulfate in skeletal development, growth, and pathology: The case of hereditary multiple exostoses. *Dev Dyn* 2013;242:1021-1032.
86. Sinha R, Mundy C, Bechtold T, et al: Unsuspected osteochondroma-like outgrowths in the cranial base of hereditary multiple exostoses patients and modeling and treatment with a BMP antagonist in mice. *PLoS Genet* 2017;13:e1006742.
87. Decker RS: Articular cartilage and joint development from embryogenesis to adulthood. *Sem Cell Dev Biol* 2017;62:50-56.
88. Decker RS, Koyama E, Pacifici M: Genesis and morphogenesis of limb synovial joints and articular cartilage. *Matrix Biol* 2014;39:5-10.
89. Longobardi L, Li T, Tagliaferro L, et al: Synovial joints: From development to homeostasis. *Curr Osteoporos Rep* 2015;13:41-51.
90. Rux D, Decker RS, Koyama E, Pacifici M: Joints in the appendicular skeleton: Developmental mechanisms and evolutionary influences. *Curr Top Dev Biol* 2019;133:119-151.
91. Salva JE, Merrill AE: Signaling networks in joint development. *Dev Dyn* 2017;246:262-274.
92. Koyama E, Shibukawa Y, Nagayama M, et al: A distinct cohort of progenitor cells participates in synovial joint and articular cartilage formation during mouse limb skeletogenesis. *Dev Biol* 2008;316:62-73.
93. Johnstone B, Alini M, Cucchiarini M, et al: Tissue engineering for articular cartilage repair. The state of the art. *Eur Cells Mater* 2013;25:248-267.

©Copyright 2021 American Academy of Orthopaedic Surgeons

10

Biology of Bone

Robert J. Majeska, PhD
Oran D. Kennedy, PhD
Mitchell B. Schaffler, PhD
Elise F. Morgan, PhD
Louis C. Gerstenfeld, PhD

Keywords: *age-related fractures; bone biology; histomorphometry; radiological assessments*

OVERVIEW OF BONE DEVELOPMENT AND FUNCTION

Bone come in a variety of shapes, sizes, and internal organizational patterns that serve a number of physiological functions with each bone uniquely suited for its functional role.

Functionally, the bony skeleton carries out three primary roles. Structurally, bone is a load-bearing scaffold providing mechanical support to the body and the load-bearing scaffold onto which the musculature is attached. It also provides protection for internal organs of the head, thorax, and abdomen. Metabolically, bone is a reserve source of minerals, particularly calcium and phosphate, for the management of mineral metabolism. Finally, bone plays a major role in organismal homeostasis by housing tissue niches that contain the postnatal stem cell populations supporting hematopoiesis, myelopoiesis, and skeletogeneis. Thus, bone tissues are integral to the regeneration of these organ systems throughout adult life. Thus, while the primary clinical focus of the orthopedic surgeon is on the restoration and maintenance of the skeleton's mechanical functions in patients, the overall clinical treatment and management of many orthopaedic problems requires an understanding that the etiology of orthopaedic problems is intimately linked to interplay among the entire spectrum of functions carried out by skeletal tissues.[1-4]

Bones arise from two embryonic sources. Those of the skull and upper mandible are derived embryonically from the neural crest, by intramembranous bone formation in which cells of embryonic mesenchyme differentiate directly into osteogenic cells. Bones of the vertebrae, ribs, aspects of the pelvis and limbs arise from various elements of the mesoderm via endochondral bone formation, in which an initial cartilage model (anlage) forms within mesenchyme. The cells surrounding the anlage then differentiate into osteoblasts which lay down bone matrix upon it, after which the cartilage is gradually replaced. Details of these developmental processes are available in most anatomy texts and reviewed in Chapter 9.

Endochondral bone formation during skeletal development has several clinically relevant implications for postnatal growth and repair. First, the growth in length of long bones depends primarily on the growth of cartilage in the growth zones; consequently, as long bones are growing in length, regions of cartilage will be evident. Bones grow in length from the first trimester of development in utero until the late adolescence. A second implication is that the majority of bones formed by endochondral processes become sites in which postnatal hematopoietic tissues are housed.

Dr. Majeska or an immediate family member has stock or stock options held in Pfizer. None of the following authors or any immediate family member has received anything of value from or has stock or stock options held in a commercial company or institution related directly or indirectly to the subject of this chapter: Dr. Kennedy, Dr. Schaffler, Dr. Morgan, and Dr. Gerstenfeld.

©Copyright 2021 American Academy of Orthopaedic Surgeons

CLINICAL NOTE The development of bones by the endochondral pathway depends critically on the control of cartilage differentiation and growth throughout the developmental process. As a result, many orthopaedic pathologies characterized by skeletal malformations arise from genetic or developmental deficiencies in cartilage rather than bone per se. These include instances of defective skeletal patterning (eg, polydactyly) due to altered expression of transcription factors controlling chondrocyte differentiation and various forms of dwarfism due to impaired function of chondrocytes in growth zones. It is also important to recognize that failures in these developmental processes are causal to many of the problems that impede surgical repair, fracture healing, and surgical treatments. A complete summary of the nosology of known congenital mutations effecting skeletal tissues has been cataloged.[5]

HIERARCHICAL LEVELS OF BONE STRUCTURE

In the next section, bone structure will be reviewed beginning at the anatomical level, proceeding through tissue-level organization to its underlying molecular composition.

Anatomically, the skeleton is divided into axial elements consisting in the adult of 80 bones including the skull, the vertebral column, sacrum, coccyx, and the thoracic cage. The appendicular skeleton is composed of 126 bones that include all bones of the upper and lower limbs, plus the elements of the pelvis that attach each limb to the axial skeleton. Bones may also be categorized roughly as either long or flat.[1-4] As noted, long bones such as the humerus, femur, and tibia generally form by the endochondral process, whereas flat bones, like those of the cranium, arise via intramembranous ossification. All bones contain a dense outer layer of compact or cortical bone that surrounds a network of thin trabeculae (cancellous bone), with the intratrabecular space filled with marrow. Like size and shape, the amounts and distributions of cortical bone, cancellous bone, and marrow differ greatly among individual bones and influence how they develop, age, and are prone to fracture, as will be discussed below.

The femur illustrates most of the macrostructural features of a prototypical long bone. It roughly resembles a cylinder with fluted ends (**Figure 1**) with a middle region (diaphysis) flanked by the metaphyses and the epiphyses. The diaphysis consists of a thick shell of compact cortical bone enclosing a marrow cavity with little or no cancellous bone. In the metaphyses and epiphyses, the cortices are thinner and surround a more extensive network of cancellous bone. Marrow occupies the internal spaces of the bone. As noted previously, the epiphyseal plate, or physis, separates the epiphysis from the metaphysis in growing bones, but cartilage disappears from the physeal region after growth ceases.[6-8]

Both external and internal (marrow) surfaces of bone are covered by some form of nonmineralized connective tissue. Externally, the ends of bones that form joint surfaces are covered by articular cartilage, whereas the remainder of bone is covered by the periosteum, a somewhat elastic sleeve of dense fibrous connective tissue. The periosteum includes a layer of cells near the bone surface (the cambium layer) that contains both skeletogenic stem cells and osteogenic progenitors. These cells are capable of forming bone and cartilage cells that contribute to growth, response to injury and homeostatic maintenance of bones. Internally, surfaces of both cortical and cancellous bone are covered by the bone marrow stroma, a fibrous connective tissue more loosely organized than the periosteum. Cells of the marrow stroma comprise a heterogeneous population that plays several roles in maintaining both the hematopoietic system and connective tissue elements of the bone. Hematopoietic stem cells that give rise to all blood cell types reside physically in or around the stroma, whereas connective tissue cells within the stroma produce growth factors needed to sustain the hematopoietic stem cells and to support their differentiation. In addition, bone marrow stroma contains a population of nonhematopoietic adult stem cells (marrow stromal stem cells or MSCs) capable of differentiating into bone, cartilage, tendon, and adipose tissues, among others. Like all tissues, bone is supplied by blood vessels and nerves.[8,9] These are more extensively distributed throughout the periosteum and the bone marrow than in bone itself. Vessels and nerves that supply the marrow pass through cortical bone only at limited entry points (nutrient foramina). Smaller vessels and nerves are distributed throughout cortical bone, passing through channels in the tissue termed haversian canals and Volkmann canals (discussed below). The extent of intracortical vasculature varies considerably among individual bones and certainly among species. In bones that lack haversian systems, primary vascular canals are still present, running in both longitudinal and transverse directions. **Figure 2** presents a schematic summary of this haversian cortical bone structure.

The blood vessels in bone derive from both periosteum and marrow, which supply the outer one-third and the inner two-thirds, respectively. Marrow vasculature also services trabecular bone, which itself does not contain vessels. There is a second so-called circulatory system in bone—the extravascular movement of fluids and solutes through the pericellular space between osteocytes and their processes and their bony lacunar and canalicular walls; fluid in this space moves under convective flow driven by blood pressure and by mechanical

©Copyright 2021 American Academy of Orthopaedic Surgeons

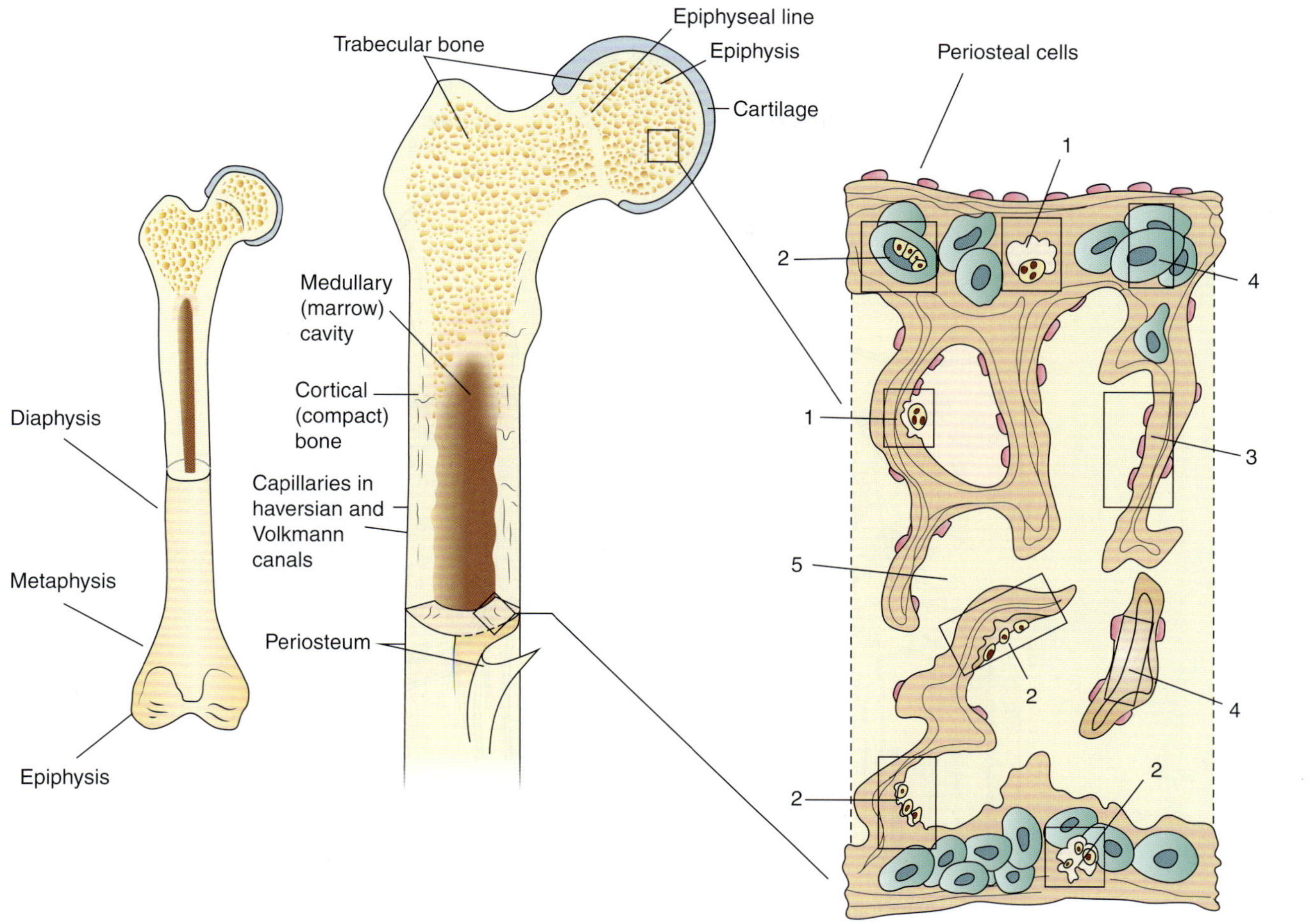

FIGURE 1 Schematic diagram of cortical and trabecular bone showing the different structures and cell types. 1 = osteoclasts, 2 = osteoblasts, 3 = bone lining cells, 4 = osteocytes, 5 = marrow space. (Reproduced with permission from Hayes WC: *Biomechanics of Cortical and Trabecular Bone: Implications for Assessment of Fracture Risk, in Basic Orthopaedic Biomechanics*. New York, NY, Raven Press, 1991, pp 93-142.)

loading. Aspects of fluid flow and tissue mechanoregulation will be further discussed below. Whether bone has lymphatic drainage remains unresolved.[9]

TISSUE-LEVEL ORGANIZATION (GROSS AND MICROSCOPIC)

Tissue-level (or intermediate) organization considers the way cells and extracellular matrix (ECM) are arranged within bone tissue at the microscopic length scale; its description is historically based largely on microscopy and histologic staining methods.[1,7,10] Cortical and cancellous bone can be characterized as either woven or lamellar. Woven bone is a poorly organized tissue in which neither the bone cells nor the fibers in their surrounding matrix exhibit any organized arrangement. Most notably, the collagen fibers in woven bone matrix are randomly oriented. Woven bone is produced during periods of rapid bone formation; for example, during development, in fracture callus, and in primary bone tumors (osteosarcomas). In nonpathologic circumstances, woven bone is a temporary or provisional tissue that is removed and replaced by more highly organized lamellar bone, which comprises effectively all adult cortical and cancellous bone tissue. Lamellar bone consists of tissue layers (lamellae) approximately 3 to 5 μm thick, in which the collagen fibers run mainly in the same direction. The orientation of fibers in adjacent lamellae, however, differs by as much as 90°, giving lamellar bone a "cross-ply" or plywood-like appearance that is particularly evident under polarized light microscopy. Biological mechanisms by which collagen fibers become arranged in successive lamellae are not understood, but have an overall significance to the mechanical strength of the tissue.

In cortical bone, lamellae are generally organized in one of several ways. (1) Circumferential lamellae extend continuously around some or a bone's entire circumference. The most prominent example is the deposition of effectively complete circumferential sheets on the periosteal surface of bone during radial growth of diaphyses ("outer circumferential lamellae"). (2) Circumferentially oriented lamellae are added to parts of

©Copyright 2021 American Academy of Orthopaedic Surgeons

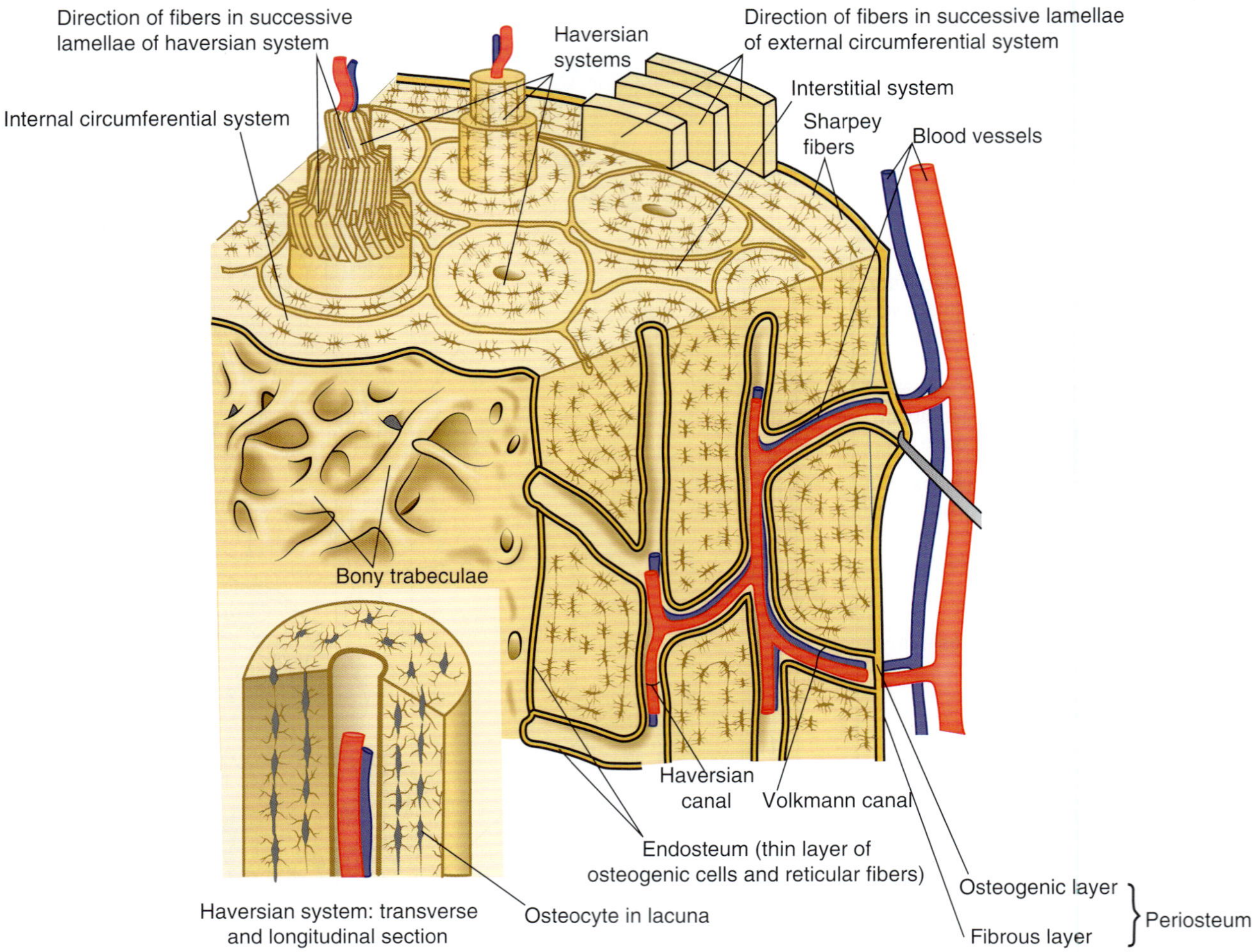

FIGURE 2 Diagram of the structure of cortical bone, showing the types of cortical lamellar bone: the internal circumferential system, interstitial system, osteonal lamellae, and outer circumferential system. The diagram also shows the intraosseous vascular system that serves the osteocytes and connects the periosteal and medullary blood vessels. The haversian canals run primarily longitudinally through the cortex, whereas the Volkmann canals create oblique connections between the haversian canals. Cement lines separate each osteon from the surrounding bone. Periosteum covers the external surface of the bone and consists of two layers: an osteogenic (inner) cellular layer and a fibrous (outer) layer. (Adapted from Miller JD, McCreadie BR, Alford AI, et al: Form and function of bone, in Einhorn TA, O'Keefe RJ, Buckwalter JA, eds: *Orthopaedic Basic Science*, ed 3. Rosemont, IL, American Academy of Orthopaedic Surgeons, 2007, pp 129-159.)

the endosteal surface as well ("inner circumferential lamellae"), although these often do not extend the full extent of the inner surface of the bone. (3) Osteonal or haversian lamellae are concentric rings of tissue that lie inside an osteon or haversian system—a cylindrical region that surrounds a vascular channel within bone. (4) Interstitial lamellae are remnants of lamellae that lie between haversian systems and can be composed of fragments of circumferential lamellar bone from earlier times in a bone's growth, or of fragments of preexisting haversian systems. The vascular canals that are roughly aligned with the long axis of the bone are termed haversian canals, whereas those that run transversely are called Volkmann canals. The borders of each osteon are delineated by a thin layer of distinctive matrix that is termed a cement line. The cement line is a bonding layer formed after the old matrix has been removed during remodeling and before new bone matrix is deposited.

CELLULAR LEVEL ORGANIZATION OF THE BONE AND THE CELLULAR ASPECTS BONE HOMEOSTASIS

All bone contains four distinct cell types: osteoblasts, osteoclasts, osteocytes, and bone lining cells. These cells are involved in the maintenance and metabolic functions of bone and carry out primarily either anabolic or catabolic functions. Osteocytes and osteoblasts synthesize and secrete the organic constituents of bone matrix and regulate its mineralization; osteoclasts degrade (resorb) bone, simultaneously breaking down mineral and matrix. Osteocytes and lining cells are bone's long-term residents that carry out day-to-day maintenance of the tissue; they are found, respectively, within the mineralized matrix and on both cortical and trabecular surfaces not being formed or resorbed.

©Copyright 2021 American Academy of Orthopaedic Surgeons

LINEAGES

Osteoblasts, lining cells, and osteocytes are part of a common mesenchymal cell lineage, differentiating from skeletal stem cells and progenitors that reside in specific tissue niches within the bone marrow and within the periosteum adjacent to bone proper. Osteocytes and lining cells are, in fact, late—and alternative—stages in the phenotypic maturation of osteoblasts. As osteoblasts lay down new matrix, some of them become buried within it and become osteocytes (some other osteoblasts die by apoptosis). When formation ceases, the last osteoblasts flatten out to cover the new matrix and become lining cells. Osteoclasts, by contrast, arise from the hematopoietic lineage,[1,2,7,10-16] specifically monocytes which are found in the marrow and recruited to potential resorption sites where they differentiate into multinucleated osteoclasts that resorb bone until the appropriate amount has been removed. Both osteoblastic and osteoclastic lineages have been extensively studied so that phenotypic markers—and in particular, critical transcription factors responsible for their distinctive gene expression patterns—have been identified for most stages of differentiation from stem cells onward (**Figure 3**, A and B). The osteoclast lineage appears to include few if any branches or reversals. On the other hand, the skeletogenic stem cells giving rise to osteogenic cells also give rise to cartilage cells, fibroblasts, and adipocytes. Moreover, cells within the osteoblastic lineage appear to have considerable plasticity and appear to be capable of phenotypic switching or reversal under differing circumstances, both in vivo and in vitro. Lining cells can be activated rapidly to become osteoblasts in vivo[17]; in addition, a substantial proportion of cells from

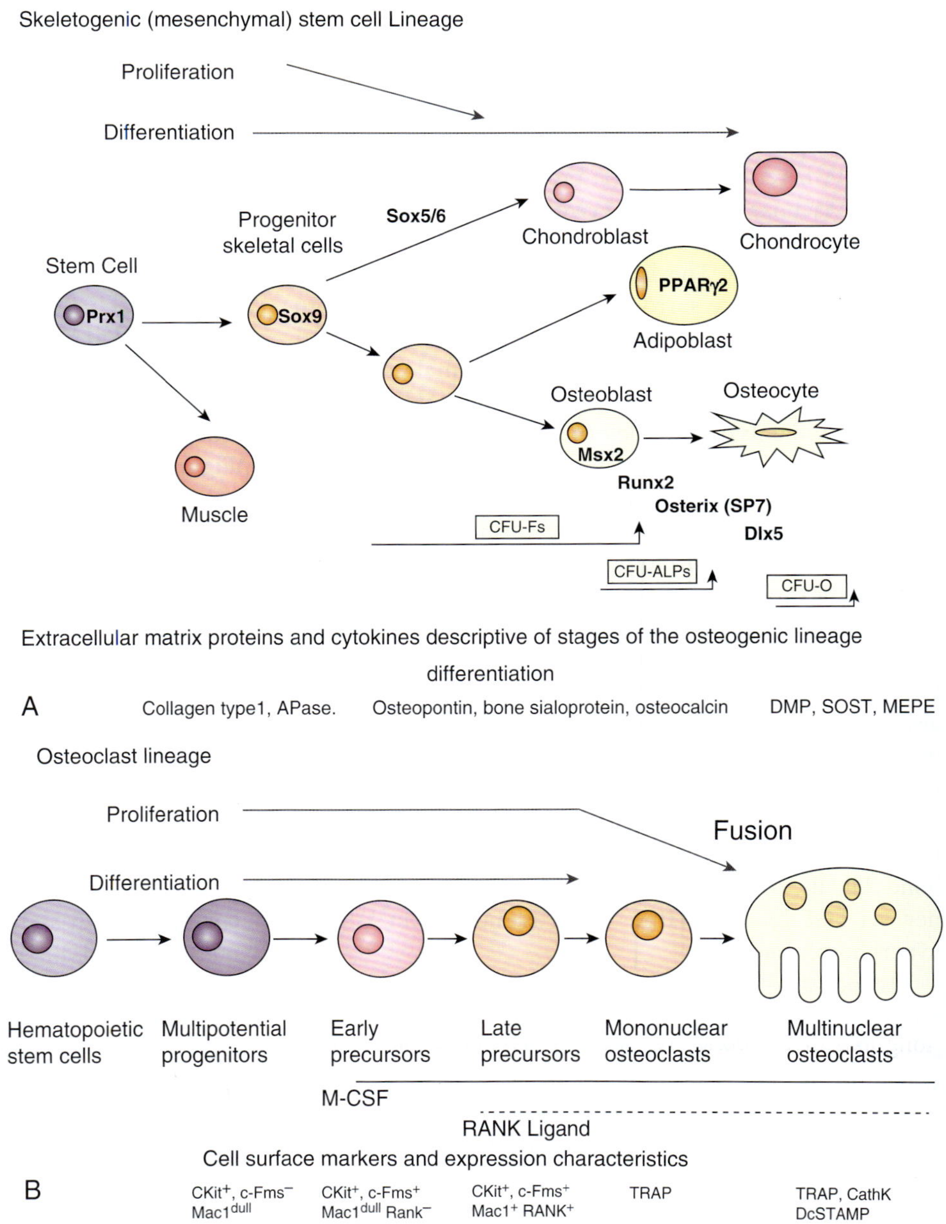

FIGURE 3 Diagram of lineage progression of osteoblasts and osteoclasts. **Panel A** depicts the currently understood progression of the skeletogenic stem cell lineage that gives rise to osteogenic cells. The major lineage stages and cell types of the lineage are shown in the diagram. The determining transcription factors that promote lineage progression are presented in bold text in the diagram. Empirically determined lineage stages defined by ex vivo culturing as colony forming unit, fibroblast, alkaline phosphatase expressing, and osteoblast/osteocyte (mineralizing) are shown relative to lineage progression. Most commonly used protein or mRNA expression features that are used to define lineage progression are highlighted. **Panel B** depicts the currently understood progression of the osteoclast lineage from the common hematopoietic stem cells (HSC). Multipotential precursors are defined as myeloid and of the monocyte/macrophage dendritic cell lineages. Early and late are defined by commitment to the monocyte/macrophage then macrophage lineages, respectively. The cell-sorting markers that are most commonly used to define osteoclast lineage progression are highlighted. Stage-specific association to macrophage colony-stimulating factor (M-CSF) and receptor activator of nuclear factor kappa-B ligand (RANKL) signaling needed for linage progression are denoted.

©Copyright 2021 American Academy of Orthopaedic Surgeons

adult bone exhibiting an osteoblastic phenotype in culture[18] were almost certainly osteocytes in vivo. Finally, osteoblast progenitors have the option to differentiate instead into adipocytes, and the propensity for each m100y change with age and/or may contribute to diminished bone-forming capability in aging and certain pathological conditions.[19]

FUNCTIONS

The function of osteoblasts, as stated previously, is to produce the organic matrix of bone and help regulate its mineralization. Details of these activities will be discussed later in the chapter. However, it should be noted that osteoblasts are post-mitotic; they do not divide. New osteoblasts are supplied from ranks of osteoblast progenitors lying "behind" the osteoblasts, away from the bone surface.

Osteocytes are the most abundant cells in bone and carry out much of the signaling throughout the tissue. Osteocytes occupy roughly ellipsoidal 300 to 500 μm^3 spaces (lacunae) and connect with each other through extensive networks of dendritic processes. These processes are located in canaliculi approximately 0.3 μm in diameter and are joined by gap junctions where they connect at process termini. In lamellar bone, the lacunae are regularly arranged and consistent with the organization of the lamellae; in woven bone, lacunae are arranged randomly. The lacunar-canalicular system (LCS), the pericellular space surrounding osteocytes and their processes, provides the major route through which fluids, nutrients, signaling molecules, wastes, and other molecules move through bone. It is hypothesized that both the fluid movement and small amounts of tissue deformation that is applied on the dendritic processes and their interconnection is how osteocytes sense mechanical loading.[11,20]

In addition to acting as mechanosensors, osteocytes have been implicated as effector cells regulating several major homeostatic functions of bone. Osteocytes upregulate the pro-osteoclastogenic cytokine RANKL in response to apoptosis induced by remodeling stimuli that include microdamage, estrogen deprivation, and mechanical unloading. Osteocytes also produce sclerostin, the Wnt antagonist that suppresses osteoblast activity. In addition, osteocytes can regulate local remodeling of the LCS in association with mineral exchange; this is especially evident in lactation and can lead to rapid, though temporary, changes in local material properties of bone. Finally, osteocytes exert systemic actions on the kidney via FGF-23 and PHEX, which is mutated in x-linked hyperphosphatemia.[21]

Osteoclasts—the cells responsible for the wholesale removal of bone at a defined site—are notably polarized cells. Osteoclasts attach to bone surfaces with specialized structures forming a resorption space that encloses a "ruffled border" of active plasma membrane. Protons generated by carbonic anhydrase within the cytoplasm are pumped into the resorption space via transport molecules in the ruffled border. Intracellular pH and ionic balance are maintained by additional ion transport systems located in the plasma membrane outside the ruffled border. The secreted protons, which render the resorption space acidic, begin to dissolve the apatite mineral salts and disrupt intramolecular and intermolecular interactions of organic constituents. Osteoclasts also secrete lysosomal enzymes including tartrate-resistant acid phosphatase (TRAP, an enzyme that has served as a convenient, histochemical marker to specifically identify osteoclasts) and proteases (most notably cathepsins B, L, and K).[12-15]

As the effector cells responsible for bone removal, osteoclasts have long been a focus of interest in understanding the mechanisms of pathologic bone loss and a target for therapeutics. The role of osteoclasts in mineral metabolism and in the homeostatic maintenance of skeletal structure throughout life is extensively reviewed in Chapter 24. Of particular importance in this regard are the pathways and mechanisms of communication between the osteoblastic and osteoclastic lineages. These include induction of osteoclast differentiation by osteocytes and osteoblasts by the obligate factors RANKL (receptor activator of NF-kappa-B ligand) and M-CSF (macrophage colony–stimulating factor) and the coupling between bone resorption and formation. Advances in understanding these processes have been exploited in the development of antiresorptive therapies to treat osteoporosis (also reviewed in Chapter 24).

MOLECULAR LEVEL OF BONE COMPOSITION AND ITS EXTRACELLULAR MATRIX

The molecular composition of bone tissue is described in **Figure 4**. It is broadly made up of organic components comprising ~30% of its mass. The organic component itself is made up of extracellular proteins comprising 98% of its mass and 2% of its mass made up of the cells found embedded within bone or on its surfaces. The other ~70% of its mass is accounted for by mineral, of which 95% is made up of a carbonated hydroxyapatite and the remainder being other trace minerals.

ORGANIC ELEMENTS OF BONE/COLLAGEN

At the molecular level bone extracellular matrix (ECM) proteins are composed of ~90% type 1 collagen and 10% noncollagenous proteins The fibers of collagen and noncollagenous proteins, in conjunction with the apatitic mineral crystals precipitated within and around the fibers, form a unique composite material. Broadly speaking, the fibrous matrix governs the tissue's tensile properties and fracture toughness whereas the mineral phase confers rigidity and compressive strength; however, this is clearly an oversimplification. The organic constituents of bone matrix can have substantial effects on bone's mechanical properties, such as resistance to fracture, and on its physiologic activities in mineral metabolism,[22-25] as well as playing a wide variety of physiological functions summarized in bottom half of **Figure 4**. As a major repository of calcium

©Copyright 2021 American Academy of Orthopaedic Surgeons

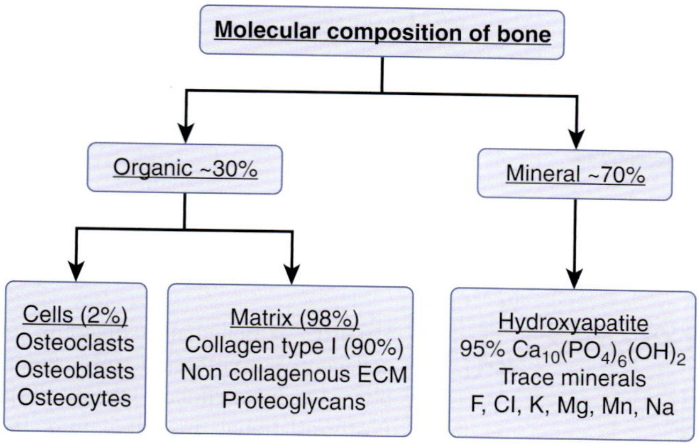

Ecm protein functions

1. Direct cell binding both osteoblasts and osteoclasts
2. Control spatial arrangement of mineral deposition
3. Control mineral nucleation +/– (temporal control)
4. Control rates and sites of mineral resorption
5. Proteolytic processing of ECM
6. Cellular signaling

FIGURE 4 Molecular composition and gunction of bone. **Upper part** of the figure depicts a schematic breakdown of the percentage composition of the major molecular component that make up bone tissue. The **low panel** summarizes the primary functional role that the proteins within the extracellular compartment of bone carry out. ECM = extracellular matrix.

and phosphate in the body, bone ECM contributes to systemic mineral metabolism.[1,3,4,22]

As stated above, type I collagen is the major collagen isotype in bone. Other collagen types found there belong to cartilage remnants from endochondral ossification (mainly types II and X), fibrous tissues of periosteum and marrow (type III), or blood vessels (type IV). Small amounts of other collagen types, including types III, V, and XI, have been identified in bone ECM, but under restricted circumstances and in association with type I fibers.[25] As the major organic component of bone, the biosynthesis and molecular structural assembly of collagen type I collagen is integral to overall structural nature of the composite material of bone. The structural unit of type I collagen is termed tropocollagen, a trimer composed of three polypeptide chains. Two are α1 (I) chains, encoded by the col1a1 gene, whereas the third, α2 (I), is encoded by the col1a2 gene. The three chains form a distinctive unit, in which the polypeptides wrap around each other for most of their length, forming a tight triple helical braid. This triple helical structure, which is not the same as the α-helix that is formed by a single polypeptide chain, is the defining structural feature of all collagens. The collagen triple helix forms because both the α1 and α2 chains contain repeated sequences of the amino acid sequence (-gly-X-Y-) where gly represents glycine, X is proline, and Y is frequently hydroxyproline. Both proline and hydroxyproline are imino acids; that is, the nitrogen that combines with adjacent amino acid to form the polypeptide backbone exists as part of a five-membered ring and is not able to rotate freely. This constrained structure imparts a tight kink in the polypeptide chain at each proline or hydroxyproline residue. The positioning of glycine, which lacks a side chain, at every third position along this repeating tripeptide sequence (and adjacent to a proline) is essential to prevent steric hindrance that would otherwise impair wrapping of the helical braid. Fibril formation is a self-assembly process, at physiologic pH, temperature, and ionic strength; monomeric tropocollagen in solution in vitro will spontaneously aggregate in a regular fashion to form fibrils. The spontaneous nature of fibril formation suggests that most or all tropocollagen will exist as part of a fibril and, moreover, that mechanisms must exist in vivo to ensure that the fibrils are of the appropriate dimensions and that fibril formation only occurs under the correct circumstances.

The triple helical region of tropocollagen comprises the central region of the molecule; the remainder includes nonhelical N- and C-telopeptides flanking the helical region on each side, as well as N- and C-terminal propeptides that are cleaved during posttranslational processing. Because the long helical region makes up most of the sequence of mature collagen molecules, each tropocollagen unit resembles a fairly stiff rod with a consistent length of approximately 300 nm. In the fibrils, the rod-like tropocollagen monomers are aligned in the same direction, but with the ends of the monomers offset by approximately 25% of their length—a quarter-stagger configuration relative to the collagen monomers immediately laterally. Thus, the tips of each tropocollagen molecule do not contact each other; rather, there are gaps (holes) between successive tropocollagen units in a line. This regular arrangement of monomers and gaps accounts for the characteristic banding patterns observed in electron microscopic images of collagen fibrils. Because of this arrangement, the addition of each new tropocollagen monomer to a growing fibril via this staggered, side-to-side interaction of monomers results in changes to the width as well as the length of the fibril. The fibrils formed by collagen can be very long, but are roughly circular in cross section and have a limited distribution of diameters that is tissue type dependent. Collagen fibril diameter appears to depend on many factors, including the association of other collagen types (minor collagens such as type V), proteoglycans, or noncollagenous proteins with the fibrils. The presence of holes within the fibril structure of collagen also has implications for the distribution of noncollagenous elements, especially mineral crystals, in bone ECM. The hole zones between the ends of tropocollagen molecules define a network of spaces that extends throughout the three-dimensional extent of the collagen fibrils and is also continuous with interfibrillar space. The basic biochemistry and biology of collagens have been extensively reviewed.[22-25] Consequently, tissue fluid and its soluble components, including noncollagenous proteins and inorganic ions, can permeate into as well as between collagen fibrils. Because of this accessibility, bone mineral crystals are

©Copyright 2021 American Academy of Orthopaedic Surgeons

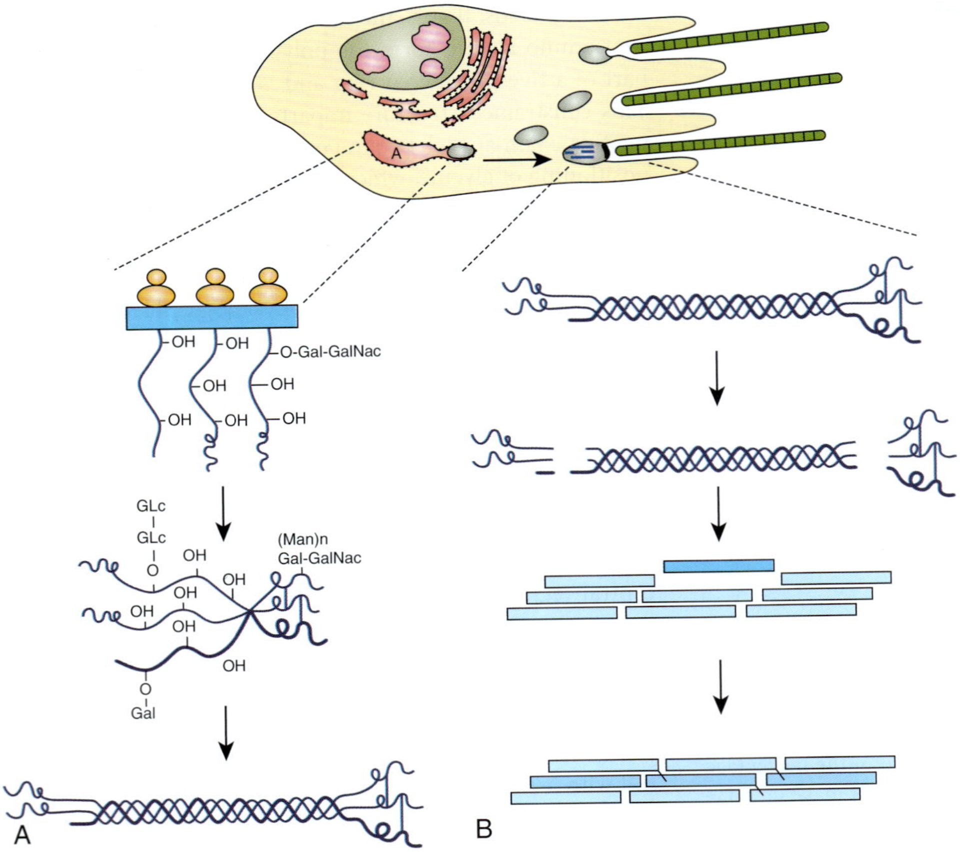

FIGURE 5 Schematic diagram of collagen biosynthesis and assembly. **A**, Intracellular events. Top: Posttranslational insertion into the endoplasmic reticulum and hydroxylation of proline and lysine. Middle: Glycosylation of hydroxylated amino acids. Bottom: Formation of procollagen by folding of the three collagen chains beginning from the C-terminal propeptide. **B**, Extracellular events. Top: Procollagen (as in part A) now at the point of secretion from the cell. Top middle: Cleavage of N- and C-propeptides from procollagen. Lower middle: Self-assembly of collagen fibrils. Bottom: Formation of cross-links between tropocollagen molecules.

closely integrated into the fibrils of bone ECM.[26] The mechanisms of collagen triple helix assembly, posttranslational modifications, fibril assembly and packing, and interactions with mineral are schematically depicted in **Figures 5** and **6**.

CLINICAL NOTE Proteolytic removal of N- and C-propeptides removal of the N- and C-terminal collagen propeptides during their biosynthesis occurs by cleavage of all three collagen chains by specific N- and C-propeptidases, respectively. This occurs as the proteins are secreted from the cell, leaving mature tropocollagen molecules with intact N- and C-telopeptides flanking the triple helix. Following cleavage, the procollagen peptides do not remain as part of the ECM; rather, they are washed out and eventually appear in the serum and finally are excreted in urine. The appearance in serum and urine of detectable amounts of collagen propeptide fragments, which are produced in equimolar amounts to collagen, has made them highly useful as biomarkers to assess collagen synthesis in vivo under normal and pathologic circumstances. Immunoassays are currently available to detect N- and C-procollagen peptides from types I and III and other collagens in serum and urine.

Collagen cross-linking: Although intracellular modifications (hydroxylation of proline and lysine) prepare tropocollagen molecules for subsequent cross-linking needed to stabilize the collagen fibrils, the cross-linking process itself occurs outside the cell.[28] Lysyl oxidase, an extracellular enzyme that converts the ε-amino groups of lysine and hydroxylysine into aldehydes via oxidative deamination, typically initiates the crosslinking process. Several nonenzymatic reactions can then occur, depending on the availability and nature of reactive side chains, leading to the formation of divalent cross-links of nearby lysine or hydroxylysine. These divalent cross-links are further converted to extremely stable trivalent cross-links by additional (nonenzymatic) reaction with a third aldehyde-bearing side chain. When any collagenous matrix is broken down as part of bone resorption or remodeling of other tissues such as tendon, ligament, or skin, the chemically complex segments of collagen chains that contain the cross-links are resistant to cleavage by protease. These resistant fragments, which contain chemically distinctive interchain links (such as pyridinoline) coupled to a few amino acids, move into the circulation and eventually are excreted in urine, similar to the propeptide products of collagen synthesis. In addition, like the procollagen peptides, the ability to detect and quantitate collagen cross-links in plasma/serum and urine has allowed them to be used as biomarkers to assess rates of collagen degradation in vivo. The limitation of these biomarker assays, of course, is that they

©Copyright 2021 American Academy of Orthopaedic Surgeons

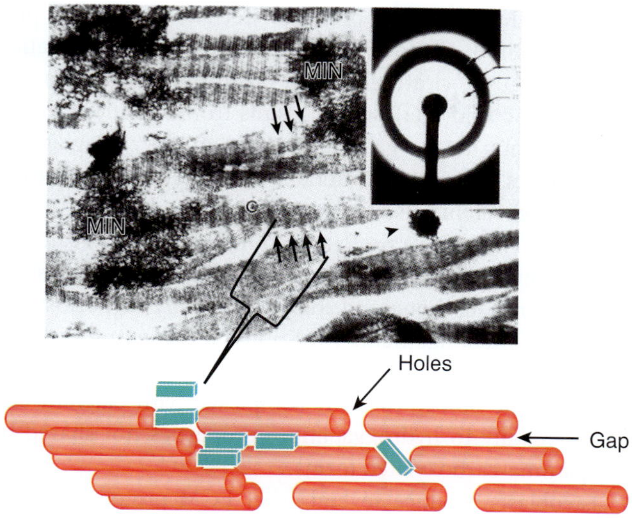

FIGURE 6 Mineral packing within collagen. **Upper** panel depicts an electron micrograph of mineralizing collagen fibrils observed in cultures of avian calvaria osteoblast. In set shows x-ray diffractions demonstrating hydroxyapatite crystals. Arrows highlight presence of apatite crystals aligned with the holes of collagen fibrils. **Lower** panel showing a schematic diagram of how collagen packing both constrains and orients apatite crystal packing within collagen fibril holes and gaps. Electron Image from Gerstenfeld et al 1988.[27]

reflect the levels of collagen synthesis or degradation from all tissues, not just bone; as a result, it is difficult to obtain specific and unambiguous information about bone matrix metabolism from these assays alone.

Congenital defects in collagen biosynthesis: Both animal and human studies of genetic alterations in collagen structure and the enzymes that modify collagen have greatly increased our understanding of collagen's role within the extracellular matrix. In this respect, long-standing clinical and biochemical investigations of patients with osteogenesis imperfecta have been especially productive. Osteogenesis imperfecta comprises a set of genetic disorders whose hallmarks include fragility of the skeleton and other type I collagen–based connective tissues. The wide range of osteogenesis imperfecta severity reflects diverse changes in the structure of col1a1 or col1a2 genes from complete ablation to single base changes in one or both copies of the collagen genes. Other forms of OI affect collagen-modifying enzymes that process collagen posttranslationally. In contrast there are many other congenital diseases that of affect connective tissues that arise through non collagen protein mutation that will alter bone skeletal tissue functions (including, but not limited to, Ehlers Danlos syndrome, Marfan syndrome, and a host of chondrodysplasias). Summary or heritable conditions of collagen may be found in Royce and Steinmann[29] that is available as free access content at https://onlinelibrary.wiley.com/doi/book/10.1002/0471221929.

ORGANIC ELEMENTS OF BONE/NONCOLLAGENOUS PROTEINS

While representing only a small fraction (~5%) of organic phase the noncollagenous proteins of bone ECM play diverse and important physiological roles in bone (summarized in **Table 1**). Early speculations that the unique nature of bone matrix might be attributable to one or two bone-specific molecules have now been largely abandoned due to extensive data showing that virtually all the bone noncollagenous proteins are expressed in many tissues.[30-32] Bone noncollagenous proteins act as structural elements, enzymes, and/or diffusible signals (cytokines) and are synthesized by several cell types and tissues (summarized in **Figure 4**). For example, some ECM proteins are synthesized and secreted by osteoblasts before mineral deposition while others are produced by osteocytes after the mineral phase is deposited. Other proteins found in bone matrix, like serum albumin and α2HS-glycoprotein, are produced by remote tissue like liver, arrive in the bone via the circulation, and subsequently become adsorbed on the surfaces within the matrix. A common feature of many noncollagenous bone ECM proteins is the ability to interact simultaneously with multiple binding partners, including cell surface receptors, other matrix macromolecules, soluble ions (in particular Ca^{2+}), and hydroxyapatite.

SIBLING (Small, Integrin-Binding LIgand, N-linked Glycoproteins), include bone sialoprotein (BSP), osteopontin (OPN), dentin matrix protein-1 (DMP-1), and matrix extracellular phosphoglycoprotein (MEPE).[20-32] These structurally related proteins possess cell-binding capability via arg-gly-asp (RGD) sequences recognized by integrin adhesion receptors, most notably integrin αVβ3. They are subject to several forms of posttranslational modification, including glycosylation, phosphorylation, and proteolytic processing. Through their integrin interactions, they serve as bridges between both osteoblasts and osteoclasts to the mineralized extracellular matrix, and various studies have suggested both roles in mediating mineral resorption and directing mineral deposition.

Proteoglycans are an extremely diverse macromolecular family of proteins characterized by their structural motif: a single polypeptide chain (the core protein) with one or more of its amino acid side chains modified by members of a specific disaccharide family, the glycosaminoglycans (GAGs). The most common GAGs are chondroitin sulfate, heparan sulfate, and keratan sulfate. As part of aggrecan, the principal cartilage proteoglycan, they have a major role in defining the cartilage matrix (see Chapter 12). Three proteoglycans specifically identified in bone are decorin, biglycan, and perlecan. Decorin and biglycan are members of the small, leucine-rich proteoglycan family, contain only one and two GAG chains per molecule, respectively, and have been suggested to regulate collagen fibril diameter. Perlecan has a larger core protein and more extensive GAG modifications and has been identified in the pericellular space of the LCS.

©Copyright 2021 American Academy of Orthopaedic Surgeons

TABLE 1 Extracellular Proteins of Bone

Collagens	**Serum Proteins**
Type I	Serum albumin
Type V, type III (trace)	α2HS-glycoprotein
Proteoglycans	**Glycoproteins**
Biglycan	BAG-75
Decorin	Alkaline phosphatase
Fibromodulin	Osteonectin (SPARC)
Perlecan	Tetranectin
Osteoglycin/mimecan	
Osteoadherin	
SIBLING Proteins	**Vitamin K–Dependent Proteins (gla-proteins)**
Osteopontin (2ar, spp1)	Osteocalcin
Bone sialoprotein	Matrix gla-protein
DMP-1 (dentin matrix protein-1)	Periostin
Dentin sialophosphoprotein	
Matrix extracellular phosphoglycoprotein (MEPE)	
RGD-Containing Proteins	**Growth Factors/Cytokines**
Fibronectin	Bone morphogenetic proteins (BMPs)
Thrombospondins	BMP antagonists (noggin, chordin)
Fibrillins (1 and 2)	Insulinlike growth factors (IGF-I, II and IGF-binding proteins)
Perlecan	Transforming growth factor-β (TGF-β) and binding proteins
	Fibroblast growth factors (FGFs)
	Sclerostin (SOST)
	LDL receptor related protein (LRP)
	Dickkopf WNT signaling pathway inhibitor 1 (DKK)
Extracellular Enzymes	
Lysyl oxidase	
Alkaline phosphatase ("tissue-nonspecific" isoenzyme, tissue nonspecific alkaline phosphatase [TNSALP])	
Matrix metalloproteinases	
Phosphate-regulating neutral endopeptidase, X-linked (PHEX)	

BAG-75 = bone acidic glycoprotein-75, RGD = arg-gly-asp, SPARC = secreted protein acidic and rich in cysteine

Vitamin K–dependent proteins: Certain bone ECM proteins contain a distinctive posttranslational modification also found in the clotting protein prothrombin: gamma carboxyglutamic acid (gla), which results from the addition of a carboxyl group to the gamma position on specific glutamic acid residues. The most abundant gla-containing protein in bone is osteocalcin (also known as bone gla-protein). A second, termed matrix gla protein, is found primarily in calcified cartilage, and a third, periostin, is produced by osteoblasts in intramembranous bone and localized mainly in periosteum and periodontal ligament. Addition of the extra carboxyl group is enzymatic, requires vitamin K, and confers on these molecules the ability to form complexes with calcium and to bind readily to hydroxyapatite—properties not shared by non–gamma-carboxylated forms.

Osteoblasts produce several other ECM proteins that are not exclusive to bone, but common to most connective tissue matrices.[23] These include fibronectin, osteonectin (also termed SPARC, or secreted protein acidic and rich in cysteine), and thrombospondin. Fibronectin is not abundant in bone, but is a major mediator of adhesion between many of the cells in bone and collagen. Fibronectin also participates in the organization of pericellular matrix by cells and is essential to the formation of several tissues during development; fibronectin-deficient mice die during gestation, even before skeletal formation. The thrombospondin family has the ability to interact simultaneously with other ECM proteins and with cell surface receptors have been described as "matricellular" proteins. Overexpression and deletion of thrombospondin isoforms in mice lead to alterations in skeletogenesis and wound healing, but overall the phenotypes are mild. In addition to OPN and BSP, bone matrix contains several other proteins that are both glycosylated and substantially phosphorylated, including bone acidic glycoprotein-75 (BAG-75), DMP-1, and MEPE. BAG-75 is characterized by an ability to self-associate into complexes that can sequester phosphate ions and so may regulate mineral deposition and/or ion exchange. DMP-1 and MEPE, in contrast to OPN and BSP, are produced in bone mainly by osteocytes rather than osteoblasts. In addition, both are subject to proteolytic cleavage. Only a small fraction of the DMP-1 in bone is intact. DMP-1 deficiency in humans and in knockout mouse models is characterized by defective bone mineralization, suggesting multiple roles in regulating the deposition and maintenance of bone mineral. MEPE overexpression in mice results in deficient mineralization, whereas MEPE deletion leads to increased bone formation. MEPE is of particular interest in that its cleavage to yield a phosphorylated, mineralization-inhibiting peptide (the ASARM peptide) is regulated by PHEX (phosphate regulating gene with homologies to endopeptidases on the X chromosome)—the osteocyte protein implicated in X-linked hypophosphatemic rickets, which results when PHEX is inactivated.[32,33]

α2HS-glycoprotein: α2HS-glycoprotein is a highly acidic protein synthesized in liver. It binds large quantities of calcium

 ©Copyright 2021 American Academy of Orthopaedic Surgeons

ions and is thought to act systemically as an inhibitor of ectopic calcification. α2HS-glycoprotein is abundant in bone, where it is likely adsorbed onto mineral crystal surfaces, and modulates calcium ion exchange with tissue fluid. Other proteins found in bone matrix include a variety of signaling molecules and enzymes necessary to carry out local modifications of matrix structure. Perhaps the best known examples of signaling molecules are the bone morphogenetic proteins (BMPs),[34] whose activities were first identified in demineralized bone matrix; others include the BMP antagonist noggin, other members of the transforming growth factor–β (TGF-β) superfamily, the TGF-β binding proteins, fibroblast growth factors (FGFs), and sclerostin.[35] Bone matrix enzymes include alkaline phosphatase (ALP), matrix metalloproteinases (MMPs), notably MMP-2, MMP-13, and MMP-14, tissue inhibitor of metalloproteinase (TIMP), and PHEX.[32,33]

CLINICAL NOTE Of these molecules, osteocalcin and ALP are often used as osteoblast phenotypic markers in vivo and in vitro, both to identify osteoblasts in heterogeneous cell populations and to assess changes in osteoblast function. ALP, a cell surface enzyme, is upregulated early in osteoblast differentiation and remains present in mature osteoblasts but is lost when the cells become osteocytes. ALP is a convenient marker as it can be detected by both biochemical and histochemical activity assays; however, it is not cell type–specific (osteoblasts express the tissue-nonspecific ALP gene). Although ALP is absent or minimally expressed in most fibroblastic cells, it is expressed by some leukocytes and other cells in bone marrow. Osteocalcin, while not as easy to assay as ALP, is considered specific for the osteoblast lineage. It appears later in the differentiation process than ALP—that is, in mature osteoblasts. Both ALP and osteocalcin can be measured in serum and are used clinically to assess the efficacy of anticatabolic and antianabolic osteoporosis therapies.[36]

INORGANIC MINERAL ELEMENTS OF BONE

The inorganic phase of bone ECM consists of mineral crystals whose structure approximates hydroxyapatite $Ca_{10}(PO_4)_6(OH)_2$ that is variably substituted by other ions, mainly Mg^{2+} and CO_3.[2-4,23] Other cations such as aluminum, lead, and strontium (as well as heavy isotopes such as thorium, plutonium, and barium) and anions such as F may also become incorporated into bone mineral (usually in trace amounts) due to diet or environmental exposure. The first mineral crystals that form under physiologic conditions are likely to differ from hydroxyapatite in structure and composition. Furthermore, crystal size and perfection may depend on metabolic circumstances (such as rate of bone turnover). However, most mineral, even in embryonic bone, is apatitic. Bone mineral is distributed throughout the organic matrix, within and between collagen fibrils as described earlier (**Figure 6**). However, the accumulation of mineral in substantial amounts does not begin until some time after the organic matrix is deposited and at a distance apart from the bone surface and its active osteoblasts. How bone mineral forms, how it is deposited so completely within the interstices of collagen fibrils, and how it is organized in a consistent fashion have yet to be fully answered. The minimum requirement for precipitation of a mineral salt is that the concentrations of its constituents are high enough so that they interact in the proper orientation to form a crystal nucleus. Subsequent growth by addition of new molecules to an existing crystal lattice is less energetically demanding. Formation and growth of crystals can be facilitated by increasing the concentrations of its constituents (either directly or by removing inhibitors that might bind to the ions and thereby reduce their effective concentration) or by heterogeneous nucleation—provision of a separate molecular entity (such as a catalyst) whose surface is a crystal nucleus and allows ions to bind in a regular arrangement and grow in a crystalline array.

Mineralization of bone uses several of these mechanisms. Bone mineralization is regulated mainly at the local level by osteoblasts and likely osteocytes.[11,31-33] Systemic levels of Ca and Pi (inorganic orthophosphate, mainly HPO_4^{2-} and $H_2PO_4^-$ at physiologic pH) are homeostatically maintained, and their overall levels in bone and other tissues are relatively constant. Pathologic changes in systemic Ca or Pi levels will affect mineralization of bone, but under normal conditions, the process is regulated locally, principally by osteoblasts. Osteoblasts produce both metabolites and macromolecules that can either favor or inhibit mineral crystal nucleation and growth. Osteoblasts produce an endogenous inhibitor of mineralization, pyrophosphate (PPi, $P_2O_7^{4-}$), by hydrolysis of trinucleotides like adenosine triphosphate (ATP) (eg, ATP → adenosine monophosphate + PPi) by enzymes both within the cytoplasm and on the cell surface. Movement of PPi from the cytoplasm to the extracellular space is performed via a transmembrane protein, ANKH, the human homolog of the mouse ank gene product that, when mutated, results in a progressive ankylosing spondylitis. On the other hand, osteoblasts also express two phosphatases, ALP on cell surfaces and PHOSPHO1 (phosphatase orphan 1) intracellularly, that cleave PPi to yield two molecules of orthophosphate (Pi, PO_4^{3-}). These enzymes promote mineralization by simultaneously removing the inhibitor PPi and also generating two molecules of the Pi required for mineral crystal formation. The balance of Pi to PPi thus is a critical determinant of matrix mineralization. In addition to these mechanisms, production and phosphorylation of matrix proteins such as osteopontin and BAG-75, which can interact with Ca ions and also with crystal surfaces, may also modulate the mineralization process. In pathologic circumstances such as osteomalacia, where bone matrix is produced but does not mineralize, the osteoid seams are wide and remain so until

©Copyright 2021 American Academy of Orthopaedic Surgeons

the condition is remedied. The analogous condition in cartilage is rickets, which is similarly characterized by widened, unmineralized epiphyseal plates. Once bone formation ceases, mineralization continues until the osteoid seam disappears and virtually the entire matrix is mineralized. The time course of mineral accumulation in bone is biphasic. Roughly, 70% of mineral deposition at a site occurs in an exponential fashion within 5 to 10 days, whereas the remaining 30% is added over the following 3 to 6 months.

RESEARCH, CLINICAL, AND PATHOLOGICAL ASSESSMENTS OF BONE TISSUES

The primary research and pathological assessments of bone tissue are made by histological and two radiological methods, computerized x-ray CT and dual-energy x-ray absorptiometry (DEXA). These different assessment modalities share a number of relatable measurement criteria and are used to obtain complementary as well as unique information regarding the development and treatment of osteoporosis and other metabolic bone diseases. Each assessment tool has its own strengths and weakness. Standardized nomenclature, sampling criteria, sample sizes, and regions or volumes of interest for each type of analysis have been defined for both radiological and histological assessments of bones that are used for research and clinical applications.[37-39]

The major limitation of histological assessments is their two-dimensional nature. For most histological assessments, multiple sections are also analyzed both from within the same clinical biopsy or segment of animal bone tissue. Histological methods by their nature are also invasive such that when used clinically most will be obtained by biopsy. Advantages of histological approaches are that they are able to provide both specific structural measurements as well as assessment of the activities of cells that give measurements of the underlying cellular mechanisms of coupled remodeling.

Two different approaches maybe used: static and dynamic. A static approach is the most common method and is used to quantify the area measurements for specific bone structures as well as bone surface areas covered by osteoblast or osteoclast as well as their numbers. As indicated above osteoclast are identified by staining for TRAP enzyme activity and their multinucleated characteristics, while osteoblasts are usually simply identified by their morphology although their phenotype may be confirmed by staining for alkaline phosphatase activity or by immunological staining for expression of any number of proteins they express, such as osteocalcin or DMP1.

Dynamic histomorphometry make use of in vivo fluorochrome labeling in which a small nontoxic compound may be ingested or injected intravenously and becomes integrated into areas of forming bone mineral. By carrying out pulse chase studies at various times, bone may be biopsied or in the case of animal studies terminally retrieved and analyzed. Dynamic bone histomorphometry assess bone formation and resorption over time and thus provides a means to measure parameters such as the mineral apposition rate, bone formation rate, and activation frequency.[37] In addition to measures of bone formation, bone histomorphometry studies typically include measures of bone volume fraction and percent-eroded surface (ES/BS), measuring rates of mineral apposition and osteoid formation. Dynamic bone histomorphometry then provides key information regarding the cellular mechanisms underlying the development and treatment of osteoporosis and other metabolic bone diseases.

In contrast to histological assessments, CT uses x-ray attenuation data acquired at multiple rotational positions to reconstruct a 3D volumetric representation of the specimen. The resulting digital image allows detailed, quantitative examination of bone microstructure and density. In both CT and histological assessments, a volume of interest that is to be assayed is first defined. For both research and clinical analysis, standardized nomenclature, sampling criteria and sample sizes have been defined.[38] **Figure 7** shows regions of interest

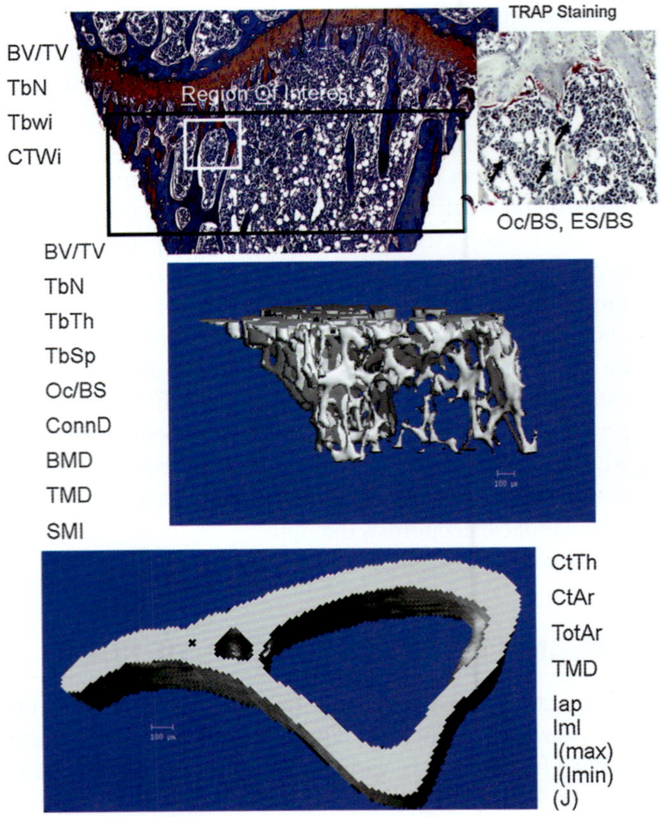

FIGURE 7 Comparison of histological and CT analysis of mouse tibia metaphyseal bone. **Upper** panel depicts the histological region of interest (ROI) in the boxed area that was analyzed. While insert box depicts matched area from a serial section stained for TRAP enzyme. **Middle and lower panel** are matched volumetric reconstructions of the same ROI analyzed by histology using microCT. The data achieved from each analysis are presented to the side of each image.

©Copyright 2021 American Academy of Orthopaedic Surgeons

TABLE 2 Common Radiological and Histological Metrics for Assessment of Bone[a,b]

Similar Values Between Histology, CT, and DEXA
TV: Total volume that is measured (CT and Histo)
BV/TV, %: Percent of total volume that is occupied by cancellous bone (both mineralized and nonmineralized). When the ratio BV/TV is low, this indicates a bone deficit in cancellous bone mass (CT and Histo)
Tb.Th: Trabecular thickness—mean distance across individual trabeculae, given in micrometers (CT and Histo)
Tb.N: Trabecular number—number of trabecular plates per unit distance (CT and Histo)
Tb.Sp: Trabecular separation—mean distance between trabeculae, given in micrometers (CT and Histo)
Ct.Wi-hist Ct Th-CT: Cortical width average width of both inner and outer cortices. In growing individuals, can be separated into periosteal perimeter and endosteal perimeter (CT and Histo)
BMD: Bone mineral density (CT and DEXA only)
BMC: Bone mineral content (CT and DEXA only)
Unique Values to CT
Conn.D: Connectivity density A measure of the degree of connectivity of trabeculae normalized by TV (CT only)
SMI: Structure model index—an indicator of the structure of trabeculae; SMI will be 0 for parallel plates and 3 for cylindrical rods (CT only)
DA: Degree of anisotropy 1¼ isotropic, >1¼anisotropic by definition; DA¼length of longest divided by shortest mean intercept length vector (CT only)
Iap: Moment of inertia about the anterior-posterior axis (CT only)
Iml: Moment of inertia about the mediolateral axis(CT only)
Imax: Maximum moment of inertia (CT only)
Imin: Minimum moment of inertia (CT only)
J: Polar moment of inertia (CT only)
Unique Static Histological Assessments
OV/BV, %: Osteoid volume—percent of a given volume of bone tissue that consists of unmineralized bone (osteoid)
OS/BS, %: Osteoid surface—percent of bone surface covered in osteoid
O.Th: Osteoid thickness—mean thickness, given in micrometers for osteoid seams
ES/BS, %: Eroded surface—percent of bone surface occupied by resorption cavities (Howships lacunae), with or without osteoclasts
Ob.S/BS: Osteoblast surface—percent of bone surface occupied by osteoblasts
Oc.S/BS: Osteoclast surface—percent of bone surface occupied by osteoclasts
Unique Dynamic Histological Assessments
Mar ¼m/d: Mineral apposition rate measurement of the linear rate of new bone deposition. It is the mean distance between the double labels, divided by the time interval between them
MS/BS, %: Mineralizing surface percent of bone surface that displays a tetracycline label reflecting active mineralization. It is calculated as the double-labeled surface plus one half of the single-labeled surface and is expressed as a function of total bone surface. It is a measure of the proportion of bone surface upon which new mineralized bone was being deposited during the period of tetracycline labeling
BFR/BS, ¼m³/¼m²/d: Bone formation rate amount of new bone formed in unit time per unit of bone surface. It is calculated by multiplying the mineralizing surface by the mineral apposition rate
Ac.F: Activation frequency provides an estimate for bone remodeling rate. It is calculated dividing the BFR/BS by wall width. The value generated represents the probability that a new remodeling cycle will be initiated at any point on the bone surface, providing a measure of the frequency at which two successive remodeling cycles are initiated at the same time on bone surface
Unique DEXA assessments
T score = (Measured BMD-Young adult mean BMD)/Young adult population SD
Z score = (Measured BMD-Age matched mean BMD)/Age matched population SD

BMP = bone morphogenetic protein, DEXA = dual-energy x-ray absorptiometry
[a]The assessment tools have been standardized by consensus committees of the American Society of Bone and Mineral Research (ASBMR).
[b]The most common assessment parameters are only summarized while the complete listing and nomenclature for all of the assessment parameters may be found in the census reports of the ASBMR.[37,38]

in the proximal tibia of a mouse, showing histological and microCT images matched to the same region of interest. The metrics that are collected from both approaches are presented in **Table 2**.

The other radiological technique that is used in the assessment of bone is DEXA. This technique only evaluates BMD and BMC by measuring the transmission of x-rays through the body at two different photon energies.[39] It application is primarily used in clinical setting, and it is limited in that is a two-dimensional projection image providing areal density measurements that are affected by bone size as well as the true volumetric density of the bone. In this regard, it cannot obtain any high-quality structural information about the bone tissues that are being assayed.

Because of the low rates of screening and poor screening protocols for osteoporosis during routine primary care health examinations, these patients are often not identified, until

©Copyright 2021 American Academy of Orthopaedic Surgeons

CLINICAL NOTE (DEXA AND TREATMENT GAP)

Current methods for evaluating fracture risk are based on measures of the average bone mineral density (BMD) by DEXA. Yet, for example, these averages explain only 50% to 70% of the variance in vertebral strength[40-45] and poorly discriminate between fracture and nonfracture cohorts.[45,46] The problem of BMD's low sensitivity and specificity in predicting fracture risk has grown acute in light of recent trends in osteoporosis treatment. Despite advances in available treatment options—namely, diphosphonates—the number of patients prescribed treatment and the number who adhere to the medication prescribed has declined.[47] The causes of this decline are multiple, but include skepticism about the utility of BMD. Better methods of identifying the individuals who are truly at high risk for fracture has therefore been identified as a key step toward resolving this treatment crisis.[48]

they have experienced one or more fractures. In this regard, up to 50% of women and 20% of men older than 50 years will experience a fragility fractures.[49] Medicare estimates are that up 65% of women older than 65 years who sustain a fragility fracture are neither worked up nor treated for osteoporosis within 6 months of their fracture. This treatment gap is recognized as a major clinical problem. Orthopedic surgeons, the initial care provider to identify these patients, are therefore positioned to initiate appropriate screening and refer these patients for definitive osteoporosis treatment and preventive fracture care. It is important to recognize this treatment gap and be aware of the evolving standards for addressing this treatment gap either through the development of fracture liaison services or practice protocol-based individual approaches for the management of these patients.[50,51]

STRUCTURAL AND METABOLIC BASIS OF SITE VARIATIONS IN METABOLIC BONE DISORDERS AND OSTEOPOROTIC FRACTURE

In the last section of this chapter, the cellular and structural basis of metabolic bone disorders and their relationship to site and age-specific variations in the occurrence of fractures will be reviewed. **Figure 8** presents a summary of the hierarchical elements, which were reviewed in the prior sections of this chapter that contribute to the overall mechanical function of a bone. A review of the contribution of the organic components of bone matrix to the overall mechanical function of bone has been recently presented.[52] All of these elements represent an interplay between underlying genetic factors that control these elements, which have variously been estimated to contribute between 20% and 40%[53,54] to the overall function of skeletal tissue and external environmental factors. As an example to the influence of the genetic influence on bone function, in humans there is sexual dimorphism in the overall size and mass of bones being less in females, thus leading to lesser mechanical robustness in women versus men.[55,56] In contrast, as an example to external factors that affect bone,

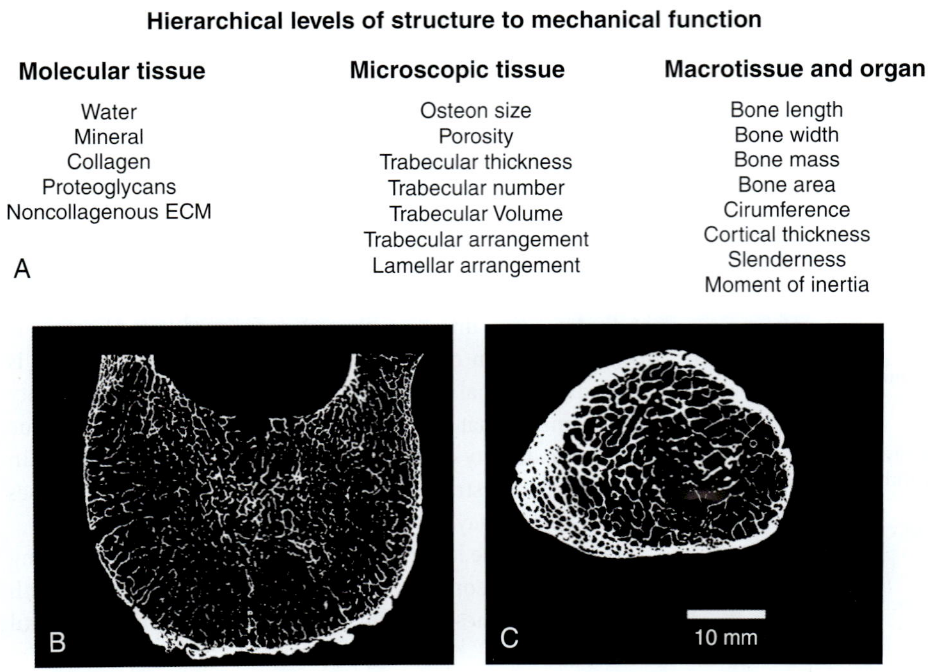

FIGURE 8 The hierarchical levels of bone composition and structure. **A**, lists the primary component elements at each of three levels of structural hierarchy. Lower panel shows cross-sections (obtained from microCT) of the human vertebra (**B**) and human femoral neck (**C**).

©Copyright 2021 American Academy of Orthopaedic Surgeons

TABLE 3 Quantitative Features of Cortical and Cancellous Bone

Index	Cortical Bone	Cancellous Bone
Fraction of skeleton (%)	80	20
Fraction of skeletal turnover (%)	50	50
Fractional tissue volume (mm^3/mm^3)	0.95	0.20
Fraction of surface undergoing resorption (%)	2	4
Fraction of surface undergoing formation (%)	8	16
Fraction of surface quiescent (%)	90	80
Surface to bone volume ratio (mm^3/mm^3)	2.5	20
Total bone volume (mm^3)	1.4×10^6	0.35×10^6
Total internal surface (mm^2)	3.5×10^6	0.35×10^6
Total number of BSU in skeleton	21×10^6	14×10^6

Adapted from Parfitt AM, Mathews CHE, Villanueva AR, Kleerekoper M, Frame B, Rao DS. Relationship between surface, volume and thickness of iliac trabecular bone in aging and in osteoporosis: implications for the microanatomic and cellular mechanisms of bone loss. *J Clin Invest* 1983;72:1396-409.

aging increases the overall width of bones thereby compensating for cortical thinning and loss of trabecular structures that occurs with aging.[57,58]

The primary metabolic bone disorders and basis of age related bone loss resides in disbalanced coupled remodeling, which was reviewed in Chapter 24 The cellular basis of this relationship is summarized **Table 3** and physiologically expressed in the age-dependent variations in fracture incidence that is summarized in **Table 4**. As can be seen in the table, even though the cortical bone represents four times more mass than cancellous bone, they show equal fractional turnover at any one time. This large difference between the masses of cortical and cancellous bone relative to their rates of turnover reflects the approximate 10-fold difference in surface to bone volume bone exposed to the marrow environment where osteoclast resides. This may be strikingly observed comparing a cross section of a human vertebrae body compared with the cross section of femoral neck in **Figure 8**. As can be seen in **Table 4**, vertebrae bodies have the smallest cortical to cancellous ratio, show the greatest prevalence of fracture, and show an increasing number of fractures across four decades of aging.[49] While the wrist shows the highest cortical to cancellous ratio and is the second most prevalent fracture, the number of fractures actually decreases with age largely, reflecting its constant rate of fracture due to falls and not to a progressive loss in bone due to coupled remodeling. In comparison, the hip, which has the next smallest cortical to cancellous ratio, has an increasing number of fractures over time. Finally comparing pelvic fractures to the hip where the cortical to cancellous ratio is almost exactly inverted to that of the hip show half the overall number of fractures and an increasing rate of fractures over time that appears to plateaus.

TABLE 4 Relationship Between Fracture Rate and Cortical to Cancellous Bone Mass

Bone Age	Cortical/ Cancellous Ratio	Percent	Fracture Rate per Thousand by Decade			
			50-64	65-74	75-84	Over 85
Vertebra	25/75	27	86,779	124,378	195,310	140,959
Hip	34/66	14	20,025	32,068	111,088	130,430
Pelvis	60/40	7	13,726	22,295	54,856	43,902
Wrist	75/25	19	63,188	89,046	76,115	37,412

Adapted from Adams J, et al: in Rosen CJ: *Primer on the Metabolic Bone Diseases and Disorders of Mineral Metabolism*. JW Wiley, 2008, pp 151-158 and Burge R, Dawson-Hughes B, Solomon DH, Wong JB, King A, Tosteson A: Incidence and economic burden of osteoporosis-related fractures in the United States, 2005–2025. *J Bone Miner Res* 2007;22(3):465-475.

©Copyright 2021 American Academy of Orthopaedic Surgeons

SUMMARY

The hierarchical nature of bone from the whole organ to molecular levels was reviewed and placed in context to the multifunctional physiological roles that bone tissues carry out. The major elements of how bone tissues are assessed for both research and clinical applications and how these assessment tools are used to deduce functional and molecular aspects of bone health and pathology were also reviewed. In the final sections of this review, the relationship between the cellular activities of how coupled remolding were linked to metabolic disorders and aging, and the structural deficiencies that develop in bones which lead to fractures was presented.

REFERENCES

1. Jee WS: Integrated bone tissue physiology: Anatomy and physiology, in Cowin SC, ed: *Bone Mechanics Handbook*, ed 2. Boca Raton, FL, CRC Press, 2001, pp 1.1-1.68.
2. Hancox NM: *Biology of Bone*. London, England, Cambridge University Press, 1972, pp 10-40.
3. Martin RB, Burr DB, Sharkey NA: *Skeletal Tissue Mechanics*. London, England, Springer-Verlag, 1998, pp 127-223.
4. Currey JD: *Bones: Structure and Mechanics*. Princeton, NJ, Princeton University Press, 2002, pp 54-124, 194-245.
5. Superti-Furga A, Unger S: Nosology and classification of genetic skeletal disorders: 2006 *Am J Med Genet* 2007;143A(1):1-18.
6. Morgan EF, Barnes G, Einhorn TA: The bone organ system: Form and function, in Marcus R, Feldman D, Nelson DA, Rosen CJ, eds: *Osteoporosis*, ed 3. Waltham, MA, Elsevier Academic Press, 2008, pp 3-22.
7. Kerr JB: *Atlas of Functional Histology*. London, England, Mosby, 1999, pp 163-184.
8. Yang Y: Skeletal morphogenesis and embryonic development, in Rosen CJ, ed: *Primer on the Metabolic Bone Diseases and Disorders of Mineral Metabolism*. Washington, DC, American Society for Bone and Mineral Research, 2009, pp 2-10.
9. Brookes M, Revell WJ: *Blood Supply of Bone*. London, United Kingdom, Springer-Verlag, 1998, pp 142-175.
10. Eriksen EF, Axelrod DW, Melsen F: *Bone Histomorphometry*. New York, NY, Raven Press, 1994, pp 3-12.
11. Dallas SL, Prideaux M, Bonewald LF: The osteocyte: An endocrine cell … and more *Endocr Rev* 2013;34(5):658-690.
12. Ross FP: Osteoclast biology and bone resorption, in Rosen CJ, ed: *Primer on the Metabolic Bone Diseases and Disorders of Mineral Metabolism*, ed 8. Wiley and Blackwell Ames, Iowa, American Society for Bone and Mineral Research, 2013, pp 49-58.
13. Tanaka S, Miyazaki T, Fukuda A, et al: Molecular mechanism of the life and death of the osteoclast. *Ann N Y Acad Sci* 2006;1068:180-186.
14. Nakamura I, Takahashi N, Jimi E, Udagawa N, Suda T: Regulation of osteoclast function. *Mod Rheumatol* 2012;22(2):167-177.
15. Suda T, Takahashi N, Udagawa N, Jimi E, Gillespie MT, Martin TJ: Modulation of osteoclast differentiation and function by the new members of the tumor necrosis factor receptor and ligand families. *Endocr Rev* 1999;20(3):345-357.
16. Teitelbaum SL, Ross FP: Genetic regulation of osteoclast development and function. *Nat Rev Genet* 2003;4(8):638649.
17. Matic I, Matthews BG, Wang X, et al: Quiescent bone lining cells are a major source of osteoblasts during adulthood. *Stem Cells* 2016 34(12):2930-2942.
18. Robey PG, Termine JD: Human bone cells in vitro. *Calcif Tissue Int* 1985;37(5):453-456.
19. de Paula FJ, Horowitz MC, Rosen CJ: Novel insights into the relationship between diabetes and osteoporosis. *Diabetes Metab Res Rev* 2010;26(8):622-630.
20. Wang Y, McNamara LM, Schaffler MB, Weinbaum S: A model for the role of integrins in flow induced mechanotransduction in osteocytes. *Proc Natl Acad Sci USA* 2007;104(40):15941-15946.
21. Quarles LD: Skeletal secretion of FGF-23 regulates phosphate and vitamin D metabolism. *Nat Rev Endocrinol* 2012;8(5):276-286.
22. Burr DB: The contribution of the organic matrix to bone's material properties. *Bone* 2002;31(1):8-11.
23. Boskey AL Robey PG: The composition of bone, in Rosen CJ, ed: *Primer on the Metabolic Bone Diseases and Disorders of Mineral Metabolism*, ed 8. Wiley and Blackwell Ames, Iowa, American Society for Bone and Mineral Research, 2013, pp 49-58.
24. Viguet-Carrin S, Garnero P, Delmas PD: The role of collagen in bone strength. *Osteoporos Int* 2006;17(3):319-336.
25. Gordon MK, Hahn RA: Collagens. *Cell Tissue Res* 2010;339(1):247-257.
26. Landis WJ, Jacquet R: Association of calcium and phosphate ions with collagen in the mineralization of vertebrate tissues. *Calcif Tissue Int* 2013;93:329-337.
27. Gerstenfeld LC, Chipman SD, Kelly CM, Hodgens KJ, Lee DD, Landis WJ: Collagen expression, ultrastructural assembly, and mineralization in cultures of chicken embryo osteoblasts *J Cell Biol* 1988;106(3):979-989.
28. Eyre DR, Weis MA, Wu J-J: Advances in collagen cross-link analysis. *Methods* 2008;45(1):65-74.
29. Royce PM, Steinmann B. *Connective Tissue and Its Heritable Disorders: Molecular, Genetic, and Medical Aspects*, ed 2. New York, NY, USA, Wiley-Liss, Inc., 2003.
30. Kalamajski S, Oldberg A: The role of small leucine-rich proteoglycans in collagen fibrillogenesis. *Matrix Biol* 2010;29(4):248-253.
31. Gorski JP: Biomineralization of bone: A fresh view of the roles of non-collagenous proteins. *Front Biosci* 2011;16:25982621.
32. Murshed M, McKee MD: Molecular determinants of extracellular matrix mineralization in bone and blood vessels. *Curr Opin Nephrol Hypertens* 2010;19(4):359-365.
33. Sapir-Koren R, Livshits G: Bone mineralization and regulation of phosphate homeostasis. *IBMS BoneKEy* 2011;8:286300.
34. Shore EM, Kaplan FS: Insights from a rare genetic disorder of extra-skeletal bone formation, fibrodysplasia ossificans progressiva (FOP). *Bone* 2008;43(3):427-433.
35. Monroe DG, McGee-Lawrence ME, Oursler MJ, Westendorf JJ: Update on Wnt signaling in bone cell biology and bone disease. *Gene* 2012;492(1):1-18.
36. Vasikaran S, Eastell R, Bruyère O, et al: Markers of bone turnover for the prediction of fracture risk and monitoring of osteoporosis treatment: A need for international reference standards. *Osteoporos Int* 2011;22(2):391-420.
37. Dempster DW, Compston JE, Drezner MK, et al: Standardized nomenclature, symbols, and units for bone histomorphometry: A 2012 update of the report of the ASBMR Histomorphometry Nomenclature Committee. *J Bone Miner Res* 2013;28(1):2.
38. Bouxsein ML, Boyd SK, Christiansen BA, Guldberg RE, Jepsen KJ, Müller R: Guidelines for assessment of bone microstructure in rodents using micro-computed tomography *J Bone Miner Res* 2010;25(7):1468-1486.
39. Blake GM, Fogelman I: Technical principles of dual-energy x-ray absorptiometry. *Semin Nucl Med* 1997;27:210-228.
40. Tabensky AD, Williams J, DeLuca V, Briganti E, Seeman E: Bone mass, areal, and volumetric bone density are equally accurate, sensitive, and specific surrogates of the breaking strength of the vertebral body: An in vitro study. *J Bone Miner Res* 1996;11:1981-1988.

©Copyright 2021 American Academy of Orthopaedic Surgeons

41. Singer K, Edmondston S, Day R, Breidahl P, Price R: Prediction of thoracic and lumbar vertebral body compressive strength: Correlations with bone mineral density and vertebral region. *Bone* 1995;17:167-174.
42. Cheng XG, Nicholson PH, Boonen S, et al: Prediction of vertebral strength in vitro by spinal bone densitometry and calcaneal ultrasound. *J Bone Miner Res* 1997;12:1721-1728.
43. Buckley JM, Loo K, Motherway J: Comparison of quantitative computed tomography-based measures in predicting vertebral compressive strength. *Bone* 2007;40:767-774.
44. Edmondston SJ, Singer KP, Day RE, Price RI, Breidahl PD: Ex vivo estimation of thoracolumbar vertebral body compressive strength: The relative contributions of bone densitometry and vertebral morphometry. *Osteoporos Int* 1997;7:142-148.
45. Cann C: Quantitative CT for determination of bone mineral density: A review. *Radiology* 1988;166:509-522.
46. Kanis JA, Johnell O, Oden A, De Laet C, Jonsson B, Dawson A: Ten-year risk of osteoporotic fracture and the effect of risk factors on screening strategies. *Bone* 2002;30:251-258.
47. Khosla S, Shane E: A crisis in the treatment of osteoporosis. *J Bone Miner Res* 2016;31:1485-1487.
48. Khosla S, Cauley JA, Compston J, et al: Addressing the crisis in the treatment of osteoporosis: A path forward. *J Bone Miner Res* 2017;32(3):424-430.
49. Burge R, Dawson-Hughes B, Solomon DH, Wong JB, King A, Tosteson A: Incidence and economic burden of osteoporosis-related fractures in the United States, 2005–2025. *J Bone Miner Res* 2007;22(3):465-475.
50. Barton DW, Griffin DC, Carmouche JJ: Orthopedic surgeons' views on the osteoporosis care gap and potential solutions: Survey results. *J Orthop Surg Res* 2019;14(1):72.
51. Barton DW, Behrend CJ, Carmouche JJ: Rates of osteoporosis screening and treatment following vertebral fracture. *Spine J* 2019;19(3):411-417.
52. Unal M, Creecy A, Nyman JS: The role of matrix composition in the mechanical behavior of bone. *Curr Osteoporos Rep* 2018;16(3):205-215.
53. Liu C-T, Karasik D, Zhou Y, et al: Heritability of prevalent vertebral fracture and volumetric bone mineral density and geometry at the lumbar spine in three generations of the Framingham study 2012;27(4):954.
54. Trajanoska K, Morris JA, Oei L, et al: Assessment of the genetic and clinical determinants of fracture risk: Genome wide association and mendelian randomisation study. *BMJ* 2018;362:k3225.
55. Gilsanz V, Wren TAL, Ponrartana S, Mora S, Rosen CJ: Sexual dimorphism and the origins of human spinal health. *Endocr Rev* 2018;39(2):221-239.
56. Seeman E: Clinical review 137: Sexual dimorphism in skeletal size, density, and strength. *J Clin Endocrinol Metab* 2001;86:4576-4584.
57. Seeman E: Pathogenesis of bone fragility in women and men. *Lancet* 2002;359:1841-1.
58. Frost HM: Bone's mechanostat: A 2003 update. *Anat Rec A Discov Mol Cell Evol Biol* 2003;275:1081-1101.
59. Parfitt AM, Mathews CHE, Villanueva AR, Kleerekoper M, Frame B, Rao DS: Relationship between surface, volume and thickness of iliac trabecular bone in aging and in osteoporosis: Implications for the microanatomic and cellular mechanisms of bone loss. *J Clin Invest* 1983;72:1396-1409.
60. Adams J, Bishop N: DXA in adults and children, in Rosen CJ, ed: *Primer on the Metabolic Bone Diseases and Disorders of Mineral Metabolism.* Hoboken, NJ, John Wiley & Sons, Inc., 2008, pp 151-158.

©Copyright 2021 American Academy of Orthopaedic Surgeons

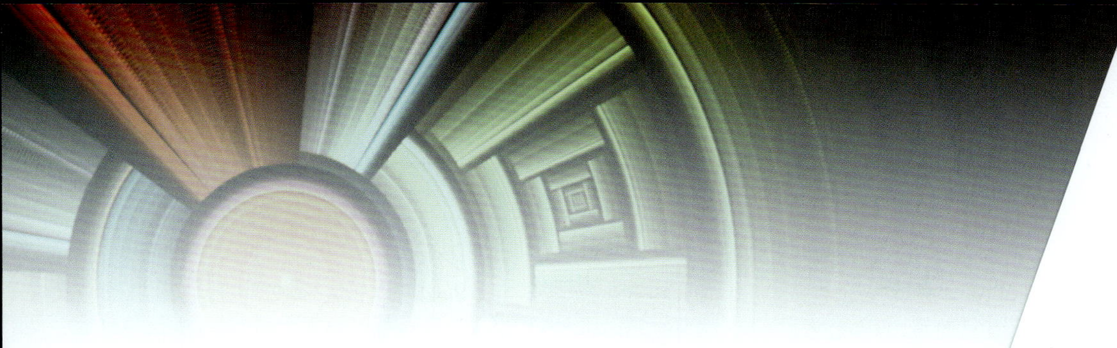

Bone Biomechanics

David B. Burr, PhD
Joseph M. Wallace, PhD

Keywords: *aging; fatigue; fracture; mechanotransduction; strain; stress*

INTRODUCTION: BASIC CONCEPTS OF BONE MECHANICS

The mechanical properties of bone are defined both by its structure (mass and architecture) and by the properties of the material of which it is made (the bone matrix). These properties can be termed structural (or extrinsic) or material (intrinsic). Extrinsic properties are usually measured by causing the bone to deform and measuring how much load it can bear before fracture. The resulting load-deformation curve is used to define the bone's *strength, stiffness,* and *energy to fracture.* When the load, or force, is adjusted for area (force/area = *stress*) and deformation is normalized by the original length of the structure (change in length/original length = *strain*), a similar curve results that defines the intrinsic properties of the tissue itself, independent of its size or geometry (**Figure 1**). This is called the *stress-strain curve,* and tissue properties analogous to structural properties can be estimated: the *ultimate stress* (tissue strength), *modulus of elasticity* (tissue stiffness), and *modulus of toughness* (fracture energy of the tissue).

Load and deformation are linearly proportional for some time, until the yield point is reached. At this point, the slope of the curve begins to decrease, meaning that lower loads are required to create substantially more deformation. The area under the linear portion of the load-deformation (or stress-strain) curve is called the elastic region because the structure will return to its original shape when the load is removed, elastically returning most of the energy required for deformation. However, the shift of fluids in the bone when it is loaded will cause some loss of elastic energy each time the bone is loaded within this range; this loss of energy is called *hysteresis.* Following yield, bone is permanently, or plastically, deformed and will not return to its original shape upon unloading. Within this postyield region, the bone has been irreversibly damaged (microcracking, slippage at cement lines, damage at the nanoscale to mineral crystals or collagen and its cross-linked structure, or combinations of these). If the load continues to increase, an *ultimate* (maximum) load is reached, and continued loading will result in fracture (the *failure load*). The brittleness of the bone is defined by the amount of strain that occurs after the yield point. Fracture after the yield point without much additional strain/deformation is typical of a brittle structure (the opposite, in which strain increases without an increase in stress, is defined as *ductility*).

The *strength* of bone may be defined as the load (or stress) at the yield point, or as the ultimate load/stress. Because there may be continued deformation after the maximum load is reached, causing the failure load to be lower than the ultimate load, it is best to use ultimate load or ultimate stress as the strength criterion. Furthermore, there is less variability in the ultimate load than in the failure load. *Stiffness* or *rigidity* is the load required to deform the bone a given amount. This is the same thing as the slope of the linear portion of the load-deformation curve. *Elastic modulus* (or *Young modulus,* named for Thomas Young [1773-1829], the physician-physicist who coined the term "modulus of elasticity") is the equivalent measurement taken from the slope of the linear portion of the stress-strain curve. The *work* or *energy* required to yield or fracture the structure is determined by measuring the area under the load-deformation curve out to the yield or failure points. The *modulus of resilience* and

Dr. Burr or an immediate family member serves as a paid consultant to or is an employee of Agnovos. Neither Dr. Wallace nor any immediate family member has received anything of value from or has stock or stock options held in a commercial company or institution related directly or indirectly to the subject of this chapter.

©Copyright 2021 American Academy of Orthopaedic Surgeons

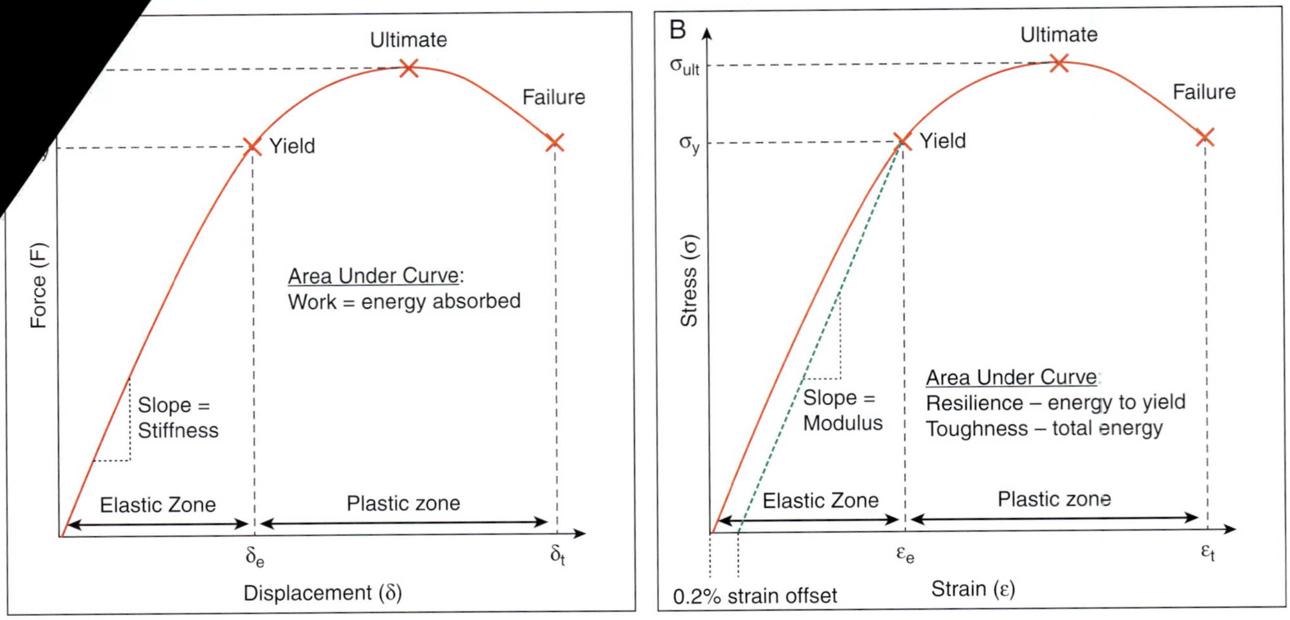

FIGURE 1 **Schematic representations of force-displacement and stress-strain curves.** In Panel A, applied load is plotted as a function of displacement. Important properties related to strength, stiffness, ductility or ability to deform, and ability to dissipate energy can be derived from this curve. An important note is that this characteristic graph represents the structural behavior of a sample and is influenced by the size and shape of the sample, as well as its material properties. By normalizing for the geometry of the sample, a complimentary stress-strain curve is obtained (panel B). Similar information can be calculated from this curve, but these parameters are estimated material properties which are no longer dependent on size and shape. Of note here is the yield point, where behavior turns from being linear-elastic to nonlinear. A typical method to locate this point is to use the 0.2% offset method in the stress-strain domain as shown.

modulus of toughness are the analogous tissue-level measurements made from the stress-strain curve.

Bone can be loaded in several different modes. When a structure is loaded in tension, it becomes longer in the load direction, and when loaded in compression, it becomes shorter. When loaded, the relationship between the change in transverse width, and the change in length is known as *Poisson ratio*. For geometric reasons, this ratio must be between 0 and 0.5 in ordinary materials. For incompressible materials (eg, cartilage), Poisson ratio is 0.5. Typical values for solids, including bone, are about 0.3, but in cortical bone the ratio can vary between 0.28 and 0.45.

Of course, human bone is seldom or never loaded in pure compression or tension, but is usually subject to bending, which produces a combination of compression and tension on different bone cortices. Under bending loads in vivo, shear stresses are also created in which one region as bone slides past an adjacent region. Bone is weaker in shear (~67 MPa for the femoral midshaft) than in either compression (~205 MPa) or tension (~135 MPa), so when bending loads are applied to bone to the point of failure, bone fracture may be accelerated by these shear stresses. This is also true when using three-point bending tests of bone ex vivo, where bone fails due to shear rather than tension or compression. One reason to use a four-point bending test is that the region between the two loading points exhibits no shear forces, and the bone fails due to tensile loading at its weakest point. In tension or compression, shear stress is maximized at a 45° angle from the direction of loading. Shear stresses are also created when bone is twisted (torsion).

CROSS-SECTIONAL PROPERTIES AS ESTIMATES OF STRENGTH AND RIGIDITY

If one can assume that the bone tissue is normal (as in osteoporosis, but perhaps not in other conditions such as osteogenesis imperfecta or types I and II diabetes), then estimates of bone's strength can be made from its geometry.

Bones are thick-walled tubes, which allows them to be strong, but not heavy. Long bones are mostly loaded in bending, and the amount that they bend under a load (their deflection) is defined by the bending moment, length of the bone, elastic modulus, and the second moment of the area (or moment of inertia) about the bending axis. For any given bending moment, the bending of the bone can be reduced by decreasing its length, making it stiffer (larger modulus), or increasing its moment of inertia. The cross-sectional moment of inertia is a measure of the distribution of material about a cross-sectional axis and is calculated as the sum of the square distance of each unit of area from the axis around which bending occurs (or the radial distance from the centroid of the section for a polar moment of inertia, which is proportional to torsional rigidity). For a circular tube, bending rigidity around

©Copyright 2021 American Academy of Orthopaedic Surgeons

a particular axis is proportional to the fourth power of its distance from the axis around which bending occurs.

$$I = \frac{\pi}{4}\left(R_o^4 - R_i^4\right)$$

where R_o is the distance from the bending axis to the periosteal surface, and R_i is the distance from the axis to the endosteal surface. Adding a small amount of bone to the periosteal surface can increase bone's bending rigidity substantially as the new material is located far away from the bending axis and, therefore, contributes more greatly to the moment of inertia (**Figure 2**). Consequently, if only one-third of the amount of bone that is removed from the endosteal surface is added to the periosteal surface, the rigidity of the bone is maintained. Thus, periosteal apposition can increase bone strength even when bone mass and bone mineral density (BMD) have declined. This also means that a small amount of bone loss near the marrow cavity may have a negligible effect on bone's overall strength and rigidity.

BONE'S MECHANICAL PROPERTIES

The mechanical properties of cortical bone vary from location to location in the skeleton, but are also determined by the direction in which the properties are measured. This is partly dependent on the orientation of osteons in cortical bone and on the orientation of lamellae within osteons and interstitial bone. Bone is stiffer in the longitudinal direction (~17 gigapascals, or GPa) than in the transverse direction (~12 GPa).[1] Materials that have different mechanical properties in different directions are termed *anisotropic* (an *isotropic* material would have the same properties in all directions; an *orthotropic* material has different properties in every direction). Bone is transversely isotropic (but also anisotropic) because its mechanical properties in all transverse directions are the same, but differ from properties measured in the longitudinal direction. Strength in the transverse direction is about 40% of that in the longitudinal direction.[1]

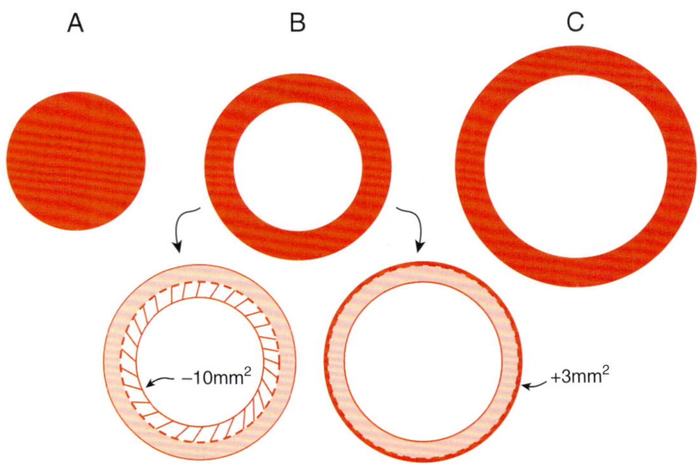

	A		B		C
Cortical Area (cm²)	1.77	1.67	1.77	1.70	1.77
Relative Axial Strength	1.00	0.94	1.00	0.96	1.00
Moment of Inertia (cm⁴)	0.25	0.61	0.64	0.64	1.13
Relative Bending Strength	1.00	2.45	2.56	2.56	4.52

FIGURE 2 Illustrations demonstrating that the rigidity of bone is partly dependent on its geometry. Cross-sections A, B, and C all have the identical cortical area, but distributed in different ways. As the outer diameter of the bone is expanded, the moment of inertia and relative bending strength increase by more than fourfold though the amount of bone has not changed. The axial strength of a bone is dependent only on the amount of bone, not its distribution, so relative axial strength does not change. The two figures in the second row demonstrate what happens when 10 mm² of bone is removed from the endocortical surface of bone (hatched area). Adding only 3 mm² of bone back onto the periosteal surface (black area) maintains the original bone bending strength, although axial strength would be slightly lower.[a]

[a]The authors wish to thank Drew Brown for his help in preparing **Figure 2**.

©Copyright 2021 American Academy of Orthopaedic Surgeons

For cancellous bone, these intrinsic properties become more difficult to measure because cancellous bone is composed of individual trabeculae, each of which may have its own stiffness. This combination of individual trabecular stiffnesses, together with the orientation of the different trabeculae (the trabecular architecture), will determine the structural stiffness of the cancellous mesh, which can vary between 0.1 and 4.5 GPa. The strength of cancellous bone, which is dependent on apparent density and orientation of the trabeculae that collectively compose it, is much less than that in cortical bone, varying between about 1 and 20 MPa.

Although strength is often equated with resistance to fracture, bone can be quite strong, but not very fracture resistant. An example is osteopetrotic bone. Although this bone is highly dense and can be loaded to a high stress, it cannot deform much before failure. Thus, it has a short post-yield region (it is *brittle*), indicating that it cannot develop damage and absorb energy efficiently before it fractures. Therefore, a strong and stiff bone is not necessarily a tough and fracture-resistant one if it is unable to absorb much energy before it breaks. In fact, great strength (or stiffness) and great toughness are often mutually exclusive[2] (**Figure 3**). These relationships also show that although there is often a close relationship between BMD and mechanical properties, the relationship between BMD and fracture risk is more complex.

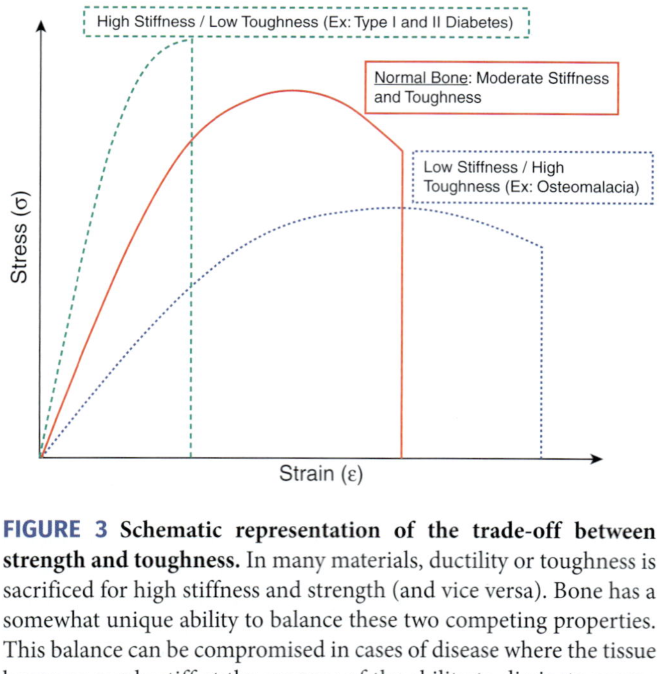

FIGURE 3 Schematic representation of the trade-off between strength and toughness. In many materials, ductility or toughness is sacrificed for high stiffness and strength (and vice versa). Bone has a somewhat unique ability to balance these two competing properties. This balance can be compromised in cases of disease where the tissue becomes overly stiff at the expense of the ability to dissipate energy and is brittle. Alternatively, some diseases have a negative impact on stiffness and strength and deform a great deal under relatively low load levels, leading to bone deformity.

THE BASIS FOR BONE'S MATERIAL PROPERTIES

Properties of the bone tissue itself (material properties) are also critical to bone's mechanical integrity. Although conventional wisdom concentrates mostly on the collagen and mineral components of the tissue, because these are the most prevalent components, noncollagenous proteins (NCPs), and water also contribute.

Bone mineral is generally considered to give bone its strength and stiffness, but the nature of the mineral crystal itself also is important. Crystallinity (the size/shape/perfection of crystals, an increase of which is associated with older tissue and/or lower bone remodeling rates) is associated with lower ultimate strain and toughness.[3,4] Carbonate replaces some of the phosphate in the hydroxyapatite crystal as the tissue ages, but the effect of this substitution is uncertain. It changes the amount of elastic and plastic deformation that occurs before fracture,[4,5] but reports about whether this increases[6] or decreases[4] elastic modulus differ. This may depend on the relationship between crystal size and crystal lattice perfection. Furthermore, too much mineral (osteopetrosis) can make the tissue brittle even though it may be strong; too little mineral (osteomalacia) will reduce elastic modulus. Both conditions impair the overall mechanical properties of bone, and increase fracture risk. Therefore, bone mineral must be kept within a fairly narrow window to achieve the best mechanical function.

The type I collagen in bone is often considered to provide bone's ductility, but equally important is the extent and manner in which the collagen fibrils are cross-linked. Two of the common trivalent (mature) cross-links, pyridinoline (PYD) and deoxypyridinoline (DPD) do not correlate with bending strength,[7,8] but the ratio of the two does correlate with increased strength and stiffness by stabilizing the collagen network.[9,10] These cross-links may also make the bone tougher,[11] because as they rupture with loading, they provide a means to dissipate energy in the tissue. Intermolecular bonds formed by nonenzymatic processes may have different effects. These cross-link-like bonds (they are not truly cross-links) result in the accumulation of advanced glycation end-products (AGEs), which are common in both types I and II diabetes and in chronic kidney disease. They make the bone tissue brittle and more likely to break.[9,12] AGEs reduce the amount of energy that can be absorbed prior to fracture by restricting movement in the collagen matrix, so may especially increase the risk of hip fractures that result from an impact such as a fall.

There are several water compartments in bone. The loosely bound water found at the mineral-collagen interface serves an important function by increasing the ductility of this interface, dissipating energy and reducing shear stresses during loading.[13] Some of this water is bound to the collagen, and some bound to the mineral, and their effects may be different. Collagen-bound water correlates positively with toughness,

©Copyright 2021 American Academy of Orthopaedic Surgeons

whereas mineral-bound water correlates negatively with elastic modulus.[14] The age-related reduction in bound water accounts for 71% of the reduction in bone toughness.[15] Some of this may be regulated by glycosaminoglycans (GAGs), which are known to be hydrophilic. One of these, biglycan, which is found in the perilacunar matrix, is thought to have shear-sensing properties. The reduction in GAGs with age may contribute to an overall 40% reduction in toughness in the later decades of life.[15,16]

Other NCPs are also known to affect mechanical properties of bone, either directly or indirectly, by regulating the mineralization process. Osteopontin and osteocalcin in particular have been noted to influence bone material properties. Osteopontin contributes to intrafibrillar sacrificial bonds that allow greater stress relaxation and more deformation prior to failure.[17,18] Genetically modified mice in which osteopontin or osteocalcin are knocked-out have lower bone toughness than those in which these NCPs are intact.[19] Greater phosphorylation of osteopontin makes cracks that develop in bone more difficult to propagate (ie, they have greater crack growth toughness).[20]

BONE FATIGUE

Measurements of bone strength and stiffness are generally made in a quasi-static fashion: a steadily increased load is placed on the bone at a constant rate until the bone yields or breaks. In real life, bone is not loaded in this way, so while providing a picture of bone's mechanical integrity, such measurements are not necessarily an accurate reflection of bone's properties when it is repetitively loaded as it is during activity. Theoretically, a bone repetitively loaded within the elastic limit will develop no damage and always return to its original shape upon unloading. However, because of microstructural features and local heterogeneities, local stresses in some areas will exceed the yield stress, and damage will occur. With repeated loading, this local damage will cause overall mechanical properties to gradually decline over time. This degradation of mechanical properties is termed *fatigue*, and precipitates bone failure at loads well below those that would normally cause it to fracture. At lower stresses (<60 MPa), the degradation is generally attributed to the initiation and growth of microcracks within the bone. At stresses above 60 MPa, fatigue is attributed to creep, which is caused by slippage at cement lines or the gradual degradation of bone's viscoelasticity.[21,22] As living bone is rarely exposed to compressive stresses greater than 40 MPa, failure in bone from cyclic loading is generally attributed to processes associated with fatigue, rather than those associated with creep.

Bone is a reasonably fatigue-resistance material, allowing cracks to initiate easily, but preventing them from growing to critical size. The lamellar and osteonal structure of bone is ideal at preventing rapid growth of cracks that occur within the cortex. In most cases, the small cracks will be repaired by remodeling before they have the chance to grow and coalesce. However, if the rate of damage accumulation exceeds the rate at which the damage can be repaired, the bone will break. Furthermore, because the remodeling process takes some time, the resorption pit that results from initial phase of remodeling may cause a stress concentration that can initiate additional damage. A common example of fatigue failure is the occurrence of a stress fracture, prevalent in athletes and military personnel. These stem from many repetitions of a high-stress activity that creates an imbalance between damage formation and its repair.

There are three phases during the fatigue process that are loosely defined by crack initiation and stable accumulation (region I), crack growth (region II), and crack coalescence/failure (region III). In the first phase, the initiation of cracks causes a rapid drop of stiffness. With about 75% of its fatigue life left, the loss of stiffness stabilizes as cracks begin to grow (region II). The growth of cracks does not cause much further stiffness loss because crack branching relieves stress concentrations within the matrix, allowing bone to absorb the energy without failure. With 90% of its fatigue life expended, coalescence of damage increases stresses within the material in a self-feeding process that again causes rapid stiffness loss and results in a catastrophic fracture (region III) (**Figure 4**).

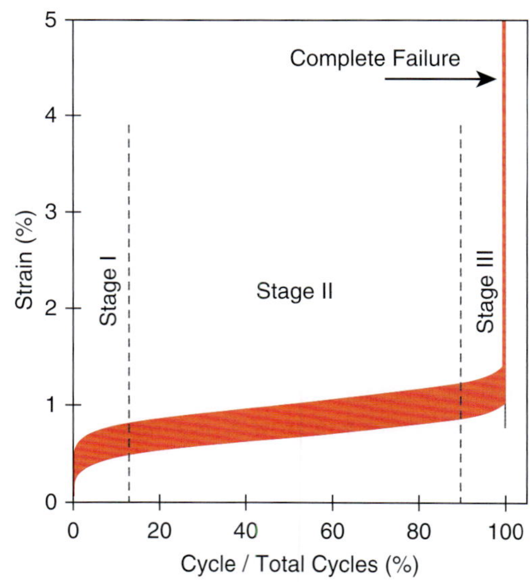

FIGURE 4 Schematic representation of fatigue response to repetitive loading. This curve shows the typical progression of fatigue to failure and was acquired during a fatigue test of a mouse femur. As a sample is cyclically loaded to a set force (typically below yield), microscopic damage accrues which leads to stiffness loss (ie, increased strain for a given load). As described in the text, the sample goes through three phases (initiation and accumulation, stable crack growth, and crack coalescence) before catastrophic failure occurs.

©Copyright 2021 American Academy of Orthopaedic Surgeons

The fatigue process can be characterized by creating an S–N curve, which plots applied stress (or strain) as a function of the number of cycles required for failure. Usually, a 30% loss of elastic modulus is the criterion for "failure," and as modulus declines with fatigue, there is a linear relationship between logS and logN. With more cycles of loading (and lower stress), an endurance limit may be reached where the stress is low enough that no matter how many cycles are applied, failure never occurs. Fatigue life (N_F), however, is nonlinearly related to applied stress. Small changes in applied stress can result in large changes in fatigue life. Based on data from Caler and Carter[23] and Pattin et al,[24] at peak physiologic strains of 2,000 microstrain (με), which can be generated during running,[25] the fatigue life of the femur is about 4.1 million cycles in tension and more than twice that in compression (9.13 million cycles).

FRACTURE MECHANICS

Bone fatigue occurs because microscopic cracks or flaws develop in the bone tissue causing its properties to degrade and reducing the amount of residual cyclic loading needed to cause fracture. Fracture mechanics is the branch of engineering that considers the conditions under which a crack can grow and result in bone fracture. Measurements of crack growth are often made by introducing a notch into a bone test specimen and then stressing that notch until failure. The notch creates a defect that causes a crack to initiate at the apex and propagate through the specimen. During the crack's propagation, various measurements of its growth can be made. One measurement is the stress intensity factor (K_c) at the crack tip, which is proportional to the stress (α) and the square root of the crack length (a):

$$K = \alpha\sqrt{a} \text{ or more correctly } K = Cs\sqrt{\pi a}$$

where C is a constant that depends on the mode of loading and the size and shape of the flaw and specimen, and s defines certain stress components. K_c is the critical stress intensity factor that defines whether the crack will propagate—if above a critical value, the crack will grow. K_c is a material property that defines the bone's *fracture toughness* (as distinct from the modulus of toughness measured from the stress strain curve). There are several modes of loading that define growth of a crack in tension (mode I), in-plane shear (mode II), or "tearing" (mode III) in which the shear loads are perpendicular to the direction of the crack growth, rather than parallel to it as in mode II. K_{Ic} (the critical stress intensity factor in mode I loading) of bone is greater than for poly methyl methacrylate (PMMA) polymers, but within the range of polycarbonate polymers or certain ceramics.[26] These values are for crack growth in the longitudinal direction; K_c values can be quite different in the transverse directions; therefore, fracture toughness is another material property that is anisotropic in bone.

It is also possible to define crack growth in terms of energy released because energy is required to create the surfaces of the crack. In this case, the mode I strain energy release rate (G_{Ic}) is defined as

$$G_{Ic} = \frac{\pi a s^2}{E}$$

where E is the elastic modulus. It turns out that these measures of crack growth are proportional to each other

$$G_I = \frac{K_I^2}{E}$$

It is worth pointing out that cracks are driven by strain energy stored in the bone tissue, and cracks can turn in any direction as they travel if this generates more elastic energy. Thus the rate of growth of a crack can be altered by the nature of the material in front of, or behind, the tip of the propagating crack through what are called "toughening mechanisms." This is the reason that cracks growing through bone can be stopped by osteonal cement lines and trapped. "Intrinsic" crack toughening mechanisms are governed by changes to the material in front of the crack, which dissipates energy and shields the crack tip by compressing the material around it. "Extrinsic" mechanisms are related to occurrences behind the crack tip, for instance, bridging of cracks by uncracked material (such as collagen fibrils or the noncollagenous protein, osteopontin).[2,27] Ligament bridging holds the surfaces of the crack together to create a "closure stress," and these must be fully broken before the tissue can completely fracture.

In healthy human bone, the stress intensity factor increases as the crack gets longer, making it more difficult for the crack to grow as it proceeds through the bone (definitely a good thing for us). The relationship between crack length and K can be plotted, and this positive relationship between length and K results in a rising R-curve (R = resistance) (**Figure 5**).

THE MECHANICAL REGULATION OF REMODELING

Although the skeleton is responsive to a wide array of hormonal and metabolic signals, its mechanical function requires that it be able to adapt to varying mechanical signals as well. This involves a threshold-driven process, that some call the "Mechanostat."[28] This functions much like the thermostat in your home—when the temperature is too high, the air conditioning turns on to bring the temperature to comfortable levels; when the temperature is too low, the furnace turns on to raise the temperature. This regulatory mechanism occurs through a series of events that are dependent both on the nature of the mechanical signals themselves, their transduction to the cell, and on the cellular processes that allow this

©Copyright 2021 American Academy of Orthopaedic Surgeons

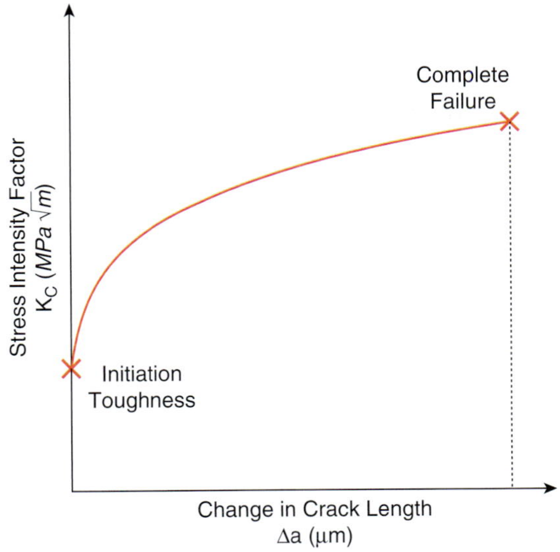

FIGURE 5 Schematic representation of rising R-curve in a fracture toughness test. This curve demonstrates the increase in fracture toughness with increased crack length that is typical in bone. As a propagating crack gets longer, toughening mechanisms inherent to the bone make it require more energy for the crack to proceed. At some point, the crack becomes too long and stable growth is no longer possible, at which time the sample fails.

signal to be received and acted upon appropriately. This series of interrelated mechanical and biological events, collectively termed mechanotransduction, can be distinguished by four separate processes.[29]

Mechanocoupling: The mechanical stimulus that initiates cellular actions. The mechanical signal may act directly by deforming the osteocyte cell wall or indirectly by generating fluid flow in osteocyte canaliculi that generate shear stress directly on the cell walls. The fluid flow may cause tension on the glycocalyx surrounding the cell processes and also may alter the diffusion of molecules that signal for certain cell responses.

Biochemical coupling: When the mechanical signal has been detected by the cell, the cell must change the signal into an intracellular biochemical reaction (probably in the sensor cell, the osteocyte) that can alter both physical (eg, integrin-cytoskeleton nuclear matrix deformation, alteration of stretch-activated protein channels) and/or biological (eg, modification of G-protein pathways, phosphorylation of proteins, or adjustment of mineral channels) regulation.

Signal transmission: Once the osteocytes have detected the signal, they must transmit the information to the cells that will resorb old bone (osteoclasts) and form new bone (osteoblasts). This can be done by transmission of a mixture of autocrine and paracrine factors through the canalicular network. This transmission is facilitated by membrane-bound proteins called connexins, primarily connexin-43, connexin-36, and mostly likely others. In the case of connexin-43, protein subunits on the cell membrane form a hexameric channel called a hemichannel or connexon. These hemichannels can open in response to stimuli (including mechanical stimuli) allowing for the rapid influx or release of signaling molecules. When hemichannels on two adjacent cells "dock," a gap junction between the cells is formed and effectively connects the cells' cytoplasm for the rapid transmission of signaling molecules between the cells.

Effector cell response: The osteoclasts and osteoblasts are the "effector" cells in that they actually do the work of resorbing and forming bone. Their response in part depends not just on the signals they have received from the osteocytes, but also on their environmental milieu (and perhaps even distant environments, such as those in the microbiome or the brain). This includes not only hormones and metabolites, but also elements of the bone matrix itself (eg, the mixture of noncollagenous proteins such as proteoglycans, osteopontin, osteocalcin, Dmp1, among many others). Ultimately, this is the response that will alter bone mass and adjust the strain back to within normal ranges.

There are a few general rules, demonstrated many times experimentally, that determine how bone does, or does not respond.

Bone response requires a dynamic load: It has been known for many years that static loads applied to bone will not create an adaptive response, regardless of how much load is applied or how much strain is developed.[30,31] This in itself suggests that strain alone is not the stimulus for bone adaptation, but that either fluid movement or the change in strain itself is the critical mechanocoupling event.

Bone adaptation is threshold driven: A series of now classic experiments demonstrated that dynamic loads below a certain strain threshold do not create an adaptive response, but strains (or strain rates) above that threshold do.[32,33] The threshold may differ for different bones, or in different locations of the same bone, and may be dependent on what the habitual strain/strain rate is in that location. It is at least interesting in this regard that the peak strains in most animals and most bones fall within the range of −1,500 to −2,500 με in compression,[34] although strains during usual submaximal activities are in a much lower range of 400 to 800 με.

Bone response occurs with short periods of loading: Again, classic experiments from Rubin and Lanyon[35] demonstrated that, once the strain threshold for cellular response is reached, adding additional cycles of loading does not create a greater response. Subsequently, Robling et al[36] demonstrated that this is because cells (either the sensor cells, or perhaps osteoblasts) become habituated to mechanical signals over time and are desensitized to those signals. Subsequent experiments[37] demonstrated that the refractory period for osteoblasts lasts about 8 to 12 hours, after which they may become fully sensitive to mechanical stimuli again. This has significant implications for the design of training and exercise programs, as well as for the prevention of stress-related fractures in bone.

©Copyright 2021 American Academy of Orthopaedic Surgeons

Compressive strains are larger than tensile strains: As mentioned above, the compressive strength and stiffness of bone is greater than its tensile strength/stiffness, so it may come as no surprise that compressive strains are generally 1.5 to 2.5 times higher than tensile strains. The reasons for this are beyond the treatment here, but in part are related to the shift of the neutral axis (the axis where strains are zero), superimposing strains generated from bending on those due to compression.

There are many aspects of the strain environment that may produce appropriate signals for bone adaptation, and it is not completely clear which of them, or which combinations of them, are the most important. These include some of the obvious—strain magnitude and rate—but also other features of the strain signal such as strain distribution, frequency, duration, and polarity.

Strain distribution: When load is placed on bone, it creates a gradient of strain across and throughout the cortex. If the distribution of that strain differs from what the bone normally experiences, or if the direction of the loading changes, new bone tissue can be formed even if the strain is lower than usual (eg, changes from high compression, to lower compression). When the strain distribution is usual, higher strains are required to cause an adaptive response than if the distribution is unusual. Clinically, this means that mechanical responses will be facilitated by loading bone in a variety of different positions, rather than by more repetitions of a usual load or loading in a single direction.

Strain duration: Duration refers to the number of loading cycles that are applied over time. As noted above, bone is responsive to very few cycles of loading if the strain is high enough and may not respond at all to many loading cycles if the strain is very low. Therefore, the number of cycles of loading seems less important than the magnitude and rate of loading.

Polarity: This refers to the mode of loading, whether compression, tension, or torsion. As stated above, most loading is in bending, which creates combinations of these types of loads. Polarity generally determines the location of the adaptive response, whereas other aspects of the strain environment determine the magnitude of the adaptation. Polarity may play a particularly important role in determining the architecture/organization of trabecular bone.

Strain magnitude, rate, and frequency: These features of the strain environment determine the magnitude of the response, and they are not independent of each other. Because we know that static loading does not create a response, whereas dynamic loading does, this suggests that some aspect of loading rate is important to the strength of the response. Consequently, those exercises that create higher rates of strain, such as running and jumping or very ballistic sports such as racquetball, tend to be more osteogenic than walking. The strain rate depends on both strain magnitude (ε) and frequency (f), the latter defined by the number of loading cycles/second. Frequency is defined in terms of Hertz (Hz), so that walking at 2 Hz means that two steps are taken per second. As strain magnitude and/or frequency increases, therefore, for a near sinusoidal wave such as that created by walking or running, strain rate increases:

$$\text{Strain rate} = 2\pi\, f\, \varepsilon_{\max} \cos(2\pi\, f\, t)$$

The relationship can be seen more easily when expressed as a strain stimulus ($S\sigma$):

$$S_\sigma = k_i \sum_{i=1}^{n} f_i \varepsilon_{\max}$$

where k is a constant and i is the number cycles. Therefore, any increase in strain magnitude or the frequency of footfall will translate into increased strain rate—suggesting that it is the combination of strain magnitude and frequency that underlie the adaptive response.

EFFECTS OF AGING ON BONE'S MECHANICAL PROPERTIES

The age-related loss of bone begins in both men and women in the fourth decade, well before the female menopause. Cortical bone is lost from the endosteal and intracortical surfaces at a rate of 2% to 5% per decade. The loss of cancellous bone is much faster, about 5% to 10% per decade on average (see Ref. 38 for a review). Between the ages of 20 and 90 years, this loss of bone results in an overall 8% reduction in elastic modulus, a 29% reduction in ultimate strain (reflecting the increased brittleness of aging bone tissue), and a 42% reduction in energy to fracture.[39] Tensile ultimate strain may decline by as much as 80% over those 7 decades.[40] At the hip, about three quarters of this decline is caused by increased porosity in the cortex of the femoral neck.[41] Removal of trabeculae in the femoral neck, on the other hand, only accounts for about 7% of the lower fracture load.[42] Decreases in toughness are much greater than this and have been estimated to decline by 30% to 40% between the ages of 50 and 80 years.[40,41] Other estimates are even higher.[43,44] Energy absorption and ultimate strain are good indicators of whether the hip will fracture from the impact of a fall.

Because of the loss of horizontal trabeculae (which act as cross-struts), and the remodeling of trabecular plates into rods as bone is lost, cancellous bone (especially in the vertebrae) becomes more anisotropic, with a preferred trabecular orientation longitudinally with respect to the direction of compressive loading in the spine. The horizontal trabeculae normally prevent buckling of those in the vertical direction, so this in itself reduces the fracture resistance of the bone. Moreover, longitudinal trabecular plates and trabecular rods have significantly lower mineralization than the horizontal plates which are lost. The combination of the loss of bone and the change in architecture leads to a reduction of nearly 70% in the failure stress of vertebral trabecular bone.[45]

©Copyright 2021 American Academy of Orthopaedic Surgeons

SUMMARY

The mechanical properties of bone are defined by both structural (extrinsic) properties and by material (intrinsic) properties. Bone's extrinsic mechanical properties, defined by a load-deformation curve, include strength, stiffness, and energy to fracture. Bone's intrinsic properties, defined by the stress-strain curve, are independent of mass and geometry and include ultimate stress, modulus of elasticity, and modulus of resilience or modulus of toughness. Bone is usually loaded in bending, which generates a combination of compressive, tensile, and shear stresses, with bone weakest in shear and strongest in compression. However, bone that is strong, by a mechanical definition, is not necessarily fracture resistant. Rather fracture resistance is defined in part by bone's ability to absorb energy before it fails. Although bone is often tested mechanically using noncyclic loads, in life, bone is loaded repetitively, and its properties may degrade over time (fatigue) if the damage created by these loads is not repaired by bone remodeling. Remodeling occurs through a series of mechanical and biochemical coupling processes that cause osteocytes to signal osteoclasts and osteoblasts to remove and replace damaged bone. This regulation is dependent on dynamic loads that create bone strains that elicit an appropriate adaptive response much like a thermostat regulates temperature.

CLINICAL NOTE

- In an osteoporotic condition, bone is more susceptible to fracture because of loss of bone mass (increased porosity) and disruption to trabecular architecture that negatively affect its extrinsic mechanical properties.
- In other conditions, such as diabetes, fracture risk is increased by a combination of structural changes and alterations to the bone tissue, such as the accumulation of AGEs that make the bone tissue less resilient and more brittle.
- The extrinsic and intrinsic properties of bone degrade during aging, partly due to increased porosity and loss of bone and partly due to negative changes to the tissue (AGE accumulation, changes in water compartments, alterations to noncollagenous proteins) that reduce bone toughness.

REFERENCES

1. Reilly RT, Burstein AH: The elastic and ultimate properties of compact bone tissue. *J Biomech* 1975;8:393-405.
2. Ritchie RO: The conflicts between strength and toughness. *Nat Mater* 2011;10:817-822.
3. Zioupos P, Currey JD: Changes in the stiffness, strength, and toughness of human cortical bone with age. *Bone* 1998 22:57-66.
4. Akkus O, Adar F, Schaffler MB: Age-related changes in physicochemical properties of mineral crystals are related to impaired mechanical function of cortical bone. *Bone* 2004;34:443-453.
5. Boskey A: Bone mineral crystal size. *Osteoporos Int* 2003;13(suppl 5):16-21.
6. Ishimoto T, Nakano T, Umakoshi Y, Yamamoto M, Tabata Y: Degree of biological apatite c-axis orientation rather than bone mineral density controls mechanical function in bone regenerated using recombinant bone morphogenetic protein-2. *J Bone Miner Res* 2013;28:1170-1179.
7. Wang X, Shen X, Li S, Agrawal CM: Age-related changes in the collagen network and toughness of bone. *Bone* 2002;31:1-7.
8. Viguet-Carrin S, Farlay D, Bala Y, Munoz F, Bouxsein ML, Delmas PD: An in vitro model to test the contribution of advanced glycation end products to bone biomechanical properties. *Bone* 2008;42:139-149.
9. Karim L, Vashishth D: Heterogeneous glycation of cancellous bone and its association with bone quality and fragility. *PLoS One* 2012;7:e35047.
10. Depalle AG, Depalle B, Duarte AG, et al: The different distribution of enzymatic collagen cross-links found in adult and children bone result in different mechanical behavior of collagen. *Bone* 2018;110:107-114.
11. Zioupos P, Currey JD, Hamer AJ: The role of collagen in the declining mechanical properties of aging human cortical bone. *J Biomed Mater Res* 1999;45:108-116.
12. Hernandez CJ, Tang SY, Baumbach BM, et al: Trabecular microfracture and the influence of pyridinium and non-enzymatic glycation-mediated collagen cross-links. *Bone* 2005;37:825-832.
13. Samuel J, Park J-S, Almer J, Wang X: Effect of water on nanomechanics of bone is different between tension and compression. *J Mech Behav Biomed Mater* 2016;57:128-138.
14. Unal M, Akkus O: Raman spectral classification of mineral- and collagen-bound water's associations to elastic and post-yield mechanical properties of cortical bone. *Bone* 2015;81:315-326.
15. Wang X, Hua R, Ahsan A, et al: Age-related deterioration of bone toughness is related to diminishing amount of matrix glycosaminoglycans (GAGS), *JBMR Plus* 2018;2:164-173.
16. Wang X, Xu H, Huang Y, Gu S, Jiang JX: Coupling effect of water and proteoglycans on the in situ toughness of bone. *J Bone Miner Res* 2016;31:1026-1029.
17. Fantner GE, Hassenkam T, Kindt JH, et al: Sacrificial bonds and hidden length dissipate energy as mineralized fibrils separate during bone fracture. *Nat Mater* 2005;4:612-616.
18. Bertassoni LE, Swain MV: The contribution of proteoglycans to the mechanical behavior of mineralized tissues. *J Mech Behav Biomed Mater* 2014;38:91-104.
19. Poundarik AA, Diab T, Sroga BE, et al: Dilatational band formation in bone. *Proc Natl Acad Sci* 2012;109:19178-19183.
20. Sroga GE, Vashishth D: Phosphorylation of extracellular bone matrix proteins and its contribution to bone fragility. *J Bone Miner Res* 2018;33(12):2214-2229. doi:10.1002/jbmr.3552.
21. Carter DR, Caler WE: A cumulative damage model for bone fracture. *J Orthop Res* 1985;3:84-90.
22. Lakes RS, Saha S: Cement line motion in bone. *Science* 1979;204:501-503.
23. Caler WE, Carter DR: Bone creep-fatigue damage accumulation. *J Biomech* 1989;22:625-635.
24. Pattin CA, Caler WE, Carter DR: Cyclic mechanical property degradation during fatigue loading of cortical bone. *J Biomech* 1996;29:69-80.

2: Structure and Function of Musculoskeletal Tissues

©Copyright 2021 American Academy of Orthopaedic Surgeons

25. Burr DB, Milgrom C, Fyhrie D, et al: In vivo measurements of human tibial strains during vigorous activities. *Bone* 1995;18:405-410.
26. Martin RB, Burr DB, Sharkey NA, Fyhrie DP: *Skeletal Tissue Mechanics*. New York, NY, Springer, 2015.
27. Launey ME, Buehler MJ, Ritchie RO: On the mechanistic origins of toughness in bone. *Annu Rev Mater Res* 2010;40:25-53.
28. Frost HM: The mechanostat: A proposed pathogenic mechanism of osteoporoses and bone mass effects of mechanical and nonmechanical agents. *Bone Miner* 1987;2:73-85.
29. Duncan RL, Turner CH: Mechanotransduction and the functional response of bone to mechanical strain. *Calcif Tiss Int* 1995;57:344-358.
30. Hert J, Liskova M, Landrgot B: Influence of the long-term continuous bending on the bone. *Folia Morph (Prague)* 1969;17:389-399.
31. Turner CH, Owan I, Takano Y: Mechanotransduction in bone: Role of strain rate. *Am J Physiol* 1995;269:E438-E442.
32. Rubin CT, Lanyon LE: Regulation of bone mass by mechanical strain magnitude. *Calcif Tiss Int* 1985;37:411-417.
33. Turner CH, Forwood M, Rho J-Y, Yoshikawa T: Mechanical loading thresholds for lamellar and woven bone formation. *J Bone Miner Res* 1994;9:87-97.
34. Rubin CT, Lanyon LE: Limb mechanics as a function of speed and gait: A study of functional strains in the radius and tibia of horse and dog. *J Exp Biol* 1982;101:187-211.
35. Rubin CT, Lanyon LE: Regulation of bone formation by applied dynamic loads. *J Bone Jt Surg* 1984;66A:397-402.
36. Robling AG, Burr DB, Turner CH: Partitioning a daily mechanical stimulus into discrete loading bouts improves the osteogenic response to loading. *J Bone Miner Res* 2000;15:1596-1602.
37. Robling AG, Burr DB, Turner CH: Recovery periods restore mechanosensitivity to dynamically loaded bone. *J Exp Biol* 2001;204:3389-3399.
38. Burr DB, Turner CH: Biomechanical measurements in age-related bone loss, in Rosen CJ, Glowacki J, Bilezikian JP, eds: *The Aging Skeleton*. San Diego, CA, Academic Press, 1999, pp 301-311.
39. Burstein AH, Reilly DT, Martens M: Aging of bone tissue: Mechanical properties. *J Bone Jt Surg* 1976;58A:82-86.
40. Morgan EF, Unnikrisnan GU, Hussein AI: Bone mechanical properties in healthy and diseased states. *Annu Rev Biomed Eng* 2018;20:119-143.
41. McCalden RW, McGeough JA, Barker MB, Court-Brown CM: Age-related changes in the tensile properties of cortical bone. The relative changes in porosity, mineralization, and microstructure. *J Bone Jt Surg* 1995;75A:1193-1205.
42. Holzer G, von Skrbensky G, Holzer LA, Pichl W: Hip fractures and the combination of cortical versus trabecular bone to femoral neck strength. *J Bone Miner Res* 2009;24:468-474.
43. Nalla RK, Kruzic JJ, Kinney JH, Ritchie RO: Effect of aging on the toughness of human cortical bone: Evaluation by R-curves, *Bone* 2004;35:1240-1246.
44. Zimmerman EA, Schaible E, Bale H, et al: Age-related changes in the plasticity and toughness of human cortical bone at multiple length scales. *Proc Nat Acad Sci* 2011;108:14416-14421.
45. Mosekilde Li: Normal age-related changes in bone mass, structure and strength – consequences of the remodeling process. *Danish Med Bull* 1993;40:65-83.

©Copyright 2021 American Academy of Orthopaedic Surgeons

12

Biology of Articular Cartilage

Rachel E. Miller, PhD
Anne-Marie Malfait, MD, PhD

2: Structure and Function of Musculoskeletal Tissues

Keywords: *aggrecan; articular cartilage; chondrocytes; collagen; extracellular matrix*

INTRODUCTION

"The fabric of the joints in the human body is a subject so much the more entertaining, as it must strike everyone that considers it attentively with an idea of fine mechanical composition. Where-ever the motion of one bone upon another is requisite, there we find an excellent apparatus for rendering that motion safe and free." Thus starts *Of the Structure and Diseases of Articulating Cartilages*, read by Scottish physician and anatomist William Hunter at a meeting of the Royal Society of London on June 2, 1743.[1] In his delightful paper, Hunter provides us with the first detailed description of articular cartilage, which is *hyaline cartilage*, one of the three major types of cartilage tissue in the body. The two other types are *elastic cartilage*, which exists in the epiglottis and the Eustachian tube, and *fibrocartilage,* which can be found in the intervertebral disks, in the meniscus of the knee, and covering the mandibular condyles in the temporomandibular joints.

Articular cartilage is the white, smooth tissue that covers the surfaces of long bones where they articulate in diarthrodial joints (**Figure 1**). Adult articular cartilage mainly consists of extracellular matrix (ECM) (15% to 40% of the wet weight) and water (60% to 85% of the wet weight), in which chondrocytes are embedded. Chondrocytes, the only cell type present in articular cartilage, are derived from mesenchymal stem cells. Chondrogenesis requires the key transcription factor, SOX9, which secures chondrocyte lineage commitment, promotes cell survival, and transcriptionally activates the genes for many cartilage-specific structural components and regulatory factors.[2]

In synovial joints, hyaline articular cartilage covers the subchondral bone underneath, and its surface faces the joint cavity and the synovial fluid.[3] Together with synovium, bone, ligaments, tendons, and—in the knee—the menisci, cartilage ensures the integrity of diarthrodial joints. Movement of the joints in daily life applies a complex set of forces to these tissues. The unique composition and structure of articular cartilage supply an almost frictionless surface for bones to move upon each other and provide tremendous load-bearing capabilities to the joint (up to several times the body weight). In addition, the unique zonal organization of cartilage as well as the interplay between the different components lends the tissue its ability to withstand shear, compression, and tensile forces.[4] Loading is integral for cartilage health, and cartilage adapts to loading patterns over time. For example, the amount of extracellular matrix molecules in cartilage varies locally depending on individual gait patterns.

Dr. Malfait or an immediate family member serves as a paid consultant to or is an employee of Merck and Vizuri; has received research or institutional support from Galapagis NV, GlaxoSmithKline; serves as a board member, owner, officer, or committee member of the Amercian College of Rheumatology, the Osteoarthritis Research Society International, and the Rheumatology Research Foundation. Neither Dr. Miller nor any immediate family member has received anything of value from or has stock or stock options held in a commercial company or institution related directly or indirectly to the subject of this chapter.

COMPOSITION OF ARTICULAR CARTILAGE

ZONAL ORGANIZATION OF ARTICULAR CARTILAGE

Chondrocytes account for approximately 1% to 5% of cartilage tissue volume,[5] and a particular feature of articular cartilage is that chondrocytes lack cell-to-cell contact. Each cell can be thought of as a functional metabolic unit, isolated from neighboring cells and responsible for the elaboration and maintenance of the ECM in its immediate vicinity.[6] The major macromolecules that make up the cartilage ECM are type II

©Copyright 2021 American Academy of Orthopaedic Surgeons

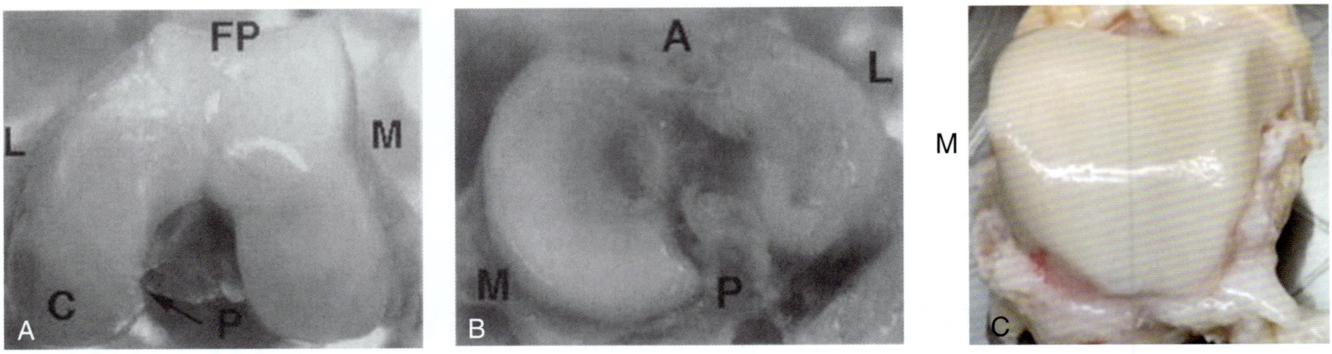

FIGURE 1 Macroscopic photographs of human knee and ankle cartilage. Legend adapted from Treppo et al: **A**, The distal femur taken inferiorly. The patellar surface of the distal femur (FP) and anterior (C) and posterior (P) of the femoral condyles with medial (M) and lateral (L) aspects labeled. **B**, The proximal tibial surface with the menisci removed (A = anterior; P = posterior). **C**, The talar surface of the talocrural joint. (A and B, reproduced with permission from Treppo S, et al: Comparison of biomechanical and biochemical properties of cartilage from human knee and ankle pairs. *J Orthop Res* 2000;18:739-748.)

collagen and the high-molecular-weight proteoglycan, aggrecan. Macroscopically, cartilage is a smooth white tissue that is resistant to compression (**Figure 1**). Microscopically, the supramolecular organization of its components changes in a depth-dependent fashion ("zones"), consistent with the differing functions of these cartilage zones (**Figure 2**, A). The first 10% of cartilage tissue underneath the surface is referred to as the superficial zone and is typified by chondrocytes that assume a flattened appearance, along with type II collagen fibers that run parallel to the cartilage surface. Proteoglycan content in the superficial zone is low.[7] A major function of the superficial zone is to support cartilage surface lubrication and low-friction joint articulation. The orientation of the collagen fibers in this zone confers tensile strength, which is important for constraining the high osmotic swelling that occurs in cartilage. In the middle or transitional zone, chondrocytes—still appearing as single cell units—assume a more rounded appearance, and type II collagen fiber orientation is no longer parallel to the surface but is random (**Figure 2**, B). The middle zone, which has the highest content of chondroitin sulfate-modified proteoglycans, helps

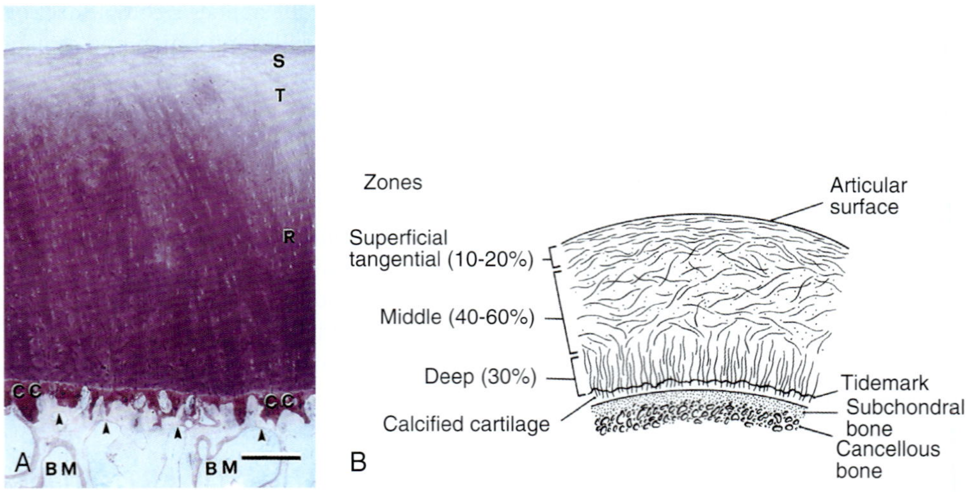

FIGURE 2 **A**, Light microscopic overview of adult human articular cartilage taken from the medial femoral condyle. By definition, the superficial (S) and transitional (T) zones each constitute 10% of the height of the articular cartilage layer, the bulk of which (80%) is represented by the radial one (R). For analytical purposes, the latter is partitioned into an upper and a lower half, each of which is further subdivided into upper and lower portions. The layer of calcified cartilage (CC) and the subchondral bone plate (arrowheads) for relatively thin strata beneath the hyaline articular cartilage tissue. BM: bone marrow space. 100-μm-thick polished section of methacrylate-embedded tissue, surface-stained with McNeil's tetrachrome, basic fuchsin, and toluidine blue O. Magnification bar = 500 μm. **B**, The collagen fiber architecture of articular cartilage is often categorized into three different zones: superficial, middle, and deep. Note that the fiber orientation is tangential in the superficial zone and radial in the deep zone, whereas it is less oriented in the middle zone. (A, Reproduced with permission from Hunziker EB, Quinn TM, Häuselmann H-J: Quantitative structural organization of normal adult human articular cartilage. *Osteoarthr Cartil* 2002;10(7):564-572. B, Reproduced with permission from Mow VC, Proctor CS, Kelly MA: Biomechanics of articular cartilage, in Noordin M, Frankel VH, eds: *Basic Biomechanics of the Musculoskeletal System*, ed 2. Philadelphia, PA, Lea & Febiger, 1989, pp 31-57).

 ©Copyright 2021 American Academy of Orthopaedic Surgeons

provide resistance to cartilage shear strain and compression. Finally, in the deep or radial zone, chondrocytes appear as vertical columns of clusters of five to eight rounded cells (**Figure 2**), whereas collagen fibers are oriented perpendicularly to the cartilage surface. This zone has the highest content of proteoglycans and correspondingly has the greatest compressive strength.

Beyond the deep zone, the "tidemark," which appears as a thin undulating basophilic line on light microscopic sections of decalcified cartilage, separates articular cartilage from a thin layer of calcified cartilage underneath. The calcified cartilage, containing hypertrophic chondrocytes, anchors the articular cartilage to the subchondral bone underneath.[8] The subchondral bone plate is vascularized, with vascular channels penetrating the calcified cartilage layer from underneath. Nerve fibers have also been shown in these vascular channels. The cartilage-bone interface is referred to as the osteochondral junction, and it is an area of active research in the context of osteoarthritis, where it has been proposed that the ingrowth of vessels and nerves at the osteochondral junction may contribute to disease pathogenesis and joint pain.[9]

CELLS OF ARTICULAR CARTILAGE: CHONDROCYTES

Articular cartilage is avascular and aneural. There is one cell type present in this tissue: chondrocytes. Cell density in adult human articular cartilage shows marked variations with tissue depth, being highest in the superficial zone, where it represents less than 10% of the tissue volume. Chondrocyte density decreases progressively in the deeper zones. In adult human femoral condyle cartilage, it has been estimated that the total number of chondrocytes in a 1 mm^2 area is 23,674.[10] In femoral condyle cartilage, the cellularity is inversely correlated with cartilage thickness, which in itself depends on the degree of load-bearing.[10,11] The weight-bearing region in adult human femoral condyle cartilage is approximately 2.4 ± 0.4 mm thick, whereas the thickness of ankle articular cartilage is approximately 1.5 ± 0.2 mm.[10,12] Cellularity and chondrocyte distribution in cartilage vary by joint, and in the ankle joint the superficial zone appears to be less distinct than in other joints, with cell numbers that are similar to the those in deep zone.[10] Although the biological implications of these variations are unknown, one may speculate that the differences in articulation in the ankle versus the knee may place different structural demands on this top tissue layer. In contrast, the deep zone appears to be the most conserved region among different joints.

Despite the low numbers of chondrocytes in cartilage, these cells are capable of producing and maintaining the extensive ECM that surrounds them (**Figure 3**). This is in contrast to other types of tissues such as bone, where distinct cell types perform the tasks of synthesis (osteoblasts) and degradation/remodeling (osteoclasts). Although chondrocytes are the only cell type in articular cartilage, their phenotype changes

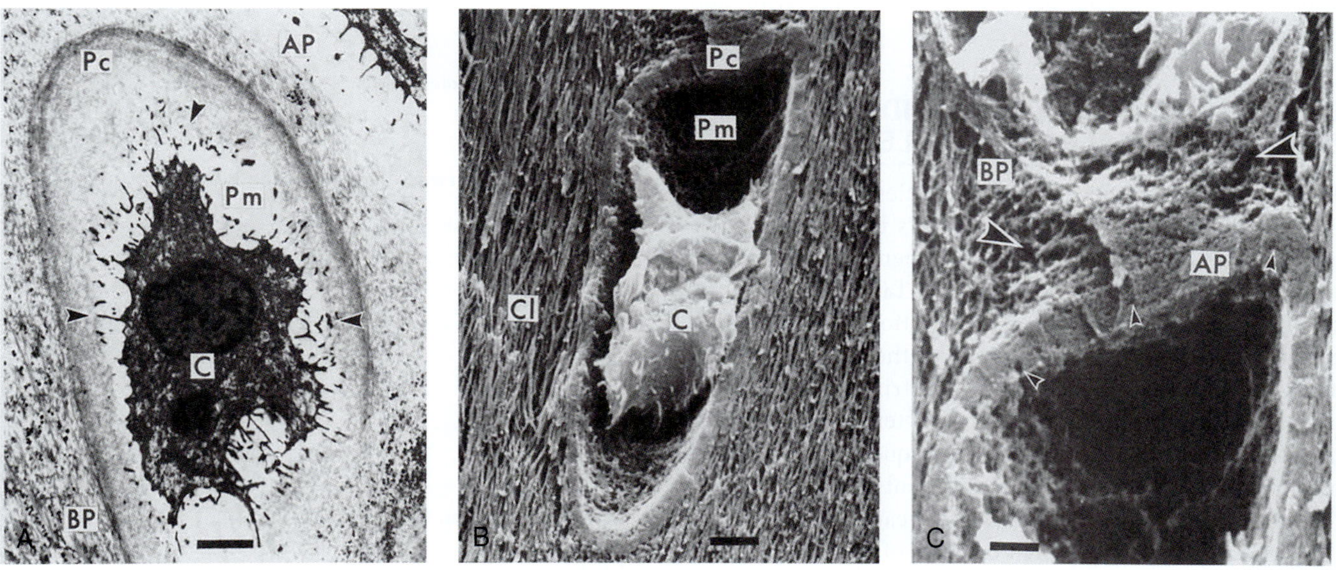

FIGURE 3 Deep layer chondrocytes. **A**, Transmission electron micrograph illustrating multiple chondrocyte cell processes (arrowheads) extending across the pericellular matrix (Pm) to the loosely woven inner border of the pericellular capsule (Pc). The articular pole (AP) forms a compacted cupola, whereas the basal pole (BP) remains loosely woven. Groups of matrix vesicles are evident at the basal pole and throughout the matrix. Head of the index phalanx. Bar = 2 μm. **B**, Scanning electron micrograph showing a chondrocyte (**C**) suspended in the pericellular matrix space (Pm) and separated from radially aligned territorial collagen fibers (Cl) by a "felt-like" pericellular capsule (Pc). Medial femoral condyle. Bar = 2 μm. **C**, Detail of B illustrating macropores (large arrowheads) formed in the loose weave at the basal pole (BP) of the chondron above and micropores (small arrowheads) formed in the dense organization of the articular pole (AP). Bar = 1 μm. (Reproduced with permission from Poole CA, Flint MH, Beaumont BW: Chondrons in cartilage: ultrastructural analysis of the pericellular microenvironment in adult human articular cartilages. *J Orthop Res* 1987;5(4):509-522.)

©Copyright 2021 American Academy of Orthopaedic Surgeons

depending on their location within the tissue. As explained above, chondrocyte morphology and ECM composition change with depth, and thus the types of molecules that chondrocytes secrete change with depth. Superficial zone chondrocytes produce a molecule called lubricin (discussed below in more detail) that helps to provide a low friction coefficient for the cartilage surface and thus aids in smooth joint articulation.[13,14] In contrast, middle and deep zone chondrocytes produce large quantities of type II collagen and aggrecan to provide structural stability and resistance to compression. Middle and deep zone chondrocytes form functional units called chondrons, which consist of the chondrocyte along with the immediately surrounding ECM, termed the pericellular matrix[15,16] (**Figure 3**).

Articular cartilage has limited intrinsic healing capacity, and cartilage injury represents a major risk factor for cartilage degeneration. In recent years, a population of cartilage-derived stem cells or progenitor cells (CSPCs), similar to those found in many other adult tissues, have been observed in human, equine, and bovine articular cartilage.[17] These cells can be isolated and characterized in vitro on the basis of their self-renewal, multilineage differentiation, and migratory abilities. It is thought that these progenitor cells emerge when cartilage is injured, migrate to the injury site, and participate in tissue repair activities. It has been proposed that these CSPCs may be a therapeutic target for cartilage injury and posttraumatic osteoarthritis, but the exact nature and origin of these cells is still uncertain and it has also been suggested that progenitor cells in the synovium play an important role.

EXTRACELLULAR MATRIX: FLUID AND STRUCTURAL MACROMOLECULES

The remarkable biomechanical properties of articular cartilage are in large part derived from its unique molecular organization and the specialized biochemical characteristics of its major constituents (listed in **Table 1**). In healthy cartilage, assembly and tissue distribution of ECM molecules vary according to the vicinity of the matrix to chondrocytes. Essentially, the cartilage matrix can be divided into three areas, the pericellular, the territorial, and the interterritorial matrix, each with its unique molecular organization (**Figure 4**). Collagen is differentially organized in these three areas. Directly surrounding each chondrocyte is the pericellular matrix, which consists of type VI collagen fibers that form a tightly woven, nest-like enclosure (2 to 4 μm thick) around each chondrocyte.[16] The 5- to 10-μm-thick zone around the pericellular matrix is the territorial matrix, where thicker collagen fibers form radial bundles around one cell or a group of cells. Finally, the interterritorial matrix contains large collagen type II bundles (described in Benninghoff's classic description as "arcades"[18]). Other proteins are also differentially expressed in these different

TABLE 1 Protein of the Cartilage Matrix

Collagens
Type II (75% of total in fetal, 90% of total in adult)
Type III (>10% in adult human cartilage)
Type IX (covalently fibril-associated collagen; 10% fetal, 1% adult)
Type X (only in hypertrophic cartilage)
Type XI (part of the fibril; 10% fetal, 3% adult)
Type VI (chondron, microfilaments; <1%)
Type XII/XIV
Type XIII (transmembrane)
Proteoglycans
Aggrecan (95% of total proteoglycan)
Biglycan
Decorin
Fibromodulin
Lumican
Asporin
Chondroadherin
Osteoadherin
Prolargin (PRELP)
Noncollagenous proteins
Fibronectin
Thrombospondins, mainly thrombospondin 5 (COMP)
Matrilin-1 (previously cartilage matrix protein)
Matrilin-2
Matrilin-3
Tenascin-C
Thrombomodulin
Chondroadherin
Cartilage intermediate layer protein (CILP)
Fibulin
Membrane proteins
Syndecan
CD44
Integrins (α1, 2, 3, 5, 6, 10; β1, 3, 5)

 ©Copyright 2021 American Academy of Orthopaedic Surgeons

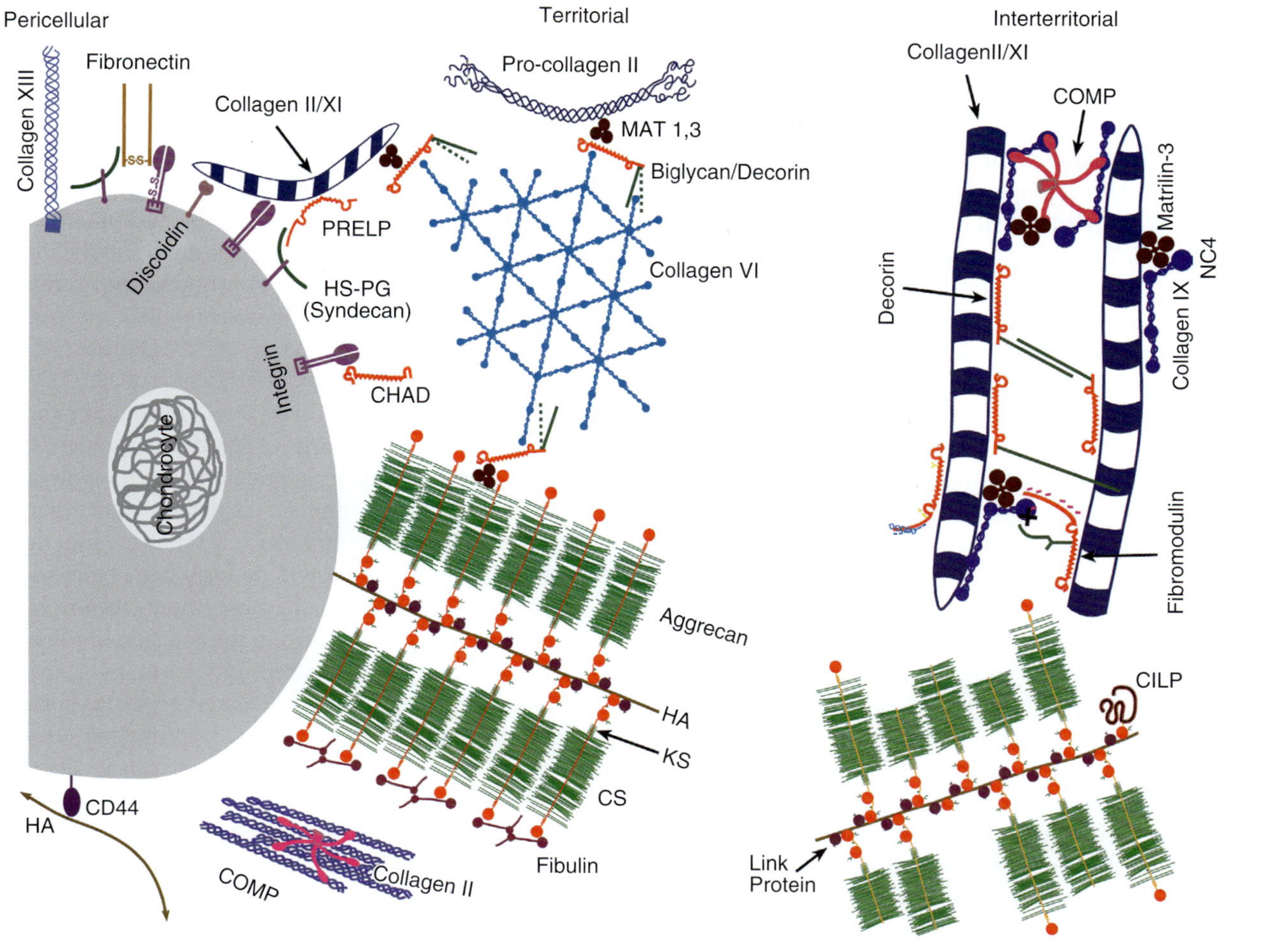

FIGURE 4 The molecular organization of normal articular cartilage. The cartilage matrix surrounding chondrocytes in healthy articular cartilage is arranged into zones defined by their distance from the cell. The pericellular matrix lies immediately around the cell and is the zone where molecules that interact with cell-surface receptors are located; for example, hyaluronan binds the receptor CD44. Next to the pericellular matrix, slightly further from the cell, lies the territorial matrix. At largest distance from the cell is the interterritorial matrix. The types of collagens and the collagen-binding proteins that form the matrices are different in each zone. Abbreviations: CILP = cartilage intermediate layer protein; COMP = cartilage oligomeric matrix protein; CS = chondroitin sulfate; KS = keratan sulfate; PRELP = proline-arginine-rich end leucine-rich repeat protein. (Reproduced with permission from Heinegard D, Saxne T: The role of cartilage matrix in osteoarthritis. *Nat Rev Rheumatol* 2011;7(1):50-56).

matrix zones. For example, the pericellular matrix is rich in fibronectin and the proteoglycans, biglycan and perlecan, which may regulate chondrocyte activity through cell-matrix interactions and growth factor sequestration.[16] Cartilage oligomeric matrix protein (COMP) is expressed solely in the interterritorial matrix, where it plays a role in collagen cross-linking.[19] Finally, the mechanical properties of these zones vary—the chondrocyte is the softest component, and these cells are softer than the pericellular matrix, which is softer than the surrounding ECM.[16] As such, the pericellular matrix likely plays an important role as a mechanotransducer by filtering mechanical signals, so the chondrocytes can respond and react to mechanical forces. One way the chondrocyte may interact with the pericellular matrix is through the primary cilium, which is an organelle that projects from the cell membrane into the surrounding matrix, where it can interact with the matrix environment through integrins and ion channels such as transient receptor potential vanilloid 4 (TRPV4).[16]

Water

Normal cartilage has a water content ranging from 65% (deep zones) to 80% (surface) of its wet weight. The flow of water through the tissue is governed by mechanical and physicochemical laws, and it is this flow that allows the transport of nutrients through this avascular tissue, in addition to providing cartilage with its biomechanical properties (please refer to the chapter[13]). Articular cartilage holds water with avidity, through contact with the major macromolecules in cartilage, type II collagen, and proteoglycans.

©Copyright 2021 American Academy of Orthopaedic Surgeons

Collagens

The shape of articular cartilage and its material strength depend heavily on its extensively cross-linked collagen network and characteristic fibrillar organization, which varies with tissue depth and distance from the cell. The main collagen in articular cartilage is type II collagen, a triple-helix composed of three identical α chains synthesized from the COL2A1 gene. Two splice variants of procollagen exist, with type IIA being characteristic for chondroprogenitors and type IIB the predominant type II collagen in adult cartilage. During biosynthesis, three identical α chains wind around each other to form collagen molecules, which then associate in a staggered alignment to form long, unbranched, banded fibrils that provide tensile strength. Transmission electron microscopy has revealed patterns of preferred fibril orientation[20]: in the surface zone of cartilage, fibrils are thin and tend to run primarily parallel to the articular surface. In the middle zones, a greater range of fibril diameters exists, and their organization appears more random. The thickest fibrils are in the deep zone, where they are perpendicular to the cartilage surface and anchored in the subchondral bone.

Type II collagen fibrils contain other types of collagen within the fibril or surrounding it. These collagens are often referred to as "minor" collagens, because of their relative amount, not their functional importance (reviewed in Ref. 21). The main functions of these minor collagens are listed in **Table 2**. Collagens II, IX, and XI form cross-linked heterotypic fibrils that form the backbone template of the collagen network in developing articular cartilage. As articular cartilage matures, the collagen framework consists mainly of type II collagen. With age, chondrocytes start to produce type III collagen, which gets superimposed in varying amounts on the original collagen fibril network. Type III collagen molecules with unprocessed N-propeptides are extensively cross-linked to type II collagen in aged joints. Because type III collagen is known to be prominent at sites of healing and repair in skin and other tissues, it has been postulated to act as a covalent modifier that may add cohesion to a weakened collagen type II fibril network as part of a chondrocyte healing response to matrix damage.[22]

Aggrecan

The hydrophilic nature of proteoglycans is what gives cartilage its affinity for water. The major proteoglycan in cartilage is aggrecan, which consists of a 220 to 250 kDa protein core, containing three globular domains, G1, G2, and G3. G1 and G2 are near the amino-terminus and separated by a short interglobular domain. The third globular domain, G3, is near the carboxy-terminus of the core protein, and the long stretch between G2 and G3 is heavily substituted with keratan sulfate and approximately 100 chondroitin sulfate glycosaminoglycan (GAG) chains (reviewed in Ref. 23) (**Figure 5**). All GAGs have repeating carboxyl (COOH) and sulfate (SO_4) groups, which are ionized (COO^- and SO_3^-) in solution and give the cartilage its negative charge. Aggrecan monomers form very large aggregates through interaction with the polysaccharide, hyaluronan. The G1 domain associates noncovalently with hyaluronan, an interaction which is stabilized by a third molecule, the 45-kDa link protein, to form high-molecular-weight aggregates (>200 MDa). Because these negatively charged aggregates are tightly packed in the collagen fibrillar network, their fixed charges are spaced only 10 to 15 Å apart, which results in extreme charge-to-charge repulsive forces. Thus, the constraining forces developed within the collagen network surrounding the trapped proteoglycan aggregates ensure a strong and cohesive matrix, which holds water avidly. The aggrecan "gel" furthermore protects cartilage collagen fibrils from degradation by collagenases. It has been demonstrated that collagen in freeze-thawed cartilage depleted of aggrecan is completely degraded following incubation with matrix metalloproteinase (MMP)-1, whereas collagen in cartilage with intact aggrecan is not. Additionally, selective aggrecanase inhibitors that do not block MMP-activity protect against aggrecan degradation as well as against collagenolysis in cartilage explants exposed to catabolic cytokines. These findings suggest that aggrecan plays a protective role in preventing pathological degradation of collagen fibrils.[24]

Other Matrix Molecules

Other noncollagenous molecules in the cartilage ECM provide functions for tissue assembly and for maintaining cartilage properties. Perlecan, a heparan sulfate proteoglycan

TABLE 2 Function of Types III, VI, IX, XI Collagen

Type III collagen	Plays a role in response of articular cartilage to matrix damage—may add cohesion to a weakened type II collagen network (in aging and in osteoarthritis).
Type VI collagen	These microfilaments are tightly woven to form a nest-like enclosure around each chondrocyte, called the chondron, thus providing communication between the cell and its microenvironment.
Type IX collagen	Decorates the surface of type II collagen fibers and forms bridges with other molecules in the ECM (for instance, fibronectin) to promote stability. Contributes to matrix assembly.
Type XI collagen	Forms a template that regulates the lateral growth of type II collagen heterofibrils.

©Copyright 2021 American Academy of Orthopaedic Surgeons

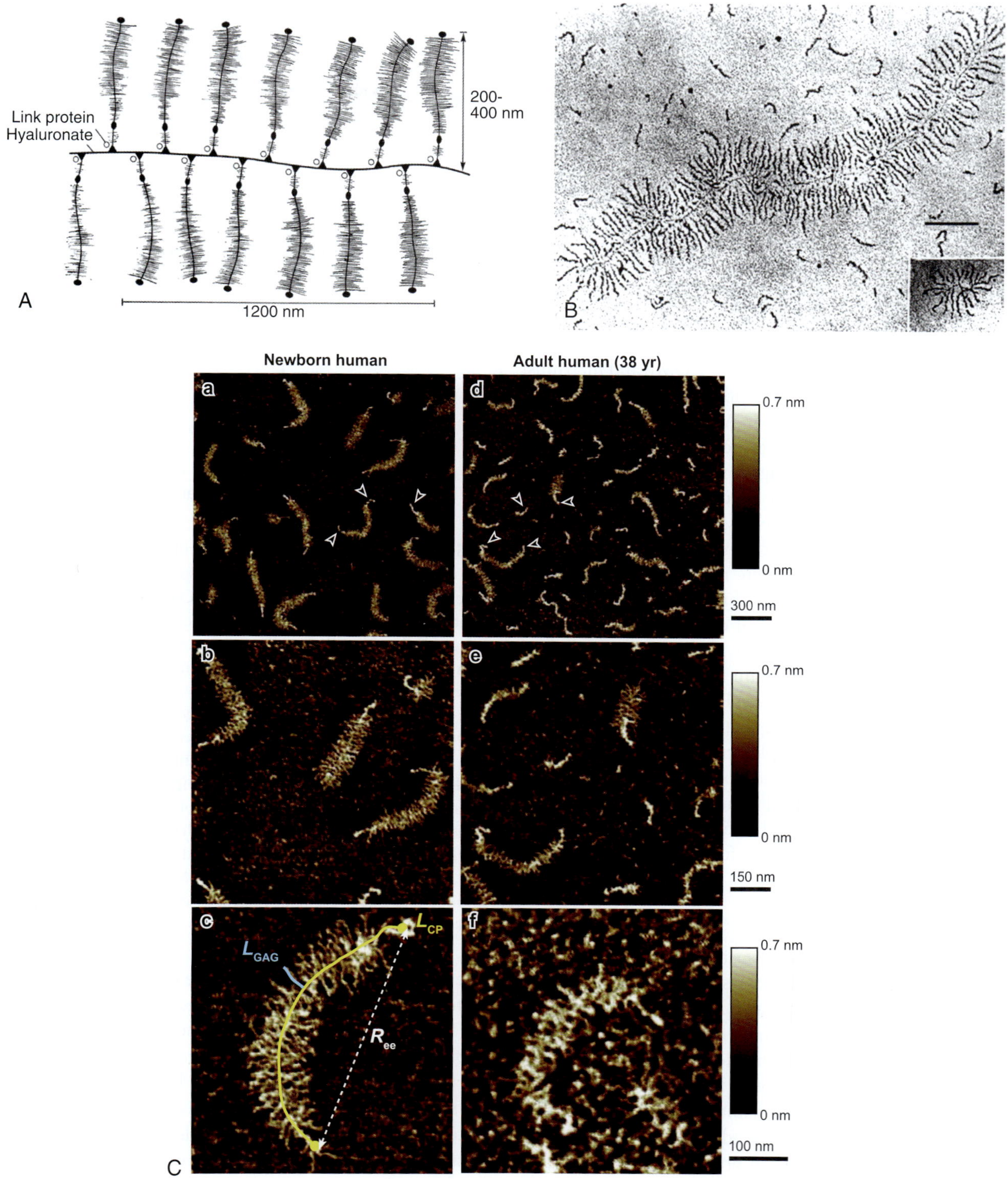

FIGURE 5 **A**, A diagram of the aggrecan molecules arranged as a proteoglycans aggregate. Many aggrecan molecules can bind to a chain of hyaluronan, forming macromolecular complexes that effectively are immobilized within the collagen network. **B**, Electron micrographs of bovine articular cartilage proteoglycans aggregates from skeletally immature calf (larger figure) and skeletally mature steer (inset). These show the aggregates to consist of a central hyaluronan filament and multiple attached monomers (bar = 500 μm). **C**, Tapping mode AFM height images of (1, 2, 3) newborn and (4, 5, 6) 38-year-old adult human aggrecan monomers. Globular domains are indicated by arrowheads (1 and 4). An example of core protein trace length, L_{CP}, end-to-end distance, R_{ee}, and GAG chain trace length, L_{GAG}, are shown in (3). (B, Reproduced with permission from Buckwalter JA, Kuettner KE, Thonar EJ: Age-related changes in articular cartilage proteoglycans: Electron microscopic studies. *J Orthop Res* 1985;3:251-257. C, Reproduced with permission from Lee, et al: Age-related nanostructural and nanomechanical changes of individual human cartilage aggrecan monomers and their glycosaminoglycan side chains. *J Struct Biol* 2013;181:264-273).

©Copyright 2021 American Academy of Orthopaedic Surgeons

present in the pericellular matrix, is important for regulating presentation of the growth factor, FGF2, to chondrocytes. In addition, the assembly of the collagen type VI network in the pericellular matrix is regulated by small leucine-rich proteoglycans (SLRPs) like decorin, biglycan, lumican, and fibromodulin. These small proteoglycans are nonaggregating and have shorter protein cores than aggrecan and, unlike aggrecans, they do not fill a large volume of the tissue. Biglycan is glycosylated with two chondroitin or dermatan sulfate chains; decorin is glycosylated with a single chondroitin or dermatan sulfate chain and fibromodulin with up to five keratan sulfate chains. Both decorin and fibromodulin can bind type I and II collagen and may have a role in organizing and stabilizing the collagen meshwork (reviewed in Ref. 23). SLRPs can further interact with other molecules, including COMP and matrilins. Matrilin 1 to 4 form a family of widely distributed proteins containing von Willebrand Factor A (vWFA) domains that are often present in proteins involved in protein interactions (reviewed in Ref. 25). In cartilage, matrilin-1 and 3 are predominantly present, where they bind different types of collagen as well as aggrecan, so they essentially support matrix assembly by connecting fibrillar components and establishing interactions between collagen networks and aggrecan (**Figure 6**). COMP (also known as thrombospondin 5) is also a part of this ingenious assembly. It consists of five identical subunits held together close to their N-terminus by a coiled-coil domain, whereas the C-termini have a globular domain that binds other matrix molecules (**Figure 6**). Most notably, through this fivefold binding capacity, one COMP molecule can rapidly bring together five collagen molecules and thus act as a catalyst for early collagen fibril formation. In osteoarthritis, COMP levels are dramatically increased, so that a single COMP molecule can occupy all binding sites on one collagen molecule, thereby hampering fibril formation and effectively hindering tissue repair.[23]

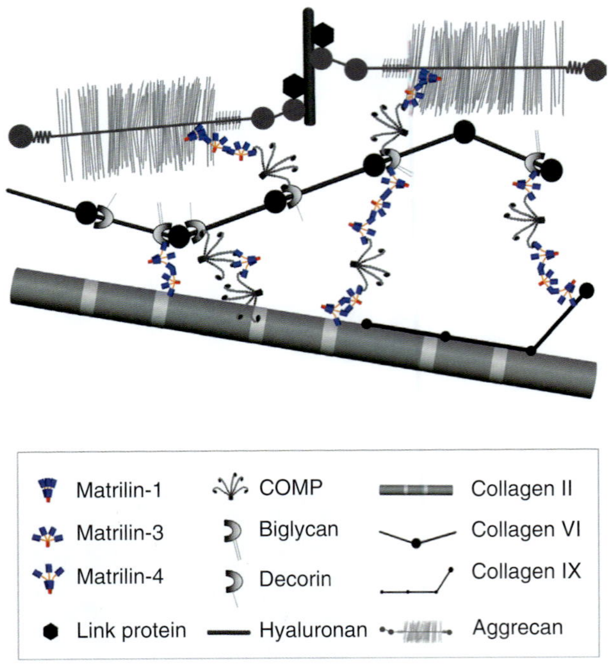

FIGURE 6 Matrilins as adaptors in cartilage matrix assembly. Model for the role of matrilins in the formation of supramolecular networks in cartilage. Matrilin-1, 3, and 4 and COMP act as adaptor molecules that interconnect D-periodically banded collagen II-containing cartilage fibrils with collagen VI-containing beaded filaments and aggrecan aggregates to generate a complex macromolecular network. The interactions may be mediated either by matrilins binding directly to the collagenous COL3 domain of collagen IX or via COMP that associates with the NC4 domain of collagen IX. The contacts of matrilin-1, 3, and 4 with collagen VI filaments are mediated by the small LRR proteoglycans decorin and/or biglycan, which preferentially bind to the filaments in the vicinity of the collagen VI N-termini, themselves acting as adaptor molecules. Note that the size of the molecules is not to scale. (Reproduced with permission from Klatt AR, Becker AK, Neacsu CD, Paulsson M, Wagener R: The matrilins: Modulators of extracellular matrix assembly. *Int J Biochem Cell Biol* 2011;43:320-330.)

Lubricin/Proteoglycan 4

To help withstand biomechanical shear forces due to articulation, articular cartilage surfaces possess an inherently low coefficient of friction, which is facilitated in part by localization of the boundary lubricant, lubricin, a mucin-like glycoprotein secreted by chondrocytes and synoviocytes (reviewed in Ref. 26). One of the primary functions of lubricin—also known as proteoglycan 4 (PRG4)—is the maintenance of joint lubrication and the prevention of cellular adhesion. Lack of lubricin expression has been connected to premature joint failure, as demonstrated in the camptodactyly-arthropathy-coxa vara pericarditis (CACP) syndrome in humans, in which genetic mutations elicit a lubricin deficit,[27] and the use of recombinant lubricin as an intra-articular biotherapeutic for osteoarthritis is being explored.[26,28] Interestingly, joint articulation stimulates the expression of lubricin, whereas pure compressive loading does not.[29] It has been speculated that the oscillating joint drags fluid into the joint space, thereby causing biophysical effects similar to those of fluid flow. Velocity magnitude of the oscillating bodies (and thus the dragged fluid) is a critical determinant for the cellular response.

Lubricin or other molecules alone, however, cannot account for the very low friction levels found at the surface of articular cartilage. Recent research has shed light on this phenomenon by suggesting that hyaluronan molecules are linked to the surface of cartilage by lubricin molecules, and hyaluronan further complexes with phospholipids to create hydration layers at the surface of the cartilage.[30]

CARTILAGE HOMEOSTASIS

Cartilage homeostasis may be defined as the processes necessary to maintain the normal function and viability of this tissue. Chondrocytes, as the only cells in cartilage, are responsible for homeostasis. Chondrocyte metabolism is strongly

©Copyright 2021 American Academy of Orthopaedic Surgeons

influenced by the unique environment of cartilage—unlike most tissues, cartilage lacks a vascular, nerve, and lymphatic supply. As a result, cartilage relies on diffusion of nutrients from the synovial fluid and from the subchondral bone, and chondrocytes get their energy primarily by the oxygen-free process of glycolysis. Overall, cartilage exists in a hypoxic state and oxygen levels within cartilage decrease with tissue depth. Under normal circumstances, chondrocytes do not divide, and overall, chondrocytes have a limited capacity to repair defects in cartilage.

TURNOVER OF MATRIX MOLECULES

In healthy cartilage, matrix turnover is slow, and the half-life of the major constituents, type II collagen and aggrecan, is very long. The half-life of type II collagen has been reported to be over 100 years,[31] and recent studies using the carbon-14 (^{14}C) bomb pulse method showed that collagen turnover in cartilage is negligible after skeletal maturity, even in individuals with osteoarthritis.[32] Using aspartic acid racemization as a marker of molecular age, it has been proposed that the half-life of the large aggrecan monomer in human cartilage is 3.4 years, whereas the free hyaluronan-binding region fragments have a half-life of 25 years. This suggests that the rate of formation and turnover of the large monomer is much more rapid than the final degradation of the free binding region fragments, which explains the accumulation of the latter in cartilage with aging (discussed below).[33] In arthritic disease, factors such as cytokines induce chondrocytes to secrete proteolytic enzymes that degrade the matrix. The aggrecanases, a disintegrin and metalloproteinase with thrombospondin motif (ADAMTS)-4 and ADAMTS-5 (reviewed in Ref. 34), cleave the aggrecan core protein at five distinct cleavage sites, thus generating multiple fragments that diffuse from the matrix into the synovial fluid. Cleavage between the amino acids Glu^{373} and Ala^{374} in the interglobular domain of the aggrecan core protein results in the loss of the bulk of the GAG-bearing portion of aggrecan from the cartilage matrix, thereby compromising its function (reviewed in Ref. 35). ADAMTS-5 has generated much interest as a target for osteoarthritis, with several companies exploring the potential disease-modifying effects of small molecules or antibodies to inhibit the activity of this enzyme.[36] ADAMTS-4 has been reported to cleave matrilin-3, and ADAMTS-7 and 12 have been reported to cleave COMP, which may all contribute to destabilization of the extracellular matrix (reviewed in Ref. 37). As these events occur, the collagen network becomes increasingly vulnerable to the action of collagenases, in particular MMP-13. The specific cleavage products that are thus generated can be monitored in the synovial fluid, and even in the urine, which has generated invaluable information on the pathogenesis of osteoarthritis.[38] There are ongoing efforts in standardizing methods to measure levels of specific matrix fragments (including fragments of collagen, aggrecan, COMP, etc.) in biological fluids, so that they can be used as biomarkers of disease.

CHONDROCYTE-MATRIX INTERACTIONS

Matrix molecules, or fragments thereof, play a key role in modulating cell behavioral responses, including cell metabolism, differentiation, and survival. For example, members of the SLRP gene family can act as signaling molecules (reviewed in Ref. 39), and soluble SLRPs can engage various cell-surface receptors, including insulin growth factor 1 receptor and epidermal growth factor receptor, triggering downstream signaling events that regulate cell behavior. In addition, these glycoproteins bind and sequester various cytokines, growth factors and morphogens (eg, transforming growth factor [TGF]-β)[40] involved in multiple signaling pathways. In healthy cartilage, TGFβ expression is regulated by biomechanical signaling and plays a role in maintaining the chondrocyte phenotype.[41] In osteoarthritis, however, TGFβ levels are elevated, which promotes fibrosis and bone changes. This upregulation of TGFβ may be due to release of bound growth factor as cartilage matrix molecules are cleaved, as well as due to increased production by other cells in the joint. In the pericellular matrix, matrix molecules interact with cell-surface receptors—for example, fibronectin can bind integrins and heparan sulfate proteoglycans such as syndecan, collagen binds discoidin domain receptors (DDRs), and CD44 acts as a hyaluronan receptor (**Figure 4**). Many molecules that bind these receptors on the surface of chondrocytes also interact with molecules in the territorial matrix, establishing communication between the matrix (sometimes far removed from the cell) and the chondrocyte. The chondrocyte can thus sense what is going on in the matrix and respond accordingly. It has been suggested that the content of matrilins in the pericellular matrix can alter the mechanical sensitivity of chondrocytes (reviewed in Ref. 25). Other proteins in the cartilage matrix (listed in **Table 1**) fulfill important roles, many of which are the subject of active research. Fibulin has been shown to be important in the supramolecular organization of the cartilage matrix, through binding of the G3 domain of aggrecan (reviewed in Ref. 23). Some proteins, like tenascin-C, are present in small amounts, but their expression goes up dramatically in osteoarthritis.[42]

As the matrix undergoes changes as part of aging or as part of a pathological process (arthritis or injury), molecular interactions and subsequent cellular responses can alter dramatically, resulting in a changed metabolic environment and often compromising cartilage function. Furthermore, molecules released from the matrix can be biologically active and have been linked to inflammation through at least two mechanisms. First, matrix molecules such as fibromodulin and COMP can activate complement and thus contribute to inflammation, which in turn generates more degradation of the matrix (reviewed in Ref. 23). Secondly, matrix components such as tenascin-C, fibronectin, and fragments of hyaluronic acid can activate toll-like receptors (TLR), expressed by many cells including chondrocytes, synoviocytes, and macrophages, resulting in the release of numerous chemokines

©Copyright 2021 American Academy of Orthopaedic Surgeons

and cytokines.[43] For example, fibronectin, a multimeric glycoprotein found in plasma and tissues, is a minor component of normal cartilage. However, osteoarthritic cartilage contains up to 10-fold more fibronectin (through synthesis and accumulation), and this is accompanied by increased levels in the synovial fluid. Products of fibronectin fragmentation can induce a catabolic phenotype in chondrocytes, and fragments have been shown to induce enzymes such as MMP-13 and ADAMTS-4/5.[44] In osteoarthritic cartilage, ADAM-8 is responsible for generating specific fibronectin fragments.[45]

Recently, a small 32-amino acid aggrecan fragment that is generated when ADAMTS-4/5 cleave the interglobular domain of the aggrecan core protein at the ^{374}ARGS cleavage site and the remaining G1-EGE^{373} stub is subsequently cleaved by MMPs at DIPEN^{341}, was also shown to signal through TLR2. This 32-mer aggrecan fragment promotes catabolic signaling in chondrocytes, macrophages, and synovial fibroblasts.[46] Interestingly, the aggrecan fragment was also shown to promote painful signaling in sensory nerves through TLR2.[47] Such observations suggest that the cartilage breakdown process can not only amplify joint damage, but also promote pain.

CHONDROCYTE-MECHANICAL LOADING INTERACTIONS

Chondrocytes are involved in the maintenance of the ECM through responding to mechanical loading by adapting the synthesis of new matrix molecules or cleavage of ECM molecules. Cartilage is subjected to a large variety of stresses in daily life, and, as has been mentioned above, the composition and arrangement of the ECM is designed to fulfill these functional requirements. For example, stair climbing, running, walking, and standing upright for long periods of time all cause different forces to be applied to the cartilage, yet cartilage has to be able to respond and protect the underlying bones from damage. Within the ECM, collagen fibers are designed to resist tensile and shear forces. In contrast, aggrecan molecules are composed of a protein core with negatively charged glycosaminoglycan side chains. This charge results in compressive strength because it causes electrostatic repulsion and osmotic swelling, allowing cartilage to resist compression and fluid flow. The collagen fibers are important for constraining the osmotic swelling properties of the proteoglycans.[5]

Chondrocytes can sense and respond to different types of mechanical loading.[4] For example, physiologic loading results in increased aggrecan production in the weight-bearing areas of knee articular cartilage, whereas injurious loading upregulates the enzymes that break down cartilage ECM. It is still not completely understood which molecules chondrocytes use to sense mechanical stimuli in the environment, but integrins and different types of ion channels have been implicated in this process. The sensation of forces then initiates downstream signaling cascades that can alter gene expression as well as protein production and modification. It was recently reported that the ion channel, TRPV4, plays an important role in the chondrocyte response to physiologic loading.[48] Two other mechanosensitive ion channels were recently discovered, Piezo1 and Piezo2, and both of these channels are expressed by chondrocytes as well as by other cell types such as sensory neurons. On chondrocytes, these channels appear to be important for sensing large forces capable of injuring cartilage (in contrast to TRPV4, which seems more important for responding to physiologic loading).[49]

AUTOPHAGY

Autophagy is a cytoplasmic mechanism used by many cells to maintain homeostasis through the removal of damaged intracellular components to adapt to environmental stresses.[50] Because chondrocytes have limited cellular turnover, autophagy is an important mechanism to clear damaged intracellular molecules and prevent the production of reactive oxygen species.[51] The superficial zone in particular has strong expression of autophagy regulators, such as ULK1, Beclin1, and LC3.[51] Histologically, autophagy can be identified in chondrocytes by the formation of autophagosomes. In addition, autophagy inhibits the production of enzymes in human chondrocytes.[52] In early osteoarthritis, autophagy pathways are upregulated, as chondrocytes are attempting to combat ECM breakdown, but in late stage osteoarthritis, autophagy pathways are decreased, promoting chondrocyte apoptosis. Because autophagy is a druggable pathway, it could be targeted in age-associated osteoarthritis.

EFFECTS OF AGING

Aging of tissues, including cartilage, can be defined as a time-dependent functional decline,[53] and aging is one of the main risk factors for osteoarthritis. Chondrocytes as well as the ECM are affected by age-related processes, which may make the tissue more vulnerable. Nine hallmarks of aging have been proposed based on common pathways that affect different tissues as a result of aging: genomic instability, telomere attrition, epigenetic alterations, loss of proteostasis, deregulated nutrient sensing, mitochondrial dysfunction, cellular senescence, stem cell exhaustion, and altered intercellular communication.[53] It has been suggested that cellular senescence and mitochondrial dysfunction, in particular, are associated with the development of primary osteoarthritis.[54] With aging and in osteoarthritis, chondrocytes have been shown to display one characteristic of senescence—increased expression of pro-inflammatory molecules (termed the senescence-associated secretory phenotype or SASP). Aging also results in decreased autophagy, which may act in concert with aging-associated mitochondrial dysfunction and oxidative stress to promote the accumulation of reactive oxygen species. Preclinical studies have suggested that selective removal of senescent chondrocytes or targeting mitochondria to limit oxidative stress could be a useful strategy to slow the development of osteoarthritis.[54]

©Copyright 2021 American Academy of Orthopaedic Surgeons

All joint tissues change with age, thus contributing to increased risk for development of osteoarthritis. The ECM of articular cartilage undergoes profound changes with aging (reviewed in Ref. 55). Formation of advance glycation end-products (AGE) affects the mechanical properties of cartilage through increased cross-linking of the collagen network and makes the cartilage too stiff. Age-related changes in GAG composition not only affect biomechanical properties of cartilage but also profoundly alter the susceptibility of the aggrecan core protein to cleavage by aggrecanases (reviewed in Ref. 34). Also, aggrecan cleavage by aggrecanases between the amino acids Glu[373] and Ala[374] in the interglobular domain generates small fragments that are retained in the matrix through the interaction of the G1 domain with hyaluronan, and thus accumulate in cartilage during the lifetime of the individual.[56] These G1-aggrecan fragments bound to hyaluronan occupy the binding sites where newly synthesized aggrecan molecules should bind, thus impeding cartilage repair.

EFFECTS OF GENETICS

Mutations in genes encoding cartilage matrix proteins are not uncommon, especially for collagen. For example, mutations in *COLII*, *COLIX*, and *COLXI* lead to chondrodysplasias and premature osteoarthritis.[57] Recent genetic association studies aiming at understanding how genetic variation in population cohorts is associated with osteoarthritis have uncovered novel insights in the function of some cartilage molecules (reviewed in Ref. 58). Genome-wide association studies (GWAS) have identified several genetic associations with knee osteoarthritis. For example, single nucleotide polymorphisms (SNPs) in double von Willebrand factor A (*DVWA*) have been associated with knee osteoarthritis in an Asian population, but this could not be replicated in a European cohort. This newly identified gene was later found to encode collagen VI alpha 4 (*COL6A4*), a collagen variant that does not appear to be expressed in articular cartilage. Hence, the importance of this SNP in relation to cartilage biology remains unknown.

Other polymorphisms of interest have been discovered, including an association between knee osteoarthritis and a polymorphism in the gene encoding the matrix molecule, asporin, which suppresses TGF-β-mediated expression of aggrecan and type II collagen. A mutation in the gene encoding matrilin-3 is associated with hand osteoarthritis. This particular point mutation (T298M) was found to have a pronounced influence on the formation of cartilage collagen fibrils in in vitro assays (reviewed in Ref. 25). Finally, among the genes that have been linked to hip osteoarthritis, a highly heritable disease, there are several that are involved in the development and maintenance of joint shape, including members of the Wingless (Wnt) and the bone morphogenetic protein (BMP) family. In particular, a SNP in *DOT1L* was strongly associated with increased risk of hip osteoarthritis, particularly in males.[58] Several features of hip joint architecture, such as acetabular dysplasia, pistol grip deformity, wide femoral neck, and altered femoral neck-shaft angle, appear to play an important role in the pathogenesis of osteoarthritis and may predate the development of clinical osteoarthritis by decades (reviewed in Ref. 59). Finally, as mentioned above, mitochondrial dysfunction in chondrocytes has been associated with aging and osteoarthritis, and mutations discovered in mitochondrial DNA have been associated with a lower risk of progression in a cohort for knee osteoarthritis.[58] In addition, there has been recent focus on epigenetic mechanisms such as DNA methylation, histone modifications, and noncoding RNAs, which may all play an important role in cartilage homeostasis and are likely important in osteoarthritis pathogenesis.[60] Indeed, the strong association between the *DOT1L* polymorphism and hip osteoarthritis spurred basic researchers to unravel the role of DOT1L, an enzyme involved in histone methylation, in cartilage homeostasis. Mechanistically, they found that the protective function of DOT1L is attributable to inhibition of Wnt signaling, a pathway that, when hyperactivated, can lead to joint disease.[61]

SUMMARY

This chapter discusses basic information on the physiology, structure, composition, biomechanical, and biochemical properties of articular cartilage. Articular cartilage is a marvelously complex tissue where one cell type, the chondrocyte, elaborates and manages an abundant avascular and aneural extracellular matrix. The biochemical characteristics of the macromolecules that build up this matrix provide the cartilage with its remarkable biomechanical properties. Significant new findings have clarified our understanding of the fine assembly of this molecular meshwork, which has important implications for lubrication and friction of the joint. This chapter also introduces emerging areas of study in cartilage homeostasis such as autophagy, senescence, genetics, and epigenetics, which collectively point toward the future of the field. Importantly, enzymatic degradation of the matrix generates fragments that are biologically active and can serve as signals to chondrocytes or a variety of other cells in the joint, including sensory neurons. These fragments can be monitored in the synovial fluid, serum, and urine and, hopefully, in the near future may be developed as functional biomarkers of cartilage health.

REFERENCES

1. Hunter WVI: Of the structure and diseases of articulating cartilages. *Clin Orthop Relat Res* 1743;42:514-521.
2. Lefebvre V, Dvir-Ginzberg M: SOX9 and the many facets of its regulation in the chondrocyte lineage. *Connect Tissue Res* 2017;58:2-14.

©Copyright 2021 American Academy of Orthopaedic Surgeons

3. Hunziker EB: Articular cartilage structure in humans and experimental animals, in Kuettner KE, Schleyerbach R, Peyron JG, Hascall VC, eds: *Articular Cartilage and Osteoarthritis.* New York, NY, Raven Press, 1991, pp 183-199.
4. Buckwalter JA, Mankin HJ, Grodzinsky AJ: Articular cartilage and osteoarthritis. *Instr Course Lect* 2005;54:465-480.
5. Maroudas A, Bayliss MT, Venn MF: Further studies on the composition of human femoral head cartilage. *Ann Rheum Dis* 1980;39:514-523.
6. Kuettner KE, Aydelotte MB, Thonar EJ: Articular cartilage matrix and structure: A minireview. *J Rheumatol Suppl* 1991;27:46-48.
7. Poole AR, Pidoux I, Reiner A, Rosenberg L: An immunoelectron microscope study of the organization of proteoglycan monomer, link protein, and collagen in the matrix of articular cartilage. *J Cell Biol* 1982;93:921-937.
8. Hoemann CD, Lafantaisie-Favreau CH, Lascau-Coman V, Chen G, Guzman-Morales J: The cartilage-bone interface. *J Knee Surg* 2012;25:85-97.
9. Mapp PI, Walsh DA: Mechanisms and targets of angiogenesis and nerve growth in osteoarthritis. *Nat Rev Rheumatol* 2012;8:390-398.
10. Quinn TM, Hauselmann HJ, Shintani N, Hunziker EB: Cell and matrix morphology in articular cartilage from adult human knee and ankle joints suggests depth-associated adaptations to biomechanical and anatomical roles. *Osteoarthr Cartil* 2013;21:1904-1912.
11. Stockwell RA: The interrelationship of cell density and cartilage thickness in mammalian articular cartilage. *J Anat* 1971;109:411-421.
12. Hunziker EB, Quinn TM, Hauselmann HJ: Quantitative structural organization of normal adult human articular cartilage. *Osteoarthr Cartil* 2002;10:564-572.
13. Flannery CR, Hughes CE, Schumacher BL, et al: Articular cartilage superficial zone protein (SZP) is homologous to megakaryocyte stimulating factor precursor and Is a multifunctional proteoglycan with potential growth-promoting, cytoprotective, and lubricating properties in cartilage metabolism. *Biochem Biophys Res Commun* 1999;254:535-541.
14. Schumacher BL, Block JA, Schmid TM, Aydelotte MB, Kuettner KE: A novel proteoglycan synthesized and secreted by chondrocytes of the superficial zone of articular cartilage. *Arch Biochem Biophys* 1994;311:144-152.
15. Poole CA: Articular cartilage chondrons: Form, function and failure. *J Anat* 1997;191(pt 1):1-13.
16. Guilak F, Nims RJ, Dicks A, Wu CL, Meulenbelt I: Osteoarthritis as a disease of the cartilage pericellular matrix. *Matrix Biol* 2018;71-72:40-50.
17. Jiang Y, Tuan RS: Origin and function of cartilage stem/progenitor cells in osteoarthritis. *Nat Rev Rheumatol* 2015;11:206-212.
18. Benninghoff A: Form und Bau der Gelenkknorpel in ihren Beziehungen zur Funktion. *Anat Entwicklungsgesch* 1925;76:43.
19. Heinegard D, Saxne T: The role of the cartilage matrix in osteoarthritis. *Nat Rev Rheumatol* 2011;7:50-56.
20. Chen MH, Broom N: On the ultrastructure of softened cartilage: A possible model for structural transformation. *J Anat* 1998;192(pt 3):329-341.
21. Eyre DR, Weis MA, Wu JJ: Articular cartilage collagen: An irreplaceable framework? *Eur Cell Mater* 2006;12:57-63.
22. Wu JJ, Weis MA, Kim LS, Eyre DR: Type III collagen, a fibril network modifier in articular cartilage. *J Biol Chem* 2010;285:18537-18544.
23. Heinegard D: Fell-Muir Lecture: Proteoglycans and more–from molecules to biology. *Int J Exp Pathol* 2009;90:575-586.
24. Pratta MA, Yao W, Decicco C, et al: Aggrecan protects cartilage collagen from proteolytic cleavage. *J Biol Chem* 2003;278:45539-45545.
25. Klatt AR, Becker AK, Neacsu CD, Paulsson M, Wagener R: The matrilins: Modulators of extracellular matrix assembly. *Int J Biochem Cell Biol* 2011;43:320-330.
26. Jay GD, Waller KA: The biology of lubricin: Near frictionless joint motion. *Matrix Biol* 2014;39:17-24.
27. Jay GD, Torres JR, Rhee DK, et al: Association between friction and wear in diarthrodial joints lacking lubricin. *Arthritis Rheum* 2007;56:3662-3669.
28. Waller KA, Chin KE, Jay GD, et al: Intra-articular recombinant human proteoglycan 4 mitigates cartilage damage after destabilization of the medial meniscus in the Yucatan minipig. *Am J Sports Med* 2017;45:1512-1521.
29. Grad S, Lee CR, Gorna K, et al: Surface motion upregulates superficial zone protein and hyaluronan production in chondrocyte-seeded three-dimensional scaffolds. *Tissue Eng* 2005;11:249-256.
30. Seror J, Zhu L, Goldberg R, Day AJ, Klein J: Supramolecular synergy in the boundary lubrication of synovial joints. *Nat Commun* 2015;6:6497.
31. Verzijl N, DeGroot J, Thorpe SR, et al: Effect of collagen turnover on the accumulation of advanced glycation end products. *J Biol Chem* 2000;275:39027-39031.
32. Heinemeier KM, Schjerling P, Heinemeier J, et al: Radiocarbon dating reveals minimal collagen turnover in both healthy and osteoarthritic human cartilage. *Sci Transl Med* 2016;8:346ra390.
33. Maroudas A, Bayliss MT, Uchitel-Kaushansky N, Schneiderman R, Gilav E: Aggrecan turnover in human articular cartilage: Use of aspartic acid racemization as a marker of molecular age. *Arch Biochem Biophys* 1998;350:61-71.
34. Tortorella MD, Malfait AM: Will the real aggrecanase(s) step up: Evaluating the criteria that define aggrecanase activity in osteoarthritis. *Curr Pharm Biotechnol* 2008;9:16-23.
35. Little CB, Fosang AJ: Is cartilage matrix breakdown an appropriate therapeutic target in osteoarthritis–insights from studies of aggrecan and collagen proteolysis?. *Curr Drug Targets* 2010;11:561-575.
36. Fosang AJ: ADAMTS-5 takes centre stage in new developments for aggrecanase inhibitors. *Osteoarthr Cartil* 2015;23:1231-1232.
37. Tortorella MD, Malfait F, Barve RA, Shieh HS, Malfait AM: A review of the ADAMTS family, pharmaceutical targets of the future. *Curr Pharm Des* 2009;15:2359-2374.
38. Lohmander LS, Neame PJ, Sandy JD: The structure of aggrecan fragments in human synovial fluid. Evidence that aggrecanase mediates cartilage degradation in inflammatory joint disease, joint injury, and osteoarthritis. *Arthritis Rheum* 1993;36:1214-1222.
39. Iozzo RV, Schaefer L: Proteoglycans in health and disease: Novel regulatory signaling mechanisms evoked by the small leucine-rich proteoglycans. *FEBS J* 2010;277:3864-3875.
40. Hildebrand A, Romarís M, Rasmussen LM, et al: Interaction of the small interstitial proteoglycans biglycan, decorin and fibromodulin with transforming growth factor beta. *Biochem J* 1994;302(pt 2):527-534.
41. van der Kraan PM: The changing role of TGFβ in healthy, ageing and osteoarthritic joints. *Nat Rev Rheumatol* 2017;13:155.
42. Hasegawa M, Yoshida T, Sudo A: Role of tenascin-C in articular cartilage. *Mod Rheumatol* 2018;28:215-220.
43. Liu-Bryan R, Terkeltaub R: Emerging regulators of the inflammatory process in osteoarthritis. *Nat Rev Rheumatol* 2015;11:35-44.
44. Ding L, Guo D, Homandberg GA: The cartilage chondrolytic mechanism of fibronectin fragments involves MAP kinases: Comparison of three fragments and native fibronectin. *Osteoarthr Cartil* 2008;16:1253-1262.
45. Zack MD, Malfait AM, Skepner AP, et al: ADAM-8 isolated from human osteoarthritic chondrocytes cleaves fibronectin at Ala(271). *Arthritis Rheum* 2009;60:2704-2713.
46. Lees S, Golub SB, Last K, et al: Bioactivity in an aggrecan 32-mer fragment is mediated via toll-like receptor 2. *Arthritis Rheumatol* 2015;67:1240-1249.
47. Miller RE, Ishihara S, Tran PB, et al: An aggrecan fragment drives osteoarthritis pain through Toll-like receptor 2. *JCI Insight* 2018;3(6). pii:95704. doi:10.1172/jci.insight.95704.
48. McNulty AL, Leddy HA, Liedtke W, Guilak F: TRPV4 as a therapeutic target for joint diseases. *Naunyn Schmiedebergs Arch Pharmacol* 2015;388:437-450.
49. Lee W, Guilak F, Liedtke W: Role of Piezo channels in joint health and injury. *Curr Top Membr* 2017;79:263-273.
50. Kroemer G: Autophagy: A druggable process that is deregulated in aging and human disease. *J Clin Invest* 2015;125:1-4.

 ©Copyright 2021 American Academy of Orthopaedic Surgeons

51. Lotz MK, Carames B: Autophagy and cartilage homeostasis mechanisms in joint health, aging and OA. *Nat Rev Rheumatol* 2011;7:579-587.
52. Rockel JS, Kapoor M: Autophagy: Controlling cell fate in rheumatic diseases. *Nat Rev Rheumatol* 2016;12:517-531.
53. Lopez-Otin C, Blasco MA, Partridge L, Serrano M, Kroemer G: The hallmarks of aging. *Cell* 2013;153:1194-1217.
54. Collins JA, Diekman BO, Loeser RF: Targeting aging for disease modification in osteoarthritis. *Curr Opin Rheumatol* 2018;30:101-107.
55. Shane Anderson A, Loeser RF: Why is osteoarthritis an age-related disease? *Best Pract Res Clin Rheumatol* 2010;24:15-26.
56. Roughley PJ, Mort JS: The role of aggrecan in normal and osteoarthritic cartilage. *J Exp Orthop* 2014;1:8.
57. WA H, JT H: Chondrodysplasias: Disorders of cartilage matrix proteins, in P R, B S, eds: *Connective Tissue and its Heritable Disorders*. New York, Wiley-Liss, Inc., 2002, pp 909-937.
58. Warner SC, Valdes AM: Genetic association studies in osteoarthritis: Is it fairytale? *Curr Opin Rheumatol* 2017;29:103-109.
59. Baker-LePain JC, Lane NE: Relationship between joint shape and the development of osteoarthritis. *Curr Opin Rheumatol* 2010;22:538-543.
60. Coutinho de Almeida R, Ramos YFM, Meulenbelt I: Involvement of epigenetics in osteoarthritis. *Best Pract Res Clin Rheumatol* 2017;31:634-648.
61. Monteagudo S, Cornelis FMF, Aznar-Lopez C, et al: DOT1L safeguards cartilage homeostasis and protects against osteoarthritis. *Nat Commun* 2017;8:15889.

©Copyright 2021 American Academy of Orthopaedic Surgeons

Biomechanics of Articular Cartilage and Its Response to Loading

Clark T. Hung, PhD
Gerard A. Ateshian, PhD

Keywords: *Articular Cartilage; Biomechanics; Chondrocyte; Diarthrodial Joint*

INTRODUCTION

This chapter aims to provide an intuitive review of articular cartilage mechanical properties and its response to loading in the context of its biochemical composition and structural organization. The implications of how changes to articular cartilage biomechanics with joint degeneration upset the normal feedback system of the chondrocyte and its ability to regulate the structure-function relationship of articular cartilage will be discussed.

PRIMARY FUNCTION OF ARTICULAR CARTILAGE

Articular cartilage is a connective tissue that lines the bony surfaces of diarthrodial joints. Its primary function is to support the loads acting across the joint while producing minimal friction and wear. More specifically, articular cartilage provides compliance to otherwise hard bony surfaces, distributing the joint contact forces over a sufficiently large area to minimize contact pressures at the articular surfaces, and stresses transmitted to the bone. In some joints, this function is further enhanced by additional soft-tissue structures that enhance joint congruence, such as menisci and labra. Since bone remodels significantly in response to stresses, whereas cartilage does not, the compliance of healthy cartilage produces suitable homeostasis in the bone remodeling process, helping to maintain normal joint anatomy. The mechanical breakdown of cartilage, however initiated, compromises this primary function, leading to a cascade of events that compromise joint health, function and anatomy.

FORCES AND MOMENTS ACROSS DIARTHRODIAL JOINTS

Forces acting across diarthrodial joints are combinations of (internal) muscle forces and external loads, including gravitational, inertial, and lifting forces. These same forces also produce moments about the joint axis of rotation, which are calculated as the product of the force times the distance from the force line of action to the axis of rotation (the moment arm). It would be a gross underestimation to assume that forces transmitted across diarthrodial joints are roughly equal to body weight (gravitational force) or loads acting on our extremities in activities of daily living (lifting forces). Due to the compactness of the musculoskeletal system, namely the proximity of muscles to the skeleton, muscles must apply much higher forces across a joint than the external forces acting on the body, to also balance the moments exerted by external forces about the joint axis of rotation.

Newton's second law of motion tells us that the sum of all forces acting on a body (including inertial forces) must be balanced. Importantly, the same law of physics tells us

---

Dr. Hung or an immediate family member has received royalties from Allosource (license) and has received research or institutional support from Musculoskeletal Transplant Foundation. Dr. Ateshian or an immediate family member has received royalties from AlloSource.

©Copyright 2021 American Academy of Orthopaedic Surgeons

that the sum of all moments acting on a body must also be balanced. Let us illustrate this basic concept by examining the force required in the biceps muscle to balance the weight of an object held in the hand (**Figure 1**). For this example, we consider that a 10 N weight (about 2 pounds) is held in the hand with the upper arm held vertically and the forearm held horizontally. The distance from the hand to the elbow joint is 30 cm (approximately 1 foot), and the distance from the biceps muscle insertion on the forearm to the elbow axis of rotation is 6 cm (approximately 2 inches). The moment exerted by the handheld weight about the elbow axis of rotation is 10 N × 30 cm = 300 N·cm. Consider that the force exerted by the biceps muscle is F; its moment about the elbow axis of rotation is $F \times 6$ cm. Accordingly, to maintain moment equilibrium about the elbow, these two moments must balance each other, $F \times 6\text{ cm} = 300\text{ N·cm}$, from which it follows that $F = 50$ N (about 10 pounds). Using force equilibrium, we conclude that the contact force exerted at the elbow joint is the difference between the muscle force and the handheld weight, thus 40 N. In other words, in this example, the force in the muscle is five times higher, and the joint contact force is four times higher, than the external force acting on the musculoskeletal system. These relations scale with the magnitude of the handheld weight; thus, for a weightlifter performing a bicep curl using a 1,000 N weight (500 N in each hand), the joint contact force in each elbow would be 2,000 N (approximately 400 pounds, or nearly three times body weight).

These multiplication factors apply across all diarthrodial joints. Lower extremity joints experience greater magnitudes of joint loads than upper extremity joints; they also typically have larger articular surfaces. Higher extremity joints are typically smaller in size, especially in the hand and wrist, and support smaller external forces; however, some joints such as the thumb and shoulder may exhibit up to 10-fold multiplication factors relating external forces to joint contact forces.[1,2] Thus, regardless of location, all diarthrodial joints transmit contact forces several times greater than the external forces acting on the musculoskeletal structures spanning those joints.

Articular cartilage distributes this contact force over a relatively large fraction of the articular surfaces. A joint contact force F distributed over a contact area A produces an average contact pressure $p=F/A$. For example, for a closed kinematic chain exercise for the knee joint (eg, squatting), the quadriceps muscle force is approximately equal to 1,600 N at 60° of flexion, producing a comparable contact force at the patellofemoral joint.[3] The resulting articular contact area is approximately 650 mm² (which is roughly half the surface area of the patellar articular layer[4]), producing an average contact pressure

$$p = \frac{1{,}600\text{ N}}{650\text{ mm}^2} = 2.5\text{ MPa}.$$

One megapascal (MPa) is equal to one hundred forty-five pounds per square inch; if a person could hang his/her weight from a single fingertip, this would be roughly equivalent to the pressure exerted on that tip. In general, activities of daily living produce average articular contact pressures in the range 1 to 6 MPa[5]; strenuous sports activities may conceivably produce contact pressures up to 12 MPa for intermittent loading durations, though the evidence for such elevated values is limited. It has been estimated from in vitro cadaver studies that cartilage and its underlying subchondral bone plate may crack when articular contact stresses exceed 15 MPa.[6] Thus, under normal loading conditions articular cartilage is well suited to support the wide range of loads acting across diarthrodial joints.

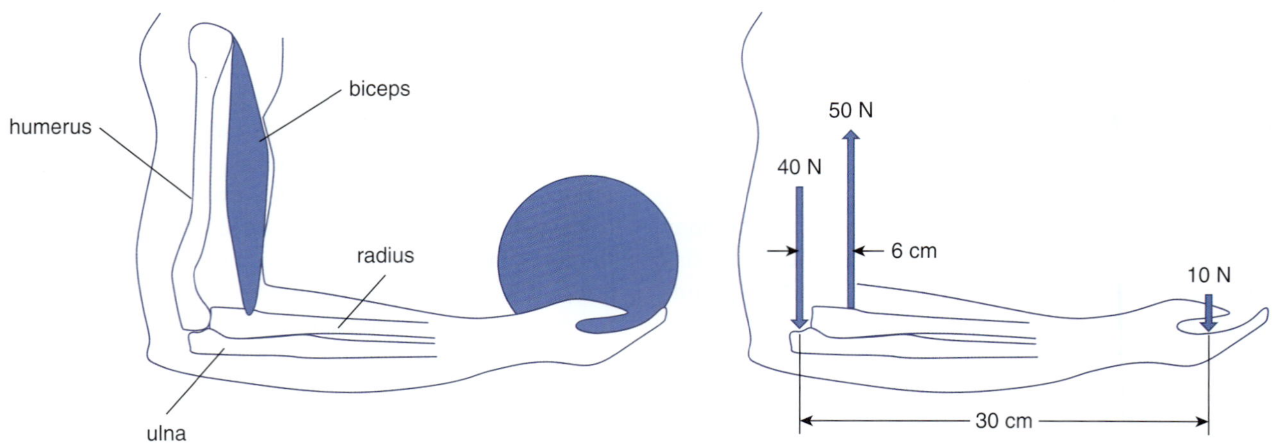

FIGURE 1 Illustration demonstrating the forces across the elbow while carrying a weight in the hand: The handheld ball weighs 10 N and the moment arm of this force is 30 cm about the elbow axis of rotation, producing a moment equal to 300 N·cm. The biceps muscle's moment arm is 6 cm, requiring a muscle force of 50 N to balance the moment applied by the ball. The elbow joint contact force is 40 N, to balance the other forces acting on the forearm. Since the line of action of the joint contact force passes through the joint's axis of rotation, it does not contribute to the moments acting across that joint.

 ©Copyright 2021 American Academy of Orthopaedic Surgeons

COMPOSITION AND ULTRASTRUCTURE

Articular cartilage is a hydrated porous permeable tissue whose interstitial fluid (water and electrolytes) contributes 60% to 85% to the tissue's weight.[7] The extracellular matrix (ECM) consists primarily of collagen (15% to 22% of the wet weight, 50% to 80% of the dry weight) and proteoglycans (4% to 7% of the wet weight, 15% to 30% of the dry weight).[8] Chondrocytes occupy less than 10% of the tissue volume. Collagen is predominantly of type II, which forms fibrils with a diameter varying between 20 and 200 nm, but not fibers. Other ECM collagens include types VI, IX, and XI. Cartilage proteoglycans have a bottle-brush appearance, with a core protein and glycosaminoglycan side chains consisting of chondroitin sulfate (CS) and keratan sulfate (KS). A link protein ties these aggrecans along a hyaluronic acid backbone, forming macromolecular complexes with molar masses on the order of millions. Both CS and KS are negatively charged in solution, thus conferring a fixed-charge density (FCD) to cartilage.[9]

The fibrillar organization and composition of the ECM varies significantly from the articular surface to the subchondral bone. The superficial zone starts at the articular surface and extends by hundreds of nanometers; it is characterized by elevated collagen and water content and very low proteoglycan content. The collagen fibrils are oriented parallel to the articular surface, with a preferential direction[10] believed to coincide with the "split-line" direction, named after the method of visualizing it by pricking the surface with a needle. The functional significance of the split-line directions remains unclear, though it appears that they coincide with directions of greatest curvature of the articular surfaces.[11,12] With increasing distance from the articular surface, collagen fibrils progressively rotate to form the middle (or transitional) zone and then become perpendicular to the cartilage-subchondral bone interface in the deep (or radial) zone. In the middle zone, the collagen fibrils are often split between two families that emanate from the superficial zone in opposite directions, eventually merging into a single family in the deep zone.[10,13] Proteoglycan content is greatest in the middle zone, followed by the deep zone, whereas collagen and water content progressively diminish from the articular surface to the subchondral bone. A tidemark delineates the interface between the deep zone and the zone of calcified cartilage where this tissue meets bone.

Other functionally significant cartilage constituents include superficial zone protein (SZP), which is believed to confer beneficial lubrication and wear properties at the articular surface.[14,15] Cartilage thickness varies approximately from less than 1 mm thick on average in smaller upper extremity joints[16] up to 3 mm thick on average in larger extremity joints.[17] Some locations in the tibial plateaus and the patella may be up to 7 mm thick.[4]

MECHANICAL PROPERTIES IN RELATION TO TISSUE FUNCTION

Unlike other connective tissues, such as tendons and ligaments which sustain tensile forces, cartilage is subjected primarily to compressive loads. It is therefore an interesting characteristic of articular cartilage that its ECM consists substantially of fibrillar collagen, a microscopically rope-like material which is best suited to resist tensile forces. As it turns out, collagen fibrils interact mechanically with the other main ECM constituents, interstitial fluid and proteoglycans, to provide the functional response that confers cartilage its remarkable load-bearing and frictional properties.

CARTILAGE PERMEABILITY

The porous ECM of articular cartilage is permeable to the interstitial fluid.[18] Upon mechanical loading of cartilage, this interstitial fluid pressurizes and flows from high pressure (loaded) to low pressure (unloaded) regions. However, the frictional resistance to this flow is very significant as fluid molecules flow past the ECM matrix constituents. Experimentally, this frictional resistance is quantitatively assessed by measuring the material property called the hydraulic permeability, represented by the symbol k. From measurements of k, it is estimated that the characteristic velocity of interstitial fluid flow in articular cartilage is on the order of 0.1 μm/s. For comparison purposes, the diameter of a chondrocyte is approximately 16 μm. In effect, interstitial fluid flows so slowly within cartilage that fluid volume loss from articular layers may be considered negligible during activities of daily living. Measurements from MRI suggest that the fluid volume loss is less than 6% of the cartilage volume in a low extremity joint subjected to strenuous exercise.[19]

INTERSTITIAL FLUID PRESSURIZATION STIFFENS CARTILAGE

The primary functional effect of interstitial fluid pressurization is to stiffen articular cartilage under dynamic loading conditions.[20] In vitro measurements performed in human patellofemoral joints show that a physiologic level of cyclical contact pressure (p = 3.3 MPa) prescribed at one cycle per second produces no more than ε = 9% cyclical change in cartilage thickness.[21] The stiffness of cartilage under cyclical compressive loading is called the dynamic compressive Young modulus E_{dyn}. Its value may be estimated from the ratio of the prescribed pressure p to the compressive strain ε; thus, for human patellofemoral joint cartilage, E_{dyn} = 37 MPa. In contrast, if the contact pressure is maintained for sufficiently long durations, the fluid pressure subsides leading to much

2: Structure and Function of Musculoskeletal Tissues

©Copyright 2021 American Academy of Orthopaedic Surgeons

larger compressive strains under physiologic pressures. This type of response is often characterized under laboratory conditions, using much smaller compressive pressures p, to yield a stiffness measure called the equilibrium compressive Young modulus, E_{eq}. Typical measurements of this equilibrium stiffness yield values on the order of E_{eq} = 0.4 MPa, nearly 100 times smaller than the dynamic modulus.[22] This comparison between dynamic and equilibrium moduli helps us better appreciate the functional importance of interstitial fluid pressurization for resisting compressive pressures and maintaining cartilage deformations to within levels not harmful to chondrocyte viability.

FUNCTIONAL ROLE OF PROTEOGLYCANS

Proteoglycans are negatively charged macromolecules enmeshed within the collagen matrix. Due to electrostatic interactions, more cations (eg, Na^+) transport into cartilage than anions (eg, Cl^-) to neutralize the proteoglycan charge. This mechanism produces a higher concentration of ions inside the tissue than in its external bathing solution, leading to an influx of water which causes the tissue to pressurize and swell. This is called Donnan osmotic swelling, and the resulting interstitial fluid pressure is the Donnan pressure. Donnan swelling effectively stiffens articular cartilage since it pressurizes the collagen matrix, similar to an inflated balloon.[23] Measurements performed in various bathing solution concentrations suggest that Donnan swelling contributes approximately 60% to the measured compressive stiffness E_{eq}.[24,25] In contrast, complete enzymatic digestion of the proteoglycans of articular cartilage has been shown to decrease its compressive equilibrium Young modulus E_{eq} by a factor of 100 (down to approximately 0.003 MPa).[25] Therefore, macromolecular proteoglycans also contribute significantly to the structural stiffness of the fiber-composite-like cartilage ECM.

FUNCTIONAL ROLE OF COLLAGEN FIBRILS

Collagen fibrils are able to sustain large tensile loads but otherwise buckle under compression. Proteoglycans enmeshed within the collagen matrix serve as a "ground matrix" that stabilizes the collagen network by helping it to resist compression.[26] The primary functional role of collagen fibrils in cartilage is to resist transverse tissue expansion upon axial compressive loading when the interstitial fluid is pressurized.[27,28] To better appreciate this functional role, assume that collagen is inextensible (infinitely stiff in tension) and consider a cylindrical plug of cartilage subjected to a compressive pressure p (**Figure 2**). Upon rapid application of this pressure, there is insufficient time for the interstitial fluid to flow out of the tissue; therefore, the fluid pressurizes and the volume of the cylindrical plug must be substantially preserved as it is being loaded (since mass must be conserved and the densities of ECM and interstitial fluid are nearly constant). If the collagen is inextensible, the cylindrical plug cannot expand in the direction transverse to loading; since its volume is to be

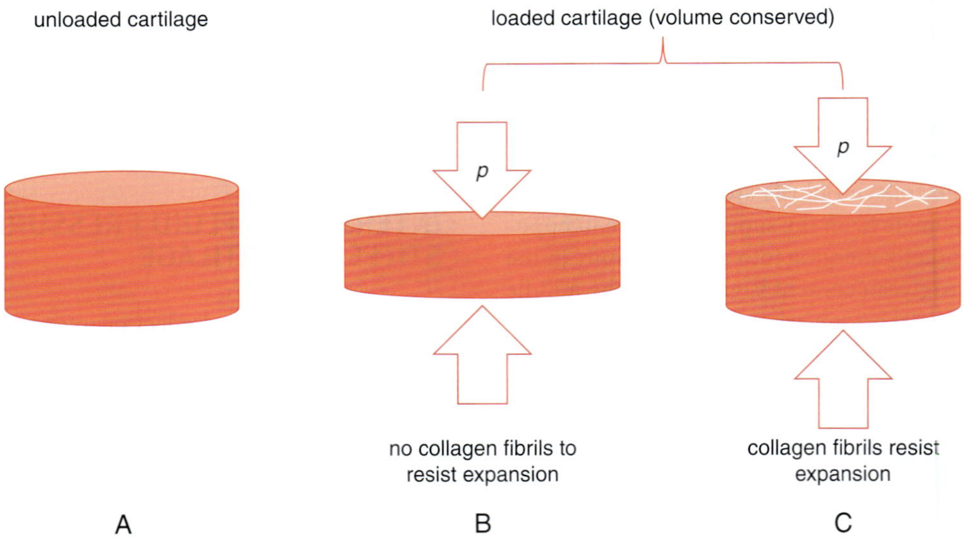

FIGURE 2 Illustrations demonstrating that collagen fibrils and interstitial fluid pressurization considerably enhance cartilage stiffness: When an unloaded cylindrical cartilage plug (**A**) is subjected to a compressive pressure p, the interstitial fluid pressurizes but the low tissue permeability limits the exudation of the fluid; consequently, the cylindrical plug's volume is substantially conserved. **B**, In the absence of collagen fibrils, the plug may expand considerably in the direction transverse to loading, leading to a substantial reduction in the plug height (large compressive strain ε). **C**, In contrast, stiff collagen fibrils oriented transversely to the direction of compressive loading resist the transverse expansion, leading to little reduction in plug height (small compressive strain ε) since the volume is conserved. As the dynamic modulus is given by $E_{dyn}=p/\varepsilon$, it follows that the presence of collagen fibrils considerably enhances E_{dyn}.

©Copyright 2021 American Academy of Orthopaedic Surgeons

preserved, the height of the plug may not change either, that is, the plug acts as an infinitely stiff spring.[29] Of course, in reality, the collagen is not perfectly inextensible so that the cartilage plug will get compressed a little (**Figure 2**, C). Nevertheless, this hypothetical example clearly shows that the tensile stiffness of the collagen matrix, when coupled with interstitial fluid pressurization, contributes considerable stiffness to cartilage under compressive loading. This mechanism explains why E_{dyn} is nearly 100 times greater than E_{eq}.

These biomechanical considerations clearly demonstrate the intricate way in which the structure of articular cartilage governs its function, namely, its ability to sustain large compressive pressures resulting from joint loads, while limiting cartilage deformation to approximately 10% of its thickness. The classic cartilage biomechanics literature has often suggested that proteoglycans are the primary structure resisting compression of articular cartilage whereas collagen resists tension. Our modern understanding of cartilage biomechanics has evolved to produce a more elaborate picture of the interaction of proteoglycans, the collagen network, and interstitial fluid pressurization when the tissue is subjected to compressive loads.

CARTILAGE STRESSES AND STRAINS

In the terminology of mechanics, stress represents a normalized measure of the forces acting inside a material which tend to pull (tension) or push (compression) on the material's molecules, or tend to shear those molecules (**Figure 3**). These forces are normalized by the surface area on which they are acting. Since stress is a measure of forces internal to a material, it cannot be measured directly, as the insertion of a putative transducer that would measure these forces would necessarily require cutting through the material and altering that measure. Strain is a normalized measure of the deformations occurring inside a material, including tensile, compressive, and shear strains (**Figure 3**). These deformations are normalized by the initial distance between the molecules. Unlike stress, strain is observable (ie, measurable) since there are a variety of noninvasive methods, such as those commonly used in medicine (radiographs, MRI, ultrasonography, etc.), that can track the positions of molecules inside the material. Since knowledge of stresses is essential for predicting the conditions under which a material gets damaged (ie, when its molecular bonds break), models are needed for calculating the stress based on measurements of the strain. These models must be validated against experimental measurements of the deformation of a material subjected to known external forces.

For articular cartilage, sophisticated models have been formulated and successfully validated, which account for the fibrillar nature of the collagen matrix, the "ground matrix" contribution of proteoglycans, and the presence of an interstitial fluid that pressurizes due to mechanical loading.[29-32] With these validated models it has been possible to investigate the state of stress in the ECM under joint contact loading, using image-based reconstructions of subject-specific joint geometry.[33] These modeling studies have yielded two interesting results: First, the contact pressure at the articular surfaces is nearly equal to the interstitial fluid pressure (**Figure 4**), implying that almost all of the contact load is supported by the pressurized interstitial fluid; second, the ECM is subjected to tensile stresses throughout the thickness of the articular layers, with the orientation of these stresses coinciding substantially with the fibrillar orientation of the collagen matrix (**Figure 5**). These findings enhance our understanding of structure-function relationships in articular cartilage, further clarifying why fibrillar collagen is needed in the ECM and why its specific orientation is ideally suited for its function under realistic contact conditions.

CARTILAGE FRICTION AND WEAR

Friction represents the force produced between two objects sliding relative to one another. The friction coefficient μ represents the ratio of the frictional force to the normal force applied when compressing these two objects. Since articular layers sustain large compressive loads while sliding, measurements of the cartilage friction coefficient have long served as a useful evaluation of this tissue's lubrication function. Several studies have demonstrated that the friction coefficient of human cartilage sliding against cartilage may be as low as 0.02, whether measurements are conducted in synovial fluid or saline.[34,35] This low value of the friction coefficient means that a joint contact force on the order of 1,000 N (approximately 200 pounds) only produces a frictional force of 20 N (4 pounds).

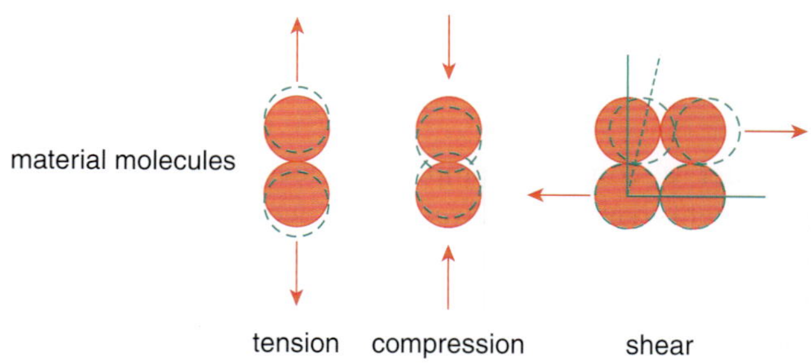

FIGURE 3 Illustration demonstrating that when a material is subjected to external loading, the molecules inside the material are subjected to tension, compression, and shear. Tensile, compressive, and shear stresses, respectively, represent the ratio of these internal tensile, compressive, and shear forces normalized by the area over which they act. Tensile and compressive strains represent the ratio of the deformations (the change in intermolecular distances) normalized by the initial intermolecular distance in the unloaded material; shear strains represent the change in angle between initially orthogonal lines.

©Copyright 2021 American Academy of Orthopaedic Surgeons

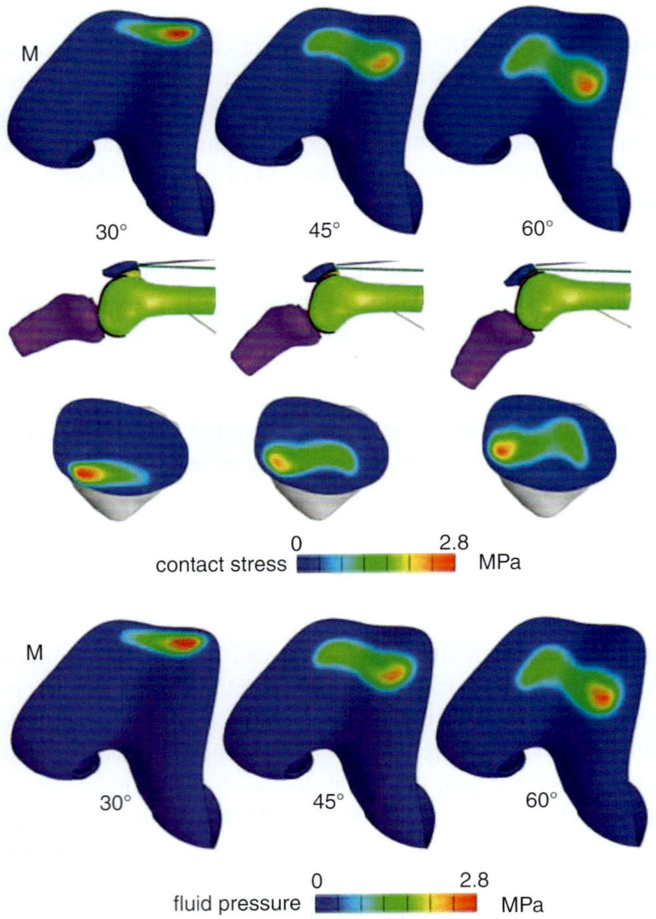

FIGURE 4 Finite element analysis of articular cartilage in the patellofemoral joint at three different flexion angles, using a cartilage model that accounts for interstitial fluid pressurization, a fibrillar collagen matrix, and a proteoglycan ground matrix: The contact stress p at the articular surfaces (top row for femur, middle row for patella) is nearly equal to the interstitial fluid pressure in the superficial zone of cartilage (bottom row for femur). (Reproduced with permission from Jones BK, Hung CT, Ateshian GA: Biphasic analysis of cartilage stresses in the patellofemoral joint. *J Knee Surg* 2016;29[2]:92-98.)

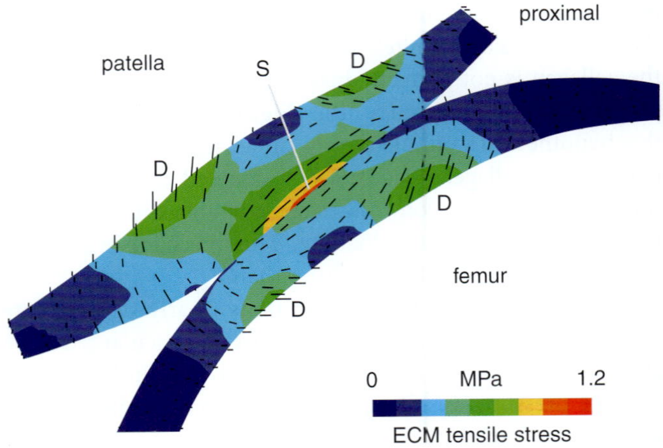

FIGURE 5 Sagittal cross-sectional view of the patellofemoral joint finite element model, showing magnitude of extracellular matrix (ECM) tensile stresses (color contours) and directions of maximum tensile stress (black dashes). The directions of maximum tensile stresses are consistent with the predominant orientation of collagen fibrils from the superficial (S) to the deep (D) zones. (Reproduced with permission from Jones BK, Hung CT, Ateshian GA: Biphasic analysis of cartilage stresses in the patellofemoral joint. *J Knee Surg* 2016;29[2]:92-98.)

Under a constant compressive load, cartilage friction experiments have also showed that μ increases over time, concomitantly as the cartilage interstitial fluid pressure subsides[36] (**Figure 6**). Based on these observations, it is now understood that interstitial fluid pressurization plays a critical role for maintaining low friction between articulating cartilage layers.[37] When a porous cartilage layer which has 80% fluid content comes into contact with another layer that also has 80% fluid content, the fraction of the contact area over which superficial zone collagen rubs against the opposing superficial zone collagen is only 4% (since the area fraction of collagen on each side is 20% and 20% × 20% = 4%). Over the remaining 96% of the contact area, pressurized interstitial fluid supports the contact force. Therefore, the only significant contribution to the frictional force across cartilage layers arises from the 4% of the contact force which is supported by collagen-contacting-collagen. If the friction coefficient of collagen-on-collagen is 0.12 (an ordinary range for many materials), the resulting cartilage friction coefficient may be as low as $0.12 \times 0.04 = 0.005$, in the limit when the interstitial fluid pressure is exactly equal to the contact pressure (**Figure 4**).

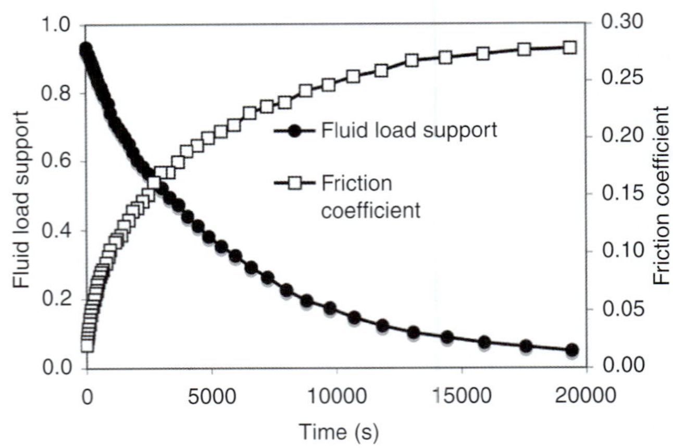

FIGURE 6 Line chart demonstrating the experimental measurement of the friction coefficient μ of a bovine articular cartilage plug sliding against glass, in unconfined compression creep. In this sample, μ increases from 0.02 to 0.28 over 20,000 s of loading. Simultaneous measurement of the interstitial fluid pressure within the cartilage plug (normalized by the prescribed contact pressure p to produce the fractional fluid load support) shows that this fluid pressure decreases concomitantly with increasing μ.[36] (Reproduced with permission from Ateshian GA: The role of interstitial fluid pressurization in articular cartilage lubrication. *J Biomech* 2009;42[9]:1163-1176.)

©Copyright 2021 American Academy of Orthopaedic Surgeons

These findings further demonstrate that the structure of articular cartilage is tightly related to its two primary biomechanical functions, namely providing compliant load bearing while also producing very low friction. Thus, despite its very low metabolic activity and repair ability in adulthood, articular cartilage is a remarkably resilient material that can withstand physiologic loads over a wide range of operating conditions.

Cartilage wear is the mechanism by which this load-bearing material degrades either mechanically or chemically to produce tissue damage and tissue loss. Different forms of mechanical wear have been described in the lubrication literature. Perhaps the most intuitive form is abrasive wear, such as that caused by rubbing sandpaper against a material, causing particulate matter loss. A less intuitive form of mechanical wear is called delamination; this mechanism occurs because the reciprocal contact loading of bearing materials produces elevated stresses at a depth slightly below the bearing surface, eventually initiating a subsurface crack that slowly propagates sideways and toward the surface, leading to the detachment of a thin layer of material (a lamina).

Recent frictional experiments conducted on articular cartilage rubbed against a variety of materials (such as glass and metal alloys used in total joint replacements) have shown that the predominant mechanism of mechanical wear is delamination, whereas particulate wear is insignificant.[38] In hindsight, this finding is not surprising since the friction coefficient of cartilage is very low, thus minimizing abrasive mechanisms, and does not increase with progression of osteoarthritis.[35] In contrast, the ECM stresses produced within the articular layers are comparable in magnitude to the contact pressure[33] (compare the results of **Figures 4** and **5**). Thus, the cyclical nature of joint loading would be consistent with a progressive mechanism of delamination wear. Based on experimental observations to date, it appears that the location where ECM delamination damage initiates is between the superficial and middle zones (**Figure 7**), where the collagen fibrillar orientation transitions from an alignment parallel to the articular surface to an alignment orthogonal to the cartilage-bone interface. Measurements of the shear modulus of cartilage through the depth of the articular layer indicate that this transitional zone is the weakest and thus most vulnerable.[39] Nevertheless, significant mechanical wear may not necessarily occur under normal loading conditions, unless it is triggered by an initiating event, such as an impact injury, which weakens the ECM.

Another likely wear mechanism in articular cartilage is enzymatic degradation (chemical wear), mediated by proteolytic enzymes released by any combination of the soft tissues present inside a joint, including cartilage, synovium, ligaments, menisci, or fat pads. The release of a larger-than-normal amount of these enzymes may be triggered by an injury, inflammatory process, or congenital condition. These enzymes will likely weaken the ECM and compromise its ability to sustain normal levels of tissue stresses, potentially leading to mechanical wear progression. Thus, neither acute nor chronic biochemical events need have drastic effects on their own; it could be their interaction with normal loading conditions that may cause further wear progression. In other words, our understanding of cartilage biomechanics provides a consistent perspective with the multifactorial nature of cartilage degenerative diseases such as osteoarthritis. Stress produced by physiologic contact loading of diarthrodial joints clearly mediates the progression of wear, but it need not be the initiating factor.

CARTILAGE DEGENERATION

Cartilage degeneration manifests itself mechanically as a loss of compressive stiffness; this loss of stiffness is accompanied or followed by increased water content and gross evidence of ECM disruption, such as surface fibrillation and swelling, then delamination and loss of proteoglycan content, and tissue thinning (**Figure 7**). The end stage of cartilage degeneration is the complete loss of this tissue, leading to bone-on-bone contact, which is often painful. This degenerative process is typically accompanied by changes in the surrounding bony structures, such as osteophyte formation, progression of the tidemark, and eburnation. Since cartilage mediates the transmission of forces across bones, and since it is well established that bone remodels in response to the stresses it sustains,[40] we can establish a simple mechanism linking cartilage degeneration to bone remodeling.

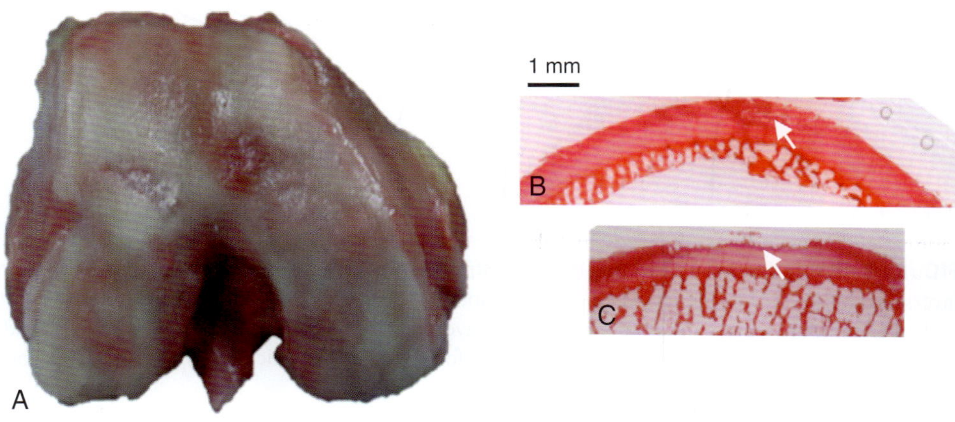

FIGURE 7 Histological cross-sections of a moderately osteoarthritic human distal femoral articular layer (**A**, photograph) show some locations with visible delamination of the articular layer between the superficial and middle zones (**B**) while other locations show complete loss of the superficial zone and cartilage thinning (**C**). (Picrosirius red staining for collagen.)

©Copyright 2021 American Academy of Orthopaedic Surgeons

As mentioned above, when a force *F* is applied across a diarthrodial joint the articular layers deform to distribute this force over a contact area *A*, producing a contact pressure $p=F/A$. This articular surface pressure is sustained by stresses within the cartilage layers and underlying bones. Under normal function, healthy articular cartilage compresses by a relatively small amount (eg, 10% compressive strain) while spreading the contact area *A* over a sufficiently large fraction of the articular surface to minimize the stresses in the underlying bones. A good analogy is the example of a good quality bed mattress placed on a hard floor. A person sleeping on this mattress has their weight distributed evenly over its surface and is unable to feel the floor underneath because the mattress compression is relatively small. Now consider that cartilage has degenerated and become softer; under the same applied load *F* the cartilage may compress by much more than 10% of its thickness, producing a smaller contact area *A* and higher contact pressure *p* (**Figure 8**). In our mattress analogy, consider that we now have a cheap foam mattress placed on the floor. A person lying on that mattress will have the back of their head and shoulders, as well as buttocks and heels digging into the mattress and feeling the hard floor underneath. It is not just the sleeper who feels these elevated pressures, the floor will also be subjected to equal and opposite forces. Thus, in the case of cartilage and bone, it becomes evident from this analysis that the softening of cartilage compromises its ability to distribute contact pressures evenly on the articular layers and the underlying bones, leading to increased bone stresses and progressive bone remodeling. As the cartilage becomes thinner, the stresses in cartilage and bone may increase further, thus producing a slow but inexorable progression of tissue degeneration.

Though we illustrated this problem by assuming initial softening of cartilage, the same mechanism may occur via iatrogenesis, such as partial or total meniscectomies, osteotomies, or other similar surgical procedures that decrease joint congruence or alter joint contact forces, leading to elevated articular contact pressures.[41,42] In summary, healthy articular cartilage under normal function is able to transmit and distribute diarthrodial joint forces such that stresses in the bone maintain remodeling homeostasis. Events that compromise the function of cartilage may disrupt this homeostasis, leading to degenerative processes that involve soft and hard tissues in those joints.

BIOLOGICAL EFFECTS OF LOADING

Cartilage is avascular and has no nerves. As such, the chondrocyte relies on nutrients from the bathing synovial fluid for its survival. Pain associated with joint degeneration is therefore not directly manifested in cartilage but from bone, ligament insertions, or the synovium that envelops the joint. The lack of blood supply is responsible for the poor reparative capacity of cartilage, as there is a lack of the typical wound healing cascades associated with vascularized tissues that exhibit healing.

Aggregates of proteoglycans are important in the development and maintenance of cartilage. Expression of the genes for aggrecan and link protein, two major components of the aggregates, can be modulated by mechanical forces as well as chemical stimuli. The biomechanical properties of articular cartilage are dependent on the integrity of the collagen network and on maintenance of a high proteoglycan content within the matrix. Chondrocytes maintain this matrix, synthesizing and secreting ECM.

Chondrocytes that reside in articular cartilage act as sensors for biophysical stimuli. They sense and interpret the environment around them, looking to maintain their environment

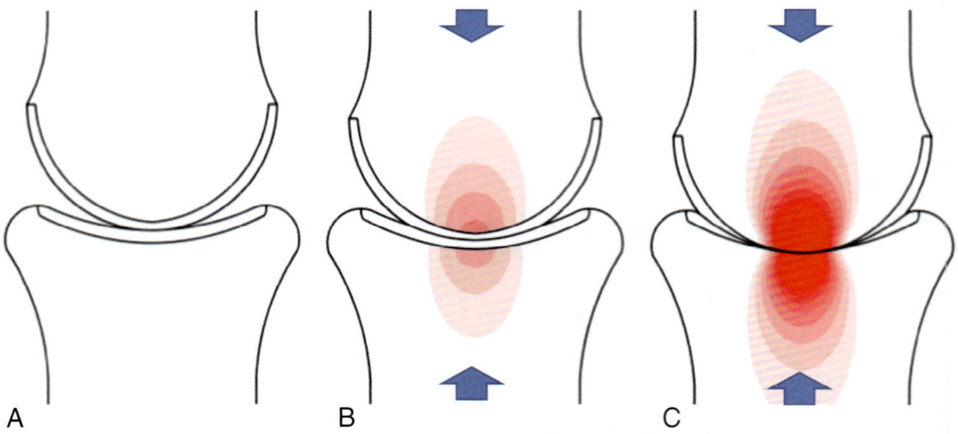

FIGURE 8 Illustrations demonstrating that bone stresses increase as cartilage becomes softer: **A**, Unloaded diarthrodial joint, showing articular layers and bones in their undeformed configuration. **B**, Loaded diarthrodial joint with healthy cartilage, showing deformed articular layers, and color contours representing the most compressive stress in the bone. **C**, Under the same load, a diarthrodial joint with degenerated (softer) cartilage shows significantly greater compressive deformation of the articular layers and higher compressive stresses (darker red contours) in the bone.

©Copyright 2021 American Academy of Orthopaedic Surgeons

in a narrow physiologic range by adjusting their local ECM through anabolic and catabolic activities to refine the stimuli that arise from joint loading. In the disease process, alterations in normal joint loading, such as arising from changes to joint motion (kinematics) or cartilage damage resulting from injury, can lead to an abnormal INPUT to the chondrocyte. Consequently, chondrocytes respond with an OUTPUT that leads to an impaired ECM. In this manner, and in the absence of any real healing capacity, the pathologic process can become recursive, spiraling to further tissue degeneration and eventually osteoarthritis.

The mechanical environment of the chondrocyte is an important factor affecting the health of articular cartilage and consequently the function of the diarthrodial joint, and the progression of joint degeneration (**Figure 9**). Deformation of the ECM during joint loading results in the generation of various physical stimuli, such as fluid and ion flows, changes to FCD, hydrostatic pressure, and cellular deformation, which may act to stimulate the anabolic and/or catabolic activities of the chondrocytes. The cell senses mechanical forces during "mechanotransduction," triggering the activation of biochemical signaling cascades that mediate downstream changes to cell function. As the total load applied to the cartilage is partitioned between the organic ECM solid phase and interstitial fluid phase, the dominant response of cartilage to loading is hydrostatic pressurization of the fluid. Accordingly, hydrostatic pressure represents not only the primary load-bearing mechanism of articular cartilage, but the main mechanical stimulus to chondrocytes. The ability of the tissue to retain this pressurized fluid is dependent on the integrity of the ECM and interactions of collagen and proteoglycans that are compromised with tissue breakdown in degenerative joint changes. In the latter, the degree of hydrostatic pressure during loading decreases, and there is a shift of load and corresponding physical stimuli to those borne by the solid matrix (including cells).

In addition to providing biophysical cues to chondrocytes, joint loading-induced deformation of cartilage facilitates the convective transport of nutrients from the synovial fluid.[43,44] Similarly, ion flow due to loading-induced fluid shifts within the charged tissue (from FCD) arises in electrokinetic phenomena, such as the streaming potential,[45] that form the basis for the use of electric fields in bone healing therapies. Attraction of positive ions in the interstitial fluid to the fixed charges associated with the aggregating proteoglycans entangled in the type II collagen fibrillar network create a more hypertonic environment for chondrocytes than for other cell types. Applied osmotic loading to isolated chondrocytes and cartilage has also been reported to modulate cell activities and tissue metabolism.[46]

Static compressive loads have been demonstrated to cause a decrease in proteoglycan synthesis and release from the ECM of articular cartilage in addition to a decrease in protein synthesis. The catabolic activity of proteoglycans has also been shown to be affected by compressive loading. Investigators using dynamic or cyclic loading conditions, corresponding to physiological loading, have also reported biosynthetic responses in articular cartilage.[47-50] These effects are strongly dependent on magnitude and frequency of the applied load, with slow-frequency loading generally resulting in suppression of proteoglycan synthesis while more rapid loading frequencies result in stimulated synthesis. Static loading is not physiologic and is not practically achievable in real life under normal conditions, as muscle firing in maintaining balance and posture results in time-varying loads on our joints.

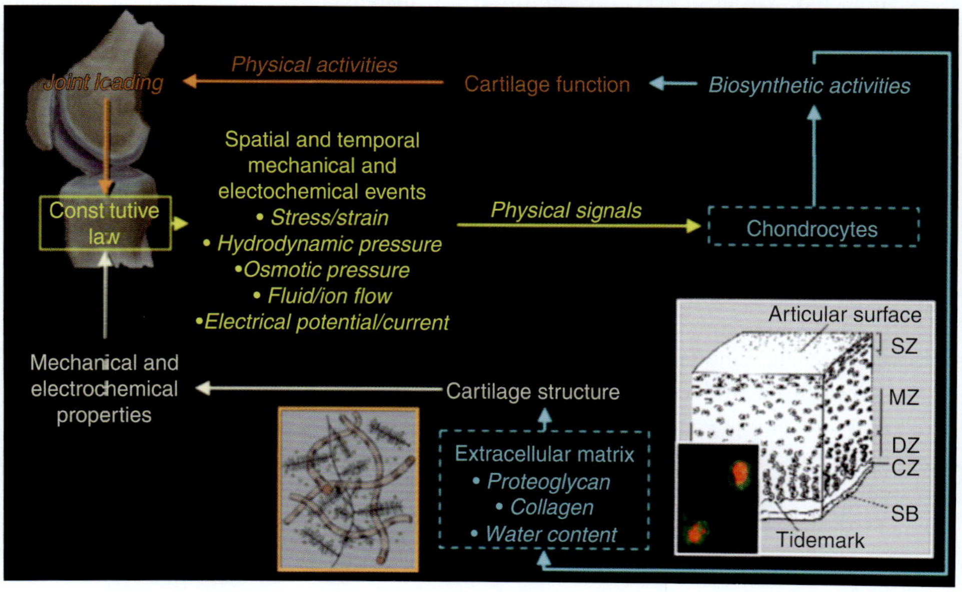

FIGURE 9 Illustration depicting the feedback system that regulates the structure and function of articular cartilage.

©Copyright 2021 American Academy of Orthopaedic Surgeons

SUMMARY

This chapter reviewed our current understanding of the biomechanics of articular cartilage as it relates to its structure and function in health and disease. Much of our understanding of cartilage structure and composition is based on decades-old investigations that have stood the test of time, though modern measurement techniques have provided increasingly more detailed insights in those respects. Similarly, measurements of cartilage mechanical properties, such as its modulus in compression or tension and its hydraulic permeability, have been reported for several decades. However, the field of cartilage biomechanics experienced major advances in our understanding of structure-function relationships once modeling frameworks started to account explicitly for the tissue's structure and composition, including interstitial fluid, fibrillar collagen network, and charged proteoglycan ground matrix, leading to the novel insights presented in this chapter. Similarly, measurement of cartilage friction dates back to the 1930s; until the 1960s, it was widely believed that synovial fluid acts as a fluid-film lubricant, just like automotive oil lubricates moving parts in a car. When models of cartilage friction based on fluid-film lubrication failed to support this mechanism, it became evident that new approaches were needed to understand cartilage lubrication and wear, leading to the findings summarized in this review.

Despite the remarkable advances in our understanding of cartilage biomechanics today, there are many open questions that remain to be addressed. From a purely mechanics perspective, we need a better understanding of cartilage damage mechanics and fatigue failure under the repetitive loading cycles to which it is subjected. We also need greater modeling insights into cartilage as a living tissue, to have a better understanding of how much damage cartilage can tolerate and repair under normal tissue maintenance conditions. As alluded to in this review, we need far greater understanding of the interaction of cartilage with other soft and hard tissue structures in diarthrodial joints, to understand if or how a disruption in any of these structures (whether mechanically or biologically mediated) may lead to a cascade of deleterious events leading to loss of joint function. Developing predictive models of tissue damage, remodeling, and repair would go a long way toward our understanding of certain surgical outcomes, and ultimately predicting outcomes of patient-specific or even novel surgical procedures prior to their actual execution.

REFERENCES

1. Cooney WP III, Chao EY: Biomechanical analysis of static forces in the thumb during hand function. *J Bone Joint Surg Am* 1977;59:27-36. https://www.ncbi.nlm.nih.gov/pubmed/833171.
2. Poppen NK, Walker PS: Forces at the glenohumeral joint in abduction. *Clin Orthop Relat Res* 1978:165-170. https://www.ncbi.nlm.nih.gov/pubmed/709928.
3. Cohen ZA, Roglic H, Grelsamer RP, et al: Patellofemoral stresses during open and closed kinetic chain exercises. An analysis using computer simulation. *Am J Sports Med* 2001;29:480-487. https://www.ncbi.nlm.nih.gov/pubmed/11476390.
4. Ateshian GA, Soslowsky LJ, Mow VC: Quantitation of articular surface topography and cartilage thickness in knee joints using stereophotogrammetry. *J Biomech* 1991;24:761-776. https://www.ncbi.nlm.nih.gov/pubmed/1918099.
5. Huberti HH, Hayes WC: Patellofemoral contact pressures. The influence of q-angle and tendofemoral contact. *J Bone Joint Surg Am* 1984;66:715-724. https://www.ncbi.nlm.nih.gov/pubmed/6725318.
6. Atkinson PJ, Haut RC: Subfracture insult to the human cadaver patellofemoral joint produces occult injury. *J Orthop Res* 1995;13:936-944. https://www.ncbi.nlm.nih.gov/pubmed/8544032.
7. Mow VC, Ratcliffe A, Poole AR: Cartilage and diarthrodial joints as paradigms for hierarchical materials and structures. *Biomaterials* 1992;13:67-97. https://www.ncbi.nlm.nih.gov/pubmed/1550898.
8. Kempson GE, Muir H, Swanson SA, Freeman MA: Correlations between stiffness and the chemical constituents of cartilage on the human femoral head. *Biochim Biophys Acta* 1970;215:70-77. https://www.ncbi.nlm.nih.gov/pubmed/4250263.
9. Carney SL, Muir H: The structure and function of cartilage proteoglycans. *Physiol Rev* 1988;68:858-910. https://www.ncbi.nlm.nih.gov/pubmed/3293094.
10. Aspden RM, Hukins DW: Collagen organization in articular cartilage, determined by X-ray diffraction, and its relationship to tissue function. *Proc R Soc Lond B Biol Sci* 1981;212:299-304. https://www.ncbi.nlm.nih.gov/pubmed/6115394.
11. Below S, Arnoczky SP, Dodds J, Kooima C, Walter N: The split-line pattern of the distal femur: A consideration in the orientation of autologous cartilage grafts. *Arthroscopy* 2002;18:613-617. https://www.ncbi.nlm.nih.gov/pubmed/12098122.
12. Kwak SD, Colman WW, Ateshian GA, Grelsamer RP, Henry JH, Mow VC: Anatomy of the human patellofemoral joint articular cartilage: Surface curvature analysis. *J Orthop Res* 1997;15:468-472. https://www.ncbi.nlm.nih.gov/pubmed/9246097.
13. Xia Y, Moody JB, Burton-Wurster N, Lust G: Quantitative in situ correlation between microscopic MRI and polarized light microscopy studies of articular cartilage. *Osteoarthr Cartil* 2001;9:393-406. https://www.ncbi.nlm.nih.gov/pubmed/11467887.
14. Flannery CR, Hughes CE, Schumacher BL, et al: Articular cartilage superficial zone protein (SZP) is homologous to megakaryocyte stimulating factor precursor and Is a multifunctional proteoglycan with potential growth-promoting, cytoprotective, and lubricating properties in cartilage metabolism. *Biochem Biophys Res Commun* 1999;254:535-541. https://www.ncbi.nlm.nih.gov/pubmed/9920774.
15. Jay GD, Torres JR, Rhee DK, et al: Association between friction and wear in diarthrodial joints lacking lubricin. *Arthritis Rheum* 2007;56:3662-3669. PMCID:PMC2688668. https://www.ncbi.nlm.nih.gov/pubmed/17968947.
16. Xu L, Strauch RJ, Ateshian GA, Pawluk RJ, Mow VC, Rosenwasser MP: Topography of the osteoarthritic thumb carpometacarpal joint and its variations with regard to gender, age, site, and osteoarthritic stage. *J Hand Surg Am* 1998;23:454-464. https://www.ncbi.nlm.nih.gov/pubmed/9620186.

©Copyright 2021 American Academy of Orthopaedic Surgeons

17. Soslowsky LJ, Flatow EL, Bigliani LU, Mow VC: Articular geometry of the glenohumeral joint. *Clin Orthop Relat Res* 1992;(285):181-190. https://www.ncbi.nlm.nih.gov/pubmed/1446435.
18. Maroudas A, Bullough P, Swanson SA, Freeman MA: The permeability of articular cartilage. *J Bone Joint Surg Br* 1968;50:166-177. https://www.ncbi.nlm.nih.gov/pubmed/5641590.
19. Eckstein F, Tieschky M, Faber SC, et al: Effect of physical exercise on cartilage volume and thickness in vivo: MR imaging study. *Radiology* 1998;207:243-248. https://www.ncbi.nlm.nih.gov/pubmed/9530322.
20. Park S, Krishnan R, Nicoll SB, Ateshian GA: Cartilage interstitial fluid load support in unconfined compression. *J Biomech* 2003;36:1785-1796. PMCID:PMC2833094. https://www.ncbi.nlm.nih.gov/pubmed/14614932.
21. Guterl CC, Gardner TR, Rajan V, Ahmad CS, Hung CT, Ateshian GA: Two-dimensional strain fields on the cross-section of the human patellofemoral joint under physiological loading. *J Biomech* 2009;42:1275-1281. PMCID:PMC2980285. https://www.ncbi.nlm.nih.gov/pubmed/19433326.
22. Froimson MI, Ratcliffe A, Gardner TR, Mow VC: Differences in patellofemoral joint cartilage material properties and their significance to the etiology of cartilage surface fibrillation. *Osteoarthr Cartil* 1997;5:377-386. https://www.ncbi.nlm.nih.gov/pubmed/9536286.
23. Maroudas A, Venn M: Chemical composition and swelling of normal and osteoarthrotic femoral head cartilage. II. Swelling. *Ann Rheum Dis* 1977;36:399-406. PMCID:PMC1000130. https://www.ncbi.nlm.nih.gov/pubmed/200188.
24. Eisenberg SR, Grodzinsky AJ: Swelling of articular cartilage and other connective tissues: Electromechanochemical forces. *J Orthop Res* 1985;3:148-159. https://www.ncbi.nlm.nih.gov/pubmed/3998893.
25. Canal Guterl C, Hung CT, Ateshian GA: Electrostatic and non-electrostatic contributions of proteoglycans to the compressive equilibrium modulus of bovine articular cartilage. *J Biomech* 2010;43:1343-1350. PMCID:PMC2900255. https://www.ncbi.nlm.nih.gov/pubmed/20189179.
26. Ateshian GA: Anisotropy of fibrous tissues in relation to the distribution of tensed and buckled fibers. *J Biomech Eng* 2007;129:240-249. PMCID:PMC2805028. https://www.ncbi.nlm.nih.gov/pubmed/17408329.
27. Cohen B, Lai WM, Mow VC: A transversely isotropic biphasic model for unconfined compression of growth plate and chondroepiphysis. *J Biomech Eng* 1998;120:491-496. https://www.ncbi.nlm.nih.gov/pubmed/10412420.
28. Soulhat J, Buschmann MD, Shirazi-Adl A: A fibril-network-reinforced biphasic model of cartilage in unconfined compression. *J Biomech Eng* 1999;121:340-347. https://www.ncbi.nlm.nih.gov/pubmed/10396701.
29. Soltz MA, Ateshian GA: A Conewise Linear Elasticity mixture model for the analysis of tension-compression nonlinearity in articular cartilage. *J Biomech Eng* 2000;122:576-586. PMCID:PMC2854000. https://www.ncbi.nlm.nih.gov/pubmed/11192377.
30. Lai WM, Hou JS, Mow VC: A triphasic theory for the swelling and deformation behaviors of articular cartilage. *J Biomech Eng* 1991;113:245-258. https://www.ncbi.nlm.nih.gov/pubmed/1921350.
31. Mow VC, Kuei SC, Lai WM, Armstrong CG: Biphasic creep and stress relaxation of articular cartilage in compression? Theory and experiments. *J Biomech Eng* 1980;102:73-84. https://www.ncbi.nlm.nih.gov/pubmed/7382457.
32. Ateshian GA, Rajan V, Chahine NO, Canal CE, Hung CT: Modeling the matrix of articular cartilage using a continuous fiber angular distribution predicts many observed phenomena. *J Biomech Eng* 2009;131:061003. PMCID:PMC2842192. https://www.ncbi.nlm.nih.gov/pubmed/19449957.
33. Jones B, Hung CT, Ateshian G: Biphasic analysis of cartilage stresses in the patellofemoral joint. *J Knee Surg* 2016;29:92-98. PMCID:PMC4747677. https://www.ncbi.nlm.nih.gov/pubmed/26641078.
34. Charnley J: The lubrication of animal joints in relation to surgical reconstruction by arthroplasty. *Ann Rheum Dis* 1960;19:10-19. PMCID:PMC1007355. https://www.ncbi.nlm.nih.gov/pubmed/13809345.
35. Caligaris M, Canal CE, Ahmad CS, Gardner TR, Ateshian GA: Investigation of the frictional response of osteoarthritic human tibiofemoral joints and the potential beneficial tribological effect of healthy synovial fluid. *Osteoarthr Cartil* 2009;17:1327-1332. PMCID:PMC2753744. https://www.ncbi.nlm.nih.gov/pubmed/19410031.
36. Krishnan R, Kopacz M, Ateshian GA: Experimental verification of the role of interstitial fluid pressurization in cartilage lubrication. *J Orthop Res* 2004;22:565-570. PMCID:PMC2842190. https://www.ncbi.nlm.nih.gov/pubmed/15099636.
37. Ateshian GA: The role of interstitial fluid pressurization in articular cartilage lubrication. *J Biomech* 2009;42:1163-1176. PMCID:PMC2758165. https://www.ncbi.nlm.nih.gov/pubmed/19464689.
38. Oungoulian SR, Durney KM, Jones BK, Ahmad CS, Hung CT, Ateshian GA: Wear and damage of articular cartilage with friction against orthopedic implant materials. *J Biomech* 2015;48:1957-1964. PMCID:PMC4492870. https://www.ncbi.nlm.nih.gov/pubmed/25912663.
39. Buckley MR, Bergou AJ, Fouchard J, Bonassar LJ, Cohen I: High-resolution spatial mapping of shear properties in cartilage. *J Biomech* 2010;43:796-800. PMCID:PMC2832609. https://www.ncbi.nlm.nih.gov/pubmed/19896130.
40. Huiskes R: If bone is the answer, then what is the question? *J Anat* 2000;197(pt 2):145-156. PMCID:PMC1468114. https://www.ncbi.nlm.nih.gov/pubmed/11005707.
41. Ahmed AM, Burke DL: In-vitro measurement of static pressure distribution in synovial joints–Part I: Tibial surface of the knee. *J Biomech Eng* 1983;105:216-225. https://www.ncbi.nlm.nih.gov/pubmed/6688842.
42. Wang VM, Sugalski MT, Levine WN, Pawluk RJ, Mow VC, Bigliani LU: Comparison of glenohumeral mechanics following a capsular shift and anterior tightening. *J Bone Joint Surg Am* 2005;87:1312-1322. https://www.ncbi.nlm.nih.gov/pubmed/15930542.
43. Albro MB, Banerjee RE, Li R, et al: Dynamic loading of immature epiphyseal cartilage pumps nutrients out of vascular canals. *J Biomech* 2011;44:1654-1659. PMCID:PMC3124764. https://www.ncbi.nlm.nih.gov/pubmed/21481875.
44. Albro MB, Cigan AD, Nims RJ, et al: Shearing of synovial fluid activates latent TGF-beta. *Osteoarthr Cartil* 2012;20:1374-1382. PMCID:PMC3448789. https://www.ncbi.nlm.nih.gov/pubmed/22858668.
45. Frank EH, Grodzinsky AJ: Cartilage electromechanics–I. Electrokinetic transduction and the effects of electrolyte pH and ionic strength. *J Biomech* 1987;20:615-627. https://www.ncbi.nlm.nih.gov/pubmed/3611137.
46. Oswald ES, Ahmed HS, Kramer SP, Bulinski JC, Ateshian GA, Hung CT: Effects of hypertonic (NaCl) two-dimensional and three-dimensional culture conditions on the properties of cartilage tissue engineered from an expanded mature bovine chondrocyte source. *Tissue Eng Part C Methods* 2011;17:1041-1049. PMCID:PMC3205796. https://www.ncbi.nlm.nih.gov/pubmed/21797756.
47. Gray ML, Pizzanelli AM, Grodzinsky AJ, Lee RC: Mechanical and physiochemical determinants of the chondrocyte biosynthetic response. *J Orthop Res* 1988;6:777-792. https://www.ncbi.nlm.nih.gov/pubmed/3171760.
48. Sah RL, Kim YJ, Doong JY, Grodzinsky AJ, Plaas AH, Sandy JD: Biosynthetic response of cartilage explants to dynamic compression. *J Orthop Res* 1989;7:619-636. https://www.ncbi.nlm.nih.gov/pubmed/2760736.
49. Guilak F, Meyer BC, Ratcliffe A, Mow VC: The effects of matrix compression on proteoglycan metabolism in articular cartilage explants. *Osteoarthr Cartil* 1994;2:91-101. https://www.ncbi.nlm.nih.gov/pubmed/11548233.
50. Palmoski MJ, Brandt KD: Effects of static and cyclic compressive loading on articular cartilage plugs in vitro. *Arthritis Rheum* 1984;27:675-681. https://www.ncbi.nlm.nih.gov/pubmed/6732884.

©Copyright 2021 American Academy of Orthopaedic Surgeons

14

Meniscus and Labrum

Taylor J. Wiley, MD
David J. Tennent, MD, MAJ MC
Chathuraka T. Jayasuriya, PhD
John Twomey-Kozak, BS
Brett D. Owens, MD

Keywords: *anatomy; labrum; meniscus*

INTRODUCTION

The knee meniscus and glenoid labrum are anatomically distinct yet analogous structures. Although the gross anatomy differs, both tissues are composed of fibrocartilage with a complex but well-organized collagen microstructure. The meniscus and labrum function to increase congruity and stability, decrease contact stresses, and distribute load across their respective joints. This chapter will outline the embryologic development, anatomy, microstructure, and function of the meniscus and labrum.

MENISCUS

NORMAL EMBRYOLOGIC DEVELOPMENT

By 8 to 10 weeks of gestation, the menisci arise from a condensation of the intermediate layer of mesenchymal tissue to form their typical shape.[1] The medial meniscus covers approximately 60% and the lateral meniscus 80% of the corresponding tibial plateau, and this proportion remains consistent throughout development.[2] During development, the vascularity arising from the periphery initially extends throughout the meniscal width, but gradually decreases to supply only the peripheral 10% to 30% of the meniscus by 10 years of age.[2] In addition, meniscal cellularity declines, whereas collagen content increases and organizes in a circumferential fashion.[2]

GROSS ANATOMY

The knee menisci are wedge-shaped fibrocartilaginous structures situated between the femoral condyles and tibial plateau. The macrostructure of the meniscus is divided into its tibial attachments at the anterior and posterior roots, the curved anterior and posterior horns, and the meniscal body at its midportion. The medial meniscus has a semicircular shape, which covers approximately 50% to 60% of the medial tibial plateau in adulthood.[3] The posterior horn averages 11 mm in the anterior-posterior dimension, whereas the anterior horn is narrower.[4] **Figure 1**, A illustrates the basic anatomy of the knee menisci and their attachments. **Figure 1**, B is a photograph diagram of a human tibial plateau with intact medial and lateral menisci. The anterior horn of the medial meniscus attaches to the tibia anterior to the anterior cruciate ligament (ACL) near the intercondylar fossa with significant variability. The transverse, or intermeniscal, ligament connects the anterior horns of the medial and lateral menisci (**Figure 1**, A). The posterior root attachment lies in the posterior intercondylar fossa between the lateral meniscus and posterior cruciate ligament.[5] In addition to its root attachments, the meniscotibial (coronary) ligament stabilizes the medial meniscus through its attachment from the inferior aspect of the posterior horn to the tibia (**Figure 1**, A).

Dr. Tennent serves as a board member, owner, officer, or committee member of the Society of Military Orthopaedic Surgeons. Dr. Owens or an immediate family member serves as a paid consultant to or is an employee of CONMED Linvatec, Flexion Therapeutics, Mitek, Musculoskeletal Transplant Foundation, and Vericel; has received research or institutional support from Hisogenics; and serves as a board member, owner, officer, or committee member of the American Orthopaedic Society for Sports Medicine. None of the following authors or any immediate family member has received anything of value from or has stock or stock options held in a commercial company or institution related directly or indirectly to the subject of this chapter: Dr. Wiley, Dr. Jayasuriya, and Dr. Twomey-Kozak.

©Copyright 2021 American Academy of Orthopaedic Surgeons

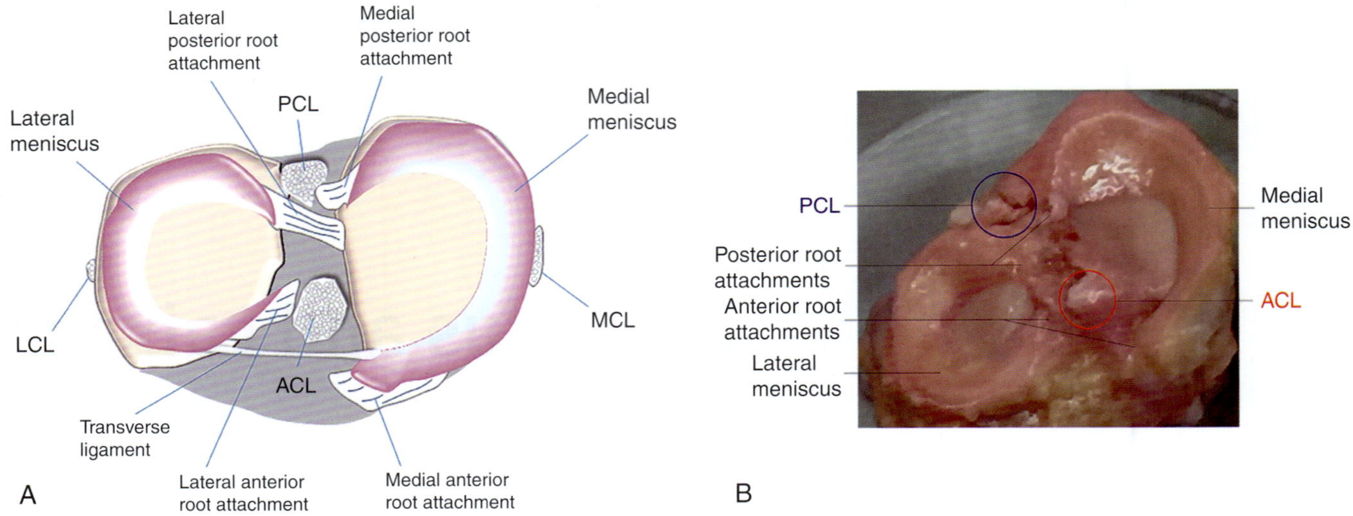

FIGURE 1 Meniscal anatomy. Illustrated diagram (**A**) and photograph diagram (**B**) of medial and lateral menisci and attachments in relation to the cruciate ligaments of the knee. ACL = anterior cruciate ligament, LCL = lateral cruciate ligament, MCL = medial collateral ligament, PCL = posterior cruciate ligament.

Peripherally, the medial meniscus is firmly attached to the deep medial collateral ligament and joint capsule, limiting its mobility.[5]

The lateral meniscus has a more circular C-shape with symmetric sizes of the anterior and posterior horns. The lateral meniscus anterior root attaches anterior to the intercondylar eminence and just lateral to the ACL insertion site on the tibia, whereas the posterior root attaches posterior to the lateral tibial spine just anterior to the medial meniscus posterior root.[3] The popliteomeniscal fascicles extend from the lateral meniscus to the posterior capsule to create the popliteal hiatus. The meniscofemoral ligaments are variably present structures which connect the posterior horn of the lateral meniscus to the medial femoral condyle. These are described by their relationship to the posterior cruciate ligament, with the ligament of Humphrey crossing anterior to the PCL and the ligament of Wrisberg posteriorly. The less continuous attachment of the lateral meniscus to the capsule allows for greater meniscal mobility. Several studies have demonstrated this, including the work of Thompson et al, which reported a mean lateral meniscus excursion of 11.2 mm versus a mean medial meniscus excursion of 5.1 mm occurring from knee extension to flexion.[6] Menisci have three zones that can be discerned based on vasculature and extracellular matrix composition (**Figure 2**). These zones are commonly described as white-white (ww), red-white (rw), and red-red (rr) zones (**Figure 2**).

VASCULAR ANATOMY

The blood supply of the menisci arises from the superior, middle, and inferior (medial and lateral) geniculate arteries as they branch from the popliteal artery. Synovial artery branches supply the anterior and posterior root attachments, whereas synovial and capsular artery branches form a perimeniscal capillary network to supply the peripheral 10% to 30% of the meniscus.[7] From the anterior and posterior horns, endoligamentous vessels branch

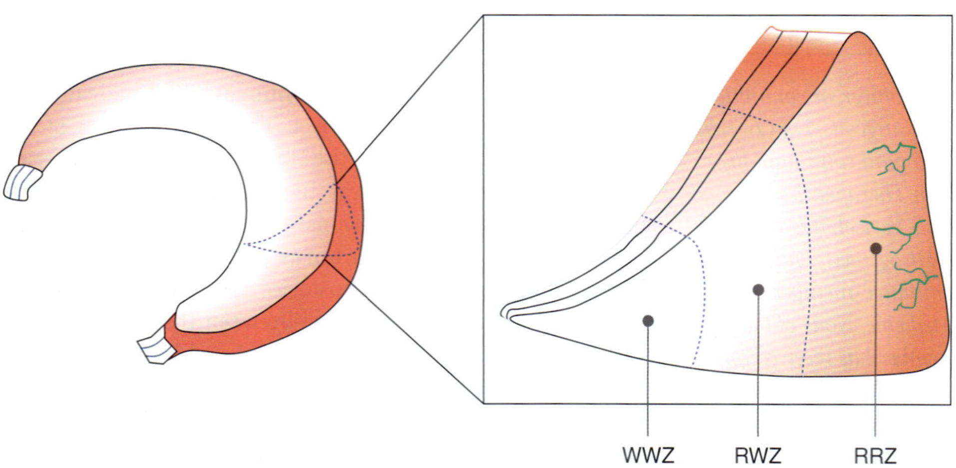

FIGURE 2 Drawing showing the meniscus zones. The inner one-third of the meniscus is avascular and called the white-white zone (WWZ). The middle zone is called the red-white zone (RWZ) because it has limited vasculature. The back one-third is called the red-red zone (RRZ) because it is the most vascularized tissue region that has access to blood supply through vessels arising from the geniculate arteries.

©Copyright 2021 American Academy of Orthopaedic Surgeons

into the substance of the menisci to perform terminal loops and provide direct nutrition over a short distance.[8] The inner one-third of the meniscus is an avascular zone which receives its nutrition from the synovial fluid via loading diffusion.[9]

NEURAL ANATOMY

The posterior articular branch of the tibial nerve innervates the knee along with contributions from the terminal branches of the obturator and femoral nerves. In addition, the recurrent peroneal branch of the common peroneal nerve supplies lateral portion of the capsule. Nerve fibers enter the capsule and peripheral portion of the menisci along a similar path as the blood supply. The highest nerve density lies in the anterior and posterior meniscal horns, whereas the peripheral third of the body has greater innervation than the middle third.[10] Three types of mechanoreceptors have been identified in the human meniscus. Ruffini endings are type 1 mechanoreceptors, which have a low threshold and adapt slowly to pressure and joint deformation. Pacinian corpuscles (type II mechanoreceptors) have a low threshold but adapt quickly to alterations in tissue tension. Golgi tendon organs (type III mechanoreceptors) have a high signal threshold and exist in a greater concentration in the posterior horns, where they play a role in neuromuscular inhibition as the knee reaches terminal flexion.[11]

COMPOSITION AND MICROSTRUCTURE

The human meniscus is a well-organized structure consisting of fibrochondrocytes dispersed among a dense extracellular matrix. As the predominant meniscal cell type, fibrochondrocytes serve to produce and maintain the extracellular matrix. The fibrochondrocytes in the superficial layer of the meniscus appear similar to fibroblasts with their fusiform shape, whereas those in the deeper portion of the meniscus are more ovoid and chondrocyte-like.[12] To assist in their matrix production function, fibrochondrocytes contain abundant endoplasmic reticulum and Golgi complexes, whereas a paucity of mitochondria suggests energy production occurs via anaerobic glycolysis.[13]

Water contained within the extracellular matrix accounts for 65% to 75% of the overall meniscal weight and volume.[3] Composing 75% of the dry weight, collagens are the predominant extracellular matrix component and function to provide tensile strength to the meniscus.[14] Type I collagen comprises the vast majority of this collagen content, with small contributions of collagen types II, III, V, and VI.[13] Random collagen fiber orientation in the most superficial layer of the meniscus provides tensile strength and resistance to shear forces. In the deeper layers, the type I collagen fibers are organized to run circumferentially within the meniscus parallel to its peripheral border. The circumferentially oriented fibers are bound together by interspersed radially oriented tie fibers providing structural support.[3] This organization allows for conversion of vertically oriented compressive forces into circumferential hoop stresses distributed throughout the meniscus.[12]

Matrix proteins other than collagen account for 8% to 13% of the meniscal dry weight.[3] Fibronectin is a matrix protein involved in cellular processes such as cell migration/adhesion and tissue repair, whereas elastin likely contributes to tissue resiliency.[13] Proteoglycans are large negatively charged molecules consisting one or more glycosaminoglycan side chains covalently bonded to a core protein. These hydrophilic molecules exist within the extracellular matrix and contribute to 1% to 2% of the dry weight, with the major type found in the meniscus being aggrecan followed by decorin, biglycan, and fibromodulin.[12] Proteoglycans play an important role in the hydration of meniscal tissue and its viscoelastic ability to resist compressive forces. The meniscal horns and inner 50% of the weight-bearing meniscus contain the highest concentration of glycosaminoglycan side chains.[15] The most common glycosaminoglycans in the adult meniscus include chondroitin-6-sulfate (40%), chondroitin-4-sulfate (10% to 20%), dermatan sulfate (20% to 30%), and keratan sulfate (15%).[14,16]

FUNCTION

Although previously believed to be a vestigial structure of the knee,[17] the meniscus has multiple important biomechanical functions crucial to the normal function of the knee. The menisci increase the contact area and congruity, in turn decreasing contact stresses, across the tibiofemoral joint.[18] Shock absorption, load transmission, stability, nutrition, joint lubrication, and proprioception are vital functions provided by the meniscus.[3]

The load-bearing function of the meniscus occurs as axial weight-bearing forces through the knee are converted to tensile forces along the circumferential collagen fibers of the meniscus.[19] The firm anterior and posterior root attachments allow these hoop stresses to be absorbed without meniscal extrusion.[20] Studies have demonstrated that 50% of the load through the medial compartment and 70% of the lateral compartment load transmission occurs through the menisci.[21] The compressive loads through the posterior horns increase during knee flexion, from 50% in extension to 85% transmission in 90° flexion.[18] Medial meniscectomy reduces the femoral condyle contact area by 50% to 70% and increases contact stress by 100%, whereas total lateral meniscectomy decreases contact area by 40% to 50% with a resultant increase in lateral compartment contact stress by 200% to 300% of normal.[22,23] The normal knee demonstrates a shock absorbing capacity roughly 20% higher than previously meniscectomized knees.[19] The clinical significance of these alterations was highlighted in a study by Pengas et al,[24] which demonstrated a statistically significant increase in osteoarthritis and a 132-fold likelihood of total knee arthroplasty in a cohort of adolescent patients after total meniscectomy at a mean follow-up of 40 years.[24]

The menisci contribute to joint stability as the concave superior meniscal surface increases the congruity between the convex femoral condyles and flat tibial plateau. This stabilizing effect has been best demonstrated in ACL-deficient knees,

©Copyright 2021 American Academy of Orthopaedic Surgeons

where medial meniscectomy has been reported to increase anterior-posterior tibial translation over 50% with the knee at 90° flexion.[25] The posterior horn of the medial meniscus has been shown to be the most essential structure to resisting anterior tibial force in the ACL-deficient knee.[26] The lateral meniscus acts as a secondary stabilizer against rotatory and valgus loads during pivot shift maneuvers in ACL-deficient knees.[27]

The menisci are thought to contribute to the nutrition and lubrication of the knee, although the mechanism for this has not been fully elucidated. Bird and Sweet used scanning electron microscopy to demonstrate a system of microcanals within the meniscus which communicated with the synovium.[28] These canals have been postulated to provide fluid transport for nutrition and joint lubrication. The menisci may reduce frictional forces through compression of synovial fluid into the articular cartilage. As noted previously, mechanoreceptors exist within the anterior and posterior meniscal horns to provide joint proprioception. The rapidly adapting Pacinian corpuscles relay joint motion, whereas the slow-adapting Ruffini endings provide joint position sense.[29]

MENISCAL INJURY AND HEALING RESPONSE

Injuries to the meniscus that occur within the peripheral one-third exist within the vascularized portion of the meniscus (rr zone) and may undergo a healing response. After injury, an initial inflammatory response is quickly followed by formation of a fibrin clot. Undifferentiated mesenchymal stem cells migrate to the zone of injury from the vasculature. A new matrix is produced and healing occurs via the formation of fibrous scar tissue.[30] The inflammatory response after meniscal injury has been investigated in multiple studies, with particular interest on its contribution to future osteoarthritis. In a rabbit model, Becker et al demonstrated increased expression of vascular endothelial growth factor (VEGF) for angiogenesis after meniscal injury.[31] Brophy et al found an increased catabolic response to meniscal injury, with elevation of several osteoarthritis-related markers including proinflammatory cytokine interleukin 1 beta (IL-1β) and several matrix metalloproteinases occurring to a greater extent in patients younger than 40 years.[32] Carter et al demonstrated increased matrix metalloproteinase activity in synovial fluid reflective of greater cartilage strain after meniscal injury.[33]

With regard to the time line for meniscal healing, a dog model previously demonstrated meniscal repair tissue attaining 80% of original strength at 12 weeks.[34] Meniscal injuries within the inner one-third, or ww zone, and within the central one-third, or rw zone, have limited capacity for healing given the avascularity of the tissue. Given this poor healing response, a multitude of research has been directed toward biologic adjuvants for meniscal repair. The earliest adjuvant was synovial abrasion with a meniscal rasp to increase vascular response, as well as trephination of the peripheral meniscus and capsule.[30] Because of the improved meniscal healing rates in the setting of concomitant ACL reconstruction, bone marrow stimulation techniques have been used to release bone marrow–derived mesenchymal cells in the setting of meniscal repair.[35] The direct application of platelet-rich plasma and/or pluripotent stem cells has been investigated in animal and human studies with variable results.[36-38] Several stem/progenitor cell sources are actively being investigated for their therapeutic healing effects that have been observed in animal models and tissue explant models of meniscus injury repair (**Table 1**). Cell sources include mesenchymal progenitor/stem cells from adipose, synovium, cartilage, and bone marrow. Cell-based therapies are promising and they are being used both by themselves and in combination with growth factors and scaffolds in preclinical settings to optimize efficacy.

LABRUM

ANATOMY

Development

During normal fetal development, the superior glenoid labrum begins to coalesce with the biceps tendon by approximately 9 weeks of gestation. Further anterior and posterior consolidations appear and transition to a highly vascular, primitive fibrocartilaginous structure with distinct transitions from glenoid to labrum from approximately 12 to 20 weeks.[39,40] However, mature labral tissue is not present until full term with a gradual transition to mature fibrocartilage over the first several years of life.[40,41] Throughout life, an increased proportion of elastin and decreased vascularity has been found to correlate with increasing age.[41]

Structure

The glenoid labrum is heavily composed of type II collagen and aggrecan, which has been suggested to help provide joint lubrication and fluid motion.[42,43] However, following injury, animal studies have shown increased levels of IL-1β, transforming growth factor beta 1, and matrix metalloproteins 3 and 13 (MMP3 and MMP13) inflammatory cytokines as well as increased proportions of type III collagen consistent with fibrocartilaginous scar formation.[44]

The microstructure of the labrum can be divided into three layers. The superficial layer is composed of a thin, woven, meshlike matrix that has been proposed to absorb compressive forces across the labrum while assisting with joint lubrication and proteoglycan storage.[43] The second intermediate layer consists of multidirectional fibrillar bundles arranged parallel to the glenoid rim and acts to resist various stresses and force vectors.[43] The deepest layer of the labrum is composed primarily of a dense core of circumferential fibers that likely helps disperse hoop stresses and tensile forces that result from glenohumeral joint compression and humeral head translation.[43] Last, the labral attachment to bone consists of cellular region of vertical and oblique interwoven collagen and

©Copyright 2021 American Academy of Orthopaedic Surgeons

TABLE 1 Current Preclinical Paradigms of Cell-Based Meniscus Repair

Cell Source (Number Used)	Animal Model (Setting)	Meniscus Injury Model	Biomaterial Used	Treatment Group	Control Group	Time Postoperative	Outcomes	Reference
Allogeneic rabbit ADSCs (0.1×10^6)	Rabbit (in vivo)	Longitudinal lesion in avascular zone	Matrigel	Suture + ADSCs suspended in Matrigel	Suture + Matrigel only	12 wk	Improved healing rate in avascular zone for acute lesions that received suture + ADSCs	Ruiz-Iban et al[37]
Autologous sheep ADSCs (20×10^6)	Sheep (in vivo)	Medial meniscectomy (and ACL resection)	N/A	Autologous chongrogenically induced ADSCs	Culture medium	6 wk	Regenerated de novo cartilage underlying meniscus	Ude et al[66]
Autologous human ADSCs (16×10^6)	Human (in vivo)	Grade II meniscal tear	Hyaluronic acid	Autologous hADSCs + PRP and hyaluronic acid injections	PRP + hyaluronic acid injections	3 mo	Reduced pain and minimal regeneration of meniscus tissue	Pak et al[67]
Human ADSCs	Bovine (explant in vitro)	Radial tear on cylindrical explant punch biopsy from inner avascular region of meniscus	Photo–cross-linked hydrogel	Hydrogel loaded with ADSCs + TGF-β3	TGF-β3 only	4 and 8 wk	Increased matrix-sulfated proteoglycan deposition and some healing of meniscus	Sasaki et al[68]
Allogeneic rabbit ADSCs	Rabbit (in vivo)	Complete meniscectomy of medial meniscus	PVA/Ch scaffold	PVA/Ch scaffold seeded with ADSCs	Scaffold seeded with articular chondrocytes OR Cell-free scaffold	7 mo	Minor meniscus regeneration for articular chondrocyte group (ADSCs had no significant contribution in healing process and lower Col II, aggrecan and Col 1)	Moradi et al[69]
Allogeneic SDSCs (50×10^6)	Pig (in vivo)	Partial meniscectomy of medial menisci	N/A	Intra-articular injection of SDSCs at 0.2 and 4 wk	Intra-articular injection of PBS	2, 4, 8, 12, and 16 wk	Resected meniscus regeneration enhanced in SDSC group based on histology and MRI + better articular cartilage protection	Hatsushika et al[70]

(Continued)

©Copyright 2021 American Academy of Orthopaedic Surgeons

TABLE 1 Current Preclinical Paradigms of Cell-Based Meniscus Repair (Continued)

Cell Source (Number Used)	Animal Model (Setting)	Meniscus Injury Model	Biomaterial Used	Treatment Group	Control Group	Time Postoperative	Outcomes	Reference
SDSCs (0.25×10^6)	Rat (in vivo)	Partial meniscectomy	N/A	SDSC aggregate	Intra-articular injection of 5×10^6 cell suspension in PBS AND 0.25×10^5 cell suspension in PBS	12 wk	Larger meniscal area and better histological scores for aggregate groups	Katagiri et al[71]
Allogeneic SDSCs (0.2×10^6 cells cultured for 3 wk to make 3D construct)	Pig (in vivo)	4 mm cylindrical defect in medial meniscus	N/A	Cultured SDSC 3D cell/matrix tissue construct (scaffold-free)	No treatment	6 mo	SDSC 3D construct group filled meniscal defect and showed improved tissue integration compared with control	Moriguchi et al[72]
Allogeneic SDSCs (2×10^6)	Rabbit (in vivo)	1.5 mm cylindrical defect in avascular zone of medial meniscus	N/A	Allogeneic SDSCs suspended in PBS	PBS only	4, 12, and 24 wk	Mixed results: Quantity of regenerated tissue significant ONLY at 4 and 12 wk. Quality of repair scores significant at 12 and 24 wk. Cells expressed type I and type II collagen at 24 wk	Horie et al[36]
Allogeneic SDSCs	Rabbit (in vivo)	Full-thickness longitudinal incision on medial meniscus	Fibrin glue/gel	Fibrin gel loaded with SDSCs + CTGF and TGF-β3	Fibrin alone OR Fibrin + CTGF	6 wk	Fibrocartilaginous tissue integration demonstrated by H&E and Saf-O fast green stain; tensile testing revealed enhanced biomechanical properties	Tarafder et al[73]

©Copyright 2021 American Academy of Orthopaedic Surgeons

Autologous BM-MSCs (6×10^6)	Sheep (in vivo)	Unilateral medial meniscectomy	Hyaff-11 (HA) scaffold construct	Autologous BM-MSCs from iliac crest in Hyaff-11 (HA) construct	BMC in HA construct	12 wk	BMC in HA construct allowed for better tissue regeneration than BM-MSCs and this group seemed to inhibit OA progression with a reduction in cartilage and meniscus inflammation. BUT subchondral bone thickness was decreased in both BM-MSC and MSC groups	Desando et al[74]
Autologous BM-MSCs (0.1×10^6)	Rabbit (in vivo)	4 mm longitudinal tear in avascular zone of medial meniscus	Hyaluronan/collagen matrix scaffold	Implantation of autologous BM-MSCs cultured and embedded in hyaluronan/collagen matrix	Suture only, cell-free matrix construct, or PRP	6 and 12 wk	BM-MSC matrix constructs initiated fibrocartilage-like repair tissue and demonstrated better integration and biomechanical properties than any control group	Zelllner et al[75]
Autologous BM-MSCs ($1\text{-}2 \times 10^6$)	Pig (in vivo)	Radial tear in the avascular zone of the meniscus	Fibrin glue	Autologous BM-MSCs + sutures and fibrin glue	No treatment OR Sutures and fibrin glue alone	8 wk	No complete healing in the no treatment group or with sutures and fibrin glue alone; complete healing was seen in three animals and incomplete healing was seen in five of the animals in the BM-MSC-treated group	Dutton et al[76]
Autologous BM-MSCs (30×10^6 cells/mL)	Goat (in vivo)	Full-thickness meniscal defect in white-white area of meniscus	Calcium alginate gel	BM-MSCs transfected with hIGF-1 + calcium alginate gel	Nontransfected BM-MSCs OR Calcium alginate gel alone OR No treatment	4, 8, and 16 wk	Defects were filled with fibrocartilage-like tissue composed of cells embedded in matrix spaces of meniscal fibers with enhanced proteoglycan levels in hIGF-1-overexpressed BM-MSCs	Zhang et al[77]

(Continued)

©Copyright 2021 American Academy of Orthopaedic Surgeons

TABLE 1 Current Preclinical Paradigms of Cell-Based Meniscus Repair (Continued)

Cell Source (Number Used)	Animal Model (Setting)	Meniscus Injury Model	Biomaterial Used	Treatment Group	Control Group	Time Postoperative	Outcomes	Reference
Human BM-MSCs (30 × 10 cells/mL)	Rat (in vivo)	Radial cut of the medial meniscus (2 × 2 mm excision)	Decellularized ECM hydrogel	Human BM-MSCs encapsulated in decellularized ECM hydrogel	PBS	8 wk	Significant tissue regeneration in BM-MSC group with higher GAG, type I and type II collagen than control group; some tissue regeneration in control animals	Yuan et al[78]
Autologous BM-MSCs	Rabbit (in vivo)	Total meniscectomy	PCL scaffold	BM-MSC-seeded PCL scaffold meniscus replacement	Cell-free scaffold, Sham operation and total meniscectomy alone	12 and 24 wk	BM-MSC-seeded PCL scaffold group had a better gross meniscus appearance with higher expression of type I, II, and III collagen and proteoglycan production found in native fibrochondrocytes + less cartilage degradation than any control group + better tensile and compressive properties in cell-seeded implant	Zhang et al[79]
Autologous BM-MSCs	Rabbit (in vivo)	Partial meniscectomy of white-red zone	Actifit scaffold	Autologous BM-MSCs loaded in a polyurethane scaffold (Actifit) and sutured into the defect	Polyurethane scaffold alone (Actifit) (No cells)	6 and 12 wk	Both cell-free and BM-MSC-loaded scaffolds led to well-integrated and stable meniscus-like repair tissue with dense vascularization; accelerated healing was achieved by the BM-MSC-loaded scaffold	Koch et al[80]
Human-derived CPCs (0.1×10^6)	Rat (ex vivo)	Radial tear in inner anterior horn	N/A	CPC line 3 + SDF-1 pretreatment OR Primary CPCs + SDF-1 pretreatment	BM-MSCs OR No cell treatment	3, 5, 10, 17, and 20 d	CPCs promoted meniscal fibrochondrocyte proliferation and native tissue integration of torn meniscal tissue; SDF-1/CXCR4 axis is required to successfully fill meniscus tissue tears	Jayasuriya et al[81]

ACL = anterior cruciate ligament, ADSC = adipose-derived stem cell, BM-MSC = bone marrow mesenchymal stem cell, BMC = bone marrow concentrate, Col = collagen, CPC = chondroprogenitor cell, CTGF = connective tissue growth factor, CXCR4 = chemokine receptor type 4, ECM = extracellular matrix, GAG = glycosaminoglycan, HA = hyaluronic acid, H&E = hematoxylin and eosin, hIGF-1 = human insulin-like growth factor, MSC = mesenchymal stem cell, OA = osteoarthritis, PBS = phosphate buffered saline, PCL = polycaprolactone, PRP = platelet-rich plasma, PVA/Ch = polyvinyl alcohol/chitosan, Saf-O = Safranin O, SDF-1 = stromal cell-derived factor 1, SDSC = synovium-derived stem cell, 3D = three dimensional, TGF-β3 = transforming growth factor beta 3

©Copyright 2021 American Academy of Orthopaedic Surgeons

fibers that insert into the superficial bone and hyaline cartilage through Sharpey fibers that function to resist multidirectional stresses.[43]

The capsulolabral soft-tissue footprint on the glenoid articular surface and neck is most prominent in the anterior/inferior region of the glenoid and ranges between 8.4 and 9.4 mm in width.[45,46] Anatomic studies have shown that double-row Bankart repairs recreate significantly more (85.9% vs 42.3%) of this native glenoid labral attachment.[46] However, biomechanical and clinical studies have not yet shown the clinical superiority of double-row labral repairs compared with the more commonly performed single row repairs.[47]

Underlying the capsulolabral footprint, the labral insertion on the glenoid has a relatively avascular 7-mm-wide calcified fibrocartilaginous footprint that allows for direct attachment of the soft tissue to the glenoid.[48] This calcified fibrocartilage is relatively avascular compared with the adjacent glenoid bone. Furthermore, the labrum overlies the glenoid articular surface between 2.5 and 4.6 mm.[48,49] Consequently, appropriate glenoid rim débridement and anchor placement on the peripheral 2 to 3 mm of the glenoid face itself may allow for a more anatomic reconstruction when performing a single-row Bankart repair for glenohumeral instability and should routinely be performed to allow for optimal healing potential.

This fibrocartilaginous footprint has also been anatomic justification for double-row labral repair. Biomechanical studies looking at the native footprint have shown a more anatomic restoration of the native labral footprint on the glenoid, an increased ultimate load to failure, and less total displacement of the osseous fragment in a bony Bankart when compared with the standard single-row labral repair.[50] However, clinical studies have not yet shown any relevant effect on clinical or functional patient outcomes.[50]

Vascular Supply

The labrum has a high propensity to heal because of its robust vascular supply. The superior and anterosuperior labrum is supplied from branches of the ascending glenoid artery, suprascapular artery, circumflex scapular artery, and muscular branches of the subscapularis. The anterior-inferior Bankart region is supplied from circumflex scapular artery, the posterior circumflex humeral artery, the circumflex scapular artery, and branches from the muscular branches of both the triceps and subscapularis. Last, the posterior labrum is supplied from branches of the suprascapular artery and muscular branches from the teres minor and infraspinatus.[51] The importance of this blood supply can partially account for the excellent outcomes of properly performed labral surgery with appropriate osseous preparation.

Neural Anatomy

The glenoid labrum contains both free sensory nerve fibers consistent with the pain response associated with labral pathology and encapsulated nerve fibers that likely play a role in the glenohumeral proprioception.[52] The most common sensory nerve endings in the labrum are Ruffini corpuscles, which are slow adapting and responsive to prolonged stimuli such as stretching and compression.[53] These nerve endings are common to those seen in the knee and resemble those seen in the meniscus and ACL. The labrum also contains fewer type 2 mechanoreceptors, which are fast adapting and responsive at the ends of motion, that are primarily located superficially at the glenolabral junction.[53]

MECHANICS

The glenoid labrum has several functions with the primary goal of providing a static constraint to the glenohumeral joint. The macroscopic structure of the labrum allows it to reduce humeral head translation on the glenoid by up to 20% when compared with those shoulders where labral resection was performed by providing a static block to motion with humeral head compression.[54,55] The labrum partially accomplishes this role by increasing the relative depth of the native glenoid in both the anterior-posterior and superior-inferior dimensions, thereby allowing a more stable structural constraint than the glenoid in isolation.[54,55]

The labrum also improves stability by increasing the total contact area of the glenohumeral joint. This allows for increased glenohumeral stability by increasing the dynamic stable range of motion. The labrum accomplishes this by increasing the surface area by which the glenoid articulates with the humeral head despite their different radii of curvature.[56] This ultimately allows for an increased functional range of motion.

Similarly, analogous to the knee meniscus, the labrum helps to disperse contact pressures across the glenohumeral joint by increasing the total surface area by which the glenoid articulates with the humeral head.[55,56] This function is evident in its microscopic structure that effectively dissipates hoop stresses as well as by studies that have shown that an incompetent labrum leads to increased glenoid contact pressures and joint overloading.[43,57] Furthermore, these pressures have been shown to decrease to their baseline, even in cases of glenoid bone loss less than 20%, following labral repair.[57]

The labrum also helps to increase glenohumeral stability by creating a negative intra-articular pressure seal that prevents glenohumeral dissociation during traction and distraction events.[58] The effect of this is most apparent following disruption of the labral seal where increased humeral translation in all directions can be seen.[58,59]

HEALING OF LABRAL INJURY

The healing potential of the labrum is directly related to its vascular blood supply at the glenolabral junction. This vascularity has been shown to decrease with increasing age and may partially account for the higher failure rates of superior labral repairs in patients older than 40 years.[60] Consequently, the importance of judicious soft tissue and bony preparation

©Copyright 2021 American Academy of Orthopaedic Surgeons

at the time of repair cannot be understated, especially in older patients. Although suggestive of playing a role in the early failure of superior labral repairs and open glenoid augmentation procedures, smoking has not yet been definitively shown to have a deleterious effect on isolated labral repairs in the absence of concomitant intra-articular pathology.[61] Following labral injury, and subsequent repair, a healing inflammatory cascade consisting of IL-1β, transforming growth factor beta 1, MMP3, and MMP13 has been seen in animal studies.[44] Consequently, some authors have suggested that the use of cyclooxygenase inhibitors may inhibit the healing response at the capsulolabral junction. Although animal studies have shown a possible relationship between decreased labral healing rates and NSAID use, clinical studies have not shown any difference in failure rates or functional outcomes between those patients receiving NSAIDs and those who did not.[62,63]

The time to labral healing has not been fully investigated and is limited to animal models that suggest that the labrum is fully healed in as few as 4 weeks.[64] However, these models are not likely fully translatable because of the more rapid healing potential of these animals when compared with humans; consequently, many surgeons primarily rely on temporal healing algorithms that also incorporates the attainment of specific range of motion and functional milestones.[65]

SUMMARY

The meniscus is a semicircular fibrocartilaginous structure with a dry weight composed predominantly of type 1 collagen. Collagen organization into circumferential hoop and radial tie fibers, along with high water content due to glycoproteins, allow the meniscus to perform its primary function of shock absorption and load transmission through the knee. The meniscus also acts as a secondary knee stabilizer by increasing tibiofemoral congruency. The peripheral third of the meniscus contains the most robust vascular supply and innervation, which is clinically relevant when considering treatment options following meniscal injury.

The glenoid labrum is a fibrocartilaginous circumferential ring, contributing to glenohumeral stability by increasing the glenoid depth and concavity. Composed primarily of type 2 collagen and aggrecan, the microstructure of the labrum consists of three layers: a superficial woven layer, an intermediate layer of multidirectional fibrillar collagen, and a deep dense core of circumferential fibers. The innervation of the labrum consists of both free nerve endings for pain as well as Ruffini corpuscles for glenohumeral proprioception. The labrum has a robust blood supply from multiple vessels, resulting in an excellent healing response after labral repair.

REFERENCES

1. Gardner E, O'Rahilly R: The early development of the knee joint in staged human embryos. *J Anat* 1968;102:289-299.
2. Clark CR, Ogden JA: Development of the menisci of the human knee joint. *J Bone Joint Surg Am* 1983;65:530.
3. Fox AJS, Bedi A, Rodeo SA: The basic science of human knee menisci: Structure, composition, and function. *Sports Health* 2012;4(4):340-351.
4. Smigielski R, Becker R, Zdanowicz U, Ciszek B: Medial meniscus anatomy: From basic science to treatment. *Knee Surg Sports Traumatol Arthrosc* 2015;23(1):8-14.
5. Johnson DL, Swenson TM, Livesay GA, Aizawa H, Fu FH, Harner CD: Insertion-site anatomy of the human menisci: Gross, arthroscopic, and topographical anatomy as a basis for meniscal transplantation. *Arthroscopy* 1995;11:386-394.
6. Thompson WO, Thaete FL, Fu FH, Dye SF: Tibial meniscal dynamics using three-dimensional reconstruction of magnetic resonance imaging. *Am J Sports Med* 1991;19:210-216.
7. Arnoczky SP, Warren RF: Microvasculature of the human meniscus. *Am J Sports Med* 1982;10:90-95.
8. Danzig L, Resnik D, Gonsalves M, Akeson WH: Blood supply to the normal and abnormal meniscus of the human knee. *Clin Orthop Relat Res* 1983;172:271-276.
9. Greis PE, Bardana DD, Holmstrom MC, Burks RT: Meniscal injury I: Basic science and evaluation. *J Am Acad Orthop Surg* 2002;10:168-176.
10. Kennedy JC, Alexander IJ, Hayes KC: Nerve supply of the human knee and its functional importance. *Am J Sports Med* 1982;10:329-335.
11. Zimny ML, Albright DJ, Dabezies E: Mechanoreceptors in the human medial meniscus. *Acta Anat* 1988;133:35-40.
12. Makris EA, Hadidi P, Athanasiou KA: The knee meniscus: Structure-function, pathophysiology, current repair techniques, and prospects for regeneration. *Biomaterials* 2011;32(30):7411-7431.
13. McDevitt CA, Webber RJ: Ultrastructure and biochemistry of meniscal cartilage. *Clin Orthop Relat Res* 1990;252:8-18.
14. Herwig J, Egner E, Buddecke E: Chemical changes of human knee joint menisci in various stages of degeneration. *Ann Rheum Dis* 1984;43:635-640.
15. Ghosh P, Taylor TKF: The knee joint meniscus: A fibrocartilage of some distinction. *Clin Orthop Relat Res* 1987;224:52-63.
16. Habuchi H, Yamagata T, Iwata H, Suzuki S: The occurrence of a wide variety of dermatan sulfate-chondroitin sulfate copolymers in fibrous cartilage. *J Biol Chem* 1973;248:6019-6028.
17. Sutton JB: *Ligaments: Their Nature and Morphology*, ed 2. London, HK Lewis, 1897.
18. Walker PS, Erkman MJ: The role of the meniscus in force transmission across the knee. *Clin Orthop Relat Res* 1975;109:184-192.
19. Voloshin AS, Wosk J: Shock absorption of meniscectomized and painful knees: A comparative in vivo study. *J Biomed Eng* 1983;5:157-161.
20. Krause WR, Pope MH, Johnson RJ, Wilder DG: Mechanical changes in the knee after meniscectomy. *J Bone Joint Surg Am* 1976;58:599-604.
21. Seedhom BB, Hargreaves DJ: Transmission of the load in the knee joint with special reference to the role in the menisci: Part II. Experimental results, discussion and conclusion. *Eng Med* 1979;8:220-228.
22. Fukubayashi T, Kurosawa H: The contact area and pressure distribution pattern of the knee: A study of normal and osteoarthritic knee joints. *Acta Orthop Scand* 1980;51:871-879.
23. Kettelkamp DB, Jacobs AW: Tibiofemoral contact area: Determination and implications. *J Bone Joint Surg Am* 1972;54:349-356.
24. Pengas IP, Assiotis A, Nash W, Hatcher J, Banks J, McNicholas MJ: Total meniscectomy in adolescents: A 40-year follow-up. *J Bone Joint Surg Br* 2012;94-B:1649-1654.
25. Markolf KL, Mensch JS, Amstutz HC: Stiffness and laxity of the knee: The contributions of the supporting structures. *J Bone Joint Surg Am* 1976;58:583-597.

 ©Copyright 2021 American Academy of Orthopaedic Surgeons

26. Shoemaker SC, Markolf KL: The role of the meniscus in the anterior-posterior stability of the loaded anterior cruciate-deficient knee: Effects of partial versus total excision. *J Bone Joint Surg Am* 1986;68(1):71-79.

27. Musahl V, Citak M, O'Loughlin PF, Choi D, Bedi A, Pearle AD: The effect of medial versus lateral meniscectomy on the stability of the anterior cruciate ligament-deficient knee. *Am J Sports Med* 2010;38(8):1591-1597.

28. Bird MDT, Sweet MBE: A system of canals in semilunar menisci. *Ann Rheum Dis* 1987;46:670-673.

29. Reider B, Arcand MA, Diehl LH, et al: Proprioception of the knee before and after anterior cruciate ligament reconstruction. *Arthroscopy* 2003;19(1):2-12.

30. Mayer SW, Bernard JA, Rodeo SA: Chapter 20: Meniscal injuries, in Miller MD, ed: *Orthopedic Knowledge Update: Sports Medicine*, ed 5. Rosemont, AAOS, 2016, pp 251-259.

31. Becker R, Pufe T, Kulow S, et al: Expression of vascular endothelial growth factor during healing of the meniscus in a rabbit model. *J Bone Joint Surg Br* 2004;86(7):1082-1087.

32. Brophy RH, Rai MF, Zhang Z, Torgomyan A, Sandell LJ: Molecular analysis of age and sex related chain expression and meniscal tears with and without a concomitant anterior cruciate ligament tear. *J Bone Joint Surg Am* 2012;94(5):385-393.

33. Carter TE, Taylor KA, Spritzer CE, et al: In vivo cartilage strain increases following medial meniscal tear and correlates with synovial fluid matrix metalloproteinase activity. *J Biomech* 2015;48(8):1461-1468.

34. Kawai Y, Fukubayashi T, Nishino J: Meniscal suture. An experimental study in the dog. *Clin Orthop Relat Res* 1989;243:286-292.

35. Freedman KB, Nho SJ, Cole BJ: Marrow stimulating technique to augment meniscal repair. *Arthroscopy* 2003;19(7):794-798.

36. Horie M, Driscoll MD, Sampson HW, et al: Implantation of allogenic synovial stem cells promotes meniscal regeneration in a rabbit meniscal defect model. *J Bone Joint Surg Am* 2012;94(8):701-712.

37. Ruiz-Iban MA, Diaz-Heredia J, Garcia-Gomez I, Gonzalez-Lizan F, Elias-Martin E, Abraira V: The effect of the addition of adipose derived mesenchymal stem cells to a meniscal repair in the avascular zone: An experimental study in rabbits. *Arthroscopy* 2011;27(12):1688-1696.

38. Griffin JW, Hadeed MM, Werner BC, Diduch DR, Carson EW, Miller MD: Platelet-rich plasma in meniscal repair: Does augmentation improve surgical outcomes? *Clin Orthop Relat Res* 2015;473(5):1665-1672.

39. Aboul-Mahasen LM, Sadek SA: Developmental morphological and histological studies on structures of the human fetal shoulder joint. *Cells Tissues Organs* 2002;170:1-20.

40. Fealy S, Rodeo SA, Dicarlo EF, O'Brien SJ: The developmental anatomy of the neonatal glenohumeral joint. *J Shoulder Elbow Surg* 2000;9:217-222.

41. Prodromos CC, Ferry JA, Schiller AL, Zarins B: Histological studies of the glenoid labrum from fetal life to old age. *J Bone Joint Surg Am* 1990;72:1344-1348.

42. Ockert B, Braunstein V, Sprecher CM, Shinohara Y, Milz S: Fibrocartilage in various regions of the human glenoid labrum. An immunohistochemical study on human cadavers. *Knee Surg Sports Traumatol Arthrosc* 2012;20:1036-1041.

43. Hill AM, Hoerning EJ, Brook K, et al: Collagenous microstructure of the glenoid labrum and biceps anchor. *J Anat* 2008;212:853-862.

44. Mulcahey MK, Marshall M, Gallacher SE, Kaback LA, Blaine TA: Factors expressed in an animal model of anteroinferior glenohumeral instability. *Orthop J Sports Med* 2015;3:2325967115599733.

45. Itoigawa Y, Itoi E, Sakoma Y, Yamamoto N, Sano H, Kaneko K: Attachment of the anteroinferior glenohumeral ligament-labrum complex to the glenoid: An anatomic study. *Arthroscopy* 2012;28:1628-1633.

46. Ahmad CS, Galano GJ, Vorys GC, Covey AS, Gardner TR, Levine WN: Evaluation of glenoid capsulolabral complex insertional anatomy and restoration with single- and double-row capsulolabral repairs. *J Shoulder Elbow Surg* 2009;18:948-954.

47. Judson CH, Voss A, Obopilwe E, Dyrna F, Arciero RA, Shea KP: An anatomic and biomechanical comparison of Bankart repair configurations. *Am J Sports Med* 2017;45:3004-3009.

48. Karns MR, Epperson RT, Baran S, Nielsen MB, Taylor NB, Burks RT: Revisiting the anterior glenoid: An analysis of the calcified cartilage layer, capsulolabral complex, and glenoid bone density. *Arthroscopy* 2018;34:2309-2318.

49. Yoshida M, Goto H, Nozaki M, et al: Quantitative analysis of attachment of the labrum to the glenoid fossa: A cadaveric study. *J Orthop Sci* 2015;20:823-829.

50. Yousif MJ, Bicos J: Biomechanical comparison of single- versus double-row capsulolabral repair for shoulder instability: A review. *Orthop J Sports Med* 2017;5:2325967117742355.

51. Alashkham A, Alraddadi A, Felts P, Soames R: Blood supply and vascularity of the glenoid labrum: Its clinical implications. *J Orthop Surg* 2017;25:2309499017731632.

52. Alashkham A, Alraddadi A, Felts P, Soames R: Histology, vascularity and innervation of the glenoid labrum. *J Orthop Surg* 2018;26:2309499018770900.

53. Witherspoon JW, Smirnova IV, McIff TE: Neuroanatomical distribution of mechanoreceptors in the human cadaveric shoulder capsule and labrum. *J Anat* 2014;225:337-345.

54. Lippitt SB, Vanderhooft JE, Harris SL, Sidles JA, Harryman DT II, Matsen FA III: Glenohumeral stability from concavity-compression: A quantitative analysis. *J Shoulder Elb Surg* 1993;2:27-35.

55. Levine WN, Flatow EL: The pathophysiology of shoulder instability. *Am J Sports Med* 2000;28:910-917.

56. Lippitt S, Matsen F: Mechanisms of glenohumeral joint stability. *Clin Orthop Relat Res* 1993:20-28.

57. Yamamoto A, Massimini DF, DiStefano J, Higgins LD: Glenohumeral contact pressure with simulated anterior labral and osseous defects in cadaveric shoulders before and after soft tissue repair. *Am J Sports Med* 2014;42:1947-1954.

58. Habermeyer P, Schuller U, Wiedemann E: The intra-articular pressure of the shoulder: An experimental study on the role of the glenoid labrum in stabilizing the joint. *Arthrosc J Arthrosc Relat Surg* 1992;8:166-172.

59. Alexander S, Southgate DF, Bull AM, Wallace AL: The role of negative intraarticular pressure and the long head of biceps tendon on passive stability of the glenohumeral joint. *J Shoulder Elb Surg* 2013;22:94-101.

60. Erickson J, Lavery K, Monica J, Gatt C, Dhawan A: Surgical treatment of symptomatic superior labrum anterior-posterior tears in patients older than 40 years: A systematic review. *Am J Sports Med* 2014;43:1274-1282.

61. Bokshan SL, DeFroda SF, Owens BD: Comparison of 30-day morbidity and mortality after arthroscopic Bankart, open Bankart, and latarjet-bristow procedures: A review of 2864 cases. *Orthop J Sports Med* 2017;5:2325967117713163.

62. Blomquist J, Solheim E, Liavaag S, Baste V, Havelin LI: Do nonsteroidal anti-inflammatory drugs affect the outcome of arthroscopic Bankart repair? *Scand J Med Sci Sport* 2014;24:e510-514.

63. Packer JD, Varthi AG, Zhu DS, et al: Ibuprofen impairs capsulolabral healing in a rat model of anterior glenohumeral instability. *J Shoulder Elbow Surg* 2018;27:315-324.

64. Abe H, Itoi E, Yamamoto N, et al: Healing processes of the glenoid labral lesion in a rabbit model of shoulder dislocation. *Tohoku J Exp Med* 2012;228:103-108.

65. Ciccotti MC, Syed U, Hoffman R, Abboud JA, Ciccotti MG, Freedman KB: Return to play criteria following surgical stabilization for traumatic anterior shoulder instability: A systematic review. *Arthrosc J Arthrosc Relat Surg* 2018;34:903-913.

66. Ude CC, Sulaiman SB, Min-Hwei N, et al: Cartilage regeneration by chondrogenic induced adult stem cells in osteoarthritic sheep model. *PLoS One* 2014;9:e98770.

67. Pak J, Lee JH, Lee SH: Regenerative repair of damaged meniscus with autologous adipose tissue-derived stem cells. *Biomed Res Int* 2014;2014:436029.

68. Sasaki H, Rothrauff BB, Alexander PG, et al: In vitro repair of meniscal radial tear with hydrogels seeded with adipose stem cells and TGF-β3. *Am J Sports Med* 2018;46:2402-2413.

©Copyright 2021 American Academy of Orthopaedic Surgeons

69. Moradi L, Vasei M, Dehghan MM, Majidi M, Farzad Mohajeri S, Bonakdar S: Regeneration of meniscus tissue using adipose mesenchymal stem cells-chondrocytes co-culture on a hybrid scaffold: In vivo study. *Biomaterials* 2017;126:18-30.
70. Hatsushika D, Muneta T, Nakamura T, et al: Repetitive allogeneic intraarticular injections of synovial mesenchymal stem cells promote meniscus regeneration in a porcine massive meniscus defect model. *Osteoarthr Cartilage* 2014;22:941-50028.
71. Katagiri H, Muneta T, Tsuji K, et al: Transplantation of aggregates of synovial mesenchymal stem cells regenerates meniscus more effectively in a rat massive meniscal defect. *Biochem Biophys Res Commun* 2013;435:603-609.
72. Moriguchi Y, Tateishi K, Ando W, et al: Repair of meniscal lesions using a scaffold-free tissue-engineered construct derived from allogenic synovial MSCs in a miniature swine model. *Biomaterials* 2013;34:2185-2193
73. Tarafder S, Gulko J, Sim KH, Yang J, Cook JL, Lee CH: Engineered healing of avascular meniscus tears by stem cell recruitment. *Sci Rep* 2018;8:8150.
74. Desando G, Giavaresi G, Cavallo C, et al: Autologous bone marrow concentrate in a sheep model of osteoarthritis: New perspectives for cartilage and meniscus repair. *Tissue Eng Part C Methods* 2016;22:608-619.
75. Zellner J, Hierl K, Mueller M, et al: Stem cell-based tissue-engineering for treatment of meniscal tears in the avascular zone. *J Biomed Mater Res B Appl Biomater* 2013;101:1133-1142.
76. Dutton AQ, Choong PF, Goh JC-H, Lee EH, Hui JHP: Enhancement of meniscal repair in the avascular zone using mesenchymal stem cells in a porcine model. *J Bone Joint Surg Br* 2010;92:169-175.
77. Zhang H, Leng P, Zhang J: Enhanced meniscal repair by overexpression of hIGF-1 in a full-thickness model. *Clin Orthop Relat Res* 2009;467:3165-3174.
78. Yuan X, Wei Y, Villasante A, et al: Stem cell delivery in tissue-specific hydrogel enabled meniscal repair in an orthotopic rat model. *Biomaterials* 2017;132:59-71.
79. Zhang ZZ, Wang SJ, Zhang JY, et al: 3D-Printed poly(∈-caprolactone) scaffold augmented with mesenchymal stem cells for total meniscal substitution: A 12- and 24-week animal study in a rabbit model. *Am J Sports Med* 2017;45:1497-1511.
80. Koch M, Achatz FP, Lang S, et al: Tissue engineering of large full-size meniscus defects by a polyurethane scaffold: Accelerated regeneration by mesenchymal stromal cells. *Stem Cell Int* 2018;2018:8207071.
81. Jayasuriya CT, Twomey-Kozak J, Newberry J, et al: Human cartilage-derived progenitors resist terminal differentiation and require CXCR4 activation to successfully bridge meniscus tissue tears. *Stem Cells* 2018;37:102-114.

©Copyright 2021 American Academy of Orthopaedic Surgeons

15

Synovium and Joint Biology

Qian Chen, PhD
Yun Gao, MD, PhD

Keywords: *cytokine; inflammation; osteoarthritis; rheumatoid arthritis; synovium*

INTRODUCTION

Joint is a multitissue organ that plays an important mechanical role in supporting daily life needs of a living human being. Synovium, a connective tissue that links various tissues in the joint, not only functions mechanically but also coordinates the chemical and biological micro-environment within the joint space. In this chapter, we describe major components of synovium and derived tissues, including synovial membrane, synovial cells, and synovial fluid. Their structure, function, and composition are described in detail at the molecular level. Furthermore, major synovial related diseases are presented including rheumatoid arthritis (RA), primary or aging associated osteoarthritis (OA), and secondary or posttraumatic osteoarthritis. Understanding the role synovium plays in the pathogenesis of these diseases is critical in developing clinical treatment, surgical and pharmacological, of these major joint diseases.

Dr. Chen or an immediate family member has stock or stock options held in NanoDe Therapeutics Inc. and serves as a board member, owner, officer, or committee member of the Orthopaedic Research Society. Neither Dr. Gao nor any immediate family member has received anything of value from or has stock or stock options held in a commercial company or institution related directly or indirectly to the subject of this chapter.

SYNOVIAL MEMBRANE

Synovium, also called the synovial membrane, is a specialized connective soft-tissue membrane that lines the inner surface of synovial joint capsules. Together with bone, articular cartilage, tendon, ligament, and fibrous capsule, it is an important component of the tissues that form an integrated joint. As such, it not only has its own specific functions but also interacts with other tissues in the joint both structurally and functionally.[1]

The function of synovium is several-fold. Structurally, it seals the inner joint cavity by physically connecting with bone, articular cartilage, capsule, and ligaments. Functionally, it enables lubrication of the joint not only through retention of the synovial fluid in the joint cavity but also through synthesis of the major lubricant in the fluid including hyaluronan and lubricin (PRG4).[2] Synovium also plays a regulatory function in the joint. Unlike the avascular articular cartilage, the other inner joint cavity surface tissue, synovium is vascularized. Therefore, it serves as an important communication channel for transport of nutrients, debris and waste removal, immune modulation, and inflammation in the joint. These specialized functions are achieved by major cell types in synovial membrane, both resident and infiltrated. The malfunction of synovial membrane, synovial cells, and synovial fluid is directly involved in major bone and joint diseases including rheumatoid arthritis, aging-associated osteoarthritis (primary OA), posttraumatic osteoarthritis (PTOA, or secondary OA), and other inflammatory joint diseases.[3] The functions of normal synovium and its diseased states are summarized in **Figure 1**.

©Copyright 2021 American Academy of Orthopaedic Surgeons

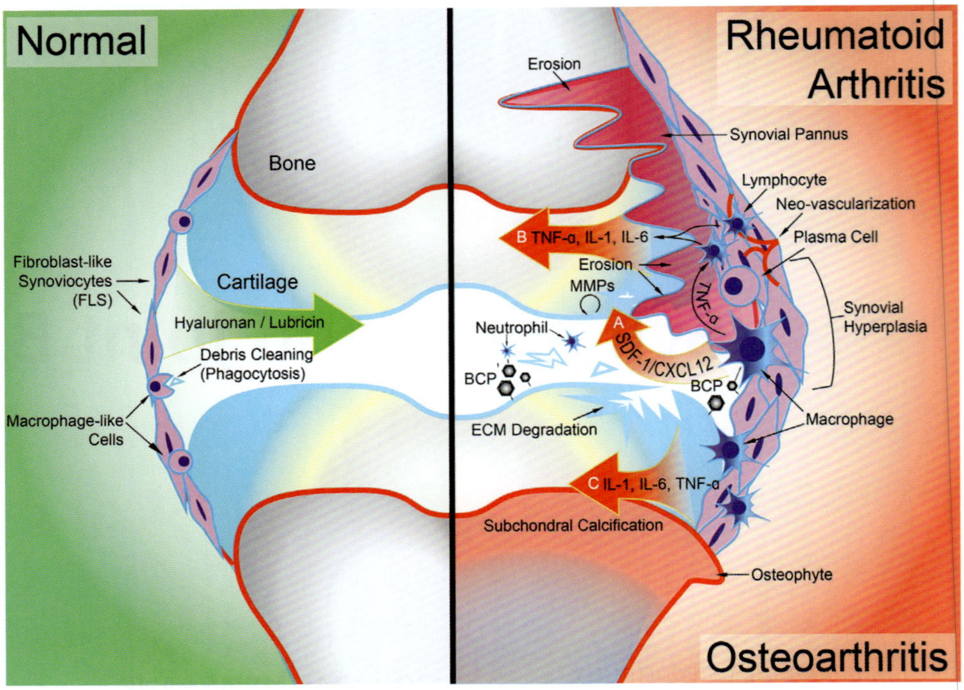

FIGURE 1 Schematic diagram of normal synovium and synovial changes under pathological conditions of rheumatoid arthritis (RA) and osteoarthritis (OA). **Left:** In normal synovial membrane, there are two major types of cells: type A macrophage-like cells, which are responsible for cleaning up debris in synovial fluid through phagocytosis, and type B fibroblast-like synoviocytes (FLS), which are responsible for synthesizing and secreting extracellular matrix in synovial fluid including hyaluronan and lubricin; **Right**: **A**, In the synovial fluid of RA patients, the concentration of stromal cell-derived factor 1 (SDF-1), also known as C-X-C motif chemokine 12 (CXCL12), is highly upregulated. C-X-C chemokine receptor type 4 (CXCR-4), the receptor of SDF-1, is distributed in the superficial zone of articular cartilage. Interaction of synovial SDF-1 with CXCR4 in human articular chondrocytes results in secretion of matrix metalloproteinase (MMP)-1, 3, 9, and 13 and ultimately the degeneration of cartilage matrix. **B**, Activated macrophages chemo-attract T cells via neovascularization through paracrine tumor necrosis factor (TNF)-α. Together with the infiltrated lymphocytes they secrete TNF-α, interleukin (IL)-1, and IL-6, major cytokines involved in RA pathogenesis. **C**, During OA pathogenesis, the major pro-inflammatory cytokines involved include IL-1, IL-6, and TNF-α. Note that while the major source of TNF-α derives from activated/infiltrated immune cells in the hyperplasic synovium and bone marrow, cartilage cells can synthesize therefore autocrine IL-1 and IL-6 under pro-inflammatory conditions.

SYNOVIAL CELLS

There are two major types of cells within the synovial membrane: type A macrophage-like cells and type B fibroblast-like synoviocytes (FLSs).[4] Type A macrophage-like cells are derived from hematopoietic monocyte lineage and account for 25% of the residential cells in synovial membrane. They are located in the inner surface of the joint cavity, responsible for removing debris in synovial fluid through phagocytosis. Mitochondria are important for synovial macrophages to fulfill this energy-consuming task. Type B FLSs are derived from mesenchymal stem cells. They are responsible for synthesizing and secreting major extracellular matrix proteins in synovial fluid including hyaluronan and lubricin (PRG4). Together with other serum proteins, hyaluronan provides viscosity of the synovial fluid, whereas lubricin lubricates the joint surface. The endoplasmic reticulum of FLS is essential for synthesizing those matrix molecules in synovial fluid. In addition, the FLS possesses some mesenchymal stem cell properties and can be used as source cells for cartilage repair.

SYNOVIAL FLUID

The synovial fluid is a specialized fluid form of synovial extracellular matrix, which serves physical, chemical, and biological functions in the joint. Physically, the fluid mechanics influence viscosity, static pressure, shear stress, and streaming potentials of the synovial fluid. Alteration of these physical factors out of the normal physiological range may induce articular surface damage, cell death, and acceleration of wear-and-tear during aging. Chemically, synovial fluid facilitates continuous exchange of oxygen, carbon dioxide, and metabolites between blood and synovial fluid. Synovial fluid also readily diffuses into articular cartilage and other soft tissues in the joint. This is especially important because it is the major source of metabolic support for articular cartilage, which is not supplied by blood vessels because of its avascular nature. Biologically, it serves as a medium for the joint tissues with which it contacts. The synovial fluid contains cells, extracellular vesicles, proteins including extracellular matrix and fragments, cytokines, chemokines, and

©Copyright 2021 American Academy of Orthopaedic Surgeons

growth factors.[5] For example, under normal conditions, synovial fluid contain <100/mL of leukocytes in which majority are monocytes. These biological components of the synovial fluid are essential for communication and coordination among tissues in the joint, which are at different anatomic locations but share common contact with synovial fluid. Such biological factors can regulate tissue growth during development as well as tissue degeneration under inflammatory conditions.[6,7]

Synovial fluid may also contain microparticles, which are endogenous crystals formed as a result of dysregulated metabolic processes. These particulates include monosodium urate crystals, which are associated with gout; calcium pyrophosphate crystals, which are associated with calcium pyrophosphate deposition disease (CPPD); and basic calcium phosphate (BCP) crystals, which are associated with osteoarthritis.[8] These particulates contribute to synovial inflammation, cartilage destruction, and subchondral bone remodeling in these synovial related joint diseases.

SYNOVIAL RELATED JOINT DISEASES

Communication between synovium and structural tissues including cartilage, bone, capsule, and ligaments is important for maintaining normal joint physiology, but also contributes to several joint disease processes. For example, BCP crystals that contain hydroxyapatite have been detected in 70% of OA cases, which correlate with the extent of cartilage degradation and lesion severity. As a "danger signal," they activate a number of joint cells including fibroblasts, macrophages, chondrocytes, and osteoclasts, which produce cartilage-degrading matrix proteinases and pro-inflammatory cytokine. Thus, it provides an intervention point for treatment of joint diseases through either physically removing or cleaning inflammation source tissues with arthroscopic surgery and joint replacement, or through blocking tissue inflammation and degeneration pathways with disease-modifying antirheumatic drugs pharmacologically. The major synovial related joint diseases are described as follows.

RHEUMATOID ARTHRITIS

An autoimmune disorder, rheumatoid arthritis is a chronic inflammatory disorder that causes joint stiffness, swelling, and pain, which ultimately results in bone erosion and joint deformity. During this pathological process, the interaction of synovium and bone and cartilage can be direct (physical) or indirect (biochemical). The direct interaction is through pannus, the hypertrophied synovium that covers, invades, and erodes contiguous cartilage and bone. Pannus tissue contains activated FLS and macrophage-like cells that release interleukin (IL)-1 and other inflammatory cytokines as well as collagenase that cause cartilage destruction and bone erosion.[9] Invasion of vascularized pannus into articular cartilage also leads to matrix removal and blood vessel growth in otherwise avascular cartilage tissue, and ultimately results in joint tissue degeneration.[10]

Secreted by inflamed synovium, cytokines and chemokines in synovial fluid can also trigger tissue degeneration through interaction with receptors in articular cartilage and bone. For example, the concentration of stromal cell-derived factor 1 (SDF-1), also known as C-X-C motif chemokine 12 (CXCL12), is highly upregulated in the synovial fluid of RA patients and to a less extent in OA patients. CXCR4, the receptor of SDF-1, is distributed in the superficial zone of articular cartilage. Interaction of synovial SDF-1 with CXCR4 in human articular chondrocytes results in secretion of matrix metalloproteinase (MMP)-1, 3, 9, and 13 and degeneration of cartilage matrix.[11] Thus, suppression of such biochemical interaction of synovium and cartilage through blocking inflammatory cytokines and chemokines signaling can also be developed into an intervention strategy for RA and OA treatment.

Such intervention strategy can be either surgical or pharmacological. Surgical synovectomy eliminates the synovium, the source of inflammatory cytokine and chemokine. Synovectomy significantly reduces serum levels of SDF-1 as well as MMP-9 and MMP-13 and is effective in both inflammatory OA and RA patients.[12] Pharmacologically, small molecules of CXCR4 antagonist inhibit interaction of SDF-1 and CXCR4 and downstream MMPs activation.[13] They have been used for intervention of RA, OA, and PTOA. Because the SDF-1/CXCR4/MMP axis is conserved in different types of cells, modulating this axis has been used not only for the treatment of arthritis but also for cancer metastasis and epiphysiodesis.[14]

Autoimmune activation in RA may involve both innate and adaptive immune system. RA synovial fluid appears turbid because of the presence of inflammatory cells, predominantly neutrophils. The volume is increased but the viscosity is decreased, resulting in a reduced ability to lubricate and protect the opposing cartilage surfaces, thus further increasing the susceptibility of cartilage to pannus attachment and matrix damage. Activated T cells and macrophages secrete tumor necrosis factor (TNF)-α, IL-1, and IL-6, which are major cytokines involved in RA pathogenesis. Antibodies to neutralize these cytokine pathways as well as small molecules to inhibit overactivation of immune cells are the first-line drugs for RA treatment.[15]

PRIMARY (AGING-ASSOCIATED) OSTEOARTHRITIS

Osteoarthritis (OA) is an aging-associated degenerative joint disease involving articular cartilage degradation, chronic inflammation, and bone remodeling.[16] Although it is a leading cause of disability in the elderly, there is no FDA-approved disease-modifying osteoarthritis drugs (DMOADs) currently. The incomplete understanding of cell and molecular mechanisms triggering inflammation and degeneration in the joint during aging hampers the development of DMOADs that can target these processes. It has been shown that joint cells including articular chondrocytes, synovial cells, and mesenchymal stem cells undergo cell senescence, telomere shortening, and SASP (senescence associated secretory phenotype) manifestation during OA.[17-19] Elimination of senescent cells in

©Copyright 2021 American Academy of Orthopaedic Surgeons

the joint genetically or pharmacologically by so-called "senolytics" inhibits OA pathogenesis in mouse models.[20] These data suggest that senescent cells can be a key target for effective treatment of OA.[21]

Although OA is not considered as a classic inflammatory disease, synovial inflammation, or synovitis, is nevertheless correlated with OA progression.[22] Synovium is mildly inflamed in early OA, which progresses in the middle phases with hypervascular changes in the synovium.[23] In late stages of OA, synovium exhibits thickening with hyperplastic cells, neo-vasculization, and villous formation. Excessively thickened synovium, filled with cells and fibrotic collagenous tissue, can physically restrict joint movement. Ultrasonography can be used to identify inflamed synovium. Pain is significantly correlated with synovial inflammation as well as bone marrow edema.[24]

In OA, the most frequently found immune cells are macrophages, T cells, and mast cells (MCs). Overall the number of cells is lower than in RA, although the number of MCs is as high as or sometimes even higher than in RA synovium. The major proinflammatory cytokines involved in OA pathogenesis include IL-1, IL-6, and TNF-α. While the major source of TNF-α comes from immune cells in synovium and bone marrow, cartilage cells can synthesize IL-1 and IL-6 under pro-inflammatory conditions. Therefore, TNF-α has been considered as a trigger of the downstream inflammatory cytokines. On the other hand, IL-1, IL-6, and MMPs are major SASPs secreted by resident senescent cells in synovium and cartilage.

Inflammatory cytokines can increase vascular permeability, attract additional mononuclear cells to inflammation site, lead to the proliferation and differentiation of lymphocytes, and stimulate downstream proinflammatory cytokine release. If the amplification of inflammation is left unchecked, tissue catabolism may take place. For instance, proinflammatory cytokines can stimulate MMP activities in synovial lining cells and can incite the development of a proliferative, erosive pannus that invades and destroys the cartilage surface. On the other hand, anti-inflammatory cytokines (eg, IL-4 and IL-10) are mainly made by lymphocytes and monocytes. Both peptides act via specific cell membrane receptors to decrease secretion of the proinflammatory cytokines in activated mononuclear cells. Therefore, the homeostasis between pro- and anti-inflammatory cytokines is critical for tissue health.

Both type A and B cells in synovium also synthesize growth factors. Growth factors are cell-secreted proteins that regulate cell proliferation and differentiation via specific binding to receptors on modulated cells to elicit intracellular signaling events. Stimulation can be autocrine, through which the secretory cell and the recipient cell are the same, or paracrine, through which the recipient cell is adjacent to the secretory cell. A major growth factor family involved in joint health and disease is TGF-β/BMP/GDF family. GDF-5 is involved in articular joint formation, whereas TGF-β plays a major role in stimulating chondrogenic differentiation and chondrogenesis of mesenchymal stem cells. On the other hand, TGF-β signaling in synovium and subchondral bone has also been shown to associate with fibrosis, bone formation, and OA pathogenesis. Bone morphogenetic protein (BMP) signaling is essential to chondrogenic and osteogenic differentiation of mesenchymal stem cells. However, excessive BMP signaling causes cartilage hypertrophy and osteophytes in osteoarthritis and heterotopic bone formation in fibrodysplasia ossificans progressiva.

POSTTRAUMATIC JOINT INJURY

PTOA is a type of secondary OA caused by physical injuries including meniscal and ligamentous injury, intra-articular fracture, chondral injury, and surgeries attempting to repair aforementioned injuries.[25,26] It accounts for 12% of all OA cases. PTOA has acute and chronic phases.[27] Inflammation including cytokines and MMP secretion is a main feature of the acute phase immediately following the traumatic injury. Between the acute and chronic phase, there can be days or months of asymptomatic phase indicating a chronic progression of pathogenesis.[28] In addition to injury, natural aging and excessive body weight also affect the disease progression. 13.9% of patients who had a history of joint injury during adulthood eventually developed knee OA.[29]

Synovium presents histopathologic changes following joint injury.[30] In the early stage, there is fibrin deposition, macrophage recruitment, and leukocyte infiltration in synovial tissue. Synovial lining cell hyperplasia and neovascularization are characteristic features that result in the outgrowth of villous projections (villi, composed of synovial lining cells, lymphocytes, macrophages, and blood vessels) from the intimal surface. In the late stage, synovial fibrosis occurs because of enhanced production of collagen, usually after the articular cartilage has been destroyed and inflammatory cells are no longer present in the synovium.[31] Reduction of inflammation with intra-articular injection of IL-1R antagonist has been shown to be effective in improving short-term outcomes of patients weeks after injury.[32] Synovial inflammation due to injury or aging also hampers movement of joint tissues, such as in "frozen shoulder." Intervention strategies may include inflammation reduction by glucocorticoid injection or by physical therapy.

CYTOKINE/GROWTH FACTOR–BASED CLINICAL THERAPEUTIC APPLICATION AND GENE THERAPY

Excessive cytokine activation or deficiency of growth factors or extracellular matrix in synovium may lead to joint diseases. Although the well-established anti-inflammatory drugs are corticosteroids and nonsteroidal anti-inflammatory drugs (NSAIDs), etc, most of the current auto-immune diseases drugs are targeting pro-inflammatory cytokines including TNF-α and IL-1β (summarized in **Table 1**).

In addition, new molecular targets and new approaches are being developed for therapeutic purposes. For example,

©Copyright 2021 American Academy of Orthopaedic Surgeons

TABLE 1 Summary of Anti-Inflammatory Drugs Approved by FDA Since 2000

Drug Name	Mechanism	Application	References
Drugs Approved in 2019			
Cimzia (certolizumab pegol)	Humanized monoclonal antibody to TNF-α	Active nonradiographic axial spondyloarthritis with inflammation	https://www.cimzia.com/
Drugs Approved in 2018			
Olumiant (baricitinib)	An inhibitor of janus kinase (JAK), blocking the subtypes JAK1 and JAK2	Adult patients with moderately to severely active RA who have had an inadequate response to TNF antagonist therapies	https://www.olumiant.com/
Drugs Approved in 2017			
Kevzara (sarilumab)	Human monoclonal antibody to IL-6 receptor	Moderately to severely active RA	https://www.kevzara.com/
Drugs Approved in 2016			
Taltz (ixekizumab)	Humanized monoclonal antibody to IL-17A	Moderate-to-severe plaque psoriasis and active psoriatic arthritis	https://www.taltz.com/
Drugs Approved in 2013			
Actemra (tocilizumab)	Recombinant humanized monoclonal antibody to human IL-6 receptor	Patients 2 yr of age and older with active polyarticular juvenile idiopathic arthritis	https://www.actemra.com
Cimzia (certolizumab pegol)	Humanized monoclonal antibody to TNF-α	Adult patients with active psoriatic arthritis; active ankylosing spondylitis	https://www.cimzia.com/
Ilaris (canakinumab)	Human monoclonal antibody to human IL-1β	Active systemic juvenile idiopathic arthritis in patients aged 2 yr and older	http://www.ilaris.com/index.jsp?usertrack.filter_applied=true&NovaId=3831502952160375928
Drugs Approved in 2012			
Xeljanz (tofacitinib)	An inhibitor of the enzyme JAK1 and JAK 3	Adult patients with moderately to severely active RA who have had an inadequate response or intolerance to methotrexate	https://www.xeljanz.com/
Drugs Approved in 2011			
Duexis	Proprietary formulation of NSAID ibuprofen	RA and OA with risk of developing upper GI ulcers in patients taking ibuprofen	https://www.duexis.com/
Actemra (tocilizumab)	Recombinant humanized monoclonal antibody to human IL-6 receptor	Active systemic juvenile idiopathic arthritis in patients aged 2 yr and older	https://www.actemra.com
Drugs Approved in 2010			
Vimovo (naproxen + esomeprazole)	Proprietary formulation of NSAID naproxen	OA, RA, and ankylosing spondylitis with risk of developing gastric ulcers in patients taking NSAID	http://www.vimovo.com/
Actemra (tocilizumab)	Recombinant humanized monoclonal antibody to human IL-6 receptor	Adult patients with moderately to severely active RA who have had an inadequate response to TNF antagonist therapies	https://www.actemra.com
Drugs Approved in 2009			
Pennsaid	Diclofenac sodium topical solution 2% w/w	OA with pain	https://www.pennsaid.com/

(Continued)

©Copyright 2021 American Academy of Orthopaedic Surgeons

TABLE 1 Summary of Anti-Inflammatory Drugs Approved by FDA Since 2000 (Continued)

Drug Name	Mechanism	Application	References
Cimzia (certolizumab pegol)	Humanized monoclonal antibody to TNF-α	Adults moderately to severely active RA	https://www.cimzia.com/
Simponi (golimumab)	Human monoclonal antibody that binds to both the soluble and transmembrane bioactive forms of human TNF-α	Adult patients with moderately to severely active RA: in combination with methotrexate; adult patients with active psoriatic arthritis: alone or in combination with methotrexate; adult patients with active ankylosing spondylitis	https://www.simponi.com/
Stelara (ustekinumab)	Human IgG1k monoclonal antibody that binds with high affinity and specificity to the p40 protein subunit used by both the IL-12 and IL-23 cytokines	Adult patients with moderate to severe plaque psoriasis who are candidates for phototherapy or systemic therapy; active psoriatic arthritis: alone or in combination with methotrexate	https://www.stelarainfo.com/
Drugs Approved in 2006			
Rituxan (rituximab)	Chimeric monoclonal antibody to cell surface protein CD20 cytolytic antibody	Adult patients with moderately to severely active RA who have inadequate response to one or more TNF antagonist therapies: in combination with methotrexate	https://www.rituxan.com/
Drugs Approved in 2002			
Humira (adalimumab)	Recombinant monoclonal antibody to human IgG1	Adult patients with moderately to severely active RA who have had an inadequate response to one or more disease-modifying antirheumatic drugs (DMARDs)	https://www.humira.com/
Remicade (infliximab)	Chimeric monoclonal antibody to TNF-α	RA: in combination with methotrexate	https://www.remicade.com/
Drugs Approved in 2001			
Kineret	Modified human interleukin 1 receptor antagonist protein by inhibiting the binding of IL-1 to the IL-1 receptor	RA: adults who have failed one or more DMARDs	https://www.kineretrx.com/
Remicade (infliximab)	Chimeric monoclonal antibody to IgG1k by neutralizing the biological activity of TNF-α through binding with high affinity to the soluble and transmembrane forms of TNF-α and inhibiting binding of TNF-α with its receptors	Adult patients with moderately to severely active RA who have had an inadequate response to methotrexate: in combination with methotrexate	https://www.remicade.com/
Drugs Approved in 2000			
Mobic (meloxicam)	NSAID, a selective inhibitor of COX-2 over COX-1	RA and OA with inflammation and pain	https://www.drugs.com/pro/meloxicam.html https://docs.boehringer-ingelheim.com/Prescribing%20Information/PIs/Mobic/MobicTabs7-5-15mg.PDF

GI = gastrointestinal, IL = interleukin, NSAID = nonsteroidal anti-inflammatory drug, OA = osteoarthritis, RA = rheumatoid arthritis, TNF = tumor necrosis factor

The detailed information of the approved drugs has been listed on the respective website in the rightmost column of the table.

Modified from FDA Approved Drugs in Rheumatology. CenterWatch. https://www.centerwatch.com/drug-information/fda-approved-drugs/therapeutic-area/19/rheumatology. Accessed July 16, 2019.

©Copyright 2021 American Academy of Orthopaedic Surgeons

mutations in lubricin (PRG-4) gene result in camptodactyly-arthropathy-coxa vara-pericarditis syndrome (CACP), an autosomal recessive disorder that develops joint failure with advancing age.[33] In addition, lubricin is also degraded following anterior cruciate ligament injury and contribute to PTOA pathogenesis. Joint degeneration can be attenuated by intra-articular supplementation of lubricin protein as well as PRG4 gene delivery via gene therapy. Because the half-lives of protein are often short in the joint cavity, gene therapy has an added advantage of long-term effects. For example, IL-1 receptor antagonist (or IL-1Ra), a naturally occurring soluble IL-1 blocking protein, binds to the signaling IL-1 receptor (type I IL-1R) with high affinity, thereby blocking its biological response.[34,35] Intra-articular administration of IL-1Ra fails to modify OA disease phenotype, probably because of its short half-life.[36] However, gene therapy with IL-1Ra gene has been shown to be effective in modifying OA either alone or in combination with PRG4 gene in large animal models of OA.[37,38] Clinical trials to determine safety of gene therapy in human OA are underway.

SUMMARY

In this chapter, the mechanical and biological roles of synovium have been described at the molecular details. Major players fulfilling mechanical lubrication and cushion functions of synovial joint include hyaluronan and lubricin. Synoviocytes, one of the major cells in synovium, are a main site for synthesis of these extracellular matrices (ECMs) in synovial fluid. In addition to their structural functions, we also described the biological regulatory roles played by synovial and cartilage-derived ECMs and their fragments. Macrophage-like cells are the second major type of cells in the synovial membrane, which are responsible for phagocytosis of tissue debris in the joint space. Together with lymphocytes and neutrophils infiltrated during neovascularization of the synovium, these immune cells are responsible for secretion of major cytokine and chemokines including TNF-a, IL-1, IL-6, and SDF-1/CXCL12, which are involved in joint inflammation, ECM degradation in cartilage and subchondral bone sclerosis, and osteophyte formation. Intercepting these autoimmune or SASP cytokine signaling transduction pathways in the joint has been a chief and successful strategy of developing treatment of major joint diseases including rheumatoid arthritis in the last 20 years. New treatment including nucleic acid therapeutics is being developed in addition to small molecule chemicals and biologics including cytokine-targeting monoclonal antibodies. This is particular exciting for developing the first disease-modifying drug for osteoarthritis, which seems within reach in the foreseeable future.

REFERENCES

1. Mescher AL: *Junqueira's Basic Histology: Text and Atlas*, ed 12. McGraw Hill Professional, 2009, p 480.
2. Waller KA, Zhang LX, Elsaid KA, Fleming BC, Warman ML, Jay GD: Role of lubricin and boundary lubrication in the prevention of chondrocyte apoptosis. *Proc Natl Acad Sci USA* 2013;110(15):5852-5857. doi:10.1073/pnas.1219289110. PubMed PMID:23530215; PMCID:PMC3625316.
3. Snoeker BA, Bakker EW, Kegel CA, Lucas C: Risk factors for meniscal tears: A systematic review including meta-analysis. *J Orthop Sports Phys Ther* 2013;43(6):352-367. doi:10.2519/jospt.2013.4295. PubMed PMID:23628788.
4. Lafyatis R, Remmers EF, Roberts AB, Yocum DE, Sporn MB, Wilder RL: Anchorage-independent growth of synoviocytes from arthritic and normal joints. Stimulation by exogenous platelet-derived growth factor and inhibition by transforming growth factor-beta and retinoids. *J Clin Invest* 1989;83(4):1267-1276. doi:10.1172/JCI114011. PubMed PMID:2784799; PMCID:PMC303817.
5. Penatti A, Facciotti F, De Matteis R, et al: Differences in serum and synovial CD4+ T cells and cytokine profiles to stratify patients with inflammatory osteoarthritis and rheumatoid arthritis. *Arthritis Res Ther* 2017;19(1):103. doi:10.1186/s13075-017-1305-1. PubMed PMID:28526072; PMCID:PMC5437517.
6. Altobelli E, Angeletti PM, Piccolo D, De Angelis R: Synovial fluid and serum concentrations of inflammatory markers in rheumatoid arthritis, psoriatic arthritis and osteoarthitis: A systematic review. *Curr Rheumatol Rev* 2017;13(3):170-179. doi:10.2174/1573397113666170427125918. PubMed PMID:28460627.
7. Bigoni M, Turati M, Sacerdote P, et al: Characterization of synovial fluid cytokine profiles in chronic meniscal tear of the knee. *J Orthop Res* 2017;35(2):340-346. doi:10.1002/jor.23272. PubMed PMID:27107410.
8. Dunne A, Mahon O: Disease-associated particulates and joint inflammation; mechanistic insights and potential therapeutic targets. *Front Immunol* 2018;9:1145.
9. Dayer JM: The pivotal role of interleukin-1 in the clinical manifestations of rheumatoid arthritis. *Rheumatology* 2003;42(suppl 2):ii3-ii10. doi:10.1093/rheumatology/keg326. PubMed PMID:12817089.
10. Xue C, Takahashi M, Hasunuma T, et al: Characterisation of fibroblast-like cells in pannus lesions of patients with rheumatoid arthritis sharing properties of fibroblasts and chondrocytes. *Ann Rheum Dis* 1997;56(4):262-267. PubMed PMID:9166000; PMCID:PMC1752353.
11. Kanbe K, Takemura T, Takeuchi K, Chen Q, Takagishi K, Inoue K: Synovectomy reduces stromal-cell-derived factor-1 (SDF-1) which is involved in the destruction of cartilage in osteoarthritis and rheumatoid arthritis. *J Bone Joint Surg Br* 2004;86(2):296-300. PubMed PMID:15046450.
12. Wei F, Moore DC, Wei L, et al: Attenuation of osteoarthritis via blockade of the SDF-1/CXCR4 signaling pathway. *Arthritis Res Ther* 2012;14(4):R177. doi:10.1186/ar3930. PubMed PMID:22849584; PMCID:PMC3580571.
13. Kanbe K, Takagishi K, Chen Q: Stimulation of matrix metalloprotease 3 release from human chondrocytes by the interaction of stromal cell-derived factor 1 and CXC chemokine receptor 4. *Arthritis Rheum* 2002;46(1):130-137. PubMed PMID:11817585.
14. Sun X, Charbonneau C, Wei L, Yang W, Chen Q, Terek RM: CXCR4-targeted therapy inhibits VEGF expression and chondrosarcoma angiogenesis and metastasis. *Mol Cancer Ther* 2013;12(7):1163-1170. doi:10.1158/1535-7163.MCT-12-1092. PubMed PMID:23686836; PMCID:PMC3707941.
15. Kanbe K, Chen Q, Nakamura A, Hobo K: Inhibition of MAP kinase in synovium by treatment with tocilizumab in rheumatoid arthritis. *Clin Rheumatol* 2011;30(11):1407-1413. doi:10.1007/s10067-011-1833-z. PubMed PMID:21909699.

©Copyright 2021 American Academy of Orthopaedic Surgeons

16. Barg A, Pagenstert GI, Hugle T, et al: Ankle osteoarthritis: Etiology, diagnostics, and classification. *Foot Ankle Clin* 2013;18(3):411-426. doi:10.1016/j.fcl.2013.06.001. PubMed PMID:24008208.
17. Martin JA, Buckwalter JA: Telomere erosion and senescence in human articular cartilage chondrocytes. *J Gerontol A Biol Sci Med Sci* 2001;56(4):B172-B179. PubMed PMID:11283188.
18. Martin JA, Buckwalter JA: Roles of articular cartilage aging and chondrocyte senescence in the pathogenesis of osteoarthritis. *Iowa Orthop J* 2001;21:1-7. PubMed PMID:11813939; PMCID:PMC1888191.
19. Martin JA, Buckwalter JA: Aging, articular cartilage chondrocyte senescence and osteoarthritis. *Biogerontology* 2002;3(5):257-264. PubMed PMID:12237562.
20. Jeon OH, Kim C, Laberge RM, et al: Local clearance of senescent cells attenuates the development of post-traumatic osteoarthritis and creates a pro-regenerative environment. *Nat Med* 2017;23(6):775-781. doi:10.1038/nm.4324. PubMed PMID:28436958; PMCID:PMC5785239.
21. Mollano AV, Martin JA, Buckwalter JA: Chondrocyte senescence and telomere regulation: Implications in cartilage aging and cancer (a brief review). *Iowa Orthop J* 2002;22:1-7. PubMed PMID:12180600; PMCID:PMC1888369.
22. de Lange-Brokaar BJ, Ioan-Facsinay A, van Osch GJ, et al: Synovial inflammation, immune cells and their cytokines in osteoarthritis: A review. *Osteoarthr Cartil* 2012;20(12):1484-1499. doi:10.1016/j.joca.2012.08.027. PubMed PMID:22960092.
23. Favero M, Ramonda R, Goldring MB, Goldring SR, Punzi L: Early knee osteoarthritis. *RMD Open* 2015;1(suppl 1):e000062. doi:10.1136/rmdopen-2015-000062. PubMed PMID:26557380; PMCID:PMC4632144.
24. Saltzman CL, Salamon ML, Blanchard GM, et al: Epidemiology of ankle arthritis: Report of a consecutive series of 639 patients from a tertiary orthopaedic center. *Iowa Orthop J* 2005;25:44-46. PubMed PMID:16089071; PMCID:PMC1888779.
25. Brown TD, Johnston RC, Saltzman CL, Marsh JL, Buckwalter JA: Posttraumatic osteoarthritis: A first estimate of incidence, prevalence, and burden of disease. *J Orthop Trauma* 2006;20(10):739-744. doi:10.1097/01.bot.0000246468.80635.ef. PubMed PMID:17106388.
26. Nelson AJ, Collins CL, Yard EE, Fields SK, Comstock RD: Ankle injuries among United States high school sports athletes, 2005-2006. *J Athl Train* 2007;42(3):381-387. PubMed PMID:18059994; PMCID:PMC1978459.
27. Gage BE, McIlvain NM, Collins CL, Fields SK, Comstock RD: Epidemiology of 6.6 million knee injuries presenting to United States emergency departments from 1999 through 2008. *Acad Emerg Med* 2012;19(4):378-385. doi:10.1111/j.1553-2712.2012.01315.x. PubMed PMID:22506941.
28. Gelber AC, Hochberg MC, Mead LA, Wang NY, Wigley FM, Klag MJ: Joint injury in young adults and risk for subsequent knee and hip osteoarthritis. *Ann Intern Med* 2000;133(5):321-328. PubMed PMID:10979876.
29. Lohmander LS, Englund PM, Dahl LL, Roos EM: The long-term consequence of anterior cruciate ligament and meniscus injuries: Osteoarthritis. *Am J Sports Med* 2007;35(10):1756-1769. doi:10.1177/0363546507307396. PubMed PMID:17761605.
30. Punzi L, Galozzi P, Luisetto R, et al: Post-traumatic arthritis: Overview on pathogenic mechanisms and role of inflammation. *RMD Open* 2016;2(2):e000279. doi:10.1136/rmdopen-2016-000279. PubMed PMID:27651925; PMCID:PMC5013366.
31. Siqueira MB, Frangiamore S, Klika AK, Gajewski N, Barsoum WK, Higuera CA: Comparison of synovial fluid cytokine levels between traumatic knee injury and end-stage osteoarthritis. *J Knee Surg* 2017;30(2):128-133. doi:10.1055/s-0036-1583269. PubMed PMID:27123668.
32. Kraus VB, Birmingham J, Stabler TV, et al: Effects of intraarticular IL1-Ra for acute anterior cruciate ligament knee injury: A randomized controlled pilot trial (NCT00332254). *Osteoarthr Cartil* 2012;20(4):271-278. doi:10.1016/j.joca.2011.12.009. PubMed PMID:22273632.
33. Iqbal SM, Leonard C, Regmi SC, et al: Lubricin/proteoglycan 4 binds to and regulates the activity of toll-like receptors in vitro. *Sci Rep* 2016;6:18910. doi:10.1038/srep18910. PubMed PMID:26752378; PMCID:PMC4707532.
34. Hannum CH, Wilcox CJ, Arend WP, et al: Interleukin-1 receptor antagonist activity of a human interleukin-1 inhibitor. *Nature* 1990;343(6256):336-340. doi:10.1038/343336a0. PubMed PMID:2137200.
35. Smith DE, Hanna R, Della F, et al: The soluble form of IL-1 receptor accessory protein enhances the ability of soluble type II IL-1 receptor to inhibit IL-1 action. *Immunity* 2003;18(1):87-96. PubMed PMID:12530978.
36. Chevalier X, Goupille P, Beaulieu AD, et al: Intraarticular injection of anakinra in osteoarthritis of the knee: A multicenter, randomized, double-blind, placebo-controlled study. *Arthritis Rheum* 2009;61(3):344-352. doi:10.1002/art.24096. PubMed PMID:19248129.
37. Smeets RL, van de Loo FA, Joosten LA, et al: Effectiveness of the soluble form of the interleukin-1 receptor accessory protein as an inhibitor of interleukin-1 in collagen-induced arthritis. *Arthritis Rheum* 2003;48(10):2949-2958. doi:10.1002/art.11234. PubMed PMID:14558102.
38. Stone A, Grol MW, Ruan MZC, et al: Combinatorial Prg4 and Il-1ra gene therapy protects against hyperalgesia and cartilage degeneration in post-traumatic osteoarthritis. *Hum Gene Ther* 2019;30(2):225-235. doi:10.1089/hum.2018.106. PubMed PMID:30070147; PMCID:PMC6383580.

©Copyright 2021 American Academy of Orthopaedic Surgeons

16

Joint Cross-talk Among Bone, Synovium, and Articular Cartilage

Courtney M. Mazur, BS
Karsyn N. Bailey, BS
Tamara Alliston, PhD

Keywords: *articular cartilage; joint cross-talk; osteoarthritis; subchondral bone; synovium*

INTRODUCTION

Diarthrodial joints facilitate smooth motion and load transfer through integrated function of multiple tissues, including articular cartilage, bone, ligaments, tendons, synovium, and menisci. Under normal conditions, the biological and mechanical activities of these tissues are exquisitely coordinated. They develop together, often share a blood supply, exchange signaling molecules, and mechanically load each other almost constantly throughout life. While cross-talk among these tissues in healthy joints supports homeostasis, it can alternatively drive a positive-feedback loop of joint destruction if any of the joint components become perturbed by injury or diseases, such as osteoarthritis (OA) (**Figure 1**).

OA is now considered a "whole-joint" disease, in recognition of the coordinated degradation and interaction of multiple tissues within the joint. Examining OA through the lens of joint cross-talk sheds light on disease origin and progression, joint pain, and therapeutic strategies. Though evidence supports the cross-talk of muscle, ligaments, menisci, nerves, and gut microbiota with joint tissues, this chapter will focus on the interactions among bone, synovium, and articular cartilage in the most common joint disease, OA. This chapter will review evidence for cross-talk at the whole-joint level and the cellular level, relying on data from humans unless otherwise noted, discuss some possible mechanisms of cross-talk among these tissues, and conclude with a discussion of therapies in development for joint disease that attempt to harness these tissue interactions.

Dr. Alliston or an immediate family member is a member of a speakers' bureau or has made paid presentations on behalf of Orthofix, Inc. Neither of the following authors nor any immediate family member has received anything of value from or has stock or stock options held in a commercial company or institution related directly or indirectly to the subject of this chapter: Ms. Mazur and Ms. Bailey.

CLINICAL EVIDENCE OF CROSS-TALK

BONE AND CARTILAGE CROSS-TALK

Bone Marrow Lesions

Bone marrow lesions (BMLs), also known as bone marrow edema or bone bruises, appear in injured subchondral bone and serve as markers of the pathological joint cross-talk observed in OA. BMLs are detected noninvasively by MRI, where they appear as areas of ill-defined hyperintense signal in fluid-sensitive, fat-saturated image sequences (**Figure 2**). In T1-weighted images, they appear as areas of low signal intensity. There is some evidence that lesions detectable by both types of sequence are more severe than those detectable by fluid-sensitive sequences only.[1] The presence of BMLs is clinically important because they forecast joint pain and osteoarthritic cartilage changes.

BMLs, while primarily a feature of bone, are strongly associated with OA severity in human joints in in vivo and ex vivo studies. Relative to healthy joints, osteoarthritic knees have more BMLs, excessive trabecular bone, and a

©Copyright 2021 American Academy of Orthopaedic Surgeons

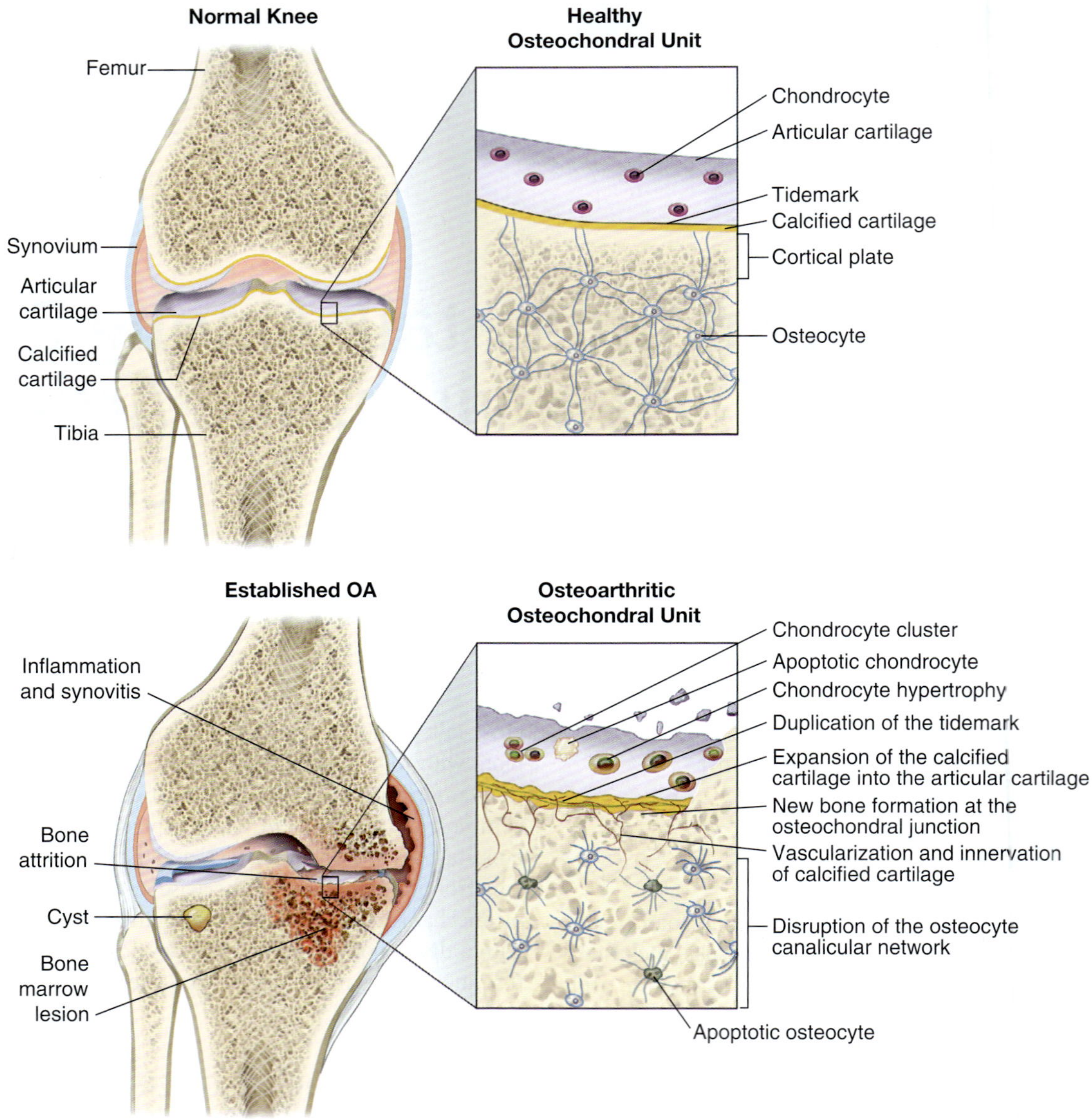

FIGURE 1 Schematic figure of the many tissue and cell types in healthy and osteoarthritis (OA) joints. (Adapted with permission from Goldring SR, Goldring MB: Changes in the osteochondral unit during osteoarthritis: structure, function, and cartilage-bone crosstalk. *Nat Rev Rheumatol* 2016;12[11]:632-644.)

thicker subchondral plate. The severity of BMLs in knees and hips also correlates with histologic evidence of OA severity such as scores on the OARSI Osteoarthritis Cartilage Histopathology Assessment System, tidemark duplication, and cartilage volume.[2] Interestingly, BMLs are detectable in some asymptomatic patients, suggesting that they may precede other signs of OA.

BMLs can be monitored noninvasively over time, making them a useful clinical tool. In longitudinal imaging studies spanning 6 weeks to 30 months, individual BMLs have been observed to appear, grow, shrink, or resolve.[3,4] BMLs that grew were strongly predictive of nearby cartilage loss, whereas patients with no BMLs had minimal cartilage loss. Improvement of BMLs is associated with less frequent and less severe pain.[5] Therefore, it is possible that future treatments for OA could be assessed based on their ability to shrink BMLs.

Although additional research is needed to evaluate the mechanisms by which BMLs arise or resolve, current evidence suggests that both biological and mechanical factors participate in BML formation. BMLs are frequently located in the overloaded medial compartment of varus-aligned knees and in the lateral compartment of valgus-aligned knees. Altered joint loading may also render the subchondral bone more susceptible to microfractures and to infiltration of synovial fluid or vasculature. Whether BMLs causally contribute to cartilage degradation remains to be determined. Nevertheless, BMLs reveal pathologic cross-talk between cartilage and subchondral bone and may be useful for early identification of OA, especially following joint injury.

©Copyright 2021 American Academy of Orthopaedic Surgeons

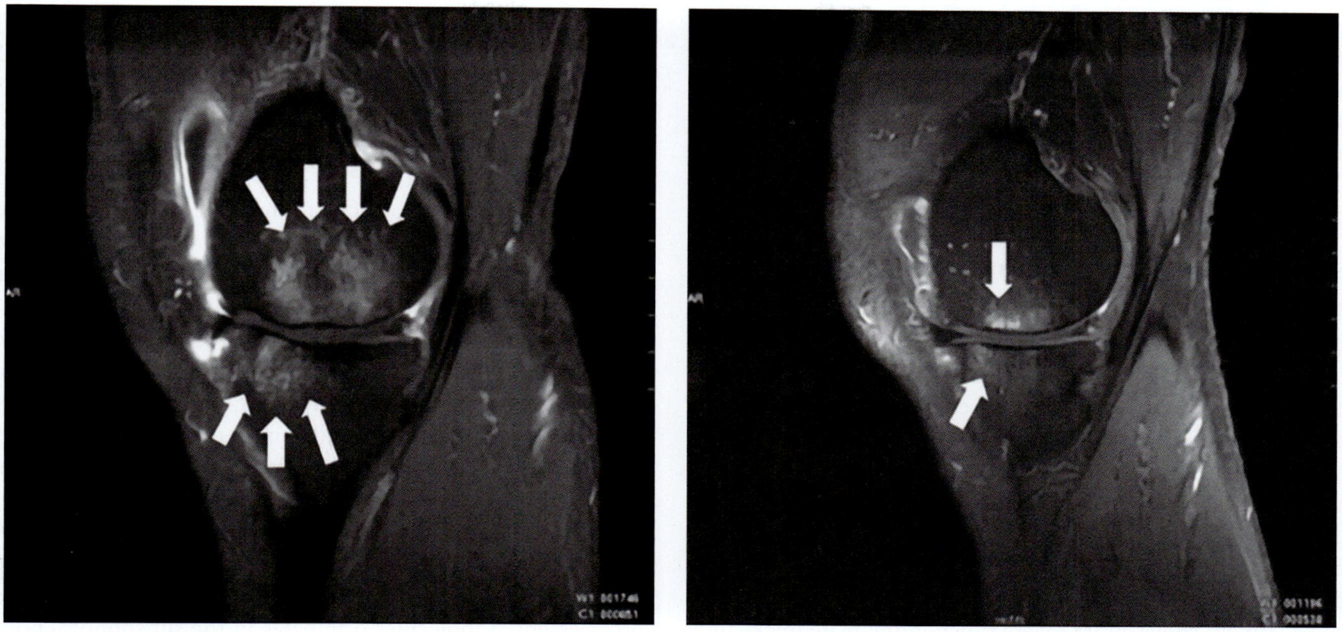

FIGURE 2 Bone marrow lesions, denoted by arrows, are visible in the subchondral bone of human joints by magnetic resonance (MR) imaging. Here they are seen as areas of diffuse hyperintense signal in the distal femur and proximal tibia. (Reproduced with permission from Alliston T, Hernandez CJ, Findlay DM, et al: Boen marrow lesions in osteoarthritis: What lies beneath. *J Orthop Res* 2018;36[7]:1818-1825.)

Subchondral Changes in Osteoarthritis

In addition to cartilage fibrillation and loss, osteoarthritic joints undergo a multiphasic process of subchondral remodeling, which in turn affects cartilage homeostasis. Beneath the articular cartilage lies a layer of highly mineralized calcified cartilage, followed by the subchondral plate, and finally the subchondral trabecular (or cancellous) bone. Each of these layers undergoes distinct changes in early and late-stage OA, so it is important to consider their roles separately. Better understanding of cross-talk between subchondral bone and cartilage may improve the success of efforts to regenerate or replace articular cartilage, which often overlook the concomitant changes in these underlying tissues.

Trabecular Bone Microarchitecture

The subchondral trabecular bone, which lies between the subchondral plate and the epiphyseal plate, is responsible for transmitting loads from the joint to the skeleton. Both the rods, the elongated cylindrical trabeculae, and the plates, the large flatter trabeculae, are essential for this function. In early OA, the remodeling rate in trabecular bone increases, meaning that newly deposited organic bone matrix does not have as much time to accumulate mineral before being resorbed again.[6] Thus, in early OA, trabecular bone experiences a net loss of bone volume and bone mineral, and it becomes more easily deformable. In late-stage OA, a persistent imbalance in bone remodeling has led to reports of both increased and decreased subchondral trabecular bone volume. These apparently different findings may result in part from methodologic differences in timepoints, experimental systems (eg, species, in vivo or ex vivo), or imaging technologies (eg, dual-energy x-ray absorptiometry [DXA] or computed tomography [CT]) for collecting outcomes in this dynamic disease process. These distinctions must be considered carefully when comparing studies.

To better understand the association of subchondral trabecular bone changes with cartilage degradation, several imaging techniques have been used to evaluate human joints. With high-resolution peripheral quantitative CT (pQCT) scans performed ex vivo, the morphology of trabecular plates and rods can be analyzed separately. In subchondral bone, trabecular plate structures contribute to the overall stiffness of the joint more than rods. In OA subchondral bone, there is a shift in the ratio of plate to rod number beneath degenerated and intact cartilage, providing a mechanical link between trabecular microarchitecture and cartilage degradation.[7] Dynamic contrast-enhanced MRI studies demonstrate that OA subchondral bone has reduced perfusion and venous outflow consistent with venous stasis.[8] Reduced perfusion may cause subchondral bone hypoxia, suggesting a biological cause for changes in bone remodeling rate. Several studies collectively suggest that, in a subset of OA, cartilage degeneration results from primary defects in bone, arising from differences in genetics, mechanics, injury, or other factors.

Studies with animal models of OA strengthen the hypothesis that trabecular bone remodeling precedes changes to cartilage. Dunkin-Hartley guinea pigs spontaneously develop OA after 3 months of age, but the plate-rod ratio increases at 2 months of age.[7] Strain 13 guinea pigs, on the other hand, have consistently high bone mass but do not develop OA. This suggests that a simple change in bone mass is not likely a causal driver of end-stage OA, but that a change in homeostatic maintenance of stable

©Copyright 2021 American Academy of Orthopaedic Surgeons

trabecular bone volume and increased bone remodeling may disrupt healthy bone-cartilage cross-talk. Along these lines, studies using antiresorptives before inducing OA in animal models often show less cartilage pathology. However, mixed results overall, especially in human trials (discussed more later) suggest that there is a critical time window in which preventive therapy could be effective.

Subchondral Plate Remodeling

The subchondral plate, the thick, corticalized layer of bone between the subchondral trabecular bone and the calcified cartilage, also undergoes dynamic remodeling in OA. In early OA, the increase in bone remodeling rate causes thinning of the subchondral plate. In late-stage OA, the subchondral plate thickens, usually in the condyle with more joint space narrowing. This strong spatial association between subchondral plate thickening and cartilage degeneration also occurs in animal models of induced OA. For example, following meniscal destabilization in mice or varus/valgus tibial angulation in rabbits, the overloaded compartment shows more severe subchondral plate thickening and cartilage lesions.[6] However, insertion of a metal rod into the subchondral bone of sheep to immediately induce subchondral stiffening did not lead to cartilage deterioration even after five years.[9] Therefore, as in trabecular bone, the process of subchondral plate remodeling may be more important for cross-talk with cartilage than its resultant change in thickness.

One of the hallmarks of OA is calcified cartilage advancement, during which this highly mineralized layer expands into the uncalcified cartilage layer, leaving telltale tidemark duplications. As a result, the remaining uncalcified cartilage layer becomes thinner, while the surface beneath it becomes much thicker and denser. The combination of thicker subchondral plate and expanded layer of calcified cartilage creates a zone of highly mineralized tissue in late-stage OA referred to as subchondral bone sclerosis. In addition, in the rare disease alkaptonuria and in human OA, highly mineralized subchondral plate protrusions extend into the calcified and uncalcified cartilage[10] (**Figure 3**). The calcified cartilage helps to transform shear stresses on the cartilage into compressive and tensile forces on the whole joint, so these protrusions and changes in thickness cause stress concentrations that can contribute to cartilage degradation.

At the border of cartilage and bone, the formation of osteophytes is another hallmark of OA. Stem cells from the periosteum or synovial lining undergo endochondral ossification, effectively expanding the subchondral bone and the cartilage surface. Osteophytes can be detected radiographically before joint space narrowing and are often a source of pain and limited mobility. While osteophyte size does not predict OA progression, their removal causes joint instability, perhaps indicating that they arise to stabilize a joint in the early stages of disease.[6,11] In addition to the knee and hip, osteophytes are also common in hand OA (**Figure 4**), which occurs twice as often in women as in men. Women are at higher risk for OA overall, but the anatomic, hormonal, and other differences causing this discrepancy are not well studied. In summary, detection of subchondral bone changes prior to gross changes in cartilage indicates that bone remodeling might causally contribute to cartilage pathology, but whether its effects are reversible remains to be determined.

Subchondral Bone Porosity

While the uncalcified articular cartilage is nonvascularized and noninnervated, human subchondral bone is perforated by channels containing blood vessels and nerves (10 to 30 μm diameter) that extend as far as the calcified cartilage. Larger pores containing fat or marrow (30 to 100 μm diameter) and nonmineralized pathways between osteocytes and chondrocytes (5 to 50 nm diameter) have also been identified. Under normal conditions, the size and density of these channels vary within the joint, and studies with fluorescein tracers show that they are functional pathways for diffusion of small molecules between the general circulation, the subchondral bone, and the uncalcified cartilage[12,13] (**Figure 5**). In humans, it is believed that nearly 50% of the cartilage supply of glucose, oxygen, and other essential molecules originates in the subchondral bone vasculature, with the remainder diffusing from the synovial fluid. In OA, changes to subchondral plate porosity occur at each length scale and may contribute to disease progression by altering bone-cartilage cross-talk.

Early in OA, elevated bone remodeling causes widening of existing channels and plate thinning, ultimately increasing subchondral plate porosity.[13] Formation of microcracks also creates new conduits for solute movement. In late disease, vascular and nerve invasion into the subchondral bone and calcified cartilage—sometimes as far as the tidemark—further increases solute delivery to the cartilage[14,15] (**Figure 6**). In particular, widening of channels in the subchondral plate increases transportation of large molecules (up to 70 kDa) 30% to 100% over what would be possible in healthy bone.[16] While therapeutic microfracture has been utilized in an attempt to deliver mesenchymal stem cells and other factors to the site of an articular cartilage lesion, increasing vascular access to articular cartilage may actually exacerbate an underlying disease process. At the same time, in two mouse models of OA, both chondrocyte-chondrocyte and chondrocyte-osteocyte diffusion was slowed, likely due to increased mineralization of the calcified cartilage or the degeneration of osteocyte canalicular channels in bone.[13]

In addition to pores connecting cartilage and bone, canalicular channels (500 nm diameter) form a rich network within bone connecting osteocytes to one another and to the vasculature. To maintain this network and control bone mineralization, osteocytes secrete proteases and acid to resorb their surrounding extracellular matrix and then replace it in a process called perilacunar/canalicular remodeling (PLR).[17] Relative to bone from healthy cadaveric joints, osteocytes in subchondral bone from osteonecrotic (ON) and OA human joints show diminished connectivity through canaliculi, suggesting a functional defect in PLR in ON and OA.[18,19] Experimental suppression of osteocyte PLR mimics the canalicular defects in human OA and

©Copyright 2021 American Academy of Orthopaedic Surgeons

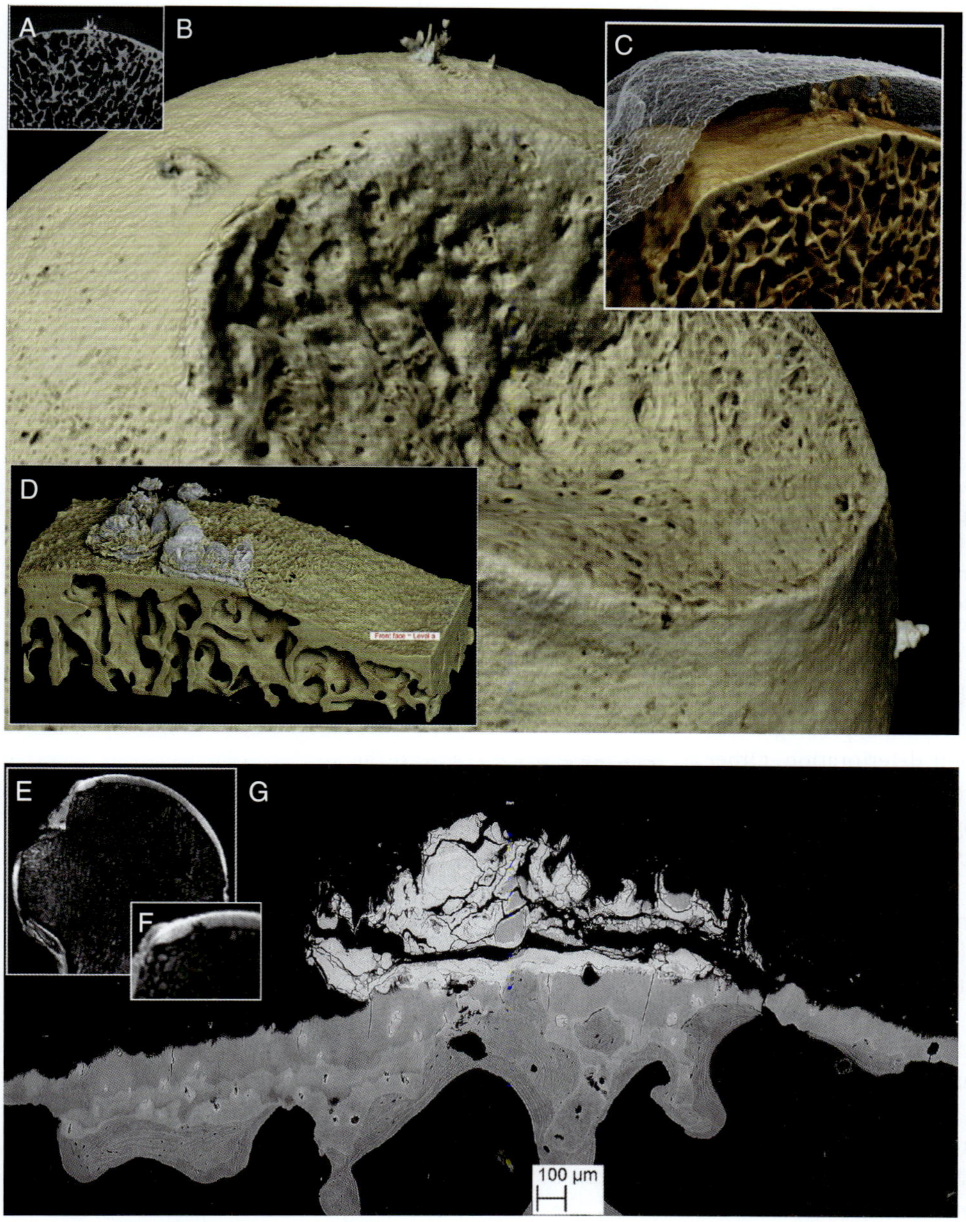

FIGURE 3 High-density mineralized protrusions from the subchondral bone into the overlying cartilage are detectable by x-ray microcomputed tomography (**A** to **D**), MRI (**E** to **F**), and scanning electron microscopy (**G**) in alkaptonuria and in osteoarthritis. (Reproduced with permission from Boyde A, Davis GR, Mills D, et al: On fragmenting, densely mineralised acellular protrusions into articular cartilage and their possible role in osteoarthritis. *J Anat* 2014;225[4]:436-446.)

ON subchondral bone and produces signs of joint disease in mouse models. Though the mechanisms remain unknown, PLR suppression could impact cartilage through impaired solute transport through the canalicular network as well as through changing the mechanical properties of subchondral bone. Thus, osteocyte PLR is an important process for the biological and mechanical homeostasis of bone, and its suppression has meaningful consequences for cross-talk within the joint.

SYNOVIAL CONTRIBUTIONS TO JOINT HOMEOSTASIS

Healthy synovium protects the joint by preventing adherence of the synovial capsule to the cartilage, by producing synovial fluid, hyaluronic acid, and lubricin, and by removing metabolites and products of matrix degradation.[20] Unlike cartilage, healthy synovium is highly vascularized and contains nociceptive fibers for pain reception, and thus serves as a nutrient and sensory source for the joint.[21] The intima, the inner layer of synovial tissue, contains type A and type B synoviocytes. Type A synoviocytes resemble macrophages and phagocytes, and type B cells are secretory fibroblasts.[20]

Synovitis, much like subchondral bone remodeling, is actively involved in OA and often precedes detectable cartilage damage.[20] This inflamed synovium, considered a source of pain in OA, produces granulation tissue that covers the synovial joint, also known as a pannus, which can then invade the subchondral bone (**Figure 7**). During inflammation, synoviocytes increase in number and size and recruit mononuclear lymphocytes and macrophages.[21,22] This cellular influx,

©Copyright 2021 American Academy of Orthopaedic Surgeons

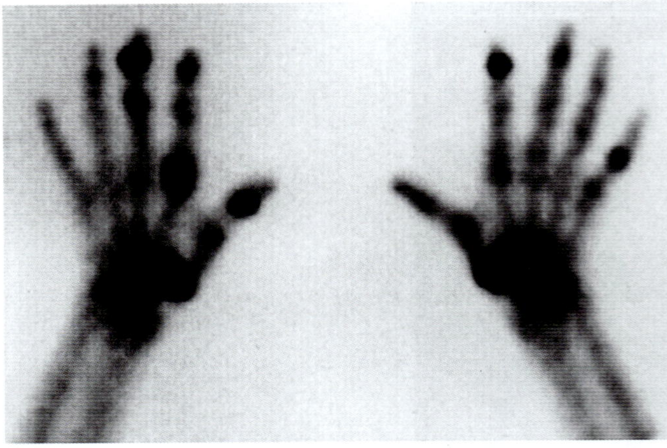

FIGURE 4 Four-hour bone scan of hand osteoarthritis demonstrates that isotope uptake correlates with osteophytes, which often appear before detectable joint space narrowing. (Reproduced with permission from Buckland-Wright C: Subchodnral bone changes in hand and knee osteoarthritis detected by radiography. *Osteoarthr Cartil* 2004;12:S10-219.)

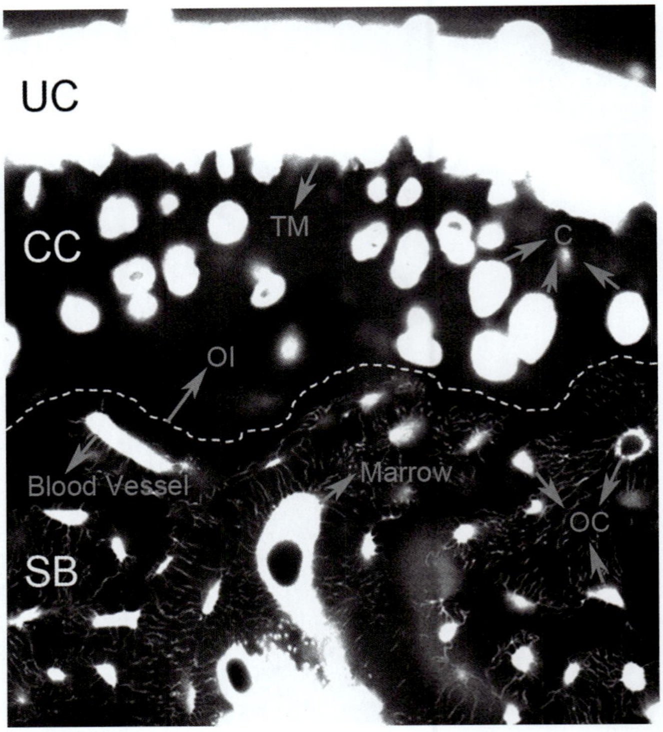

FIGURE 5 Ex vivo tracer distribution profile illustrating perfusion of mouse femur results in inhomogeneous staining throughout the joint, demonstrating variable diffusion throughout the uncalcified cartilage (UC), chondrocytes (C), calcified cartilage (CC), osteocytes (OC), subchondral bone (SB), tidemark (TM), and osteochondral interface (OI, dashed line). (Adapted with permission from Pan J, Zhou X, Li W, et al: In situ measurement of transport between subchondral bone and articular cartilage. *J Orthop Res* 2009;27[10]:1347-1352.)

coupled with the production of catabolic and proinflammatory mediators, such as cytokines, nitric oxide, prostaglandin E2, and neuropeptides, can propel joint deterioration. Other hallmarks of synovitis include an increase in angiogenesis and an increased production of proangiogenic vascular endothelial growth factor (VEGF) within the synovium. Each of these factors has well-established effects on other joint tissues.

The most prominent proinflammatory cytokines in the pathogenesis of OA are interleukin-1β (IL-1β) and tumor necrosis factor-α (TNF-α).[21,22] These cytokines can directly result in cartilage destruction or trigger their own production or the production of other cytokines, thus resulting in a feedforward cascade of joint destruction. Proinflammatory mediators can also attract other immune cells, which can in turn secrete more cytokines. The acute inflammatory response can result in a phenotypic shift in chondrocytes, causing chondrocytes to produce additional cytokines and proteolytic enzymes that increase cartilage degeneration and induce further synovial inflammation.[22] Additionally, molecules from degraded articular cartilage released into the synovial cavity can directly induce synovitis.

In addition to contributing to cartilage degeneration through release of catabolic cytokines and inducing pain in OA, inflamed synovium interacts directly with subchondral bone in OA by triggering macrophages within the synovium to differentiate into osteoclasts.[21] As these macrophages differentiate, they cause bony erosions, one possible mechanism through which bone resorption is increased in early stages of OA.

The exact cause of synovitis in OA is unclear and may be etiology-specific. For instance, posttraumatic OA that develops following joint injury often results in acute synovial inflammation.[23,24] Conversely, diseases that increase chronic systemic inflammation, such as obesity or metabolic syndrome, can induce synovial inflammation by synergizing with other inflammatory mechanisms in OA.[22] And finally, some conditions that affect the articular cartilage directly can increase synovitis as a result of the synovium detecting cartilage breakdown products.

Because there are few techniques to detect synovitis clinically, the longitudinal progression of synovitis in OA in humans is largely unknown. A histologic study of human OA revealed changes in cellular infiltration and proinflammatory cytokines with OA progression.[25] Another technique to clinically identify synovitis is detecting inflammatory mediators within the synovial fluid, but these could come from cartilage, subchondral bone, or synovium.

Since MRI and ultrasonography can visualize synovial changes, they can help to dissect the relationship between synovitis and OA clinically. Clinical imaging reveals that synovitis often presents in areas close to cartilage degeneration.[22] Contrast-enhanced MRI can allow for the visualization of synovial hypertrophy, synovial fluid volume, and level of synovial enhancement.[22] As noncontrast MRI cannot distinguish these features, it may underestimate the degree of synovitis.[26] Optimizing imaging techniques to detect synovitis, whether through MRI or ultrasonography, presents a noninvasive option to monitor the progression of synovitis with OA.

 ©Copyright 2021 American Academy of Orthopaedic Surgeons

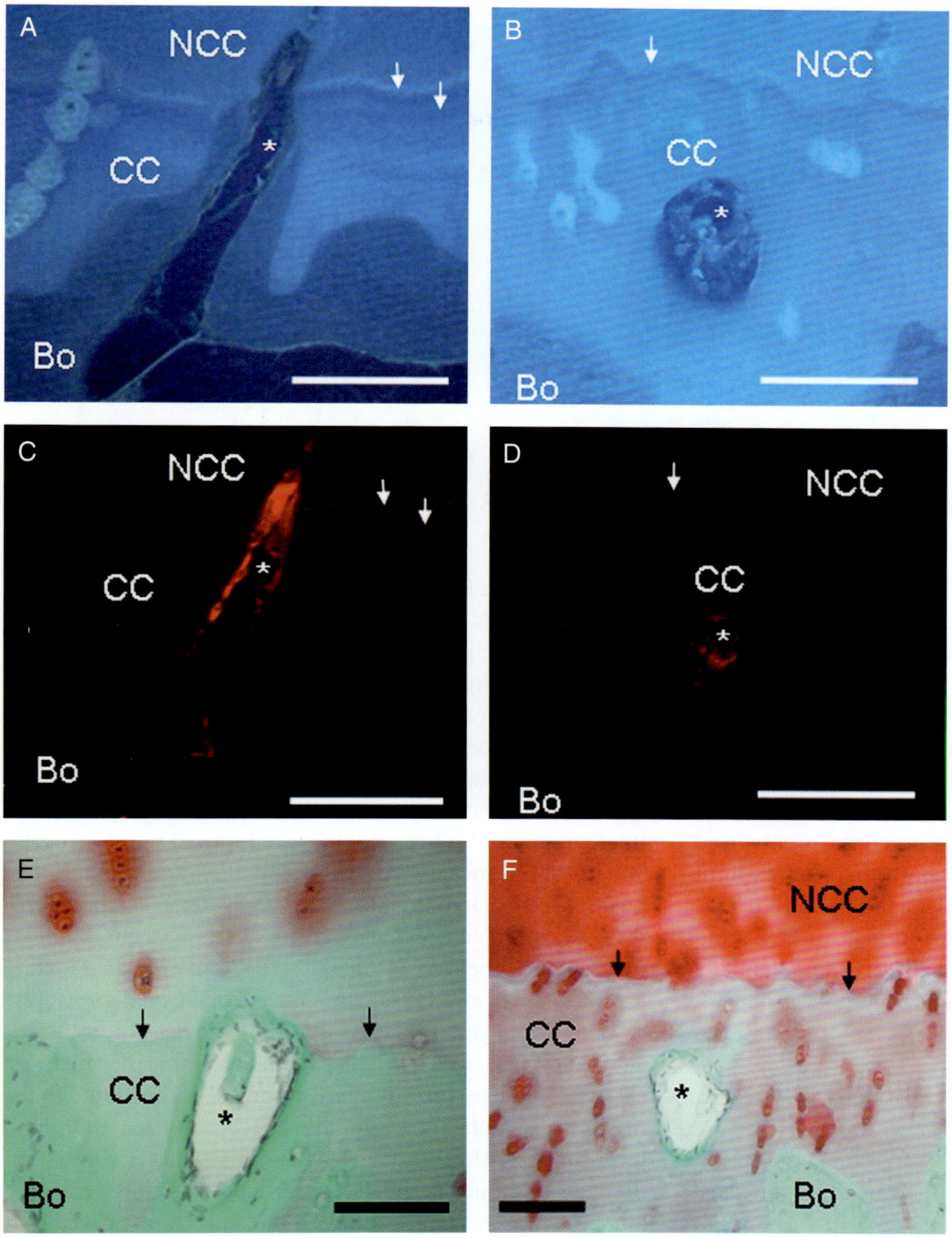

FIGURE 6 Histological specimens of the medial tibial osteochondral junction show that vasculature, demonstrated by red CD34+ endothelial cells (**C** and **D**), from bone (Bo) and calcified cartilage (CC), invades noncalcified cartilage (NCC) in osteoarthritis (**A**) more than in healthy specimens (**B**). Vascularization in osteoarthritic joints corresponds with adjacent loss of proteoglycan staining (**E**), compared with normal proteoglycan content in healthy joints (**F**). (Adapted with permission from Walsh DA, Bonnet CS, Turner EL, et al: Angiogenesis in the synovium and at the osteochondral junction in osteoarthritis. *Osteoarthr Cartil* 2007;15[7]:743-751.)

As illustrated earlier, synovium independently engages in cross-talk with articular cartilage through production of synovial fluid in joint homeostasis and through production of catabolic proinflammatory mediators in joint disease. Additionally, synovium independently interacts with subchondral bone in OA by triggering the differentiation of synovial macrophages into osteoclasts, thus inducing bone resorption. Evidence of whole-joint cross-talk in OA includes the significant association of synovitis with BMLs.[26] Synovial thickening, as detected using contrast-enhanced MRI, accompanies joint space narrowing, osteophyte formation, and BML severity. Likewise, histologic evidence of synovitis correlates with BMLs, subchondral bone cysts, and subchondral bone loss observed by MRI.[27] Dissecting the precise contribution of each of these tissue compartments in OA and their temporal relationship is critical for the development of successful therapeutics.

While animal models allow causal exploration of OA mechanisms, most clinical studies analyze either end-stage OA tissues collected after joint arthroplasty or cross-sectional MRI data. Two prospective observational studies of knee OA advance our understanding of synovitis in OA. Evaluation of the MRI outcomes in one patient cohort demonstrated that cartilage lesions, meniscal damage, synovitis, and BMLs were all risk factors for OA.[28] Even after adjusting for confounding cartilage and meniscal damage, synovitis was independently associated with incident OA. Because synovitis can occur as a result of cartilage or meniscal damage, identifying synovitis as an independent contributor brings promise to potential

©Copyright 2021 American Academy of Orthopaedic Surgeons

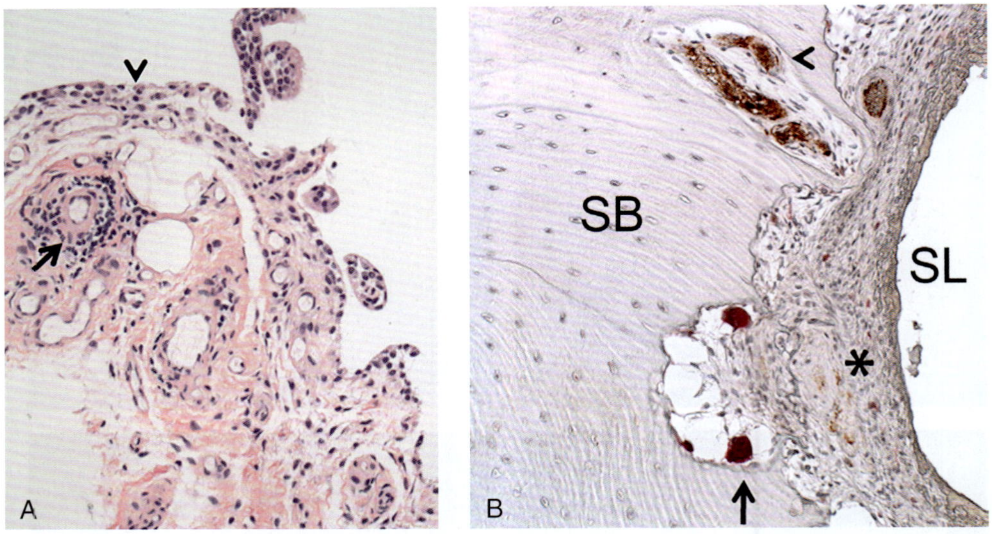

FIGURE 7 Histological specimens of synovitis in knee OA (**A**) shows histological evidence of hyperplasia with multiple layers of synovial lining cells (arrowhead) and perivascular inflammatory cell infiltration (arrow). Synovial lining (SL) pannus in OA (**B**) demonstrates inflammatory cell infiltration (asterisk) eroding the subchondral bone (SB), CD34^{+} neoangiogenesis (arrowhead), and TRAP^{+} osteoclast formation (arrow). (Adapted with permission from Hügle T, Geurts J: What drives osteoarthritis?–synovial versus subchondral bone pathology. *Rheumatology* 2016;56[9]:1461-1471.)

treatments that specifically target synovial inflammation. Similar findings held true in a different cohort, which found that synovitis and medial meniscal damage can predict radiographic OA 2 years later.[3] This was especially notable since detection of cartilage damage by MRI did *not* predict OA, thus emphasizing the role of noncartilaginous tissues in early OA.

Synovitis and pain in OA are closely linked, but the precise contributions of synovitis to pain in OA are still unknown. Increased levels of synovitis measured on contrast-enhanced MRI associate with increased pain,[26] but other factors limit the strength of this relationship.[21] Understanding the contexts in which synovitis directly contributes to pain in OA could give rise to synovitis treatments with analgesic, and potentially disease-modifying, benefits.

POSSIBLE MECHANISMS OF CROSS-TALK

Having highlighted the numerous changes to bone and synovium that occur in concert with changes to cartilage in OA, we now discuss the mechanisms by which these tissues might interact. In general, these fall into biological or mechanical categories.

BIOLOGICAL FACTORS

A critical concept in understanding joint cross-talk is the compartment- and cell-type-specific effects of each biological regulator in the healthy joint. Chondrocytes in cartilage explants are more resistant to apoptosis when cocultured with a bone explant, even if the tissues are physically separated, showing that cross-talk is often beneficial.[6] However, efforts to unravel this cross-talk reveal that factors required for homeostatic function in one compartment can drive the progression of OA in another. For example, matrix metalloproteinase-13 (MMP-13) is one of the proteases necessary for maintenance of the canalicular network in bone, but it is also the primary protease that cleaves type II collagen in cartilage. In OA, not only are the expression levels of these biological factors disrupted, but with changes to subchondral porosity and joint loading, so is their localization. Here we focus on key biological pathways implicated in joint cross-talk, including inflammation, hypoxia, and Wnt and transforming growth factor-β (TGF-β) signaling.

While not as pronounced as in rheumatoid arthritis, inflammatory pathways play a central role in OA, since TNF-α, interleukins, and other cytokines are induced in synoviocytes and in chondrocytes. As detailed earlier, the uncontrolled positive feedback of inflammatory processes exacerbates protease secretion and cartilage erosion. The subsequent release of alarmins, chemokines, and cartilage matrix degradation products such as fibronectin, small leucine-rich proteoglycans, and collagen fragments into the synovial fluid can activate integrins, which further stimulates this degenerative cycle.[29] Osteoblasts from sclerotic bone also contribute to the inflammatory phenotype in chondrocytes by secreting high levels of IL-6, IL-8, and prostaglandin E2 that act on chondrocytes to induce MMP-13 expression.[6] Additional cartilage and bone fragments including CTX-II (protease-cleaved type II collagen fragments), ARGS (aggrecanase-cleaved aggrecan fragments), and NTX-I (cathepsin K-degraded type I collagen fragments) are detectable in serum and urine;[30] however, their diagnostic utility remains unclear. Thus, control of inflammation throughout the joint is a necessary aspect of potential OA treatments.

Hypoxia-inducible factors (HIFs) also play an important role in OA. Normal chondrocytes exist in a state of hypoxia and express HIF-1α, which protects them from apoptosis.[31] Increased oxygen, due to vascularization and permeability of OA subchondral bone, may be sufficient to change chondrocyte behavior. Chondrocytes cultured in normoxia express less HIF-1α, type II collagen, and aggrecan and more MMP-13 and aggrecanase MMP-3 than those in hypoxic conditions.[29] When exposed to IL-1α and TNF-α, normoxic chondrocytes express more of the proinflammatory mediators, nitric oxide

©Copyright 2021 American Academy of Orthopaedic Surgeons

and prostaglandin E2, than hypoxic cells. Inhibition of HIF-1 in mice promotes cartilage degradation and osteophyte formation. HIF-2α, however, is highly expressed in osteoarthritic cartilage and induces expression of aggrecanases and MMPs.[32] Therefore, the shift from HIF-1α to HIF-2α in chondrocytes may be a critical event influencing whole-joint catabolism. For osteoblasts, however, hypoxia in subchondral bone during early OA induces changes to cell behavior that likely contribute to bone remodeling and cartilage degeneration.[33] In addition to stimulating the angiogenesis associated with OA, osteoblasts in a hypoxic environment secrete more TGF-β1, insulin-like growth factor-1 (IGF-1), and collagen I and are more susceptible to apoptosis and necrosis. Thus, changes in oxygenation of joint tissues is a key biological stimulus for cartilage and bone.

Tight control of Wnt signaling in bone and cartilage is critical for joint homeostasis. Canonical Wnt signaling through β-catenin is a potent agonist for bone formation, and its activity is regulated by several secreted Wnt antagonists. For example, sclerostin is expressed by osteocytes and chondrocytes in a mechanosensitive manner to suppress inappropriate bone formation. Overloading of the joint in OA may contribute to sclerostin downregulation, abnormal Wnt activation, and eventually subchondral bone sclerosis in OA.[34] In chondrocytes, expression of β-catenin is required for formation of primary and secondary ossification centers, and Wnt signaling acts as a survival signal for chondrocytes by inhibiting apoptosis.[35] However, high levels of Wnt signaling have been detected in synovial fibroblasts and chondrocytes from OA patients, and returning Wnt signaling levels to normal in a mouse model reduced cartilage degeneration and synovitis. Wnt signaling plays an essential role in development of bones and cartilage, and its expression must be carefully controlled to maintain joint homeostasis.

TGF-β signaling also plays a carefully calibrated role in cartilage and bone homeostasis. In bone, osteoclasts liberate TGF-β ligand during bone resorption, which promotes osteoprogenitor recruitment and proliferation. However, TGF-β represses terminal osteoblast differentiation and matrix mineralization. Accordingly, TGF-β inhibition in mice increases trabecular bone density. These findings inform our understanding of the joint phenotype in a surgical model of mouse OA, in which high levels of active TGF-β in subchondral bone accompany cartilage degradation, increased subchondral bone remodeling, and low trabecular bone mass.[36] In this OA model, a neutralizing TGF-β antibody helped to preserve the healthy cartilage and subchondral bone phenotype. These findings are clinically encouraging, especially because elevated levels of TGF-β in synovial tissue are associated with OA severity.[27]

On the other hand, inhibition of TGF-β signaling in chondrocytes exacerbates OA, in part because TGF-β normally stimulates the production of essential cartilage matrix components collagen II and aggrecan and restrains the expression of proteases like MMP-13.[37] This mechanism is likely responsible for the association with OA of human mutations in the TGF-β effector Smad3. As discussed in the following section, the TGF-β pathway is also mechanosensitive and can regulate material properties of joint tissues. While many questions remain about the multiple mechanisms of TGF-β action in joint tissues, clinical strategies to treat OA must carefully consider the distinct roles of this and other growth factors in each joint compartment.

MECHANICAL CROSS-TALK

The tissues of the joint are comprised of complex extracellular matrices which allow the joint to withstand unique mechanical demands, and the cells within these tissues are highly mechanosensitive. Physical cues, including applied mechanical load, tissue stiffness, osmolarity, and fluid flow, directly affect cells in each joint tissue. To elicit their downstream responses, mechanical cues stimulate a suite of activity on extracellular matrix proteins, ligands, receptors, intracellular effectors, and transcriptional regulators.[38] As joint tissues undergo development or disease, the changing physical environment impacts cellular activity in ways that alter the biological and mechanical homeostasis of the joint.

A precise amount of mechanical stimulation is required for proper function of joint tissues from development onward. In utero, embryonic muscle contractions guide bone shape and connectivity to tendons and ligaments. In cartilage, low-intensity cyclic loading induces aggrecan, represses protease expression, and mitigates the catabolic response of chondrocytes to inflammatory cytokines. Relative to static controls, knee joints undergoing passive motion secrete more hyaluronan into the synovial fluid to lubricate the joint.[39]

Since these mechanosensitive functions are carefully calibrated for a physiologic range of forces, either increases or decreases in normal mechanical stimulation can contribute to a disease phenotype. Humans exposed to bed rest or microgravity rapidly lose bone mass. Hind limb immobilization in rodents induces OA with reduced cartilage proteoglycan content and increased aggrecanase expression. Chondrocytes exposed to injurious load exhibit an inflammatory response, with elevated synthesis of MMP-13, IL-1β, nitric oxide synthase, and prostaglandins.[39] Additionally, changes in the stiffness of extracellular matrix can prime cells for a robust or muted response to ligands like TGF-β.[38] Therefore, both the increased loads associated with joint injury and the offloading of a joint due to pain contribute to the disruption of mechanical homeostasis in joint disease.

In OA, bone remodeling and cartilage degeneration alter the basal mechanical environment of the cell, which elicits changes in cellular signaling through integrins. After binding extracellular matrix proteins, transmembrane integrins assemble an intracellular protein complex, called a focal adhesion. Active signaling complexes at focal adhesions allow integrins to calibrate cellular mechanics, signaling, and function to changes in the physical environment. The protective effects of physiological load on chondrocytes are integrin-dependent, as the response is lost after integrin inhibition and in OA.[39]

©Copyright 2021 American Academy of Orthopaedic Surgeons

Thus, integrin sensing of the mechanical environment has direct effects on cellular activity in the joint.

In addition to aiding the convection of soluble factors between tissues, fluid flow due to mechanical loading serves as a stimulus itself. TRPV4 is a mechanosensitive nonselective, calcium-permeable cation channel that is expressed in cartilage, bone, and synovium. As cartilage is loaded and unloaded in normal locomotion, fluid leaves and enters the tissue causing large fluctuations in osmotic pressure that activate TRPV4 signaling.[40] Mechanosensitive calcium influx through TRPV4 can suppress catabolic and proinflammatory factors and induce Col2a1 gene expression. Systemic loss of TRPV4 function in mice leads to cartilage fibrillation and proteoglycan loss, likely through disruption of joint cross-talk. TRPV4 channels localized at specialized organelles, primary cilia, are particularly important for cellular mechanotransduction.

Articular cartilage, calcified cartilage, and subchondral bone together form a composite that deflects to absorb the energy of applied loads. However, increased thickness of the stiff calcified cartilage and subchondral bone layers during OA limits deflection of these layers, which changes the stress concentrations in the underlying bone and overlying cartilage.[9] A 10% decrease in joint compliance elevates compressive stresses in cartilage by 15% to 20%, potentially shifting chondrocytes from homeostatic mechanosensation to injury responses. As with orthopaedic implants, stiffening of the subchondral plate in OA shields the underlying trabecular bone from stress, which stimulates bone resorption due to its perceived unloading. Changes to trabecular bone volume and the plate-rod ratio ultimately disrupt dissipation of joint loads throughout the skeleton. Accordingly, sites of aberrant subchondral plate thickness and mineralization colocalize with cartilage lesions. Bone marrow lesions also occur most often in the overloaded side of a joint, further supporting mechanical cross-talk among joint tissues.

One unanswered question in OA research is whether posttraumatic OA develops slowly as a result of altered joint biomechanics or in an inflammatory cascade that begins immediately after a mechanical insult. Joint injuries including meniscal tears, ligamentous tears, and intra-articular fractures predispose a joint to osteoarthritic changes nearly 30 years before age-related OA presents.[41] Acute injury causes overloading, inflammation, and tissue degradation, but with or without reconstructive surgeries, instability and chronic low-grade synovitis may persist for years, altering biochemical and mechanical joint cross-talk. Twelve years after anterior cruciate ligament (ACL) rupture, nearly 50% of male and female former soccer players had joint space narrowing and osteophytes regardless of reconstructive surgery, suggesting that the injury matters more than the destabilization.[41] However, multiple studies in animal models suggest that mechanical destabilization of the joint may be sufficient to cause cartilage degradation and bone remodeling. It is likely that with the numerous tissues involved in OA, disruption of any one of them can undermine the normal cross-talk required to keep the entire joint healthy.

HARNESSING JOINT CROSS-TALK FOR THERAPEUTIC TARGETS

Given the evidence of joint cross-talk in the pathogenesis of OA and the current dearth of disease-modifying osteoarthritis drugs (DMOADs), the search for new therapies has increasingly shifted from cartilage to other affected joint tissues, including subchondral bone and synovium. Additionally, radiographic evidence of OA, such as joint space narrowing, poorly correlates with pain,[42] suggesting that clinical improvements in some widely used clinical outcome measures of OA may not be sufficient to achieve a therapeutic benefit to patients.

TREATING JOINT DISEASE BY TARGETING SUBCHONDRAL BONE

In light of the evidence of subchondral bone changes preceding cartilage degeneration in OA, particularly an increase in bone remodeling in the early stages of the disease, clinical trials have targeted bone resorption to mitigate OA severity. Many randomized controlled trials (RCTs) have been conducted using diphosphonates, antiresorptive drugs that inhibit osteoclast-mediated bone resorption. We discuss these results in detail because diphosphonates are already in clinical use for treatment of osteoporosis. Therefore, success in RCTs could allow diphosphonates to quickly be employed to treat OA.

Once-daily oral risedronate has been shown to improve pain, function, and stiffness in patients with knee OA, with a trend toward attenuation of joint space narrowing.[43] These patients also demonstrated significantly reduced markers of cartilage degradation and bone resorption, suggesting an arrest of pathologic joint remodeling. A separate study, however, similarly tested the effect of oral risedronate on knee OA, but found that risedronate did not significantly reduce radiographic progression of OA, and while it did reduce pain by 20%, this was also true of patients treated with placebo.[30] While this study also observed a dose-dependent reduction in urinary cartilage degradation markers, it was in the absence of any other observed improvement in OA, demonstrating potential diagnostic limitations of urinary cartilage degradation markers.

The effect of another diphosphonate, zoledronic acid, has been tested in the setting of a single intravenous infusion in patients with knee OA.[44] This study reports temporal effects of diphosphonates on pain and BML size. Pain scores were significantly reduced in patients receiving zoledronic acid compared with placebo after 6 months, but not after 3 or 12 months. Additionally, reduction in total BML area was greater in patients who received zoledronic acid compared with placebo after 6 months, with a trend after 12 months. As mentioned above, BMLs and OA progression are closely linked, so a clinically meaningful reduction in BML area may be a good surrogate outcome for OA progression and indicate potential

©Copyright 2021 American Academy of Orthopaedic Surgeons

efficacy for treatment. Interestingly, the findings from this study were specific to one of two pain scales, highlighting the relative subjectivity of these scales and emphasizing the importance of the chosen pain scale in evaluating drug efficacy.

While these studies reinforce the importance of joint cross-talk and show clinical promise on their own, a meta-analysis of RCTs showed that diphosphonate treatment of OA provides no significant benefit over placebo in pain relief, functional improvement, or prevention of radiographic progression.[45] It did find, however, that diphosphonates displayed no significant differences in adverse outcomes relative to placebo groups. These mixed results might reflect the need to identify the subset of OA patients with a disease course that may benefit from targeting bone resorption. If used earlier in OA progression in patients with a specific etiology, diphosphonates may show more success and could be a good DMOAD option given their safety profile.

Two phase III clinical trials of symptomatic knee OA testing the efficacy of treating OA with oral calcitonin also had mixed results.[46] Calcitonin, also an antiresorptive, inhibits bone resorption by binding to and activating the calcitonin receptor on osteoclasts. Each of these clinical trials demonstrated a comparable reduction in pain, function, and stiffness scores in the treatment and placebo groups, with no effect on joint space narrowing. The modest effects of calcitonin on markers of cartilage degradation and bone resorption did not correspond with changes in other OA outcomes.

Strontium ranelate, also used as an osteoporosis drug, inhibits bone resorption and induces bone formation. In an RCT, patients with knee OA received daily strontium ranelate for three years to observe its effect on OA progression. Strontium ranelate limited joint space narrowing over the course of the study and improved pain outcomes.[47] Further stratification of patients from this study identified a relationship between BMLs, a pathologic feature that predicts OA progression to total knee arthroplasty, and efficacy of strontium ranelate.[48] As strontium ranelate reduced BML size, this treatment may limit joint deterioration enough to protect or delay some OA patients from requiring a total knee arthroplasty.

Studies employing antiresorptives to treat OA in clinical trials have provided mixed results at best. With our current understanding of OA progression, antiresorptives would be most effective in early disease, a time at which patients may be asymptomatic. This poses a challenge of identifying patients to treat and suggests that some patients in these clinical trials may have OA that is too advanced to benefit from antiresorptive therapy. Longitudinal data on patients undergoing antiresorptive treatment are needed to answer these questions.

TREATING JOINT DISEASE BY TARGETING SYNOVIUM

Due to the association of synovitis with OA development, as well as the relative success in targeting local and systemic inflammation in the treatment of rheumatoid arthritis, clinical trials have tested the effect of inflammation-suppressing drugs, such as corticosteroids, on OA. Despite the hypothesis that reducing synovitis may attenuate OA, an RCT that administered intra-articular triamcinolone every 12 weeks for 2 years found that, relative to placebo, this corticosteroid failed to reduce knee pain and exacerbated cartilage loss.[49] Although intra-articular corticosteroid injection is commonly used clinically for short-term pain relief, treating OA with sustained intra-articular corticosteroids is not effective and could instead worsen the disease.

An RCT studying the effect of chondroitin sulfate, a glycosaminoglycan with both anti-inflammatory effects and direct effects on chondrocytes in vitro, found that patients who received chondroitin sulfate had significantly reduced BML area and cartilage volume loss than those who received placebo.[50] Interestingly, between treated and control groups, no differences were detected in synovial thickness or pain, as assessed by two different pain scores. These findings reinforce the discordance between radiographic outcomes, such as BMLs and cartilage volume, and the experience of pain. Successful therapeutics will need to consider each of these outcomes to demonstrate efficacy in treating OA. Better understanding of the role of the synovium in OA could advance the development of new therapies that more effectively prevent cartilage degeneration while improving joint pain.

TREATING JOINT DISEASE BY TARGETING PAIN

The complex relationship between cartilage degeneration and joint pain poses a significant problem for the development of DMOADs.[42] Some clinical trials have, instead of targeting cartilage, bone, or synovium, specifically treated OA pain using nonsteroidal anti-inflammatory drugs (NSAIDs) or inhibitors of nerve growth factor. Meta-analysis of NSAID treatment for OA, specifically considering the cyclooxygenase-2 prostaglandin synthase inhibitor celecoxib, demonstrates a small improvement in pain.[51] This benefit was no longer significant when the meta-analysis considered only high-quality clinical trials. Other pain-specific treatments have targeted nerve growth factor, which is produced in the synovium in OA and is stimulated by IL-1β and TNF-α to further induce proliferation of the synovium.[21] Expression of nerve growth factor by osteoclasts in osteochondral channels is also strongly associated with pain in OA.[52] Tanezumab, a humanized monoclonal antibody that binds to and inhibits nerve growth factor, has been tested as an analgesic for knee OA. Patients who received tanezumab had a reduction in joint pain and improvement in function when compared with placebo, with mild and moderate adverse events.[53] Radiographic OA progression was not assessed.

While some treatments effectively reduce pain, none meaningfully prevent or delay OA progression. In fact, the combined use of NSAIDs with inhibitory nerve growth factor antibodies increased the prevalence of rapidly progressive OA.[54] These findings reinforce the idea that pain is an

©Copyright 2021 American Academy of Orthopaedic Surgeons

important physiological process, and specifically reducing pain in the absence of other disease-modifying benefits may paradoxically worsen OA. Analysis of serological biomarkers is underway in patients from the tanezumab study, in an effort to predict which patients will benefit and which may be predisposed to rapidly progressive OA.[54]

TREATING JOINT DISEASE BY INCREASING BONE-CARTILAGE CROSS-TALK

Microfracture, a technique in which small holes are drilled through a cartilage defect and into the subchondral plate, is used in some cases of OA and osteochondral defects to surgically induce physical cross-talk within the joint.[55] These holes permit the exchange of marrow contents into the joint, and synovial fluid into the marrow space, in a procedure that stimulates formation of a "superclot" within the cartilage defect. This migration of marrow stromal cells and growth factors yields a largely fibrocartilaginous repair tissue within the cartilage defect. However, microfracture has been shown to increase bone tissue overgrowth, subchondral bone cyst formation, and subchondral plate fragility. While patients can experience short-term functional improvements, microfracture has not demonstrated long-term efficacy and patients still often require total joint arthroplasty.

IMPROVING THERAPEUTIC APPROACHES

Many of the above-mentioned treatments have attenuated the phenotype of OA in animals, but none have successfully delayed or prevented OA in humans. These paradoxical findings highlight the need for further research, especially to elucidate the mechanisms of cross-talk among tissues in the healthy joint and in OA. The lack of success in developing DMOADs brings to light a few key areas for improvement.

Even though OA is considered one disease, it can arise from several originating causes, including joint injury, obesity, and age, among others. Joint cross-talk is one of the processes that may result in a common disease outcome, as dysregulation of any individual tissue can trigger pathological behaviors in others. Given the multiple OA phenotypes, certain therapeutic approaches may be more efficacious in some etiologies than in others. Additional research is needed to better understand these OA phenotypes, diagnose them in humans, and stratify treatments accordingly.

While it is becoming increasingly important to elucidate the longitudinal disease progression to determine the appropriate time of intervention, current radiographic standards are unable to detect the relative stage of OA. Additionally, patients often present at the clinic with prolonged pain, at which point OA may have progressed past the opportunity for successful interventional treatment. Longitudinal MRI tracking of joint outcomes, such as BMLs and synovitis, may improve detection of early OA in time for patients to benefit from certain therapeutics.

The limitations of observing disease progression in humans underscore the importance of animal studies to test the causal role of joint cross-talk mechanisms. However, current outcomes of OA in animals may not be representative of disease in humans. For instance, histologic evidence of cartilage degeneration tracks with OA severity in animal models, but not necessarily in humans, where a reduction in cartilage degradation has little to no relationship to pain.[30] Development of OA animal models that better recapitulate human disease is needed.

Finally, pain is a fundamental symptom of joint disease that plays a complex, and incompletely understood, role in OA. Consequently, current outcome measures in clinical trials, such as pain assessment scores, radiographic joint space narrowing, or cartilage volume, may not be appropriate to determine if a given therapeutic is disease-modifying. Radiologic assessment of OA and pain are poorly correlated,[42] and placebo can result in a marked amelioration of pain. Furthermore, RCTs have employed distinct pain scores to evaluate pain improvement, which can complicate drawing conclusions about the effect of a specific treatment on pain, especially in meta-analyses. The design of future basic and clinical research requires further consideration of OA pain, and its causes and treatments.

SUMMARY

In conclusion, the multiple tissues in the joint interact through sophisticated mechanisms of biological and mechanical cross-talk. In the healthy joint, this cross-talk coordinates the function of each tissue to work together as an integrated whole. However, in joint disease, this cross-talk is one mechanism by which damage to one tissue can lead to the progressive cycle of joint destruction that causes OA. With an improved understanding of these cross-talk mechanisms, the ability to therapeutically intervene in this degenerative cycle will be improved, especially in early stage OA.

REFERENCES

1. Muratovic D, Cicuttini F, Wluka A, et al: Bone marrow lesions detected by specific combination of MRI sequences are associated with severity of osteochondral degeneration. *Arthritis Res Ther* 2016;18:54. doi:10.1186/s13075-016-0953-x.
2. Taljanovic MS, Graham AR, Benjamin JB, et al: Bone marrow edema pattern in advanced hip osteoarthritis: Quantitative assessment with magnetic resonance imaging and correlation with clinical examination, radiographic findings, and histopathology. *Skelet Radiol* 2008;37:423-431. doi:10.1007/s00256-008-0446-3.
3. Roemer FW, Kwoh CK, Hannon MJ, et al: What comes first? Multitissue involvement leading to radiographic osteoarthritis: Magnetic resonance imaging-based trajectory analysis over four years in the osteoarthritis initiative. *Arthritis Rheumatol* 2015:67;2085-2096. doi:10.1002/art.39176.
4. Felson DT, Parkes MJ, Marjanovic EJ, et al: Bone marrow lesions in knee osteoarthritis change in 6-12 weeks. *Osteoarthr Cartil* 2012;20:1514-1518. doi:10.1016/j.joca.2012.08.020.

©Copyright 2021 American Academy of Orthopaedic Surgeons

5. Callaghan MJ, Parkes MJ, Hutchinson CE, et al: A randomised trial of a brace for patellofemoral osteoarthritis targeting knee pain and bone marrow lesions. *Ann Rheum Dis* 2015;74:1164-1170. doi:10.1136/annrheumdis-2014-206376.
6. Goldring SR, Goldring MB: Changes in the osteochondral unit during osteoarthritis: Structure, function and cartilage bone crosstalk. *Nat Rev Rheumatol* 2016;12:632-644. doi:10.1038/nrrheum.2016.148.
7. Chen Y, Hu Y, Yu YE, et al: Subchondral trabecular rod loss and plate thickening in the development of osteoarthritis. *J Bone Miner Res* 2018;33:316-327. doi:10.1002/jbmr.3313.
8. Aaron RK, Racine JR, Voisinet A, Evangelista P, Dyke JP: Subchondral bone circulation in osteoarthritis of the human knee. *Osteoarthr Cartil* 2018;26:940-944. doi:10.1016/j.joca.2018.04.003.
9. Burr DB, Gallant MA: Bone remodelling in osteoarthritis. *Nat Rev Rheumatol* 2012;8:665-673. doi:10.1038/nrrheum.2012.130.
10. Boyde A, Davis GR, Mills D, et al: On fragmenting, densely mineralised acellular protrusions into articular cartilage and their possible role in osteoarthritis. *J Anat* 2014;225:436-446. doi:10.1111/joa.12226.
11. Felson DT, Gale DR, Elon Gale M, et al: Osteophytes and progression of knee osteoarthritis. *Rheumatology* 2005;44:100-104. doi:10.1093/rheumatology/keh411.
12. Duncan H, Jundt J, Riddle JM, Pitchford W, Christopherson T: The tibial subchondral plate. A scanning electron microscopic study. *JBJS* 1987;69.
13. Pan J, Wang B, Li W, et al: Elevated cross-talk between subchondral bone and cartilage in osteoarthritic joints. *Bone* 2012;51:212-217. doi:10.1016/j.bone.2011.11.030.
14. Walsh DA, Bonnet CS, Turner EL, et al: Angiogenesis in the synovium and at the osteochondral junction in osteoarthritis. *Osteoarthr Cartil* 2007;15:743-751. doi:10.1016/j.joca.2007.01.020.
15. Suri S, Walsh DA: Osteochondral alterations in osteoarthritis. *Bone* 2012;51:204-211. doi:10.1016/j.bone.2011.10.010.
16. O'Hara BP, Urban JP, Maroudas A: Influence of cyclic loading on the nutrition of articular cartilage. *Ann Rheum Dis* 1990;49:536-539.
17. Bonewald LF: The amazing osteocyte. *J Bone Miner Res* 2011;26:229-238. doi:10.1002/jbmr.320.
18. Fowler TW, Acevedo C, Mazur CM, et al: Glucocorticoid suppression of osteocyte perilacunar remodeling is associated with subchondral bone degeneration in osteonecrosis. *Sci Rep* 2017;7:44618. doi:10.1038/srep44618.
19. Jaiprakash A, Prasadam I, Feng JQ, et al: Phenotypic characterization of osteoarthritic osteocytes from the sclerotic zones: A possible pathological role in subchondral bone sclerosis. *Int J Biol Sci* 2012;8(3):406-417. doi:10.7150/ijbs.4221.
20. Hügle T, Geurts J: What drives osteoarthritis?—synovial versus subchondral bone pathology. *Rheumatology* 2016;56(9):1461-1471. doi:10.1093/rheumatology/kew389.
21. Sellam J, Berenbaum F: The role of synovitis in pathophysiology and clinical symptoms of osteoarthritis. *Nat Rev Rheumatol* 2010;6:625-635. doi:10.1038/nrrheum.2010.159.
22. Mathiessen A, Conaghan PG: Synovitis in osteoarthritis: Current understanding with therapeutic implications. *Arthritis Res Ther* 2017;19:18. doi:10.1186/s13075-017-1229-9.
23. Furman BD, Kimmerling KA, Zura RD, et al: Articular ankle fracture results in increased synovitis, synovial macrophage infiltration, and synovial fluid concentrations of inflammatory cytokines and chemokines. *Arthritis Rheumatol* 2015;67:1234-1239. doi:10.1002/art.39064.
24. Elsaid KA, Fleming BC, Oksendahl HL, et al: Decreased lubricin concentrations and markers of joint inflammation in the synovial fluid of patients with anterior cruciate ligament injury. *Arthritis Rheum* 2008;58:1707-1715. doi:10.1002/art.23495.
25. Benito MJ, Veale DJ, FitzGerald O, van den Berg WB, Bresnihan B: Synovial tissue inflammation in early and late osteoarthritis. *Ann Rheum Dis* 2005;64:1263-1267, doi:10.1136/ard.2004.025270.
26. Krasnokutsky S, Belitskaya-Lévy I, Bencardino J, et al: Quantitative magnetic resonance imaging evidence of synovial proliferation is associated with radiographic severity of knee osteoarthritis. *Arthritis Rheum* 2011;63:2983-2991. doi:10.1002/art.30471.
27. Yusup A, Kaneko H, Liu L, et al: Bone marrow lesions, subchondral bone cysts and subchondral bone attrition are associated with histological synovitis in patients with end-stage knee osteoarthritis: A cross-sectional study. *Osteoarthr Cartil* 2015;23:1858-1864. doi:10.1016/J.JOCA.2015.05.017.
28. Felson DT, Niu J, Neogi T, et al: Synovitis and the risk of knee osteoarthritis: The MOST study. *Osteoarthr Cartil* 2016;24:458-464. doi:10.1016/J.JOCA.2015.09.013.
29. Houard X, Goldring MB, Berenbaum F: Homeostatic mechanisms in articular cartilage and role of inflammation in osteoarthritis. *Curr Rheumatol Rep* 2013;15:375, doi:10.1007/s11926-013-0375-6.
30. Bingham CO, Buckland-Wright JC, Garnero P, et al: Risedronate decreases biochemical markers of cartilage degradation but does not decrease symptoms or slow radiographic progression in patients with medial compartment osteoarthritis of the knee: Results of the two-year multinational knee osteoarthritis structural arthritis study. *Arthritis Rheum* 2006;54:3494-3507. doi:10.1002/art.22160.
31. Schipani E, Ryan HE, Didrickson S, et al: Hypoxia in cartilage: HIF-1alpha is essential for chondrocyte growth arrest and survival. *Genes Dev* 2001;15:2865-2876. doi:10.1101/gad.934301.
32. Yang S, Kim J, Ryu J-H, et al: Hypoxia-inducible factor-2α is a catabolic regulator of osteoarthritic cartilage destruction. *Nat Med* 2010;16:687-693. doi:10.1038/nm.2153.
33. Aaron RK, Racine J, Dyke JP: Contribution of circulatory disturbances in subchondral bone to the pathophysiology of osteoarthritis. *Curr Rheumatol Rep* 2017;19:49. doi:10.1007/s11926-017-0660-x.
34. Jia H, Ma X, Wei Y, et al: Loading-induced reduction in sclerostin as a mechanism of subchondral bone plate sclerosis in mouse knee joints during late-stage osteoarthritis. *Arthritis Rheumatol* 2018;70:230-241, doi:10.1002/art.40351.
35. De Santis M, Di Matteo B, Chisari E, et al: The role of Wnt pathway in the pathogenesis of OA and its potential therapeutic implications in the field of regenerative medicine. *BioMed Res Int* 2018;2018:7402947. doi:10.1155/2018/7402947.
36. Zhen G, Wen C, Jia X, et al: Inhibition of TGF-beta signaling in mesenchymal stem cells of subchondral bone attenuates osteoarthritis. *Nat Med* 2013;19:704-712. doi:10.1038/nm.3143.
37. Chen CG, Thuillier D, Chin EN, Alliston T: Chondrocyte-intrinsic Smad3 represses Runx2-inducible matrix metalloproteinase 13 expression to maintain articular cartilage and prevent osteoarthritis. *Arthritis Rheum* 2012;64:3278-3289, doi:10.1002/art.34566.
38. Rys JP, Monteiro DA, Alliston T: Mechanobiology of TGFbeta signaling in the skeleton. *Matrix Biol* 2016;52-54:413-425, doi:10.1016/j.matbio.2016.02.002.
39. Leong DJ, Hardin JA, Cobelli NJ, Sun HB: Mechanotransduction and cartilage integrity. *Ann N Y Acad Sci* 2011;1240:32-37. doi:10.1111/j.1749-6632.2011.06301.x.
40. Phan MN, Leddy HA, Votta BJ, et al: Functional characterization of TRPV4 as an osmotically sensitive ion channel in porcine articular chondrocytes. *Arthritis Rheum* 2009;60:3028-3037. doi:10.1002/art.24799.
41. Roos EM: Joint injury causes knee osteoarthritis in young adults. *Curr Opin Rheumatol* 2005;17:195-200. doi:10.1097/01.bor.0000151406.64393.00.
42. Claessens AA, Schouten JS, van den Ouweland FA, Valkenburg HA: Do clinical findings associate with radiographic osteoarthritis of the knee? *Ann Rheum Dis* 1990;49:771-774.
43. Spector TD, Conaghan PG, Buckland-Wright JC, et al: Effect of risedronate on joint structure and symptoms of knee osteoarthritis: Results of the BRISK randomized, controlled trial [ISRCTN01928173]. *Arthritis Res Ther* 2005;7:R625-R633. doi:10.1186/ar1716.
44. Laslett LL, Doré DA, Quinn SJ, et al: Zoledronic acid reduces knee pain and bone marrow lesions over 1 year: A randomised controlled trial. *Ann Rheum Dis* 2012;71:1322-1328. doi:10.1136/annrheumdis-2011-200970.
45. Vaysbrot EE, Osani MC, Musetti MC, McAlindon TE, Bannuru RR: Are bisphosphonates efficacious in knee osteoarthritis? A meta-analysis of randomized controlled trials. *Osteoarthr Cartil* 2018;26:154-164. doi:10.1016/J.JOCA.2017.11.013.

©Copyright 2021 American Academy of Orthopaedic Surgeons

46. Karsdal MA, Byrjalsen I, Alexandersen P, et al: Treatment of symptomatic knee osteoarthritis with oral salmon calcitonin: Results from two phase 3 trials. *Osteoarthr Cartil* 2015;23:532-543. doi:10.1016/J.JOCA.2014.12.019.

47. Reginster J-Y, Badurski J, Bellamy N, et al: Efficacy and safety of strontium ranelate in the treatment of knee osteoarthritis: Results of a double-blind, randomised placebo-controlled trial. *Ann Rheum Dis* 2013;72:179-186. doi:10.1136/annrheumdis-2012-202231.

48. Pelletier J-P, Roubille C, Raynauld J-P, et al: Disease-modifying effect of strontium ranelate in a subset of patients from the phase III knee osteoarthritis study SEKOIA using quantitative MRI: Reduction in bone marrow lesions protects against cartilage loss. *Ann Rheum Dis* 2015;74:422-429. doi:10.1136/annrheumdis-2013-203989.

49. McAlindon TE, LaValley MP, Harvey WF, et al: Effect of intra-articular triamcinolone vs saline on knee cartilage volume and pain in patients with knee osteoarthritis. *J Am Med Assoc* 2017;317:1967. doi:10.1001/jama.2017.5283.

50. Wildi LM, Raynauld J-P, Martel-Pelletier J, et al: Chondroitin sulphate reduces both cartilage volume loss and bone marrow lesions in knee osteoarthritis patients starting as early as 6 months after initiation of therapy: A randomised, double-blind, placebo-controlled pilot study using MRI. *Ann Rheum Dis* 2011;70:982-989. doi:10.1136/ard.2010.140848.

51. Gregori D, Giacovelli G, Minto C, et al: Association of pharmacological treatments with long-term pain control in patients with knee osteoarthritis. *J Am Med Assoc* 2018;320:2564. doi:10.1001/jama.2018.19319.

52. Aso K, Shahtaheri SM, Hill R, et al: Associations of symptomatic knee osteoarthritis with histopathologic features in subchondral bone. *Arthritis Rheumatol* 2019;71:916-924. doi:10.1002/art.40820.

53. Lane NE, Schnitzer TJ, Birbara CA, et al: Tanezumab for the treatment of pain from osteoarthritis of the knee. *N Engl J Med* 2010;363:1521-1531. doi:10.1056/NEJMoa0901510.

54. Karsdal MA, Verburg KM, West CR, et al: Serological biomarker profiles of rapidly progressive osteoarthritis in tanezumab-treated patients. *Osteoarthr Cartil* 2019;27:484-492. doi:10.1016/J.JOCA.2018.12.001.

55. Green CJ, Beck A, Wood D, Zheng MH: The biology and clinical evidence of microfracture in hip preservation surgery. *J Hip Preserv Surg* 2016;3:108-123. doi:10.1093/jhps/hnw007.

©Copyright 2021 American Academy of Orthopaedic Surgeons

17

The Intervertebral Disk

Jeffrey C. Lotz, PhD
Aaron J. Fields, PhD
Andrew K. Chan, MD
Alexander M. Ballatori, BS

Keywords: *degenerative disk disease; disk degeneration; intervertebral disk; IVD; pathophysiology of intervertebral disk degeneration*

INTRODUCTION

The intervertebral disk (IVD) is a fibrocartilaginous joint in the vertebral column that serves unique functional roles. It allows for multiaxial movement, while supporting the compressive forces exerted onto the spine. IVD degeneration is age-associated and can be accelerated by multiple, integrated mechanical and biological mechanisms. IVD degeneration is thought to be a leading cause of back pain, either directly as a pain generator or indirectly via diminished biomechanical properties and consequent alterations in adjacent tissue stresses. The goal of this chapter is to provide a summary of the fundamental characteristics of the IVD and processes involved with physiologic (age-related) and pathologic (painful) degeneration.

Dr. Lotz or an immediate family member has received royalties from Relievant MedSystems; has stock or stock options held in Bioniks, LLC, ISTO Technologies, Nocimed, LLC, Relievant MedSystems, and SMC Biotech; and has received research or institutional support from DePuy, A Johnson & Johnson Company, and Orthofix, Inc. Dr. Chan has received nonincome support (such as equipment or services), commercially derived honoraria, or other non–research-related funding (such as paid travel) from Orthofix, Inc. Dr. Ballatori or an immediate family member serves as a board member, owner, officer, or committee member of the American Academy of Orthopaedic Surgeons. Neither Dr. Fields nor any immediate family member has received anything of value from or has stock or stock options held in a commercial company or institution related directly or indirectly to the subject of this chapter.

ANATOMY

The spinal column is composed of 33 vertebrae comprising five distinct regions: the cervical, thoracic, lumbar, sacral vertebrae, and the coccyx. At the most cephalad extent, the cervical spine is composed of seven vertebrae and assumes a lordotic curvature. Below that, the thoracic spine is composed of 12 vertebrae and assumes a kyphotic curvature. Caudally, the lumbar spine is composed of five vertebrae and assumes a lordotic curvature. Together, these regions give rise to the "S"-shaped characteristic curve of the spinal column. Next, the five, fused sacral vertebrae form a portion of the pelvis. At the most caudal extent of the spinal column, four small, fused vertebrae form the coccyx. Each vertebra is composed of an anterior portion (vertebral body) and a posterior arch which is formed by the pedicle, facet, lamina, and spinous process (**Figure 1**, A). The vertebral body is composed of an inner region of cancellous bone surrounded by a thin shell of cortical bone.

Each successive vertebra is connected via multiple points: anteriorly via the IVD (separating the vertebral bodies) (**Figure 1**, B) and posteriorly via the facet joints. Additional soft-tissue structures provide passive support, including the anterior longitudinal ligament, the posterior longitudinal ligament, the ligamentum flavum, the facet joint capsule, the interspinous ligament, and the supraspinous ligaments (**Figure 1**, C). The spinal column is also stabilized by a set of paraspinal muscles that include the erector spinae that runs longitudinally on the dorsal surface of the spinal column and functions to extend the spine; the psoas that runs longitudinally on the ventrolateral surface of the spinal column and serves to flex the hip (bilateral contraction) or laterally bend the trunk (unilateral contraction); and the multifidus that connects intersegmentally to stabilize the spine by acting like a bowstring to maintain lordosis.

©Copyright 2021 American Academy of Orthopaedic Surgeons

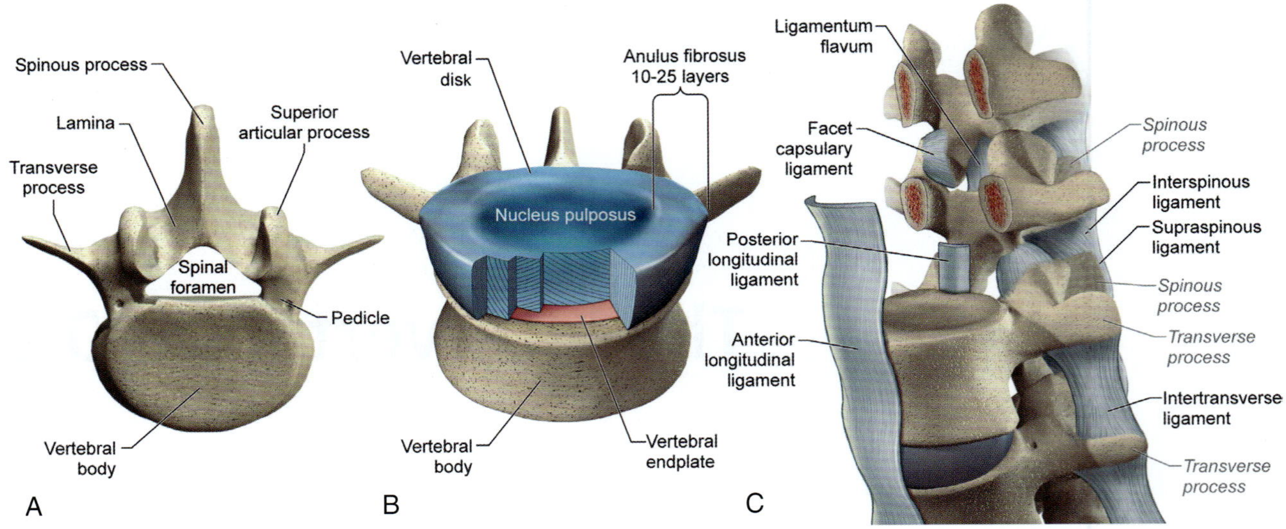

FIGURE 1 Anatomic illustrations of the human intervertebral disk (IVD) and vertebral body. **A**, Cranial-caudal view of the lumbar vertebra depicting the vertebral body and posterior arch. **B**, IVD with partially removed anulus fibrosus (AF) revealing the cartilage end plate. **C**, Spinal segment demonstrating the multiple ligaments that facilitate proper alignment during multiaxial movement.

Except between the atlas (C1) and the axis (C2), the IVD separates each successive vertebral body and provides a unique combination of compressive stiffness and flexibility to support normal spine biomechanics. It is composed of an inner nucleus pulposus (NP) and an outer ring termed the anulus fibrosus (AF) (**Figure 1**, B). The NP serves as an osmotic pump to attract water and generate hydraulic pressure when subjected to significant loads during activities of daily living. The AF encapsulates the gelatinous NP and provides the mechanical support to both contain NP pressure and constrain intervertebral rotations. The outer AF is integrated with the vertebral rim via a fibrocartilage enthesis that consists of a thin layer of calcified cartilage, or "tidemark." The end plate (EP) is a bilayer of cartilage and bone that separates the disk from adjacent vertebrae.[1] The cartilage EP integrates with the inner AF to fully encapsulate the NP. The EP facilitates important but potentially conflicting biophysical functions: it must be strong and thick to resist significant loads but must also be permeable to favor chemical transport and disk cellular vitality.[1]

COMPOSITION

The disk extracellular matrix (ECM) is maintained by a mixed population of cells and is finely tuned to meet disk biomechanical demands. Although the basic biochemical components of the NP, the AF, and the EP are generally the same, that is, water, proteoglycans (PG), and collagens, their relative proportions differ between structural domains (**Table 1**),[2] although these proportions change dramatically with aging and disk degeneration. The composition of the healthy ECM varies gradually along the radial direction with the central NP having the highest water/PG and lowest collagen/elastin content and the outer AF having the lowest water/PG and highest collagen/elastin content. Moving cranially and caudally, the EP has the lowest water/PG and the highest collagen content.

TABLE 1 Approximate Relative Proportion of the Four Main Extracellular Matrix (ECM) Components of the Adult Human IVD.

	Nucleus Pulposus (%)	Anulus Fibrosus (%)	Cartilage End Plate
Water	77	60	55%
Proteoglycan	14	5	8%
Collagen	4	15	25%
Elastin	<1	<10	<1%

Data from Urban JP, Roberts S: Chemistry of the intervertebral disc in relation to functional requirements. *Grieve's Mod Man Ther* 1994:163-75.

The major PG of the IVD is aggrecan, a large molecule with a molecular weight ranging from 3,000 to 7,000 kDa. Aggrecan structure is comprised of a linear core protein with large numbers of sulfated glycosaminoglycan (GAG) side chains, which carry a net negative charge. These GAGs bind mobile ions (mostly sodium) and thereby generate an osmotic pressure that attracts water and produces physical pressure to support spinal compression. The tendency of the PG network to swell and generate osmotic pressure is resisted circumferentially by tension in the network of collagen fibrils in the AF, which holds the NP together and anchors the periphery of the disk to the subchondral bone. The fraction of aggrecans decreases with degeneration, as proteolytic degradation of the link protein by matrix metalloproteinases (MMPs) increases PG fragmentation.

©Copyright 2021 American Academy of Orthopaedic Surgeons

Collagen type I and II make up approximately 90% of total IVD collagen.[3] Each molecule consists of three polypeptide chains, or alpha chains, twisted into a triple helix (300 nm long, 1.5 nm diameter). Individual molecules assemble end-on-end and side-by-side to form microfibrils. The NP, EP, and inner AF consist almost exclusively of type II fibrils, which are very fine (10 to 100 nm in diameter) in comparison to the larger type I fibrils (100 to 200 nm in diameter) that predominate in the AF and increase in relative proportion peripherally. The differences in the relative proportions of type I and type II collagen among the NP, AF, and EP hint at the predominant loading experienced by each structure of the disk: collagen type I is usually found in tensile structures such as ligaments, whereas collagen type II is normal in compressed tissues like articular cartilage. In the NP, the collagen fibers are irregularly oriented and outnumber PGs by approximately 20:1; in the AF, they are organized into 10 to 25 unidirectionally aligned concentric lamellae, which encircle the NP and attach to the cartilage EP in the inner zone and to the vertebral EP in the outer zone (**Figure 1**, B). Alignment alternates between +30° and −30° with respect to the circumferential direction of the IVD.

The cartilage EP is typically between 0.1 and 2.0 mm thick[4]; however, its thickness is known to vary with position and level, being thinner centrally and in the upper levels of the spine than peripherally and in the lower levels of the spine.[4] The nature of the structural integration between the EP and the surrounding tissues also varies with position. Peripherally, the collagen fibers in the lamellae of the AF are continuous with the collagen fibers in the EP, whereas centrally, the integration between collagen fibers in the NP and the EP is more convoluted.[4] The collagen fibers of the cartilaginous and bony components of the EP are completely separate.[4]

Elastin is the third and relatively less abundant structural protein in the disk. These fine, extensible fibers predominate in the AF, where they are organized in a crisscross pattern between neighboring lamellae (**Figure 2**). This pattern suggests that elastin helps resist radial expansion of the NP during disk compression by regulating interlamellar sliding or shearing movements.

Advanced glycation end-products (AGEs), often called nonenzymatic "cross-links," play structural and biological roles with increasing importance in the aging disk. One pathway of cross-link formation is via nonenzymatic glycation of

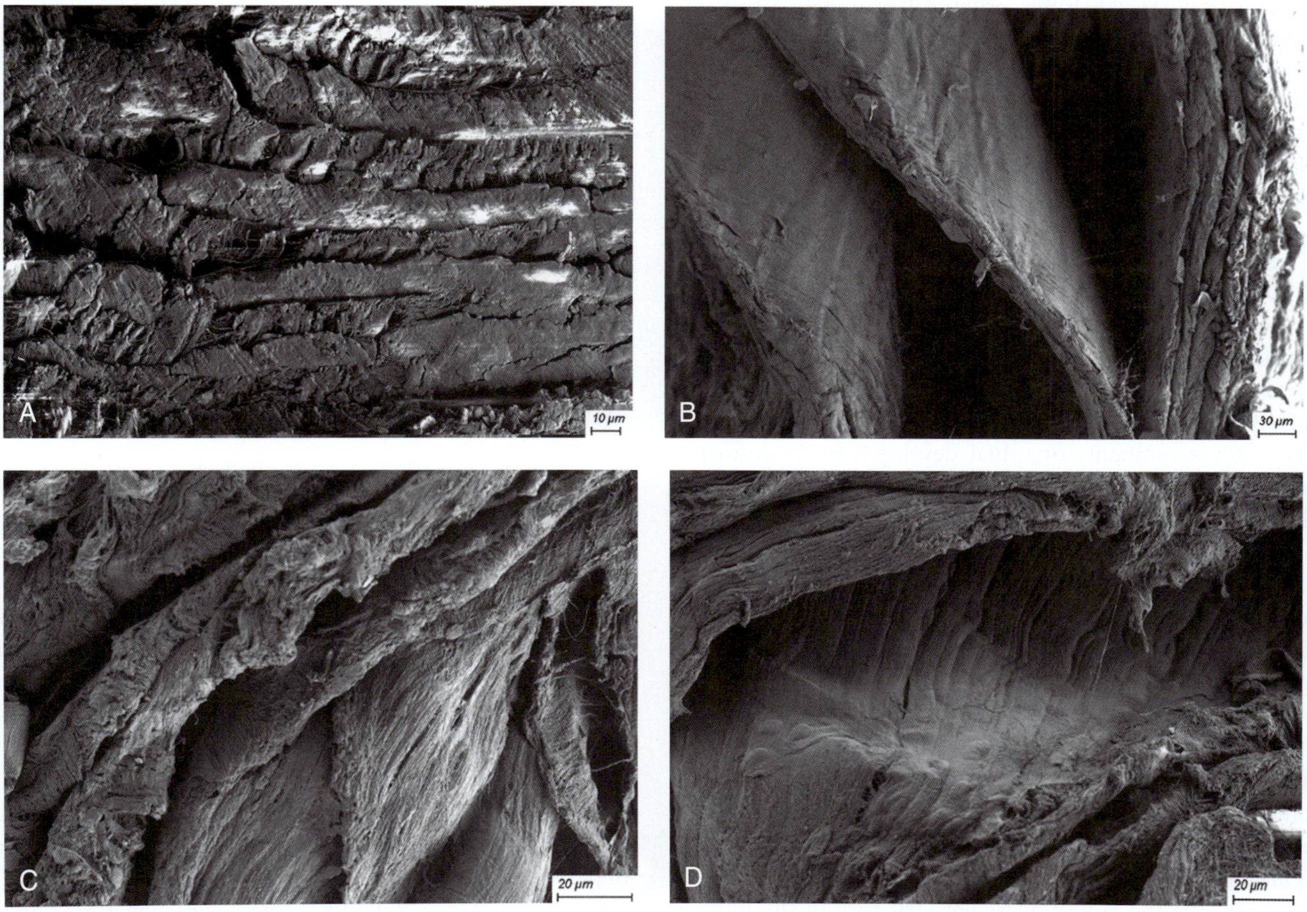

FIGURE 2 High-resolution scanning electron microscopy (SEM) images illustrating lamellar structure within the anulus fibrosus (AF) of a rat coccygeal disk. **A**, Transverse cut through the AF showing alternating type I collagen fibril orientations between adjacent lamellae. **B**, Lamellae with fine elastin cross-bridges. **C** and **D**, Oblique cut through the AF showing highly aligned intralamellar collagen fibrils.

©Copyright 2021 American Academy of Orthopaedic Surgeons

the free amino groups of proteins and lipids by reducing sugars. The cross-link formation is irreversible, and thus, long-lived proteins like collagen are especially susceptible to AGE accumulation. In normal disks, AGE accumulation has been shown to increase with age, trigger catabolic actions within disk cells, reduce disk hydration, and increase disk tissue stiffness.[5] Hyperglycemic conditions like diabetes accelerate the ordinarily slow rate of endogenous glycation by increasing the availability of sugars that can attach to the amino groups leading to accelerated disk degeneration.[5]

The most abundant nonstructural proteins in the IVD are the families of MMPs (matrix-metalloproteinases), TIMPs (tissue inhibitors of metalloproteinases), and ADAMTS (A Disintegrin and Metalloproteinase with Thrombospondin Motifs). These zinc-dependent proteinases, which are regulated in part by cytokines, increase during disk degeneration, leading to increased cleavage of the ECM.

Degenerative processes compromise both the biological and mechanical functions of the ECM. Enzymatic degradation of NP PG reduces osmotic pressure. This is typically concurrent with increased collagen production and increased AGE levels that combine to decrease swelling and water content. These ECM changes associate with age and can be accelerated by excessive physical loading,[6] where adverse tissue stress can damage matrix and trigger altered biological activities, that in turn cause NP fibrosis and disorganization of the AF architecture. ECM biochemical changes and damage accumulation can stimulate inflammatory cellular responses that promote a cascade of further structural modifications that progressively compromise disk biomechanics.

BIOLOGY

Compared with other tissues, relatively few disk cells maintain an extensive ECM. IVD cells are a mixed population across the NP, AF and EP.[7] At birth, the NP contains notochordal cells that are remnants of spinal development. In humans, notochordal cells are gradually replaced by chondrocyte-like cells over the first two decades of life. This conversion is initiated by notochordal cell apoptosis caused by a combination of increased pressure from gravity loading, plus decreases in nutrition secondary to changes in adjacent vertebral perfusion.[8] Subsequently, cells from either the cartilage EP or inner anulus migrate to fill the NP.[9]

NP cells are chondrocytic and synthesize aggrecan and collagen II as the main structural proteins. By contrast, AF cells are fibrocytic and make type I, II, III, and VI collagen along with chondroitin and keratin sulfate. The cartilage EP is mainly composed of chondrocyte-like cells that mainly secrete PG and type II collagen.

The IVD is the largest avascular structure in the human body, with a distance of up to 6 to 8 mm between cells and the nearest blood supply.[10] Therefore, nutrient supply and drainage of metabolic products rely on diffusion between the IVD cells and the capillary endings of the vascular network that terminates in the outer AF and in the bony EP. The diffusion rate depends on the microstructure and composition of the transport route, the rate of cellular consumption, and on the biochemical properties of the solute (size, shape, and charge). The EP has a higher permeability in the central NP zone, which is essential to maintain a sustainable metabolite transport to and from the NP cells. Competition for nutrients limits cell density to approximately 1,600 cells/mm.[3] Because the disk tissue oxygen levels are low (0.5% to 5%), disk cells create energy via glycolysis, which utilizes glucose and generates lactic acid. Disk dehydration and EP sclerosis impair diffusion, as these changes reduce the effective pore size of the ECM and hinder solute transport.[11,12] Impaired diffusion promotes cell death and disk degeneration because of nutrient deprivation, mainly oxygen and glucose, and accumulation of metabolic products, mainly lactic acid.

In addition to nutrient availability and the accumulation of metabolic waste products, disk cell function is influenced by spinal load and consequent matrix deformations. The healthy disk nucleus is largely water and, consequently, is subjected to hydrostatic pressure during spinal loading. NP cells can rapidly detect and respond to fluctuations in hydrostatic pressure. By contrast, the outer AF in the healthy disk is generally subjected to biaxial loading and AF cells are exquisitely sensitive to stretch. Matrix loading also stimulates cells indirectly by compacting matrix, which decreases tissue permeability, water content, oxygen tension, and pH. These changes can alter both PG and collagen synthesis. Data from both organ- and cell-level studies suggest the existence of optimal loading regimens, where both excessive and negligible pressure/stretch responses are catabolic, which may underlie the U-shaped relationship between physical exposure and back pain, where both low and high exposures are observed to be detrimental.

BIOMECHANICS

The spinal column supports the torso mass and facilitates trunk movement. By itself, the spinal column is inherently unstable, and it will buckle under axial compressive loading. In life, the column's static and dynamic stability is determined by synergy between passive constraints (defined by osteoligamentous tissues such as the vertebra, facet joints, IVD, and intervertebral ligaments) and active constraints (defined by muscles such as the psoas, erector spinae, and multifidus). The passive constraints transmit the forces generated by muscle contraction. Additionally, the passive constraints provide for muscular antagonism, which enables the force of muscle contraction to re-elongate their antagonists. The contribution of passive and active stiffness varies at each spinal level.[13] The clinical importance of active stiffness is demonstrated by the fact that the cross-sectional area of the paraspinal muscles is smaller in low back pain patients compared with healthy subjects.[14] This may be because muscle weakness and fatigue leads

©Copyright 2021 American Academy of Orthopaedic Surgeons

to changes in muscle recruitment patterns, increases in spinal force, and decreases in spinal stability.

The combined action of muscle contraction and gravity cause the lumbar disks to be among the most highly loaded tissues in the body. These disks routinely experience compressive pressures in the 2 MPa range and as high as 3 MPa under extreme activities such as weight lifting during flexion.[15] Diurnal fluctuations can be significant. For example, during sleep, pressures decrease to 0.1 MPa, and during quiet standing 0.5 MPa[15] (**Figure 3**). Disk loading also compacts adjacent vertebral bone and creates a multiaxial stress state in the EP that involves biaxial tensile stretching in the transverse plane.[16] Bone tissue is inherently weaker in tension than in compression, which may partly explain why the EP is the "weak link" during excessive spinal compression.

Together, nuclear pressure plus EP and AF tension support spinal loads and provide resistance to bending, torsion, and shear. Yet, the pressure/tension balance is time-dependent because the EP is semi-permeable and allows water movement out of the disk when spinal stress exceeds nuclear swelling

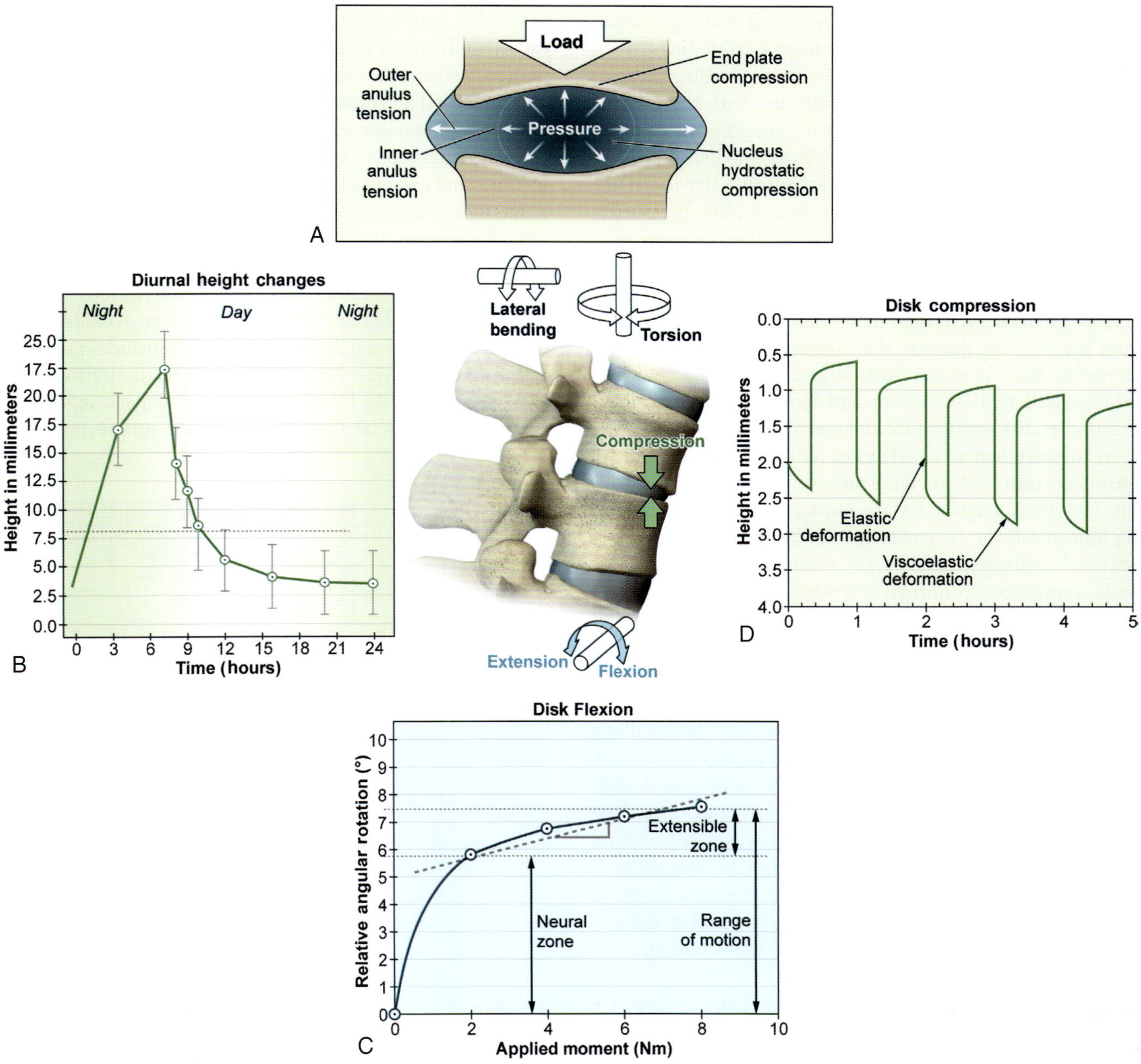

FIGURE 3 Experimental data examples. **A**, The multiaxial biomechanical behaviors of the intervertebral disk (IVD) are nonlinear and time dependent. **B**, Diurnal fluctuations of load and corresponding effects on disk height—height gain at night when osmotic pressure exceeds spine stress and vice versa. **C**, The spine response to bending is nonlinear, with increasing stiffness with increasing bending angle. **D**, Cyclic compression and unloading of the disk demonstrates an immediate elastic height loss followed by a viscoelastic deformation when the load held constant.

©Copyright 2021 American Academy of Orthopaedic Surgeons

pressure, and vice versa.[17] Additionally, the disk's extracellular solid-fluid interactions further contribute to time-varying (viscoelastic) behavior that underlie diurnal variations (**Figure 3**) in disk water content, disk height, and spinal flexibility. For example, sustained compression during activities of daily living results in loss of stature of 15 to 25 mm, contributed in large part by decreases in spine length. Even low-impact activities, such as gentle walking, have been shown to decrease stature significantly, although more strenuous exercise, work-related activities, and high body mass exacerbate this loss.[18,19] These stature changes are primarily attributed to the redistribution of the fluid, which compacts the disk matrix. At night, when the spine is relatively unloaded, the elevated swelling pressure of the disk causes it to imbibe water from surrounding tissues, increasing stature. As disk tissue rehydrates, swelling pressure falls until it again approaches equilibrium with the external mechanical load. These diurnal loading changes cause significant daily variations in disk volume (approximately 10%).

In addition to governing biomechanical behavior at the whole disk level, the interplay between nucleus pressurization and annular stretching is critical for tissue homeostasis. Static loads induce fluid shifts that reduce NP volume, which causes the AF to function more as a compression-bearing strut than as a biaxially stretched membrane.[20] As fluid is expelled from the PG-rich nucleus, the matrix and cells consolidate, ultimately leading to deregulated gene expression,[20] including increased MMP activation, and apoptosis.[21] These cellular effects alter disk architecture and mechanics.

In contrast, beneficial effects of NP pressurization and AF tension are observed when the disk is subjected to cyclic loading. Low load magnitudes are most amenable to maintaining homeostatic stress environments in the NP and AF over extended loading durations. For example, under low cyclic loads comparable to normal activities, NP cells exhibit little alteration in expression of genes that would lead to matrix remodeling, regardless of loading frequency. Similarly, AF cells undergo a low level of apoptosis and exhibit depressed expression of certain catabolic factors such as MMPs and ADAMTSs.[22] High magnitudes of stress can be similarly accommodated for brief durations and frequencies, near 1 Hz. However, if applied at low frequency or long durations, high compression magnitudes lead to a shift in cell function and tissue morphology. Under these circumstances, NP cells respond via upregulation of genes associated with ECM remodeling,[23] leading to decreases in disk height and mechanical stability. In the AF, lower loading frequencies also cause a shift in the balance of gene expression toward a more catabolic profile.

PATHOPHYSIOLOGY

IVD degeneration involves a permanent alteration to the rates of matrix production and degradation such that the NP and AF are impaired in their ability to perform their physiologic biomechanical functions. Clinically, disk degeneration seen on MRI or radiographic imaging oftentimes associates with pain, stiffness, or progressive regional dysfunction of the spine and is observed at higher rates in individuals with known risk factors (**Figure 4**). As mentioned above, coupled alterations in the mechanical and biological environments of the NP or AF trigger a cascade of aberrant cellular responses, including dedifferentiation of NP and AF cells and altered matrix metabolism that further compromises the mechanical environment.

Disk degeneration is a physiologic, age-related chronic matrix remodeling process. It generally begins in the second decade of life coincident with the disappearance of notochordal cells from the NP, and reductions in GAG typically progress at 3% to 4% per year, being fastest at the lowest level, L5/S1, where biomechanical demands are the greatest. Degeneration of at least one level is present in almost all elderly (eg, >60 years) individuals.

The earliest and most conspicuous feature of disk degeneration is loss of nuclear water due to reductions in swelling pressure. Dehydration, in turn, triggers a cascade of effects both intrinsic and extrinsic to the disk. Nuclear dehydration causes reductions of disk height, stress shielding of the inner AF, redistribution of compressive stress over the vertebral EP, motion segment hypermobility, and facet overloading. Over time, the NP and inner AF become indistinct as the nucleus becomes more fibrotic while the AF lamellae denature. Annular weakening leads to internal disk disruption that includes radial and circumferential fissures plus EP cartilage disruptions/erosions and avulsions, bony EP fractures, and tidemark separations (**Figure 5**). As disk continues to degenerate, progressive height

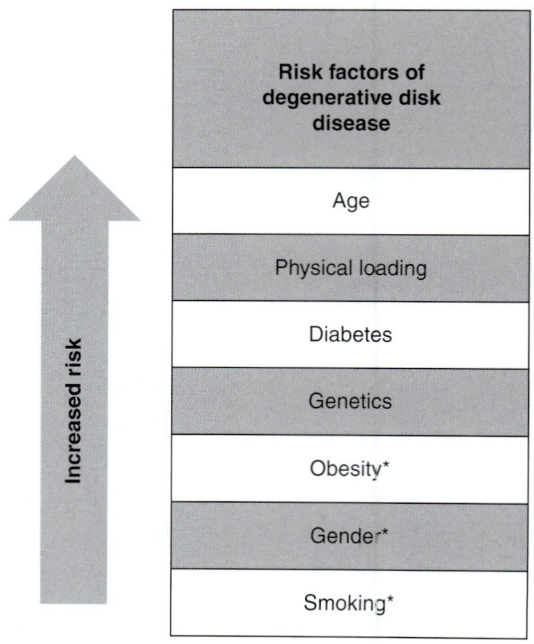

FIGURE 4 Illustration depicting the known risk factors of degenerative disk disease (DDD) in increasing order of the strength of evidence (lowest at the bottom, highest at the top). Risk factors with an asterisk (*) possess conflicting evidence in literature but have shown positive associations with DDD.

©Copyright 2021 American Academy of Orthopaedic Surgeons

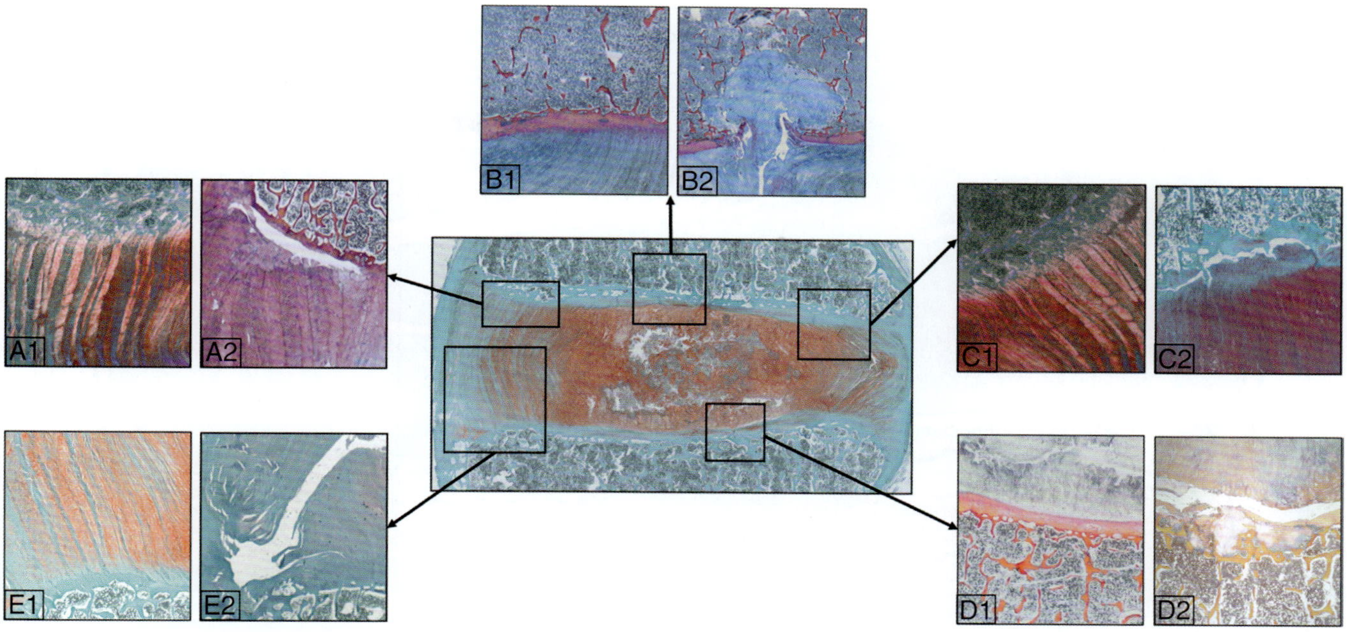

FIGURE 5 Decalcified, paraffin embedded histology. Characteristics of a healthy intervertebral disk (IVD) (center) include cut in the sagittal plane that demonstrates a clear distinction between the organized fibers of the anulus fibrosus (AF) (blue) and central nucleus pulposus (NP) (red); a continuous cartilage and bony end plate (EP) at the interface of the vertebral body and disk; and uniform haematopoietic bone marrow. Each pair of images represents the normal/healthy structure (1) left of degenerative change that can occur at the corresponding anatomic position (2). **A**, Tidemark avulsion of the anulus. **B**, Schmorl node—herniation of NP into the trabecular bone of the vertebral body. **C**, Avulsion of the cartilage EP. **D**, Erosion of the cartilage EP. **E**, Fissure of the anulus.

loss and hypermobility can cause facet arthritis and spinal ligament hypertrophy. Ultimately, dehydration, tissue crosslinking, and disk height loss lead to stiffening and restabilization.

Sustained changes in disk water content and height simultaneously impact disk cell biology in ways that may accelerate disk degeneration. For example, fluctuations in water content also impact load distributions, tissue pH, osmolality, and fixed charge density. Disk cells are highly sensitive to variations in these environmental parameters and may respond by decreasing production of important matrix proteins and increasing production of proinflammatory and catabolic factors. In general, in vitro studies suggest that for both nucleus and anulus cells, low pressure (0.2 to 1.0 MPa) tends to increase expression of anabolic matrix genes and enzyme inhibitors[24] with a parallel reduction of catabolic factors. However, high pressure (1 to 4 MPa) tends to reduce matrix production and increase catabolic[25] and inflammatory factors.[24] In the anulus, cyclic tension of low magnitude (1% strain) and physiologic frequencies (1 Hz) are homeostatic, while excessive strain (above 5% strain) turns catabolic.

Fundamentally, degeneration happens because the rate of matrix damage exceeds the disk cells' ability to repair. NP cells progressively lose their capacity to secrete aggrecan and collagen and begin to produce matrix degrading enzymes and cytokines, ultimately becoming senescent and apoptotic. These problems may be exacerbated by poor disk perfusion, as the vertebral capillary network deteriorates with age, or by fibrosis of the cartilage EP[12] (**Figure 6**). Deficient solute transport across the EP not only limits disk cell nutrition, but also causes the accumulation of degraded matrix fragments that interact with cells to trigger further catabolic behaviors. Paradoxically, decreased disk cell density is not consistently observed with advanced degeneration, which may be due to shortened diffusion distances accompanying losses in disk height.

PAIN

While disk degeneration underlies many spinal disorders, such as disk herniation, degenerative spondylolisthesis, spinal stenosis, foraminal stenosis, spondylosis, spondyloptosis, facet arthritis, and degenerative scoliosis, not all disk degeneration is symptomatic. In fact, there is a high prevalence of age-related degeneration[26] that is not associated with painful symptoms. Yet, the disk is believed to be a pain generator in approximately half of chronic LBP cases.[27]

The outer layers of the disk are innervated by mechanoreceptors that are believed to be important for proprioception. In the healthy disk, these nerve fibers are limited to the outer three annular layers and primarily consist of small myelinated (group-III or A-delta fibers in the size range of 1 to 5 μm) and unmyelinated (group-IV or C-fibers in the size range of 0.5 to 2 μm) fibers. Disk nerves are afferent axons whose cell bodies reside outside the central nervous system and within the dorsal root ganglia. Therefore, nociceptive signals are transmitted from the disk to the spinal cord via dorsal root ganglia neurons.

©Copyright 2021 American Academy of Orthopaedic Surgeons

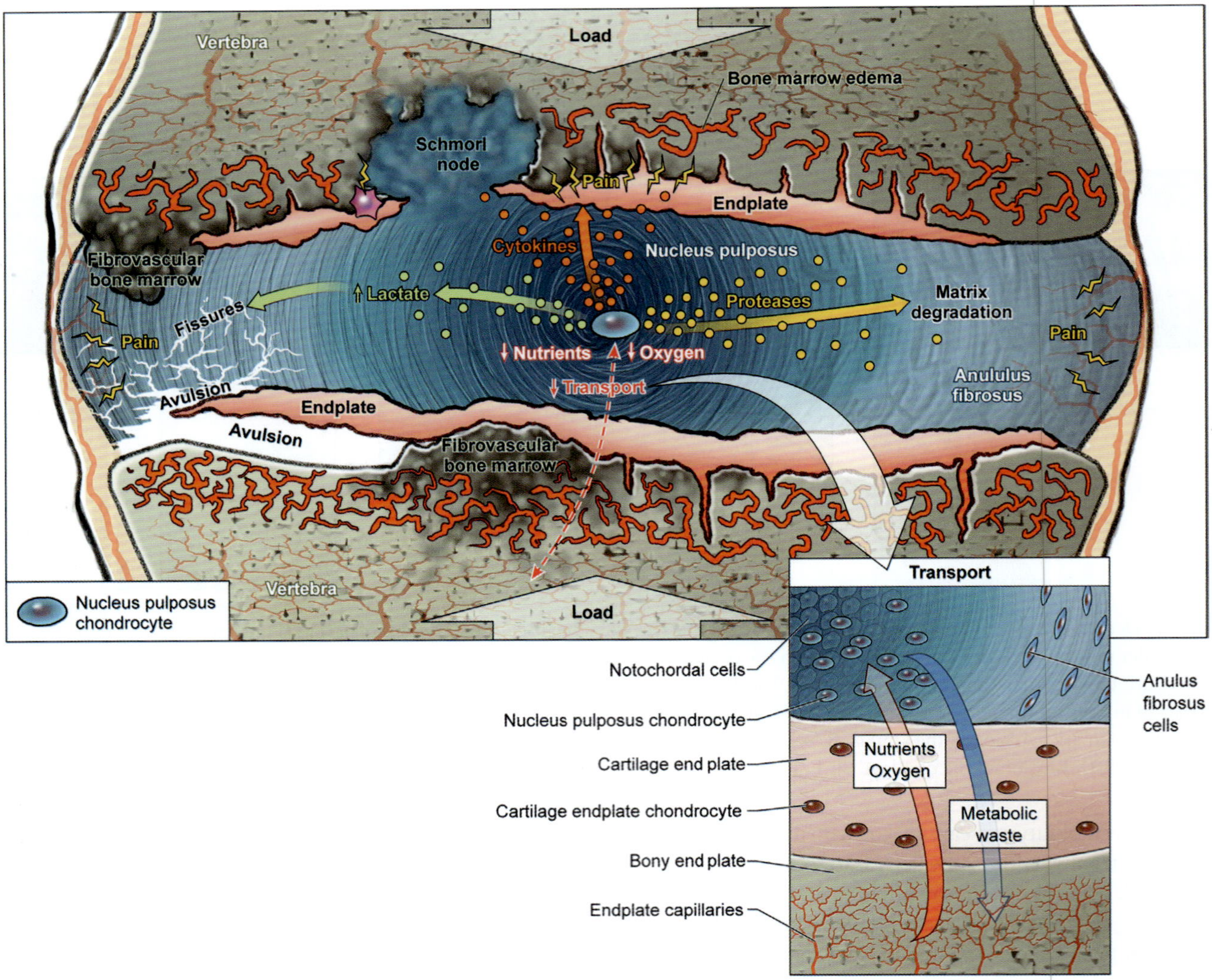

FIGURE 6 Illustration showing nutrient and waste exchange of intervertebral disk (IVD) across the cartilage and bony end plate (EP) is critical for normal disk and nucleus pulposus (NP) cell function. Transport can be adversely influenced by load, hypoxia, and nutrient deprivation. In response, NP cells can secrete lactate (green), cytokines (orange), and proteases (yellow). These factors can cause end plate erosions, fibrovascular bone marrow changes, nociceptor sensitization, and exacerbation of adverse effects of diminished transport. Sensitized nociceptors can, in turn, be stimulated by tissue stress to cause pain in the affected areas.

Immunocytochemical studies demonstrate that there are two paths between the anulus and the dorsal root ganglia—one from the sinuvertebral nerve and another along the paravertebral sympathetic trunk. The sinuvertebral nerve is a recurrent branch of the ventral primary ramus of the spinal nerve; that is, a portion of the spinal nerve at each spinal level connects back to the posterior disk. The sympathetic trunk is a paired chain of ganglia that runs along the ventrolateral borders of the spine. Axons from the sympathetic trunk course through the gray rami communicantes to the spinal nerve.

In addition to the peripheral portion of the anulus, the disk is innervated at the vertebral EP via the basivertebral nerve (thought to be a branch of the sinuvertebral nerve) that enters the vertebra through the posterior neurovascular foramen. Adjacent to the EP, bone marrow sensory and sympathetic fibers are frequently associated with blood vessels and consist of both fast myelinated fibers (group III or A-delta fibers with diameters ranging from 1 to 5 µm) that transmit sharp pain and slow unmyelinated fibers (group IV or C-fibers with diameters ranging from of 0.5 to 2 µm) that transmit dull or aching pain. The density of end plate innervation is comparable to and in many cases higher than that of the peripheral anulus.[28] Normally, these nerves do not penetrate deep into the disk due to high pressures and PG that repel nerve ingrowth.

A theoretical requirement for disk-related pain is pathologic innervation. Areas of annular and EP damage foster increased production of growth factors such as basic fibroblast growth factor (bFGF), insulin-like growth factor-1 (IGF-1), and platelet-derived growth factor (PDGF) that encourage granulation tissue formation.[29] Increased production of IL-1 by disk cells leads to secretion of neurotropic factors, such as nerve growth factor (NGF) and brain-derived neurotrophic

©Copyright 2021 American Academy of Orthopaedic Surgeons

factor (BDNF) that, along with decreases in GAG, encourage neoinnervation and neovascularization at the vertebral EP and peripheral annulus.[30] Inflammatory and neurotrophic factors may also trigger nociceptor sensitization. Consequently, imaging evidence of EP and/or annular edema and neovascularization are highly specific for predicting diskogenic pain.

Provocation diskography (PD) is considered by many as the benchmark for diagnosing diskogenic pain. The procedure consists of injecting a contrast agent into disks of a lightly sedated patient while monitoring the injected volume, pressure, contrast distribution pattern, and patient's pain response. This test can reveal internal disk disruption and also identify which disks are painful and may be appropriate for treatment. Although not without controversy regarding its usefulness and safety,[31] PD results can be quite accurate (specificity of 0.94 and a false-positive rate of 6%) if performed using low-pressure technique.[32] Yet, there are conflicting data regarding PD validity and its correlation with postoperative outcomes. For example, false-positive responses may be due to concordant pain from pressure increases in an adjacent sensitive disk. And, while some reports show greater symptom improvement when PD is used to guide surgery, others do not.

The role of EP in back pain is indicated by the strong association between PD-confirmed diskogenic pain and EP bone marrow abnormalities. There are three types of vertebral bone marrow lesions (BML) noted on MRI. Modic type I changes (fibrovascular replacement) show decreased signal intensity on T1-weighted images and increased signal intensity on T2-weighted images. Histopathology of Modic type I changes shows an active inflammatory stage that coincides with disruption and fissuring of the EP and vascularized granulation tissue within the marrow. Modic type II changes show increased signal intensity on T1-weighted images and an iso- or slightly hyperintense signal on T2-weighted images. Modic type II changes correlate with fatty marrow replacement (**Figure 7**). Both types of Modic changes (MC) are dynamic in that type I changes can convert to Modic type II or back to normal marrow, and similarly, Modic type II can convert back to type I.[33] Modic type III changes are represented by decreased signal intensity on both T1- and T2-weighted images that correlate with dense woven bone (sclerosis).

Data from multiple independent studies suggest that Modic type I and II changes adjacent to the EP are among the most specific of all MRI observations for predicting concordant PD-induced pain.[34] Not surprisingly, increased EP innervation has been reported for EP with MC.[28] However, the presence of Modic changes are not very sensitive (15% to 65%) to PD-confirmed disk pain.[35] Poor sensitivity may reflect the categorical and subjective techniques used to classify BML, rather than ones that are quantitative and objective. It may also be that innervated EP damage is not well visualized using standard MRI techniques.

The precise etiology of BML is not well understood, but it appears to involve autoimmune and inflammatory responses to chemicals produced by disk cells. These include proinflammatory and neurogenic factors such as interleukin-1, -6, and -8; tumor necrosis factor-α, prostaglandin E_2, monocyte chemotactic protein-1, and NGF. These nucleus-derived chemicals can both sensitize existing nerves and promote new nerve growth. Additionally, EP nerves can be irritated via accumulated by-products of disk cell anaerobic metabolism, such as lactic acid.[36]

A predisposing factor for enhanced communication between the nucleus and vertebral marrow is EP damage. Various forms of EP defects have been clinically associated with disk degeneration and axial back pain. These include Schmorl nodes, fractures, avulsions/erosions, and calcifications. Small EP defects are difficult to observe radiographically, and they are thought to be a common component of normal aging[37] (**Figure 8**). Schmorl nodes are large, focal EP indentations that represent herniations of nucleus into adjacent vertebrae and are significantly associated with disk degeneration severity. Because it can be challenging to distinguish between nodes that arise prior to skeletal maturity (eg, at sites of cartilage defects that remain after notochord regression and epiphyseal plate closure) and nodes that form traumatically secondary to age-related subchondral weakening, the results from clinical studies relating Schmorl nodes to symptoms are mixed. For example, Schmorl nodes are relatively common in asymptomatic individuals.[38] However, in cases where the nodes associate with chronic low back pain (LBP), MRI shows evidence of BML and fibrovascular bone marrow changes, which suggests a traumatic etiology. Cadaveric studies relating different types

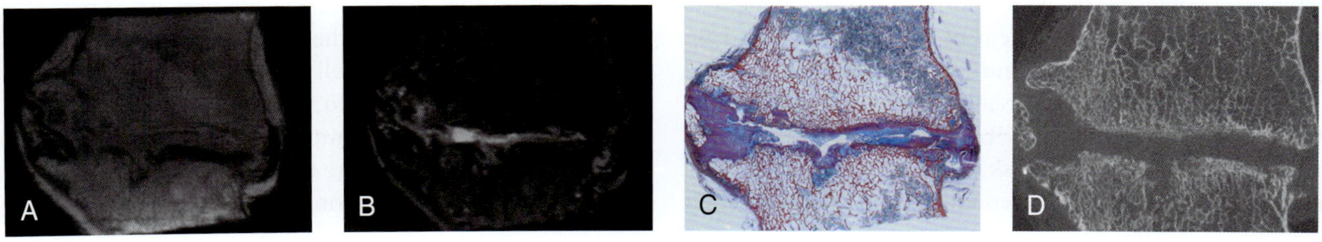

FIGURE 7 Vertebral bone marrow signal changes seen on MRI are known as modic changes (MC). Modic changes are commonly observed in patients with low back pain. Modic type II changes observed, from left to right, with (**A**) T1- and (**B**) T2-MRI, (**C**) histology, and with (**D**) μCT.

2: Structure and Function of Musculoskeletal Tissues

©Copyright 2021 American Academy of Orthopaedic Surgeons

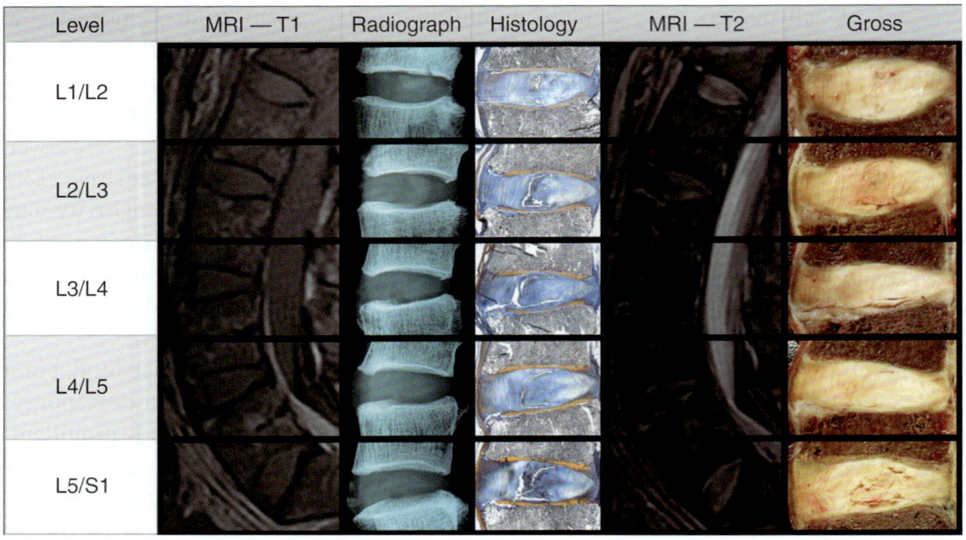

FIGURE 8 Sagittal images of the same human lumbar disks using multiple modalities. From left to right, images were taking using T1-weighted MRI, radiograph, histology, T2-weighted MRI, and macroscopic visualization. Compared with histology, each imaging modality can discriminate different features with varying detail.

of EP defects to back pain history demonstrated a clear dose effect: larger lesions were associated with more severe degeneration and more frequent back pain (odds ratio 1⁄4 17.88).[39]

DIAGNOSTICS

In the context of back pain, the main objective of clinical imaging is to rule out significant pathology (eg, tumors, fractures, stenosis) and to classify degeneration to facilitate treatment planning. Radiographic detection of disk degeneration via the Thompson grading scale is a commonly used method, but it can only detect gross morphological deformities. While CT diskography has been used to improve surgical outcome, it is an invasive study requiring placement of needle through the annular fibers and injection of fluid, and there are high incidences of false positives.[40] MRI is considered the benchmark for clinically assessing the disk, because it can provide fine anatomic detail. MRI precision is influenced by field strength (eg, 1.5 vs 3.0 T) and pulse sequence parameters (eg, T1-weighted vs T2-weighted) because these factors directly affect image resolution, signal-to-noise, and contrast-to-noise ratios. In conventional (T2-weighted) magnetic resonance (MR) images, the healthy NP appears bright and the healthy cartilage EP is invisible due to its short T2 relaxation time. The widely used classification system of Pfirrmann is based on T2-weighted MR images[41] (**Figure 9**). Grades between I and V are assigned to the disk, based on structural morphology (eg, homogeneity within the NP, distinction between the NP and AF, signal intensity, and disk height). Some recent studies based on large populations have shown that disk degeneration on MRI is significantly associated with a history of LBP history in adults, and such an association increases according to the global severity of disk degeneration (ie, degenerative disk disease score).[42] Additionally, disk degeneration severity in asymptomatic individuals may be predictive for future first-time LBP episodes. That being said, because disk degeneration is commonly observed in asymptomatic individuals, the use of MRI has not yet been shown to improve outcomes in chronic LBP patients. Instead, MRI can increase the identification of incidental findings that can trigger a "cascade effect" leading to further diagnostic procedures or treatments that can be costly and may pose additional risk to the patient. Consequently, current consensus recommends against the routine use of MRI except in cases with suspected structural pathology when progress is not being made with conservative care.

Other MRI findings, such as the previously mentioned MC, may provide more clinically relevant information. MC are significantly associated with chronic LBP. Modic type I changes appear to be especially painful and correlate with persistence of symptoms.[43]

New, advanced imaging techniques can reveal subtle chemical biomarkers that may be useful for localizing painful disks. For example, T1-rho MRI, T2-mapping, magnetization transfer MRI, sodium MRI, and MR spectroscopy highlight chemical changes that occur with disk degeneration that may represent biomarkers of pathological change.[44] Such approaches may help clinicians identify painful spinal levels as well as sensitively monitor novel biologic therapies meant to rejuvenate pathologic disks.[45] However, more research into the natural history of these biomarkers is needed before they can be confidently incorporated into clinical decision making.

 ©Copyright 2021 American Academy of Orthopaedic Surgeons

Pfirrmann grade	I	II	III	IV	V
Sagittal T2-MRI	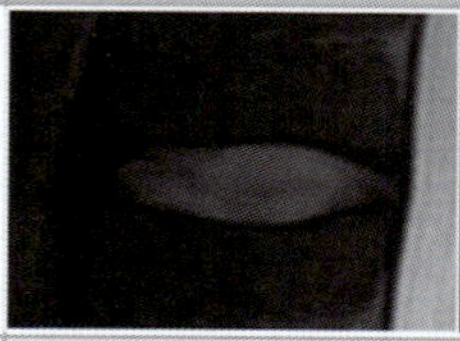	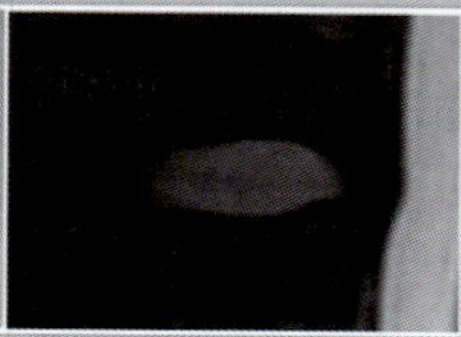	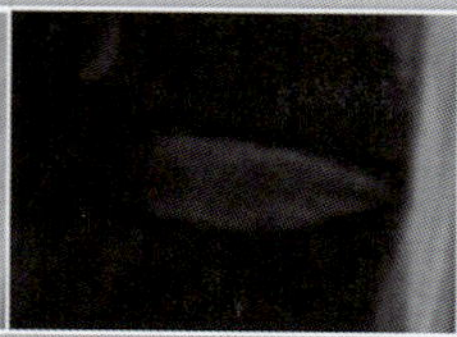	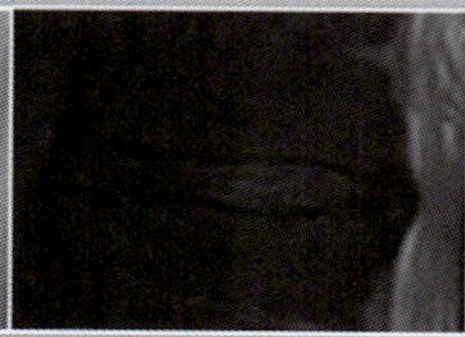	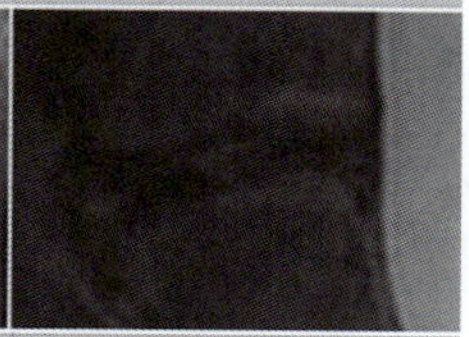
Structure	Homogenous, white	Inhomogenous, with or without horizontal bands	Inhomogenous, grey	Inhomogenous, grey to black	Inhomogenous, black
Distinction of nucleus and anulus	Clear	Clear	Unclear	Lost	Lost
Signal intensity	Hyperintense, isointense to cerebrospinal fluid	Hyperintense, isointense to cerebrospinal fluid	Intermediate	Intermediate to hypointense	Hypointense
Height of intervertebral disk	Normal	Normal	Normal to slightly decreased	Normal to moderately decreased	Collapsed disk space

FIGURE 9 Illustration demonstrating Pfirrmann grading scale of lumbosacral disk degeneration with T2-MRI. Pfirrmann grading ranges from I-V, with Pfirrmann grade V representing severely degenerated disks. (Images reproduced with permission from Pfirrmann CWA, Metzdorf A, Zanetti M, et al: Magnetic resonance classification of lumbar intervertebral disc degeneration. *Spine* 2001;26[17]:1873-1878. doi:10.1097/00007632-200109010-00011.)

SUMMARY

The IVD is composed of three primary tissues, the NP and surrounding EP and AF. The disk contains cells that have a very slow turnover and, as such, has impaired repair/healing due to lack of vascularization. The disk serves important biomechanical functions that support spinal compression forces and works synergistically with the facet joints and paraspinal muscles to support multiaxial movement. Disk degeneration is an age-related chronic matrix remodeling process. It generally begins in the second decade of life coincident with the disappearance of notochordal cells from the NP. Though disk degeneration underlies many spinal disorders, not all disk degeneration is clinically symptomatic. Current imaging techniques, such as MRI, can aid in the diagnosis and treatment of diskogenic back pain. Improved understanding of disk pain mechanisms is guiding development of novel diagnostic tools, such as advanced MRI and spectroscopy sequences, that aim to improve the accurate identification of clinically relevant disk pathology.

REFERENCES

1. Lotz JC, Fields AJ, Liebenberg EC: The role of the vertebral end plate in low back pain. *Glob Spine J* 2013;3(3):153-163. doi:10.1055/s-0033-1347298.
2. Urban JP, Roberts S: Chemistry of the intervertebral disc in relation to functional requirements, in *Grieve's Modern Manual Therapy: The Vertebral Column*. Churchill Livingstone, Edinburgh, 1994, pp 163-175.
3. Le Maitre C, Pockert A, Buttle D, et al: Matrix synthesis and degradation in human intervertebral disc degeneration. *Biochem Soc Trans* 2007;35(4):652-655. doi:10.1042/bst0350652.
4. Roberts S, Menage J, Urban JPG: Biochemical and structural properties of the cartilage end-plate and its relation to the intervertebral disc. *Spine* 1989;14(2):166-174. doi:10.1097/00007632-198902000-00005.
5. Fields AJ, Berg-Johansen B, Metz LN, et al: Alterations in intervertebral disc composition, matrix homeostasis and biomechanical behavior in the UCD-T2DM rat model of type 2 diabetes. *J Orthop Res* 2015;33(5):738-746. doi:10.1002/jor.22807.
6. Adams MA, Freeman BJC, Morrison HP, Nelson IW, Dolan P: Mechanical initiation of intervertebral disc degeneration. *Spine* 2000;25(13):1625-1636. doi:10.1097/00007632-200007010-00005.
7. Chelberg MK, Banks GM, Geiger DF, et al: Identification of heterogeneous cell populations in normal human intervertebral disc. *J Anat* 1995;186(pt 1):43-53.
8. Guehring T, Nerlich A, Kroeber M, et al: Sensitivity of notochordal disc cells to mechanical loading: An experimental animal study. *Eur Spine J* 2009;19(1):113-121. doi:10.1007/s00586-009-1217-0.
9. Kim K-W, Lim T-H, Kim JG, et al: The origin of chondrocytes in the nucleus pulposus and histologic findings associated with the transition of a notochordal nucleus pulposus to a fibrocartilaginous nucleus pulposus in intact rabbit intervertebral discs. *Spine* 2003;28(10):982-990. doi:10.1097/01.brs.0000061986.03886.4f.

©Copyright 2021 American Academy of Orthopaedic Surgeons

10. Urban JP, Smith S, Fairbank JC: Nutrition of the intervertebral disc. *Spine* 2004;29(23):2700-2709.
11. Rajasekaran S1, Babu JN, Arun R, et al: ISSLS prize winner: A study of diffusion in human lumbar discs: A serial magnetic resonance imaging study documenting the influence of the endplate on diffusion in normal and degenerate discs. *Spine* 2004;29(23):2654-2667.
12. Wong J, Sampson S, Bell-Briones H, et al: Nutrient supply and nucleus pulposus cell function: Effects of the transport properties of the cartilage endplate and potential implications for intradiscal biologic therapy. *Osteoarthr Cartil* 2019;27(6):956-964. doi:10.1016/j.joca.2019.01.013.
13. Kiefer A, Shirazi-Adl A, Parnianpour M: Synergy of the human spine in neutral postures. *Eur Spine J* 1998;7(6):471-479. doi:10.1007/s005860050110.
14. Hides J, Gilmore C, Stanton W, et al: Multifidus size and symmetry among chronic LBP and healthy asymptomatic subjects. *Man Ther* 2008;13(1):43-49. doi:10.1016/j.math.2006.07.017.
15. Wilke HJ, Neef P, Caimi M, et al: New in vivo measurements of pressures in the intervertebral disc in daily life. *Spine* 1999;24(8):755-762.
16. Fields AJ, Lee GL, Keaveny TM: Mechanisms of initial endplate failure in the human vertebral body. *J Biomech* 2010;43(16):3126-3131.
17. Hukins DWL: Disc structure and function, in Ghosh P, ed: *The Biology of the Intervertebral Disc*. CRC Press, Inc, Boca Raton, Florida, 1988, pp 1-39.
18. Rodacki AL, Fowler NE, Provensi CL, et al: Body mass as a factor in stature change. *Clin Biomech* 2005;20(8):799-805.
19. McGill SM, van Wijk MJ, Axler CT, et al: Studies of spinal shrinkage to evaluate low-back loading in the workplace. *Ergonomics* 1996;39(1):92-102.
20. Lotz JC, Chin JR: Intervertebral disc cell death is dependent on the magnitude and duration of spinal loading. *Spine* 2000;25(12):1477-1483.
21. Chin JR, Court C, et al: Compression-induced apoptosis in the 863 mouse intervertebral disc is time and stress dependent. 45th Annual 864 Meeting, Orthopaedic Research Society 1999.
22. Maclean JJ, Lee CR, Alini M, et al: Anabolic and catabolic mRNA levels of the intervertebral disc vary with the magnitude and frequency of in vivo dynamic compression. *J Orthop Res* 2004;22(6):1193-1200. doi:10.1016/j.orthres.2004.04.004.
23. Maclean JJ, Lee CR, Alini M, et al: The effects of short-term load duration on anabolic and catabolic gene expression in the rat tail intervertebral disc. *J Orthop Res* 2005;23(5):1120-1127. doi:10.1016/j.orthres.2005.01.020.
24. Sowa G, Coelho P, Vo N, et al: Determination of annulus fibrosus cell response to tensile strain as a function of duration, magnitude, and frequency. *J Orthop Res* 2011;29(8):1275-1283. doi:10.1002/jor.21388.
25. Maitre CLL, Frain J, Millward-Sadler J, et al: Altered integrin mechanotransduction in human nucleus pulposus cells derived from degenerated discs. *Arthritis Rheum* 2009;60(2):460-469. doi:10.1002/art.24248.
26. Brinjikji W, Luetmer P, Comstock B, et al: Systematic literature review of imaging features of spinal degeneration in asymptomatic populations. *Am J Neuroradiol* 2014;36(4):811-816. doi:10.3174/ajnr.a4173.
27. Boos N, Weissbach S, Rohrbach H, et al: Classification of age-related changes in lumbar intervertebral discs. *Spine* 2002;27(23):2631-2644. doi:10.1097/00007632-200212010-00002.
28. Fields AJ, Liebenberg EC, Lotz JC: Innervation of pathologies in the lumbar vertebral end plate and intervertebral disc. *Spine J* 2014;14(3):513-521. doi:10.1016/j.spinee.2013.06.075.
29. Peng B, Hao J, Hou S, et al: Possible pathogenesis of painful intervertebral disc degeneration. *Spine* 2006;31(5):560-566.
30. Johnson WE, Caterson B, Eisenstein SM, et al: Human intervertebral disc aggrecan inhibits nerve growth in vitro. *Arthritis Rheum* 2002;46(10):2658-2664.
31. Carragee EJ, Don AS, Hurwitz EL, et al: 2009 ISSLS prize winner: Does discography cause accelerated progression of degeneration changes in the lumbar disc: A ten-year matched cohort study. *Spine* 2009;34:2338-2345.
32. Wolfer LR, Derby R, Lee JE, et al: Systematic review of lumbar provocation discography in asymptomatic subjects with a meta-analysis of false-positive rates. *Pain Physician* 2008;11:513-538.
33. Marshman LA, Trewhella M, Friesem T, et al: Reverse transformation of Modic type 2 changes to Modic type 1 changes during sustained chronic low-back pain severity. Report of two cases and review of the literature. *J Neurosurg Spine* 2007;6:152-155.
34. Weishaupt D, Zanetti M, Hodler J, et al: Painful lumbar disk derangement: Relevance of endplate abnormalities at MR imaging. *Radiology* 2001;218:420-427.
35. O'Neill C, Kurgansky M, Kaiser J, et al: Accuracy of MRI for diagnosis of discogenic pain. *Pain Physician* 2008;11:311-326.
36. Keshari KR, Lotz JC, Link TM, et al: Lactic acid and proteoglycans as metabolic markers for discogenic back pain. *Spine* 2008;33:312-317.
37. Coventry MB, Ghormley RK, Kernohan JW: The intervertebral disc: Its microscopic anatomy and pathology. *J Bone Joint Surg Br* 1945;27:460-474.
38. Mok FP, Samartzis D, Karppinen J, et al: Modic changes of the lumbar spine: Prevalence, risk factors, and association with disc degeneration and low back pain in a large-scale population-based cohort. *Spine J* 2016;16(1):32-41.
39. Wang Y, Videman T, Battié MC: ISSLS prize winner: Lumbar vertebral endplate lesions: Associations with disc degeneration and back pain history. *Spine* 2012;37:1490-1496.
40. Ala-Kokko L: Genetic risk factors for lumbar disc disease. *Ann Med* 2002;34(1):42-47.
41. Pfirrmann CWA, Metzdorf A, Zanetti M, et al: Magnetic resonance classification of lumbar intervertebral disc degeneration. *Spine* 2001;26(17):1873-1878. doi:10.1097/00007632-200109010-00011.
42. Samartzis D, Karppinen J, Chan D, et al: *The association of disc degeneration based on magnetic resonance imaging and the presence of low back pain. Presented at: World Forum for Spine Research: Intervertebral Disc,* Montreal, Canada, July 5-8, 2010.
43. Jarvinen J, Karppinen J, Niinimaki J, et al: Association between changes in lumbar Modic changes and low back symptoms over a two-year period. *BMC Musculoskelet Disord* 2015;16:98.
44. Lotz JC, Haughton V, Boden SD, et al: New treatments and imaging strategies in degenerative disease of the intervertebral disks. *Radiology* 2012;264(1):6-19.
45. Gornet MG, Peacock J, Claude J, et al: Magnetic resonance spectroscopy (MRS) can identify painful lumbar discs and may facilitate improved clinical outcomes of lumbar surgeries for discogenic pain. *Eur Spine J* 2019;28(4):674-687. doi:10.1007/s00586-018-05873-3.

©Copyright 2021 American Academy of Orthopaedic Surgeons

18

Tendons and Ligaments

Matthew M. Counihan, MD
Louis J. Soslowsky, PhD

Keywords: *ligament anatomy and functional properties; tendon anatomy and functional properties; tendon and ligament injuries; tendon and ligament repair and reconstruction*

INTRODUCTION

Tendons and ligaments are complex connective tissues and essential components of the musculoskeletal system, aiding in locomotion and assisting in both dynamic and static joint stabilization. The burden of musculoskeletal injuries in the United States continues to expand. The proportion of the population reporting these injuries increased from 76.0 million from 1996 to 1998 to 102.5 million from 2009 to 2011, with a disproportionate amount of this increase occurring among those aged 45 to 64 years. The aggregate economic impact of these injuries from 2009 to 2011 was estimated at $796.3 billion.[1] Because tendon and ligament disorders are especially common and are significant contributors to this musculoskeletal injury burden, a clear understanding of their function in health, as well as their dysfunction in pathology and treatment mechanisms, is essential.

Tendon and ligament are frequently discussed together because of their many similarities they share and despite their significant differences. Both have elastic and viscoelastic properties that contribute to their ability to resist a variety of loading scenarios. These behaviors are a result of their complex composition and structural characteristics at each level of organization that lead to their response to joint function.

This chapter will provide an overview of the preclinical concepts behind clinical conditions involving tendon and ligament, highlighting anatomic considerations; gross morphology, microanatomy, and biology; their biomechanical function in the body; relevant injuries; considerations in tendon and ligament repair; and current concepts in tissue engineering for tendon and ligament injuries.

TENDON

CLASSIFICATION AND ANATOMY

Tendons can be classified through multiple schema, according to anatomic considerations: specifically, shape (round or flat), anatomic location (intra-articular or extra-articular; intra-articular soft-tissue injuries have a lower likelihood of healing),[2] or the surrounding layer of connective tissue (paratenon or synovium, which acts to reduce friction and allows for tendon gliding).

GROSS MORPHOLOGY, HISTOLOGY, MICROANATOMY, AND CELL BIOLOGY

The connection of the tendon between muscle and its point of origin or insertion at the bone requires several complex anatomic and morphologic characteristics that are continued through the microscopic and molecular level. Primarily, this

Dr. Counihan or an immediate family member serves as a paid consultant to or is an employee of Jazz Pharmaceuticals, Sun Pharmaceuticals, CSL Behring, Biomotive and has stock or stock options held in Merck. Dr. Soslowsky or an immediate family member has received research or institutional support from Embody, Marine Polymer Technology, and Orthofix, Inc.

This chapter is adapted from Reuther KE, Gray CF, Soslowsky LJ: Form and function of tendon and ligament, in O'Keefe RJ, Jacobs JJ, Chu CR, Einhorn TA, eds: *Orthopaedic Basic Science*, ed 4. Rosemont, IL, American Academy of Orthopaedic Surgeons, 2013, pp 213-228.

©Copyright 2021 American Academy of Orthopaedic Surgeons

connection allows for the transfer of force from muscle to bone and enables highly specific motion by the musculoskeletal system. Not all muscles have a tendon; those that do primarily provide motion at a joint or need to provide force either over a distance or in a tightly confined space. Tendons provide a mechanical advantage for muscle by focusing or redirecting force, lengthening a lever arm, or acting around a pulley (such as in the flexor hallucis longus tendon).

The round or flat shape of the tendon is associated with specific functional consequences. Classic examples of round tendons include the flexor digitorum tendons of both the upper and lower extremities; flat tendons include the rotator cuff tendons and the Achilles tendon. Most round tendons behave similarly and are biomechanically subjected to a consistent environment. They are accustomed to high tensile loads and are capable of a high degree of motion, or gliding. The flat tendons are less easily categorized. They are generally subject to less glide but are capable of bearing high tensile loads (as in the quadriceps tendon) in addition to more complex loads such as compression and shear. Consequently, these different functions are represented in the structure of these tendons.

Further investigation of tendons reveals a complex composition with more functional implications. At the most basic level, tendon composition is organized consistently throughout the body, despite its often-differing superstructure. Like most connective tissue, the main functional components of tendon are water and collagen. Water is the primary constituent, comprising approximately 50% to 60% of tendon weight. Collagen makes up approximately 75% of the dry weight with 95% type I collagen and a small amount of type III and other collagens. Tendon is also composed of tendon cells, referred to as tenocytes, and proteoglycans. Proteoglycans are composed of a core protein covalently bound to one or more glycosaminoglycan (GAG) chains. GAGs are thought to play an important role in mechanics, specifically viscoelastic properties, through their association with water. The major subcategory of proteoglycans in tendon is the small leucine-rich proteoglycans (SLRPs). The most abundant SLRPs in tendon are decorin and biclycan, also known as class I SLRPs. Other SLRPs, though not as common, are also well described, such as fibromudulin and lumican (class II). Both classes have been found to play significant roles in tendon growth, regulation, and homeostasis. These molecules have been shown to bind to collagen and have significant impact on the hierarchical organization of tendon and its mechanical properties.[3] Several investigators have suggested a role for these proteins in tendinopathy, although the specific mechanisms of this relation remain unclear.

At the molecular level, tendons are arranged in a hierarchy starting with the triple helix of collagen, then microfibrils, fibrils, fascicles, and ultimately the tendon itself (**Figure 1**). The mediated assembly and cross-linking of collagen into these microfibrils is critical for the mechanical strength of the tissue. This process is largely dependent on the family of extracellular SLRPs, which can dictate the overall thickness and quality of fibril assembly.[4] Another important element of collagen assembly and structure is crimp. Crimp is evident ultrastructurally and appears as "crimped" lines in the tendon when viewed at the microscopic level. This crimping results from the specific orientation of the microfibrils in the tendon and contributes important mechanical properties that are discussed later in this chapter.

The superstructure of tendons is the progressive organization of fibrils into larger fascicles that group to yield a functional tendon, as well as supporting connective tissue that preserves local anatomic and physiologic relationships. These groups of fascicles are separated and bound together by a thin connective tissue layer known as the endotenon. Contiguous with the endotenon is the epitenon, which envelops the entire tendon. Some tendons are then wrapped with a paratenon

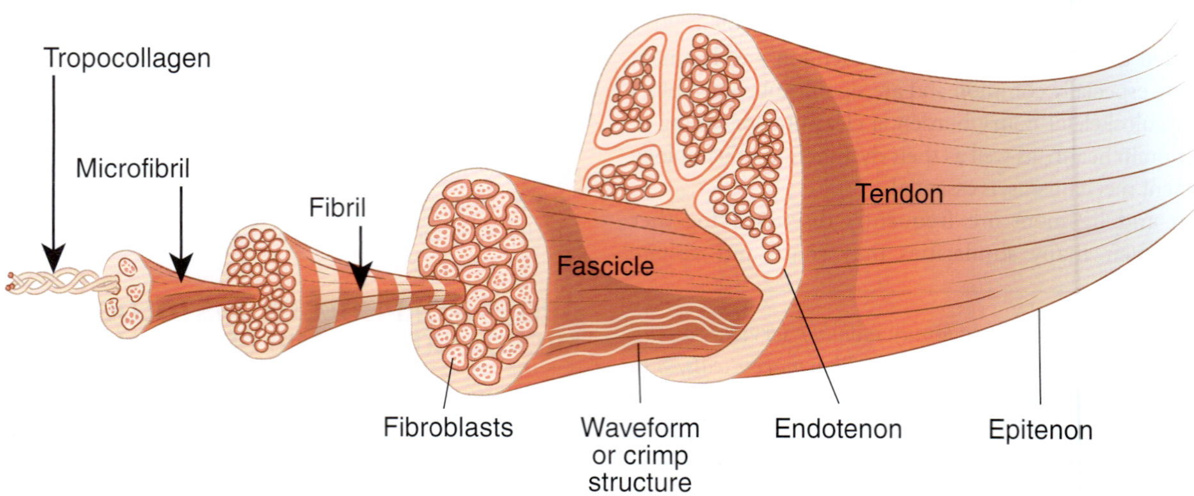

FIGURE 1 Representative illustration of a tendon. Tendon has a hierarchical structure, with collagen molecules assembled into progressively larger bundles, until the level of the tendon itself is reached. Note the endotenon (surrounding the fascicle) and epitenon (surrounding the tendon), containing the neurovasculature of the tendon.

©Copyright 2021 American Academy of Orthopaedic Surgeons

(eg, Achilles tendon), and some are covered with synovium (eg, flexor tendons), depending on the degree of gliding required. The endotenon and epitenon serve to permeate the tendon with vasculature, lymphatics, and nerves.

Another aspect of tendon's morphology and functional relationships are its origin and insertion (its junctions). As the tissue that bridges muscle to bone, tendon has two junction regions: the myotendinous junction, where the muscle transitions to tendon, and the bone-tendon junction, where the tendon transitions to bone. Each is differentially organized and contributes to the varying properties along the length of the muscle-tendon-bone unit. The myotendinous junction is composed of the interdigitations of end sarcomeres and connective tissue elements. An end portion of the sarcomere, known as the z-line, which is arranged in a staggered organization with the next sarcomere, splits and gives rise to myofilament bundles that insert directly onto collagen fibrils. This arrangement minimizes stress to the myotendinous junction with forceful contractions.

At the bone-tendon junction, known as the enthesis, there are two typical arrangements with different biomechanical roles: direct or indirect insertions. Direct, or fibrocartilaginous, insertions have been classically characterized by a four-layer transition from tendon to bone: tendon, fibrocartilage, mineralized fibrocartilage, and bone (**Figure 2**). These insertions are typical in regions where the tendon-bone unit is subject to high tensile loads (such as the rotator cuff).[5,6] In an indirect insertion, which is less common than the direct insertion, the tendon fibers insert directly into the periosteum. The fibers that interdigitate with the periosteal tissue have commonly been referred to as Sharpey fibers. These transitions are more common in areas where tensile loading at the tendinous insertion does not predominate (such as the distal head of the rectus femoris).

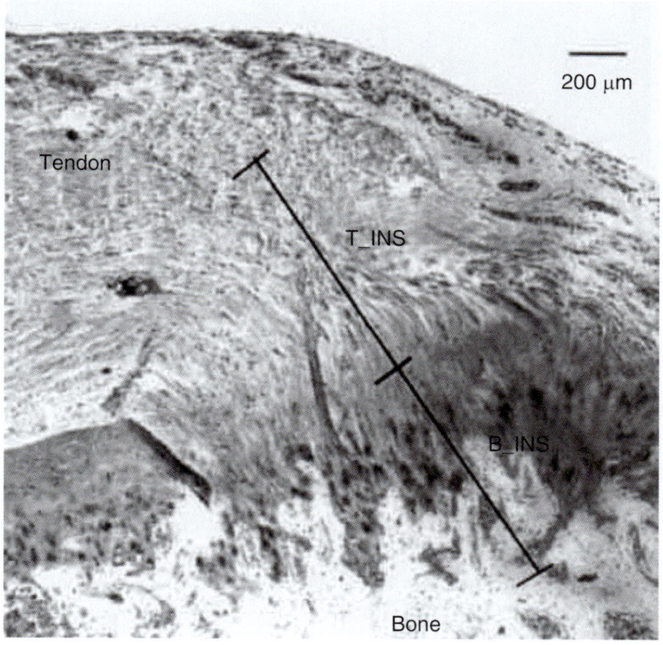

FIGURE 2 Histology of the normal rat supraspinatous tendon. The four transition zones that make up the direct tendon insertion: tendon, uncalcified fibrocartilage, calcified fibrocartilage, and bone, as seen in a rat supraspinatus tendon insertion site. This transition enables transfer of load from a compliant (tendon) to a stiff (bone) material (B_INS = bony insertion, T_INS = tendinous insertion). (Reproduced with permission from Thomopoulos S, Williams GR, Gimbel JA, Favata M, Soslowsky LJ: Variation of biomechanical, structural, and compositional properties along the tendon to bone insertion site. *J Orthop Res* 2003;21[3]:413-419.)

At the cellular level there are also considerations that have implications for structure and function. Tendon is often classified as relatively hypocellular, yet recent evidence connects tenocytes with a highly defined role in maintenance of tendon structure.[7] Tenocytes maintain the extracellular milieu that allows the normal function of tendon by secreting the extracellular matrix, synthesizing collagen and the proteoglycans. They possess long cellular processes that envelop and interdigitate with the collagen fibrils and other tenocyte processes and cell bodies. They are responsive to mechanical loading and can communicate with adjacent tenocytes through gap junctions at their interface as well as by production of inflammatory mediators under stress.[7]

BLOOD SUPPLY AND INNERVATION

Although tendon is considered largely hypovascular, blood flow has important consequences for tendon in health and disease. The blood supply and innervation of tendon, as mentioned previously, is primarily through the endotenon and epitenon. The tendon is fed primarily through vasculature that enters through the paratenon or at the bony insertions and continues to travel throughout the endotenon. The situation is more complex in sheathed tendons, in which blood supply must enter the tendon through mesotenon in vincula, defined as redundancies of the synovium that tether the tendon to its sheath in certain locations, analogous to the mesentery of the peritoneum (**Figure 3**). Sheathed tendon is also thought to receive some nutrition through diffusion via the synovial fluid. In addition to tendon's hypovascularity, there are specific regions of relative avascularity between vascular zones, which are thought to be at particular risk for rupture. These hypovascular areas have been identified in the supraspinatus tendon, long head of the biceps tendon, Achilles tendon, and patellar tendon, all of which are prone to rupture.[8]

Innervation in tendon includes several types of nerve endings with different functions. Tendon is typically innervated by the same nerve as its muscle. The various special organs include Golgi organs, which provide steady-state information when undergoing large stimulations for prolonged periods; Pacinian corpuscles, which are considered sensitive, fast-adapting mechanoreceptors; and Ruffini endings, which are also very sensitive but can relay information for prolonged periods similar to Golgi organs. These end-organs are typically localized to the myotendinous region. Free nerve endings, responsible for nociception, on the other hand, tend to be clustered at the enthesis.

©Copyright 2021 American Academy of Orthopaedic Surgeons

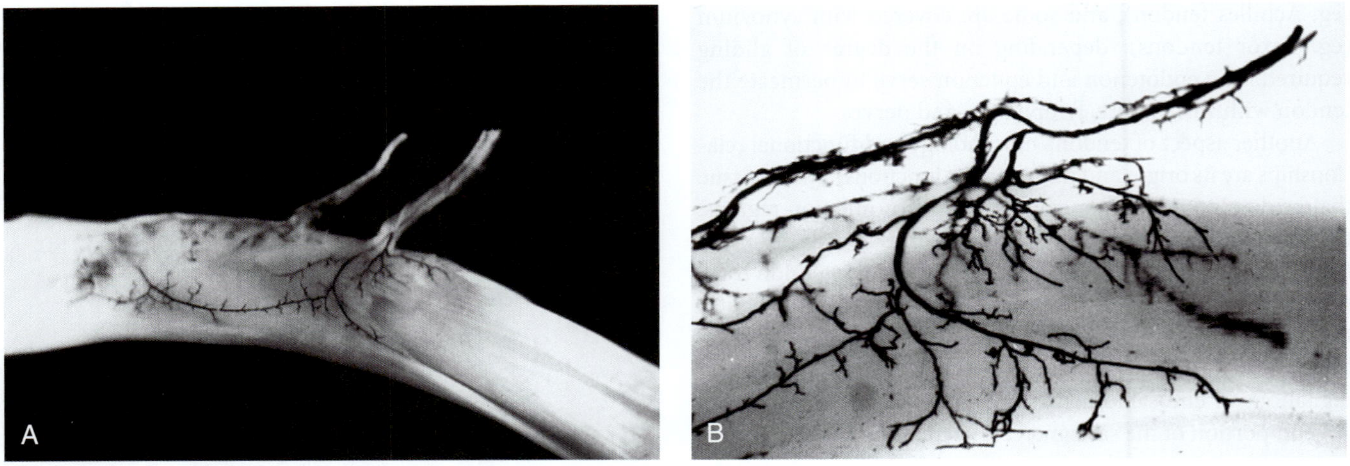

FIGURE 3 **A**, Photograph of a human flexor digitorum profundus tendon, injected with India ink, highlighting the contribution of the vinculum (a bandlike structure connecting the flexor tendon and the phalanges) to tendon blood supply. **B**, Close-up of the tendon demonstrating the extent of the vinculum blood supply. (Reproduced with permission from Woo SL, An KN, Frank CB, et al: Anatomy, biology, and biomechanics of tendon and ligament, in Buckwalter JA, Einhorn TA, Simon SR, eds: *Orthopaedic Basic Science*, ed 2. Rosemont, IL, American Academy of Orthopaedic Surgeons, 2000, p 585.)

TENDON FUNCTIONS

Tendon serves the primary purpose of allowing the transmission of force from muscle to bone, providing the capacity for locomotion, as well as allowing dynamic joint stability in concert with ligament, which provides more static restraint to joint translation. This is accomplished through an intricately designed and executed structure that enables these certain biomechanical properties. The relationship between structure and function is paramount.

Mechanical

The mechanical function of tendon is to orchestrate a fine balance between mobility and stability. The most obvious aspect of this function is the transmission of muscle-derived force to bone, which provides volitional control of the skeleton. Tendon also possesses the ability to elastically store and transfer energy. This dual ability has protective implications for the musculoskeletal system, as tendon can help absorb force and protect surrounding tissue. The composition of tendon as primarily water and collagen enables it to function viscoelastically, with its stiffness changing in response to loading. This viscoelastic behavior will be discussed later in the chapter.

Another important mechanical function of tendon is to provide secondary restraint to joint motion and add stability to the musculoskeletal system. The insertion of a tendon just distal to the joint on which it primarily acts enables the tendon to buttress against translation of the articular surfaces. A classic example of this function is the hamstring mechanism as a secondary stabilizer of the knee, protecting against anterior tibial translation in the setting of anterior cruciate ligament (ACL) deficiency.

These functional properties of tendon are derived from material and structural properties of the constituents and intrinsic tendon properties as well as the characteristics of the muscle-tendon-bone interface. The intrinsic tendon properties are referred to as material properties because they describe characteristics that are specific to the tendon material itself. This differentiates material properties from the structural properties, which are not normalized by tendon area or length, and thus describe qualities of the whole structure.

Three essential components of tendon function, and both its material and structural properties, are its nonlinear anisotropy and its elastic and viscoelastic behavior. The term nonlinear anisotropy means that tendon mechanical properties differ depending on the direction of applied force and have different values depending on the degree of force applied. Viscoelasticity describes a propensity of many biologic tissues, in which a tissue's mechanical properties are different depending on the time and recent history of loading the tissue.

Nonlinear anisotropic properties that are important when discussing tendon can be derived from two experimental scenarios. The first, representing structural properties, is called a load-elongation study. In this setting, the tendon-bone unit is elongated while the resultant load developed in the construct is measured (**Figure 4**, A). At low loads, the tendon is stretched easily (low slope) with nonlinear behavior; this is known as the toe region. This stretching has been attributed to the recruitment and realignment of crimped collagen fibrils (**Figure 5**). Following the toe region, there is a linear region, where rate of load development is constant. Finally, there is a failure region, at which point load drops off, and stretching is easily accomplished. From this test, the following properties can be derived: stiffness, represented by the slope of the curve in the linear region; ultimate load, represented by the load value at failure; and energy absorbed to failure, represented

©Copyright 2021 American Academy of Orthopaedic Surgeons

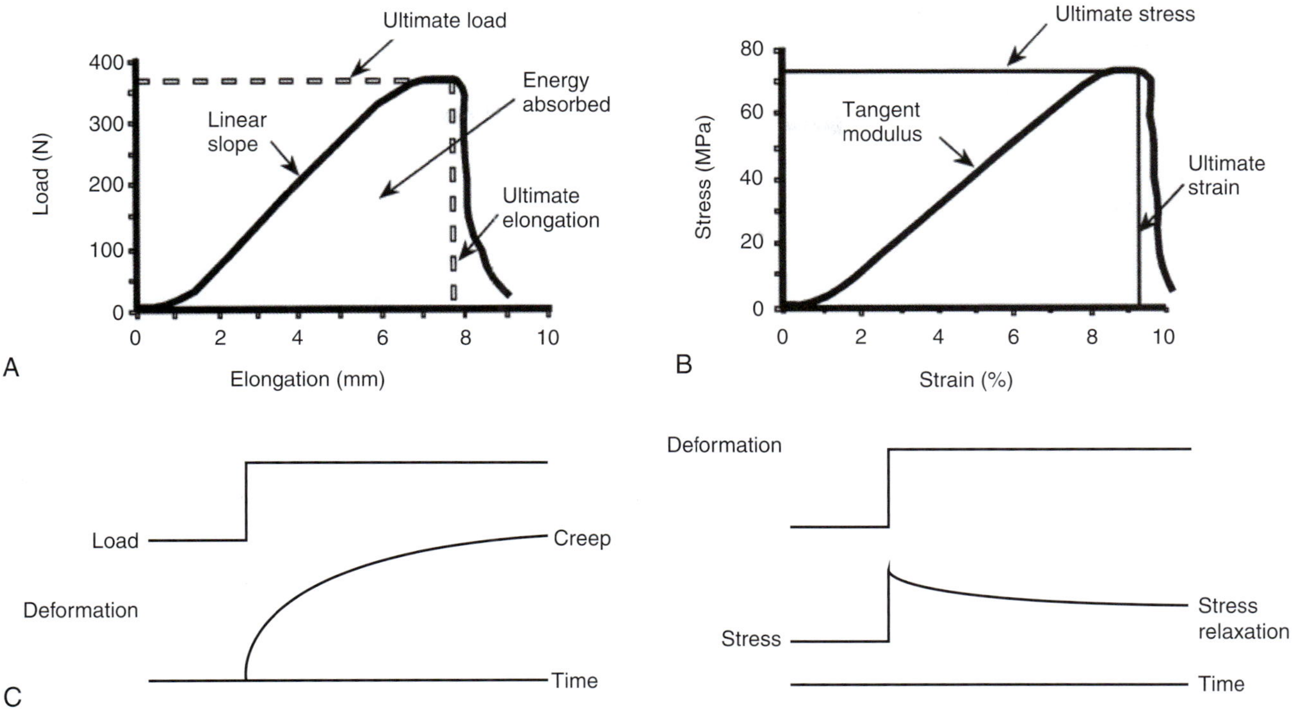

FIGURE 4 Graphic representation of the load-elongation curve of tendon, with load as the dependent variable and elongation as the independent variable. **A**, Various material properties can be derived from this curve. **B**, Stress-strain curve of tendon. This curve normalizes properties to tendon parameters, including length and area. **C**, Viscoelastic behavior of tendon, demonstrating the response to load history. For a creep test (left), load is held constant, and amount of deformation is measured. For a stress relaxation test (right), the deformation is held constant while developed stress is measured. (**B**, Reproduced with permission from Woo SL, Debski RE, Withrow JD, Janaushek MA: Biomechanics of knee ligaments. *Am J Sports Med* 1999;27[4]:533-543. **C**, Adapted with permission from Brinker MR, O'Connor DP, Almekinders LC, et al: Physiology of injury to musculoskeletal structures, in Drez D Jr, DeLee JC, Miller MD, eds: *Orthopaedic Sports Medicine: Principles and Practice*. Philadelphia, PA, WB Saunders, 2007.)

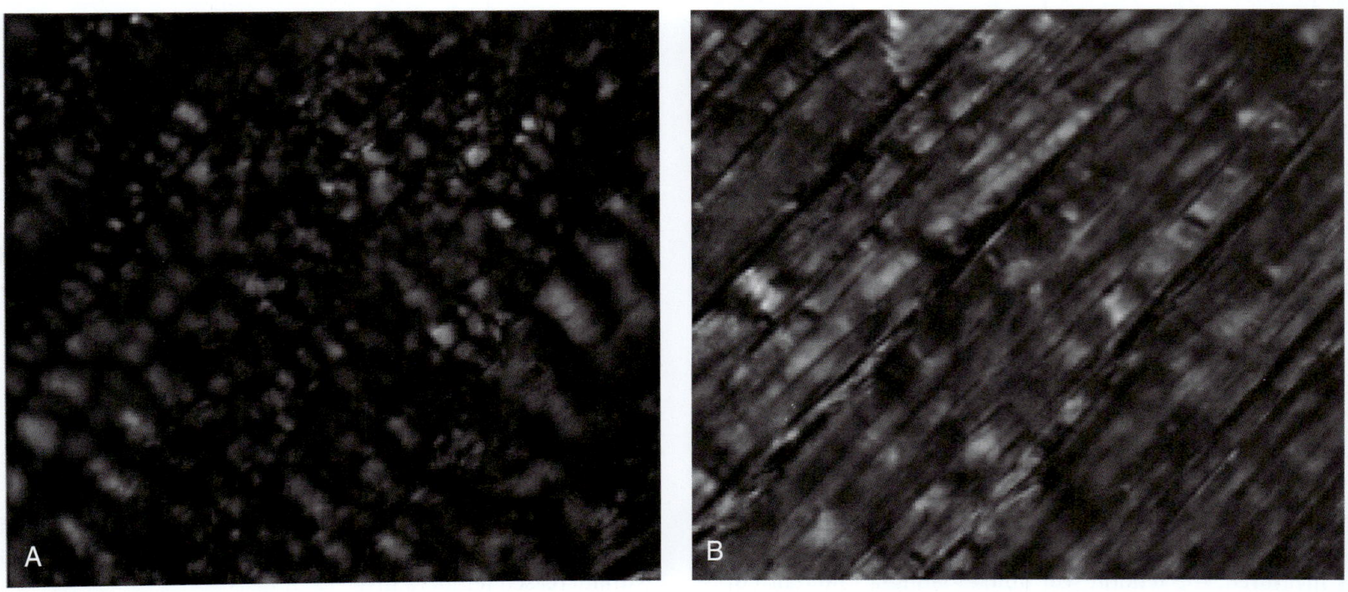

FIGURE 5 Polarized light microscopy of collagen fibril crimp in mouse supraspinatus tendon (90 days old) (**A**). Under applied tensile loading, the collagen fibrils become uncrimped (**B**). (Reproduced with permission from Miller K, Connizzo B, Feeney E, Soslowsky L: Characterizing local collagen fiber re-alignment and crimp behavior throughout mechanical testing in a mature mouse spraspinatus tendon model. *J Biomech* 2012;45[11]:1861-2060.)

©Copyright 2021 American Academy of Orthopaedic Surgeons

by the area under the curve. These parameters are useful in understanding the overall performance of the enthesis in a given experimental setting.

A more refined measure of the tendon material properties is obtained by the normalization of these structural properties to tendon area and length. This analysis yields a curve known as a stress-strain curve (**Figure 4**, B). Strain, which represents change in length of the tendon relative to total tendon length, is derived in several ways, the discussion of which is beyond the scope of this chapter. This curve is also nonlinear and represents uniaxial tensile loading of the tendon per area. Several parameters can be determined, including modulus, which is the slope of the curve; tensile strength, which is the stress value at failure; ultimate strain; and strain energy density, represented by the area under the curve.

Both structural and material properties are important in experimental evaluation of tendon and its enthesis, especially when considering tendon repair and healing. It should be recognized that an increase in stiffness alone might not be a positive indicator of repair strength; if there has been a substantial increase in cross-sectional area of the tendon, stiffness may increase while modulus decreases. This is a scenario indicative of an increase in quantity, not quality, of tendon tissue and may not represent successful reconstitution of tendon properties.

Viscoelastic

The viscoelastic properties of tendon are essential to understanding how tendon structure contributes to its function. Viscoelasticity can be defined as mechanical behavior that is time- and history-dependent, with material classified by both viscous properties (resisting deformation under stress) and elastic properties (indicating a tendency to resume its original shape when stress is removed). Stated differently, a viscoelastic material subjected to stress will undergo an initial deformation, but the same stress will cause less deformation with time. Tendon behavior tends to be dominated by viscous properties at low loads and more elastic behavior at high loads.

Viscoelastic behavior can be characterized by creep, stress relaxation, hysteresis, and strain rate sensitivity parameters (**Figure 4**, C). Under a constant applied load, tendon will undergo initial deformation and then continue to elongate at a much slower rate, without any further increase in applied load. This tendency is known as creep. Another aspect of this phenomenon can be seen in the case of a constant elongation. In this scenario, the elongation is the independent variable, held constant. The load in the tendon is the measured, dependent variable. With time, the load will decrease. This behavior is known as stress relaxation. Tendon also displays a behavior responsive to its loading history. If tendon is cyclically elongated to a set length and allowed to relax, and the load is measured, the tendon will unload along a different curve than in loading. The area between the two curves represents dissipated energy and is known as hysteresis. Furthermore, repeated cycling will give rise to progressively smaller loads in the tissue, consistent with stress relaxation, in a pattern known as cyclic load relaxation. In addition, when a repeated stress is applied, nonlinear changes occur in the deformation, resulting in cyclic creep.

Proprioception

Tendon has been shown to have excellent innervation for the purpose of proprioception, or the sensing of joint position in space. This ability enables tendon to contribute more effectively to biomechanical function. Clinically, an appreciation of proprioception is relevant because of tendon repair and transfer surgeries. If proprioception is not reestablished, tendon repair outcomes seem to be diminished. As an example, the outcome of teres major transfer to the supraspinatus insertion for massive rotator cuff tear is dramatically improved if the teres can be retrained to function as an arm abductor, which requires preservation of proprioception in the teres tendon.[9]

Biologic Factors Influencing Tendon Properties

Several biologic factors have significant effects on tendon properties, including age, presence of comorbidities, activity level, and anatomic location. Specifically, studies have shown that tendons from older individuals are prone to increased incidence of tendon injury.[10,11] Additionally, medical comorbidities can lead to in vivo degradation of tendon; diabetes, hypercholesterolemia, and kidney disease each have been identified. Exercise can also profoundly affect tendon, with exercised tendons showing increased modulus compared with age-matched control tendons.[12] Anatomic location also significantly affects tendon tensile strength. As shown previously, tendon from the erector spinae muscles have modulus values an order of magnitude higher than the rotator cuff tendons.[13] These factors apply to most connective tissue and will be discussed in more detail in the Ligament section.

Experimental Factors Influencing Tendon Properties

Several technical aspects must be considered when performing experimental measurements as a method to determine tendon mechanical properties. These include the appropriate testing environment, specimen type and orientation, strain rate, and specimen storage, as well as biologic conditions; samples must be similar in age at the moment of harvest and these must be similar in size and diameter.

Testing Environment

The environment for testing has a significant effect on mechanical properties. Specifically, the hydration and temperature of the tissue should be taken into consideration. For example, studies have shown that tendon stiffness decreases with increased temperature.[13]

Specimen Type and Orientation

As described previously, tendon is composed of a bone-tendon-muscle complex. To examine the structural properties,

©Copyright 2021 American Academy of Orthopaedic Surgeons

the entire complex is often tested experimentally. The specimen is typically positioned in an anatomic orientation, so that the amount of fibers engaged along the longitudinal axis during loading is maximized. In addition, to examine material properties, the attachments to the tendon are often removed and the tendon is tested independently of the bone. In each of these situations, the specimens must be gripped differently to determine tensile properties. To minimize the error as a result of slipping and stress concentrations at the grips, the tendon should have a high length versus width ratio, defined as an aspect ratio.

Finally, the rate of loading applied experimentally and proper specimen storage also have significant effects on tendon properties. These factors are characteristic of most soft tissues and will be discussed in more detail in the Ligament section.

CLINICALLY RELEVANT INJURIES

Tendon injuries are an important aspect of musculoskeletal medical conditions. There are several types of tendon injury, ranging from overuse injuries (such as tendinosis) to rupture, with different clinical consequences. Tendon ruptures are classified into direct and indirect ruptures based on mechanism: direct injuries involve direct trauma to the tendon causing a tear, whereas indirect injuries result from forceful loading of the muscle-tendon-bone unit to the point of tendon failure.

Tendinopathy is an umbrella term for a group of syndromes on the same spectrum, considered to be overuse injuries, resulting in pain and varying degrees of loss of function of the tendon. Tendinosis has largely replaced the term tendinitis in the orthopaedic literature to describe the chronic overuse injury to tendon, as true inflammation is generally absent in these patients. These injuries are characterized by persistent pain and radiographic evidence of intrasubstance tendon degeneration.[14] Upon histologic examination, the hallmarks of tendinosis include disrupted and disorganized collagen, increased extracellular matrix, increased tenocyte population, and neovascularization. Tendinosis, in addition to being a clinical problem itself, can lead to more severe injury, such as complete tendon rupture. Direct and indirect ruptures of tendons remain an important orthopaedic problem, with ongoing management challenges. Injury to the flexor tendons of the upper extremity is the most common and highly characterized of the direct tendon injuries. Penetrating trauma is usually responsible, with stab wounds making up a large portion of these injuries. These tendons typically have no preexisting condition that predisposes them to injury. The tendon is lacerated and retracts because of its muscular attachment. Additionally, the tendon sheath is violated, introducing the risk of infection into a hypovascular space and depriving the tendon of the normal synovial fluid, through which it obtains a portion of its nutrition.[15]

By contrast, indirect tendon injuries are more common and occur through overloading of the bone-tendon-muscle unit. The underlying tendon is predisposed to injury from a variety of etiologies.[16] As described previously, tendinosis has been identified as a likely factor predisposing to rupture, in addition to location in a hypovascular vascular zone, which is also a likely etiology. Several tendons are prone to indirect rupture and are a common orthopaedic injury, including the rotator cuff tendons, long head and distal biceps tendons, hamstring tendon, quadriceps and patellar tendons, and Achilles tendon.

As discussed previously, the material and structural properties of tendon are finely organized to maximize stability and mobility at minimal risk of injury. In the setting of tendinosis, the behavior of tendon is disturbed, and injury becomes a threat. The mechanism of this injury is classically an eccentric contraction, in which there is forced lengthening of the myotendinous unit during contraction. This condition puts maximum stress through the tendon and leads to rupture at a site of weakening, disabling the naturally protective qualities of tendon discussed previously, including viscoelastic behaviors.

TENDON REPAIR

Healing Processes, Principles, and Deficiencies

Tendon healing processes are characterized by a reactive scar formation that results in tissue that is biologically and mechanically inferior to native tissue. In some instances the healing is functional, producing tissue that adequately substitutes for native tissue, whereas in other instances the tissue is nonfunctional, leading to further tendon injury and sometimes joint instability and altered joint function.

Paratenon-covered tendon healing primarily follows the generalized healing process for connective tissues, occurring in three overlapping phases: inflammation, proliferation, and remodeling. During the inflammatory phase, inflammatory cells and erythrocytes migrate to the site of injury and the gap between the tendon ends is filled. Next, resorption of the initial hematoma is initialized by monocytes and macrophages that enter the lesion. Various vasoactive and chemotactic factors increase vascularity and recruit more inflammatory cells, triggering both degradative and reparative processes, to remove and replace damaged material. During the final stages of inflammation, tenocytes begin to migrate to the injury site and the synthesis of type III collagen begins.[17]

The proliferative phase follows. Within a few days after injury, matrix and cellular proliferation predominate at the injury site. This stage is characterized by continuous collagen production and deposition, creating a scarlike fibrous tissue (**Figure 6**, A). The synthesis of type III collagen is maximal during this stage, and cellularity remains high.

The remodeling phase begins approximately 6 weeks following injury and is characterized by a gradual decrease in cellularity and vascularity and the continually increasing organization and maturation of scar tissue over time. During this phase, collagen fibers, along with fibroblasts, attempt to reorient themselves along the length of the tendon (**Figure 6**, B).

©Copyright 2021 American Academy of Orthopaedic Surgeons

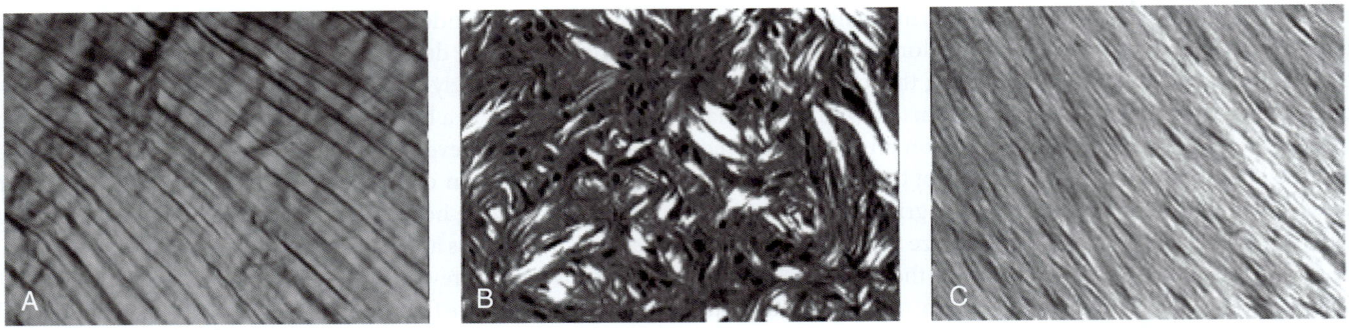

FIGURE 6 Polarized light histology of the supraspinatus tendon in the rat for uninjured control (**A**), 1 week postinjury (**B**), and 16 weeks postinjury (**C**). The uninjured control demonstrates aligned collagen fibers and collagen crimp, as observed in normal tendon. After 1 week postinjury, the tendon displays an increase in collagen disorganization and by 16 weeks, the collagen organization improves. (Reproduced with permission from Gimbel JA, Van Kleunen JP, Mehta S, Perry SM, Williams GR, Soslowsky LJ: Supraspinatus tendon organizational and mechanical properties in a chronic rotator cuff tear animal model. *J Biomech* 2004;37[5]:739-749.)

In addition, the synthesis of type I collagen, the main collagen present in uninjured tendons, predominates.[17] Each of these steps in the remodeling phase represents a significant attempt during the healing process to return to normal tendon characteristics (**Figure 6**, C). Tendon healing occurs by two mechanisms, each of which has both drawbacks and benefits to function. As previously mentioned, tendons heal by deposition of scar tissue at the site of injury. Although this scar tissue may allow for functional healing, deposition of scar tissue is often harmful to the tissue when it impedes tendon gliding and ultimately tendon function. This is particularly apparent in tendons encapsulated with a synovial sheath, such as zone II in the flexor tendon system of the hand. Two mechanisms of tendon healing have been proposed: intrinsic and extrinsic. The extrinsic mechanism involves cells from the periphery invading the injury site, whereas the intrinsic mechanism involves cells within the tendon itself (**Figure 7**). It is likely that a combination of the two mechanisms occurs clinically; however, the extrinsic mechanism has been implicated as the primary source of adhesions between the tendon and surrounding structures. Because of these adhesions, outcomes after tendon repair, particularly of sheathed tendons, are often less than desirable. Although the ability to restore function after tendon injury has been greatly improved by advanced suture techniques and rehabilitation protocols, development of gene therapies, cell therapies, and tissue bioengineering approaches will likely be necessary to yield further clinical improvements in these outcomes in the future.[15]

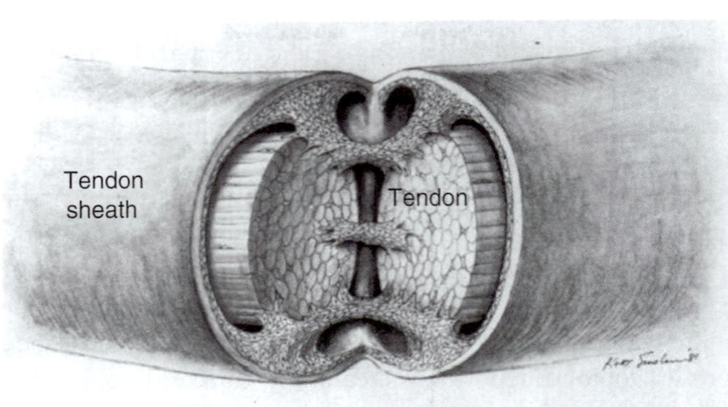

FIGURE 7 Illustration of extrinsic and intrinsic healing processes in a sheathed tendon. Adhesions may result from activation of the extrinsic process, inhibiting tendon gliding within the synovial sheath. (Adapted with permission from Gelberman RH, Vande Berg JS, Lundborg GN, Akeson WH: Flexor tendon healing and restoration of the gliding surface: An ultrastructural study in dogs. *J Bone Joint Surg Am* 1983;65[1]:70-80.)

Clinically Relevant Variables Affecting Tendon

Repair optimization of tendon repair by enhancing both stability and mobility is essential for adequate joint function. Rehabilitation regimens, specifically immobilization and early postoperative motion, are important factors in enhancing stability and mobility, respectively. However, these regimens are conflicting, with immobilization leading to increased stiffness that limits mobility and early postoperative motion potentially disrupting the initial stability of the repair. Thus, optimal treatment must consider careful balance of the two.

Numerous suture techniques, including various configurations, quantities, and materials of sutures, have also been developed in an attempt to optimize the mechanical strength of the tendon.[15] Increasing the strength of the construct may allow for a more aggressive prescribed postoperative protocol.

As mentioned previously, tendons are extremely sensitive to their mechanical environment, and therefore specific rehabilitation protocols for injured tendons are critical for healing. For uninjured tendons, the mechanical properties tend to increase with increased loading (during exercise) and decrease with decreased loading (during immobilization). However, conflicting evidence exists regarding the optimal rehabilitation treatment of healing tissues. Several studies have shown benefits to increased loading,[18] whereas others have shown negative effects. Although it is generally believed that low loading regimens seem to promote healing, and high-intensity

©Copyright 2021 American Academy of Orthopaedic Surgeons

loading regimens may be more likely to have detrimental effects,[19] more recent evidence suggests that early, higher intensity rehabilitation protocols may promote improved patient outcomes for certain tendon injuries, such as ruptures of the Achilles tendon.[20] Further evidence is needed to elucidate the optimal rehabilitation techniques after injury and repair of various tendons.

Chronic tendon injuries caused by overuse and excessive loading have limited propensity for healing because of irrecoverable degeneration of the tendon tissue. Previous work has shown that tendons with chronic injuries demonstrate decreased collagen organization, increased cellularity, altered cell shape (eg, more rounded), and decreased mechanical properties, indicative of a degenerative tissue.[21] In addition, chronic rotator cuff tears are clinically characterized by fatty degeneration and atrophy of the rotator cuff muscles, which alter the healing response and limit the success of rotator cuff tendon repairs. The difficulties associated with healing of chronic injuries may be a result of the lack of inflammation and the failed healing response associated with the degenerative tissue.[22,23] As a result of these findings, it has been shown that the quality of the tissue must be assessed before prescribing both surgical treatment and postoperative protocols.

LIGAMENT

CLASSIFICATION AND ANATOMY

Like tendons, ligaments are classified as dense bands of fibrous connective tissue characterized by closely packed collagen fibers. Despite their gross similarities, ligaments and tendons differ in their function, mechanical properties, and biochemical composition. Most noticeably, ligaments both originate and insert onto bone, whereas tendons connect muscle to bone. Ligaments also have different inherent properties based on their function and anatomic location. In general, the basic function of ligaments is to guide joint kinematics, maintain joint stability, and prevent abnormal displacement of bones. Anatomically, they are classified according to their attachment sites on bone, which are critical for the distribution and dissipation of joint forces. Capsular ligaments, which are located within the articular capsule that surrounds synovial joints, are anatomically less discrete than extracapsular ligaments but also function to provide stability to the joint.

GROSS MORPHOLOGY, HISTOLOGY, MICROANATOMY, AND CELL BIOLOGY

Ligament is composed of collagenous connective tissue arranged in a hierarchical manner, as in tendon. In general, ligament is characterized as relatively avascular. A thin layer of connective tissue, the epiligament, surrounds the ligament and is analogous to the tendon epitenon. Similar to tendon, the epiligament carries nerves, blood vessels, and lymphatics and is thought to play a role in ligament healing. Morphologically, collagen fiber interactions in ligaments are defined as being more highly cross-linked than tendon and more intertwined in comparison with the generally parallel-oriented tendon fibers. Ligaments also contain more metabolically active fibroblast cells that are incorporated between the collagen fibers. In addition to differences in cell morphology, ligaments also have more type III collagen than tendon but in general have less total collagen.

Different ligaments have different properties and structure according to their anatomic location, based on their interaction with joint synovial fluid (whether they are intra-articular or extra-articular). For example, the intra-articular ACL has cells that are more chondroid in appearance and are classified as less biologically active than those of the medial collateral ligament (MCL), which is extra-articular (**Figure 8**).

Within a ligament, there are also important regional differences in collagen fiber orientation and composition and cell shape between the midsubstance and bony insertion sites. The morphology of the insertion site has two different forms:

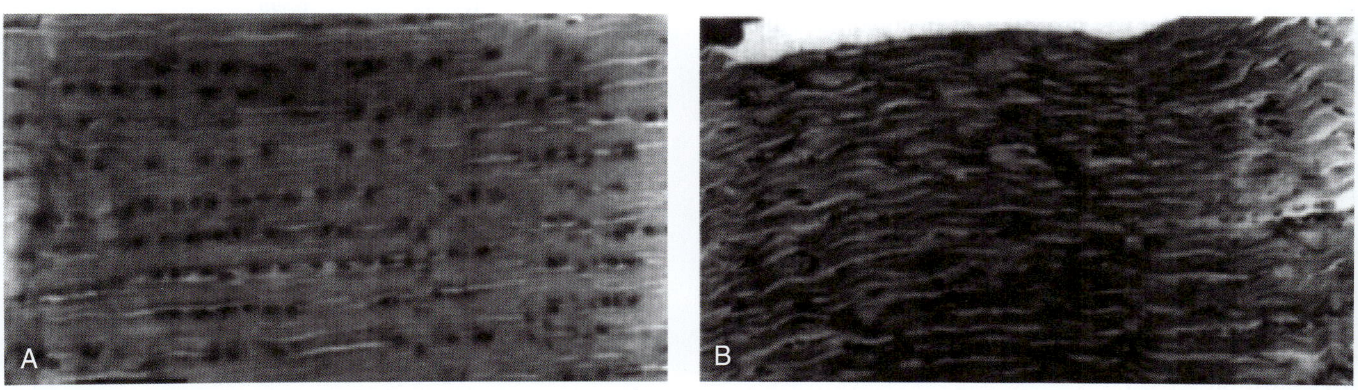

FIGURE 8 Histology showing differing morphology of intra-articular anterior cruciate ligament (ACL) cells (**A**) and extra-articular medial collateral ligament (MCL) cells (**B**) in the New Zealand white rabbit. ACL cells are chondroid in appearance, whereas the MCL cells appear more elongated. (Reproduced with permission from Frank CB: Ligament injuries: Pathophysiology and healing, in Zachazewski JE, Magee DJ, Quillen WS, eds: *Athletic Injuries and Rehabilitation*. Philadelphia, PA, WB Saunders, 1996.)

©Copyright 2021 American Academy of Orthopaedic Surgeons

direct and indirect. As with tendon, direct insertions are most common and are characterized by four zones: ligament, fibrocartilage, calcified fibrocartilage, and bone. Indirect insertions, such as the tibial insertion site of the MCL, are anchored directly to the bone by calcified collagen fibers, called Sharpey fibers, that merge with the periosteum and bone. In the midsubstance, cells appear elongated in shape, whereas at the insertion the cells appear to be more rounded. This cellular transition and change in collagen composition is a reflection of the distribution and dissipation of stresses during loading.

The composition of ligament is similar to that of tendon. The primary constituents are water, collagen, elastin, proteoglycans, and cells. Water comprises approximately 60% to 70% of the total weight, whereas approximately 80% of the dry weight is attributed to collagen. Type I collagen is the main collagen present in ligaments (approximately 90% of the collagen present). A significantly smaller portion is type III collagen with the addition of many other types including V, VI, XI, and XIV. Proteoglycans represent approximately 1% of the ligament dry weight and function in ligament hydration and viscoelastic behavior. The relative proportions of proteoglycans vary according to ligament anatomic location and function, specifically whether there is a significant compressive load-bearing responsibility in addition to its primary tensile load-bearing function. Another component that appears in ligament in a small proportion (approximately 1% of dry weight) is the fibrillar protein elastin. Elastin functions in ligament elasticity and in its return to a prestretched length after loading. The primary cell type found in ligament is fibroblasts, which are oriented longitudinally within the collagen fiber framework. These cells synthesize the collagen and extracellular matrix that constitute ligament structure.

Blood Supply and Innervation

Vascularity is crucial for nutrient supply and healing of ligaments. Despite its generally sparse vasculature, ligament has an organized and distinct microvasculature system. As described previously, the epiligamentous plexus, surrounding the ligament, gives rise to most ligament vasculature; in general, ligaments exhibit regional differences, with a denser distribution near the insertion sites.[24] Ligaments also accommodate different sensory nerve endings near their insertion sites. These nerves have different capabilities as nociceptive pain sensors as well as proprioceptive position sensors, which both contribute to the functional stability of the joint.[25]

LIGAMENT FUNCTIONS

Mechanical

Ligaments serve as the primary static stabilizers in joints. They connect bone to bone and act as passive restraints, guiding joint motion. In addition, ligaments are also characterized as having both dominant and load-sharing functions. For example, the knee joint is stabilized by the interaction of several ligaments, particularly the ACL and MCL, which have an interdependent load-sharing relationship. When one structure is deficient, the force in the complementary structure increases significantly to compensate.[26] However, in general, individual ligaments can be characterized by their dominant functions and their ability to resist unique abnormal displacements (eg, the role of the ACL in resisting anterior tibial translation).

Ligament mechanical properties are directly influenced by their structure, collagen composition, and fiber orientation. As with tendon at low loads, ligaments tend to behave in a nonlinear viscous-dominated manner, whereas at high loads ligaments are more elastic-dominated. As previously mentioned, ligaments have a more disorganized collagen orientation compared with the highly aligned tendon. Thus, the toe region is typically elongated in ligament because it takes more time to align the ligament collagen fibers in the direction of loading.

Some individual ligaments also have a unique functional anatomy, consisting of distinct bands serving specific functions (**Figure 9**). These bands are recruited differently throughout the entire joint range of motion. For example, the ACL can be divided into two distinct bands, the anteromedial

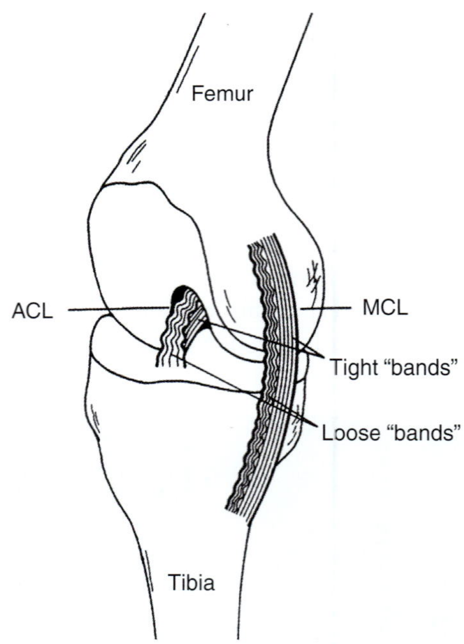

FIGURE 9 Schematic of the distinct, functional bands in the anterior cruciate ligament (ACL) and medial collateral ligament (MCL) of the knee. Positioning of the joint determines which band is under tension, and each contributes specifically to joint rotation and translation. (Reproduced with permission from Frank CB: Ligament injuries: Pathophysiology and healing, in Zachazewski JE, Magee DJ, Quillen WS, eds: *Athletic Injuries and Rehabilitation*. Philadelphia, PA, WB Saunders, 1996.)

 ©Copyright 2021 American Academy of Orthopaedic Surgeons

and posterolateral, with dominant roles in preventing anterior tibial translation and resisting rotation in knee extension, respectively.[27] Thus, the position of the joint determines which band is most tightly engaged and therefore most susceptible to damage.

Viscoelastic

As in tendon, ligaments also express viscoelastic behavior (time- and history-dependent behavior). This is due in part to the complex interaction between collagen, water, and other extracellular matrix components. Proteoglycans and associated negatively charged GAGs play a major role in water retention and have been identified as factors that contribute to soft-tissue viscoelasticity. However, the role of GAGs remains controversial—some studies have shown that GAGs may have no direct contribution to ligament viscoelasticity.[28] The primary viscoelastic properties of ligaments are measured, as with tendon, during a stress relaxation test, where under constant elongation, the tissue will relax and the load will decrease over time, and during a creep test, where under constant load, the deformation will increase over time.

Proprioception

As previously mentioned, ligaments have proprioceptive nerve endings that play a key role in joint function and dynamic stability. Histologic evidence in the knee and shoulder has identified the presence of mechanoreceptors in the ligaments. In addition, several techniques have been used to quantify joint proprioceptive function in vivo, including joint position sense and threshold to detection tests. Specifically, it has been shown that in an ACL-deficient knee, proprioceptive function is less than that found in a normal knee and that in general, decreased proprioceptive function correlates with a decreased amount and subsequent disruption of mechanoreceptors.[29] Thus, these mechanoreceptors may play an afferent role in providing the central nervous system with joint proprioceptive information.[30]

Biologic Factors Influencing Ligament Properties

As in tendon, many biologic factors influence ligament properties. Biologic factors that lead to ligament variation include skeletal maturation and aging, anatomic location, and sex, as well as variation in tissue response associated with immobilization and exercise.

Skeletal Maturation and Aging

The tensile properties of both skeletally immature and mature ligaments have also been examined. In general, ligament structural properties, including stiffness, ultimate load, and energy absorbed at failure, increase over time but remain relatively constant after skeletal maturation. In addition, the mode of failure in skeletally mature specimens is typically localized to the midsubstance, whereas immature specimens often undergo avulsion-type failure, most likely a result of the weaker open epiphyses.[31]

Ligament properties are also found to change with aging. In human cadaver knees and shoulders, studies have shown that these same structural properties of stiffness, ultimate load, and energy absorbed at failure of the ligaments decrease with aging. Similar to the difference between skeletally mature and immature specimens, it has also been noted that older specimens have a higher incidence of midsubstance failure than younger specimens.[32,33]

Anatomic Location

Ligaments also have different properties based on anatomic location. For example, the shoulder joint experiences a larger range of motion than the knee joint, and therefore the mechanical behavior of these ligaments varies as a result of their different functions.

Sex

Sex-specific and hormone-related variables have also been implicated as potential biologic factors influencing ligament properties. Studies have shown that females are two to eight times more likely to damage their ACL than males.[34,35] This is due, in part, to the increased dynamic valgus and abduction loads experienced by females during physical activity,[36] which may be a result of anatomic differences between males and females. Changes in hormone levels have also been implicated, although evidence suggests that ligament mechanical properties are not influenced by alterations in estrogen, the primary female sex hormone.[37] Recent evidence found that another female hormone, relaxin, which has been reported to affect collagen synthesis, may decrease connective tissue mechanical properties, including load to failure and stiffness.[38] One study demonstrated that when treated with excess relaxin hormone, the ACL was found to be significantly weaker.[39] These results suggest that reduced mechanical properties caused by increased serum relaxin levels may place the joint at higher risk for injury.

Immobilization

As previously mentioned, stress deprivation due to immobilization has profound morphologic, biochemical, and biomechanical effects on synovial joints. Some changes include the development of synovial adhesions (which leads to increased joint stiffness), disruption of ligament collagen and cellular organization, disruptions in the ligament insertion sites (caused by osteoclastic resorption of bone), and in general, decreased ligament structural properties.[40] As in tendon, remobilization in the ligament reveals a slow but significant improvement of the detrimental effects following immobilization. However, incomplete recovery occurs at the insertion sites, and ligament properties do not return to normal.[41]

©Copyright 2021 American Academy of Orthopaedic Surgeons

Exercise

Ligament properties following exercise have also been extensively evaluated, and evidence suggests that short-term exercise regimens increase ligament mechanical and structural properties, including strength and stiffness.[42-44] For example, one study demonstrated that failure load of the MCL was significantly increased in an exercise group compared with a decreased activity group.

Experimental Factors Influencing Ligament Properties

Similar to tendon, many experimental factors, including strain rate, specimen storage, and appropriate testing environment, in addition to the unique bone-ligament-bone complex specific to ligaments, also influence ligament properties. In general, the tensile properties of ligaments slightly increase with increased extension rates.[45] In addition, the effect of freezing ligaments, which is necessary to preserve ligament tissue, has displayed no significant difference in the ligament structural or mechanical properties in comparison with fresh ligament tissue.[46] In contrast to tendon, structural properties of ligaments are characterized by the bone-ligament-bone complex. When tested in various orientations, the structural properties and modes of failure significantly differ in the ligament,[33,47] suggesting that a standard for experimental testing should be followed.

CLINICALLY RELEVANT INJURIES

Ligament injuries are typically the result of traumatic joint injury and are often classified according to severity of the injury (grade I, II, or III). Grade I injuries are characterized as a mild sprain in which fibers are overstretched but not actually torn, grade II injuries are classified as partial disruption of ligament fibers, and grade III injuries involve complete rupture of the ligament. Grade II and III ligament tears may have serious implications, putting patients at an increased risk for concomitant injuries of the MCL, posterior cruciate ligament, posterolateral corner, and menisci. One study showed a significant association between complete meniscal root tears and high grade (II or III) ACL injuries compared with grade I ACL injuries.[48] These injuries have serious implications for quality of life, especially for the young athlete. Although studies have shown the majority of athletes return to some level of sport after an ACL injury, only 65% can return to their preinjury level, and only 38% can remain at that level for multiple years after the time of injury. In addition, ligament tears are associated with increased joint instability and in some cases, the development of debilitating chronic conditions. For instance, multiple studies have shown an increased risk in the development of osteoarthritis of the knee after ACL tears, whether managed surgically or nonsurgically, and this risk further increases in subjects with combined injuries.[49]

Traumatic joint injuries often involve multiple ligaments, such as the combination of ACL and MCL ruptures in the knee. Combined ligamentous injuries cause dramatic instability in the joint, decreasing the propensity for spontaneous healing. Ligament replacement or repair is often required to prevent or delay the progression of damage to the joint, caused by chronic joint laxity and instability.

LIGAMENT REPAIR

Healing Processes, Principles, and Deficiencies

The healing process of ligaments is analogous to that of the tendons, occurring in three phases: inflammation, matrix and cellular proliferation, and remodeling and maturation. In general, severe (complete) ligament injuries lead to poor healing because of retraction of torn ends. Various biologic alterations occur during ligament healing including the alteration of proteoglycan and collagen content, specifically increased expression of types III and V collagen.[50] Healing ligaments are also characterized by their increased vascularization[51] and discontinuities within their cellular connections and organization.[52]

Despite the various healing challenges, experimental evidence suggests that in some cases natural healing is possible. When the gap created by the retraction of the torn ligament ends is minimal, certain ligaments have the potential to develop local repair responses, in an attempt to "bridge the gap." Cellular components recruited to the area synthesize collagen and other extracellular matrix components at the injury site. The result is the formation of a collagen-rich scar and matrix that slowly remodel to align with the ligament tissue. Ultimately, the healed ligament is mechanically inferior to native tissue, reaching only 30% to 50% of native tissue quality.[53]

Clinically Relevant Variables Affecting Ligament Repair: Strategies to "Heal"

Because of the MCL's ability to heal spontaneously, it has often been used as a model system to understand ligament healing and the effect of various treatment modalities on ligament repair. For instance, nonsurgical treatment of an isolated MCL injury has been found in some studies to produce better results than surgical intervention.[53] In addition, immobilization after ligament injury was found to lead to increased collagen disorganization as well as decreased structural and mechanical properties, including ultimate load and maximum energy adsorbed and stress-strain behavior, respectively.[40] As a result of these findings, clinical management of MCL tears has shifted to nonsurgical treatment with early controlled remobilization.[2]

Biochemical interventions have also been evaluated as potential methods to improve scar tissue quality and composition. Extrinsic factors including growth factors, hyaluronic acid, platelet-rich plasma, and prolotherapy have all been implicated as potential strategies to assist in ligament healing. However, controversy exists over the quality of evidence to

©Copyright 2021 American Academy of Orthopaedic Surgeons

support these interventions and therefore their effectiveness has not been clearly defined. As previously mentioned, gap size is another clinically relevant variable affecting ligament repair. Evidence suggests that the natural healing ability of ligament is variable and that the amount of retraction by the torn ends can be highlighted as a causative factor.

TENDON AND LIGAMENT GRAFTING AND REPLACEMENT

OVERVIEW: REPAIR VERSUS RECONSTRUCTION

As discussed previously, tendon and ligament injuries occur as a result of acute trauma or chronic overuse and are among the most common musculoskeletal injuries. The understanding of the pathogenesis of these conditions continues to improve; however, treatment regimens remain suboptimal. Both ACL and rotator cuff tendon tears do not heal spontaneously and the success of nonsurgical management in active patients is limited. Therefore, these soft tissues must undergo either repair or reconstruction to prevent joint instability, which may lead to the development of chronic pain, disability, and osteoarthritis.

Several factors influence the standards for surgical treatment including the tissue's anatomic location and the severity of the injury. Typically, intrasynovial tissues have limited ability to heal and therefore the common standard for surgical treatment is reconstruction with a local autograft or allograft. The standard treatment of extrasynovial tissues, on the other hand, is often direct repair. For instance, ACL tears are typically treated by reconstruction, whereas rotator cuff tendon tears are usually treated with direct repair. In addition, the severity of the injury must also be taken into consideration when determining the appropriate surgical treatment. In cases where the tissue has a chronic or massive tear, surgical reconstruction or repair with augmentation is almost always necessary to achieve optimal results.

GRAFTING USING NORMAL TISSUES

Currently, the standard of care for tendon and ligament repair and reconstruction is grafting connective tissue within the same individual (autograft) or from another individual postmortem (allograft). These tissues have become main sources for harvestable grafts because of their potentially expendable roles. Xenografts (taken from a different species) are also useful for tissue grafting but currently have no clinical use in tendon or ligament reconstruction.

For reconstruction, the primary role of the replacement graft is to reproduce the anatomy and function of the native tissue. The most commonly used grafts for reconstruction include the bone–patellar tendon–bone complex and the semitendinosus or gracilis of the hamstring. For repair, the primary role of the graft is to augment the natural healing process while maintaining the mechanical properties of the native tissue. Whether for repair or reconstruction, the material type, graft placement, initial graft tension, and graft fixation are all significant factors that will alter joint kinematics, graft forces in situ, and articular compressive loads. For ACL reconstruction, various graft/fixation options include bone–patellar tendon–bone grafts and hamstring tendon grafts, either of which can be autograft or allograft, fixed by various methods, including interference screws, pin fixation, or an Endobutton (Acufex, Microsurgical Inc, Mansfield, MA). Additionally, the amount of graft tensioning before fixation could decrease the amount of graft elongation following fixation and therefore its optimization for ACL reconstruction remains a heavily researched and controversial topic.[54] Despite the increased understanding of ideal techniques for grafting, the results are still suboptimal, and under cyclic loading, grafts have a tendency to elongate and migrate leading to deterioration of the initial stability of the reconstruction.[55] In addition, no grafting technique has been able to mimic the function of the native tissue, and as a result, the standard for grafting using normal tissues remains a highly debated and heavily researched topic.

FUNCTIONAL TISSUE ENGINEERING: CURRENT CONCEPTS

Studies have shown that neither spontaneous healing, soft-tissue repair, nor reconstruction has the ability to generate native quality tissue after injury; as a result, restoring the normal function remains a significant challenge. Therefore, new treatment modalities are being considered to improve the properties of healing ligaments and tendons. As tissue engineering and regeneration techniques become more readily available, increased focus has been placed on utilization of these techniques as tools to enhance ligament and tendon healing.

With recent advances in tissue engineering, tendon and ligament grafts have taken a comprehensive role, acting as both a source of mechanical stability and a biologic environment with the ability to regenerate and incorporate living tissue (**Figure 10**). A variety of biologic and synthetic materials can act as scaffolds, however, regardless of type; each of these scaffolds should have specific characteristics. These characteristics include biocompatibility and high porosity to permit cell permeation and growth. Some biologic materials used include collagen derivatives and as mentioned in the previous section, normal tissues such as allografts, autografts, and xenografts. In addition, current synthetic materials being considered include resorbable polyesters, such as poly(lactic-co-glycolic) acid and silk, and nonresorbable materials, such as carbon, polytetraethylene, and polytetrafluoroethylene. Ultimately, the goal of the tissue-engineered construct is to replicate the mechanical and biologic properties of the native tissue.

©Copyright 2021 American Academy of Orthopaedic Surgeons

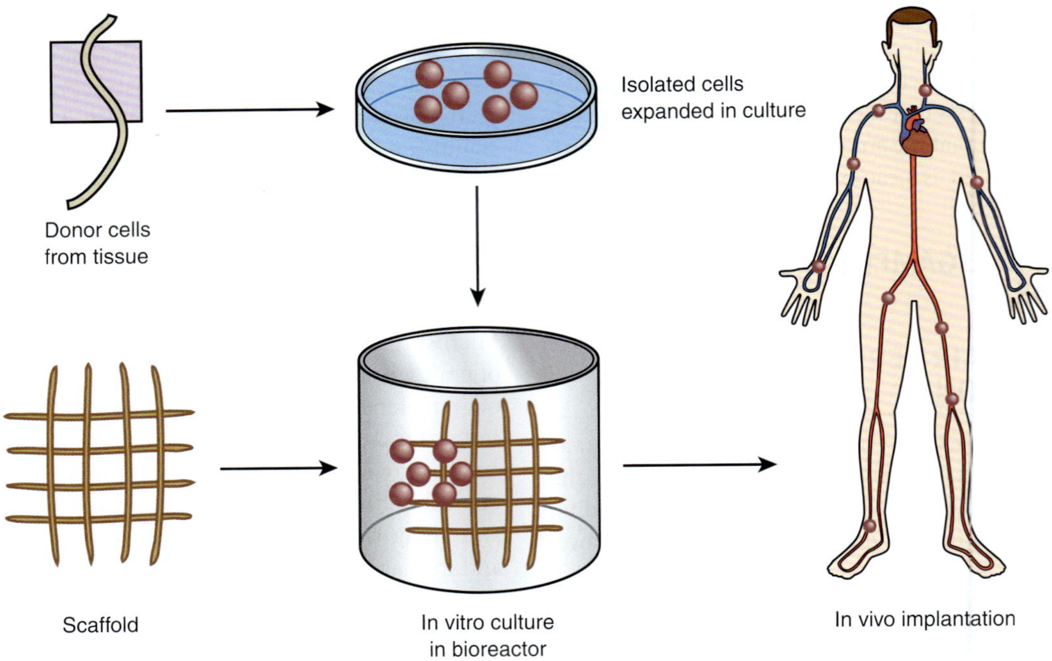

FIGURE 10 Illustration of functional tissue-engineering approaches for tendon and ligament that include the use of biologic scaffolds and methods to replicate the native tissue properties using cell seeding and mechanical stimulation techniques.

In addition to scaffold material, with advances in molecular biology and biochemistry, several novel therapeutic approaches have been identified for both in vitro and in vivo augmentation of tendon and ligament grafts. These techniques include the incorporation of growth factors (such as transforming growth factor-β, platelet-derived growth factor, fibroblast growth factor, and endothelial growth factor), the incorporation of native cells (such as mesenchymal stem cells and fibroblasts), and gene therapy (which involves altering protein synthesis to induce expression of specific proteins). To prepare the graft for the appropriate mechanical environment, mechanical stimulation techniques have been used to align the collagen fibers and fibroblasts in a physiologic manner. In addition, various vascularization strategies (including the application of vascular endothelial growth factor, basic fibroblast growth factor) have been used to replicate the native vascularized biologic environment.

Despite recent advances in functional tissue engineering, optimal constructs have not been developed for tendon or ligament and further progress must be made. While this is an extremely robust area of research and novel techniques are actively being pursued and refined, no one tissue engineering modality in the area of ligament or tendon repair has been adopted for routine clinical use. Despite this, we remain hopeful that tissue engineering techniques will have a significant, positive impact on tendon and ligament repair and healing in the future.

It should be noted that successful tissue-engineering approaches have been developed and are currently in routine use in a related connective tissue, the skin. Skin substitutes such as Integra (Integra Lifesciences, Plainsboro, NJ), Dermagraft (Smith and Nephew, Largo, FL), and Apligraf (Organogenesis, Canton, MA) have been approved by the US FDA to treat burn victims and/or heal skin wounds, and each has proved successful.

The recent advances in functional tissue-engineering approaches and successes achieved by marketed skin substitutes elucidate the potential of connective tissue constructs in general. With further improvements, tissue-engineered products have the potential to provide immediate, economical treatments of ligament and tendon injuries.

SUMMARY

Tendons and ligaments are connective tissues that are functionally and biologically diverse. As with most connective tissues, tendons and ligaments have a complex structure that affects their mechanical behavior. In addition, tendons and ligaments are capable of biologically adapting to altered loading and disease states. However, in chronic conditions or after severe injury, the modified tissue is often inadequate and fails to restore joint function. As a result, increased focus has been placed on reconstruction and regenerative techniques such as functional tissue engineering in an attempt to enhance tendon and ligament healing. In the near future, research and clinical trials will help in the understanding of pathologic and physiologic events after nonsurgical or surgical treatment.

©Copyright 2021 American Academy of Orthopaedic Surgeons

REFERENCES

1. Yelin E, Weingstein S, King T: The burden of musculoskeltal diseases in the United States. *Semin Arthritis Rheum* 2016;46(3):259-260.
2. Indelicato PA: Isolated medial collateral ligament injuries in the knee. *J Am Acad Orthop Surg* 1995;3(1):9-14.
3. Robinson KA, Sun M, Barnum CE, et al: Decorin and biglycan are necessary for maintaining collagen fibril structure, fiber realignment, and mechanical properties of mature tendons. *Matrix Biol* 2017;64,81-93.
4. Kalamajski S, Oldberg A: Homologous sequence in lumican and fibromodulin leucine-rich repeat 5-7 competes for collagen binding. *J Biol Chem* 2009;284(1):534-539.
5. Thomopoulos S, Genin GM, Galatz LM: The development and morphogenesis of the tendon-to-bone insertion: What development can teach us about healing. *J Musculoskelet Neuronal Interact* 2010;10(1):35-45.
6. Cooper RR, Misol S: Tendon and ligament insertion: A light and electron microscopic study. *J Bone Joint Surg Am* 1970;52(1):1-20.
7. Cook JL, Feller JA, Bonar SF, Khan KM: Abnormal tenocyte morphology is more prevalent than collagen disruption in asymptomatic athletes' patellar tendons. *J Orthop Res* 2004;22(2):334-338.
8. Cheng NM, Pan WR, Vally F, Le Roux CM, Richardson MD: The arterial supply of the long head of biceps tendon: Anatomical study with implications for tendon rupture. *Clin Anat* 2010;23(6):683-692.
9. Steenbrink F, Nelissen RG, Meskers CG, van de Sande MA, Rozing PM, de Groot JH: Teres major muscle activation relates to clinical outcome in tendon transfer surgery. *Clin Biomech* 2010;25(3):187-193.
10. Langberg H, Olesen J, Skovgaard D, Kjaer M: Age related blood flow around the Achilles tendon during exercise in humans. *Eur J Appl Physiol* 2001;84(3):246-248.
11. Abate M, Silbernagel KG, Siljeholm C, et al: Pathogenesis of tendinopathies: Inflammation or degeneration? *Arthritis Res Ther* 2009;11(3):235.
12. Arnoczky SP, Lavagnino M, Egerbacher M, Caballero O, Gardner K, Shender MA: Loss of homeostatic strain alters mechanostat "set point" of tendon cells in vitro. *Clin Orthop Relat Res* 2008;466(7):1583-1591.
13. Mow VC, Rik AH: *Basic Orthopaedic Biomechanics and Mechano-Biology*. Philadelphia, PA, Lippincott Williams & Wilkins, 2005.
14. Mishra A, Woodall J Jr, Vieira A: Treatment of tendon and muscle using platelet-rich plasma. *Clin Sports Med* 2009;28(1):113-125.
15. Graham JG, Wang ML, Rivlin M, Beredjiklian PK: Biologic and mechanical aspects of tendon fibrosis after injury and repair. *Connect Tissue Res* 2018;60(1):1-11.
16. McMaster PE: Tendon and muscle ruptures: Clinical and experimental studies on the causes and location of subcutaneous ruptures. *J Bone Joint Surg Am* 1933;15(3):18.
17. Sharma P, Maffulli N: Tendon injury and tendinopathy: Healing and repair. *J Bone Joint Surg Am* 2005;87(1):187-202.
18. Gelberman RH, Woo SL, Lothringer K, Akeson WH, Amiel D: Effects of early intermittent passive mobilization on healing canine flexor tendons. *J Hand Surg Am* 1982;7(2):170-175.
19. Thomopoulos S, Williams GR, Soslowsky LJ: Tendon to bone healing: Differences in biomechanical, structural, and compositional properties due to a range of activity levels. *J Biomech Eng* 2003;125(1):106-113.
20. Frankewycz B, Krutsch W, Weber J, Ernstberger A, Nerlich M, Pfeifer CG: Rehabilitation of Achilles tendon ruptures: Is early functional rehabilitation daily routine? *Arch Orthop Trauma Surg* 2017;137(3):333-340.
21. Dourte LM, Perry SM, Getz CL, Soslowsky LJ: Tendon properties remain altered in a chronic rat rotator cuff model. *Clin Orthop Relat Res* 2010;468(6):1485-1492.
22. Kovacevic D, Rodeo SA: Biological augmentation of rotator cuff tendon repair. *Clin Orthop Relat Res* 2008;466(3):622-633.
23. Carpenter JE, Thomopoulos S, Flanagan CL, DeBano CM, Soslowsky LJ: Rotator cuff defect healing: A biomechanical and histologic analysis in an animal model. *J Shoulder Elbow Surg* 1998;7(6):599-605.
24. Bray RC, Fisher AW, Frank CB: Fine vascular anatomy of adult rabbit knee ligaments. *J Anat* 1990;172:69-79.
25. Johansson H, Sjölander P, Sojka P: A sensory role for the cruciate ligaments. *Clin Orthop Relat Res* 1991;268:161-178.
26. Lujan TJ, Dalton MS, Thompson BM, Ellis BJ, Weiss JA: Effect of ACL deficiency on MCL strains and joint kinematics. *J Biomech Eng* 2007;129(3):386-392.
27. Petersen W, Zantop T: Anatomy of the anterior cruciate ligament with regard to its two bundles. *Clin Orthop Relat Res* 2007;454:35-47.
28. Lujan TJ, Underwood CJ, Jacobs NT, Weiss JA: Contribution of glycosaminoglycans to viscoelastic tensile behavior of human ligament. *J Appl Physiol* 2009;106(2):423-431.
29. Adachi N, Ochi M, Uchio Y, Iwasa J, Ryoke K, Kuriwaka M: Mechanoreceptors in the anterior cruciate ligament contribute to the joint position sense. *Acta Orthop Scand* 2002;73(3):330-334.
30. Grandis A, Spadari A, Bombardi C, Casadio Tozzi A, De Sordi N, Lucchi ML: Mechanoreceptors in the medial and lateral glenohumeral ligaments of the canine shoulder joint. *Vet Comp Orthop Traumatol* 2007;20(4):291-295.
31. Woo SL, Ohland KJ, Weiss JA: Aging and sex-related changes in the biomechanical properties of the rabbit medial collateral ligament. *Mech Ageing Dev* 1990;56(2):129-142.
32. Lee TQ, Dettling J, Sandusky MD, McMahon PJ: Age related biomechanical properties of the glenoid-anterior band of the inferior glenohumeral ligament-humerus complex. *Clin Biomech* 1999;14(7):471-476.
33. Woo SL, Hollis JM, Adams DJ, Lyon RM, Takai S: Tensile properties of the human femur-anterior cruciate ligament-tibia complex: The effects of specimen age and orientation. *Am J Sports Med* 1991;19(3):217-225.
34. Arendt E, Dick R: Knee injury patterns among men and women in collegiate basketball and soccer: NCAA data and review of literature. *Am J Sports Med* 1995;23(6):694-701.
35. Stevenson H, Webster J, Johnson R, Beynnon B: Gender differences in knee injury epidemiology among competitive alpine ski racers. *Iowa Orthop J* 1998;18:64-66.
36. Krosshaug T, Nakamae A, Boden BP, et al: Mechanisms of anterior cruciate ligament injury in basketball: Video analysis of 39 cases. *Am J Sports Med* 2007;35(3):359-367.
37. Warden SJ, Saxon LK, Castillo AB, Turner CH: Knee ligament mechanical properties are not influenced by estrogen or its receptors. *Am J Physiol Endocrinol Metab* 2006;290(5):E1034-E1040.
38. Pearson SJ, Burgess KE, Onambélé GL: Serum relaxin levels affect the in vivo properties of some but not all tendons in normally menstruating young women. *Exp Physiol* 2011;96(7):681-688.
39. Dragoo JL, Padrez K, Workman R, Lindsey DP: The effect of relaxin on the female anterior cruciate ligament: Analysis of mechanical properties in an animal model. *Knee* 2009;16(1):69-72.
40. Akeson WH, Amiel D, Abel MF, Garfin SR, Woo SL: Effects of immobilization on joints. *Clin Orthop Relat Res* 1987;219:28-37.
41. Woo SL, Gomez MA, Sites TJ, Newton PO, Orlando CA, Akeson WH: The biomechanical and morphological changes in the medial collateral ligament of the rabbit after immobilization and remobilization. *J Bone Joint Surg Am* 1987;69(8):1200-1211.
42. Tipton CM, James SL, Mergner W, Tcheng TK: Influence of exercise on strength of medial collateral knee ligaments of dogs. *Am J Physiol* 1970;218(3):894-902.
43. Cabaud HE, Chatty A, Gildengorin V, Feltman RJ: Exercise effects on the strength of the rat anterior cruciate ligament. *Am J Sports Med* 1980;8(2):79-86.
44. Noyes FR, Torvik PJ, Hyde WB, DeLucas JL: Biomechanics of ligament failure: II. An analysis of immobilization, exercise, and reconditioning effects in primates. *J Bone Joint Surg Am* 1974;56(7):1406-1418.
45. Woo SL, Peterson RH, Ohland KJ, Sites TJ, Danto MI: The effects of strain rate on the properties of the medial collateral ligament in skeletally immature and mature rabbits: A biomechanical and histological study. *J Orthop Res* 1990;8(5):712-721.
46. Viidik A, Lewin T: Changes in tensile strength characteristics and histology of rabbit ligaments induced by different modes of postmortal storage. *Acta Orthop Scand* 1966;37(2):141-155.

©Copyright 2021 American Academy of Orthopaedic Surgeons

47. Figgie HE III, Bahniuk EH, Heiple KG, Davy DT: The effects of tibial-femoral angle on the failure mechanics of the canine anterior cruciate ligament. *J Biomech* 1986;19(2):89-91.
48. Song GY, Zhang H, Liu X, et al: Complete posterolateral meniscal root tear is associated with high-grade pivot-shift phenomenon in non-contact anterior cruciate ligament injuries. *Knee Surg Sport Traumatol Arthrosc* 2017;25(4):1030-1037.
49. Sepúlveda F, Sánchez L, Amy E, Micheo W: Anterior cruciate ligament injury: Return to play, function and long-term considerations. *Curr Sports Med Rep* 2017;16(3):172-178.
50. Niyibizi C, Kavalkovich K, Yamaji T, Woo SL: Type V collagen is increased during rabbit medial collateral ligament healing. *Knee Surg Sports Traumatol Arthrosc* 2000;8(5):281-285.
51. Bray RC, Leonard CA, Salo PT: Correlation of healing capacity with vascular response in the anterior cruciate and medial collateral ligaments of the rabbit. *J Orthop Res* 2003;21(6):1118-1123.
52. Lo IK, Ou Y, Rattner JP, et al: The cellular networks of normal ovine medial collateral and anterior cruciate ligaments are not accurately recapitulated in scar tissue. *J Anat* 2002;200(pt 3):283-296.
53. Weiss JA, Woo SL, Ohland KJ, Horibe S, Newton PO: Evaluation of a new injury model to study medial collateral ligament healing: Primary repair versus nonoperative treatment. *J Orthop Res* 1991;9(4):516-528.
54. Figueroa D, Calvo R, Vaisman A, Meleán P, Figueroa F: Effect of tendon tensioning: An in vitro study in porcine extensor tendons. *Knee* 2010;17(3):245-248.
55. Staerke C, Möhwald A, Gröbel KH, Bochwitz C, Becker R: ACL graft migration under cyclic loading. *Knee Surg Sports Traumatol Arthrosc* 2010;18(8):1065-1070.

©Copyright 2021 American Academy of Orthopaedic Surgeons

19

Form and Function of Skeletal Muscle

Johnny Huard, PhD
Hajime Utsunomiya, MD, PhD
Sudheer K. Ravuri, PhD
Marc J. Philippon, MD

Keywords: *atrophy; extracellular matrix; fibrosis; losartan; musculoskeletal tissue; myofibrils; PRP; stem cells*

INTRODUCTION

Muscle injuries are extremely common, and they tend to recur. The intrinsic ability of the skeletal muscle to repair after injury because of the activation of muscle progenitor cells often leads to the development of fibrotic tissue at the original site of injury. Fibrotic tissue consequently limits force production and predisposes the muscle to reinjury. This chapter reviews the basic anatomy and physiology of skeletal muscle, the basic mechanisms of muscle growth and adaptation, the types of muscle injuries, and the stages of the healing process. Recent achievements in biological approaches to improve muscle healing after injury include methods for enhancing muscle regeneration and reducing muscle fibrosis. Other useful and less studied strategies to enhance skeletal muscle repair include gene therapy, exercise, neuromuscular electrical stimulation, blood flow restriction, and, potentially, massage therapy. It is clear that basic science and preclinical studies must be performed to ensure the safety of such therapies before they can become part of standard orthopaedic care.

TYPES OF SKELETAL MUSCLE

Skeletal muscles can be categorized based on the distribution of myofibers and their insertion into the tendons. Muscles with parallel fibers are most common. These parallel muscles can produce a substantial change in length with relatively little force, but their relatively small cross-sectional area means that total force production is relatively small. A unipennate muscle has fibers that insert on only one side of a tendon, thus creating a relatively large cross section and greater strength but less change in length. Fibers in a bipennate muscle consolidate on two sides of the inserting tendon, increasing relative cross section, allowing greater strength than a unipennate muscle, with smaller changes in length.

Dr. Huard or an immediate family member serves as a board member, owner, officer, or committee member of ORS and Orthopaedic Research Society. Dr. Philippon or an immediate family member has received royalties from Arthrex, Arthrosurface, Bledsoe, CONMED Linvatec, and DonJoy; serves as a paid consultant to or is an employee of Smith & Nephew, MIS; has stock or stock options held in Arthrosurface, MIS, MJP Innovations, LLC, and Vail Valley Surgery Center; has received research or institutional support from Smith and Nephew, Ossur, Arthrex, Siemens, and Vail Vally Medical Center; has received nonincome support (such as equipment or services), commercially derived honoraria, or other non–research-related funding (such as paid travel) from Smith & Nephew; and serves as a board member, owner, officer, or committee member of ASIAM, the International Society for Hip Arthroscopy, the American Orthopaedic Society for Sports Medicine, the Steadman Philippon Research Institute, the Vail Health Services, and the Vail Valley Surgery Center Governing Council. Neither of the following authors nor any immediate family member has received anything of value from or has stock or stock options held in a commercial company or institution related directly or indirectly to the subject of this chapter: Dr. Utsunomiya and Dr. Ravuri.

©Copyright 2021 American Academy of Orthopaedic Surgeons

THE STRUCTURE OF SKELETAL MUSCLE

GROSS STRUCTURE

Skeletal muscle is enclosed by fascia (a smooth sheath of connective tissue that allows the muscle to slide past surrounding tissues). A muscle is composed of bundles of muscle fibers called fascicles, which are connected by a delicate connective tissue called epimysium. Fascicles are composed of hundreds of muscle fibers enclosed by endomysium, and each individual fiber (myofiber) is enveloped by perimysium. Each myofiber is a long, thin, tubular structure, often many centimeters long and usually running the entire length of the muscle.

CELL STRUCTURE

The skeletal muscle cell has a plasma membrane called the sarcolemma, which is surrounded by several layers of tissue including a connective tissue basement membrane, a reticular layer, and the extracellular matrix. These surrounding layers make up the endomysium. The skeletal muscle fiber contains multiple nuclei, typically situated at the periphery of the cell just beneath the sarcolemma. The unique structure of the sarcolemma makes the muscle fiber an efficient contractile apparatus. The sarcolemma extends into the cell, surrounding the contractile elements of the muscle cell (myofibrils) and forming transverse tubules. Smaller longitudinal tubules extend from the transverse tubules to interact with the sarcoplasmic reticulum, which is a system of membrane-bound organelles that stores calcium. The sarcoplasmic reticulum contains several enzymes to regulate calcium sequestering and release; the intracellular concentration of calcium turns the contractile apparatus on and off. The permeating design of the sarcolemma and sarcoplasmic reticulum increases the cross-sectional area, permits quick transmission of action potentials to the contractile elements, and provides a reservoir of calcium ions close to the contraction.

SARCOMERES

The myofibrils are a highly ordered set of proteins arranged in parallel along the axis of the cell. This arrangement ensures a cumulative effect of contractions. A distinct banding pattern produces the characteristic striated appearance of alternating light and dark bands seen under the microscope. Myofibrils are divided into contractile units called sarcomeres. The dark band (the A band) represents thick filaments centered around interconnecting proteins (the M line). The thick filaments are primarily composed of myosin, which is a large protein made up of a long, insoluble helical portion and two globular portions called cross-bridges. The globular portions are capable of binding the thin filaments and hydrolyzing high-energy adenosine triphosphate (ATP) to release stored chemical energy. The thick filaments also contain C protein, M protein, myosin, titin, and creatine kinase.

The thin filaments attach to an interconnecting set of structural proteins (the Z line) and extend into the middle of the sarcomere. The thin filaments are primarily composed of the protein actin as well as troponin and tropomyosin. Additional proteins at the Z line include desmin, α-actinin, and filamin. The overlap of actin and myosin allows binding between the proteins and subsequent contraction of the myofibrils.

MUSCLE CONTRACTION

Muscular contraction is produced by interaction between the thick and thin filaments. The myosin molecules in the thick filaments form cross-bridges with the actin molecules of the thin filaments. The globular domain of the myosin molecule hydrolyzes ATP to adenosine diphosphate, causing a conformational change in the myosin molecule that pushes the filaments past each other. The myosin molecule quickly releases the actin molecule and returns to its original conformation. This ATP-dependent cycle repeats in rapid succession to cause the thick and thin filaments to pull toward each other. Because of the relative polarities of the thick and thin filaments, active cross-bridging results only in a sliding of the thick and filament complexes toward each other and a shortening or resistance to stretching of the sarcomere.

Cross-bridge cycling is modulated by intracellular calcium through the regulatory proteins troponin and tropomyosin. Tropomyosin is a molecule on the thin filament that prevents myosin-actin interaction. Troponin is a calcium-dependent regulatory protein with three domains: the troponin-C subunit binds calcium, troponin-T binds tropomyosin, and troponin-I is inhibitory to the actin-myosin interaction. When troponin-C binds calcium, the molecule changes conformation, relieving the troponin-I and tropomyosin inhibition of myosin-actin cross-bridging. Therefore, when intracellular calcium levels are high, cross-bridge cycling is active, and the myofibrils contract.

Each myofibril is stimulated by one nerve axon, but one axon can branch and stimulate multiple myofibrils. All of the myofibrils contacted by one axon constitute a motor unit. When the motor unit is activated, its entire muscle fibers contract. The number of muscle fibers in a motor unit ranges from approximately 10 to 1,000; in general, muscles that require fine motor control have relatively few fibers per motor unit. The neuromuscular junction is the site at which the nervous system controls muscular contraction. The neuromuscular junction is composed of the presynaptic axon, the synaptic cleft, and the postsynaptic muscle cell.

During the conversion of neuronal depolarization to muscular contraction, an action potential from the motor neuron reaches the axon terminal, releasing acetylcholine into the synaptic cleft. Acetylcholine binds to postsynaptic receptors, which respond by increasing permeability to sodium and depolarizing the sarcolemma. This depolarization spreads through the transverse tubules, stimulating the sarcoplasmic reticulum to release calcium into the cell. Calcium binds to the

©Copyright 2021 American Academy of Orthopaedic Surgeons

protein troponin, allowing myosin filaments to slide past actin filaments in an ATP-dependent process and shorten the muscle fiber. Contraction ceases when acetylcholine is degraded at the postsynaptic receptor, the membrane repolarizes, and calcium is pumped back into the sarcoplasmic reticulum.

A single action potential results in a quick contraction followed by relaxation. The length of the contraction ranges from approximately 7.5 ms (for fast myofibers) to 100 ms (for slow myofibers). Unlike nerve tissue, muscle tissue has no refractory period for the contractile mechanism; a rapid sequence of depolarizations results in a continuous, tetanic contraction.

TYPES OF CONTRACTIONS

Muscular contractions typically are described as shortening the muscle in a concentric contraction. Several other types of contractions also exist. In an eccentric contraction, myosin-actin cross-bridges are formed, but the opposing force is greater than the force created by the muscle and the muscle therefore lengthens. In an isometric contraction, the force of contraction equals the opposing force, and the length does not change.

THE RELATIONSHIP BETWEEN LENGTH AND TENSION

The structural makeup of skeletal muscle creates unique properties of force production based on muscle length (**Figure 1**). The length of the sarcomere at the time of contraction affects the amount of force produced, because of the amount of overlap between actin and myosin molecules. The overlap is greatest at resting length; as a result, more cross-bridging occurs, and greater force is achieved. The force of contraction drops off exponentially as a muscle fiber is shortened or lengthened.

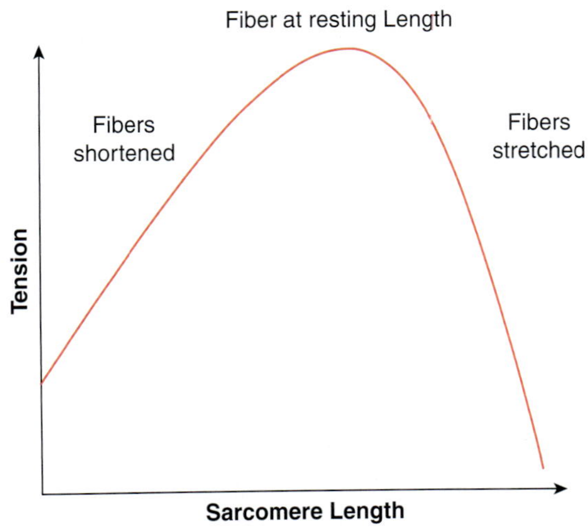

FIGURE 1 Illustration showing the relationship between tension and sarcomere length. The greatest tension is attained at the normal muscle fiber length, when the overlap between actin and myosin is greatest.

These anatomic properties of skeletal muscle are significant in determining biomechanical strength, running speed, and jumping height.

THE RELATIONSHIP BETWEEN FORCE AND VELOCITY

The force-velocity relationship also is a property of skeletal muscle mechanics. As originally described by Hill in isometrically stimulated amphibian muscle, the velocity of a muscle contraction is related to the load placed on the muscle (**Figure 2**).[1] The larger the load, the lower the velocity at which the muscle can contract. In contrast, muscle velocity increases with a light load. This relationship applies only to the initial concentric action after isometric stimulation. In eccentric contraction, the force-velocity curve is different; an eccentrically loaded muscle lengthens rather than shortens. Because muscle becomes stiffer when it resists shortening, a large change in load results in a smaller change in velocity. Eccentric contractions produce more force at the same movement velocity and therefore require less energy expenditure, which is clinically important. For example, in normal gait, the quadricep is most active eccentrically during heel strike, while the knee is flexing, and is most active concentrically during knee extension.

FIBER TYPES

Skeletal muscle is a heterogeneous tissue. The myofibers frequently are grouped based on their contraction speed and predominant energy pathways. This heterogeneity is the result of different structural and metabolic properties of the fibers. Variability in isoforms of the contractile and structural proteins can result in different fiber types. Most important are the types of myosin adenosine triphosphatase, which produce different shortening speeds (the fast and slow forms of myosin).

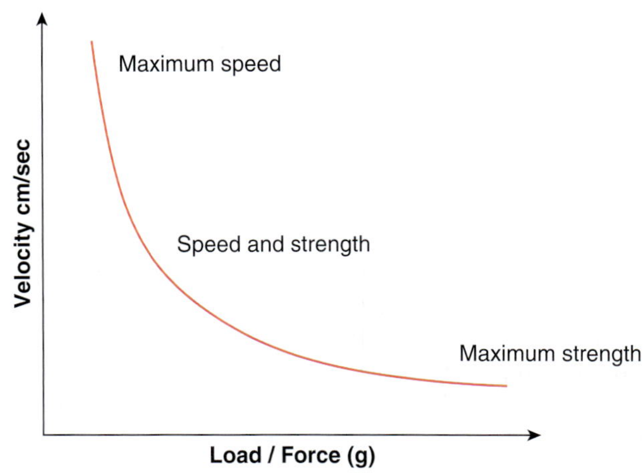

FIGURE 2 Illustration showing the relationship between force and velocity in isometric skeletal muscle contraction. The smaller the load, the more rapid is the muscle response.

©Copyright 2021 American Academy of Orthopaedic Surgeons

The three general fiber types are slow oxidative (type I), fast oxidative-glycolytic (type IIA), and fast glycolytic (type IIB). Type I fibers are smaller, contract more slowly, and produce less force than type II fibers, but are fatigue resistant. Type II fibers are larger, contract more quickly and forcefully, and are more easily fatigued. Type IIA is considered intermediate; type IIB is the fastest, most powerful, and most fatigable type. When motor units are activated by the central nervous system, the smallest motor units (predominantly type I), are recruited first; the larger type IIA and IIB units are recruited when more intense contractions are required.

ENERGY PATHWAYS

ATP is the common energy source for muscle contraction. The intracellular stores of ATP are limited, however. ATP is regenerated to supply energy for contracting muscle through three pathways. Creatine phosphate is dephosphorylated by mitochondrial creatine kinase to convert adenosine diphosphate to ATP. Creatine phosphate reserves are adequate for short-duration (10 to 20 s), high-intensity contractions, as required for sprinting. After a maximum of 30 seconds of exercise, muscle glycogen is converted to ATP through anaerobic glycolysis, and lactate is produced. In sustained exercise of more than approximately 1 minute, aerobic oxidation of glucose and fatty acids predominates, allowing a much more efficient energy yield. While anaerobic oxidation yields 2 ATP per molecule of glucose, aerobic oxidation yields 32 per molecule. Cardiac output and total ventilation increases dramatically to provide the oxygen required to support aerobic oxidation. The endurance limit (approximately 370 W in elite athletes) is the maximum sustainable energy output, as restricted by the rate of oxygen delivery and aerobic oxidation. Beyond this limit, anaerobic glycolysis can temporarily compensate through the rapid production of lactate. Increasing lactate and H^+ ion production causes a systemic drop in pH, inhibiting the reactions that drive muscular contraction. At a plasma lactate level of approximately 4 mmol/L, the anaerobic threshold is reached; at this point, performance declines, and rapid fatigue ensues.

MUSCLE GROWTH AND ADAPTATION

DEVELOPMENT

Skeletal muscle arises from mesodermal somite tissue. Early muscle progenitor cells are called myoblasts, and the fusiform cells that eventually fuse into multinucleated cells are called myotubes. Many contractile elements appear in the cell at the approximate time of myotube formation. Further differentiation occurs with muscle-specific expression of contractile proteins, elements of the metabolic pathways, and connections to the extracellular matrix.

During normal development, skeletal muscle grows in volume and length. To accommodate skeletal growth, total muscle length increases but sarcomere length remains constant. Additional sarcomeres are added in series near the region of the myotendinous junction. This mechanism persists at skeletal maturity, when muscles immobilized under stretch increase in length. Initially, the myofibrils and sarcomeres of a stretched muscle are lengthened. Over a period of weeks, additional sarcomeres are added so that resting sarcomere length is restored, but the entire muscle remains at the new, stretched length. The mechanical properties of a lengthened muscle also change; the length-tension curve shifts to produce peak tension at a greater length and to produce less passive force when stretched. Conversely, greater passive force is generated by the same stretch if a muscle is shortened for a prolonged period of time. Clinically, the mutability of muscle length has been advantageously applied in surgical limb-lengthening and muscle transfer procedures.

IMMOBILIZATION

Muscle undergoes several changes in response to immobilization or disuse. When skeletal muscle is immobilized, atrophy quickly ensues because of many factors including reduced protein synthesis and hormonal contributions. The result is a loss of cross-sectional area, leading to decreased muscle strength. Fatigability increases, partly because of diminished energy stores and metabolic efficiency. The response to immobilization depends on muscle length, however. Atrophy, loss of extensibility, and loss of force production are more pronounced in muscle immobilized without tension than in muscle immobilized under stretch. When muscles are stretched in immobilization, the loss of strength is partially compensated for by the growth in length, with formation of new sarcomeres and contractile proteins. Stretched muscle also produces less tension from stretch and maintains its extensibility. Although prolonged immobilization should be avoided, attention to joint position and muscle length can optimize future function.

ATROPHY

Skeletal muscle atrophies during periods of decreased muscle stimulation or systemic illness, as during immobilization or bed rest (eg, in burn treatment or surgery). The mechanisms driving disuse atrophy are a decrease in muscle protein synthesis and an increase in muscle protein breakdown.[2] As the body ages, skeletal muscle atrophies and muscle function gradually declines with decreased force production, contraction velocity, and impaired relaxation.[3] Sarcopenia (degenerative loss of skeletal muscle) was found in approximately 25% of people aged 65 to 70, and 40% of those older than 80 years.[4] Resistance exercise training and nutritional supplementation have been shown to improve the results of rehabilitation and to reduce muscle wasting in disuse, aging, or disease states.[5]

 ©Copyright 2021 American Academy of Orthopaedic Surgeons

TRAINING

Under the demands of physical training, the skeletal musculature undergoes a range of adaptations to improve muscle performance. The types of training and their primary effects can be simplified into three categories: motor learning, endurance training, and resistance training. Motor learning to improve the accuracy and performance of motor skills primarily results in nervous system adaptations such as the timing and rate of contractions. Endurance training (eg, in distance running) focuses on increasing the oxidative capacity of slow-twitch (type I) fibers, mainly by increasing mitochondrial density and cardiac output. Resistance training (eg, in weight lifting) uses relatively short, powerful contractions and requires training the fast-twitch (type II) fibers. Adaptations result from increases in the cross-sectional area of the muscle as well as improved neural activation.

MUSCLE INJURY

Muscle injury commonly occurs during physical activities and in almost all patients with skeletal trauma. Muscle injury usually is found with a strain, contusion, or laceration. Regardless of the mechanism of injury, the pattern of biologic response is muscle degeneration and inflammation followed by regeneration and fibrous scar formation (**Figure 3**).

DEGENERATION AND INFLAMMATION

In a contusion or laceration injury, a compressive force or direct tear causes tissue degeneration close to the injury site. In a muscle strain injury, tensile force along the muscle typically causes rupture near the musculotendinous junction.[6] Mechanical injury usually disrupts the myofiber across its entire cross section, and necrosis can develop along the entire length of the long, threadlike muscle cell. However, condensations of cytoskeleton called contraction bands contain the injury at regular intervals.[7] The plasma membrane defect is sealed off within hours. Blood vessels are also damaged, and hematoma develops. Inflammatory cells enter the injury site directly through the damaged blood vessels and are recruited via chemoattractants.[8] The extracellular matrix stores growth factors that are released when the extracellular matrix is disrupted.[9] Local macrophages and fibroblasts produce growth factors, cytokines, and chemokines in response to injury. Neutrophils are the predominant inflammatory cell during the acute period, and an influx of monocytes follows 1 day after the injury. These monocytes mature into macrophages that phagocytose the necrotic tissue before tissue repair.

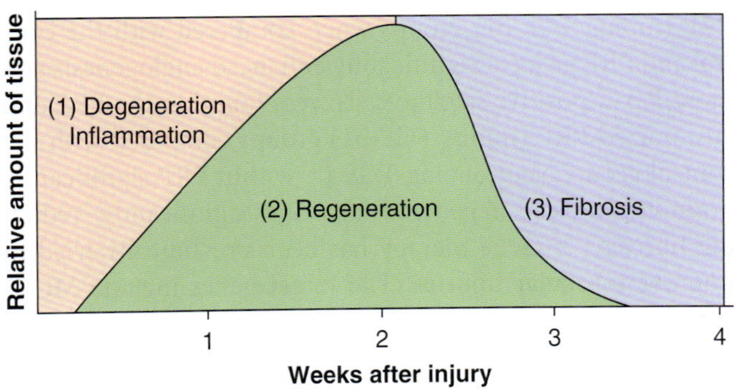

FIGURE 3 Illustration showing the general process of skeletal muscle repair.

REGENERATION

Myofiber regeneration occurs approximately 1 to 4 weeks after the injury. Myofibers are terminally differentiated, but skeletal muscle also contains cell populations capable of forming new muscle tissue.[10] Satellite cells are a well-defined population of undifferentiated cells found underneath the basal lamina of myofibers. The proliferation of satellite cells is stimulated when inflammatory cells release stimulatory growth factors such as the fibroblast growth factors, insulinlike growth factor 1 (IGF-1) and hepatocyte growth factor.[11] These cells differentiate into myoblasts, which fuse with the injured myofibers. Additional progenitor cells have been found to be critical in contributing to regeneration, including cells present in muscle tissue (muscle-derived stem cells), as well as cells from blood vessels, bone marrow, connective tissues, and mesenchymal tissues.[12]

FIBROSIS

Fibrosis (the formation of a connective tissue scar) begins with the cross-linking of fibrin and fibronectin within the hematoma to create early granulation tissue. Fibroblasts anchor to the granulation tissue and synthesize extracellular matrix components. Early strength and elasticity are provided to the granulation tissue by fibronectin, followed by type III collagen. After several days, fibroblasts produce type I collagen, the major component of mature scar tissue, thereby increasing the tensile strength of the muscle. Any rupture that occurs later is at the scar-myofiber interface.[13]

REVASCULARIZATION AND REINNERVATION

The vascular supply must be restored to allow full recovery of the injured muscle. Early myotubes possess few mitochondria and function largely on anaerobic metabolism. In late regeneration, however, aerobic metabolism is predominant. New capillary ingrowth appears to be necessary to provide the level of oxygen required for aerobic metabolism and full regeneration.[14] Similarly, new myofibers require reinnervation for full recovery after nerve injury. After myotubes are formed in denervated muscle, the new myofibers will atrophy in the absence of subsequent innervation.[15] When the nerve axon is disrupted, regrowth of the distal axon segment must be completed to ensure full reinnervation and muscle regeneration.

©Copyright 2021 American Academy of Orthopaedic Surgeons

BIOLOGICAL APPROACHES TO IMPROVE MUSCLE HEALING

RICE PROTOCOL

The acute treatment of muscle injuries generally includes **r**est, **i**ce, **c**ompression, and **e**levation (the **RICE** protocol). These immediate measures reduce bleeding at the injury site. Immobilization prevents retraction of the muscle edges, reduces further hematoma formation, and reduces the size of the fibrotic scar.[16] Although immobilization is beneficial immediately after injury, after more than a few days it is detrimental to muscle regeneration. Immobilization causes muscle fiber atrophy, loss of strength, and excessive connective tissue deposition. In a mouse laceration model, 5 days of immobilization decreased histologic and functional healing.[17] Return to function can be maximized by relatively early mobilization (approximately 3 to 5 days after injury), followed by progressive strengthening, stretching, and a graduated return to activity.

MODULATION OF INFLAMMATION

Nonsteroidal anti-inflammatory drugs (NSAIDs) are commonly used to control pain after muscle injury, but their effect on muscle healing is not well understood. To further examine the validity of using these drugs after muscle injury, we investigated the working mechanism of NS-398, acyclooxygenase-2-specific inhibitor.[18] In vitro experiments showed that NS-398 inhibited the proliferation and maturation of differentiated myogenic precursor cells, suggesting a detrimental effect on skeletal muscle healing.[18] Using a mouse laceration model, we analyzed the in vivo effect of NS-398 on skeletal muscle healing at time points up to 4 weeks after injury. The in vivo results revealed delayed muscle regeneration at early time points after injury in the NS-398-treated mice. Compared with controls, lacerated muscles treated with NS-398 expressed higher levels of transforming growth factor-beta1, which corresponded with increased fibrosis.[18] In addition, transforming growth factor-beta1 co-localized with myostatin, a negative regulator of skeletal muscle growth. We also found reduced neutrophil and macrophage infiltration in treated muscles, indicating that the delayed skeletal muscle healing observed after NS-398 treatment could be influenced by the anti-inflammatory effect of NS-398. Our findings suggest that the use of cyclooxygenase-2-specific inhibitors to treat skeletal muscle injuries warrants caution because they may interfere with muscle healing through delaying muscle regeneration and increasing fibrotic deposition.[19]

IMPROVING MUSCLE REGENERATION

Although the established treatments of muscle injury are limited, biologic approaches to improving muscle regeneration and repair are evolving. These approaches include the addition of stimulatory growth factors, gene therapies, cell therapies, and antifibrotic agents. Growth factors serve a variety of roles during muscle regeneration.[20] In mice, direct injections of the stimulatory growth factors IGF-1, basic fibroblast growth factor, and (to a lesser extent) nerve growth factor were found to enhance muscle regeneration and muscle strength after laceration, contusion, or strain.[21,22] Direct injection of recombinant growth factors is safe and easy. However, a high concentration of these recombinant proteins is required to generate a substantial effect, and therefore they have limited efficacy. Growth factors have a dose-dependent effect on myoblast proliferation and differentiation in vitro, but measurable enhancement of skeletal muscle healing in mice usually requires multiple consecutive injections of a relatively high concentration of IGF-1, basic fibroblast growth factor, and nerve growth factor (100 ng/injection for each growth factor).[23] Short biologic half-life and rapid clearance from the bloodstream may explain the need for high concentrations of growth factor.

The injection of platelet-rich plasma (PRP), which provides local delivery of a wide variety of growth factors, is increasingly common in treating musculoskeletal injury. PRP injection in a rat model of muscle strain led to functional improvement.[24] Meanwhile, clinical data provide limited scientific support for the use of PRP in muscle strain injuries. A double-blinded, placebo-controlled randomized trial showed no significant differences between leukocyte-poor PRP and placebo groups; no effects on quick recovery[25] or muscular status at 1-year follow-up was found.[26] Two single-blinded randomized controlled trials reported shorter time to return to sports in the PRP groups[27,28]; recent meta-analyses also concluded that PRP might shorten return to play, but there seemed to be no long-term improvement. PRP contains beneficial growth factors for skeletal muscle repair; however, it also contains deleterious cytokines and growth factors, such as TGF-β1, that can cause fibrosis and inhibit optimal muscle healing. We have recently tested if neutralizing the action of TGF-β1 within PRP, through neutralization antibodies, could improve PRP's beneficial effect on skeletal muscle repair. A significant increase in the number of regenerative myofibers was observed in the PRP and customized PRP (minus TGF-β1) groups compared with the untreated control. A significant decrease in collagen deposition was observed in customized PRP (minus TGF-β1) groups when compared with the control and PRP groups. Significantly enhanced angiogenesis and more Pax-7 positive satellite cells were found in the PRP and customized PRP (minus TGF-β1) groups compared with the control group. Neutralizing TGF-β1 within PRP significantly promotes muscle regeneration while significantly reducing fibrosis.[29-32] Gene therapy has been preclinically tried to improve muscular injuries. The target genes include MG53 gene,[33] insulin-like growth factor 1 gene,[34] and sonic hedgehog.[35] Gene therapy can be a novel approach for the treatment of muscle injuries,[36] but numerous limitations have hindered their use to improve muscle healing including immune response and cytotoxicity.

©Copyright 2021 American Academy of Orthopaedic Surgeons

Cell therapy involves the use of mesenchymal stem cells (MSCs), including muscle-derived stem cells (MDSCs). MDSCs are multipotent stem cells that are isolated from skeletal muscle.[37] Injection of MDSCs 4 days after injury is shown to significantly increase angiogenesis and reduce scar tissues through higher expression of vascular endothelial growth factor in a mouse model.[38]

PREVENTION OF MUSCLE FIBROSIS

The formation of connective tissue scaring at the site of muscle injury interferes with complete muscle regeneration. TGF-β1 plays a role in the formation of fibrosis in some tissues and muscle diseases, and strong expression of TGF-β1 has been observed in injured skeletal muscle.[39] TGF-β1 plays an important role in the development of fibrosis after muscle injury. Antifibrotic agents that block the effects of TGF-β1 include a neutralizing TGF-β1 antibody or receptor blocker,[40] decorin,[41] suramin,[42] relaxin,[43] interferon-γ,[44] and losartan (an angiotensin II blocker).[45] By blocking the stimulation of TGF-β1 production by the US Food and Drug Administration–approved antihypertensive drug losartan, we have shown to significantly decrease fibrosis and increase muscle fiber regeneration in mice. Based on these data, we have conducted a case study on two hamstring injury patients and found that losartan treatment was well tolerated and possibly improved recovery time.[46] We believe this medication holds great promise to optimize muscle repair in humans. Neutralization of TGF-β1 is a promising treatment option for muscle injuries by reducing scar tissue formation.

COMBINATION OF BIOLOGICAL APPROACHES TO IMPROVE MUSCLE HEALING AFTER INJURY

Furthermore, combined use of losartan and MDSCs,[47] losartan and PRP,[31] and customized PRP with TGF-β1 neutralization antibody[32] have shown to significantly promote the scarless healing of skeletal muscle after injuries, in preclinical studies. These combinatorial approaches can target different stages of muscle healing, that is, MDSC promote muscle repair while losartan blocks fibrosis, and therefore can act synergistically to improve muscle healing after injury. It would be important in the future to determine whether controlling inflammation would improve the benefit of enhancing regeneration and/or preventing fibrosis for optimal muscle healing after injuries. Blood flow restriction (BFR) training is another technique shown to be safe and effective at increasing muscular strength and endurance in healthy fitness populations and is under study for its use in postinjury rehabilitation.[48] BFR stimulates muscular strength and hypertrophy gains at much lower loads than traditional methods, allowing patients to begin the rehabilitation process much sooner. Incorporating tourniquet-assisted blood flow restriction with rehabilitation programs and other biological approaches, an exciting combinatorial approach that can improve strength, endurance, and function after muscle injuries has been found.

SUMMARY

The skeletal muscles represent a large part of body mass and can efficiently regenerate after injury because of the presence of endogenous muscle progenitor cells. However, the regeneration process declines with aging or the progression of muscle diseases such as muscular dystrophies. The phases of muscle recovery are remarkably similar after different injuries. The interrelated and overlapping stages of muscle repair involve degeneration of injured muscle fibers, an inflammatory phase, muscle regeneration, and the development of fibrosis. Acute muscle injuries usually are treated with the RICE protocol, and NSAIDs often are used to control pain. Muscle healing may be impaired by the use of NSAIDs. Biologic approaches to modulating muscle repair use a combination of stem cell populations including muscle-derived stem cells; cell growth–promoting biologic products such as IGF-1, basic fibroblast growth factor, and PRP; antifibrotic agents such decorin, suramin, and losartan; and gene therapy. These therapies may become effective for improving muscle healing. Other useful strategies to enhance skeletal muscle repair through increased vascularization may include exercise, neuromuscular electrical stimulation, BFR, and, potentially, massage therapy. Based on recent studies showing an accelerated recovery of muscle function from intense eccentric exercise through massage-based therapies, we believe that this treatment modality offers a practical and noninvasive form of therapy for skeletal muscle injuries.[49] However, the biological mechanism(s) behind the beneficial effect of massage are still unclear and require further investigation using animal models and potentially randomized, human clinical studies.[49] It is clear that basic science and preclinical studies must be performed to ensure the safety of such therapies before they can become part of standard orthopaedic care.

REFERENCES

1. Hill AV: The heat of shortening and the dynamic constants of muscle. *Proc R Soc Lond B Biol Sci* 1938;126(843):136-195.
2. Marimuthu K, Murton AJ, Greenhaff PL: Mechanisms regulating muscle mass during disuse atrophy and rehabilitation in humans. *J Appl Physiol* 2011;110(2):555-560.
3. Ryall JG, Schertzer JD, Lynch GS: Cellular and molecular mechanisms underlying age-related skeletal muscle wasting and weakness. *Biogerontology* 2008;9(4):213-228.

©Copyright 2021 American Academy of Orthopaedic Surgeons

4. Baumgartner RN, Koehler KM, Gallagher D, et al: Epidemiology of sarcopenia among the elderly in New Mexico. *Am J Epidemiol* 1998;147(8):755-763.
5. Phillips SM: Physiologic and molecular bases of muscle hypertrophy and atrophy: Impact of resistance exercise on human skeletal muscle (protein and exercise dose effects). *Appl Physiol Nutr Metab* 2009;34(3):403-410.
6. Järvinen TA, Järvinen TL, Kääriäinen M, Kalimo H, Järvinen M: Muscle injuries: Biology and treatment. *Am J Sports Med* 2005;33(5):745-764.
7. Hurme T, Kalimo H, Lehto M, Järvinen M: Healing of skeletal muscle injury: An ultrastructural and immunohistochemical study. *Med Sci Sports Exerc* 1991;23(7):801-810.
8. Tidball JG: Inflammatory cell response to acute muscle injury. *Med Sci Sports Exerc* 1995;27(7):1022-1032.
9. Rak J, Kerbel RS: bFGF and tumor angiogenesis: Back in the limelight? *Nat Med* 1997;3(10):1083-1084.
10. Péault B1, Rudnicki M, Torrente Y, et al: Stem and progenitor cells in skeletal muscle development, maintenance and therapy. *Mol Ther* 2007;15(5):867-877.
11. Chargé SB, Rudnicki MA: Cellular and molecular regulation of muscle regeneration. *Physiol Rev* 2004;84(1):209-238.
12. Nombela-Arrieta C, Ritz J, Silberstein LE: The elusive nature and function of mesenchymal stem cells. *Nat Rev Mol Cell Biol* 2011;12(2):126-131.
13. Velnar T, Bailey T, Smrkolj V: The wound healing process: An overview of the cellular and molecular mechanisms. *J Int Med Res* 2009;37(5):1528-1542.
14. Järvinen M: Healing of a crush injury in rat striated muscle: 3. A micro-angiographical study of the effect of early mobilization and immobilization on capillary ingrowth. *Acta Pathol Microbiol Scand* 1976;84(1):85-94.
15. Rantanen J, Ranne J, Hurme T, Kalimo H: Denervated segments of injured skeletal muscle fibers are reinnervated by newly formed neuromuscular junctions. *J Neuropathol Exp Neurol* 1995;54(2):188-194.
16. Järvinen MJ, Lehto MU: The effects of early mobilisation and immobilisation on the healing process following muscle injuries. *Sports Med* 1993;15(2):78-89.
17. Menetrey J, Kasemkijwattana C, Fu FH, Moreland MS, Huard J: Suturing versus immobilization of a muscle laceration: A morphological and functional study in a mouse model. *Am J Sports Med* 1999;27(2):222-229.
18. Shen W, Li Y, Tang Y, Cummins J, Huard J: NS-398, a cyclooxygenase-2-specific inhibitor, delays skeletal muscle healing by decreasing regeneration and promoting fibrosis. *Am J Pathol* 2005;167(4):1105-1117.
19. Shen W, Prisk V, Li Y, Foster W, Huard J: Inhibited skeletal muscle healing in cyclooxygenase-2 gene-deficient mice: The role of PGE2 and PGF2alpha. *J Appl Physiol* 2006;101(4):1215-1221.
20. Huard J, Li Y, Fu FH: Muscle injuries and repair: Current trends in research. *J Bone Joint Surg Am* 2002;84(5):822-832.
21. Kasemkijwattana C, Menetrey J, Somogyl G, et al: Development of approaches to improve the healing following muscle contusion. *Cell Transplant* 1998;7(6):585-598.
22. Kasemkijwattana C, Menetrey J, Bosch P, et al: Use of growth factors to improve muscle healing after strain injury. *Clin Orthop Relat Res* 2000;370:272-285.
23. Menetrey J, Kasemkijwattana C, Day CS, et al: Growth factors improve muscle healing in vivo. *J Bone Joint Surg Br* 2000;82(1):131-137.
24. Hammond JW, Hinton RY, Curl LA, Muriel JM, Lovering RM: Use of autologous platelet-rich plasma to treat muscle strain injuries. *Am J Sports Med* 2009;37(6):1135-1142.
25. Reurink G, Goudswaard GJ, Moen MH, et al: Plate-rich plasma injections in acute muscle injury. *N Engl J Med* 2014;370(26):2546-2547.
26. Reurink G, Goudswaard GJ, Moen MH, et al: Rationale, secondary outcome scores and 1-year follow-up of a randomised trial of platelet-rich plasma injections in acute hamstring muscle injury: The Dutch hamstring injection therapy study. *Br J Sports Med* 2015;49(18):1206-1212.
27. A Hamid MS, Mohamed Ali MR, Yusof A, George J, Lee LP: Platelet-rich plasma injections for the treatment of hamstring injuries: a randomized controlled trial. *Am J Sports Med* 2014;42(10):2410-2418.
28. Rossi LA, Romoli ARM, Altieri BAB, Flor JAB, Scordo WE, Elizondo CM: Does platelet-rich plasma decrease time to return to sports in acute muscle tear? A randomized controlled trial. *Knee Surg Sports Traumatol Arthrosc* 2017;25:3319-3325.
29. Grassi A, Napoli F, Romandini I, et al: Platelet-rich plasma (PRP) effective in the treatment of acute muscle injuries? A systematic review and meta-analysis. *Sports Med* 2018;48(4):971-989.
30. Sheth U, Dwyer T, Smith I, et al: Does platelet-rich plasma lead to earlier return to sport when compared with conservative treatment in acute muscle injuries? A systematic review and meta-analysis. *Arthroscopy* 2018;34(1):281-288.
31. Terada S, Ota S, Kobayashi M, et al: Use of an antifibrotic agent improves the effect of platelet-rich plasma on muscle healing after injury. The combined use of losartan and muscle-derived stem cells significantly improves the functional recovery of muscle in a young mouse model of contusion injuries. *J Bone Joint Surg Am* 2013;95(11):980-988.
32. Li H, Hicks JJ, Wang L, et al: Customized platelet-rich plasma with transforming growth factor 1 neutralization antibody to reduce fibrosis in skeletal muscle. *Biomaterials* 2016;87:147-156.
33. He B, Tang RH, Weisleder N, et al: Enhancing muscle membrane repair by gene delivery of MG53 ameliorates muscular dystrophy and heart failure in delta- Sarcoglycan-deficient hamsters. *Mol Ther J Am Soc Gene Ther* 2012;20(4):727-735.
34. Schertzer JD, Lynch GS: Comparative evaluation of IGF-I gene transfer and IGF-I protein administration for enhancing skeletal muscle regeneration after injury. *Gene Ther* 2016;13(23):1657-1664.
35. Piccioni A, Gaetani E, Neri V, et al: Sonic hedgehog therapy in a mouse model of age-associated impairment of skeletal muscle regeneration. *J Gerontol A Biol Sci Med Sci* 2014;69(3):245-252.
36. Stihano RS, Martins L, Ingham SJM, Pesquero JB, Huard J: Gene and cell therapy for muscle regeneration. *Curr Rev Musculoskeletal Med* 2015;8(2):182-187.
37. Ota S, Uehara K, Nozaki M, et al: Intramuscular transplantation of muscle-derived stem cells accelerates skeletal muscle healing after contusion injury via enhancement of angiogenesis. *Am J Sports Med* 2011;39(9):1912-1922.
38. Li Y, Huard J: Differentiation of muscle-derived cells into myofibroblasts in injured skeletal muscle. *Am J Pathol* 2002;161(3):895-907.
39. Li Y, Foster W, Deasy BM, et al: Transforming growth factor-beta1 induces the differentiation of myogenic cells into fibrotic cells in injured skeletal muscle: A key event in muscle fibrogenesis. *Am J Pathol* 2004;164(3):1007-1019.
40. Burks TN, Cohn RD: Role of TGF-β signaling in inherited and acquired myopathies. *Skelet Muscle* 2011;1(1):19.
41. Li Y, Li J, Zhu J, et al: Decorin gene transfer promotes muscle cell differentiation and muscle regeneration. *Mol Ther* 2007;15(9):1616-1622.
42. Nozaki M, Li Y, Zhu J, et al: Improved muscle healing after contusion injury by the inhibitory effect of suramin on myostatin, a negative regulator of muscle growth. *Am J Sports Med* 2008;36(12):2354-2362.
43. Li Y, Negishi S, Sakamoto M, Usas A, Huard J: The use of relaxin improves healing in injured muscle. *Ann N Y Acad Sci* 2005;1041:395-397.
44. Foster W, Li Y, Usas A, Somogyi G, Huard J: Gamma interferon as an antifibrosis agent in skeletal muscle. *J Orthop Res* 2003;21(5):798-804.
45. Bedair HS, Karthikeyan T, Quintero A, Li Y, Huard J: Angiotensin II receptor blockade administered after injury improves muscle regeneration and decreases fibrosis in normal skeletal muscle. *Am J Sports Med* 2008;36(8):1548-1554.
46. Gharaibeh B, Chun-Lansinger Y, Hagen T, et al: Biological approaches to improve skeletal muscle healing after injury and disease. *J Birth Defects Res C Embryo Today* 2012;96(1):82-94.

©Copyright 2021 American Academy of Orthopaedic Surgeons

47. Kobayashi M, Ota S, Terada S, et al: The combined use of losartan and muscle-derived stem cells significantly improves the functional recovery of muscle in a young mouse model of contusion injuries. *Am J Sports Med* 2016;44(12):3252-3261.

48. Yow BG, Tennent DJ, Dowd TC, Loenneke JP, Owens JG: Blood flow restriction training after achilles tendon rupture. *J Foot Ankle Surg* 2018;57(3):635-638.

49. Best TM, Gharaibeh B, Huard J: Stem cells, angiogenesis and muscle healing: A potential role in massage therapies? *Br J Sports Med* 2013;47(9):556-560.

©Copyright 2021 American Academy of Orthopaedic Surgeons

Structure and Physiology of Peripheral Nerves

Emily A. Van Kouwenberg, MD
Michael Hausman, MD

Keywords: *anatomy; peripheral nerve; physiology; structure*

INTRODUCTION

Peripheral nerves comprise afferent and efferent pathways and autonomic control fibers. A complex connective tissue lattice is responsible for protecting the nerve cells and maintaining homeostasis that is crucial to normal nerve function. Peripheral nerve dysfunction can result from degenerative conditions, nerve compression, or extremity trauma. The degree of nerve recovery after these insults will determine the ultimate functionality of the affected limbs. Understanding the macroscopic structure, microscopic structure, and physiology of peripheral nerves is necessary to understand the effects of nerve injury.

MACROSCOPIC STRUCTURE OF PERIPHERAL NERVES

The central nervous system includes the brain and spinal cord, while the peripheral nervous system is composed of peripheral nerves and their spinal nerve derivatives, cranial nerves, and the peripheral autonomic nervous system. Peripheral nerves consist of motor, sensory, and postganglionic autonomic nerve fibers that serve to communicate between the spinal cord and the rest of the body. Motor axons that exit the ventral horn and sensory axons that enter the dorsal horn of the spinal cord distally form the ventral and dorsal rootlets, respectively; these combine to form mixed spinal nerves as they pass through the spinal foramen. Spinal nerves then split into dorsal and ventral rami, which contribute to plexuses and peripheral nerves that supply different areas of the body (**Figure 1**). For example, the ventral rami of C5 through T1 form the brachial plexus, while the dorsal rami at these levels supply the posterior neck and trunk. The motor neuron cell bodies of peripheral nerves are located in the ventral horn of the spinal cord, and the sensory neuron cell bodies are located in the dorsal root ganglia just outside of the spinal cord in the intervertebral foramina. Understanding the distinct locations of motor versus sensory cell bodies is critical to accurately diagnose and localize conditions such as a brachial plexus injury. For example, nerve avulsion from the spinal cord constitutes a postganglionic injury to the motor nerve fibers, but a preganglionic injury to the sensory nerve fibers since the connections between the sensory cell bodies in the dorsal root ganglion and the axons are not severed.

Peripheral nerves are composed of organized groups of nerve fascicles that form nerve branches to innervate end organs. Fascicles within a nerve are larger and fewer in number in more proximal locations and smaller and greater in number distally. In the proximal extremity, the nerve fibers that supply the proximal limb tend to be more superficially located within the nerve to facilitate branching to their target, compared with more distally directed fibers that are distributed over multiple fascicles.[1,2] As the nerve reorganizes distally, nerve fibers with the same distal target join the same fascicles. Fascicles become superficially positioned before branching, and terminal branches are often monofascicular.[2] Distally, fascicles are

Dr. Hausman or an immediate family member is a member of a speakers' bureau or has made paid presentations on behalf of Trimed; serves as an unpaid consultant to Skeletal Dynamics; and has stock or stock options held in Checkpoint SurgicalNDI MedicalSPR Therapeutics Neither Dr. Van Kouwenberg nor any immediate family member has received anything of value from or has stock or stock options held in a commercial company or institution related directly or indirectly to the subject of this chapter.

©Copyright 2021 American Academy of Orthopaedic Surgeons

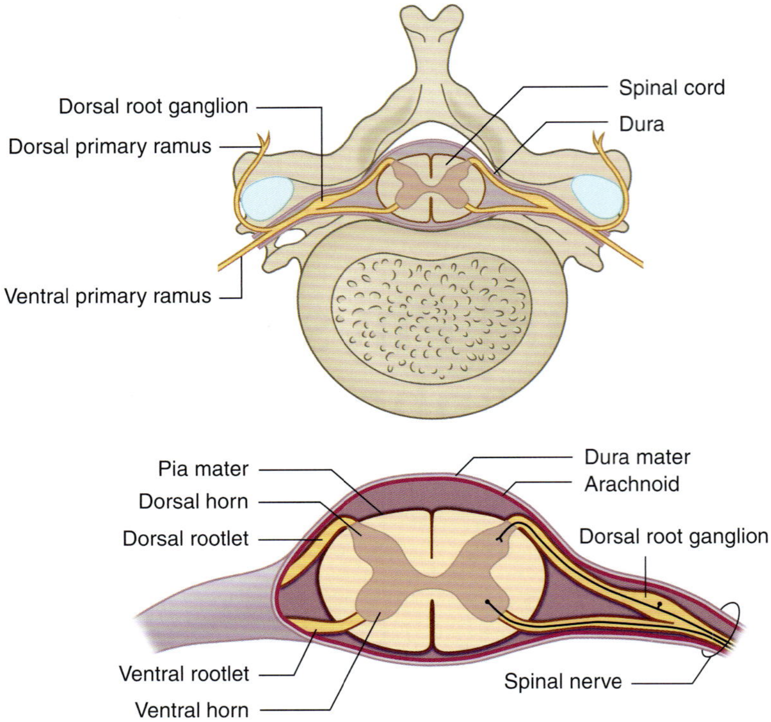

FIGURE 1 Illustration showing that motor axons that exit the ventral horn of the spinal cord form ventral rootlets, and sensory axons that enter the dorsal root ganglia form dorsal rootlets. Ventral and dorsal rootlets combine to form mixed spinal nerves, which then split into ventral and dorsal rami. (Reproduced with permission from Farnebo S, Thorfinn J, Dahlin LB: Peripheral nerve injuries of the upper extremity, in Neligan PC, ed: *Plastic Surgery Volume Six: Hand and Upper Extremity*, Elsevier, 2018.)

cable-like and can be followed proximally for a considerable distance with consistent somatic organization. Eventually, fascicles will begin to intermingle with other fascicles proximally and will become less discrete[3]. The ability to follow well-defined fascicles for a substantial distance proximally is the basis for nerve transfer surgery. Historically, it was thought that fascicles frequently redistribute by branching and uniting with other fascicle branches, resulting in a constantly changing plexiform architecture.[2,4] Sunderland believed that any given fascicular pattern would not persist for more than 1.5 cm.[5] More recent studies, however, have shown that although nerve fascicles intermingle proximally, there is far less intermingling than previously reported by Sunderland. These more recent works have also shown that nerve fibers that innervate specific end organs typically remain together along much of the nerve course, even throughout fascicular rearrangements proximally[3,6-8].

Although major peripheral nerves are generally well protected, there are anatomic sites where they are vulnerable to injury, including sites where they pass through narrow channels, run across bony structures, or travel at sharp angles. Compressive and tensile forces sustained in various positions and with various motions can impact blood flow to the nerve, axonal transport, and conduction of action potentials. Biomechanical properties of peripheral nerves allow them to tolerate these forces to an extent.[9] With increased tensile stress during range of motion, nerves are able to lengthen as a result of viscoelastic properties. Nerves are also able to glide during excursion toward the site of elongation to relieve some of the tension.[9] With normal range of motion, the brachial plexus has a total excursion of about 50 mm with shoulder motion. The median and ulnar nerves have about 7.3 and 9.8 mm of excursion, respectively, at the elbow and 14.5 and 13.8 mm of excursion, respectively, at the wrist.[1,10] Mobility is more restricted at sites of nerve branching and vessel penetration.[11]

MICROSCOPIC STRUCTURE OF PERIPHERAL NERVES

The neuron is the smallest functional unit of nerves and is composed of a cell body with cytoplasmic extensions, including multiple dendritic processes to receive information (afferent) and a single axonal process to transmit information (efferent)[12] (**Figure 2**). Inside of the cell body, otherwise known as the soma, is the nucleus, neurofilaments, mitochondria, lysosomes, and Nissl bodies surrounded by cytoplasm.[12,13] The cell bodies of peripheral nerves are sometimes located within the central nervous system.[14] The axon originates from the soma at a site called the axon hillock and travels distally as a peripheral extension.[1,11] Each axon has a thin outer layer called the axolemma, which is the cell membrane that encloses the axoplasm and extends from the cell body along the entire length of the axon.[11] The axoplasm acts as a conduit for transport of substances from the cell body to the distal nerve terminals, and vice versa.[11] Within the axon there are many structures supporting its function, including mitochondria, endoplasmic reticulum, lysosomes, vesicles, microtubules, and neurofilaments[11] (**Figure 3**). Schwann cells wrap around the axons and lay down myelin along the axolemma.[11]

©Copyright 2021 American Academy of Orthopaedic Surgeons

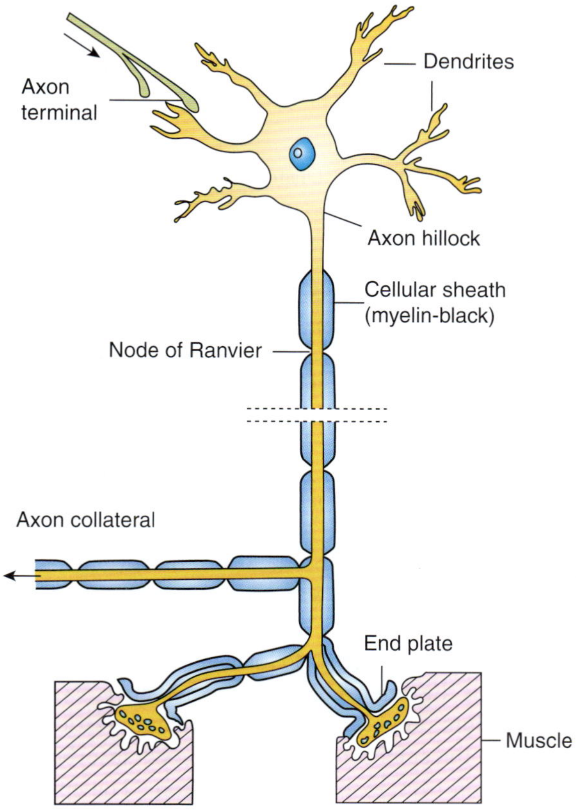

FIGURE 2 Diagram of a neuron, which is the smallest functional unit of peripheral nerves. The dendrites receive information (afferent) and the axon transmits information (efferent) to other neurons or to end organs such as motor end plates. The axon hillock is the site where the axon originates from the cell body. Each axon is covered by a cellular sheath, otherwise known as the axolemma. Myelinated nerve fibers have axons that are surrounded by a series of Schwann cells, each wrapped around the axon many times to form the myelin sheath. The segments of axon between Schwann cells are called nodes of Ranvier. Axons can form branches at the nodes of Ranvier, allowing a single cell body to innervate multiple end organs. (Reproduced with permission from Kuczynski K: Functional micro-anatomy of the peripheral nerve trunks. *Hand* 1974;6[1]:1-10.)

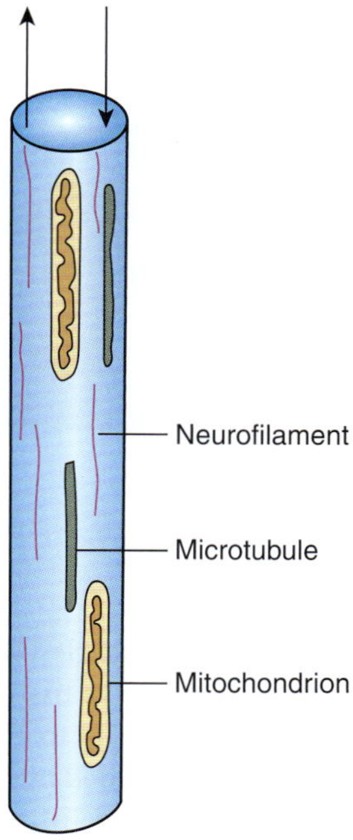

FIGURE 3 Illustration of internal axonal structure with neurofilaments, microtubules, and mitochondria supporting bidirectional transport. (Reproduced with permission from Kuczynski K: Functional micro-anatomy of the peripheral nerve trunks. *Hand* 1974;6[1]:1-10.)

Axons with their associated Schwann cells form nerve fibers. Myelinated nerve fibers are composed of a series of adjacent Schwann cells that surround and wrap around a single axon, covering it with multiple compact layers of plasma membrane to form a myelin sheath.[9,15] The segments of axon covered by Schwann cells and myelin are called internodes, whereas the small segments of axon between Schwann cells are called nodes of Ranvier[9,11] (**Figures 4** and **5**). Nodes of Ranvier are about 1 μm in length and occur about every 1 mm along the length of the axon.[4] Axons can form branches at the nodes of Ranvier, allowing a single cell body to innervate multiple end organs.[14] The myelin sheath extends along the length of the nerve fiber, beginning just after the axonal hillock and terminating 1 to 2 μm from the end of the axon.[11] Unmyelinated nerve fibers contain several axons that are surrounded as a group by a single layer of Schwann cells, without the formation of multiple, compacted plasma membrane layers seen in myelinated nerve fibers[9,15] (**Figure 6**). In both myelinated and unmyelinated nerve fibers, Schwann cells are surrounded by an associated basal lamina.[4] Myelinated nerve fibers tend to be larger than unmyelinated nerve fibers, with myelin typically found in those greater than 2 μm and absent in those smaller than 2 μm; myelinated nerve fibers usually range 2 to 14 μm while unmyelinated fibers range 0.2 to 3 μm in size.[9,11,16]

Most peripheral nerves contain both myelinated and unmyelinated nerve fibers.[3,14] Nerve fibers can be classified by their size and function. The largest myelinated nerve fibers are classified as group A fibers and have the fastest conduction velocity. Myelinated autonomic and preganglionic fibers are group B fibers, and thin nonmyelinated fibers are group C fibers.[1,13]

Nerves comprise many nerve fibers arranged and held into groups by connective tissues, including the endoneurium, perineurium, and epineurium (**Figures 7** and **8**). These connective tissues provide nerves with protection, framework, and compartmentalization to maintain specialized environments.[4,15] The connective tissue surrounding each individual nerve fiber is called the endoneurium, which encases longitudinally oriented type I and type II collagen fibers, fluid, and cells such as fibroblasts, macrophages, and mast cells along with the nerve fiber.[9] In larger nerve fibers, the endoneurium can be divided into two layers, including a thin inner layer that covers Schwann cells and comes into close contact with the nodes of Ranvier and an outer layer that does not approach the nodes of Ranvier.[11]

©Copyright 2021 American Academy of Orthopaedic Surgeons

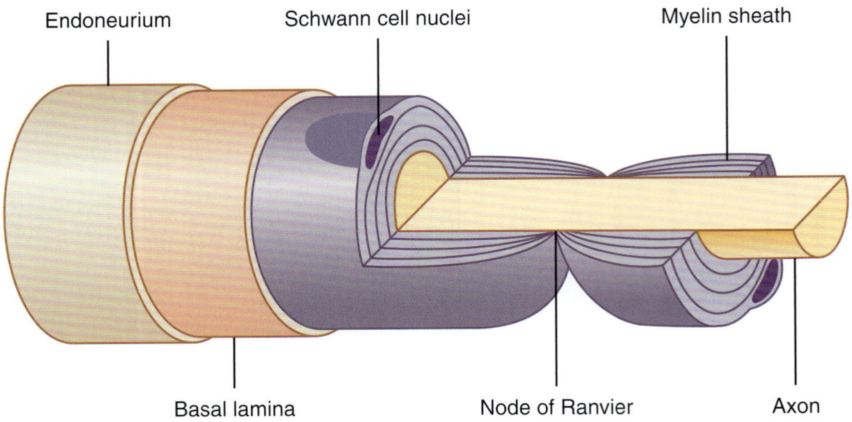

FIGURE 4 Diagram of a myelinated axon surrounded by a series of Schwann cells, each wrapped around the axon multiple times to form the myelin sheath. Nodes of Ranvier are the segments of axon between the Schwann cells. (Reproduced with permission from Farnebo S, Thorfinn J, Dahlin LB: Peripheral nerve injuries of the upper extremity, in Neligan PC, ed: *Plastic Surgery Volume Six: Hand and Upper Extremity*, Elsevier, 2018.)

Nerve fibers are bundled into fascicles, which are bound by a relatively thin but dense connective tissue sheath called the perineurium. This sheath includes up to 15 concentric layers of flattened polygonal cells surrounded by basal laminas, with collagen and elastic fibers arranged in varying orientations between the perineurial cells. The perineurium can be subdivided into internal, intermediate, and external zones.[4,9,14] The internal zone is typically comprised of a single layer of tightly interconnected perineurial cells called the perilemma, while the intermediate and external zones are comprised of multiple cell layers.[9] The tight cellular junctions of the internal zone contribute to the blood-nerve barrier, resulting in diffusion properties that preserve intrafascicular pressures and protect the nerve fibers against infection.[3,11,17] The external zone is not easily distinguished from the epineurium and contains type I and type II collagen fibers and elastic fibers arranged in longitudinal, oblique, and circumferential orientations between the cell layers; these fibers contribute to the biomechanical properties of the perineurium.[9,14] Collagen in the perineurium has a wavy arrangement similar to the epineurium, but a relatively smaller period of the waves (6 vs 39 μm), possibly due to smaller fibril diameter (60 vs 80 nm).[4,18,19] The perineurium functions to provide tensile strength to the nerve and is thicker at sites more vulnerable to strain, such as across joints or at nerve bifurcations.[9] The perineurium is under a degree of longitudinal tension at baseline, which is why nerve ends retract after transection.[4,20] As fascicles reach terminal nerve branches, the surrounding perineurium transitions into a single layer that is continuous with muscle spindle and end organ capsules.[11]

Fascicles are held together to form a nerve trunk by epineurium, which is the outermost layer of connective tissue. While the perineurium provides tensile strength and elasticity to tolerate stretch, the epineurium acts as a shock-absorber to provide protection from external compression.[2] The epineurium is formed by longitudinally oriented bundles of type I and type III collagen fibers, elastic fibers, and adipose tissue, and contains abundant fibroblasts and scattered mast cells.[9,11] The adipose tissue helps to protect the nerve from compression and is often reduced in diabetics; this potentially explains the increased vulnerability to compression injuries seen in diabetic patients.[4] The fibroblasts within the epineurium are responsible for fibrosis after nerve injury, which can limit mobility and thereby increase the risk for additional injury by stretch or compression forces.[4] The epineurium can be divided into epifascicular and interfascicular components. The epifascicular epineurium is the outer nerve sheath and is surrounded by a layer of loose areolar tissue called the mesoneurium, which loosely attaches to adjacent soft tissues and allows movement of peripheral nerves along their courses.[3,11,13,15,18] This tissue is

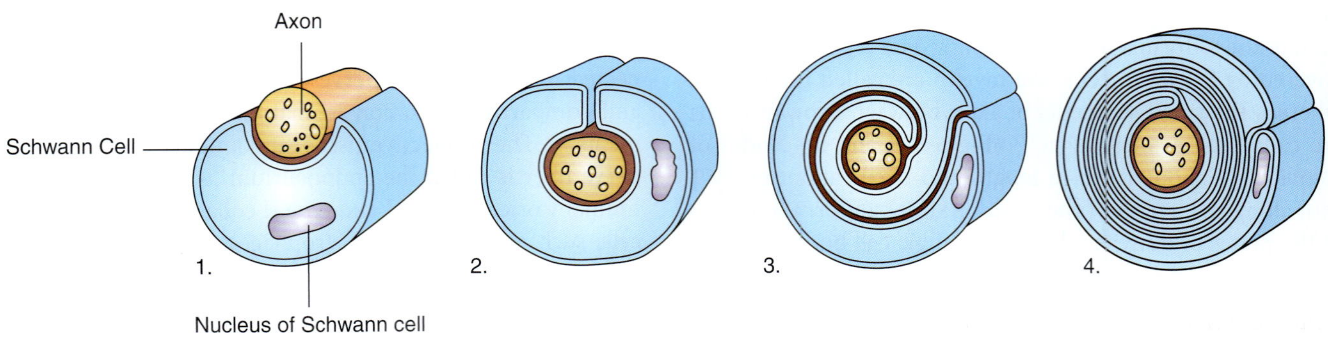

FIGURE 5 Illustrations demonstrating the formation of the myelin sheath as the Schwann cell wraps around the axon multiple times, as seen by sequential illustrations 1-4. (Modified from Kuczynski K: Functional micro-anatomy of the peripheral nerve trunks. *Hand* 1974;6[1]:1-10.)

©Copyright 2021 American Academy of Orthopaedic Surgeons

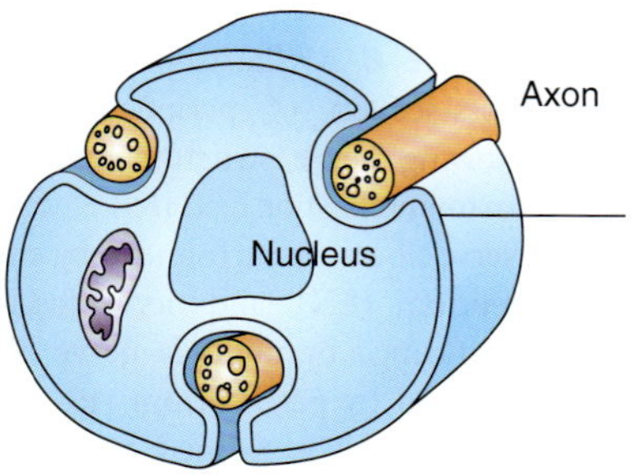

FIGURE 6 Diagram of multiple unmyelinated axons surrounded by a single Schwann cell. (Reproduced with permission from Kuczynski K: Functional micro-anatomy of the peripheral nerve trunks. *Hand* 1974;6[1]:1-10.)

sometimes confused with adipose tissue, which has led to the popular misconception that fat is a good environment for a damaged nerve. In actuality, fat can scar to the epineurium, and the mesoneurium is more complex with a tenosynovial-like gliding property that is lacking in fat. The interfascicular epineurium allows gliding between the fascicles and contains collagen fibers in wavy arrangements to accommodate stretch.[9,15,18] Nerves composed of many smaller fascicles tend to have more total epineurium than those composed of larger and fewer fascicles and are therefore better protected from compression forces.[2,17] The epineurium tends to be proportionally thicker in larger nerves and where nerves cross joints.[4,13]

The connective tissue layers of peripheral nerves are continuous with the central nervous system meninges: the epineurium is continuous with the dura mater, the outer perineurium with the arachnoid mater, and the inner perineurium with the pia mater.[9,17] The endoneurial space is continuous with the subarachnoid space, with communication between the endoneurial fluid and cerebrospinal fluid.[9] Nerve roots lack both epineurium and perineurium and have a less substantial endoneurium, resulting in greater susceptibility to injury from compression or traction.[2] Understanding this regional variation of structure along the course of the nerve can help the surgeon make an accurate assessment of the degree of damage and, hence, the prognosis for recovery.

The connective tissue within nerves is innervated by the nervi nervorum, which supplies vasomotor sympathetic fibers and sensory fibers with nociceptive properties that can result in hypersensitivity after nerve injury.[9,14]

The vascular network of the nerve can be divided into a segmental extrinsic system that enters from the mesoneurium and a longitudinal intrinsic system present in the epineurium, perineurium, and endoneurium[4,15]. The macrocirculation, or vasa nervorum, consists of segmental vessels that enter the epineurium and split into ascending and descending branches that travel along the length of the nerve.[1] These vessels lie in a coiled orientation with excess length, which prevents vessel injury during nerve gliding and excursion.[1] The segmental vessels anastomose within the interfascicular epineurium and send branches through the perineurium and endoneurium to supply the microcirculation of the endoneurial space.[9] The density of capillaries found within the endoneurial space is

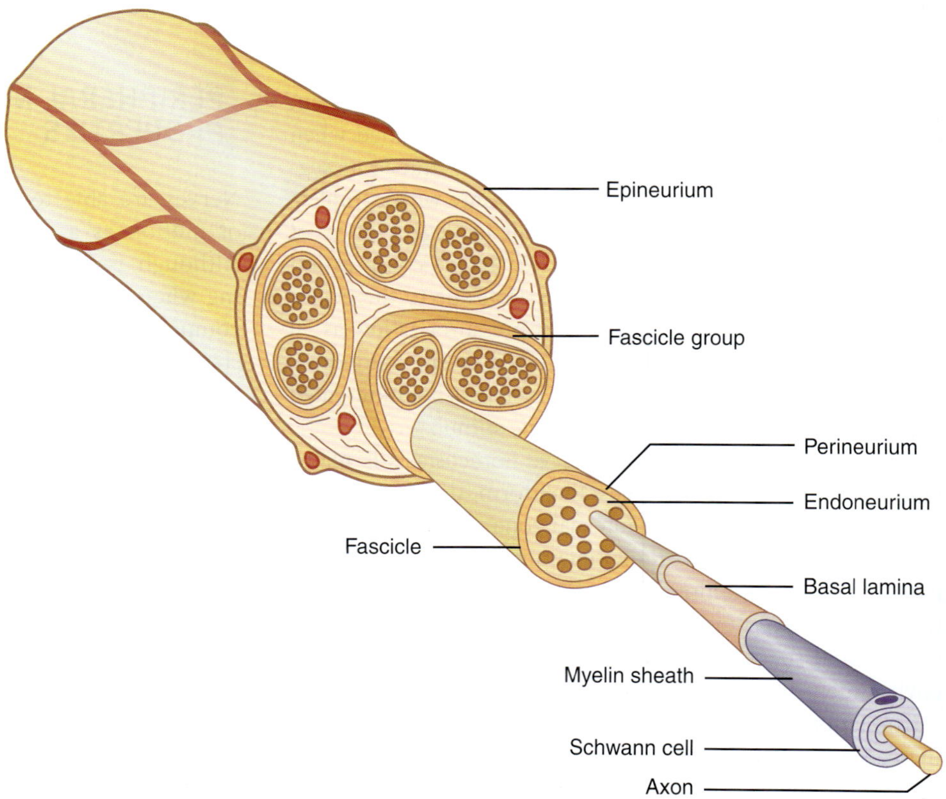

FIGURE 7 Diagram of peripheral nerve structure and compartmentalization. Each nerve fiber is composed of an axon and surrounding Schwann cells. The endoneurium surrounds individual nerve fibers, the perineurium encloses groups of nerve fibers to form fascicles, and the epineurium encloses groups of fascicles to form nerve trunks. (Reproduced with permission from Farnebo S, Thorfinn J, Dahlin LB: Peripheral nerve injuries of the upper extremity, in Neligan PC, ed: *Plastic Surgery Volume Six: Hand and Upper Extremity*, Elsevier, 2018.)

©Copyright 2021 American Academy of Orthopaedic Surgeons

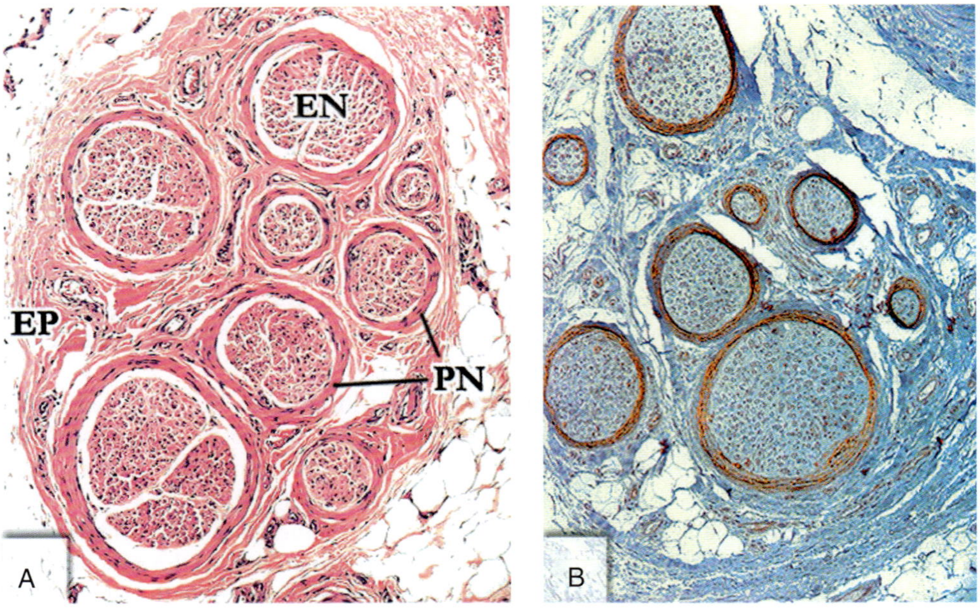

FIGURE 8 **A**, Electron micrograph cross-section of peripheral nerve, showing nerve structure and compartmentalization (H&E, 100×). Nerve fibers are surrounded by endoneurium (EN), and nerve fascicles are formed by multiple nerve fibers enclosed by perineurium (PN). The nerve trunk is formed by multiple fascicles enclosed by the epineurium (EP). The epifascicular epineurium is the outer nerve sheath while the interfascicular epineurium is found between fascicles. **B**, Epithelial membrane antigen (EMA) staining of the perineurium (100×). (Reproduced with permission from Piña-Oviedo S, Ortiz-Hidalgo C: The normal and neoplastic perineurium: A review. *Adv Anat Pathol* 2008;15[3]:147-164.)

proportional to the local metabolic demands, with fewer capillaries supplying peripheral nerves compared with sites of neuronal cell bodies.[9] Lymphatic vessels travel adjacent to blood vessels within the epineurium.[11] Epineurial arterioles and venules are permeable to macromolecules, allowing them to enter the epineurial interstitial space where they are removed by lymphatics.[4]

The extrinsic system accounts for about 50% of total circulation to nerve fibers and is especially important to more superficial nerve fibers, while more central nerve fibers within fascicles rely more heavily on the intrinsic system.[4] Nerve mobilization usually has little or no effect on intrinsic flow, and the effect on the extrinsic perfusion depends on the extent of mobilization. Extrinsic flow is relatively maintained when small vessels are sacrificed over short distances due to its segmental nature.[2,4,21] In contrast, epineurectomy with complete removal of epineurial vessels will result in degeneration of superficial nerve fibers within fascicles.[4] Nerve compression results in a similar pattern of degeneration due to the occlusion of epineurial vessels occurring at pressures as low as 30 mm Hg.[4] The extrinsic system is affected by the autonomic nervous system, whereas the intrinsic system is not innervated and therefore is unaffected by adrenergic stimuli.[4]

The blood-nerve barrier and nerve homeostasis is maintained by the endothelial cells that form the endoneurial capillaries together with the internal zone perineurial cells.[4,9] These groups of cells have tight junctions that only allow small ions to pass, maintaining a hypertonic electrolyte concentration and positive fluid pressure of 2 to 3 mm Hg within the endoneurial space.[1,4,9] Maintenance of the endoneurial ionic environment is essential to conduction of action potentials.[9] Introduction of local anesthetics into an area can result in an increased perineurial permeability, affecting the ionic environment of the endoneurial space and thus conduction.[4] The constant positive endoneurial fluid pressure prevents inflow of fluid into the endoneurial space, despite positive oncotic pressure that would otherwise promote inflow. This is a critical function as excess endoneurial fluid increases endoneurial pressure and can lead to nerve hypoperfusion and dysfunction, and over time demyelination.[4,9] Due to lack of endoneurial lymphatics, such fluid is slow to dissipate.[9] Although edema can rapidly accumulate in the epineurial space following nerve injury, the fascicles remain relatively protected as a result of the perineurial diffusion barrier.[1,4]

PERIPHERAL NERVE BIOMECHANICAL PROPERTIES

Nerves are able to glide and elongate with normal range of motion as a result of their biomechanical properties.[2] Although peripheral nerves accept a degree of lengthening when placed on stretch, excessive nerve elongation can compromise intrafascicular microcirculation and result in structural nerve damage.[2] Nerves exhibit a nonlinear resistance to stretch, with an increasing resistance to elongation as increased tension is applied.[20,22] The perineurium is the primary provider of tensile strength, with a minor contribution from the endoneurium.[20]

The first line of protection from tensile forces is the slack inherently present in nerve fibers as a result of their coiled arrangements within their compartments. When the nerve trunk and fascicles are maximally lengthened, the residual slack in nerve fibers allows the traction forces to be absorbed by the outer structures.[2] With continued force, the perineurium functions to resist further elongation to protect the nerve from injury. Once a yield point is reached, nerve fibers rupture at multiple locations along the nerve; this is followed

©Copyright 2021 American Academy of Orthopaedic Surgeons

by longitudinal tearing within the perineurium, nerve fiber herniation, and loss of perineurial elasticity.[20] Injury to the perineurium results in a disrupted diffusion barrier, with increased permeability and intrafascicular edema that can lead to fibrosis over time.[20] Stretch also leads to decreased circulation along the nerve and impaired conduction, first affecting sensory fibers followed by motor fibers.[20] Although multiple studies have evaluated the threshold elongation that a nerve can withstand, there still is not an agreed upon critical limit; some studies suggest that injury can occur with as little as 4% nerve elongation.[20,22,23] The amount of elongation that a nerve can tolerate depends on the nerve fascicular structure as well as the direction, magnitude, rate, and duration of the deforming force.[2,23] There is also regional variation along the length of a nerve, with different degrees of stretch tolerated at different locations.[23] Although nerves are vulnerable to acute tensile forces, they are able to tolerate gradual stretch as seen with limb lengthening procedures.[20] When a nerve is stretched over a period of time, it will eventually begin to relax as a result of nerve viscoelastic properties.[20]

PERIPHERAL NERVE PHYSIOLOGY

ACTION POTENTIALS

Nerves transmit signals through action potentials, by creating a transient reversal of electrical potential across cell membranes. Membrane potential describes the transmembrane distribution of charge, or in other words, the relative charge inside of the cell compared with the charge outside of the cell.[24] The resting membrane potential of a neuronal cell is −70 mV, with a relatively high concentration of sodium (Na^+) and chloride (Cl^-) ions in the extracellular fluid and a relatively high concentration of potassium (K^+) ions in the intracellular fluid. To initiate an action potential, a stimulus causes Na^+ channels in the plasma membrane to open, resulting in passive inflow of positively-charged Na^+ ions into the cell and an increased (ie, less negative) membrane potential. Stimulus initiating this process can come from multiple sources, including neurotransmitters that bind to and open ligand-gated Na^+ channels, or physical stimulus such as pressure that is detected by sensory receptors and opens mechanical-gated Na^+ channels.[24,25] If the threshold potential of −55 mV is reached, voltage-gated Na^+ channels open, allowing additional Na^+ ions to passively enter the cell driven by the concentration gradient. The resulting membrane depolarization results in an action potential; the positive current created passively travels down the axon, resulting in a series of membrane depolarizations along the axon by the same process.[9,24]

Soon after membrane depolarization, Na^+ channels inactivate after a predetermined period of time (approximately 1 ms) due to a conformational change that blocks further passage of Na^+ ions through the open voltage-gated channels.[24] As a result of depolarization, voltage-gated K^+ channels also open; these channels require a higher threshold to activate than voltage-gated Na^+ channels and are therefore slower to open.[24] Once K^+ channels open, positively charged K^+ ions passively move out of the cell driven by concentration gradient, resulting in membrane repolarization and eventually hyperpolarization. Repolarization causes the voltage-gated Na^+ and K^+ channels to deactivate and close; hyperpolarization occurs because K^+ channels are relatively slow to deactivate.[24] Additional action potentials are difficult to initiate until after K^+ channels close (relative refractory phase) and cannot occur until after Na^+ channels recover from transient inactivation (absolute refractory phase).[9] These refractory phases ensure that action potentials are not able to propagate in retrograde fashion.[24] An active sodium-potassium pump is required to restore the ionic composition of the resting cell membrane, using adenosine triphosphate (ATP) energy to move Na^+ ions out of the cell and K^+ ions in, both against their concentration gradients.[12]

The rate that action potentials propagate down an axon, or conduction velocity, is affected by the presence or absence of myelin sheath and the nerve fiber diameter, with faster conduction occurring in myelinated nerve fibers with greater diameters.[11] The myelin sheath acts as insulation, preventing loss of current and increasing the speed of travel. Conduction in myelinated fibers occurs by salutatory travel, during which action potentials skip rapidly from node of Ranvier to node of Ranvier.[9,11] Larger nerve fibers have longer internodes, resulting in increased distances of conduction between each node of Ranvier during saltatory travel, which further increases conduction velocity.[11] Myelinated fibers conduct at approximately 4.6 to 6 m/s/mm diameter, with larger diameter axons conducting at greater velocities, compared with unmyelinated fibers at approximately 1.7 m/s/mm diameter.[9]

AXONAL TRANSPORT

Neurons rely on transport of nutrients and other substances along the axon by axoplasmic flow. Axonal transport occurs both anterograde and retrograde along microtubules. Proteins synthesized within the neuron and organelles such as mitochondria, endoplasmic reticulum, neurofilaments, and microtubules are transported along the axon from the cell body toward the terminal nerve fiber in an antegrade fashion, to support nerve fiber growth and metabolic activity.[1,4,11] Retrograde transport returns materials to the cell body to be recycled or degraded, as well as materials that provide information to the cell body regarding the peripheral environment.

Direction of axonal transport is guided by the orientation of the microtubules, with the positive ends directed away from the cell body and the negative ends directed towards the cell body.[9] Fast anterograde transport is directed toward the positive ends of the microtubules, carrying synaptic vesicle precursors and mitochondria down the axon toward the

©Copyright 2021 American Academy of Orthopaedic Surgeons

axon terminal. This process is powered by kinesin family ATPase motor molecules and occurs at an approximate rate of 410 mm/d for both sensory and motor nerves; rate of axonal transport is not affected by nerve fiber size, in contrast to conduction velocity.[9,11,26] Cytoskeleton proteins also travel anterograde, but by slow transport at an approximate rate of 1 mm/d (0.1 to 30 mm/d), similar to that of axonal regeneration after injury.[1,9,27] Slow transport occurs by peristalsis of the nerve fiber membrane, rather than by microtubules.[14] In contrast to anterograde transport, fast retrograde transport is directed toward the negative ends of microtubules, carrying neurotrophins produced by peripheral targets, proteins, and organelles such as mitochondria back to the cell body via dynein family motors at a rate of about 300 mm/d.[1,9,11] Retrograde return of these substances to the cell body is thought to help regulate protein synthesis in the neuron through a negative feedback system, with unregulated synthesis occurring after nerve transection.[11] Disruption of axonal transport due to interruption or compression of the axon leads to accumulation of neurofilaments and microtubules at the proximal axon.[4]

EFFERENT AND AFFERENT SYSTEMS

The efferent system includes motor innervation to skeletal and smooth muscle, with large myelinated axons that release acetylcholine at neuromuscular junctions. A motor unit is a group of skeletal muscle fibers innervated by a single neuron. During muscle contraction, the smallest motor units are the first to fire, and additional motor units are recruited in order of increasing size until adequate force is generated; this recruitment can be observed with electromyography.[9] Smaller muscles tend to have smaller motor units to allow fine motor control.[9]

The afferent system includes sensory innervation, translating various forms of stimuli into electrical signals. Sensory receptors can be rapidly adapting, with a short response to a maintained stimulation, or slowly adapting, with a response that lasts until stimulation ceases.[9] A receptive field is the cutaneous area that a single neuron innervates; areas with smaller receptive fields, such as the fingertips, have superior stimuli discrimination.[9] Tactile mechanoreceptors are present in the dermis, fascia, and periosteum and allow interpretation of physical stimuli such as pressure, vibration, and position. These include slowly adapting Merkel cells that sense constant touch, quickly adapting Meissner corpuscles that sense moving touch, and quickly adapting Pacinian corpuscles that sense vibration. Innervation density can be evaluated with static and moving two-point discrimination to evaluate Merkel cells and Meissner corpuscles, respectively. Threshold sensory detection can be evaluated with tuning forks to assess threshold vibration detected by Pacinian corpuscles and with Semmes-Weinstein monofilaments to assess threshold touch detected by Merkel cells.[28] Proprioceptive receptors provide feedback regarding position, such as muscle spindles, Golgi tendon organs, and Ruffini endings in joint capsules.[9] Nociceptors interpret pain and thermoreceptors interpret temperature.

PERIPHERAL NERVE INJURY

PERIPHERAL NERVE INJURY PATHOPHYSIOLOGY

Immediately after axonal injury, the axon distal to the site of trauma degenerates by a process called Wallerian degeneration, described in 1850 by Augustus Waller.[4,15] Degeneration also occurs within the proximal stump for a variable distance.[12] Schwann cells and macrophages are recruited to the area and phagocytize the myelin and axonal debris over the course of three to six weeks, reducing tension within endoneurial tubes and the cross-sectional areas of fascicles.[2,4,15] Such changes can be evaluated histologically by various techniques, such as the benchmark resin-embedded semithin section treated with toluidine blue staining[29] (**Figure 9**). The basement membranes of Schwann cells associated with the endoneurial tubes are left behind, and proliferating Schwann cells align themselves along these basement membranes.[15] The persistence of the basal lamina serves as a conduit during regeneration of nerve fibers, guiding axons toward the appropriate end organs.[4] During this process, the epineurial tissue does not undergo significant change.[2]

The cell body undergoes a process called chromatolysis as early as several hours following nerve injury, during which there is swelling of the cell body and nucleolus,

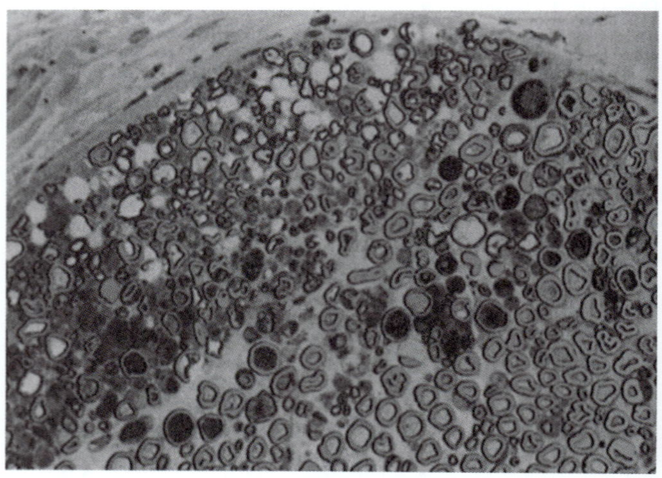

FIGURE 9 Light micrograph of rat sciatic nerve fibers stained with para-phenylenediamine, undergoing Wallerian degeneration with darkly stained axoplasm, attenuated myelin sheaths, and endoneurial edema. (Reproduced with permission from Myers RSR, James HE, Powell HC: Laser injury of peripheral nerve: A model for focal endoneurial damage. *J Neurol Neurosurg Psychiatry* 1985;48[12]:1265-1268.)

©Copyright 2021 American Academy of Orthopaedic Surgeons

morphologic changes of the nucleus, and changes in cellular metabolism.[15] The primary goal of metabolism transitions from supporting nerve signal transmission to supporting nerve regeneration, with an increase in synthesis of RNA, growth-associated proteins (eg, GAP-43, tubulin, actin, etc.), lipids, and enzymes that peaks two to three weeks following injury.[14,15,30] Axons at the site of injury sprout into multiple regenerating axons; timing of sprouting depends on the severity of injury.[12,15] Neurotropism is the phenomenon in which neurotropic factors present at the distal nerve stump of an injured nerve attract regenerating axons to their appropriate targets.[2,31] Although this process can help guide regeneration in physically separated nerve ends, it is less effective after nerve repair; once nerve ends are reapproximated, regenerating axons typically take the path of least resistance.[2]

Following injury of motor nerve fibers, the perimysium and epimysium thicken and spindle cells atrophy over two to six weeks.[15] As fibrosis forms around motor nerve fibers, they eventually fragment and lose synaptic contact with muscle fibers.[15] Motor end plate atrophy typically occurs within 12 to 24 months after injury, at which point motor reinnervation is no longer possible.[15]

PERIPHERAL NERVE INJURY CLASSIFICATION

Following Wallerian degeneration, intact structural nerve components can help guide regenerating axons to their appropriate targets. For this reason, the continuity or discontinuity of nerve structural components helps to define the severity of peripheral nerve injury and predict functional outcomes.[2] If axons do not reach their appropriate end organ, or at least a functionally similar end organ, then regeneration does not result in functional recovery. Significant nerve injury can occur without transection by processes of ischemia, contusion, stretch, or compression that result in physiological conduction block and/or failure of axonal transport that maintains nerve integrity and function.[11]

The mildest form of nerve impairment is a temporary physiologic conduction block without physical nerve damage, often occurring as the result of moderate nerve compression that interferes with intraneural microcirculation.[1,2] Nerve conduction will continue both proximal and distal to the lesion, but not across it. Nerve dysfunction is immediately reversible if the compression is removed within a short time period; however, extended compression leads to edema and increased endoneurial fluid pressure that can impact nerve conduction for hours to days.[1] Compression of 20 to 30 mm Hg reduces venous flow in the epineurium, which impairs endoneurial circulation and results in oxygen depletion; if hypoperfusion persists, the permeability of endoneurial capillaries will increase and lead to endoneurial edema.[1] After 2 to 8 hours, sustained compression will result in inhibition of both anterograde and retrograde axonal transport.[1] Lack of effective axonal transport results in a shortage of supplies that the axon relies on, which increases susceptibility of the nerve to the effects of compression at other sites; when a secondary compression occurs, this is known as double-crush syndrome.[1]

Greater magnitudes of compression can result in localized damage to the myelin sheath in addition to microcirculatory changes.[1] Total intraneural ischemia occurs at about 80 mm Hg, depending on systolic blood pressure.[1,32] Schwann cells are relatively sensitive to ischemia and can undergo degeneration resulting in nerve fiber demyelination; complete conduction block occurs if the insult is widespread.[4] Such localized nerve damage without axonal discontinuity is described as a neurapraxia in the Seddon classification, or a first-degree injury in the Sunderland classification[2,33] (**Figure 10**; **Table 1**). Because the axons are intact, neuropraxias are generally reversible with spontaneous return to prior function within three months.[1] While decompression will immediately resolve simple metabolic conduction blocks, fibers with neurapraxia take longer to recover.[1] Histologic inspection of nerves that have undergone Schwann cell degeneration and subsequent recovery have an onion bulb appearance due to duplicate layers of Schwann cell basal lamina; the basal lamina persists after Schwann cell degeneration, and subsequent regeneration results in additional layers.[4] Areas of remyelination can also be identified by proportionally thinner areas of myelin compared with the uninjured areas of the axon.[4] Nonmyelinated nerve fibers are relatively resistant to compression, and among myelinated nerves, thicker nerve fibers are more resilient to compression than thinner fibers.[1]

With crush or traction forces, axons can rupture resulting in Wallerian degeneration distal to the site of the lesion, followed by regeneration of axons. If the surrounding connective tissues are intact, they can act as a guide for accurate axonal regeneration. Injuries that are limited to the axons with preserved endoneurial and perineurial sheaths are classified as axonotmesis in the Seddon classification and as second-degree injuries in the Sunderland classification.[2,15,33] Intact endoneurial tubes contain and guide regenerating axons back to their appropriate targets, resulting in restoration of the original pattern of innervation and function.[2] The persistent basal laminas of degenerated Schwann cells also serve as conduits to guide regenerating axons toward their appropriate end organs.[4] These injuries rarely require intervention. Regeneration will occur in a proximal to distal fashion, in contrast to random recovery seen in neuropraxias. Recovery can be monitored by an advancing Tinel sign, which represents nerve regeneration and typically occurs at a rate of approximately 1 mm/d; a Tinel sign will not occur in injuries without axonal damage such as neuropraxias.[15] It can sometimes be difficult to clinically differentiate a neurapraxia from axonotmesis, and this may require a period of observation. A nerve injury that recovers within three months is likely a neurapraxia, whereas an injury that recovers at the expected rate of axonal regeneration with

©Copyright 2021 American Academy of Orthopaedic Surgeons

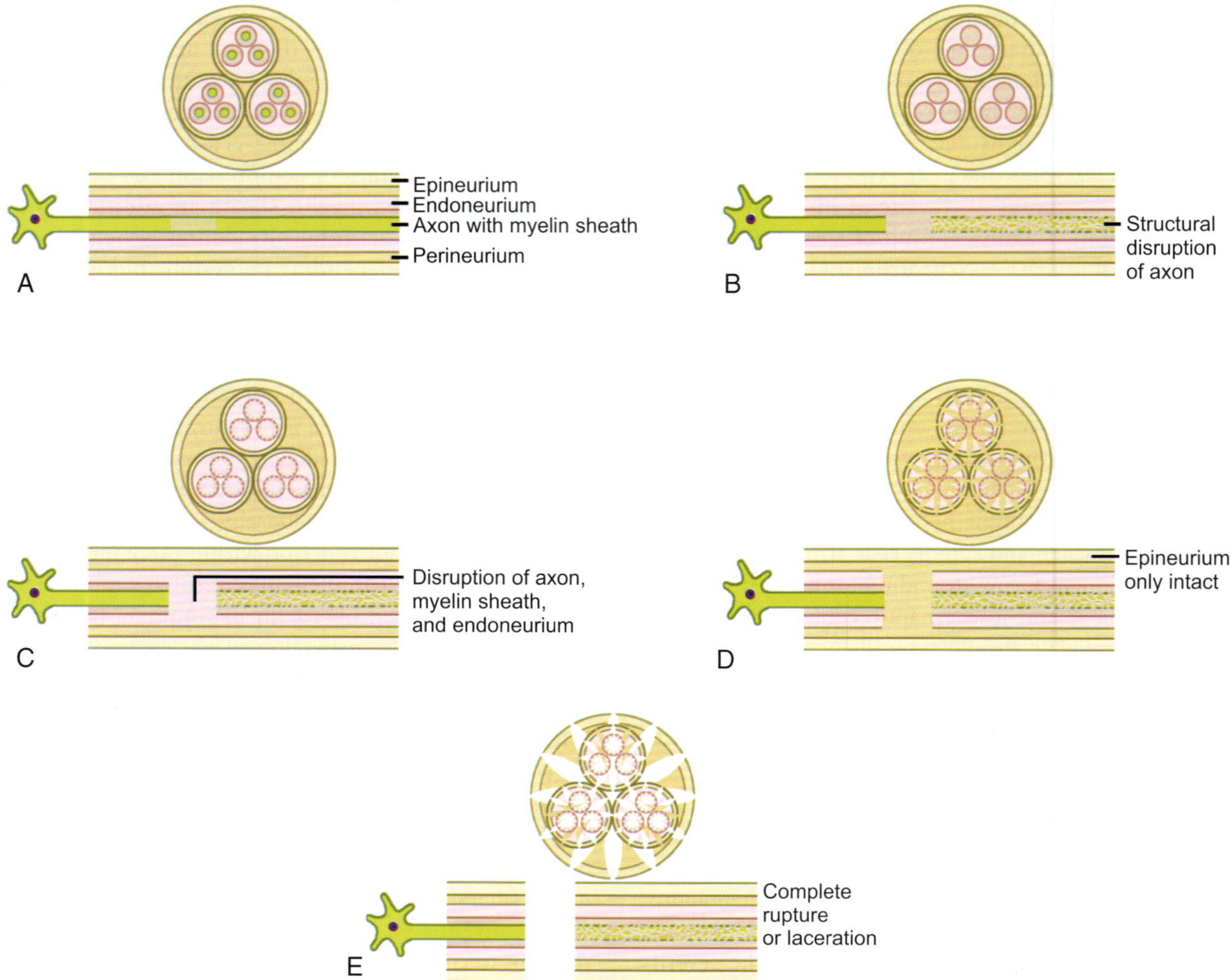

FIGURE 10 Illustrations showing Seddon and Sunderland nerve injury classifications. **A**, Neurapraxia (Seddon) is a grade I injury (Sunderland) resulting in areas of myelin loss but with all structures intact. Axonotmesis (Seddon) occurs when there is structural damage to the axon. This is further divided in the Sunderland classification into grade II injury limited to the axon (**B**), grade III injury with damage to the endoneurium (**C**), and grade IV injury with damage to the endoneurium and perineurium (**D**). Neurotmesis (Seddon) is a grade V injury (Sunderland) that also includes damage to the epineurium with complete nerve transection (**E**). (Reproduced with permission from Wiesel SW, ed: *Operative Techniques in Orthopaedic Surgery*, 2nd ed. Philadelphia, Wolters Kluwer, 2016, vol 3, Figure 70-3.)

TABLE 1 Seddon and Sunderland Nerve Injury classifications

Seddon	Sunderland	Injury
Neurapraxia	Grade I	Focal segmental demyelination
Axonotmesis	Grade II	Axon damaged with intact endoneurium
Axonotmesis	Grade III	Axon and endoneurium damaged with intact perineurium
Axonotmesis	Grade IV	Axon, endoneurium, and perineurium damaged with intact epineurium
Neurotmesis	Grade V	Complete nerve transection
	Grade VI (MacKinnon and Dellon)	Mixed levels of injury along the nerve

Reproduced with permission from Menorca RMG, Fussell TS, Elfar JC: Peripheral nerve trauma: mechanisms of injury and recovery. *Hand Clin* 2013;29(3):317-330.

©Copyright 2021 American Academy of Orthopaedic Surgeons

an advancing Tinel sign is likely an axonotmesis.[15] Nerve conduction studies can also assist with differentiation, as muscle fibrillations and denervation potentials can be seen after axonotmesis but are not present after neurapraxia.

A Sunderland third-degree nerve injury occurs when there is complete disruption of nerve fibers, including both axons and their endoneurial sheaths. Loss of endoneurial tube guidance results in axonal regeneration that is less specific, and axons often fail to reach their intended end organs.[2,15] If axons regenerate to end organs with similar function to their original target then the consequences are minimal; however, if axons regenerate to end organs with unrelated function then the resulting dysfunction is more pronounced.[2] Endoneurial disruption can also lead to intrafascicular fibrosis, which can further complicate axonal regeneration by blocking or diverting axonal growth and preventing normal function of regenerated axons.[2] If the nerve is not completely transected and some connective tissue elements remain intact, a neuroma-in-continuity may form. This occurs when damaged axons within a partially injured nerve undergo abnormal regeneration and fail to reach their target, forming a painful mass within the nerve; although the nerve appears intact, the damaged portion of the nerve will no longer transmit signals.[34] Regeneration of third-degree injuries occurs at a similar rate as second-degree injuries, but is less-predictable.[15] Recovery is incomplete and highly variable, influenced by the degree of endoneurial fibrosis and the potential for crossing of motor and sensory fibers in mixed nerves.[15] Intervention is sometimes required for third-degree injuries, including neurolysis or resection and reconstruction of the injured segment.[2,11,15]

Injury resulting in complete disruption of fascicles including the perineurium is classified as a Sunderland fourth-degree injury.[2] The nerve remains in continuity as a result of intact epineurium, but loss of perineurial continuity leads to diffuse fibrosis that causes further disorganization and obstruction of regenerating axons.[2,15] Although a Tinel sign can be present at the site of injury, intraneural scarring will prevent axonal regeneration and therefore advancement of the Tinel sign.[15] These injuries require resection of the damaged segment and reconstruction.[2] A Sunderland fifth-degree injury, or neurotmesis in the Seddon classification, occurs when there is complete transection of the nerve trunk, including the epineurium.[2,33] These injuries have no potential for recovery without surgical reconstruction.[2]

Mixed nerve injuries can occur, in which nerve fibers within a nerve trunk are injured to varying degrees of severity and therefore have various patterns of recovery; this is described as a sixth-degree injury.[2,15] Similarly, partial nerve injuries can occur in which only some nerve fibers are affected within a nerve trunk.[2] When partial nerve injuries occur more proximally, the affected nerve fibers often belong to various distal nerve branches and injury can be difficult to localize or even detect.[2] This is in contrast to more distal partial injuries, where adjacent nerve fibers often have similar end organ targets and injury results in a more localized nerve dysfunction.[2]

SUMMARY

Peripheral nerves function to communicate between the central nervous system and the rest of the body, consisting of motor, sensory, and postganglionic autonomic nerve fibers. Nerve fibers are arranged into groups by connective tissues that also provide protection and maintain specialized compartmental environments. The endoneurium surrounds individual nerve fibers, the perineurium encloses groups of nerve fibers to form fascicles, and the epineurium encloses groups of fascicles to form nerve trunks.

Neurons transmit signals by creating a transient reversal of cell membrane electrical potential that results in an action potential. To maintain neuronal function, axonal transport is necessary to supply nutrients from the cell body to the axon and to subsequently return materials to the cell body to be recycled or degraded. Compressive and tensile forces sustained by nerves can impact blood flow, axonal transport, and conduction of action potentials. Nerve injury can occur with these forces, or as the result of blunt or penetrating trauma. Following nerve injury, the continuity or discontinuity of nerve structural components helps to define the severity of injury, predict functional outcomes, and guide treatment. Peripheral nerve injuries require accurate identification of the nature of the injury and treatment strategy that is specific to the underlying pathology.

REFERENCES

1. Lundborg G, Dahlin LB: Anatomy, function, and pathophysiology of peripheral nerves. *Hand Clin* 1996;12(2):185-193.
2. Sunderland S: The anatomy and physiology of nerve injury. *Muscle Nerve* 1990;13:771-784.
3. Stewart JD: Peripheral nerve fascicles: Anatomy and clinical relevance. *Muscle Nerve* 2003;28:525-541.
4. Myers RR: Anatomy and microanatomy of peripheral nerve. *Neurosurg Clin N Am* 1991;2(1):1-20.
5. Sunderland S: *Nerves and Nerve Injuries*. Edinburgh, E. & S. Livingstone Ltd., 1968.
6. Brushart TME: Central course of digital axons within the median nerve of Macaca mulatta. *J Comp Neurol* 1991;311:197-209.
7. Jabaley MF, Wallace WH, Heckler FR: Internal topography of major nerves of the forearm and hand: A current view. *J Hand Surg* 1980;5:1-18.
8. Urushidani H: The funicular pattern of the sciatic nerve in Japanese adults. *Arch Jpn Chir* 1974;43:254-275.
9. Topp KS, Boyd BS: Peripheral nerve: From the microscopic functional unit of the axon to the biomechanically loaded macroscopic structure. *J Hand Ther* 2012;25:142-152.
10. Wilgis S, Murphy R: The significance of longitudinal excursions in peripheral nerves. *Hand Clin* 1986;2:761.
11. Battista A, Lusskin R: The anatomy and physiology of the peripheral nerve. *Foot Ankle Int* 1986;7(2):65-70.
12. Omer GE: Anatomy of peripheral nerve function and regeneration: An introduction. *Instr Course Lect* 1984;33:461-463.

©Copyright 2021 American Academy of Orthopaedic Surgeons

13. Matloub HS, Yousif J: Peripheral nerve anatomy and innervation pattern. *Hand Clin* 1992;8(2):201-214.
14. Kuczynski K: Functional micro-anatomy of the peripheral nerve trunks. *Hand* 1974;6(1):1-10.
15. Flores AJ, Lavernia CJ, Owens PW: Anatomy and physiology of peripheral nerve injury and repair. *Am J Orthoped* 2000;167-173.
16. Ochoa J, Mair WG: The normal sural nerve in man. I. Ultrastructure and numbers of fibres and cells. *Acta Neuropathol* 1969;13(3):197:216.
17. Estebe JP, Atchabahian A: The nerve: A fragile balance between physiology and pathophysiology. *Eur J Anaesthesiol* 2017;34:118-126.
18. Stolinski C: Structure and composition of the outer connective tissue sheaths of peripheral nerves. *J Anat* 1995;186:123-130.
19. Gamble HJ, Eames RA: An electron microscope study of the connective tissues of human peripheral nerves. *J Anat* 1964;98(4):655-663.
20. Grewel R, Xu J, Sotereanos DG, Woo SL: Biomechanical properties of peripheral nerves. *Hand Clin* 1996;12(2):195-204.
21. Lundborg G: The intrinsic vascularization of human peripheral nerves: Structural and functional aspects. *J Hand Surg* 1979;4(1):34-41.
22. Rydevik BL, Kwan MK, Myers RR, et al: An in vitro mechanical and histological study of acute stretching on rabbit tibial nerve. *J Orthop Res* 1990;8(5):694-701.
23. Mahan M, Yeoh S, Light A, et al: Rapid stretch injury to peripheral nerves: Biomechanical results. *Neurosurgery* 2018;0:1-8.
24. Barnett MW, Larkman PM: The action potential. *Pract Neurol* 2007;7:192-197.
25. College, OpenStax. *Anatomy and Physiology*. Rice University: OpenStax CNX, 2013.
26. Ochs S: Rate of fast axoplasmic transport in mammalian nerve fibers. *J Physiol* 1972;227:627-645.
27. Jacob JM, McQuarrie JG: Assembly of microfilaments and microtubules from axonally transported actin and tubulin after axotomy. *J Neurosci Res* 1996;43:412-419.
28. Gelberman RH, Szabo RM, Williamson RV, Dimick M: Sensibility testing in peripheral-nerve compression syndromes. *J Bone Jt Surg* 1983;65A(5):632-638.
29. Carriel V, Garzón I, Alaminos M, Cornelissen M: Histological assessment in peripheral nerve tissue engineering. *Neural Regen Res* 2014;9(18):1657-1660.
30. Fu SY, Gordon T: The cellular and molecular basis of peripheral nerve regeneration. *Mol Neurobiol* 1997;14(1-2):67-116.
31. Menorca RMG, Fussell TS, Elfar JC: Peripheral nerve trauma: Mechanisms of injury and recovery. *Hand Clin* 2013;29(3):317-330.
32. Rydevik B, Lundborg G, Bagge U: Effects of graded compression on intraneural blood flow. An in vitro study on rabbit tibial nerve. *J Hand Surg* 1981;6:3.
33. Seddon HJ: Three types of nerve injuries. *Brain* 1943;66:237.
34. Mavrogenis AF, Pavlakis K, Stamatoukou A, et al: Current treatment concepts for neuromas-in-continuity. *Injury* 2008;39 suppl(3):S43-S48.

©Copyright 2021 American Academy of Orthopaedic Surgeons

3

PATHOPHYSIOLOGY AND ORTHOPAEDIC MEDICINE

SECTION EDITORS

Roy K. Aaron, MD
Robert H. Brophy, MD

Venous Thromboembolic Disease and Fat Embolism Syndrome

Vincent D. Pellegrini Jr, MD

Keywords: *anticoagulants; aspirin; deep vein thrombosis; hypercoagulability; pulmonary embolism*

INTRODUCTION

Venous thromboembolic disease (VTED) and the fat embolism syndrome (FES) have a similar underlying pathophysiology that depends on intravasation of the adipose tissue of the bone marrow into the vascular tree. Marrow fat is an intense activator of the clotting cascade and is responsible for the hypercoagulable state following long bone trauma and instrumentation of the intramedullary canal during total hip and knee replacement. In both conditions, the lung acts as an essential filter in clearing the embolic material from the bloodstream and determining the nature of the body's response to the embolic insult. The differences in the clinical presentation of the two conditions depend upon the size and aggregate volume of the embolus as well as the nature of the embolic material invoking a response from the lung. The embolic material in VTED primarily is clotted blood, and in fat embolism syndrome, it consists of fat globules enmeshed in platelets. Considering that musculoskeletal injury and related surgical procedures often involve disruption of the marrow fat, it is no wonder that these clinical conditions can uniquely complicate the course of orthopaedic treatment. Orthopaedic surgeons must understand the pathophysiology and treatment of these conditions not only for effective patient care and communication with consulting physicians but, even more importantly, to place the specific treatment of these complications into the context of overall management of the patient. Only the orthopaedic surgeon is best positioned to balance the risks of pulmonary embolism with those of perioperative bleeding when prescribing VTED prophylaxis after total joint arthroplasty.

Dr. Pellegrini or an immediate family member is a member of a speakers' bureau or has made paid presentations on behalf of DePuy, A Johnson & Johnson Company; has received research or institutional support from Synthes; and serves as a board member, owner, officer, or committee member of the American Orthopaedic Association, the Association of American Medical Colleges, Board of Directors, Chair, the Council of Faculty and Academic Societies, AAMC, the Health Volunteers Overseas/Orthopaedics Overseas, Board of Directors, and the South Carolina Orthopaedic Association, Board of Directors.

VENOUS THROMBOEMBOLIC DISEASE

Historically, the most significant perioperative threat to the life of a patient undergoing arthroplasty is VTED, and specifically pulmonary embolism (PE). In a series of 7,959 total hip arthroplasties (THAs) from 1962 to 1973, the overall incidence of PE was 7.89% and the incidence of fatal PE was 1.04%.[1] As Charnley[2] stated, "The possibility of fatal pulmonary embolism after total hip replacement is a hip surgeon's constant worry…no matter how rare this might be." Additionally, bleeding complications related to VTED prophylaxis have become the most common cause of hospital readmission after hip or knee replacement. It is no wonder that VTED remains one of the most controversial topics in contemporary orthopaedics.

Deep vein thrombosis (DVT) is the most common precursor of PE. The predominant form of DVT after total knee arthroplasty (TKA) is in the calf distal to the trifurcation, probably initiated by stasis. Proximal DVT after TKA

©Copyright 2021 American Academy of Orthopaedic Surgeons

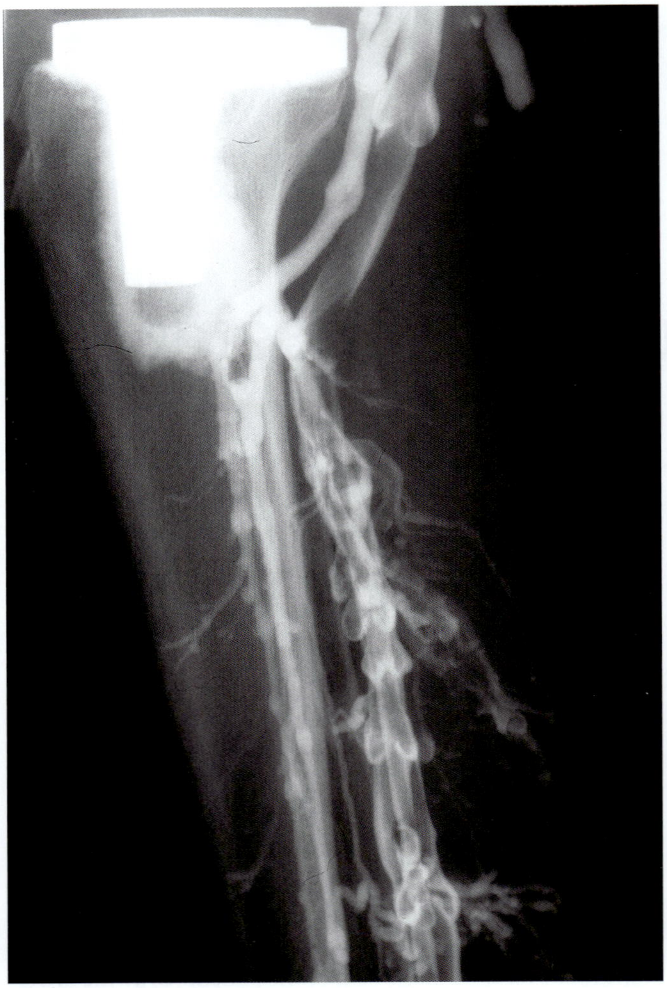

FIGURE 1 Contrast venogram showing calf thrombosis extending proximally to the popliteus vein after total knee arthroplasty (TKA).

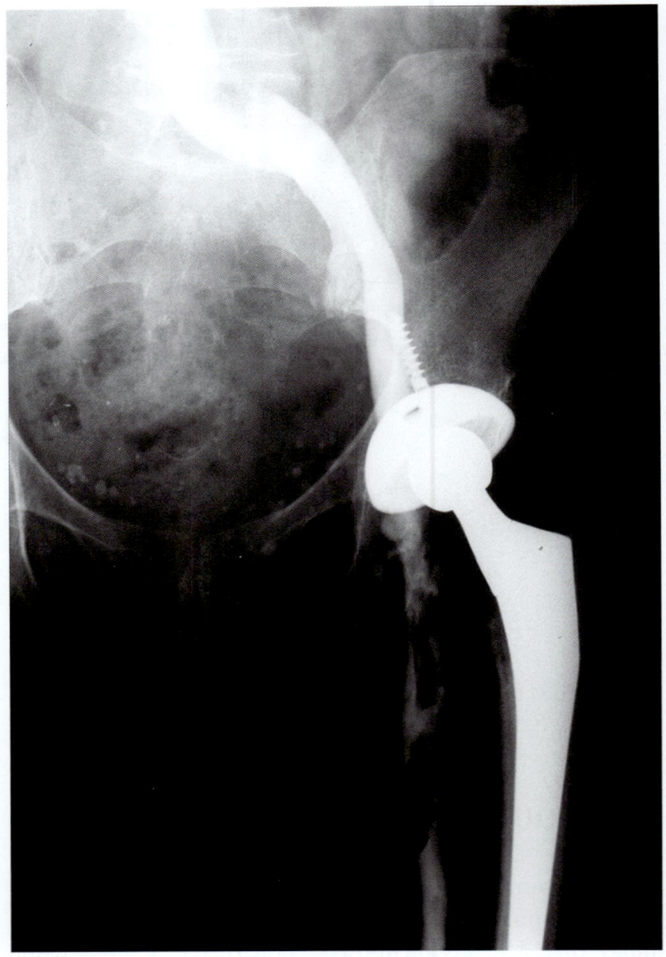

FIGURE 2 Contrast venogram showing segmental proximal femoral vein thrombosis at the level of the lesser trochanter after total hip arthroplasty (THA).

typically results from propagation of a calf clot (**Figure 1**). Proximal thrombi, specifically segmental clots in the femoral vein at the level of the lesser trochanter, predominate after THA and are likely initiated by intimal injury resulting from torsion of the vein during femoral preparation (**Figure 2**). PE traditionally was diagnosed by pulmonary arteriography (**Figure 3**) but now is most sensitively identified by CT of the chest. In the general population, the frequency of autopsy-proven fatal PE is 2.5 times that of symptomatic nonfatal PE.[3] Independently, DVT is responsible for morbidity related to chronic venous insufficiency. Five years after surgery, signs and symptoms of postthrombotic syndrome were found in 67% of patients with asymptomatic, venographically confirmed DVT, compared with 32% of patients who had a negative postoperative venogram. Moreover, postthrombotic morbidity is more common after idiopathic than after postoperative DVT,[4] probably because postoperative thrombosis is typically nonocclusive and flow past the thrombus is maintained.

EPIDEMIOLOGY

BEFORE ROUTINE PROPHYLAXIS

Historically, the risk of DVT in an unprotected patient was 70% to 84% after THA or TKA; the risk of symptomatic PE approached 15%, and the risk of fatal PE was 1% to 3.4%.[5,6] Coventry et al[5] reported a 3.4% fatal PE rate after 2,012 consecutive THAs from 1969 to 1971; the average duration of surgery was 2.4 hours, the average blood loss was 1,650 mL, patients were on bed rest for 1 week, and the mean postoperative hospital stay was 3 weeks. Since that time, the incidence of VTED after total joint arthroplasty has steadily declined, the reasons for which are widely accepted as being the adoption of routine pharmacologic and/or mechanical prophylaxis regimens as well as improved surgical techniques, earlier mobilization, and anesthetic management.[7,8] Data from two studies with a 3- to 6-month follow-up revealed a fatal PE rate as low as 0.12% to 0.35% in 4,594 patients who underwent THA without any type of chemoprophylaxis.[8,9] Compared with earlier studies,

©Copyright 2021 American Academy of Orthopaedic Surgeons

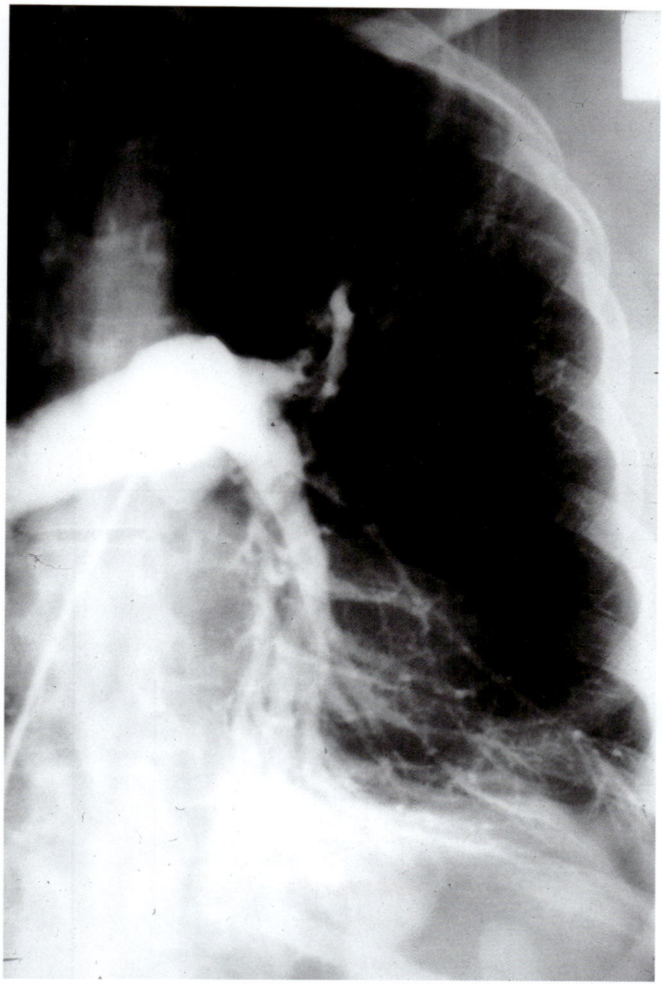

FIGURE 3 Pulmonary arteriogram revealing the presence of pulmonary emboli.

these patients benefited from more rapid postoperative mobilization and a shorter length of hospital stay. To achieve further reduction in the likelihood of fatal PE by using potent anticoagulants, it is necessary to balance the incremental benefit of eliminating PE against the increased risk of bleeding complications.[10]

AFTER ROUTINE PROPHYLAXIS

Routine prophylaxis for VTED after THA or TKA became the standard of care in North America after it was endorsed by the National Institutes of Health (NIH) Consensus Conference in 1986.[11] Low-intensity warfarin was the agent most commonly used by orthopaedic surgeons during the past three decades[12,13]; while its use has considerably reduced the incidence of DVT, screening venography revealed persistent asymptomatic venous thrombi in 15% to 25% of patients after THA and in 35% to 50% after TKA.[7] A smaller reduction in venographic DVT after TKA than after THA has been observed with the use of newer anticoagulant agents, resulting in an overall risk of DVT that is two to three times greater after TKA than after THA despite use of contemporary prophylaxis.[7] Clinically important bleeding events in patients on warfarin prophylaxis were reduced with acceptance of low-intensity anticoagulation from 8% to 12% with a prothrombin time index of 2.0 to 1% to 2% with a prothrombin time index target of 1.3 to 1.5 (International Normalized Ratio [INR] 2.0 to 2.5).[14] Although these data suggest that VTED is more refractory to standard prophylaxis after TKA than after THA, 85% to 90% of thrombi after TKA occur in the deep calf veins below the venous trifurcation, and the immediate risk of embolization is much smaller.[6] In contrast, the distribution of DVT after THA historically was 40% proximal and 60% distal.[4,7] Recent studies suggest less than 10% of thrombi after THA are proximal in location, and 85% to 90% of all DVTs after THA or TKA now occur in the calf with current prophylaxis[15-17] Yet, longitudinal surveillance studies found that 17% to 23% of these distal thrombi extend to the more proximal veins of the thigh, where they acquire considerable embolic potential.[18,19] The considerable embolic potential of postoperative calf thrombi suggests that anticoagulant prophylaxis should be continued for several weeks after surgery.[15]

PATHOGENESIS

Virchow triad, consisting of stasis, hypercoagulability, and damage to the intimal wall, remains the basis of our conceptual understanding of the mechanism of coagulation. Perturbations in elements of the triad are responsible for the abnormalities of thrombosis after musculoskeletal injury, disease, or surgery. Recent discoveries and improved understanding of the clotting cascade form the basis of new approaches to prevent and treat thrombotic disease (**Figure 4**).

FAMILIAL THROMBOPHILIA AND FACTOR V LEIDEN

Familial thrombophilia is the heritable tendency to develop severe and recurrent VTED, often spontaneously. This condition has not been adequately explained by any deficiency of circulating anticoagulants; levels of proteins C and S as well as antithrombin III were rarely found to be low in patients with familial thrombophilia. Mutations in genetic material encoding proteins C and S or antithrombin III were found to account for fewer than 5% of all incidences of familial thrombophilia.[20] In 1994, a single amino acid substitution of glutamine for arginine in the protein C cleavage region of factor V was reported to occur in 50% of patients with familial thrombophilia, compared with 3% to 7% of the general population.[21] This single nucleotide substitution, known as factor V Leiden, is responsible for resistance of activated factor V to cleavage inactivation by protein C, which normally provides a physiologic check on the clotting cascade.

Variable phenotypic expression of factor V Leiden is now accepted as being responsible for a host of clinical disease

©Copyright 2021 American Academy of Orthopaedic Surgeons

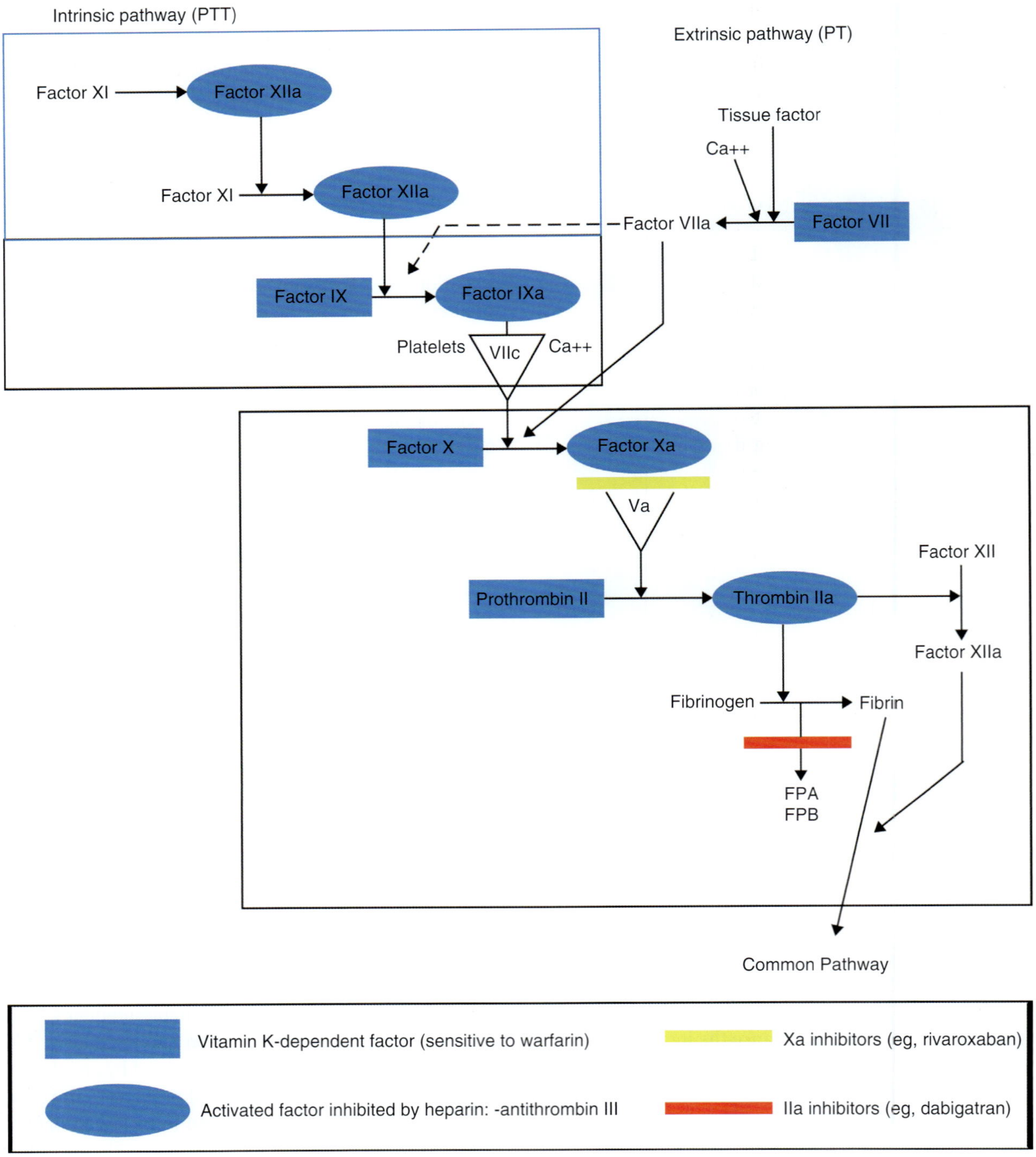

FIGURE 4 Schematic diagram showing the clotting cascade, with critical points of interference by anticoagulant agents. FPA = fibrinopeptide A; FPB = fibrinopeptide B; HMWK = high-molecular-weight kallikrein; KAL = kallikrein; PT = prothrombin time; PTT = partial thromboplastin time. (Adapted with permission from Stead RB: Regulation of hemostasis, in Golhaber SZ, ed: *Pulmonary Embolism and Deep Venous Thromboembolism*. Philadelphia, PA, WB Saunders, 1985, p 32.)

states related to thrombosis. More than half of all individuals with factor V Leiden will develop DVT in the presence of a single additional risk factor, such as a long bone fracture or total joint arthroplasty. The incidence of factor V Leiden was 26% among men older than 60 years with primary spontaneous DVT. Mixed findings have been reported from preliminary investigations of activated protein C resistance and VTED after total joint arthroplasty, and two North American studies of patients who had undergone THA or TKA found no correlation between the presence of factor V Leiden (or depletion of any other circulating anticoagulant) and the occurrence of VTED.[22,23] This negative observation

©Copyright 2021 American Academy of Orthopaedic Surgeons

can be explained by the effect of a potent thrombogenic stimulus associated with violation of the medullary canal during total joint arthroplasty, which is intense enough to overshadow any heritable predisposition to thrombosis imparted by factor V Leiden.

THROMBOGENESIS AFTER MUSCULOSKELETAL INJURY

It has long been recognized that VTED is more refractory to standard prophylaxis after orthopaedic procedures than after general surgical procedures. This phenomenon was first recognized as the inefficacy of subcutaneous heparin for DVT prevention after THA, despite the successful use of subcutaneous heparin after major abdominal or chest surgery. The discrepancy was found to be secondary to a decline in circulating levels of antithrombin III (a binding intermediary necessary for the heparins to be clinically effective), that occurred in conjunction with a decline in several other acute-phase reactants after skeletal injury or manipulation of the medullary canal (as occurs during total joint arthroplasty).[24]

The findings by Geerts et al[25] in a series of polytrauma patients with multiple injuries and an injury severity score higher than 9 underscore the influence of skeletal trauma on the clotting cascade. Contrast venography of 349 patients showed an overall DVT prevalence of 58% and a proximal DVT rate of 18%. Like patients who undergo total joint arthroplasty, most of these patients were asymptomatic; only 3 of 201 DVTs (1.5%) were clinically evident. The influence of fracture on the clotting cascade was shown by a DVT incidence of 61% with pelvic fracture, 77% with tibial shaft fracture, and 80% with femoral shaft fracture; isolated femoral or tibial shaft fracture was associated with a relative DVT risk almost five times as high as that of the overall group. Spinal cord injury was associated with an 81% incidence of DVT and an odds ratio of 8.5, compared with the total group.[25]

The same investigators subsequently studied the impact of VTED prophylaxis on 344 patients with polytrauma who were randomly assigned to one of two anticoagulant protocols.[26] Patients receiving unfractionated heparin had an overall DVT incidence of 44% (60 of 136 patients), compared with 31% of those receiving enoxaparin (40 of 129 patients, $P = 0.014$); the rates for proximal DVT were 15% (20 of 136) and 6% (8 of 129), respectively ($P = 0.012$). These findings highlight the relative ineffectiveness of unfractionated heparins for clinical thromboprophylaxis when circulating levels of antithrombin III have been reduced. Major bleeding complications were five times more common with enoxaparin therapy (2.9%) than with heparin (0.6%, $P = 0.12$). Because of their propensity for causing increased bleeding, fractionated heparins should be used cautiously for VTED prophylaxis in patients with polytrauma and especially in those with closed head trauma, a visceral injury, or an expectation of delayed surgical fracture repair (especially if the pelvis is involved).

THROMBOGENESIS DURING ANESTHESIA AND TOTAL JOINT ARTHROPLASTY

It is now accepted that the principal thrombogenic stimulus associated with THA occurs intraoperatively. More specifically, femoral preparation is closely linked with intense activation of the clotting cascade as well as torsion or complete obstruction of the femoral vein. Sharrock et al[27] measured markers of thrombin generation and fibrin formation in circulating blood during THA and found that the process of thrombosis does not begin immediately but is delayed until preparation of the femoral canal. Elevation of prothrombin F1.2, thrombin-antithrombin complexes, fibrinopeptide A, and D-dimer was most pronounced during insertion of the cemented femoral implant and continued to increase throughout the first hour after surgery. Mean values for three of the four markers were significantly higher after insertion of a cemented femoral implant than after insertion of a noncemented component. Mean pulmonary artery pressures peaked and central venous oxygen tension reached a nadir after reduction of the hip. These measurements suggest the delayed collection of embolic medullary contents in the lung resulting from kinking of the femoral vein during component insertion. Mechanical manipulation while the limb is being positioned for femoral preparation also is likely to cause local intimal injury to the femoral vein, may cause the unique finding of segmental femoral thrombi after total hip arthroplasty, and completes an across-the-board disturbance in the Virchow triad (along with hypercoagulability and stasis) in this high-risk scenario.

A subsequent investigation of the efficacy of short-acting anticoagulants for blunting the intraoperative activation of the clotting cascade during THA found that standard heparin administered intravenously after socket implantation significantly inhibited fibrin formation at 10 units/kg and completely suppressed fibrin formation at 20 units/kg.[28] With a 30- to 40-minute half-life, the dose of unfractionated heparin in theory briefly increased the bleeding risk, but no additional intraoperative bleeding was clinically evident. This anticoagulation strategy targets primary prevention of intraoperative clot formation rather than secondary prevention of the postoperative extension of existing thrombi. Epidural anesthesia, when evaluated by contrast venography as an outcome measure for DVT, has a similarly beneficial influence on thrombogenesis and VTED prophylaxis.[28,29] The mechanism for reducing the risk of venous thromboembolism with epidural anesthesia or epidural analgesia has been the subject of much conjecture. Inhibition of platelet and leukocyte adhesion and stimulation of endothelial fibrinolysis have been proposed as mechanisms but have not been substantiated by controlled studies. Rather, the sympathectomy effect of epidural blockade, resulting in increased lower extremity blood flow and mitigating the adverse effects of stasis, is most likely to be responsible for reducing the risk of venous thrombosis. Regardless of the type of anticoagulant prophylaxis, several clinical studies found an incremental 40% to 50% reduction in the risk of venographic

©Copyright 2021 American Academy of Orthopaedic Surgeons

DVT when regional anesthesia was used compared with general anesthesia.[30] The incidence of fatal PE also is reduced when epidural anesthesia is used rather than general anesthesia; a retrospective review of THA and TKA by Sharrock et al[31] reported a 0.12% rate of fatal in-hospital PE (7 of 5,874 patients) when general anesthesia was used between 1981 and 1986, compared with a 0.02% rate (2 of 9,685 patients, $P = 0.03$) when epidural anesthesia was used between 1987 and 1991. Continued use of the epidural catheter for postoperative analgesia was found to benefit VTED prophylaxis. In another study which utilized warfarin exclusively as VTE prophylaxis, 322 consecutive patients undergoing THA who received epidural anesthesia and 48-hour postoperative epidural analgesia demonstrated an overall venographic DVT rate of 8.9%, with proximal thrombi in 2.3% of patients.[29] Both aspirin, as an antiplatelet agent, and regional anesthesia have been observed to decrease expression of VTED (specifically, clinical PE) after total joint arthroplasty.[28-31]

THROMBOPROPHYLAXIS

Several issues have clouded the introduction of safe and effective antithrombotic prophylaxis—(1) industry-sponsored drug trials, (2) uncertainty of surrogates for clinically meaningful events, and (3) debate between the American Academy of Orthopaedic Surgeons (AAOS) and the American College of Chest Physicians (ACCP) with each emphasizing different aspects of anticoagulation efficacy. During the past 30 plus years, many relatively selective anticoagulant drugs have been introduced, but the evidence for prevention of fatal PE after THA and TKA has changed very little. The Institute of Medicine has identified this area as a priority for comparative effectiveness research, and the Agency for Healthcare Research and Quality Evidence-based Practice Center project[32,33] twice, in 2012 and 2017, noted a paucity of high-quality studies with lack of clear consensus and a clear tradeoff between lowered VTE risk and increased frequency of major bleeding after major orthopaedic surgery. Specifically noted was the difficulty in separating surrogate outcomes from clinically meaningful events. Most studies evaluated "total DVT" despite its questionable clinical significance. Nonetheless, the Joint Commission and Surgical Care Improvement Project now mandate VTE prophylaxis for all patients undergoing THA or TKA, according to prevailing guidelines.[34]

The guidelines of the ACCP historically have been based on the goal of reducing the frequency of DVT (as a surrogate for fatal PE), using prospective randomized clinical studies for the underlying data set.[35] From 1992 until 2012, the ACCP guidelines endorsed the use of fractionated heparins, full-intensity warfarin (INR 2.0 to 3.0), and synthetic pentasaccharide and specifically recommended *against* the use of aspirin for VTE prophylaxis. The guideline of the AAOS was intended to reduce the incidence of clinical PE while avoiding bleeding that could result in wound hematoma and secondary infection, both of which can require revision surgery and prosthesis removal. In the first AAOS clinical practice guideline on the subject, released in 2007 and published in 2009,[36] patients were stratified into four risk groups, with a recommendation for the elective use of ACCP-recommended agents. The use of aspirin or low-intensity warfarin was endorsed for patients at high risk of bleeding by the AAOS, because the rates of clinical PE with these agents are comparable to those of ACCP-recommended agents, and rates of bleeding are lower. Both ACCP and AAOS supported the use of adjunctive pneumatic compression.[36]

These disparate recommendations are predicated on studies utilizing vastly different scientific methodologies[37] Prospective randomized clinical trials found a reduction in the incidence of lower limb clots discovered on contrast venography with the use of potent new anticoagulants but were unable to confirm a commensurate reduction in fatal PEs.[15-17] These studies were insufficiently powered for discerning a difference in bleeding events, however, and may have had bias related to industry funding. Observational studies found low PE event rates, comparable to those with newer ACCP-endorsed agents, with the use of aspirin,[28,38-40] low-intensity warfarin (INR 2.0),[14,41,42] and multimodal prophylaxis regimens predicated on use of mechanical compression devices. In 2011, the AAOS released the second, and still current, version of its clinical practice guideline for VTE prophylaxis after THA and TKA,[43] and less than 6 months later, the ACCP released the ninth edition of its guidelines for antithrombotic therapy and thrombosis prevention,[44] which loosely defined a compromise middle ground.[45,46] The AAOS no longer specifically endorsed aspirin, and the ACCP awarded aspirin the same level of recommendation as every other form of chemoprophylaxis, including unfractionated heparin. The AAOS provides no recommendation for any single chemoprophylaxis agent, and the ACCP's level 1-B endorsement of all agents was equally nondiscriminating. The ACCP considered effectiveness in preventing clinical thromboembolic events to be tempered by a new appreciation of patient-perceived importance of bleeding. An ongoing study, The Comparative Effectiveness of Pulmonary Embolism Prevention after Hip and Knee Replacement (PEPPER) trial, is a large pragmatic study funded by the Patient-Centered Outcomes Research Institute (PCORI) comparing aspirin, warfarin, and rivaroxaban in 25,000 patients undergoing THA or TKA.[47] The two primary endpoints are an aggregate of clinical DVT, PE, and all-cause mortality, and clinically important bleeding events; patient-reported outcomes will align clinical results after operation with types of VTED prophylaxis. These end points represent clinically relevant surrogates, rather than thrombi discovered on venography or lung imaging of asymptomatic patients, and the large sample size of the PEPPER trial allows concurrent study of both anticoagulant effectiveness in preventing clots and safety in avoidance of untoward bleeding events. The ideal prophylaxis is yet to be determined, but it must represent a balance between the risk of fatal PE and the morbidity of anticoagulation-associated bleeding.

©Copyright 2021 American Academy of Orthopaedic Surgeons

MECHANICAL MODALITIES

External pneumatic compression devices are inherently attractive because they increase venous return, decrease stasis, and enhance endothelium-derived fibrinolysis without creating a bleeding risk. Sequential calf and thigh sleeves were associated with a reduction in calf DVT but had a variable effect on high-risk proximal clots after THA. Plantar foot compression combined with aspirin was found to reduce the incidence of proximal DVT after TKA when compared with aspirin alone. External pneumatic devices alone have not been shown to be as effective as pharmacologic prophylaxis after THA, but they may offer an advantage when used in combination with pharmacologic prophylaxis. Although the use of graduated compression stockings is widely accepted, some studies comparing warfarin with pneumatic compression sleeves alone after THA found a complementary decrease in distal DVT and a worrisome increase in proximal DVT when pneumatic sleeves were used.[5,48,49] This finding suggests that thigh-high pneumatic compression sleeves alone are less efficacious for specifically preventing proximal thrombosis than warfarin prophylaxis.

Pneumatic compression during the acute postoperative period has been endorsed as the sole means of thromboprophylaxis after TKA or THA (a level-1B or level-1A recommendation, respectively), if the bleeding risk with pharmacologic agents is unacceptably high.[35,44] The ACCP guidelines further recommend that chemoprophylaxis be added to, or substituted for, mechanical modalities as soon as the period of elevated bleeding risk has passed.

CHEMOPROPHYLAXIS

Aspirin

During the 1990s, the use of aspirin for VTE prophylaxis regained popularity among orthopaedic surgeons. This development was based not on new efficacy data but was largely attributable to the greater perceived safety and lower bleeding risk associated with aspirin in comparison with the fractionated heparins introduced during the same decade. Some authors found that all-cause mortality among patients who received potent anticoagulants such as low-molecular-weight heparin (LMWH) after THA or TKA was more than twice that of patients treated with aspirin, pneumatic compression devices, and regional anesthesia.[50] Since 2006, observational data from three large single-center studies and a national joint arthroplasty registry analysis have provided support for aspirin as an effective prophylaxis for clinically evident PE after total joint arthroplasty, especially when used in conjunction with regional anesthesia.[28,38,39,51] Reexamination of data from the Pulmonary Embolism Prevention study likewise resulted in an endorsement of aspirin in the ninth edition of the ACCP practice guidelines for thromboprophylaxis after THA and TKA.[44] The Pulmonary Embolism Prevention study primarily involved 13,356 patients with hip fracture but also included 4,088 patients undergoing elective THA or TKA.[40] Prophylaxis consisted of aspirin (160 mg daily for 35 days) or placebo, and outcome measures were in-hospital clinical PE-VTE morbidity and 35-day mortality. Aspirin use resulted in a 34% reduction in the overall incidence of PE and DVT compared with placebo (2.3% vs 1.6%, $P = 0.003$) after hip fracture, but there was no difference in overall PE-DVT incidence or mortality in the patients undergoing arthroplasty. Since its publication in 2000, the Pulmonary Embolism Prevention (PEP) study has been interpreted as not supporting the use of aspirin for VTE prophylaxis after THA or TKA. This original interpretation was based on perceived critical methodologic flaws in the PEP trial. A more recent interpretation of the trial as a pragmatic study considered comparative clinical effectiveness, and was more tolerant of the methodologic flaws.[44] In the patients with hip fracture, aspirin use resulted in a 43% reduction in PE and a 29% reduction in DVT, and it prevented four fatal PEs for every 1,000 patients.[40] In the patients undergoing arthroplasty, aspirin use resulted in an overall 19% reduction in aggregate VTE end points (1.15% vs 1.4%). Several recent observational studies have supported the use of aspirin as effective VTED prophylaxis, but a flaw that permeates many of these reports is selection bias of the surgeon. Risk stratification affects the intensity of anticoagulation felt necessary for effective prophylaxis, and observational databases are complicated by bias in selecting predominantly low-risk patients as being appropriate for aspirin as was specified by clinical practice guidelines in force at the time of these studies. Those at traditional (high) risk simply by virtue of undergoing THA or TKA, but without additional risk factors such as a personal history of prior DVT or PE, are the customary recipients of aspirin prophylaxis. Typically, such observational series from single institutions report that between 85% and 95% of patients receive aspirin, while 5% to 15% are "high risk" and receive more potent anticoagulation such as warfarin or fractionated heparin.[28,38,39,52] A recent report involving nearly 42,000 primary TKA procedures from 29 institutions in the Michigan Arthroplasty Collaborative declared aspirin was noninferior to more traditional anticoagulants as VTED prophylaxis with a noninferiority margin of 0.3.[53] However, only 30.9% of patients received aspirin alone and 13% received aspirin in combination with an anticoagulant. With less than 44% of patients receiving aspirin, a strong selection bias is evident with only the healthiest and lowest risk patients receiving aspirin. In a favorable report of 11,459 patients undergoing THA, TKA, or unicompartmental knee arthroplasty (UKA), a 16-month audit showed that 90.4% received aspirin alone for 6 weeks and 8.2% received warfarin or LMWH.[52] Clinical events were audited at 90 days; PE incidence was 0.6% and 1.47% after THA and TKA, respectively, with corresponding all-cause mortality of 0.39% and 0.44% after THA and TKA. Leading causes of death were ischemic heart disease and respiratory failure; like other recent reports from the United Kingdom, PE accounted for only 18% of deaths. Aspirin dosing is variable; one study suggested that 81 mg bid was not inferior to 325 mg bid, with a 0.25% noninferiority margin, in a nonconsecutive selected

©Copyright 2021 American Academy of Orthopaedic Surgeons

series of patients undergoing THA or TKA. Patients deemed to be at "high risk" by the surgeon were excluded from the aspirin protocol.[54]

Concurrent with these favorable observational reports using aspirin, two prospective trials cast serious doubt on its effectiveness and safety. Woller et al, from Intermountain Health, prematurely stopped a trial of aspirin compared with warfarin utilizing AAOS risk stratification guidelines after 700 patients undergoing THA or TKA because of a ninefold increased risk of PE (0.65% vs 4.6%; $P = 0.01$) and a sevenfold increased risk of VTED (1.1% vs 7.9%; $P = 0.001$) in the aspirin group.[55] Anderson et al reported a clinical noninferiority trial involving 3,753 THA and TKA procedures from 15 centers in Canada with patients randomized to receive either aspirin or rivaroxaban, after both groups received 5 days of rivaroxaban from the time of surgery, with a large noninferiority margin of 1.0%.[56] While not adequately powered to discern differences between the groups, 90-day VTED events were similar in the groups, but relative risk of a major bleeding event was 1.6-fold greater in the aspirin than the rivaroxaban group (0.47% vs 0.29%). These varying results suggest that there is a continuing and compelling need for a randomized clinical study to rigorously investigate the effectiveness and safety of aspirin for orthopaedic VTE prophylaxis.

Warfarin

Warfarin has remained the single most commonly used agent for total joint arthroplasty thromboprophylaxis in the United States over the past four decades, interrupted only by a transient surge in popularity of the fractionated heparins during the 1990s and a recent increase in aspirin use following its guideline acceptance in 2012.[12,13] Warfarin is an orally administered vitamin K antagonist that blocks synthesis of related procoagulant factors (factors II, VII, IX, and X) and physiologic anticoagulants (proteins C and S) in the liver. Despite the need for regular monitoring, some observers feel that warfarin represents the best therapeutic compromise between efficacy and safety and between VTE prevention and bleeding, compared with other chemoprophylaxis agents. The critics of warfarin have been more concerned about untoward bleeding associated with its use than with its efficacy.

Early warfarin studies reported bleeding rates of 8% to 12%, with occasional life-threatening events. In a landmark study, Coventry et al[5] delayed prophylactic anticoagulation therapy until the fifth postoperative day, presumably because of a concern over bleeding during the early postoperative period, but still observed untoward bleeding in 4.1% of patients on warfarin. In a similar report, Amstutz[57] administered warfarin prophylaxis for 3 weeks postoperatively and observed overall bleeding complications in 1.5% of 3,000 patients undergoing THA. Bleeding was noted in 4.7% of the first 405 patients, but closer monitoring and lowering of the target prothrombin time from between 18 and 20 seconds to between 16 and 18 seconds resulted in a reduction in the bleeding rate to 1% in the subsequent patients. Of the 44 major bleeding complications, 36 were wound hematomas and 8 involved the gastrointestinal or genitourinary tracts. Noncemented stems were independently associated with a bleeding rate of 2.3%. Contemporary recommendations favoring reduced-intensity anticoagulation with a prothrombin time ratio of 1.3 to 1.5 times control (INR 2.0 to 2.5) have been associated with markedly lower rates of bleeding, ranging from 1.2% to 3.7%.[14] In a meta-analysis of DVT prophylaxis after hip replacement, Imperiale and Speroff[58] identified a six times greater risk of clinically important bleeding with the use of LMWH compared with patients without chemoprophylaxis and a 50% greater risk compared with warfarin. Colwell et al[59] compared clinically evident VTE after THA in patients receiving adjusted-dosage warfarin or LMWH (enoxaparin; 30 mg every 12 hours) for an average of 6.5 days; clinically important bleeding was significantly more frequent with enoxaparin (1.3%) than with warfarin (0.5%).

Low-intensity warfarin prophylaxis (INR 2.0) resulted in overall venographic DVT rates of 9% to 26% and proximal clot rates of 2% to 5% after THA[41] and in overall DVT rates of 35% to 55% and proximal clot rates of 2% to 14% after TKA.[42] Moreover, warfarin was shown to have a peculiar propensity for reducing the incidence of proximal DVT compared with distal calf thrombosis after THA. Consistent with most reports on the effects of regional anesthesia, recent evidence suggests that 48 hours of warfarin combined with continuous epidural anesthesia-analgesia is associated with an additional 50% reduction in residual DVT rates in comparison with a combination of warfarin and general anesthesia.[7,29]

Very convincing are observational data from centers using extended low-intensity warfarin prophylaxis. A two-decade review studied 3,293 patients undergoing THA or TKA for a 6-month period after hospital discharge.[41,42] Contrast venography was used for routine surveillance before discharge, and all patients with negative venograms were discharged home without further prophylaxis. Patients with documented VTE received standard heparin and warfarin therapy. During the first decade of the study, patients not completing venography were discharged without further anticoagulant prophylaxis. Because of observed readmissions related to embolic events in these patients, during the second decade all patients not completing venography received empirical low-intensity warfarin for 6 weeks after discharge. Readmissions for VTE, DVT, PE, or a bleeding complication within 6 months of surgery were audited by communication with the patient or primary care physician. The overall readmission rate for VTE was 1.6% in patients who underwent THA (32 of 1,972 patients, including 14 with PE and 18 with DVT),[41] compared with 0.6% after TKA (8 of 1,321 patients, including 3 with PE and 5 with DVT, $P = 0.009$).[42] The readmissions affected 2.2% of the patients who underwent THA and had negative venography with no further anticoagulation therapy (19 of 880 patients), compared with 0.28% of patients who underwent THA and received outpatient warfarin (1 of 360 patients, $P = 0.013$). In the combined population of patients undergoing THA or TKA, 6 weeks of warfarin therapy eliminated the risk of PE (0 of 844 patients vs 17 of

©Copyright 2021 American Academy of Orthopaedic Surgeons

2,449 patients, $P = 0.01$) and significantly reduced the VTE-related readmission rate (2 of 844 patients [0.2%] vs 38 of 2,449 patients [1.6%], $P = 0.0015$) compared with patients who did not continue warfarin therapy after hospital discharge. Three bleeding events (in 3 of 3,292 patients [0.1%]) led to one death from intracranial bleeding while on warfarin and two revision surgeries necessitated by hematoma while on fractionated heparin. Routine surveillance, even with contrast venography, was a poor predictor of the need for continued anticoagulant prophylaxis after discharge. Extended warfarin as a method of secondary prophylaxis eliminated PE-related deaths and reduced the rate of VTE-related readmission after THA or TKA.

Extending low-intensity warfarin (INR 1.5 to 2.0) for 4 to 6 weeks after surgery is a highly effective and time-honored method of prophylaxis; VTE-related readmission is necessary in only 0.3% of patients after THA and 0.2% after TKA; the major bleeding rate is 0.1%; and a residual incidence of DVT is less than 10% in conjunction with sustained epidural anesthesia after THA.[41,42,57] The optimal use of warfarin begins the evening before surgery because of its 48-hour latency to onset of anticoagulant effect. The combination of preoperative warfarin and epidural anesthesia has been found safe and effective. Moreover, warfarin use prevents VTE-related morbidity and mortality, as judged by late PE-related readmission or death, even in patients with a tendency to form thrombi in the face of primary warfarin prophylaxis.[41,42]

Newer Selective Anticoagulants—Heparinoids and Direct Oral Anticoagulants

The newer anticoagulants (fractionated heparins,[18,59] synthetic pentasaccharide,[60] factor Xa,[16,17,61,62] and direct thrombin inhibitors[63]) all have greater demonstrated efficacy than older agents for reducing venographic thrombosis when used as primary chemoprophylaxis after THA or TKA. However, these newer agents are also uniformly associated with a considerably increased risk of perioperative bleeding.[64,65] In contrast, low-intensity warfarin (INR 2.0) and aspirin have been associated with an incidence of residual venographic clotting as much as five times higher than that of the newer agents, but with a comparable clinical PE rate. As evidence of the clotting-bleeding tradeoff, the risk of major bleeding complications with low-intensity warfarin and aspirin is two to three times less than with the more potent anticoagulants.[58]

Rivaroxaban, an orally administered direct inhibitor of activated factor X (factor Xa), is the most extensively studied (in 12,729 patients) anticoagulant after both THA and TKA in direct comparison with enoxaparin, using clinical end points and venographic screening.[16,61,62] A pooled analysis of two hip arthroplasty studies (7,050 patients) and two knee arthroplasty studies (5,679 patients) showed a 58% reduction in combined all-cause mortality and symptomatic VTE (0.6% vs 1.3%, $P < 0.001$).[66] However, the use of rivaroxaban was associated with an increase in major or clinically relevant nonmajor bleeding events (3.2% vs 2.6%, $P = 0.039$) as well as increase in return to the operating room to manage bleeding complications.[67]

Dabigatran, an oral direct inhibitor of activated factor II (thrombin), is in use for thromboprophylaxis around the world and is approved in the United States for cardiovascular anticoagulation, specifically atrial fibrillation. Dabigatran (220 mg or 150 mg once daily) has efficacy comparable to that of enoxaparin for all-cause mortality, total VTE prevention, and major bleeding rates after THA, when compared with enoxaparin (40 mg once daily). Dabigatran had similar efficacy and safety after TKA when compared with the European dosage of enoxaparin (40 mg once daily) but was inferior in efficacy to the North American enoxaparin regimen (30 mg twice daily).[63] Despite their superior efficacy, these newer, more specific agents have been associated with a risk of bleeding frequently greater than that of fractionated heparin, which itself carries a greater bleeding risk than low-intensity warfarin or aspirin.

FAT EMBOLISM SYNDROME

Posttraumatic fat embolization, specifically the fat embolism syndrome, has been a source of interest since the original description by Zenker in 1861 in a patient with a thoracoabdominal crush injury.[68] The fat embolism syndrome can be practically defined as a complex alteration in coagulation homeostasis that occurs as an infrequent complication of fracture of the pelvis and long bones and is clinically manifested as acute respiratory insufficiency. The full-blown clinical syndrome is evident in 0.5% to 2% of patients after an isolated long bone fracture and in 5% to 10% of patients with multiple fracture and pelvic injury after polytrauma.[68] In contrast, fat embolization occurs as a subclinical event after every fracture and every instrumentation of the medullary canal with release of fatty marrow during total joint arthroplasty. The likelihood of fat embolization resulting in the clinical syndrome characterized by florid respiratory failure is determined by the quantity of fat intravasated into the systemic circulation and the ability of the patient's cardiopulmonary system to withstand the filtration of this material by the lung.

PATHOPHYSIOLOGY

Disruption of the intramedullary canal, whether accidentally through trauma or iatrogenically during surgical instrumentation, results in liberation of marrow fat from its protected position within the long bones. Neutral fat and tissue thromboplastin released from the fracture site enter the systemic circulation and activate the clotting cascade and platelet aggregation. Suppression of the fibrinolytic system in the injured patient aggravates the ongoing accumulation of aggregates of fat macroglobules, marrow elements, platelets, erythrocytes, fibrin, and leukocytes. These heterogeneous emboli passively concentrate in the lung as a result of the filtering action of the lung on venous blood before it returns to the systemic circulation (**Figure 5**).

When the fat emboli become lodged in the pulmonary bed, a biphasic reaction ensues within the lung.[68,69] The pulmonary

©Copyright 2021 American Academy of Orthopaedic Surgeons

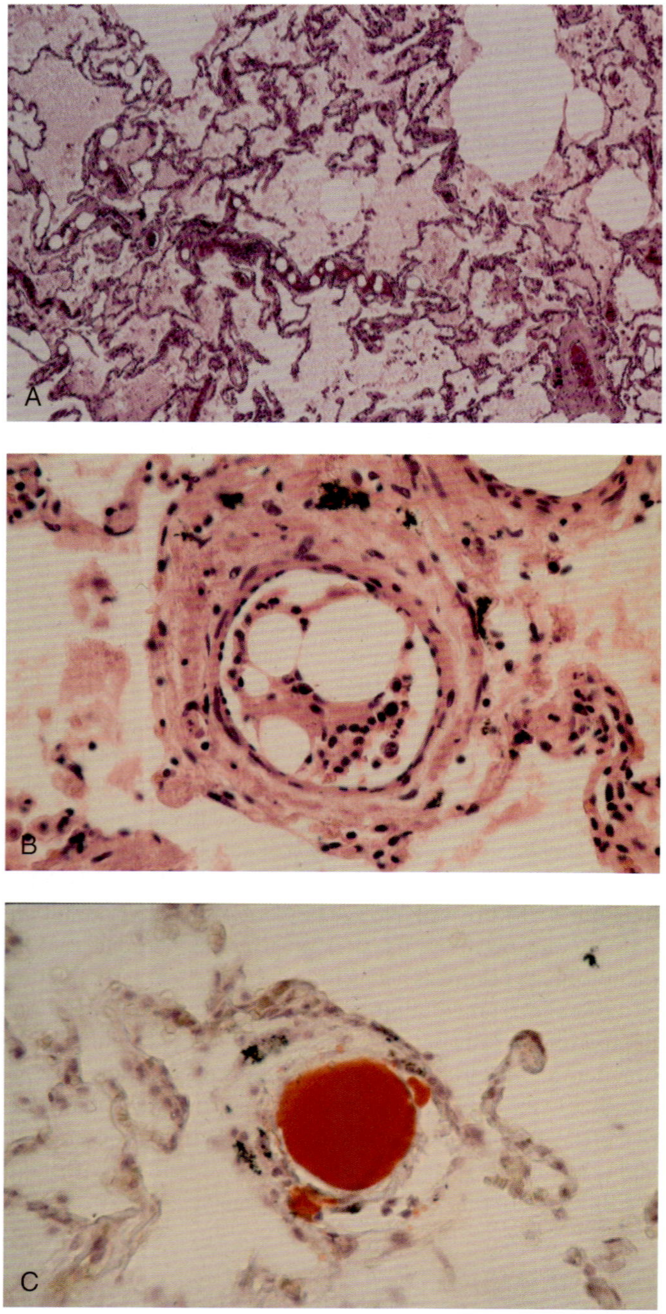

FIGURE 5 Histologic images of postmortem embolic material from the lung of a patient with a fatal fat embolism syndrome. **A**, Fat globules in a pulmonary arteriole, with prominent exudate in the air spaces (17× magnification). **B**, Embolic marrow elements and fat in a pulmonary arteriole (110× magnification). **C**, Oil Red O stain showing fat in a pulmonary arteriole (110× magnification).

circulation normally is a low-pressure, low-resistance system; observations from acute PE suggest that 80% of the pulmonary circulation must be obstructed to create a significant hemodynamic effect. Massive fat embolization to the lungs therefore can result in elevation of right heart pressures and, in extreme circumstances, acute cor pulmonale and death. Such

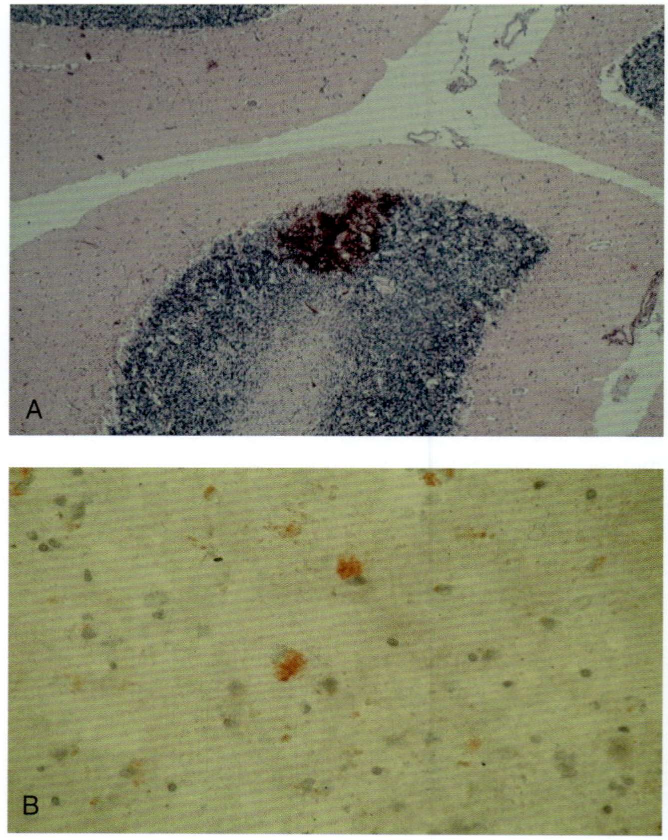

FIGURE 6 Histologic images of postmortem brain tissue from a patient with systemic fat embolization. **A**, Petechial hemorrhage in the cerebellum (17× magnification). **B**, Oil Red O stain showing fat in the brain (43× magnification).

a dramatic circulatory collapse has been found in animals but is rare in humans. The situation can be further aggravated if the patient has a patent foramen ovale, in which a right-to-left shunt bypassing the lung filter allows immediate systemic embolization of fat to the arterial circulation with clinical consequences such as stroke and digital ischemia (**Figure 6**).

Subacute or delayed clinical manifestations of fat embolization most commonly are seen in patients with the fat embolism syndrome.[69] The primary defect is in arterial oxygenation, with severe hypoxemia resulting from a large ventilation-perfusion shunt. This clinical scenario has been reproduced in animals immediately after injection of fatty acids or within 72 hours after injection of neutral fat; a rise in serum lipase is observed concurrent with the lung changes after neutral fat injection.[70] Peltier[69] promoted a theory of pulmonary failure after fracture in humans, in which neutral marrow fat becomes lodged in the lung, where it is broken down by lipase produced locally by pneumatocytes in response to the embolic material. The resulting free fatty acids chemically inactivate existing surfactant and are toxic to the alveolar type II cells that synthesize surfactant in the lung. This theory of free fatty acid liberation in the lung is controversial, but it is supported by an observed increase in serum lipase and free fatty acids before a decrease

©Copyright 2021 American Academy of Orthopaedic Surgeons

in oxygenation in patients with fulminant fat embolism syndrome. It is not necessary to implicate the local conversion of neutral marrow fat to free fatty acids in the lung to explain the profound respiratory collapse characteristic of fat embolism syndrome. Aggregates of fat, fibrin, platelets, and leukocytes alone are capable of disturbing oxygen diffusion in the lung by inciting release of numerous vasoactive substances that result in increased pulmonary capillary permeability and impaired gas exchange. Regardless of the particular insult to the lung, whether by fatty acid conversion and toxicity, leukocyte lysosomal enzymes, or complement activation from intravascular marrow fat, it is evident that the final common pathway of pulmonary injury leads to acute respiratory distress syndrome, which is characterized by so-called wet lung and life-threatening impairment of oxygen exchange.

CLINICAL PRESENTATION AND TREATMENT

It is important to distinguish between fat embolization, which is a common subclinical event occurring after fracture or medullary canal instrumentation, and fat embolism syndrome, which is a rare clinical event of respiratory failure after fracture or polytrauma. The initial insult after embolic fat reaches the lungs is characterized by increased right heart pressures and cardiovascular collapse. Although this condition rarely is clinically evident in humans,[68] it has been reported after cementation of the femoral implant during THA[71] (especially for femoral neck fracture in an elderly osteoporotic patient) or after intramedullary nailing of the femur for an impending pathologic fracture with concurrent filling of the medullary canal with methyl methacrylate cement. Embolic marrow elements have been found postmortem in the capillary bed of the brain in such patients, suggesting that an overwhelmed lung filter allowed overflow of embolic material into the systemic circulation.[68] Transient aphasia and even death have been observed after major orthopaedic procedures in patients later found to have a patent foramen ovale with a documented embolic intracerebral event.[72]

The typical fat embolism syndrome is delayed in its appearance. Clinical signs and symptoms develop in 60% of patients within 24 hours and in 85% of patients within 48 hours after fracture or medullary canal instrumentation.[68,69] This delay is believed to be secondary to the evolving effects of vasoactive substances in the lung and the resulting decrement in gas exchange. The clinical manifestations are primarily cardiopulmonary in nature and include arterial hypoxemia; oxygen desaturation, sinus tachycardia, and fever are the classic triad of early findings.[69] Nonspecific changes of pulmonary congestion can be seen on the chest radiograph in one-third of patients, and the electrocardiogram may show ST segment elevation consistent with ischemia or right heart strain. Alterations in cognition are common, ranging from lethargy to delirium and possibly seizures; it is unclear whether these findings are more related to hypoxemia or fat embolization to the brain. Petechiae develop in 50% to 60% of patients, typically in the axilla (**Figure 7**), over the chest and base of the neck, and in the conjunctivae; often they appear after 24- to 48-hour delay and are transient in nature. Despite the frequency of abnormalities in laboratory coagulation markers, a clinical bleeding disorder rarely is a component of fat embolism syndrome.[68,69] This constellation of findings is uncommon after musculoskeletal trauma, but the mortality rate approaches 10% to 15% in patients developing full-blown fat embolism syndrome, and a high index of suspicion is necessary for early identification and proper treatment.

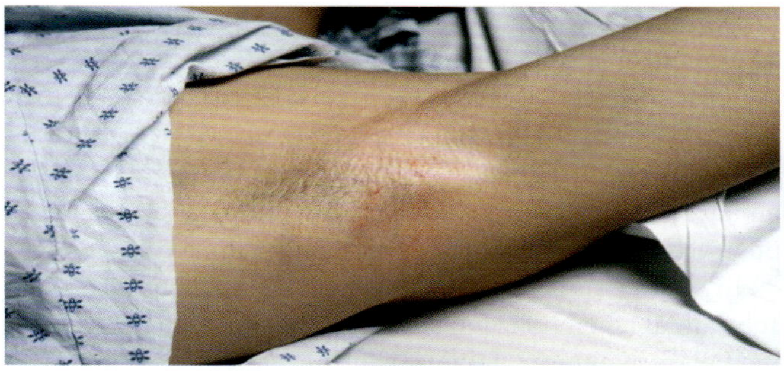

FIGURE 7 Photograph showing petechiae, as are commonly seen in the axilla, in a patient with a fat embolism syndrome after a closed femoral shaft fracture.

Intramedullary nailing soon after injury has been promoted as critical for early mobilization and avoidance of the pulmonary and thromboembolic complications of recumbency.[73,74] However, early fracture nailing has been criticized as adding insult to lung injury in a patient with polytrauma, and delayed intramedullary fixation has been considered if the patient has compromised pulmonary function from the index injury. The consensus in North America is that patients with isolated long bone fracture or polytrauma without lung injury should be treated with early intramedullary nailing to facilitate mobilization but that intramedullary fracture fixation should be delayed 5 days, or until pulmonary function improves, for patients with polytrauma and lung dysfunction. Preparation of the femoral canal during total hip arthroplasty or intramedullary nailing for an impending pathologic fracture has been associated with cardiopulmonary dysfunction, especially if cement is being used.[71] In the operating room, this first phase of clinically important fat embolization leading to cardiopulmonary dysfunction may manifest as hypotension, right heart strain, bradycardia, and cardiovascular collapse, and postoperatively it typically appears as hypoxemia and self-limiting confusion and changes in cognition.[70] Distal venting of the femoral canal with direct suction is advisable, particularly during cementing of a long stem for fracture fixation or nailing of the femur in a patient with metastatic disease and multiple lytic lesions. The purpose is to reduce intramedullary pressures and subsequent embolization of fat to the lungs and thereby to reduce the likelihood of pulmonary complications. During bilateral TKA, when the medullary canals of four bones are instrumented and the volume of intravasated fat can be large, it is unwise to operate on both knees concurrently.[75] Instead, it is more prudent to complete the arthroplasty on one

3: Pathophysiology and Orthopaedic Medicine

©Copyright 2021 American Academy of Orthopaedic Surgeons

knee and note whether there is a substantial drop in oxygen saturation or systolic pressure after tourniquet release; if so, the second-knee surgery should be deferred. Bilateral total knee arthroplasty with extramedullary instrumentation that did not violate the medullary canals was not found to offer an advantage over intramedullary instrumentation related to observed fat embolization and pulmonary function.[76]

In elective surgery, the most effective treatment is to avoid substantial fat embolization. It also is advisable to delay intramedullary nailing of fractures in the presence of lung dysfunction, to vent the femur when cementing a stem or nail in a patient with osteoporosis or metastatic disease, and to perform sequential rather than concurrent bilateral TKAs. Supportive care is critical for a patient with florid respiratory failure secondary to fat embolism syndrome. In the absence of specific therapies, the mainstays of treatment are mechanical ventilation with airway pressure support, volume repletion, and judicious use of steroids to stabilize the pulmonary capillary and improve gas exchange.[77]

SUMMARY

Thromboembolic phenomena resulting from instrumentation of the intramedullary canal of long bones are common and potentially serious complications of major orthopaedic procedures; these must be understood by every orthopaedic practitioner. Intravasation of marrow fat activates the clotting cascade and is responsible for the uniquely high prevalence of venous thromboembolism observed after total hip and total knee arthroplasty as well as hip fracture repair. In its most severe form, massive pulmonary embolism may result in sudden death following any of these procedures as well as long bone fixation, repair of ankle fracture, and even anterior cruciate ligament reconstruction. While there is consensus agreement on the routine use of prophylaxis for venous thromboembolism after total hip and knee arthroplasty and hip fracture, there is no agreement on which agents or methods provide the optimal balance between efficacy, in preventing fatal PE, and safety, in avoiding excessive bleeding complications. Additional prospective randomized clinical trials, free of surgeon selection bias directed by prevailing clinical guidelines for aspirin use, are essential to provide data on the effectiveness and safety of aspirin as primary VTED prophylaxis. Likewise, massive embolization of marrow fat droplets from the medullary canal to the pulmonary capillary bed may cause acute cardiovascular collapse as well as late manifestations of hypoxemia attributable to the adult respiratory distress syndrome. Optimal timing of long bone fracture fixation may help to avoid this condition, and high-dose steroids may blunt life-threatening signs and symptoms once the fat embolism syndrome is evident.

REFERENCES

1. Johnson R, Green JR, Charnley J: Pulmonary embolism and its prophylaxis following the Charnley total hip replacement. *Clin Orthop Relat Res* 1977;127:123-132.
2. Charnley J: *Low Friction Arthroplasty of the Hip: Theory and Practice.* Berlin, Germany, Springer-Verlag, 1979.
3. Surgeon General's call to action to prevent deep vein thrombosis and pulmonary embolism. Available at: http://www.surgeongeneral.gov/topics/deepvein/calltoaction/call-to-action-on-dvt-2008.pdf.
4. Prandoni P, Lensing AW, Prins MR: The natural history of deep-vein thrombosis. *Semin Thromb Hemost* 1997;23(2):185-188.
5. Coventry MB, Nolan DR, Beckenbaugh RD: "Delayed" prophylactic anticoagulation: A study of results and complications in 2,012 total hip arthroplasties. *J Bone Joint Surg Am* 1973;55(7):1487-1492.
6. Stulberg BN, Insall JN, Williams GW, Ghelman B: Deep-vein thrombosis following total knee replacement: An analysis of six hundred and thirty-eight arthroplasties. *J Bone Joint Surg Am* 1984;66(2):194-201.
7. Pellegrini VD Jr, Sharrock NE, Paiement GD, Morris R, Warwick DJ: Venous thromboembolic disease after total hip and knee arthroplasty: Current perspectives in a regulated environment. *Inst Course Lect* 2008;57:637-661.
8. Seagroatt V, Tan HS, Goldacre M, Bulstrode C, Nugent I, Gill L: Elective total hip replacement: Incidence, emergency readmission rate, and postoperative mortality. *BMJ* 1991;303(6815):1431-1435.
9. Warwick D, Williams MH, Bannister GC: Death and thromboembolic disease after total hip replacement: A series of 1162 cases with no routine chemical prophylaxis. *J Bone Joint Surg Br* 1995;77(1):6-10.
10. Murray DW, Britton AR, Bulstrode CJ: Thromboprophylaxis and death after total hip replacement. *J Bone Joint Surg Br* 1996;78(6):863-870.
11. Prevention of venous thrombosis and pulmonary embolism. *Natl Inst Health Consens Dev Conf Consens Statement* 1986;6(2):1-8.
12. Markel DC, York S, Liston MJ Jr, Flynn JC, Barnes CL, Davis CM III; AAHKS Research Committee: Venous thromboembolism: Management by American Association of Hip and Knee Surgeons. *J Arthroplasty* 2010;25(1):3-9, e1-e2.
13. Anderson FA Jr, Huang W, Friedman RJ, et al: Prevention of venous thromboembolism following hip or knee arthroplasty: Findings from a 2008 survey of US orthopaedic surgeons. *J Arthroplasty* 2012;27(5):659-666.e5.
14. Hirsh J, Levine MN: The optimal intensity of oral anticoagulant therapy. *JAMA* 1987;258:2723-2726.
15. Eikelboom JW, Quinlan DJ, Douketis JD: Extended-duration prophylaxis against venous thromboembolism after total hip or knee replacement: A meta-analysis of the randomised trials. *Lancet* 2001;358(9275):9-15.
16. Eriksson BI, Borris LC, Friedman RJ, et al: Rivaroxaban versus enoxaparin for thromboprophylaxis after hip arthroplasty. *N Engl J Med* 2008;358(26):2765-2775.
17. Kakkar AK, Brenner B, Dahl OE, et al: Extended duration rivaroxaban versus short-term enoxaparin for the prevention of venous thromboembolism after total hip arthroplasty: A double-blind, randomised controlled trial. *Lancet* 2008;372(9632):31-39.
18. Kakkar VV, Howe CT, Flanc C, Clarke MB: Natural history of postoperative deep-vein thrombosis. *Lancet* 1969;2(7614):230-232.
19. Pellegrini VD Jr, Langhans MJ, Totterman S, Marder VJ, Francis CW: Embolic complications of calf thrombosis following total hip arthroplasty. *J Arthroplasty* 1993;8(5):449-457.
20. De Stefano V, Leone G, Mastrangelo S, et al: Clinical manifestation and management of inherited thrombophilia: Retrospective analysis and follow-up after diagnosis of 238 patients with congenital deficiency of antithrombin III, protein C, protein S. *Thromb Haemost* 1994;72(3):352-258.
21. Bertina R, Keoleman B, Koster T, et al: Mutation in blood coagulation factor V associated with resistance to activated protein C. *Nature* 1994;369:64-67.

©Copyright 2021 American Academy of Orthopaedic Surgeons

22. Woolson S, Zehnder JL, Maloney WJ: Factor V Leiden and the risk of proximal venous thrombosis after total hip arthroplasty. *J Arthroplast* 1998;13(2):207-210.
23. Ryan D, Crowther MA, Ginsberg JS, Francis CW: Relation of factor V Leiden genotype to risk for acute deep venous thrombosis after joint replacement surgery. *Ann Intern Med* 1998;128(4):270-276.
24. Dahl OE, Pedersen T, Kierulf P, et al: Sequential intrapulmonary and systemic activation of coagulation and fibrinolysis during and after total hip replacement surgery. *Thromb Res* 1993;70:451-458.
25. Geerts WH, Code KI, Jay RM, Chen E, Szalai JP: A prospective study of venous thromboembolism after major trauma. *New Engl J Med* 1994;331:1601-1606.
26. Geerts WH, Jay RM, Code KI, et al: A comparison of low-dose heparin with low-molecular weight heparin as prophylaxis against venous thromboembolism after major trauma. *NEJM* 1996;335:701-707.
27. Sharrock NE, Go G, Harpel PC, Ranawat CS, Sculco TP, Salvati EA: Thrombogenesis during total hip arthroplasty. *Clin Orthop Relat Res* 1995;319:16-27.
28. González Della Valle A, Serota A, Go G, et al: Venous thromboembolism is rare with a multimodal prophylaxis protocol after total hip arthroplasty. *Clin Orthop Relat Res* 2006;444:146-153.
29. Dalldorf PG, Perkins FM, Totterman S, Pellegrini VD Jr: Deep venous thrombosis following total hip arthroplasty: Effects of prolonged postoperative epidural anesthesia. *J Arthroplasty* 1994;9(6):611-616.
30. Modig J, Borg T, Karlström G, Maripuu E,and Sahlstedt B. Thromboembolism after total hip replacement: Role of epidural and general anesthesia. *Anesth Analg* 1983;62:174-180.
31. Sharrock NE, Cazan MG, Hargett MJL, Williams-Russo P, Wilson PD Jr: Changes in mortality after total hip and knee arthroplasty over a ten-year period. *Anesth Analg* 1995;80:242-248.
32. Sobieraj DM, Coleman CI, Tongbram V, et al: *Venous Thromboembolism in Orthopedic Surgery*. Rockville, MD, Agency for Healthcare Research and Quality, March 2012. www.effectivehealthcare.ahrq.gov/reports/final.cfm.
33. Balk EM, Ellis AG, Di M, Adam GP, Trikalinos TA: *Venous Thromboembolism Prophylaxis in Major Orthopedic Surgery*. Rockville, MD, Agency for Healthcare Research and Quality, June 2017. www.effectivehealthcare.ahrq.gov/reports/final.cfm.
34. Centers for Medicare and Medicaid Services: *Medicare and Medicaid move aggressively to encourage greater patient safety in hospitals and reduce never events [press release]*. July 31, 2008. http://www.cms.gov/apps/media/press/release.asp?Counter=3219. Accessed March 27, 2012.
35. Geerts WH, Bergqvist D, Pineo GF, et al: Prevention of venous thromboembolism: American College of Chest Physicians evidence-based clinical practice guidelines (8th edition). *Chest* 2008;133(6 suppl):381S-453S.
36. Johanson NA, Lachiewicz PF, Lieberman JR, et al: Prevention of symptomatic pulmonary embolism in patients undergoing total hip or knee arthroplasty. *J Am Acad Orthop Surg* 2009;17(3):183-196.
37. Eikelboom JW, Karthikeyan G, Fagel N, Hirsh J: American Association of Orthopedic Surgeons and American College of Chest Physicians guidelines for venous thromboembolism prevention in hip and knee arthroplasty differ: What are the implications for clinicians and patients? *Chest* 2009;135(2):513-520.
38. Cusick LA, Beverland DE: The incidence of fatal pulmonary embolism after primary hip and knee replacement in a consecutive series of 4253 patients. *J Bone Joint Surg Br* 2009;91(5):645-648.
39. Lotke PA, Lonner JH: The benefit of aspirin chemoprophylaxis for thromboembolism after total knee arthroplasty. *Clin Orthop Relat Res* 2006;452:175-180.
40. Pulmonary Embolism Prevention (PEP) Trial: Prevention of pulmonary embolism and deep vein thrombosis with low dose aspirin. *Lancet* 2000;355(9212):1295-1302.
41. Pellegrini VD Jr, Donaldson CT, Farber DC, Lehman EB, Evarts CM: Prevention of readmission for venous thromboembolic disease after total hip arthroplasty. *Clin Orthop Relat Res* 2005;441:56-62.
42. Pellegrini VD Jr, Donaldson CT, Farber DC, Lehman EB, Evarts CM: Prevention of readmission for venous thromboembolism after total knee arthroplasty. *Clin Orthop Relat Res* 2006;452:21-27.
43. American Academy of Orthopaedic Surgeons: *Clinical Guideline on Preventing Venous Thromboembolic Disease in Patients Undergoing Elective Hip and Knee Arthroplasty*. September 2011. http://www.aaos.org/research/guidelines/VTE/VTE_guideline.asp. Accessed June 8, 2019.
44. Falck-Ytter Y, Francis CW, Johanson NA, et al: Prevention of VTE in orthopaedic surgery patients: Antithrombotic Therapy and Prevention of Thrombosis, 9th ed: American College of chest physicians evidence-based clinical practice guidelines. *Chest* 2012;141(2 suppl):e278S-e325S.
45. Lieberman JR: American College of Chest Physicians evidence-based guidelines for venous thromboembolic prophylaxis: The guideline wars are over. *J Am Acad Ortho Surg* 2012;20(6):333-335.
46. Lieberman JR, Heckmann N: Venous thromboembolism prophylaxis in total hip arthroplasty and total knee arthroplasty patients: From guidelines to practice. *J Am Acad Orthop Surg* 2017;25(12):789-798.
47. Comparative Effectiveness of Pulmonary Embolism Prevention after Hip and Knee Replacement (PEPPER). US National Library of Medicine, Clinical Trials.gov identifier: NCT02810704.
48. Francis CW, Pellegrini VD Jr, Marder VJ, et al: Comparison of warfarin and external pneumatic compression in prevention of venous thrombosis after total hip replacement. *JAMA* 1992;267(21):2911-2915.
49. Paiement G, Wessinger SJ, Waltman AC, Harris WH: Low-dose warfarin versus external pneumatic compression for prophylaxis against venous thromboembolism following total hip replacement. *J. Arthroplasty* 1987;2:23-26.
50. Sharrock NE, Gonzalez Della Valle A, Go G, Lyman S, Salvati EA: Potent anticoagulants are associated with a higher all-cause mortality rate after hip and knee arthroplasty. *Clin Orthop Relat Res* 2008;466(3):714-721.
51. Jameson SS, Charman SC, Gregg PJ, Reed MR, van der Meulen JH: The effect of aspirin and low molecular weight heparin on venous thromboembolism after hip replacement. A nonrandomized comparison from information in the National Joint Registry. *JBJS Br* 2011;93B:1465-1470.
52. Ogonda L, Hill J, Doran E, Dennison J, Stevenson M, Beverland D: Aspirin for thromboprophylaxis after primary lover limb arthroplasty. *Bone Joint J* 2016;98-B:341-348.
53. Hood BR, Cowen ME, Zheng HT: Association of aspirin with prevention of venous thromboembolism in patients after total knee arthroplasty compared with other anticoagulants. A noninferiority analysis. *JAMA Surg* 2019;154(1):65-72.
54. Parvizi J, Huang R, Restrepo C, et al: Low-dose aspirin is effective chemoprophylaxis against clinically important venous thromboembolism following total joint arthroplasty. *JBJS Am* 2017;99:91-98.
55. Woller SC, Bertin KC, Stevens SM, et al: A prospective comparison of warfarin to aspirin for thromboprophylaxis in total hip and total knee arthroplasty. *J Arthroplasty* 2012;27(1):1-9.
56. Anderson DR, Dunbar M, Murhaghan J, et al: Aspirin or rivaroxaban for VTE prophylaxis after hip or knee arthroplasty. *NEJM* 2018;378:699-707.
57. Amstutz HC, Friscia DA, Dorey F, Carney BT: Warfarin prophylaxis to prevent mortality from pulmonary embolism after total hip replacement. *J Bone Joint Surg* 1989;71-A:321-326.
58. Imperiale TF, Speroff T: A meta-analysis of methods to prevent venous thromboembolism following total hip replacement. *JAMA* 1994;271(22):1780-1785.
59. Colwell CW Jr, Collis DK, Paulson R, et al: Comparison of enoxaparin and warfarin for the prevention of venous thromboembolic disease after total hip arthroplasty: Evaluation during hospitalization and three months after discharge. *J Bone Joint Surg Am* 1999;81(7):932-940.
60. Turpie AGG, Gallus AS, Hoek JA: A synthetic pentasaccharide for the prevention of deep vein thrombosis after total hip replacement. *NEJM* 2001;344:619-625.
61. Lassen MR, Ageno W, Borris LC, et al: Rivaroxaban versus enoxaparin for thromboprophylaxis after total knee arthroplasty. *N Engl J Med* 2008;358(26):2776-2786.

©Copyright 2021 American Academy of Orthopaedic Surgeons

62. Turpie AG, Lassen MR, Davidson BL, et al: Rivaroxaban versus enoxaparin for thromboprophylaxis after total knee arthroplasty (RECORD4): A randomised trial. *Lancet* 2009;373(9676):1673-1680.
63. Friedman RJ, Dahl OE, Rosencher N, et al: Dabigatran versus enoxaparin for prevention of venous thromboembolism after hip and knee arthroplasty: A pooled analysis of three trials. *Thromb Res* 2010;126:175-182.
64. Burnett RS, Clohisy JC, Wright RW, et al: Failure of the American College of Chest Physicians-1A protocol for lovenox in clinical outcomes for thromboembolic prophylaxis. *J Arthroplasty* 2007;22(3):317-324.
65. Francis CW, Pellegrini VD Jr, Totterman S, et al: Prevention of deep-vein thrombosis after total hip arthroplasty: Comparison of warfarin and dalteparin. *J Bone Joint Surg Am* 1997;79(9):1365-1372.
66. Turpie AGG, Lassen MR, Eriksson BI, et al: Rivaroxaban for the prevention of venous thromboembolism after hip or knee arthroplasty. Pooled analysis of four studies. *Thromb Haemost* 2011;105:444-453.
67. Jensen CD, Steval A, Partington PF, Reed MR, Muller SD: Return to theatre following total hip and knee replacement, before and after the introduction of rivaroxaban. *JBJS British* 2011;93B:91-95.
68. Gossling HR, Pellegrini VD Jr: Fat embolism syndrome: A review of the pathophysiology and physiological basis of treatment. *Clin Orthop Relat Res* 1982;(165):68-82.
69. Peltier LF: Fat embolism: A current concept. *Clin Orthop Relat Res* 1969;66:241-253.
70. Tornabene VW, Fortune JB, Wagner PD, Halasz NA: Gas exchange after pulmonary fat embolism in dogs. *J Thorac Cardiovasc Surg* 1979;78:589-599.
71. Herndon JH, Bechtol CO, Crickenberger DP: Fat embolism during total hip replacement: A prospective study. *J Bone Joint Surg Am* 1974;56(7):1350-1362.
72. Della Valle CJ, Jazrawi LM, DiCesare PE, Steiger DJ: Paradoxical cerebral embolism complication a major orthopaedic operation. A report of two cases. *JBJS* 1999;81:108-110.
73. Bone LB, Johnson KD, Weigelt J, Scheinberg R: Early versus delayed stabilization of femoral fractures: A prospective randomized study. *J Bone Joint Surg Am* 1989;71(3):336-340.
74. Pinney SJ, Keating JF, Meek RN: Fat embolism syndrome in isolated femoral fractures: Does timing of nailing influence incidence? *Injury* 1998;29(2):131-133.
75. Kim YH: Incidence of fat embolism syndrome after cemented or cementless bilateral simultaneous and unilateral total knee arthroplasty. *J Arthroplasty* 2001;16(6):730-739.
76. O'Connor MI, Brodersen MP, Feinglass NG, Leone BJ, Crook JE, Switzer BE: Fat emboli in total knee arthroplasty: A prospective randomized study of computer-assisted navigation vs standard surgical technique. *J Arthroplasty* 2010;25:1034-1040.
77. Habashi NM, Andrews PL, Scalea TM: Therapeutic aspects of fat embolism syndrome. *Injury* 2006;37(suppl 4):S68-S73.

©Copyright 2021 American Academy of Orthopaedic Surgeons

22

Biology and Diagnosis of Skeletal Infection

Alexus M. Cooper, BS
Karan Goswami, MD, MRCS
Javad Parvizi, MD, FRCS

Keywords: *musculoskeletal infection; osteomyelitis; periprosthetic joint infection (PJI); septic arthritis; surgical site infection*

INTRODUCTION

Healthcare-associated infection (HAI) affects 1 in 31 hospitalized patients at any given time and costs the US healthcare system an estimated $9.8 billion annually, making it a major public health concern.[1,2] Among the five major HAI subtypes, surgical site infection (SSI) contributes the most toward this cost and 33% of SSI cases occur in patients who have undergone orthopaedic procedures.[1] Overall, bacteria from the *Staphylococcus* genera have been identified as the most common pathogens causing SSI, along with *Enterobacteriaceae, Streptococci,* and *Enterococci.*[3,4] Drug-resistant organisms, such as methicillin-resistant *Staphylococcus aureus* (MRSA) and vancomycin-resistant *Enterococci* (VRE), that can colonize patients are becoming an increasing concern because of their impact on quality of life, length of stay (LOS), and overall cost of care.[5-7] Of note, orthopaedic SSI following inpatient procedures has been reported to prolong hospital LOS by a median of 2 weeks per patient, double the readmission rates, and more than triple overall healthcare costs.[8]

Targeted prevention of musculoskeletal infection depends on risk factor assessment and the subsequent incorporation of appropriate interventions. Of 99,152 spine surgery cases from the American College of Surgeons National Surgical Quality Improvement Program (NSQIP) database, 2.3% were complicated by SSI.[4] Among this cohort of infected patients, the significant risk factors for SSI and wound dehiscence included increased surgical time, body mass index (BMI) ≥ 30, smoking, and wound classification ≥ II.[4] Conversely, previous studies have found the infection rate for total joint arthroplasty (TJA) to range from 1% to 2.5%.[9] Risk factors for infection after total hip arthroplasty and total knee arthroplasty (TKA) include male gender, cardiac disease, and LOS.[10] Other modifiable risk factors for SSI and PJI across the orthopaedic subspecialties include high alcohol intake, diabetes, previous joint surgery, and high Charlson Comorbidity Index (CCI).[11] Knowledge of such risk factors has led to targeted and evidence-based measures in the medical management of orthopaedic patients and generated new endeavors in research focused at SSI/PJI risk mitigation.

Dr. Parvizi or an immediate family member has received royalties from Corentec; serves as a paid consultant to or is an employee of CeramTec, ConvaTec, Corentec, Ethicon, Heron, Tenor, TissueGene, and Zimmer; has stock or stock options held in Alphaeon, Ceribell, Corentec, Cross Current Business Intelligence, Hip Innovation Technology, Intellijoint, Invisible Sentinel, Joint Purification Systems, MDValuate, MedAp, MicroGenDx, Parvizi Surgical Innovations, Physician Recommended Nutriceuticals, and PRN-Veterinary; and serves as a board member, owner, officer, or committee member of Eastern Orthopaedic Association and Muller Foundation. Neither of the following authors nor any immediate family member has received anything of value from or has stock or stock options held in a commercial company or institution related directly or indirectly to the subject of this chapter: Dr. Cooper and Dr. Goswami.

©Copyright 2021 American Academy of Orthopaedic Surgeons

BIOLOGIC PRINCIPLES OF SKELETAL INFECTIONS

ETIOLOGY

Pathogenic organisms include bacteria, viruses, parasites, and fungi. Of these, bacteria are the most common source of musculoskeletal infection. Bacteria are prokaryotic organisms, which lack an enveloped nucleus and instead have a nucleoid of genetic material located in the cytoplasm. Bacteria also do not have membrane-bound organelles such as mitochondria and lysosomes. A consistent feature exclusive to prokaryotes is the presence of a cell wall, which allows bacteria to resist osmotic stress. Cell wall complexity can differ between species and bacteria are dichotomized into two major groups: gram-positive and gram-negative. This designation is contingent upon cell wall response of bacterium to crystal violet indium dye after an alcohol rinse. Gram-positive bacteria retain the dye and appear violet under light microscopy. Gram-negative bacteria only retain the safranin O counter-stain and appear pink under light microscopy. Additional classification based on bacteria phenotype can be done with bacteria being labeled as round (cocci) and rod-shaped (bacilli).

Bacteria can resist microbial treatment through innate or extrinsic mechanisms, creating a major challenge in the treatment of musculoskeletal infection. Innate resistance mechanisms that bacteria inherently possess preclude the action of an antibiotic against it. Examples of intrinsic resistance mechanisms that allow bacteria to evade pharmacologic therapy include enzyme-mediated destruction of antibiotics, changes in cell-wall permeability, alterations to structure, mutations in efflux mechanisms, and bypass of metabolic pathway. These aforementioned mechanisms may also be combined to enable resistance as well.

Extrinsic antibiotic resistance strategies are those that an organism acquires, for example, resistance to an antibiotic to which it was previously susceptible. This can take place because of a chance mutation in the genetic material of the microbial cell, or via the acquisition of drug-resistant genes from another drug-resistant cell through a process known as transformation. Transformation-acquired resistance is usually mediated via plasmids, small circles of double-stranded DNA which carry genes for specialized functions such as antimicrobial resistance.

BIOMATERIALS AND BIOFILM

Biomaterials such as indwelling catheters and orthopaedic prostheses are inert nonliving surfaces that can serve as an adherence site for bacteria, leading to the development of a structure known as biofilm. Biofilm is a highly structured community of bacteria cells that adopts a distinct phenotype and can be troublesome to eradicate because of its ability to respond and adapt to stressors.[12] Cell-cell communication known as quorum sensing plays a key regulatory role in the biofilm life cycle, thereby influencing motility, adhesion, cell-to-cell aggregation, virulence, and metabolic activity.[13-15] These advanced capabilities make biofilm less susceptible to hostile environmental changes in pH, osmolarity, and temperature. Compared with planktonic bacterial cells, bacteria in biofilm are less accessible to antibiotic agents and even host immune responses. Efficient surface modification of biomaterials to prevent biofilm formation and the attachment of microorganisms is an ongoing focus of translational research.

The four-stage growth cycle of biofilm involves initiation, maturation, maintenance, and dispersion.[13] The initiation phase of biofilm development involves adherence of the bacteria to a surface and formation of microcolonies. Bacteria subsequently produce extracellular polysaccharides which form a glycocalyx that bacterial cells embed themselves within. Other microorganisms are attracted to the surface of the substratum by physical forces including van der Waals forces, hydrophobic interactions, and gravitational forces. Chemical interactions such as ionic, hydrogen, and covalent bonding play a role as well.

Bacterial adherence is influenced by the chemical composition of the biomaterial and surface properties. Roughness, hydrophobicity/hydrophilicity, porosity, pore topology, and other surface conditions are the key factors for microbial adhesion.[16] In vivo studies have identified a higher rate of bacterial adherence to stainless steel over titanium.[17] Tantalum appears to be more resistant to *S aureus* adherence.[18] When a biomaterial is implanted, its surface becomes coated with a film of plasma and extracellular matrix molecules such as fibrinogen, laminin, fibronectin, and collagen. Bacterial surface receptors facilitate adhesion via interaction with these matrix molecules. Bacterial pili and flagella are also involved in this process, particularly in gram-negative organisms.[19]

PRINCIPLES OF ANTIMICROBIALS

Successful treatment of musculoskeletal infection requires the utilization of appropriate surgical modalities in conjunction with targeted antimicrobial therapy. An antimicrobial is any substance of natural, semisynthetic, or synthetic origin that kills or inhibits the growth of a microorganism but causes little or no host damage. It is important to consider factors such as infection type, pathogen susceptibility, and virulence. Important patient factors include their health and nutritional status, and potential for adverse drug effects. Antibiotics are used for prophylaxis for patients with open wounds/fractures or in a preoperative setting, and to eradicate infections after their onset. They can be delivered orally, intramuscularly, intravenously, locally via antibiotic beads, powder, or spacers, or via an osmotic pump.

Successful antimicrobial therapy requires knowledge of an antimicrobial's spectrum of activity, distribution pharmacokinetics, toxicity, synergy and antagonism with other antimicrobials, and cost. The spectrum of activity is also an important consideration when choosing an antimicrobial

©Copyright 2021 American Academy of Orthopaedic Surgeons

directed against a specific pathogen. First, the physician must identify the pathogen(s) causing the infection. Once isolated, an antimicrobial with activity against the organism(s) causing disease can be chosen. During the selection process, it is important to consider antibiotic distribution and pharmacokinetics, because an antimicrobial's activity against a particular bacterium can be hampered if a subtherapeutic concentration reaches the site of infection. The benefits of an antimicrobial must also outweigh the risks of use for patients, particularly in cases where risk of medicinal toxicity can outweigh the benefit of a medication's therapeutic effects.

Other qualities of antimicrobials include their ability to produce additive (synergistic) and counteracting (antagonistic) effects when used together. For example, bacteriostatic antimicrobials can slow the killing rate of a bactericidal antimicrobial. In life-threatening infections, cost will not play a major role in choosing antimicrobial therapy; however, for mild infections such as cystitis or for antimicrobial prophylaxis, regimens may vary 10-fold in cost. Therefore, the clinician must have some understanding of the cost of various antimicrobials.

Although a current recommendation suggest a prolonged course of IV antimicrobial therapy may be necessary for musculoskeletal infection, a recent randomized control trial found oral antibiotic therapy to be noninferior to intravenous antibiotic therapy when used during the first 6 weeks for complex orthopaedic infection, as assessed by treatment failure at 1 year.[20] Emergent findings such as this may influence the recommendations for antibiotic treatment of musculoskeletal infection in the future.

HOST-RELATED RISK FACTORS

A number of musculoskeletal infections may be preventable through the identification and treatment of modifiable risk factors.[4,11,21,22] Some of these risk factors include disease states such as HIV, rheumatoid arthritis, diabetes, and other local or distant infections such as urinary tract infections[23] (**Table 1**). Other modifiable patient risk factors include obesity, malnutrition, smoking, and poor oral health. By being aware of these factors, particularly those that are modifiable, patient optimization before surgery can be conducted to reduce the risk of infection.

Evidence-based risk stratification metrics such as those created by Tan et al[24] can help inform perioperative risk as well. Among TJA patients, host-related factors such as history of previous surgery, substance abuse, HIV, and a revision procedure were found to put patients at significant risk for infection. Additional risk factors included coagulopathy, renal disease, congestive heart failure, psychosis, rheumatologic disease, diabetes, anemia, male sex, liver disease, and smoking.[24]

For elective TJA, centers often implement a multifaceted and evidence-based approach to SSI prevention. This process typically commences with a structured preoperative risk evaluation and targeting risk factor optimization. In keeping with current literature, institutions may advocate for smoking cessation; weight loss before surgery if patients have a BMI >40 kg/m^2; optimizing diabetic control until HbA1c <8% or Fructosamine <292 μmol/L; and assessing nutritional parameters in selective high-risk patients.[21] Other risk factors that may be addressed before elective orthopaedic surgery include disease-modifying agents and immunosuppressive medications, which should be stopped 2 to 4 weeks before surgery.[11]

PERIOPERATIVE RISK FACTORS

SKIN PREPARATION

Preoperative skin preparation plays an important role in reducing the risk for SSI in patients undergoing orthopaedic surgical procedures. Bacteria found in skin flora include *Staphylococci*, diphtheroid organisms, *Pseudomonas*, and *Propionibacterium*.[25] Before being admitted for elective procedures, the Centers for Disease Control (CDC) recommends patients shower or bathe their entire body with soap (antimicrobial or nonantimicrobial) or an antiseptic agent at least one day before surgery. Per additional recommendation from the CDC, skin decolonization should take place before incision with a bactericidal antiseptic solution.[25-27] The ideal skin preparation solution should prevent the growth of pathogens for at least 6 hours after application. Previous studies, however, have found that this process may only remove up to 80% of skin flora.[28,29]

Antiseptic skin preparation agents include iodine povacrylex and isopropyl alcohol, povidone-iodine (PI), and chlorhexidine gluconate (CHG) with isopropyl alcohol.[26,30] Current literature lacks evidence to support the use of one solution over another for SSI prevention, but there is an overall consensus that it should contain isopropyl alcohol.[26] In one study of patients undergoing shoulder surgery, preoperative cleansing with 2% CHG impregnated cloth led to the least amount of microbial growth on incision cultures compared with those who used PI or water.[31] These findings were in agreement with those from an earlier study that also demonstrated superior performance for CHG over iodophor, isopropyl alcohol, and PI.[32] On the other hand, there is evidence in the literature which shows no difference in the effectiveness of CHG compared to PI.[33]

HAIR REMOVAL

Preoperative hair removal is another component of perioperative infection control. Although high-quality evidence for or against preoperative hair removal is lacking, the practice remains commonplace in orthopaedics. The rationale for this practice is a reduced risk of hair entering, contaminating, and irritating the open wound.[34] When hair removal is considered necessary, it should not be accomplished by shaving because

©Copyright 2021 American Academy of Orthopaedic Surgeons

TABLE 1 Summary of Risk Factors Associated With Development of Surgical Site Infection/Periprosthetic Joint Infection by Level of Evidence

Modifiable host factors	*Factors with limited evidence of associations with SSI/PJI*
• BMI—Strong	• Age (as a continuous exposure)—Limited
• Smoking—Strong	• Hispanic ethnicity—Limited
• High alcohol intake (alcohol abuse)—Strong	• Native American and Eskimo ethnicity—Limited
• Low income—Strong	• Asian race—Limited
• Malnutrition (low serum albumin)—Strong	• History of drug abuse—Limited
• History of DM—Strong	• Rural location vs. nonrural location—Limited
• History of CVD—Moderate	• Underweight—Limited
• History of CHF—Strong	• History of hypertension—Limited
• History of cardiac arrhythmia—Strong	• History of osteoarthritis—Limited
• History of PVD—Strong	• History of posttraumatic arthritis—Limited
• Chronic pulmonary disease—Strong	• Low- or high-risk dental procedures—Limited
• Chronic obstructive pulmonary disease—Strong	• History of UTI—Limited
• History of renal disease—Strong	• History of dementia—Limited
• History of liver disease/cirrhosis—Strong	• Hypercholesterolemia—Limited
• History of RA—Strong	• Peptic ulcer disease—Limited
• History of cancer/malignancy—Strong	• Valvular disease—Limited
• History of osteonecrosis—Strong	• Metastatic tumor—Limited
• History of depression—Strong	• History of coagulopathy—Limited
• History of psychosis—Strong	• History of venous thromboembolism—Limited
• History of HIV/AIDS—Strong	• Pulmonary circulatory disorders—Limited
• Neurologic disease (hemiplegia, paraplegia)—Moderate	• Hypothyroidism—Limited
• History of corticosteroid administration—Strong	• Hepatitis (B or C)—Limited
• History of intra-articular corticosteroid injection—Moderate	• Electrolyte imbalance—Limited
• Previous joint surgery—Strong	• Autogenous blood transfusion—Limited
• Revision arthroplasty—Strong	
• Previous joint infection—Moderate	
• Frailty—Moderate	
• Preoperative anemia—Strong	
• ASA grade >2—Strong	
• Charlson Comorbidity Index (High)—Strong	
• Preoperative hyperglycemia and high HbA1c—Moderate	
• Allogeneic blood transfusion—Strong	
• Prophylaxis with warfarin or low-molecular-weight heparin—Moderate	
Nonmodifiable host factors	
• Age (≥75 yr)—Moderate	
• Male sex—Strong	
• Black race—Strong	
• TKA vs THA—Strong	

BMI = body mass index, CHF = congestive heart failure, CVD = cardiovascular disease, DM = diabetes mellitus, PJI = periprosthetic joint infection, PVD = peripheral vascular disease, RA = rheumatoid arthritis, SSI = surgical site infection, THA = total hip arthroplasty, TKA = total knee arthroplasty, UTI = urinary tract infection

Reproduced with permission from Zainul-Abdin S, Amanatullah DF, Anderson MB, et al: General assembly, prevention, host related general: Proceedings of international consensus on orthopedic infections. *J Arthroplasty* 2018;34:S13-S35.

of concern for microscopic trauma to the epidermis that can become nidus for SSI.[35,36] Instead, a depilatory or electric clipping immediately before surgery should be used.[37-39]

OPERATING ROOM ENVIRONMENT

In implant surgery, air and surface contamination are important factors in postoperative wound infection. Infection rates have been shown to correlate with the number of airborne bacteria within 30 cm of the wound, which is influenced by intraoperative factors such as the number of operating room personnel, their clothing, and the type of ventilation system used.[40,41] In one study, a high contamination rate of gowns was attributed to gown packs having been left opened for too long. It has therefore been hypothesized that some infections can be avoided if single gown packs are used, because multiple-gown packs result in delay and increased traffic around the table, providing additional potential sources of infection.[42] Although appropriate use of drapes during invasive procedures is widely recommended to minimize contamination of the surgical field, the independent efficacy of this practice at reducing SSI has not been assessed by scientific studies. It has been found that bacteria easily penetrate woven reusable fabrics within 30 minutes,[30,43] whereas disposable, nonwoven drapes have been

©Copyright 2021 American Academy of Orthopaedic Surgeons

proven to be impermeable. Thus, the use of nonwoven disposable drapes or woven drapes with an impermeable operating tray in all surgical cases is recommended.

Healthcare personnel are an important contributing source to the aerosolized bacteria which exist in the operating room environment.[44] The quantity of environmental bacteria is directly related to the amount of bacteria shed by personnel (10^6 skin scales loaded with bacteria per day) and the number of people present.[45] One study found that when the number of operating room personnel rises from 8 to 16, the rate of SSIs increases from 1.5% to 3.8%.[18,46] Since 30% of healthcare personnel are estimated to be colonized by *S aureus*, this is an area of concern that should not go unnoticed.[47] With the widespread use of hand-held devices, it is not surprising that *S aureus* is one of the most commonly isolated organisms from operating room devices used by healthcare personnel.[48,49] There are limited data pertaining to the impact of these devices in the operating room; however, it is advised that they are routinely disinfected to reduce their colonization by organisms of pathogenic potential.[41]

Several other factors relating to the air in the operating room can significantly affect bacterial counts. One such factor is the position of the door and how often it opens.[41,45] In one study, the average colony-forming units (CFUs) per square foot per hour with closed doors was 13.3, versus 24.8 with open doors, and 19.4 with swinging doors.[50] The type of airflow in the operating room has also been shown to affect the status of air particle contamination. Laminar airflow (LAF) systems have been shown to reduce the number of airborne particles by 80% and down to 1 CFU per cubic meter when used in conjunction with body exhaust suits.[51-55] It is critical to acknowledge that LAF must be used properly because impedance of airflow may increase the amount of downwind bacterial contamination around the wound.[51] Thus the International Consensus Meeting on Musculoskeletal Infection states it is not necessary to perform a clean orthopedic surgery procedure, including elective joint replacement surgery, in an operating theater equipped with LAF systems because of the lack of recent literature demonstrating their ability to reduce SSI or PJI in orthopedic surgery.[56]

PROCEDURE-RELATED RISK FACTORS

A recent study from Wang et al has demonstrated that increased surgical time may increase a patient's risk for PJI.[57] Among their cohort of over 17,000 patients undergoing primary TKA, those with a surgical time >90 minutes had a significantly higher incidence of SSI and PJI (2.1% and 1.4%, respectively). These rates were greater compared with those with a case duration of 60 to 90 minutes (1.1% and 0.7%), and ≤60 minutes (0.9% and 0.7%, $P < 0.01$). Though these findings are specific to TKA, efforts to optimize surgical time without compromising quality of care are essential.

Before closure, intraoperative irrigation of deep or subcutaneous tissue may also help with the prevention of SSI. The World Health Organization (WHO), CDC, and International Consensus Group (ICG) all advocate for the use of an aqueous iodophor solution such as dilute betadine for irrigation before closure for SSI prophylaxis.[27,58]

DIAGNOSTIC MODALITIES

CLINICAL EVALUATION

The cardinal signs of inflammation are calor, dolor, tumor, and rubor (temperature), pain, swelling, and erythema. Pathogens at the site of infection are recognized by the immune system. The characteristic response of the immune cells leads to local and systemic changes including increased local blood flow and vascular permeability. Local signs such as joint effusion or wound drainage may also be present. When determining the cause of an infection, it is important to consider distant anatomic locations as the source. A thorough clinical examination of the pulmonary, urinary, gastrointestinal, and cardiovascular systems is essential. In addition, the existence of any secondary symptoms of infection, such as fever or chills, accompanied by the location, quality, and onset of pain should also be closely considered.[59]

LABORATORY EVALUATION

Serum Biomarkers

In a patient with osteomyelitis or septic arthritis, the erythrocyte sedimentation rate (ESR) and C-reactive protein (CRP) may be elevated while the white cell count may be near normal or elevated. Combination testing of CRP and ESR can have utility for PJI screening purposes per AAOS recommendations.[60,61] Recent work also suggests the utility of serum D-dimer and IL-6 testing as a parameter in the diagnosis of infection, but further investigation is needed for validation.[62,63]

Synovial Fluid Testing

Synovial fluid aspiration is necessary for definitive diagnosis of septic arthritis. This fluid should be analyzed for white cell count and Gram stain, as well as microbiological culture. Fluid should also be analyzed for the presence of crystals, as crystal arthropathy can mimic septic arthritis. Synovial protein levels greater than 40 mg/dL but less than the serum protein are likely to be consistent with a diagnosis of septic arthritis. Furthermore, the glucose level in synovial fluid is typically lower than serum glucose in the setting of joint infection.

On examination, joint aspirate may demonstrate gross pus. Features of infection include an elevated synovial white blood cell count (>50,000/mm^3) and percentage of polymorphonuclear leukocytes (>75%). A white cell count of great than 50×10^9/L is concerning for septic arthritis.[64] Intraoperative Gram stains are only positive in 30% to 50% of cases, and synovial fluid cultures are positive in around 50% to 80% of cases.[65] A neutrophil differential of >90% is highly suggestive of

©Copyright 2021 American Academy of Orthopaedic Surgeons

infection. Values for the diagnosis of infection in arthroplasty differ from these and are discussed later in this chapter.

Synovial fluid cultures can help reach a definitive diagnosis and are useful for determining antimicrobial susceptibility, with a sensitivity for diagnosis of nongonococcal septic arthritis of 75% to 90%. The sensitivity for Gram staining is between 50% and 75%.[66] Specific culture media are needed for the growth of certain fastidious microorganisms, such as *Mycobacterium tuberculosis* or fungi. PCR can also be implemented to detect a diagnosis of *Borrelia burgdorferi* or *Neisseria gonorrhoeae*. The diagnostic yield for gonococcal synovial fluid cultures tends to be lower, particularly in the setting of disseminated infection. In this scenario, it is imperative to also obtain cultures from the primary site of mucosal infection.

MICROBIOLOGY

Optimal medical therapy for a patient with infection requires the identification of causative microorganisms and their in vitro antimicrobial susceptibility. If possible, antimicrobial agents should be withheld until specimens are collected for culture. Accurate tissue diagnosis can allow for prompt rationalization of antibiotics, particularly in the context of resistant organisms. Joint aspiration with immediate Gram stain and microscopy followed by culture and sensitivity remains the mainstay for diagnosis of septic arthritis.[67] In suspected osteomyelitis, definitive diagnosis can be obtained with bone biopsy specimens obtained via punch biopsy, needle biopsy, or curettage of deep tissue.[68]

The Infectious Disease Society of America (IDSA) recommends that synovial fluid specimens for culture be transported at room temperature in sterile containers. When ample amounts are available, additional procurement should be made in blood culture bottles (aerobic and anaerobic if there is enough specimen volume) alongside traditional culture methods in an effort to increase culture yield.[69]

DIAGNOSTIC IMAGING

The use of CT, MRI, or nuclear medicine can potentially unveil the extent of soft-tissue/bone involvement in patients with PJI. Furthermore, these imaging modalities can help to delineate the extent of bone and soft-tissue involvement and may guide bone resection.

Plain radiography is the initial modality for imaging in musculoskeletal infections. Orthogonal radiographs should be taken to evaluate the site in question. In PJI, radiographs may reveal periosteal reaction, bone cysts, and focal resorption indicative. Although radiographs rarely detect osteomyelitis during the early stages, they may identify adjacent soft-tissue swelling, joint effusion, and/or erosion related to adjacent septic arthritis. Radiographs may also show subluxation or dislocation of the joint in severe infection. In the later stages of osteomyelitis, frank bone destruction and sequestered bony necrosis may be evident.

Radionuclide imaging is a sensitive, but nonspecific, modality for infection. There are three main methods available: the technetium 99m bone scan, the gallium 67 scan, and the labeled white blood cell scan. Bone scans may show a decreased uptake, or cold scan, early in the disease process and an increased uptake, that is,, hot scan, at later stages. Combined leukocyte–bone marrow imaging is a nuclear imaging technique that may be useful in the setting of infection. Although leukocytes do not usually accumulate at sites of increased bone mineral turnover in the absence of infection, they do accumulate in the bone marrow which may be disturbed by the implantation of orthopaedic hardware. As a result, native leukocytes in the bone marrow may be difficult to decipher from those that are present secondary to periprosthetic infection.

This problem can be overcome by performing complementary bone marrow scintigraphy with Tc-99m sulfur colloid. With this technique, labeled leukocytes and sulfur colloid accumulate in the marrow, whereas only leukocytes accumulate in infection. For instances where images have similar distribution of two radiotracers, leukocyte uptake involving the marrow is implied. When there is activity on the leukocyte image without corresponding activity on the bone marrow image, leukocyte uptake is due to infection. The specificity of this dual radiotracer technique has been found to exceed 90%.[70]

CT can be used to detect or localize a source of infection. CT findings in osteomyelitis include cortical bone destruction, periosteal new bone formation, intraosseous gas, increased attenuation of the marrow, narrowing of the medullary cavity, serpentine drainage tracts, and the presence of an involucrum or sequestrum.[70] The presence of a punctate area of increased attenuation, with a region of focal cortical destruction, suggests a sequestrum and is very specific for an infective process.

MRI is another diagnostic imaging modality that can be used to diagnose musculoskeletal infection.[71] In osteomyelitis, marrow space of the involved bone demonstrates decreased signal of T1-weighted images and increased signal on T2-weight images. Cortical destruction or thickening and edema or abscess formation in the soft tissues can also be demonstrated on MRI. Although both an abscess and edema will have low signal on T1-weighted images and high signal on T2-weighted images, a well-demarcated border and a rim of decreased intensity are more characteristic of an abscess. The penumbra sign is a feature of subacute osteomyelitis found with MRI. The sign can be identified on unenhanced T1-weighted spin echo images by its discrete peripheral zone of marginally higher signal intensity compared with the central bony abscess cavity and a surrounding lower signal intensity of the reactive new bone and edema.[72] In chronic osteomyelitis, findings that favor chronic infection on T2-weighted images include thickening of the cortex, a relatively sharp interface between diseased and normal marrow, and a well-defined soft-tissue abnormality.[71]

Ultrasonography of a septic joint, especially the hip, can detect an effusion and aid in aspiration. The use of ultrasonography has been described in the emergency department setting

 ©Copyright 2021 American Academy of Orthopaedic Surgeons

to rapidly evaluate the patient with suspected septic arthritis, particularly in the pediatric setting.[71] Ultrasonography can also detect features of osteomyelitis such as deep soft-tissue swelling, periosteal thickening, and early subperiosteal fluid collection.[71]

Fluorine-18 (F-18) fluorodeoxyglucose-positron emission tomography (FDG-PET) is a modality for imaging musculoskeletal infection which has the potential to play an important role in the evaluation of chronic osteomyelitis and spinal infection.[71] FDG-PET has the ability to diagnose both acute and chronic infection of the axial and appendicular skeletons. PET imaging can be useful in patients with metallic implants because FDG uptake is not hampered by metallic artifacts (unlike MRI and CT). PET/CT involves the combination of PET and a low-dose or full-dose diagnostic CT. This modality provides exact anatomical correlation of bone and joint lesions and increases the accuracy of the test compared with PET alone. This imaging test should be reserved for patients in whom PJI is suspected but when other tests are inconclusive, such as patients with dry aspiration of the joint.[70]

SUMMARY

Skeletal infection is a highly morbid and potentially fatal condition which has the potential to inflict irreversible damage on the musculoskeletal system. Consequently, it is critical to initiate a diagnostic workup promptly when there are concerns for infection. The chronology of events leading up to patient presentation, knowledge of patient-related risk factors, and examination findings should be used to inform an evidence-based diagnostic workup for skeletal infection. In the absence of definitive laboratory or radiographic findings, continued investigation for a course of infection should be pursued when clinical suspicion is high. Furthermore, the emergence of drug-resistant organisms and biofilm adherence to orthopedic hardware remains an area of increasing concern in surgical patients. As a result, precautionary measures should be adhered to diligently reduce the risk of postoperative skeletal infection.

REFERENCES

1. Zimlichman E, Henderson D, Tamir O, et al: Health care–associated infections: A meta-analysis of costs and financial impact on the US health care system. *JAMA Intern Med* 2013;173(22):2039-2046.
2. HAI Data | CDC. Available at: https://www.cdc.gov/hai/data/index.html. Published October 25, 2018. Accessed January 5, 2019.
3. Mirzashahi B, Chehrassan M, Mortazavi SMJ: Intrawound application of vancomycin changes the responsible germ in elective spine surgery without significant effect on the rate of infection: A randomized prospective study. *Musculoskelet Surg* 2018;102(1):35-39.
4. Nasser R, Kosty JA, Shah S, Wang J, Cheng J: Risk factors and prevention of surgical site infections following spinal procedures. *Global Spine J* 2018;8(4 suppl):44S-48S.
5. Anderson DJ, Kaye KS, Chen LF, et al: Clinical and financial outcomes due to methicillin resistant Staphylococcus aureus surgical site infection: A multi-center matched outcomes study. *PLoS One* 2009;4(12):e8305.
6. Coello R, Charlett A, Wilson J, Ward V, Pearson A, Borriello P: Adverse impact of surgical site infections in English hospitals. *J Hosp Infect* 2005;60(2):93-103.
7. Badia JM, Casey AL, Petrosillo N, Hudson PM, Mitchell SA, Crosby C: Impact of surgical site infection on healthcare costs and patient outcomes: A systematic review in six European countries. *J Hosp Infect* 2017;96(1):1-15.
8. Whitehouse JD, Friedman ND, Kirkland KB, Richardson WJ, Sexton DJ: The impact of surgical-site infections following orthopedic surgery at a community hospital and a university hospital adverse quality of life, excess length of stay, and extra cost. *Infect Control Hosp Epidemiol* 2002;23(4):183-189.
9. Mistry J, Naqvi A, Chughtai M, et al: Decreasing the incidence of surgical-site infections after total joint arthroplasty. *Am J Orthop* 2017;46(6):E374-E387. Available at: https://www.amjorthopedics.com/article/decreasing-incidence-surgical-site-infections-after-total-joint-arthroplasty. Accessed January 6, 2019.
10. Kurtz SM, Lau EC, Son M-S, Chang ET, Zimmerli W, Parvizi J: Are we winning or losing the battle with periprosthetic joint infection: Trends in periprosthetic joint infection and mortality risk for the medicare population. *J Arthroplast* 2018;33(10):3238-3245.
11. Zainul-Abidin S, Amanatullah DF, Anderson MB, et al: General assembly, prevention, host related general: Proceedings of international consensus on orthopedic infections. *J Arthroplast* 2019;34(2 suppl):S13-S35.
12. Costerton JW: Overview of microbial biofilms. *J Ind Microbiol* 1995;15(3):137-140.
13. Bazaka K, Jacob MV, Crawford RJ, Ivanova EP: Efficient surface modification of biomaterial to prevent biofilm formation and the attachment of microorganisms. *Appl Microbiol Biotechnol* 2012;95(2):299-311.
14. Davies DG, Parsek MR, Pearson JP, Iglewski BH, Costerton JW, Greenberg EP: The involvement of cell-to-cell signals in the development of a bacterial biofilm. *Science* 1998;280(5361):295-298.
15. Bjelland AM, Sørum H, Tegegne DA, Winther-Larsen HC, Willassen NP, Hansen H: LitR of Vibrio salmonicida is a salinity-sensitive quorum-sensing regulator of phenotypes involved in host interactions and virulence. *Infect Immun* 2012;80(5):1681-1689.
16. Saeed K, McLaren AC, Schwarz EM, et al: 2018 international consensus meeting on musculoskeletal infection: Summary from the biofilm workgroup and consensus on biofilm related musculoskeletal infections. *J Orthop Res* 2019;37(5):1007-1017.
17. Sheehan E, McKenna J, Mulhall KJ, Marks P, McCormack D: Adhesion of *Staphylococcus* to orthopaedic metals, an in vivo study. *J Orthop Res* 2004;22:39-43.
18. Schildhauer TA, Robie B, Muhr G, Köller M: Bacterial adherence to tantalum versus commonly used orthopedic metallic implant materials. *J Orthop Trauma* 2006;20(7):476.
19. O'Toole GA, Kolter R: Flagellar and twitching motility are necessary for *Pseudomonas aeruginosa* biofilm development. *Mol Microbiol* 1998;30(2):295-304.
20. Li H-K, Rombach I, Zambellas R, et al: Oral versus intravenous antibiotics for bone and joint infection. *N Engl J Med* 2019;380(5):425-436.
21. Jiranek W, Kigera JWM, Klatt BA, et al: General assembly, prevention, host risk mitigation – general factors: Proceedings of international consensus on orthopedic infections. *J Arthroplasty* 2019;34(2 suppl):S43-S48.
22. Florschutz AV, Fagan RP, Matar WY, Sawyer RG, Berrios-Torres SI: Surgical site infection risk factors and risk stratification. *J Am Acad Orthop Surg* 2015;23 suppl:S8.

©Copyright 2021 American Academy of Orthopaedic Surgeons

23. International Consensus Group: *Proceedings of the Second International Consensus Meeting (ICM) on Musculoskeletal Infection.* Data Trance Publishing Company, 2018.
24. Tan TL, Maltenfort MG, Chen AF, et al: Development and evaluation of a preoperative risk calculator for periprosthetic joint infection following total joint arthroplasty. *J Bone Joint Surg* 2018;100(9):777-785.
25. Dumville JC, McFarlane E, Edwards P, Lipp A, Holmes A, Liu Z: Preoperative skin antiseptics for preventing surgical wound infections after clean surgery. *Cochrane Database Syst Rev* 2015;(4):CD003949.
26. Akins GJ, Alberdi MT, Beswick A, et al: General assembly, prevention, surgical site preparation: Proceedings of international consensus on orthopedic infections. *J Arthroplast* 2018;34(2 suppl):S85-S92.
27. Berríos-Torres SI, Umscheid CA, Bratzler DW, et al: Centers for disease control and prevention guideline for the prevention of surgical site infection, 2017. *JAMA Surg* 2017;152(8):784-791.
28. Selwyn S, Ellis H: Skin bacteria and skin disinfection reconsidered. *Br Med J* 1972;1(5793):136-140.
29. Rezapoor M, Parvizi J: Prevention of periprosthetic joint infection. *J Arthroplasty* 2015;30(6):902-907.
30. Markatos K, Kaseta M, Nikolaou VS: Perioperative skin preparation and draping in modern total joint arthroplasty: Current evidence. *Surg Infect* 2015;16(3):221-225.
31. Murray MR, Saltzman MD, Gryzlo SM, Terry MA, Woodward CC, Nuber GW: Efficacy of preoperative home use of 2% chlorhexidine gluconate cloth before shoulder surgery. *J Shoulder Elbow Surg* 2011;20(6):928-933.
32. Saltzman MD, Nuber GW, Gryzlo SM, Marecek GS, Koh JL: Efficacy of surgical preparation solutions in shoulder surgery. *J Bone Joint Surg Am* 2009;91(8):1949-1953.
33. Savage JW, Weatherford BM, Sugrue PA, et al: Efficacy of surgical preparation solutions in lumbar spine surgery. *J Bone Joint Surg Am* 2012;94(6):490-494.
34. Lefebvre A, Saliou P, Lucet JC, et al: Preoperative hair removal and surgical site infections: Network meta-analysis of randomized controlled trials. *J Hosp Infect* 2015;91(2):100-108.
35. Greene LR: Guide to the elimination of orthopedic surgery surgical site infections: An executive summary of the association for professionals in infection control and epidemiology elimination guide. *Am J Infect Control* 2012;40(4):384-386.
36. Daines BK, Dennis DA, Amann S: Infection prevention in total knee arthroplasty. *J Am Acad Orthop Surg* 2015;23(6):356-364.
37. Mangram AJ, Horan TC, Pearson ML, Silver LC, Jarvis WR: Guideline for prevention of surgical site infection, 1999. Centers for disease control and prevention (CDC) Hospital Infection Control Practices Advisory Committee. *Am J Infect Control* 1999;27(2):97-132; quiz 133-134; discussion 96.
38. Parvizi J, Cavanaugh PK, Diaz-Ledezma C: Periprosthetic knee infection: Ten strategies that work. *Knee Surg Relat Res* 2013;25(4):155-164.
39. Tanner J, Norrie P, Melen K: Preoperative hair removal to reduce surgical site infection. *Cochrane Database Syst Rev* 2011;(11):CD004122.
40. Gosden PE, MacGowan AP, Bannister GC: Importance of air quality and related factors in the prevention of infection in orthopaedic implant surgery. *J Hosp Infect* 1998;39(3):173-180.
41. Baldini A, Blevins K, Del Gaizo D, et al: General assembly, prevention, operating room – personnel: Proceedings of international consensus on orthopedic infections. *J Arthroplasty* 2018;34(2 suppl):S97-S104.
42. Kong KC, Sheppard M, Serne G: Dispensing surgical gloves onto the open surgical gown pack does not increase the bacterial contamination rate. *J Hosp Infect* 1994;26(4):293-296.
43. Blom A, Estela C, Bowker K, MacGowan A, Hardy JR: The passage of bacteria through surgical drapes. *Ann R Coll Surg Engl* 2000;82(6):405-407.
44. Illingworth KD, Mihalko WM, Parvizi J, et al: How to minimize infection and thereby maximize patient outcomes in total joint arthroplasty: A multicenter approach. *J Bone Joint Surg Am* 2013;95(8):e50.
45. Rezapoor M, Alvand A, Jacek E, Paziuk T, Maltenfort MG, Parvizi J: Operating room traffic increases aerosolized particles and compromises the air quality: A simulated study. *J Arthroplasty* 2018;33(3):851-855.
46. Pryor F, Messmer PR: The effect of traffic patterns in the OR on surgical site infections. *AORN J* 1998;68(4):649-660.
47. Bethune DW, Blowers R, Parker M, Pask EA: Dispersal of *Staphylococcus aureus* BY patients and surgical staff. *Lancet* 1965;1(7383):480-483.
48. Shakir IA, Patel NH, Chamberland RR, Kaar SG: Investigation of cell phones as a potential source of bacterial contamination in the operating room. *J Bone Joint Surg* 2015;97(3):225-231.
49. Murgier J, Coste J-F, Cavaignac E, et al: Microbial flora on cell-phones in an orthopedic surgery room before and after decontamination. *Orthop Traumatol Surg Res* 2016;102(8):1093-1096.
50. Ritter MA: Operating room environment. *Clin Orthop Relat Res* 1999;(369):103-109.
51. Salvati EA, Robinson RP, Zeno SM, Koslin BL, Brause BD, Wilson PD: Infection rates after 3175 total hip and total knee replacements performed with and without a horizontal unidirectional filtered air-flow system. *J Bone Joint Surg Am* 1982;64(4):525-535.
52. Lidwell OM: Air, antibiotics and sepsis in replacement joints. *J Hosp Infect* 1988;11 suppl C:18-40.
53. Howorth FH: Prevention of airborne infection during surgery. *Lancet* 1985;1(8425):386-388.
54. Lidwell OM, Lowbury EJ, Whyte W, Blowers R, Stanley SJ, Lowe D: Effect of ultraclean air in operating rooms on deep sepsis in the joint after total hip or knee replacement: A randomised study. *Br Med J* 1982;285(6334):10-14.
55. Hooper GJ, Rothwell AG, Frampton C, Wyatt MC: Does the use of laminar flow and space suits reduce early deep infection after total hip and knee replacement?: The ten-year results of the New Zealand joint registry. *J Bone Joint Surg Br* 2011;93(1):85-90.
56. Aalirezaie A, Akkaya M, Barnes CL, et al: General assembly, prevention, operating room environment: Proceedings of international consensus on orthopedic infections. *J Arthroplasty* 2019;34(2 suppl):S105-S115.
57. Wang Q, Goswami K, Shohat N, Aalirezaie A, Manrique J, Parvizi J: Longer operative time results in a higher rate of subsequent periprosthetic joint infection in patients undergoing primary joint arthroplasty. *J Arthroplasty*. 2019;34(5):947-953.
58. Alsadaan M, Alrumaih HA, Brown T, et al: General assembly, prevention, operating room - surgical field: Proceedings of international consensus on orthopedic infections. *J Arthroplast* 2019;34(2):S127-S130.
59. Tande AJ, Patel R: Prosthetic joint infection. *Clin Microbiol Rev* 2014;27(2):302-345.
60. Lee YS, Koo K-H, Kim HJ, et al: Synovial fluid Biomarkers for the diagnosis of periprosthetic joint infection: A systematic review and meta-analysis. *J Bone Joint Surg Am* 2017;99(24):2077-2084.
61. Parvizi J, Della Valle CJ: AAOS clinical practice guideline: Diagnosis and treatment of periprosthetic joint infections of the hip and knee. *J Am Acad Orthop Surg* 2010;18(12):771-772.
62. Xie K, Dai K, Qu X, Yan M: Serum and synovial fluid interleukin-6 for the diagnosis of periprosthetic joint infection. *Sci Rep* 2017;7(1):1496.
63. Shahi A, Kheir MM, Tarabichi M, Hosseinzadeh HRS, Tan TL, Parvizi J: Serum D-dimer test is promising for the diagnosis of periprosthetic joint infection and timing of reimplantation. *J Bone Joint Surg Am* 2017;99(17):1419-1427.
64. Carpenter CR, Schuur JD, Everett WW, Pines JM: Evidence-based diagnostics: Adult septic arthritis. *Acad Emerg Med* 2011;18(8):781-796.
65. Weston V, Jones A, Bradbury N, Fawthrop F, Doherty M: Clinical features and outcome of septic arthritis in a single UK Health District 1982–1991. *Ann Rheum Dis* 1999;58(4):214-219.
66. Swan A, Amer H, Dieppe P: The value of synovial fluid assays in the diagnosis of joint disease: A literature survey. *Ann Rheum Dis* 2002;61(6):493-498.
67. Mathews CJ, Kingsley G, Field M, et al: Management of septic arthritis: A systematic review. *Ann Rheum Dis* 2007;66(4):440-445.

 ©Copyright 2021 American Academy of Orthopaedic Surgeons

68. Peel TN, Dylla BL, Hughes JG, et al: Improved diagnosis of prosthetic joint infection by culturing periprosthetic tissue specimens in blood culture bottles. *MBio* 2016;7(1):e01776-01715.
69. Abdel MP, Akgün D, Akin G, et al: Hip and knee section, diagnosis, pathogen isolation, culture: Proceedings of international consensus on orthopedic infections. *J Arthroplasty* 2019;34(2 suppl):S361-S367.
70. Diaz-Ledezma C, Espinosa-Mendoza R, Gallo J, et al: General assembly, diagnosis, imaging: Proceedings of international consensus on orthopedic infections. *J Arthroplast* 2019;34(2 suppl):S215-S223.
71. Pineda C, Espinosa R, Pena A: Radiographic imaging in osteomyelitis: The role of plain radiography, computed tomography, ultrasonography, magnetic resonance imaging, and scintigraphy. *Semin Plast Surg* 2009;23(2):80-89.
72. Davies AM, Grimer R: The penumbra sign in subacute osteomyelitis. *Eur Radiol* 2005;15(6):1268-1270.

©Copyright 2021 American Academy of Orthopaedic Surgeons

23

Treatment of Skeletal Infections

Alexus M. Cooper, BS
Karan Goswami, MD, MRCS
Javad Parvizi, MD, FRCS

Keywords: *musculoskeletal infection; osteomyelitis; periprosthetic joint infection; septic arthritis; surgical site infection*

INTRODUCTION

Success in treating musculoskeletal infection requires an aggressive surgical approach and optimized antimicrobial therapy. The type of infection, the virulence and antimicrobial susceptibilities of the involved microorganism, potential adverse effects of the proposed antimicrobial therapy, alternative antimicrobial therapies, and the patients' general health should be considered prior to initiation of treatment. Antimicrobials can be used for prophylaxis or treatment of infection. Antimicrobials can be delivered systemically, in the form of oral or parenteral dosing, or locally, in the form of topical solutions or local delivery devices such as antibiotic beads, powder, or spacers. The local delivery of antimicrobial agents to the site of orthopaedic infection is based on the need for high concentrations of these drugs to kill planktonic and biofilm-based bacteria. Many musculoskeletal infections require prolonged systemic antimicrobial therapy, often administered on an outpatient basis under the guidance of an infectious disease specialist in close collaboration with an orthopaedic surgeon.

ANTIMICROBIALS

BIOAVAILABILITY

Evidence in the literature on antibiotic therapy for patients with antimicrobial-resistant surgical site infection or periprosthetic joint infection (SSI/PJI) is not conclusive. When selecting antibiotics for patients, patient comorbidities, mode of administration, risk of *Clostridium difficile*, need for monitoring, allergy profile of the patient, intolerance, regional resistance patterns, cost, and availability should all be considered.[1] The selected antibiotic for treatment should also have good bone and soft-tissue penetration and activity against biofilm.

Using an intravenous route for antimicrobial administration has the greatest quantitative potential, as it permits a mass balance approach to be applied to distribution, clearance, and the body processes associated with excretion and metabolic elimination (eg, renal, hepatic). The administration of a drug by other routes, notably oral, introduces an uncertainty that reflects the unknown fraction that is actually absorbed.

The most important property of any nonintravenous microbial intended to treat systemic infection is its ability to distribute active ingredients to the bloodstream in an amount sufficient to cause the desired response. This

Dr. Parvizi or an immediate family member has received royalties from Corentec; serves as a paid consultant to or is an employee of CeramTec, ConvaTec, Corentec, Ethicon, Heron, Tenor, TissueGene, and Zimmer; has stock or stock options held in Alphaeon, Ceribell, Corentec, Cross Current Business Intelligence, Hip Innovation Technology, Intellijoint, Invisible Sentinel, Joint Purification Systems, MDValuate, MedAp, MicroGenDx, Parvizi Surgical Innovations, Physician Recommended Nutriceuticals, and PRN-Veterinary; and serves as a board member, owner, officer, or committee member of the Eastern Orthopaedic Association and the Muller Foundation. Neither of the following authors nor any immediate family member has received anything of value from or has stock or stock options held in a commercial company or institution related directly or indirectly to the subject of this chapter: Dr. Cooper and Dr. Goswami.

©Copyright 2021 American Academy of Orthopaedic Surgeons

property of a dosage form has historically been identified as physiologic availability, biologic availability, or bioavailability. Bioavailability captures two essential features, namely how fast the drug enters the systemic circulation (rate of absorption) and how much of the nominal strength enters the body (extent of absorption). Given that the therapeutic effect is a function of the drug concentration in a patient's blood, these two properties of nonintravenous dosage forms are, in principle, important in identifying the response to a drug dose.

Bioavailability following oral doses of antimicrobials may vary due to patient-related or dosage-form-related factors such as the nature and timing of meals, age, disease, genetic traits, and gastrointestinal physiology. Such factors include (1) the chemical form of the drug (eg, salt vs acid), (2) its physical properties (eg, crystal structure, particle size), and (3) an array of formulation (eg, nonactive ingredients) and manufacturing (eg, tablet hardness) variables. Furthermore, doses need to be weight-adjusted.

ELUTION CHARACTERISTICS OF ANTIBIOTIC-LOADED CEMENT SPACERS

The current standard of care for infected joint arthroplasty is considered to be two-stage revision arthroplasty including: removal of the prosthesis and cement, thorough débridement, placement of an antibiotic-impregnated cement spacer, a course of intravenous antibiotics, and a delayed second-stage revision arthroplasty. The choice of the spacer, either articulating or nonarticulating, is based on many factors, including the amount of bone loss, the condition of the soft tissues, the need for joint motion, the availability of prefabricated spacers or moulding methods, and antibiotic selection. Additionally, in nonarthroplasty infections, bone cement beads may be used to deliver antibiotics to the local area after surgical débridement.

The elution of antibiotics from bone cement depends on several factors including the type of antibiotic, amount and number of antibiotics, porosity and type of cement, and surface area of the spacer.[2] Masri et al investigated the long-term elution of antibiotics from poly methyl methacrylate (PMMA) bone cement in vivo in 40 patients. Their study found that effective levels of tobramycin remained four months after the surgery.[3] This observation is consistent with the suggestion that at least 3.6 grams (g) of tobramycin per 40 g of bone cement, with 1 g of vancomycin, is an effective antibiotic regimen. As effective levels of vancomycin were not present four months after the surgery, Masri et al also determined that the two antibiotics acted synergistically with one another to increase the elution rates but vancomycin should not be used alone.[3] This finding was consistent with the results of an in vitro study that showed that combining tobramycin and vancomycin in PMMA bone cement improved the elution rates of both antibiotics.[4]

The preparation of an antibiotic-loaded cement spacer can also impact its performance. Antibiotic release from hand-mixed and vacuum-mixed cement was found to be decreased compared with commercially available antibiotic-loaded cement; however, cost implications and the need for specific antimicrobials tailored to specificity may offset this issue.[5] Unlike antibiotics that are commercially mixed in cement, hand-mixed antibiotics do not have a homogeneous distribution in the cement, which decreases their rate of elution from a given surface area.[6] Vacuum-mixing decreases the porosity of the cement, which also decreases the rate of elution of the antibiotics.[7] The elution of antibiotics from PMMA bone cement is determined by a combination of surface area and porosity.[7] One study showed that increasing the surface area of PMMA bone cement by 40% resulted in a 20% higher rate of elution of vancomycin.[8] Dextran has been added to cement to enhance porosity and increase antibiotic elution rates. Kuechle et al found that the addition of 25% dextran to cement increased the release of antibiotics in the first 48 hours approximately four times compared with that associated with routine preparation.[9]

APPROACH TO TREATMENT

SURGICAL DÉBRIDEMENT AND LAVAGE

The most important determinant for success of treatment for acute or chronic orthopaedic infections is the quality the surgical débridement. The primary goal of débridement is to achieve a clean viable wound with minimal trauma to the remaining soft tissue. Among a cohort of patients with chronic osteomyelitis, aggressive débridement with a wide margin (>5 mm) was found to eradicate infection in almost all cases.[10] For an acute infection, the most straightforward method of débridement is incision and drainage, coupled with copious lavage. In chronic infection, a more aggressive approach is required, often due to local and systemic compromise of the host, presence of foreign bodies, and adherent biofilms.[11]

Incisions should be made through the previous incision site, or perpendicular to the site, to avoid wound edge necrosis. In the context of osteomyelitis, all necrotic bony tissue must be excised leaving only viable bone.[11] If 70% or more of the original cortical bone at the level of débridement is intact, the risk of fracture is low. If a more extensive débridement is required, it may be necessary to stabilize the bone with an external or internal fixator.[11] Management of the resultant "dead space" created by débridement may involve local myoplasty, free tissue transfers, and the use of antibiotic-impregnated beads to eradicate any remnant pathogens. Soft-tissue procedures have also been developed to improve local blood flow and antibiotic delivery.

For cases of musculoskeletal infection in spine surgery, primary goals are contingent upon the overall status of the patient. When neurologic deficits, pain, or spinal instability have manifested secondary to infection, evaluation for

©Copyright 2021 American Academy of Orthopaedic Surgeons

surgical intervention should be promptly considered and geared toward decompressing the spinal canal, débridement of infectious foci, and stabilizing vertebrae.[12]

TYPES OF MUSCULOSKELETAL INFECTION

OSTEOMYELITIS AND SEPTIC ARTHRITIS

Septic arthritis is a condition characterized by infection of the synovium and the joint space which causes an intense inflammatory reaction and release of proteolytic enzymes, leading to the rapid destruction of the articular cartilage.[13] Though uncommon among the general population, the occurrence of septic arthritis among pediatric patients, with or without subsequent occurrence of osteomyelitis, is increasing.[14-16]

Septic arthritis in combination with osteomyelitis is common in children, with the metaphysis of long bones the most commonly affected location. Patients usually present within several days to one week after the onset of symptoms. In addition to local signs of inflammation and infection, patients have signs of systemic illness, including fever, irritability, and lethargy. Typical clinical findings include tenderness over the involved bone and decreased range of motion in adjacent joints. Kocher criteria can be used to distinguish patients presenting with septic arthritis from those with transient synovitis[17] (**Table 1**). Based on a 2004 study validating Kocher criteria for septic arthritis risk based on presence of predictors is as follows—0 predictors: 2.0% risk, 1 predictor: 9.5%, 2 predictors: 35.0%, 3 predictors: 72.8%, 4 predictors: 93.0%.[17]

Acute hematogenous infection is the most common etiology for osteomyelitis and septic arthritis in children. This may be attributed to anatomic characteristics of pediatric bones such as thin cortex, loose periosteum, and directly communicating blood vessels to the metaphysis and epiphysis giving pathogens access to the joint space.[18] In the shoulder, elbow, hip, and ankle joints, the capsule overlaps a portion of the adjoining metaphysis. If the focus of osteomyelitis breaks through the metaphyseal bone, it can directly infect the joint and lead to concurrent septic arthritis. Septic arthritis can also occur in patients with a history of intravenous drug use, bacteremia, gonococcal disease, and after arthroscopic procedures.[13]

TABLE 1 Kocher Criteria

Clinical Findings	Predictor Scoring
Non–weight bearing	Yes: +1 No: 0
Temperature > 38.5°C/101.3°F	Yes: +1 No: 0
ESR[a] > 40 mm/hr	Yes: +1 No: 0
WBC count[b] > 12,000 cells/mm^3	Yes: +1 No: 0

[a]ESR, erythrocyte sedimentation rate.

[b]WBC count, white blood cell count.

Adapted with permission from Kocher MS, Mandiga R, Zurakowski D, Barnewolt C, Kasser JR: Validation of a clinical prediction rule for the differentiation between septic arthritis and transient synovitis of the hip in children. *J Bone Joint Surg Am* 2004;86-A(8):1629-1635.

PATHOPHYSIOLOGY

With septic arthritis, proteolytic enzymes released from synovial cells lead to destruction of the articular cartilage.[19] Interleukin-1 (IL-1) triggers the release of proteases from chondrocytes and synoviocytes in response to polymorphonuclear leukocytes and bacteria. Smith et al. showed that cartilage destruction starts to occur as early as 8 hours after infection.[20] Early administration of antibiotics helps to slow down the process, but even if intravenous antibiotic therapy is started within the first 24 hours of infection, significant glycosaminoglycan destruction and collagen disruption occurs. Degradation results in the loss of proteoglycans from the articular cartilage by 5 days and loss of collagen by 9 days.[21] Impairment of the intracapsular vascular supply secondary to elevation of the intracapsular pressure and thrombosis of the vessels also play a role in the destruction of the articular cartilage.[22] The common sites of involvement in children are the hip and knee, but in the adult, about 85% of cases are monoarticular, the knee being the most common.[13]

Subacute and chronic osteomyelitis typically occurs in adults. The diagnosis of osteomyelitis is usually made by a combination of clinical findings, radiography, bone scans, and magnetic resonance scans, along with the aspiration of purulent discharge from the involved area and positive blood cultures. In chronic osteomyelitis, radiographic signs of necrotic bone (sequestrum) and periosteal new bone formation (involucrum) are evident. Generally, this type of infection occurs secondary to an open wound, most often an open injury to bone and surrounding soft tissue. Bone pain, erythema, and drainage around the affected area are frequently present along with deformity, instability, local signs of impaired vascularity, limited range of motion, and altered neurologic status. The incidence of deep musculoskeletal infection from open fractures has been reported to be approximately 23%, with a 6% of cases resulting in osteomyelitis.[23] A further study divided patients with open fractures into subgroups according to comorbidities and reported a host-dependent infection rate ranging from 4% to 30%.[24] Factors such as altered neutrophil defense, humoral immunity, and cell-mediated immunity can increase the risk of osteomyelitis.

TREATMENT

The treatment for septic arthritis involves antibiotic therapy in conjunction with prompt consideration for surgical drainage of the affected joint via arthroscopy, arthrocentesis, or arthrotomy. In a major review done in 1990, Shaw and Kasser described open surgical drainage as the "benchmark" of treatment for acute septic arthritis.[18] More recent publications have

©Copyright 2021 American Academy of Orthopaedic Surgeons

demonstrated effective use of arthroscopic techniques, particularly with copious irrigation, for the management of septic arthritis.[13] Though a critical "time to treatment" has not been defined yet, it is imperative that treatment be delivered expeditiously as delayed treatment may lead to undesirable outcomes.[25]

After the initial evaluation and staging of infection, treatment of osteomyelitis includes antimicrobial therapy based on cultured organism susceptibility, débridement with management of resultant dead space, and, if necessary, stabilization of bone. In most patients with osteomyelitis, early antibiotic therapy is administered over a 4-6-week period for optimal outcomes. To reduce costs, parenteral antibiotic administration (via a peripherally inserted central catheter line) on an outpatient basis or the use of oral antibiotics can be considered. Initial first-line antibiotic choice is determined by the patient's history and sensitivities of the isolated organism(s). Most the time, osteomyelitis can be effectively treated with antibiotics and pain medications alone. In more severe cases such as chronic osteomyelitis, aggressive débridement may be necessary. If there is an area of localized abscess, this may need to be opened, washed out, and drained. For instances where there is damaged soft tissue or bone is removed, grafting and/or stabilization may also be performed during surgery.

PERIPROSTHETIC JOINT INFECTION

Overview

Periprosthetic joint infection (PJI) is a rare, but dreaded, complication in orthopaedic surgery affecting patients that undergo arthroplasty. Unwanted effects of this complication include increased cost and utilization of medical resources and physical/emotional distress that place a taxing strain on patients and the healthcare system.[26] With the projected prevalence of patients with prosthetic joints expected to rise and there not yet being a "benchmark" for the diagnosis of PJI, concerted efforts to mitigate the risk and impact of this complication are in full force. Organizations such as the American Association of Orthopaedic Surgeons (AAOS), Centers for Disease Control (CDC), World Health Organization (WHO), Musculoskeletal Infection Society (MSIS), and the International Consensus Group on Musculoskeletal Infection (ICM) have developed practice guidelines for clinicians to follow based on evidence from the literature and multidisciplinary consensus drawn from experts in orthopaedic surgery and infectious disease.

Diagnosis

Clinical history and physical examination are critical for determining the risk of periprosthetic infection. A good history identifying the specific presentation, duration and localization of symptoms, predisposing factors, and response to treatments may render an early diagnosis (see Chapter 22 Table 2). In 2018, diagnostic criteria for hip and knee PJI was developed, validated, and compared with previous criteria set by the MSIS and Internal Consensus Meeting (ICM) on Musculoskeletal Infection (**Figure 1**). Sensitivity of these new diagnostic criteria was found to be 97.7% compared with the MSIS (79.3%) and ICM (86.9%) while the specificity for these three diagnostic criteria was 99.5%.[27] After categorizing patients' diagnostic criteria into major and minor groupings, patients are assigned a composite score and categorized

Major criteria (at least one of the following)	Decision
Two positive cultures of the same organism	Infected
Sinus tract with evidence of communication to the joint or visualization of the prosthesis	

		Minor Criteria	Score	Decision
Preoperative diagnosis	Serum	Elevated CRP *or* D-Dimer	2	≥6 Infected **2-5 Possibly infected [a]** 0-1 Not infected
		Elevated ESR	1	
	Synovial	Elevated synovial *WBC count or LE*	3	
		Positive alpha-defensin	3	
		Elevated synovial PMN (%)	2	
		Elevated synovial CRP	1	

	Inconclusive pre-op score *or* dry tap [a]	Score	Decision
Intraoperative diagnosis	Preoperative score	-	≥6 Infected **4-5 Inconclusive [b]** ≤3 Not infected
	Positive histology	3	
	Positive purulence	3	
	Single positive culture	2	

FIGURE 1 Illustration demonstrating new scoring-based definition for periprosthetic joint infection (PJI). Proceed with caution in adverse local tissue reaction, crystal deposition disease, and slow growing organisms. For patients with inconclusive minor criteria, surgical criteria can also be used to fulfill definition for PJI. Consider further molecular diagnostics such as next-generation sequencing. CRP = C-reactive protein, ESR = erythrocyte sedimentation rate, LE = leukocyte esterase, PMN = polymorphonuclear, WBC = white blood cell. (Reproduced with permission from. Parvizi J, Tan TL, Goswami K, et al: The 2018 definition of periprosthetic hip and knee infection: An evidence-based and validated criteria. *J Arthroplasty* 2018;33[5]:1309-1314.e2.)

©Copyright 2021 American Academy of Orthopaedic Surgeons

as infected, inconclusive, or not infected[27] (**Figure 1**). Based on this validated definition of PJI, patients with preoperative diagnostic scores greater than or equal to 6 are deemed to have infection while patients with scores ranging from 2 to 5 may be possibly infected and must be diagnosed intraoperatively. Some of the key diagnostic parameters used to assess for PJI include the presence of a sinus tract, two positive cultures, elevated inflammatory markers such as serum erythrocyte sedimentation rate (ESR) and serum/synovial C-reactive protein (CRP), and elevated synovial white blood cell (WBC) count. Diagnostic criteria for shoulder PJI have been recently published as well which use similar markers as part of the evaluation process.[25]

Extensive research has been done on the diagnostic parameters utilized in the assessment and diagnosis of PJI. Previous work has shown that blood leukocyte count and differential is neither sensitive nor specific to PJI, whereas synovial fluid leukocyte count and differential is a rapid and accurate assay for predicting PJI.[28] Although they are generally nonspecific markers of inflammation, ESRs, and CRP are also commonly used for initial screening test of infection due to their reported sensitivity being high.[29] Both of these markers normally rise after surgery, with CRP returning to normal within 3 weeks. ESR, however, takes up to 6 weeks to reach normal values with some diurnal variation present even at that time.[30] Elevation of these markers after 3 months is considered abnormal and may indicate the development of PJI. As noted in the previously mentioned study on the 2018 evidence-based definition of PJI, cut-offs for serum CRP and ESR are >1 mg/dL and >30 mm/hr, respectively.[27] New developments from a recent study found the sensitivity of serologic ESR and CRP to vary based on the virulence of the infectious organism present. Considering this, it is important to understand that laboratory values may be falsely "negative" in the presence of organisms with low virulence such as coagulase-negative *Staphylococcus* and *Cutibacterium acnes*.[29]

Synovial fluid markers found validated in the diagnosis of PJI include elevated synovial fluid WBC count (acute, >3,000 cells/μL; chronic, >3,000 cells/μL), alpha-defensin (signal-to-cutoff ratio >1), positive leukocyte esterase (LE; ++), polymorphonuclear (PMN) percentage (acute, >90%; chronic, >80%), and synovial CRP (6.9 mg/L).[27] More recently, serum levels of interleukin-6 (IL-6) (an inflammatory marker produced by monocytes and macrophages) greater than 10 pg/mL have been shown to correlate with infection and improve diagnostic accuracy for PJI.[31,32] Alpha defensin is another emerging marker that has been shown to have utility in the diagnosis of PJI. This naturally occurring peptide has antimicrobial properties, is released as part of the innate immune system response and is unaffected by prior antibiotic administration.[33] Though it has proven to be highly accurate as a diagnostic tool, its cost has limited its accessibility at this time.[34]

Next-generation sequencing (NGS) is an emergent diagnostic technology with potential to revolutionize the diagnosis of periprosthetic joint infection.[33] This technique involves "open" non-Sanger-based high-throughput DNA sequencing which may produce complete analysis of all potential microbes (fungi, bacteria, viruses, parasites, yeast) that might be present in an infected tissue sample. Further studies are needed to validate this methodology; however, there has been preliminary data, which suggest 16s-amplicon targeted NGS in particular can play a role in diagnosing PJI caused by pathogens unidentified with standard culture techniques.[33,35,36]

Treatment

Suppressive Antimicrobial Therapy

Treatment for PJI may allow retention of the prosthesis or require exchange arthroplasty depending on the circumstances. Patients with contraindications to surgery such as those at high risk for local or systemic complications, suspected failure at previous surgical attempt to treat infection, or those with insufficient antibiotic/surgical therapy may be treated with suppressive antimicrobial therapy (SAT). The reported outcomes of SAT have varied widely, with treatment success rates ranging from 18% to 86%.[37-39] Treatment should ideally be lifelong, though studies have indicated treatment withdrawal after an average of 23 months due to risk for adverse drug reactions.[40] This treatment option should only be considered for low virulence infections around well-fixed implants, for which effective oral antibiotics are easily accessible. The presence of an additional uninfected foreign body, such as another joint prosthesis or mechanical heart valve, is a relative contraindication for SAT. Antimicrobial agents should be selected based upon susceptibility testing and with the assistance of an infectious disease specialist.

Débridement, Antibiotics, and Implant Retention

Débridement, antibiotics, and implant retention (DAIR) is another implant-retaining treatment strategy that may be used to treat infection. While the indications for its use are narrow, irrigation and débridement remains the standard intervention for patients presenting with acute periprosthetic infection during the early postoperative period or with late hematogenous infection.[41] Though exchange arthroplasty is considered to be the "benchmark" for treating PJI, prosthesis débridement with antibiotic therapy and implant retention (DAIR) is a viable alternative in uncomplicated cases where acute presentation is within 4 weeks of initial surgery.[42]

One-Stage and Two-Stage Revision Arthroplasty

Some indications for implant removal include late-occurring PJI appearing chronic in nature, instances of infection with loose components, and severe systemic manifestations of infection (sepsis). With septic cases in particular, expedited implant removal to quickly reduce the bioburden and improve hemodynamic stability is necessary. Exchange arthroplasty should also be considered for acute infections with a highly virulent organism, in a compromised host, or after failed eradication with débridement alone.

©Copyright 2021 American Academy of Orthopaedic Surgeons

Exchange arthroplasty may be performed either as a direct exchange in a single-stage or as a two-stage procedure with interim placement of an antibiotic-eluting spacer to allow for a period of treatment with parenteral antibiotics prior to reimplantation. In the United States, two-stage exchange has traditionally been considered the most appropriate and time-tested method for the management of PJI. However, direct exchange has been used with a high rate of success by the majority of surgeons in Europe. As no study has been sufficiently convincing in asserting the superiority of one particular approach, most surgeons choose to engage in the treatment method with which they have had the most experience in training.

With two-stage exchange, reimplantation does not occur during the initial treatment of active infection with prosthesis removal and débridement. Instead, a temporary antibiotic-laden cement spacer is placed to allow for a period of local and systemic antibiotic treatment to eradicate residual infection prior to secondary reimplantation. One of the major advantages of this technique is that successful eradication may be verified during an antibiotic-free period before reimplantation is even considered. However, some patients may not be medically fit for the morbidity associated with undergoing multiple surgeries for definitive treatment.

Two-stage exchange is indicated for nearly all long-standing or late PJIs, including many of those for which direct exchange is contraindicated. There is no established limit as to the number of exchange procedures that may be attempted; however, a salvage procedure may be a more suitable option after multiple previous failures or in patients at exceptionally high risk for infection recurrence (**Table 2**). Exchange arthroplasty should also be avoided in patients who are unlikely to achieve a functional outcome.

Antibiotic-Impregnated Cement Spacers

Use of antibiotic-impregnated PMMA bone-cement spacers is now considered to be the standard of care for patients with a chronic infection at the site of a total joint replacement. These spacers provide direct local delivery of antibiotics while preserving patient mobility and facilitating reimplantation surgery. This surgical treatment decreases cost and improves patient outcomes as well as addresses some of the disadvantages of two-stage revision procedures in which spacers are not used. There are two types of antibiotic-impregnated cement spacers that are typically used in two-stage revisions of total hip and knee arthroplasties: nonarticulating (**Figure 2**) and articulating[43,44] (**Figure 3**).

Nonarticulating spacers allow local delivery of a high concentration of antibiotics and at the same time function to maintain joint space for future revision procedures. Disadvantages of nonarticulating spacers include limited range of motion of the joint after the surgery, possibly resulting in quadriceps or abductor shortening. In contrast, articulating spacers permit more joint motion and can improve function prior to the second-stage reimplantation.[43] From a technical perspective, improved joint function and decreased scar formation after resection arthroplasty can facilitate exposure during reimplantation. Although the distinction between articulating and nonarticulating spacers is somewhat controversial, use of a well-molded, well-fitted articulating spacer that restores soft-tissue tension and allows a greater degree of joint motion has been reported to have better outcomes than use of a nonarticulating spacer, specifically in terms of improved range of motion and functional knee scores without concomitant increases in infection rate and bone loss.

TABLE 2 Criteria for Device Salvage in Periprosthetic Infection

Acute infection for <14-28 d
Stable implant
Clear diagnosis
Susceptible organism
Effective antimicrobial preferably bactericidal
Compliant patient

Arthrodesis

The most functional salvage procedure is an arthrodesis; however, resection arthroplasty and amputation may also be utilized on a limited basis. The most common indication for performing arthrodesis is for a patient with multiple previous failures of infection eradication or an unacceptably high risk for infection recurrence, such as those with multidrug-resistant organisms, severe immunocompromise, or intravenous drug users.[45] Patients with an unreconstructible knee joint, such as those with irreparable extensor mechanism disruption or an inadequate soft-tissue envelope, may also be more appropriately treated with arthrodesis. On the contrary, knee arthrodesis is a poor solution for patients with significant dysfunction of the contralateral limb or ipsilateral hip or ankle, as these patients would be unable to ambulate. Adequate bone stock must also be available for successful fusion.

Resection Arthroplasty

Resection (excision) arthroplasty involves the resection of the infected prosthesis and thorough débridement without consideration of reimplantation. The indications for resection arthroplasty as definitive treatment are quite limited. Patients with low physical demand or those that are medically complex may be served well by resection arthroplasty. It allows patients to sit more comfortably after surgery compared with those who undergo arthrodesis. However, patients without functional limitations prior to surgery are likely to find the significant loss of function, instability, and persistent pain to be troublesome.[46]

©Copyright 2021 American Academy of Orthopaedic Surgeons

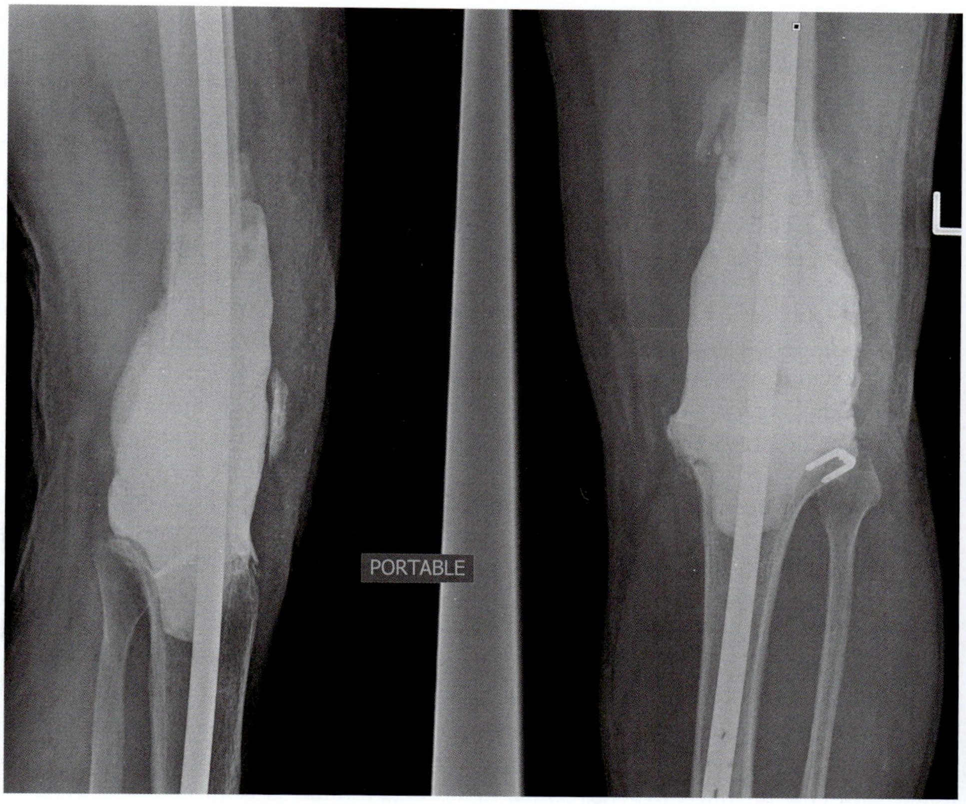

FIGURE 2 Radiographs showing intramedullary rods with antibiotic cement for treating infected knees that provide joint stability in the light of periprosthetic joint infection (PJI). (Reproduced with permission from Chen AF, Heller S, Parvizi J: Prosthetic joint infections. *Surg Clin North Am* 2014;94[6]:1265-1281.)

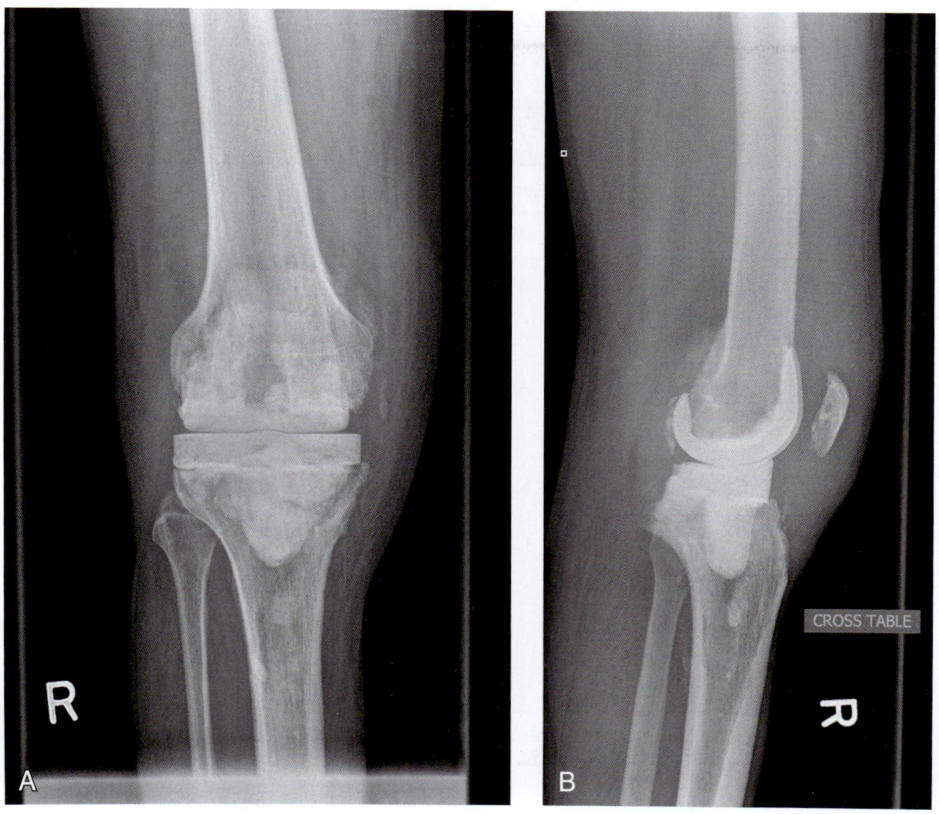

FIGURE 3 Articulating spacer in which the antibiotic cement is shaped into a femur and tibia for a knee that allows for improved motion in the immediate postoperative period between stages. **A**, AP radiograph; **B**, lateral radiograph. (Reproduced with permission from Chen AF, Heller S, Parvizi J: Prosthetic joint infections. *Surg Clin North Am* 2014;94[6]:1265-1281.)

©Copyright 2021 American Academy of Orthopaedic Surgeons

Amputation

In cases where all other treatment options have been considered but are not ideal, amputation may be the final remedy to eradicate persistent. Typically, massive bone loss or soft-tissue erosion precludes an additional attempt at reconstruction or even arthrodesis. Amputation may also be necessary after a significant vascular or nerve injury, necrotizing fasciitis, or severe life-threatening sepsis.[45]

SPINE

Spine infections can result in significant morbidity and even mortality. Smoking, obesity, malnutrition, diabetes, immunodeficiency, or local radiation treatment can predispose to infection. Medical comorbidities associated with increased SSI risk following procedures of the cervical and thoracolumbar spine include neurological disorders, cardiac disease, substance abuse, pulmonary disease, hypertension, and psychiatric disorders.[47,48] Unique to thoracolumbar spine surgery, cancer was also found to be a statistically significant risk factor for SSI. Additional risk factors for SSI include estimated blood loss (EBL) greater than one liter (L), history of previous SSI at the surgical site, obesity, longer procedural times (more than five hours), smoking, ASA score of three or more, dependent functional status, perioperative hyperglycemia, suboptimal timing of antibiotic prophylaxis, and two or more surgical residents participating in the surgical procedure.[47,48] Pyogenic infections are most commonly caused by *Staphylococcus aureus*, although *Staphylococcus epidermidis*, *Streptococcus spp*., and *Escherichia coli* infections may also occur. Granulomatous infections may be caused by *Mycobacterium tuberculosis* and rarely, fungi.

Symptoms of spine infection include back pain that may be accompanied by radicular pain. Less common symptoms include neurological disability with sensory disturbance and motor weakness. Systemic manifestations of spine infection include malaise, weight loss, and altered mental status. The mainstay of treatment is antimicrobial therapy typically for 6 weeks; however, response to therapy can be monitored using serial ESR and CRP.[12]

Surgery is indicated if the infection is refractory to appropriate nonsurgical treatment. Spinal cord decompression should be performed promptly in the context of an emerging neurological deficit, sepsis, spinal epidural abscess, spine instability, or deformity. Major factors associated with poor outcomes include neurologic deficits prior to intervention lasting greater than 36 hours, include age older than 60 years, CRP greater than or equal to 100 g/L, and presence of multiple medical comorbidities on admission.[12,49]

Mycobacterial tuberculosis (TB) of the spine may arise secondary to primary tuberculosis in another organ system. Spinal TB has five stages: implantation, early destruction, advanced destruction/collapse, neurologic involvement, and residual deformity. During the early stages of spinal TB, patients may report dull back pain and muscle spasms, while clinical radiographs demonstrate loss of spinal curvature. As the disease process progresses, diminished disk space, paradiskal erosion, increased vertebral involvement, and kyphotic changes (kyphosis <10° [K1], kyphosis 11° to 60° [K2] or gibbus >60° [K3]) will manifest. Patients affected by spinal tuberculosis may experience neurologic deficits categorized by patient-reported symptoms (weakness/walking) and examination findings (motor, sensory, autonomic).[50] Based on these findings, their paraplegia is graded on a scale of 1 to 4 (**Table 3**).

TABLE 3 Classification of Paraplegia in Tuberculosis of Spine

Grade of Paraplegia	Complaints/Symptom		Examination/Neurological Deficit		
	Weakness	Walking	Motor	Sensory	Autonomic
1	Negligible or weakness appearing after exercise	Able to walk without support	Extensor plantar ± brisk ankle jerks, muscle power grade IV to V	Nil	Nil
2	Mild or feels weakness	Able to walk with support	Motor weakness, brisk tendon jerks, ill sustained muscle clonus, muscle power grade III	Sensory dulling or paresthesia	Nil
3	Moderate or weakness is more marked	Not able to walk Confined to bed Can move limbs	Brisk tendon jerks, sustained muscle clonus, muscle power grade I to II	Hypoesthetic or anesthetic patches	May be present
4	Severe or complete loss of power and control	Not able to move the limbs even in the bed	**a.** Paraplegia in extension, power grade 0 **b.** Paraplegia in flexion, power grade 0, flaccid paralysis	Total loss	Complete loss of bladder and bowel control and incontinence

Adapted with permission from Kumar K: Spinal tuberculosis, natural history of disease, classifications and principles of management with historical perspective. *Eur J Orthop Surg Traumatol* 2016;26(6):551-558. doi:10.1007/s00590-016-1811-x.

©Copyright 2021 American Academy of Orthopaedic Surgeons

TABLE 4 AO/EBJIS Consensus Definition of Fracture-related Infection

Confirmatory Criteria	Suggestive Criteria
Fistula, sinus, or wound breakdown	Clinical signs: Local or systemic (pain, redness, fever, swelling, warmth)
Purulent wound drainage or presence of pus during surgery	Radiological signs (bone lysis, implant loosening, nonunion, sequestration)
Phenotypically indistinguishable pathogens identified by culture in at least TWO separate deep tissue/implant specimens	New-onset joint effusion
Presence of microorganisms in deep tissue specimens, confirmed by histopathological examination	Persistent or new-onset wound drainage
	ONE single positive culture result from a deep tissue/implant/sonicate fluid culture
	Elevated serum inflammatory markers (ESR, WBC, CRP)

CRP = C-reactive protein, ESR = erythrocyte sedimentation rate, WBC = white blood cell
Adapted with permission from Metsemakers W, Morgenstern M, McNally MA, et al: Fracture-related infection: A consensus on definition from an international expert group. *Injury* 2018;49(3):505-510.

Conservative antimicrobial treatment of spinal TB is achieved with RIPE (rifampicin, isoniazid, pyrazinamide, and ethambutol) therapy. The advantage of this is that it also treats the nidus for the primary TB infection which spread to the spine. In instances where drug resistance to RIPE therapy exists, patients must be managed at specialized centers with capacity to treat such cases.[50] If neurologic deficits progress to the point where they are severe, surgical decompression of the spinal cord may be necessary. Procedures such as single-stage anterior and posterior stabilization, extrapleural anterior stabilization of the dorsal spine, and endoscopic thoracoscopic surgery (video-assisted thoracoscopic surgery [VATS]) have been shown to reduce the morbidity and mortality of spinal TB.[51]

INFECTED NONUNION AND FRACTURE-RELATED INFECTION

While definitions vary, infected nonunion has been defined as persistence of an infection at the fracture site and the surrounding tissue with failure of bone healing for 8 months. It is often associated with a severe open fracture, extensive comminution and segmental bone loss, or after internal fixation of a comminuted closed fracture. Risk factors associated with an infected nonunion include exposed bone devoid of vascularized periosteal coverage for more than six weeks, purulent discharge, a positive microbiological culture from the wound, and histological evidence of necrotic bone containing empty lacunae.[52]

Recent collaborative efforts have formulated a standardized definition for fracture-related infection after consensus opinion from 2,000 international trauma experts.[53] Four "confirmatory" criteria were suggested (infection definitely present) and six "suggestive" criteria (**Table 4**). The four confirmatory criteria include fistula, sinus, or wound breakdown; purulent drainage from the wound; phenotypically similar pathogens identified by culture from at least two separate deep tissue/implant specimens; and the presence of pathogens in deep tissue confirmed on histopathological examination.

Treatment and long-term outcomes of infected nonunion are commonly complicated by soft-tissue problems including multiple sinuses, osteomyelitis, osteopenia, complex deformities with limb-length discrepancy, and adjacent joint stiffness. In addition, motor and sensory dysfunction of the limb, chronic pain, and biopsychosocial factors may lead to considerable physical, social, financial, and mental impact on the life of affected patients.

Traditionally, patients have been categorized into two groups. Type A involves infected nonunion of long bones with nondraining (quiescent) infection, with or without implant in situ while type B involves infected nonunion of long bones with draining (active) infection. Both are classified further into two subtypes: nonunion with a bone gap <4 cm or nonunion with a bone gap >4 cm. Single-stage débridement and bone grafting with fracture stabilization are the methods of choice for type A1 infected nonunions. Adequate débridement, fracture stabilization, and second-stage bone grafting gives desirable results in type B1 infected nonunions. Distraction histiogenesis is the preferred procedure for type A2 and B2. The autogenous nonvascularized fibular graft, posterolateral bone grafting for the tibia, and centralization of the ulna over distal radial remnant (single bone forearm) may be good treatment options in selected cases.[54]

©Copyright 2021 American Academy of Orthopaedic Surgeons

SUMMARY

Skeletal infection may be treated with pharmacologic and/or surgical intervention. Treatment should be initiated with broad-spectrum antimicrobial coverage and narrowed down once cultures and sensitivities of specimens from the affected site are obtained. With regard to surgical intervention for infection, adequate débridement remains a crucial step in the treatment process. Furthermore, inflammation may destroy the integrity of orthopaedic hardware, which may be evident on physical, radiographic, or intraoperative examination. The decision to replace or retain hardware may also be contingent on the integrity of both native and artificial structures, distribution of infection, chronicity of infection, and response to previous débridement when applicable. In current practice, some clinicians have also incorporated local antibiotic delivery with products such as antibiotic beads, powder, or cement into their practice. These may be beneficial, particularly in cases where hardware is to be removed and implanted at a later time once the infection has cleared. When such efforts fail, patients may need to be treated with long-term antibiotic therapy or more aggressive modalities such as arthrodesis or amputation. Given the significant morbidity and mortality associated with skeletal infection, early diagnosis and initiation of treatment are fundamental.

REFERENCES

1. Bondarenko S, Chang CB, Cordero-Ampuero J, et al: General assembly, prevention, antimicrobials (systemic): Proceedings of international consensus on orthopedic infections. *J Arthroplasty* 2019;34(2S):S61-S73.
2. Anagnostakos K, Meyer C: Antibiotic elution from hip and knee acrylic bone cement spacers: A systematic review. *BioMed Res Int* 2017;2017:4657874.
3. Masri BA, Duncan CP, Beauchamp CP: Long-term elution of antibiotics from bone-cement: An in vivo study using the prosthesis of antibiotic-loaded acrylic cement (PROSTALAC) system. *J Arthroplasty* 1998;13(3):331-338.
4. Penner MJ, Masri BA, Duncan CP: Elution characteristics of vancomycin and tobramycin combined in acrylic bone-cement. *J Arthroplasty* 1996;11(8):939-944.
5. Kuehn K-D, Ege W, Gopp U: Acrylic bone cements: Mechanical and physical properties. *Orthop Clin N Am* 2005;36(1):29-39.
6. Nelson CL, Griffin FM, Harrison BH, Cooper RE: In vitro elution characteristics of commercially and noncommercially prepared antibiotic PMMA beads. *Clin Orthop Relat Res* 1992;(284):303-309.
7. Neut D, van de Belt H, van Horn JR, van der Mei HC, Busscher HJ: The effect of mixing on gentamicin release from polymethylmethacrylate bone cements. *Acta Orthop Scand* 2003;74(6):670-676.
8. Greene N, Holtom PD, Warren CA, et al: In vitro elution of tobramycin and vancomycin polymethylmethacrylate beads and spacers from Simplex and Palacos. *Am J Orthop* 1998;27(3):201-205.
9. Kuechle DK, Landon GC, Musher DM, Noble PC: Elution of vancomycin, daptomycin, and amikacin from acrylic bone cement. *Clin Orthop Relat Res* 1991;(264):302-308.
10. Simpson AHRW, Deakin M, Latham JM: Chronic osteomyelitis: The effect of the extent of surgical resection on infection-free survival. *J Bone Joint Surg Br Vol* 2001;83-B(3):403-407.
11. Jerzy K, Francis H: Chronic osteomyelitis – bacterial flora, antibiotic sensitivity and treatment challenges. *Open Orthop J* 2018;12:153-163.
12. Duarte RM, Vaccaro AR: Spinal infection: State of the art and management algorithm. *Eur Spine J* 2013;22(12):2787-2799.
13. Ross JJ: Septic arthritis of native joints. *Infect Dis Clin N Am* 2017;31(2):203-218.
14. Boff D, Crijns H, Teixeira MM, Amaral FA, Proost P: Neutrophils: Beneficial and harmful cells in septic arthritis. *Int J Mol Sci* 2018;19(2):1-28.
15. Castellazzi L, Mantero M, Esposito S: Update on the management of pediatric acute osteomyelitis and septic arthritis. *Int J Mol Sci* 2016;17(6):855.
16. Montgomery NI, Epps HR: Pediatric septic arthritis. *Orthop Clin North Am* 2017;48(2):209-216.
17. Kocher MS, Mandiga R, Zurakowski D, Barnewolt C, Kasser JR: Validation of a clinical prediction rule for the differentiation between septic arthritis and transient synovitis of the hip in children. *J Bone Joint Surg Am* 2004;86-A(8):1629-1635.
18. Shaw BA, Kasser JR: Acute septic arthritis in infancy and childhood. *Clin Orthop Relat Res* 1990;(257):212-225.
19. Dingle JT: The role of lysosomal enzymes in skeletal tissues. *J Bone Joint Surg Br* 1973;55(1):87-95.
20. Smith RL, Schurman DJ, Kajiyama G, Mell M, Gilkerson E: The effect of antibiotics on the destruction of cartilage in experimental infectious arthritis. *J Bone Joint Surg Am* 1987;69(7):1063-1068.
21. McCarthy JJ, Dormans JP, Kozin SH, Pizzutillo PD: Musculoskeletal infections in children: Basic treatment principles and recent advancements. *Instr Course Lect* 2005;54:515-528.
22. Morrey B, Bianco A, Rhodes K: Suppurative arthritis of the hip in children. *J Bone Joint Surg Am* 1976;58(3):388-392.
23. Khatod M, Botte MJ, Hoyt DB, Meyer RS, Smith JM, Akeson WH: Outcomes in open tibia fractures: Relationship between delay in treatment and infection. *J Trauma* 2003;55(5):949-954.
24. Bowen TR, Widmaier JC: Host classification predicts infection after open fracture. *Clin Orthop Relat Res* 2005;(433):205-211.
25. International Consensus Group: *Proceedings of the Second International Consensus Meeting (ICM) on Musculoskeletal Infection*. Data Trance Publishing Company, 2018.
26. Kurtz SM, Lau EC, Son M-S, Chang ET, Zimmerli W, Parvizi J: Are we winning or losing the battle with periprosthetic joint infection: Trends in periprosthetic joint infection and mortality risk for the medicare population. *J Arthroplast* 2018;33(10):3238-3245.
27. Parvizi J, Tan TL, Goswami K, et al: The 2018 definition of periprosthetic hip and knee infection: An evidence-based and validated criteria. *J Arthroplast* 2018;33(5):1309-1314.e2.
28. Lee YS, Koo K-H, Kim HJ, et al: Synovial fluid biomarkers for the diagnosis of periprosthetic joint infection: A systematic review and meta-analysis. *J Bone Joint Surg Am* 2017;99(24):2077-2084.
29. Kheir MM, Tan TL, Shohat N, Foltz C, Parvizi J: Routine diagnostic tests for periprosthetic joint infection demonstrate a high false-negative rate and are influenced by the infecting organism: *J Bone Joint Surg Am* 2018;100(23):2057-2065.
30. Bauer TW, Parvizi J, Kobayashi N, Krebs V: Diagnosis of periprosthetic infection. *J Bone Joint Surg Am* 2006;88(4):869-882.
31. Berbari E, Mabry T, Tsaras G, et al: Inflammatory blood laboratory levels as markers of prosthetic joint infection: A systematic review and meta-analysis. *J Bone Joint Surg Am* 2010;92(11):2102-2109.
32. Xie K, Dai K, Qu X, Yan M: Serum and synovial fluid interleukin-6 for the diagnosis of periprosthetic joint infection. *Sci Rep* 2017;7(1):1496.
33. Goswami K, Parvizi J, Maxwell Courtney P: Current recommendations for the diagnosis of acute and chronic PJI for hip and knee—cell counts, alpha-defensin, leukocyte esterase, next-generation sequencing. *Curr Rev Musculoskelet Med* 2018;11(3):428-438.

©Copyright 2021 American Academy of Orthopaedic Surgeons

34. Kasparek MF, Kasparek M, Boettner F, Faschingbauer M, Hahne J, Dominkus M: Intraoperative diagnosis of periprosthetic joint infection using a novel alpha-defensin lateral flow assay. *J Arthroplasty* 2016;31(12):2871-2874.
35. Tarabichi M, Alvand A, Shohat N, Goswami K, Parvizi J: Diagnosis of Streptococcus canis periprosthetic joint infection: The utility of next-generation sequencing. *Arthroplasty Today*. 2017;4(1):20-23.
36. Tarabichi M, Shohat N, Goswami K, et al: Diagnosis of periprosthetic joint infection: The potential of next-generation sequencing. *J Bone Joint Surg Am* 2018;100(2):147-154.
37. Bengtson S, Knutson K: The infected knee arthroplasty. A 6-year follow-up of 357 cases. *Acta Orthop Scand* 1991;62(4):301-311.
38. Hanssen AD, Rand JA: Evaluation and treatment of infection at the site of a total hip or knee arthroplasty. *Instr Course Lect* 1999;48:111-122.
39. Rao N, Crossett LS, Sinha RK, Le Frock JL: Long-term suppression of infection in total joint arthroplasty. *Clin Orthop Relat Res* 2003;(414):55-60.
40. O'Toole P, Osmon D, Soriano A, et al: Oral antibiotic therapy. *J Arthroplasty* 2014;29(2 suppl):115-118.
41. De Man FHR, Sendi P, Zimmerli W, Maurer TB, Ochsner PE, Ilchmann T: Infectiological, functional, and radiographic outcome after revision for prosthetic hip infection according to a strict algorithm. *Acta Orthop* 2011;82(1):27-34.
42. Argenson JN, Arndt M, Babis G, et al: Hip and knee section, treatment, debridement and retention of implant: Proceedings of international consensus on orthopedic infections. *J Arthroplast* 2019;34(2 suppl):S399-S419.
43. Anagnostakos K: Therapeutic use of antibiotic-loaded bone cement in the treatment of hip and knee joint infections. *J Bone Jt Infect* 2017;2(1):29.
44. Chen AF, Heller S, Parvizi J: Prosthetic joint infections. *Surg Clin North Am* 2014;94(6):1265-1281.
45. Lichstein P, Gehrke T, Lombardi A, et al: One-stage vs two-stage exchange. *J Arthroplasty* 2014;29(2 suppl):108-111.
46. Falahee MH, Matthews LS, Kaufer H: Resection arthroplasty as a salvage procedure for a knee with infection after a total arthroplasty. *J Bone Joint Surg Am* 1987;69(7):1013-1021.
47. Chitale R, Campbell PG, Yadla S, Whitmore RG, Maltenfort MG, Ratliff JK: International classification of disease clinical modification 9 modeling of a patient comorbidity score predicts incidence of perioperative complications in a nationwide inpatient sample assessment of complications in spine surgery. *J Spinal Disord Tech* 2015;28(4):126-133.
48. Radcliff KE, Neusner AD, Millhouse PW, et al: What is new in the diagnosis and prevention of spine surgical site infections. *Spine J* 2015;15(2):336-347.
49. Kwon J-W, Hyun S-J, Han S-H, Kim K-J, Jahng T-A: Pyogenic vertebral osteomyelitis: Clinical features, diagnosis, and treatment. *Korean J Spine* 2017;14(2):27-34.
50. Kumar K: Spinal tuberculosis, natural history of disease, classifications and principles of management with historical perspective. *Eur J Orthop Surg Traumatol* 2016;26(6):551-558.
51. Agrawal V, Patgaonkar PR, Nagariya SP: Tuberculosis of spine. *J Craniovertebr Junction Spine* 2010;1(2):74-85.
52. Jain AK, Sinha S: Infected nonunion of the long bones. *Clin Orthop Relat Res* 2005;(431):57-65.
53. Metsemakers W, Morgenstern M, McNally MA, et al: Fracture-related infection: A consensus on definition from an international expert group. *Injury* 2018;49(3):505-510.
54. Struijs PAA, Poolman RW, Bhandari M: Infected nonunion of the long bones. *J Orthop Trauma* 2007;21(7):507-511.

©Copyright 2021 American Academy of Orthopaedic Surgeons

24

Sex and Gender Differences in Clinical and Preclinical Studies

Laura L. Tosi, MD
Austin P. Gillies, BA
Rolanda A. Willacy, BA
Barbara D. Boyan, PhD

Keywords: *bone loss; inflammation; musculoskeletal development; osteoarthritis; osteoporosis; peak bone mass; sarcopenia; sex differences; sexual dimorphism*

Dr. Tosi or an immediate family member serves as a board member, owner, officer, or committee member of American Orthopaedic Association, Osteogenesis Imperfecta Foundation, and US Bone & Joint Initiative. Dr. Boyan or an immediate family member is a member of a speakers' bureau or has made paid presentations on behalf of TitanSpine, Inc.; serves as a paid consultant to or is an employee of National Institutes of Health (NIAMS & NICHD), Spineology Inc., and Titan Spine, LLP; serves as an unpaid consultant to Institut Straumann AG, and Musculoskeletal Transplant Foundation; has stock or stock options held in SpherIngenics, and Titan Spine; has received research or institutional support from Institut Straumann AG, Musculoskeletal Transplant Foundation, and Titan Spine LLC; has received nonincome support (such as equipment or services), commercially derived honoraria, or other non-research-related funding (such as paid travel) from LifeNet, Musculoskeletal Transplant Foundation, and Titan Spine, LLP; and serves as a board member, owner, officer, or committee member of Commonwealth Center for Advanced Logistics Systems, Commonwealth Center for Advanced Manufacturing, Virginia Academy of Science, Engineering, and Medicine, and Virginia Bio. Neither of the following authors nor any immediate family member has received anything of value from or has stock or stock options held in a commercial company or institution related directly or indirectly to the subject of this chapter: Mr. Gillies and Ms. Willacy.

INTRODUCTION

The US National Institutes of Health (NIH) define "sex" as biological differences between females and males, including chromosomes, sex organs, and hormonal profile. "Gender" is defined as socially constructed as well as enacted roles and behaviors within a historical and cultural context.[1] Musculoskeletal health is one of the areas of medicine in which differences between men and women—in morphological, physiological, and behavioral characteristics—are most evident. Although there is a higher incidence of acute traumatic injuries among men, women tend to be disproportionately more disabled by musculoskeletal conditions. Examples of conditions leading to disability with higher incidence in the female population, as compared with their male counterpart, include anterior cruciate ligament (ACL) injuries and spinal deformities during adolescence, stress fractures during adulthood, osteoarthritis, rotator cuff tears, reduced bone density, and osteoporotic fragility fractures. However, the study of the impact of sex on these differences has mostly focused on epidemiological aspects, and the biological basis of sexual dimorphism has only recently begun to be elucidated.[2]

For most of the last century, researchers believed that in higher vertebrates genetic sex determination dictated the sex of the gonads and that hormonal secretions produced by the gonads then determined the sexual phenotype of the rest of the body as well as behavior. Over the past two decades, genome-wide analyses of gene expression have provided a much better understanding of the genes located on the sex chromosomes, their evolution, and their

©Copyright 2021 American Academy of Orthopaedic Surgeons

function. This research has not only confirmed that there are extensive phenotypic differences between the sexes, but has also revealed that there is an equally extensive amount of divergence in gene expression. Moreover, the inherent inequality of the amount of genetic material in the X and Y chromosomes in the two sexes has effects throughout the body, not just on the gonads. Thus, although males and females share a common genome, genes that differ in expression between the sexes, or sex-biased genes, lead to variation in phenotypic traits.[3]

Despite these discoveries, progress in the recognition of sex differences has been slow. Before the 1990s, biomedical research was centered on the male model, and this belief was grounded in the ideology that male biology (excluding the reproductive system) was representative of the species. It was not until 1985 that the US Public Health Service noted that the lack of knowledge of female biology compromised the health of women. And it was not until 1993 that Congress passed the NIH Revitalization Act mandating that women and minorities be included in all clinical research. Additionally, this Act required that data from phase III clinical trials be analyzed by sex.

A major step forward was taken in 2001 when the Institute of Medicine Committee on Understanding the Biology of Sex and Gender Differences published the report titled "*Exploring the biological contributions to human health: Does sex matter?*", which stated that "every cell has a sex" and that research should account for sex differences from "womb to tomb."[4] Researchers then began to realize that every organ in the body, not just in the reproductive system, responds differently on the basis of sex due to chromosomal differences and to sex-specific hormonal regulation. A male cell is not the same as a female cell, and sex chromosome-linked genes can be expressed in the somatic cells as well as germline. However, as noted above, it was primarily the explosion of genomic data that has underscored the importance of this report.

In 2014, the NIH issued a mandate stating that all funded preclinical studies had to include both females and males (animals, tissues, or cells).[5] The rationale behind this mandate was the idea that the failure to consider sex and sex-related differences in cellular biology and pathology played a role in the lack of reproducibility in biomedical studies and in the literature.

Two years later, an initiative implemented by the NIH included sex as a biological variable (SABV).[1] This policy was designed to improve the reproducibility of studies by requiring that sex be factored into the design, analysis, and reporting of human and vertebrate animal research. It was also designed to increase the attention that was given to the role of sex in cell physiology, biologic function, and disease symptoms and manifestations.

Since the issuance of these recommendations and guidelines, the inclusion of "sex" in research analyses has led to groundbreaking discoveries in areas such as medication dosing and also to a greater understanding of diseases such as multiple sclerosis (MS), Parkinson disease, schizophrenia, and stroke, underscoring the importance of sex as a biological variable.[1] The inclusion of "gender" is far more nuanced. In the past, many authors have used the term incorrectly, likely because of their discomfort in using the term "sex." However, this is no longer acceptable and, as more individuals begin to acknowledge that they have chosen to assume a gender role that is different from the sex they were assigned at birth, it is clear that additional research is needed to ensure that their health needs are also met.

This chapter will explore the wide heterogeneity of musculoskeletal growth, development, and pathological traits due to sex differences and the opportunities to improve healthcare through recognition of sex as a biological variable.

SEXUAL DIMORPHISM IN THE DEVELOPMENT OF THE MUSCULOSKELETAL SYSTEM

Men and women have fundamentally different strategies for building mechanically functional bone. Jepsen and colleagues have demonstrated that, on average, women build more slender bones (narrow relative to length) for their body size, with less cortical area and only slightly more cortical bone mineral density (BMD), compared with the more robust bones of men.[6] Differences in the way these traits covary with sex is consistent for both Caucasian and African-American cohorts. As discussed below, female femurs are not just a more slender version of male femurs; their differences have far-reaching clinical implications for developing sex-specific diagnostic and treatment strategies to reduce fragility fractures.

Bone structural integrity is a function of a multitude of complex and interrelated traits of the bone matrix, microstructure, macroscopic bone morphology, and bone density.[7] Research data support the concept that bone traits coadapt to functional loading in a complex multivariate manner and that these complex traits differ between the sexes and vary with age. In both sexes, elegant coadaptation for a myriad of traits—at all of bone's hierarchical levels of organization—functions to maintain adequate biomechanical properties in the face of ever-changing, and sometimes competing, physiological and mechanical demands. Evidence of sex-specific genetic effects on a number of fragility-related traits, taken together with physiological differences between men and women throughout life, indicate that important differences exist in the genetic regulation of bone formation. Historically, male mice have been used to study these traits, but Jepsen et al. have called this practice into question as females were shown to build stronger and more robust bones than their male counterparts in a study of inbred mice.[6] This also raises the issue of whether murine models are appropriate for modeling human sexual dimorphism in the musculoskeletal system.

 ©Copyright 2021 American Academy of Orthopaedic Surgeons

SEXUAL DIMORPHISM IN THE DEVELOPMENT OF PEAK BONE MASS

Peak bone mass (PBM), the maximum amount of bone accrued at the end of the growth period, is an important predictor of future risk of osteoporosis and fracture. Phenotypic sex differences are found in bone diameter and cortical index (a ratio of cortical thickness over bone diameter) at a very early age and continue throughout most of life. Sexual dimorphism in summed cortical thickness and bone length, however, is not evident until shortly after the pubertal growth spurt. The greatest gain in bone mass occurs during the rapid bone growth period associated with puberty[8] (**Figure 1**). During skeletal growth, males display increased periosteal apposition, bone diameter, and cortical thickness. However, females at puberty display inhibited periosteal apposition and increased cortical thickness through the formation of endosteal bone formation, which decreases the endosteal perimeter[9] (**Figure 2**).

Lifestyle choices affect 20% to 40% of adult PBM.[10] However, genomic investigations of BMD in young individuals (ie, prior to attaining PBM) indicate that between a third and a half of the variations in bone growth and mineral accretion are influenced by common genetic variants. Liu et al failed to find a gene by sex interaction effect on BMD in adults[11]; however, a recent genome-wide association study (GWAS) in children participating in the Bone Mineral Density in Childhood Study (BMDCS) found two unexpected results: sex specificity of two loci and large effect size.[12] Moreover, the signals identified in this study do not reside on the X chromosome, adding to the mounting evidence for autosomal sex-specific effects.

This study is particularly interesting because the effect sizes reported for the GWAS associations were higher (sometimes

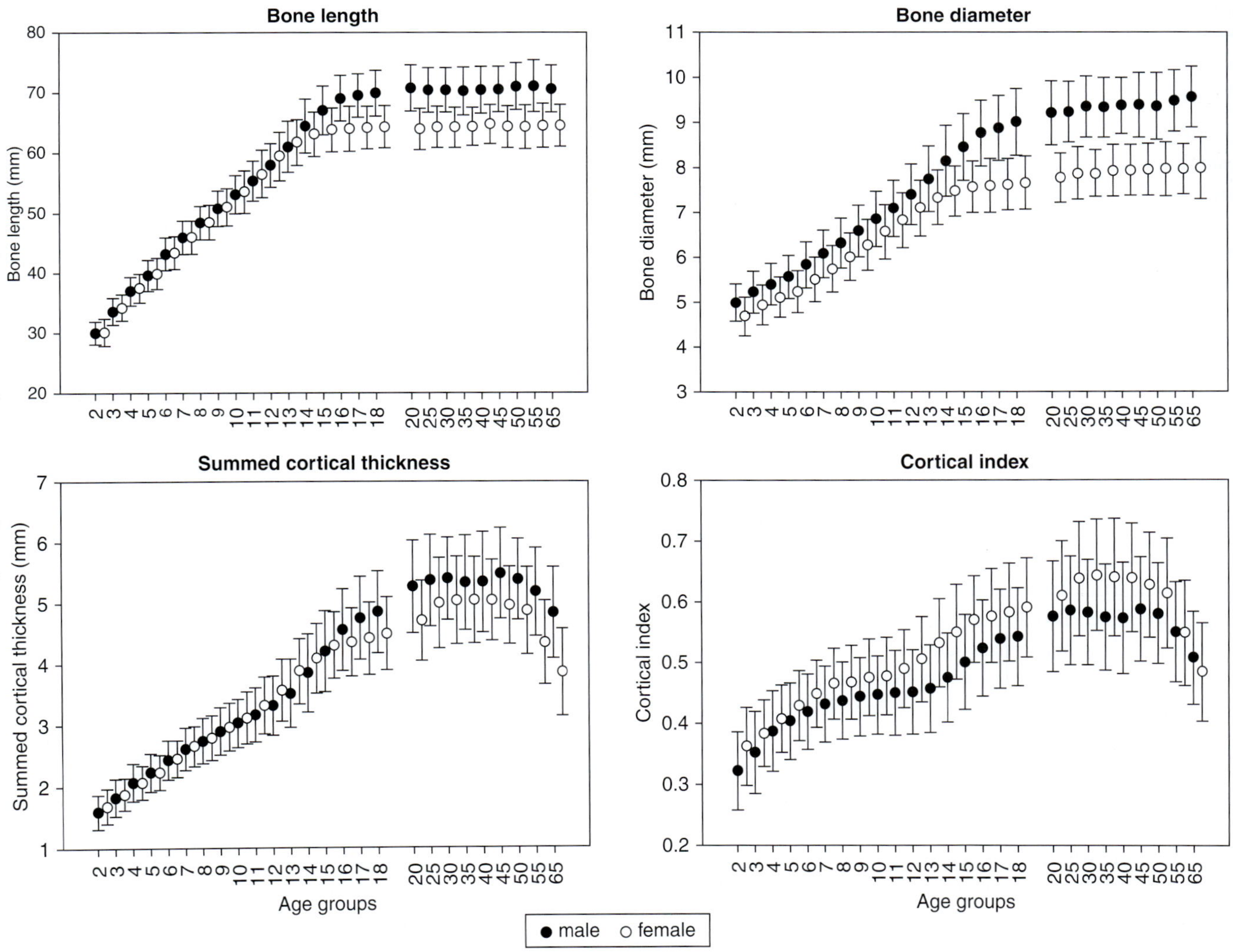

FIGURE 1 Scatter plot of the phenotypic landscape of second metacarpal (1) bone length, (2) bone diameter, (3) summed cortical thickness, and (4) cortical index across the life span. Circles indicate means; whiskers indicate SD. Black circles are male; white circles are female. (Reproduced with permission from Duren DL, Seselj M, Froehle AW, Nahhas RW, Sherwood RJ: Skeletal growth and the changing genetic landscape during childhood and adulthood. *Am J Phys Anthropol* 2013;150[1]:48-57.)

©Copyright 2021 American Academy of Orthopaedic Surgeons

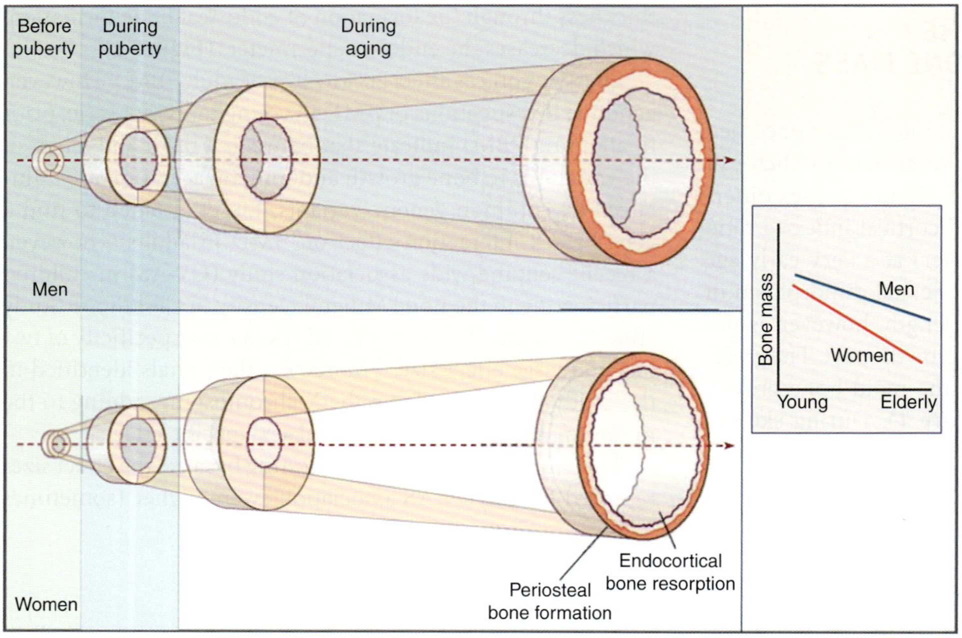

FIGURE 2 Diagram of the differences between men and women in periosteal apposition and net bone loss during aging. (Reproduced with permission from Seeman E: Periosteal bone formation- a neglected determinant of bone strength. *N Engl J Med* 2003;394[4]: 320-323.)

by an order of magnitude) than those reported in larger adult meta-analyses.[13] The authors noted that while this could be an effect of the "winner's curse" or Beavis effect (statistical terms that refer to the possible overestimation of effect size of a quantitative trait locus as the result of small sample size), it is plausible that genetic variation exerts a stronger influence in children, in whom cumulative exposure to environmental factors is lower than in adults.[14] They suggested that this age-specificity may explain why they could not find strong evidence of replication for many of the pediatric signals in the publicly available datasets for BMD in adults (which also are not stratified by sex).

EXERCISE

Numerous articles have sought to analyze lifestyle factors that might optimize PBM and strength and reduce the risk of osteoporosis or low bone mass later in life. Perhaps the greatest interest has been in the area of exercise. During periods of growth, increased body weight and muscle strength and longitudinal bone growth lead to increased loads placed on the skeletal structure. As a result of the high levels of bone modeling and remodeling that occur, it has been suggested that these periods of growth are ideal to positively affect bone mass. Observational studies have reported higher areal bone mineral content (aBMC) and areal bone mineral density (aBMD) in physically active children compared with sedentary children.[15]

In the early 1990s, observational studies began to report higher bone density among physically active children. Unfortunately, subsequent randomized trials were less convincing than observational studies. There are several explanations for this, and they are typically not consistent among studies. Results from observational studies, in which children or young adults with high activity levels were likely to have been more active throughout their lifetime, indicate that increased bone density may have been a reflection of cumulative effects of activity on bone, whereas in randomized trials exercise is for shorter time periods. Inconsistencies among exercise trials may be explained in part by sex and maturity differences in the bone response to loading.

Unfortunately, the majority of trials do not report results by sex and have either been completed in single sex groups or have combined both sexes in the analyses. However, a recent report by McVeigh et al underscores the influence of organized sports activity on PBM as well as highlights the challenge that fewer females are likely to achieve "consistent sport participation."[16] Future studies need to report separate results for women and men, and the data need to be analyzed in the context of estrogen-driven bone packing in females during puberty and extending into the reproductive years, as well as bone responsiveness.

HORMONES AND PEAK BONE MASS

Estrogens and androgens act as promoters of accrual of bone mass during puberty, and low levels of these hormones play a role in the initiation of the pubertal growth spurt. Sex hormones indirectly regulate this period of skeletal growth via growth hormone (GH) and insulinlike growth factor I (IGF-I).[17] The result of differential initiation of puberty in boys in girls can be seen as a greater length of time for prepubertal appendicular growth in boys, which contributes to height differences between sexes. In girls, elevated levels of estrogen limit the expansion of periosteal bone, but stimulate endocortical

©Copyright 2021 American Academy of Orthopaedic Surgeons

apposition. During puberty, boys experience significant effects of both estrogens and androgens, which stimulate periosteal bone expansion and higher rates of cortical bone growth.[18] At the end of puberty, estrogen contributes to the closing of epiphyseal plates, slowing longitudinal growth. Thus, there is a differential rate in longitudinal bone growth between the sexes. These hormonal changes can be observed as complex multivariate interactions between the hormone milieu found in the bone environment and mechanical loading.

Estrogen is produced by the action of aromatase on testosterone.[19] Therefore, the pathways for synthesis of estrogen and androgens are closely related to each other, which causes some difficulty when attempting to study the individual impact of hormones on bone homeostasis. The role of estrogen receptors (ERs) and androgen receptors (ARs) in the response of cells to these hormones has been widely studied through the use of animal models with the use of germline or tissue-specific knockouts. Although these models do not fully explain the phenotypes of sex hormone deficiency, much has been learned concerning their mechanism of action. In females, increased estrogen serum levels at puberty have a number of effects on bone cell activity. Estrogen acts via estrogen receptor alpha (ERα) to inhibit periosteal apposition, endosteal bone resorption, and chondrocyte remodeling, which result in epiphyseal closure and attenuated periosteal expansion. In contrast, in males at puberty, estrogen stimulates periosteal expansion via ERα and androgen acts via the androgen receptor (AR) to increase trabecular bone formation.[18]

Sex hormones bind to nuclear hormone receptors to act upon target cells. In addition, many steroid hormones, including estrogen can act on target cells via membrane-associated receptors. Compared with the sex steroid receptors ER and AR, less is known about the role of progesterone and the progesterone receptor (PR) in bone cell metabolism. Similar to the action of estrogen and testosterone, the biological effects of progesterone are mediated by interaction with membrane-associated receptors as well as intracellular receptors. Selective inhibition of PR signaling in mesenchymal stem cells (MSCs) and particularly in osteoprogenitor cells but not mature osteoblasts, significantly affects pathways involving immunomodulation, bone remodeling, extracellular signaling, and matrix interactions.[19] Most importantly, these effects are only seen in males. These findings suggest that PR signaling in MSCs may intrinsically regulate sex differences in health and disease conditions.

The pubertal period is routinely the most active time for bone changes, and the size, shape, and mass of long bones are arguably the most outwardly identifiable phenotypic sex differences in the skeleton. Some of these differences can be seen as early as two years of age. By the age of two years, boys already show significantly greater bone diameter than girls, and girls possess a concomitantly greater proportion of cortical bone than boys.[8] These differences are magnified during puberty, when the pubertal hormone surge elicits different responses from the growing bones in girls and boys. Both boys and girls are experiencing an earlier onset of puberty and a connected acceleration in bone maturation than several decades ago.

Using data from the FELS Study, the world's largest and longest running study of human and growth development, Duren et al. have recently demonstrated sex-specific secular changes in skeletal maturation, and that individual processes underlying the bone age phenotype may be differentially affected by this secular trend.[20] Specifically they found that over the past century, the age at epiphyseal fusion initiation and the age at epiphyseal fusion completion have gradually decreased by as much as 6.7 and 6.8 months in males and 9.8 and 9.7 months in females, respectively.[21] This is important for clinical management, including treatment timing, of orthopaedic patients, because children today exhibit a different pattern of maturation than children on whom original maturity assessments were based, including both the FELS Method or the Greulich-Pyle Atlas.[22]

INFLUENCE OF SEXUAL DIMORPHISM ON THE DEVELOPMENT OF MUSCULOSKELETAL CONDITIONS DURING CHILDHOOD, ADOLESCENCE, AND YOUNG ADULTHOOD

PREMATURE OSTEOARTHRITIS

Femoroacetabular impingement (FAI) and developmental dysplasia of the hip (DDH) are the leading causes of premature osteoarthritis of the hip joint. Females are uniquely predisposed to DDH, and there is frequently a history of left-sided disease and breech presentation. In DDH, a shallow acetabulum causes an increase in mechanical stress on the cartilage matrix, with failure of the acetabular labrum that progresses to degeneration and osteoarthritis.

In the nondysplastic hip, repetitive abnormal contact of the femoral head-neck junction and the anterior rim of the acetabular labrum during dynamic hip motion results in damage to both the joint cartilage and the labrum. The morphology and pattern of disease is very distinct and results in variable patterns of joint injury. Asphericity of the head and loss of offset at the head-neck junction, combined with focal or global overcoverage of the acetabulum, results in repetitive collisions and microtrauma to the chondrolabral complex with terminal hip range of motion.

Even though these abnormalities affect both genders, FAI is more common in males and more likely to be bilateral. In addition, several authors have noted that the hip morphology is more similar between the two sides in this non-DDH group. This suggests that adolescent dysplasia may be caused by malformation of the entire pelvis, which is different from infant DDH. The etiology of FAI remains undefined, but sex- and sport-specific differences in prevalence and morphology suggest adaptive changes in the immature musculoskeletal system in response to mechanical stresses. In addition, recent studies

©Copyright 2021 American Academy of Orthopaedic Surgeons

have demonstrated that there are demographic differences between patients diagnosed with hip dysplasia in infancy versus adolescence/adulthood, and there is a growing consensus that these represent distinct forms of dysplasia. In both, there is a familial tendency toward hip disease with a higher incidence of arthroplasty in the adolescence/adulthood dysplasia group's family members and higher frequency of infantile dysplasia in the DDH group's family members.[23]

ANTERIOR CRUCIATE LIGAMENT INJURIES

ACL injuries of the knee are common in women, with an incidence of two to eight times higher than in men, in sports such as basketball, soccer, and handball. Women more commonly exhibit an anteriorly rotated pelvis, contralateral pelvic drop, internal hip rotation and adduction, knee valgus, tibia external rotation, and foot pronation. The sex-based bony architecture differences in osseous morphology such as plateau dimensions and femoral condyle geometry, hip version, and length of the femur, as compared with the pelvic width, notch width index (NWI), and tibial slope, have all been associated with increased risk of functional knee instability and ACL injury. However, no causal relationship has been proven to this point. Recent studies have investigated proximal and distal anatomical differences in the kinetic chain, including restricted hip range of motion and its impact on the compensatory stresses and risk of ACL injury. The recognition of variable anatomy and, perhaps more importantly, the understanding of the etiology of these differences is of paramount importance in injury prevention and rehabilitation.[24] Females land with a more upright and erect posture than males, and this subjects the knees to forces that lead to anterior tibial translation. Also in females, greater external rotation may predispose them to increased rates of ACL injury because of increased laxity of the knee. Differences have also been reported in the functional adaptation of females to sports biomechanics notably, jumping and landing, which may be learned behaviors.

SEX DIFFERENCES IN COMMON MUSCULOSKELETAL DISORDERS SUCH AS SCOLIOSIS AND CLUBFOOT—THE POLYGENIC THRESHOLD AND THE CARTER EFFECT

Clubfeet are 2.5 to 4 times more common in men than women, whereas adolescent idiopathic scoliosis is 10 times more common in females than in males. This suggests a polygenic inheritance mode with a dimorphic sex threshold for the affected phenotype, which is commonly termed the Carter effect.[25] Thus, women require a greater number of, or more potent, susceptibility genes than men to inherit clubfoot. It would be predicted that women should have a higher rate of transmission of the affected phenotype to their children, but this has not yet been demonstrated.[26] In scoliosis, however, a study of over 200 multiplex families in which there was more than one individual affected with scoliosis revealed that men were most likely to transmit this disorder to their children and to have siblings with adolescent idiopathic scoliosis.[27]

SEXUAL DIMORPHISM IN ADULT/MIDDLE AGE CONDITIONS

IMMUNE-MEDIATED DISEASES

Sex differences occur in both innate and adaptive immune responses and are evolutionarily conserved across diverse species. In the human, sex differences in immune responses change throughout life and are influenced by both the age and reproductive status of an individual. Sex chromosome genes and sex hormones, including estrogens, progesterone, and androgens, contribute to the differential regulation of immune responses between the sexes. Environmental factors, including nutrition status and the composition of the microbiome, also alter the development and functioning of the immune system differently in males and females. Sex differences in immune responses result in differential susceptibility of males and females to autoimmune diseases, malignancies, and infectious diseases, as well as affecting the outcome of vaccination.[28]

Autoimmune diseases (ADs) affect approximately 10% of the world's population, and 80% of those individuals are females[29] (**Figure 3**). The average onset of AD is between 40 and 50 years of age, although many ADs commonly appear in childhood and adolescence. There are more than 20 ADs that are strongly sex-biased in women, including rheumatoid arthritis (RA), multiple sclerosis (MS), systemic lupus erythematosus (SLE), Sjogren syndrome, and systemic sclerosis. Only a few ADs are more common in men, particularly ankylosing spondylosis, with the remaining diseases demonstrating no observable sex bias.

For example, RA is a chronic, inflammatory disorder that presents with progressive joint damage. It often results in loss of physical function, decreased quality of life, and reduced lifespan. The disease affects the small joints of the wrists, hands, ankles, and feet, and radiographically, there is bony erosion of the insertion site of inflamed synovium. The incidence of RA is four- to fivefold higher in women than in men younger than 50 years; however, after the age of 70 years, this ratio is reduced to approximately 2:1.[30] The recent development of biologic therapies has been a boon for numerous individuals with autoimmune disorders. Unfortunately, in RA, women report significantly increased fatigue and worse function scores compared with men.[31] This difference underscores the need for sex-specific therapies in some autoimmune disorders.

Ankylosing spondylitis (AS) is a systemic inflammatory condition that occurs primarily in men and presents with back pain, peripheral arthritis, and functional limitation. In many cases, there is a delay in the onset of symptoms at the time the diagnosis is made. Furthermore, the presence of sacroiliitis on

©Copyright 2021 American Academy of Orthopaedic Surgeons

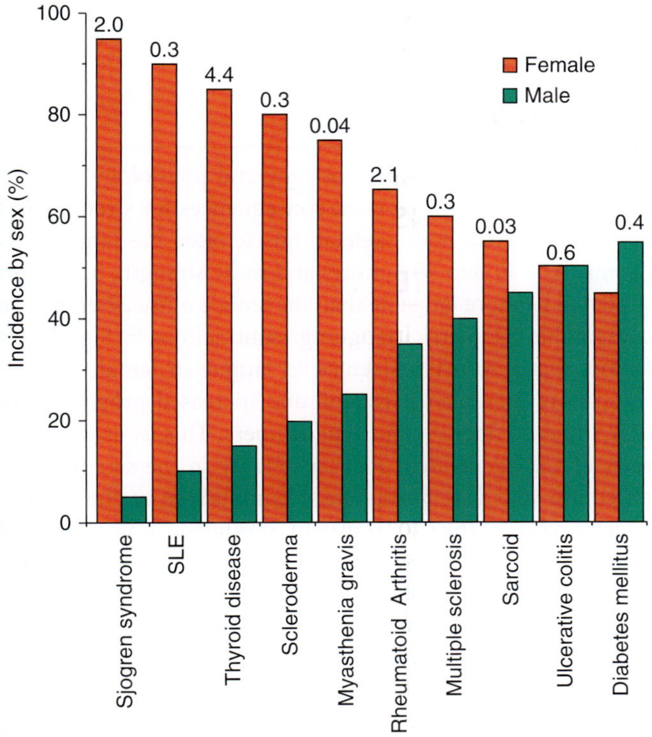

FIGURE 3 Bar graph of the sex differences in autoimmune conditions (the sex distribution of the major autoimmune diseases). The numbers above the bars refer to the total number of disease cases in millions in the United States. SLE = systemic lupus erythematosus. (Reproduced with permission from Billi AC, Kahlenberg JM, Gudjonsson JE: Sex bias in autoimmunity. *Curr Opin Rheumatol* 2019;31[1]:53-61.)

plain radiographs, which is required as part of the 1984 diagnostic criteria, is not a sensitive method to identify this condition. New diagnostic criteria do not include radiographic sacroiliitis, but rather MRI evidence of sacroiliac inflammation or HLA-B27 in the appropriate clinical setting.[32] While AS is predominantly a male condition, with a male to female ratio that is roughly 2:1, axial spondyloarthropathy has a similar incidence in both sexes. The symptoms of axial spondyloarthropathy include pain and stiffness, predominantly of the axial skeleton, as well as sacroiliitis, which is a diagnostic hallmark. Here too, the symptoms are frequently missed, particularly in women.

Other disorders such gout, sepsis, and postsurgery infections display higher incidence and severity in men. These changes also occur at an accelerated rate in men as compared with women.[31] Two risk factors for infection and multiple organ failure are male gender and increased age. Inflammation is a line of defense that aids in maintaining homeostasis following trauma and infection. This inflammatory process results in pro- and anti-inflammatory mechanisms. Previous studies have found significant reduction in immune-competent cells in postsurgical men. Furthermore, Offner et al demonstrated that male sex is an independent risk factor. It has been hypothesized that sexual dimorphism is likely due to increased expression of pro- and anti-inflammatory cytokines such as interleukin (IL)-6, IL-8, IL-10, and tumor necrosis factor-α (TNF-α).[33]

CANCER

Sexual dimorphism of musculoskeletal tumors depends on both hormonal and genetic factors governing bone mineralization and remodeling. The Surveillance, Epidemiology, and End Results (SEER) cancer registry statistics demonstrate that primary bone tumors are more prevalent in males than in females with a ratio of 1.35:1.[34] Osteoid osteoma and osteoblastoma favor males more than 2 to 1, while giant cell tumor and parosteal/periosteal osteogenic sarcoma are more common in females at a ratio of around 2:1.[35]

Hormonal differences in bone development at the cellular and molecular levels result in sexual dimorphism in the presentation of bone and joint cancers. For example, osteogenic sarcoma develops 2 years earlier in females versus males. New data suggest relative levels of ERα and ERβ have important clinical implications in bone cancer, with greater ERα expression correlated with the absence of metastases at presentation and better event-free survival.[36] ERβ expression, which is more frequent in males, is elevated in extra-abdominal fibromatosis, which is more prevalent in female patients and has been responsive to adjuvant antiestrogen therapy. Studies also suggest that sex-specific differences occur in cell death programs. In general, male and female cells (XY and XX, respectively) have a different response to cellular stressors. The same stressor can induce apoptosis in male cells while female cells survive by induction of autophagy. XX and XY cells also have a different level of susceptibility to cytotoxic agents. For example, while XY neurons have a higher sensitivity to excitotoxicity, XX neurons have a greater likelihood to undergo staurosporine-induced apoptosis.

In addition, there is growing evidence that sexual dimorphism in cancer incidence may be independent of hormones and directly related to genetic differences. X-inactivation is a phenomenon in which one of the two X chromosomes is silenced epigenetically in every cell. However, in up to 15% of cases, X-linked genes escape X-inactivation, leading to a second functional copy of genes located in the X-chromosome inactivation (XCI)-escaper region. Dunford et al have found that there are tumor suppressor genes among the escaper genes, which when mutated, have a significant association with cancer in males.[37] This suggests that the second copy of the gene in the XCI-escaper region has a protective role in females. Moreover, it is possible that the protection provided by the second copy in the XCI-region does not last throughout the lifespan. Reports demonstrate that around 55 years of age, age-related preferential inactivation of one X-chromosome occurs, which can result in increased morbidity. Patterns of XCI are altered in women's cancers, which can result in inactivation of tumor suppressor genes.[38]

©Copyright 2021 American Academy of Orthopaedic Surgeons

Epigenetic factors, such as microRNAs (miRs) have also been shown to play a role in cancer development. miRs play an essential role in posttranscriptional gene regulation of cell proliferation and cell death. These short noncoding RNAs bind directly to the 3′ untranslated regions (UTRs), resulting in translational repression or mRNA degradation. The X chromosome has a significantly higher number of miRs than the Y chromosome: the X and Y chromosomes contain 118 and 2 miRs, respectively. miRs have tumorigenic as well as tumor suppressor functions.[39] Additionally, miRs are involved in immunosurveillance against the development of tumor growth. One example is the role that miRNAs play in immunotherapies of the PD-1/PD-L1 pathway blockade. In vivo experiments have been conducted which confirm that miR-142-5p can inhibit pancreatic cancer growth.[40]

There is evidence of sex-specific differences in cancer progression. Cancer metastasis to the bone is the most common cause of bone cancer and severe cancer pain. Currently, 60% to 80% of patients with metastatic breast, lung, and prostate cancer develop bone metastases.[36] In breast cancer, bone is the most common site of metastasis and represents the first location of relapse in nearly half of patients. In breast cancer bone metastasis formation, in addition to signaling via an ERα66 and an ERα variant ERα36, signaling via ERβ also appears to play a role. Although XX and XY cells both possess ERα36, signaling by this ERα "variant" is not operational in male cells.[41]

Estrogen influences the bone microenvironment, creating and conditioning a favorable niche for colonization and breast cancer progression. For lung cancer, studies support the hypothesis that females have a more favorable bone microenvironment for metastasis formation. For prostate cancer, a decrease in the relative androgen to estrogen balance or a "feminization" of bone marrow favors bone metastasis formation, with a potentially important role for ERβ that may be similar to that in breast cancer.[36,41] Long-term estrogen administration or androgen blockade in males may feminize the bone marrow niche to one more favorable for bone metastases in prostate cancer. Administration of androgens in females, especially combined with mastectomy, may reduce risk of developing bone metastatic breast cancer.

The response to chemotherapeutic treatment also displays sex-linked differences in musculoskeletal oncology. An analysis of patients with high-grade osteosarcoma of the trunk or limbs treated with surgery and chemotherapy found females responded better to chemotherapy than males. This translated into superior outcomes for females, as can be seen in the probability of 10-year event-free survival (60.9% for females, 54.5% for males).[34] Similar results have been reported for soft-tissue sarcomas and are supported by overall SEER survival rates. Drug metabolism and pharmacokinetics also differ by sex, and despite these sexually dimorphic differences, the increased efficacy of certain chemotherapeutic agents in female patients may be accompanied by a simultaneous increase in complications or severity of complications. For example, there is greater toxicity in females who undergo isolated-limb perfusion for soft-tissue sarcoma than in males (22% compared with 7%).[34]

SEXUAL DIMORPHISM IN AGING—WHEN DO WE START LOSING GROUND?

SKELETAL MUSCLE LOSS

Sexual dimorphism in the anatomy and physiology of adult skeletal muscle has important consequences for strength and fatigability. While male skeletal muscle often has larger mass (as much as 30% to 40% more) and more strength, it has also shown to be more fatigable than the female muscle but to have comparable isometric fatiguing contractions.[42] Significant factors that improve resistance to fatigue in female skeletal muscle are increased perfusion and increased proportion of type I muscle fibers versus type II fibers. This leads to slower rates of Ca^{2+}-dependent ATPase activity in the sarcoplasmic reticulum and less phosphate accumulation in the cytosol which preserves the Ca^{2+} transient, producing a more gradual relaxation of female muscle. Moreover, type I fibers metabolize excess lactic acid created by nearby type II fibers, further ameliorating fatigue. Differences in male and female muscle fatigability can also be mediated by external factors including cognitive stressors, which cause higher fatigability in females during sustained maximal static contractions.[42] Additional factors like the neurologic contribution of motor pools and the adverse effects of aging could be different between the sexes, but this requires further exploration.

Sarcopenia and Loss of Skeletal Muscle

Muscle mass and strength peak in early adulthood and then begin to decline from approximately the fifth decade. As the body ages, the musculoskeletal system begins a slow progression to decrease muscle mass, at a rate of 1% to 3% per year after the age of 60 years.[43] Mechanisms for this process include the gradual change from anabolic to catabolic processes, which begin to break down muscle fibers and motor units. Factors that are thought to be associated with this decline include dietary factors like malnutrition, decreased physical activity, changes in metabolic activity, or lower satellite cell numbers that perpetuates reduced neuromuscular stimulation and muscle wasting. Additionally, the relative and absolute losses of mass due to age-related sarcopenia are higher in men, possibly because estrogen has a protective effect on skeletal muscle by attenuating inflammation. This would suggest that men undergo significant changes in late adulthood and old age that bring about significant skeletal muscle loss. Although various genetic and age-related pathways can help explain muscle loss, sex hormones clearly play a critical role.

With aging and other muscle wasting diseases, men and women undergo similar pathological changes in skeletal muscle: increased inflammation, enhanced oxidative stress, mitochondrial dysfunction, satellite cell senescence, elevated apoptosis and proteasome activity, and suppressed protein synthesis and myocyte regeneration.[44] Decreased food intake and physical activity also indirectly contribute to muscle wasting. Sex hormones play important roles in maintaining

©Copyright 2021 American Academy of Orthopaedic Surgeons

skeletal muscle homeostasis, and the decline of circulating sex hormone levels results in the loss of muscle mass and integrity seen in sarcopenia.

Sex steroids aid in the growth and maintenance of muscle mass and strength but appear to do so through different pathways. While testosterone is associated with anabolic growth factors including IGF-I, which induces hypertrophy and contributes to significant protein synthesis, estrogen has been shown to have a protective effect on muscle via anti-inflammatory and anticatabolic pathways, as demonstrated by reductions in decreased expression of myostatin and interleukin genes.[45] Across the lifespan, greater decreases in testosterone in men versus women appear to contribute to the higher rates of sarcopenia, while decreases in estrogen do not have as profound effects on muscle qualities. Hormone replacement with testosterone in men has shown promise for increasing muscle size and strength, while estrogen has only shown significant protective effects on muscle in preclinical studies.

In both female and male animals, the loss of gonadal function triggers a strong biological drive toward sedentary behavior. Within 1 to 2 weeks of gonadectomy, spontaneous physical activity plummets by 30% to 80%, but can be fully rescued in males by testosterone and in females by estradiol.[42] Ultimately, treatments that help improve muscle strength and function in aging men and women could lead to reduced falls and frailty.

Sarcopenia and Frailty

Sarcopenia has significant effects in the elderly, including limiting mobility and function across sexes. A meta-analysis by Wong et al conducted in 2018 demonstrated that sarcopenia is also linked to fragility fractures, or the low-energy fractures seen in people with decreased bone mass.[46] Individuals with sarcopenia are at three times greater risk for falling, and significantly higher percentages of men were found to have sarcopenia after a fragility fracture. These numbers suggest that while osteopenia and osteoporosis may exhibit different rates between men and women, the muscle loss experienced in men could contribute to higher comorbidities with other musculoskeletal conditions.

OSTEOARTHRITIS

Osteoarthritis (OA) is a progressive disorder defined as narrowing of the joint space as a product of damage and inflammation to the cartilage, synovium, capsule, bone muscles ligaments, and tendons involved in the joint.[47] Between 2008 and 2014, 32.5 million adults in the United States reported symptoms of OA, or nearly 1 in 7.[48] While OA is significantly associated with age and race (higher rates in elderly and non-White populations), the influence of sex has been more recently attributed to differences in etiology and severity of the condition. Women make up an estimated 78% of adults with OA and experience higher rates of knee and hand involvement. Notably, only 10% of preclinical studies of OA reported "sex" or "gender" as factors in their analysis, suggesting that significant gaps still exist in the field. Here we will explore the underlying metabolic, mechanical, and physiological sexual dimorphism that can help explain these differences.

Hormonal Influences

One of the challenges in prior research has been the use of primarily male animal models and cell lines, which cannot account for the influences of sex hormones, particularly estrogen, which may play a role in the etiology of OA. Studies have demonstrated in articular cartilage that the signaling of sex hormones can promote growth and cellular matrix production, and notably, the total number of receptors is higher in females versus males.[49] In both sexes, there are androgen receptors, but the processes by which chondrocytes use them are dimorphic. While female cells are able to metabolize testosterone into estrogen, male cells use it to form dihydrotestosterone (DHT), which produces immediate membrane responses unique to male cells. Progesterone has also been found to have widespread effects in connective tissue in both sexes, yet one study associated progesterone level alterations during the menstrual cycle and joint laxity in female athletes. Another piece in the puzzle is the fluctuation in receptor levels in the knee tissue, demonstrated in animal models studying pregnancy, ovariohysterectomy, joint injury, ACL transection, and antigen-induced arthritis. While further research is needed, there is the potential to analyze multiple types of tissues for receptor and ligand levels utilizing novel techniques, with a focus on sex differences.

Mechanical Influences

The differences observed in the incidence of OA in men and women may also be influenced by mechanical factors, including limb alignment, muscle properties, and obesity. In patients with varus and valgus deformities of the lower extremities, weight bearing is distributed medially and laterally (respectively) and could factor into additional mechanical wear on knee cartilage. While studies have not demonstrated large significant odds ratios (ORs) for limb alignment contributing to the development of OA, data on the progression seem to suggest that varus knees contribute to the worsening of radiographic signs of OA (OR 3.59).[50] These data, in conjunction with the higher rates of valgus alignment in women from studies looking at lower limb alignment in various ethnic groups, suggest how weight-bearing mechanics in the lower limbs could affect knee OA prevalence. Furthermore, studies of muscle strength have demonstrated that knee extensor weakness is predictive of symptomatic, but not radiographic, OA in men and women. A significant predictive factor across multiple studies has proven to be obesity, which has been theorized to add additional stress and strain to knee joints during physical activity. Body mass index (BMI) was predictive of the development of

©Copyright 2021 American Academy of Orthopaedic Surgeons

OA in women more than men, while other specific measures of body shape or activity level did not show the same risk. Although limb alignment has been associated with obesity, studies in OA demonstrated weak links to disease onset and severity. Meniscal tears also present a risk factor for knee OA, and a separate study found such alterations to be associated with age, females, and obesity. Obesity may contribute directly to mechanical strains on the knee joint and influence OA development; however, the proinflammatory nature of obesity has also been thought to contribute to cytokine and potential metabolic influences on OA development and progression. Recent work has demonstrated that both general obesity and central obesity are associated with increased levels of cytokines. IL-1, TNF-α, and IL-6 may cause OA indirectly because they regulate the release of adiponectin and leptin from adipocytes.[51,52]

Pain and Neurological Influence

For patients with OA, some of the most important challenges to improving outcomes and quality of life are related to pain symptoms. Large studies have demonstrated that women reported higher incidence and intensity of pain post-total knee arthroplasty (TKA), but the specific reasons for this could be complex and multifaceted.[53] Notably, the level of pain is not associated with radiographic changes in OA progression and is likely related to the development of peripheral and central pain sensitization. Whether acute insult to pain nociceptors from injury, referred pain, or central associations with knee sensation and pain are contributing factors for individuals, sex does appear to have some role in OA pain. Pain signaling neurotransmitters have shown to have increased response in joints of female animal models, and opioid agonists may have variable effects in different sexes for postoperative pain. Particularly interesting are studies demonstrating upregulation of endogenous opioids after injury and the decrease in arthritic pain after intra-articular administration of naloxone, an opiate antagonist. Central nervous system processing of pain signals also seems to differ between men and women, as one study demonstrated an increased pain threshold and decreased temporal summation for conditioned pain stimuli for men, but this was not in studied in OA patients. One study observed prefrontal limbic region activation unique to patients with OA reporting spontaneous knee pain when compared with healthy controls. These dimorphic traits could prove invaluable when addressing the challenges of OA treatment. In addition, there is a growing body of literature on sex differences in psychological coping strategies.[54,55]

BONE LOSS

Sexual dimorphism in both the development of PBM as well as bone loss contributes in large part to the two to threefold greater lifetime fracture risk for women compared with

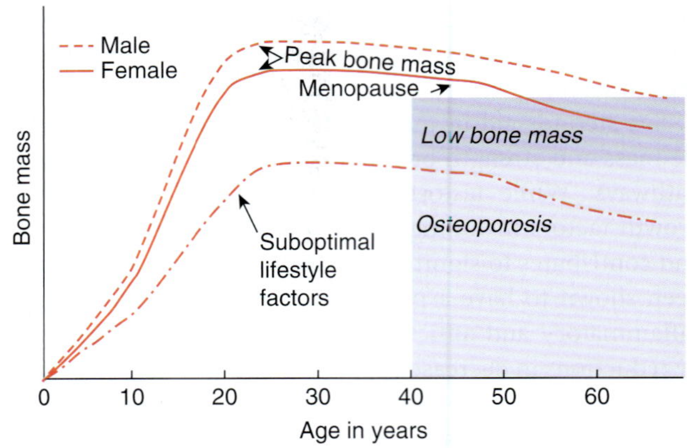

FIGURE 4 Line plot of bone mass across the lifespan with optimal and suboptimal lifestyle choices. (Reproduced with permission from Weaver CM, Gordon CM, Janz KF, et al: The National Osteoporosis Foundation's position statement on peak bone mass development and lifestyle factors: a systematic review and implementation recommendations. *Osteoporos Int* 2016;27[4]:1281-1386.)

men (**Figure 4**). Fracture incidence is higher in men than women younger than 50 years and is commonly the result of high-energy trauma; this trend reverses after the age of 50 years. A 50-year-old woman has a 39.7% remaining lifetime risk of an osteoporotic fracture, while a 50-year-old man has only a risk of 13.1%.[56] These differences are, in part, due to the marked differences between women and men in terms of the onset of sex steroid deficiency in midlife, which contributes to different patterns of bone loss in women versus men. Thus, the abrupt cessation of ovarian function in women at the time of menopause leads to a decrease in total and bioavailable estrogen, which triggers a rapid phase of bone loss leading to a greater net bone loss throughout life as compared with men. Estrogen deficiency leads to bone loss by decreasing osteoblast lifespan and increasing osteoclast lifespan.[57] In contrast, recent data from the MrOS study indicates that lower bioavailable estradiol or higher sex hormone-binding globulin (SHBG) was related to greater hip bone loss and fracture in men.[58] However, as yet, this has not proven to be clinically useful in fracture risk discrimination.[59]

As noted earlier, men build a not just a bigger but also more robust skeleton. The difference in bone mass and geometry leads to greater skeletal integrity in males, which also contributes to the lower incidence of osteoporotic fractures. During the aging process, periosteal expansion is necessary to maintain bone strength and also results in variation of adult bone width.[8] Although periosteal apposition occurs after menopause in women, it is not enough to counteract the endocortical resorption that occurs simultaneously. Increased remodeling intensity occurs during menopause, resulting in increased bone loss; the remodeling rate reduces the mineral content of bone tissue.

©Copyright 2021 American Academy of Orthopaedic Surgeons

In both sexes, trabecular bone loss begins in the 20s, whereas cortical bone is stable until midlife and then decreases. Studies using high-resolution peripheral quantitative CT (HRpQCT) have shown that over a lifetime, women lose bone volume principally due to loss of entire trabeculae, whereas men lose bone primarily due to trabecular thinning.[60] This has a significant impact on age-related changes in bone strength, because based on finite element modeling, reductions in trabecular number have a two- to fivefold greater impact on bone strength as compared with reductions in trabecular thickness that result in similar decreases in bone volume. In addition, HRpQCT studies have also demonstrated that the major effect of age on bone microarchitecture, independent of BMD by dual-energy x-ray absorptiometry (DXA), is on increasing cortical porosity. This may account for the DXA-independent effect of age on fracture risk.

Accurately estimating whole bone strength is critical for identifying individuals that may benefit from prophylactic treatments aimed at reducing fracture risk. Strength is often estimated from stiffness, but it is not known whether the relationship between stiffness and strength varies with age and sex. These results indicated that older bones tended to be significantly weaker for a given stiffness than younger bones. These results suggest that human bones exhibit diminishing strength relative to stiffness with aging and with decreasing postyield displacement (PYD).[61]

Bone's response to mechanical load is essential to maintaining skeletal integrity. A recent study revealed that deletion of a single allele of ß-catenin in mouse osteocytes stopped new bone formation in response to mechanical loads. It is currently understood that, as individuals age, the ability of the skeleton to respond to the stresses of mechanical load diminishes. The work demonstrated male and female differences that were more significant in females than in controls and that Wnt/ß--catenin signaling may be a central factor in the bone's response to mechanical loading.[62]

The chromosomal configuration (46 XY in males transitioning to females [transwomen] and 46 XX females transitioning to males [transmen]) remains unchanged when individuals chose to undertake sex-affirming therapies. Thus, these individuals also provide a unique opportunity to determine which metabolic functions are influenced by altering sex steroids, particularly bone quality. While studies of cardiovascular risk in both transmales and transfemales demonstrate a higher incidence of type 2 diabetes than the general population, hormone therapy has not been shown to have a negative effect on BMD. In transmen, masculinizing hormone therapy has not been associated with significant changes in BMD, while in transwomen feminizing hormone therapy has been associated with an increase at the lumbar spine.[63] The impact of these changes on patient-important outcomes, such as fracture risk, has yet to be determined.

SUMMARY

In summary, the many studies discussed in this chapter clearly demonstrate that genetic sex has a significant role in determining musculoskeletal health. This includes the susceptibility to disease and its severity, as well as to the effectiveness of therapeutic modalities. The effects of sex hormones are mediated by their receptors, which are present on both male and female cells, but the mechanisms involved may differ. Further complicating the actions of these hormones is the ability of the target cells to further metabolize serum hormones as well as to produce hormones locally, which is also mediated by sex-specific regulatory mechanisms. These mechanisms contribute to differential regulation of growth and development of muscle, bone, and cartilage, but they also influence sex-dependent immune modulation of these tissues in health and disease. It is clear that recognizing sex-related differences in all aspects of musculoskeletal health will be essential to accelerating improvements in patient-centered and precision medicine.

REFERENCES

1. Clayton JA: Applying the new SABV (sex as a biological variable) policy to research and clinical care. *Physiol Behav* 2018;187:2-5.
2. Tosi LL, Boyan BD, Boskey AL: Does sex matter in musculoskeletal health? The influence of sex and gender on musculoskeletal health. *J Bone Joint Surg Am* 2005;87(7):1631-1647.
3. Parsch J, Ellegren H: The evolutionary causes and consequences of sex-biased gene expression. *Nat Rev Genet* 2013;14(2):83-87.
4. Institute of Medicine (US) Committee on Understanding the Biology of Sex and Gender Differences , Wizemann TM, Pardue ML, ed: *Exploring the Biological Contributions to Human Health: Does Sex Matter?* Washington, DC, National Academy Press, 2001.
5. Collins FS, Tabak LA: Policy: NIH plans to enhance reproducibility. *Nature* 2014;505(7485):612-613.
6. Jepsen KJ, Bigelow EM, Schlecht SH: Women build long bones with less cortical mass relative to body size and bone size compared with men. *Clin Orthop Relat Res* 2015;473(8):2530-2539.
7. Nicolella DP, Bredbenner TL: Development of a parametric finite element model of the proximal femur using statistical shape and density modelling. *Comp Meth Appl Mech Eng* 2012;15:101-110.
8. Duren DL, Seselj M, Froehle AW, Nahhas RW, Sherwood RJ: Skeletal growth and the changing genetic landscape during childhood and adulthood. *Am J Phys Anthropol* 2013;150(1):48-57.
9. Seeman E: Periosteal bone formation – a neglected determinant of bone strength. *N Engl J Med* 2003;349:320-323.
10. Weaver CM, Gordon CM, Janz KF, et al: The National Osteoporosis Foundation's position statement on peak bone mass development and lifestyle factors: A systematic review and implementation recommendations. *Osteoporos Int* 2016;27:1281-1386.
11. Liu CT, Estrada K, Yerges-Armstrong LM, et al: Assessment of gene-by-sex interaction effect on bone mineral density. *J Bone Miner Res Oct* 2012;27(10):2051-2064.

©Copyright 2021 American Academy of Orthopaedic Surgeons

12. Chesi A, Mitchell JA, Kalkwarf HJ, et al: A genomewide association study identifies two sex-specific loci, at SPTB and IZUMO3, influencing pediatric bone mineral density at multiple skeletal sites. *J Bone Miner Res* 2017;32(6):1274-1281.
13. Kemp JP, Medina-Gomez C, Tobias JH, Rivadeneira F, Evans DM: The case for genome-wide association studies of bone acquisition in paediatric and adolescent populations. *BoneKEy Rep* 2016;5:796.
14. Xu S: Theoretical basis of the Beavis effect. *Genetics* 2003;165:2259-2268.
15. Specker B; Thiex NW; Sudhagoni RG: Does exercise influence pediatric bone? A systematic review. *Clin Orthop Relat Res* 2015;473:3658-3672.
16. McVeigh JA, Howie EK, Zhu K, Walsh JP, Straker L: Organized sport participation from childhood to adolescence is associated with bone mass in young adults from the raine study. *J Bone Miner Res* 2019;34(1):67-74.
17. Callewaert F, Sinnesael M, Gielen E, Boonen S, Vanderschueren D: Skeletal sexual dimorphism: Relative contribution of sex steroids, GH-IGF1, and mechanical loading. *J Endocrinol* 2010;207(2):127-134.
18. Nieves JW: Sex-differences in skeletal growth and aging. *Curr Osteoporos Rep* 2017;15(2):70-75.
19. Kot A, Zhong ZA, Zhang H, Lay YE, Lane NE, Yao W: Sex dimorphic regulation of osteoprogenitor progesterone in bone stromal cells. *J Mol Endocrinol* 2017;59(4):351-363.
20. Duren DL, Nahhas RW, Sherwood RJ: Do secular trends in skeletal maturity occur equally in both sexes? *Clin Orthop Relat Res* 2015;473:2559-2567.
21. Boeyer ME, Sherwood RJ, Deroche CB, Duren DL: Early maturity as the new normal: A century-long study of bone age. *Clin Orthop Relat Res* 2018;476(11):2112-2122.
22. Chumela WC, Roche AF, Thissen D: The FELS method of assessing the skeletal maturity of the hand-wrist. *Am J Hum Biol* 1989;1(2):175-183.
23. Duncan ST, Bogunovic L, Baca G, Schoenecker PL, Clohisy JC: Are there sex-dependent differences in acetabular dysplasia characteristics? *Clin Orthop Relat Res* 2015;473(4):1432-1439.
24. Sutton KM, Bullock JM: Anterior cruciate ligament rupture: Differences between males and females. *J Am Acad Orthop Surg* 2013;21(1):41-50.
25. Carter CO, Evans KA: Inheritance of congenital pyloric stenosis. *J Med Genet* 1969;6(3):233-254.
26. Kruse LM, Dobb MB, Gurnett CA: Polygenic threshold model with sex dimorphism in clubfoot inheritance: The carter effect. *J Bone Joint Surg Am* 2008;90:2688-2694.
27. Kruse LM, Buchan JG, Gurnett CA, Dobbs MB: Polygenic threshold model with sex dimorphism in adolescent idiopathic scoliosis: The carter effect. *J Bone Joint Surg Am* 2012;94:1485-1491.
28. Markle JG, Frank DN, Mortin-Toth S, et al: Sex differences in the gut microbiome drive hormone-dependent regulation of autoimmunity. *Science* 2013;339:1084-1088.
29. Hayter SM, Cook MC: Updated assessment of the prevalence, spectrum and case definition of autoimmune disease. *Autoimmun Rev* 2012;11:754-765.
30. Gubbels Bupp MR: Sex, the aging immune system, and chronic disease. *Cell Immunol* 2015;294(2):102-110.
31. Pace S, Sautebin L, Werz O: Sex-biased eicosanoid biology: Impact for sex differences in inflammation and consequences for pharmacotherapy. *Biochem Pharmacol* 2017;145:1-11.
32. Strand V, Rao SA, Shillington AC, Cifaldi MA, McGuire M, Ruderman EM: Prevalence of axial spondyloarthritis in United States rheumatology practices: Assessment of SpondyloArthritis International Society criteria versus rheumatology expert clinical diagnosis. *Arthritis Care Res* 2013;65:1299-1306.
33. Offner PJ, Moore EE, Biffl WL: Male gender is a risk factor for major infections after surgery. *Arch Surg* 1999;134(9):935-938.
34. Cook MB, Dawsey SM, Freedman ND, et al: Sex disparities in cancer incidence by period and age. *Cancer Epidemiol Biomarkers Prev* 2009;18(4):1174-1182.
35. Sisu AM, Stana LG, Petrescu CL, et al: On the bone tumors: Overview, classification incidence, histopathological issues, behavior and review using literature data. Histopathology-reviews and recent advances. *Intech Open Science* 2012;4:1-16.
36. Farach-Carson MC, Lin SH, Nalty T, Satcher RL: Sex differences and bone metastases of breast, lung, and prostate cancers: Do bone homing cancers favor feminized bone marrow? *Front Oncol* 2017;7:163.
37. Dunford A, Weinstock DM, Savova V, et al: Tumor-suppressor genes that escape from X inactivation contribute to cancer sex bias. *Nat Genet* 2017;49:10-16.
38. Larson NB, Fogarty ZC, Larson MC, et al: An integrative approach to assess X-chromosome inactivation using allele-specific expression with applications to epithelial ovarian cancer. *Genet Eidemiol* 2017;41:898-914.
39. Carè A, Bellenghi M, Matarrese P, Gabriele L, Salvioli S, Malorni W: Sex disparity in cancer: Roles of microRNAs and related functional players. *Cell Death Differ* 2018;25(3):477-485.
40. Jia L, Xi Q, Wang H, et al: Mir-142-5p regulates tumor cell PD-L1 expression and enhances anti-tumor immunity. *Biochem Biophys Res Commun* 2017;488:425-431.
41. Chaudhri RA, Olivares-Navarrete R, Cuenca N, Hadadi A, Boyan BD, Schwartz Z: Membrane estrogen signaling enhances tumorigenesis and metastatic potential of breast cancer cells via estrogen receptor-α36 (ERα36). *J Biol Chem* 2012;287(10):7169-7181.
42. Hunter SK: The relevance of sex differences in performance fatigability. *Med Sci Sports Exerc* 2016;48(11):2247-2256. Review.
43. Cruz-Jentoft AJ, Bahat G, Bauer J, et al: Sarcopenia: Revised European consensus on definition and diagnosis. *Age Ageing* 2019;48(1):16-31.
44. Anderson LJ, Liu H, Garcia JM: Sex differences in muscle wasting. *Adv Exp Med Biol* 2017;1043:153-197.
45. Carson JA, Manolagas SC: Effects of sex steroids on bones and muscles: Similarities, parallels, and putative interactions in health and disease. *Bone* 2015;80:67-78.
46. Wong RMY, Wong H, Zhang N, et al: The relationship between sarcopenia and fragility fracture—a systematic review. *Osteoporos Int* 2019;30(3):541-553.
47. Boyan BD, Tosi LL, Coutts RD, et al: Addressing the gaps: Sex differences in osteoarthritis of the knee. *Biol Sex Differ* 2013;4:4.
48. Hochberg MC, Cisternas MG, Watkins-Castillo SI: Osteoarthritis. The burden of musculoskeletal diseases in the United States. 2014;(4):1-6. Available at: https://www.boneandjointburden.org/fourthedition/iiib10/osteoarthritis. Accessed October 7, 2019.
49. Boyan BD, Hart DA, Enoka RM, et al: Hormonal modulation of connective tissue homeostasis and sex differences in risk for osteoarthritis of the knee. *Biol Sex Differ* 2013;4:3.
50. Nicolella DP, O'Connor MI, Enoka RM, et al: Mechanical contributors to sex differences in idiopathic knee osteoarthritis. *Biol Sex Differ* 2012;3:28.
51. Schmidt FM, Weschenfelder J, Sander C, et al: Inflammatory cytokines in general and central obesity and modulating effects of physical activity. *PLoS One* 2015;10(3):e0121971.
52. Wang T, He C: Pro-inflammatory cytokines: The link between obesity and osteoarthritis. *Cytokine Growth Factor Rev* 2018;44:38-50.
53. Sluka KA, Berkley KJ, O'Connor MI, et al: Neural and psychosocial contributions to sex differences in knee osteoarthritic pain. *Biol Sex Differ* 2012;3:26.
54. Greenspan JD, Craft RM, LeResche L, et al: Studying sex and gender differences in pain and analgesia: A consensus report. *Pain* 2007;132:S26-S45.
55. Paller CJ, Campbell CM, Edwards RR, Dobs AS: Sex-based differences in pain perception and treatment. *Pain Med* 2009;10(2):289-299.
56. Wright NC, Looker AC, Saag KG, et al: The recent prevalence of osteoporosis and low bone mass in the United States based on bone mineral density at the femoral neck or lumbar spine. *J Bone Miner Res* 2014;29(11):2520-2526.

©Copyright 2021 American Academy of Orthopaedic Surgeons

57. Clarke BL, Khosla S: Female reproductive system and bone. *Arch Biochem Biophys* 2010;503(1):118-128.

58. Hidayat K, Du X, Shi BM: Sex hormone-binding globulin and risk of fracture in older adults: Systematic review and meta-analysis of observational studies. *Osteoporos Int* 2018;29(10):2171-2180.

59. Orwoll ES, Lapidus J, Wang PY, et al: The limited clinical utility of testosterone, estradiol, and sex hormone binding globulin measurements in the prediction of fracture risk and bone loss in older men. *J Bone Miner Res* 2017;32(3):633-640.

60. Farr JN, Khosla S: Skeletal changes through the lifespan–from growth to senescence. *Nat Rev Endocrinol* 2015;11:513-521.

61. Patton DM, Bigelow EMR, Schlecht SH, Kohn DH, Bredbenner TL, Jepsen KJ: The relationship between whole bone stiffness and strength is age and sex dependent. *J Biomech* 2019;83:125-133.

62. Javaheri B, Stern AR, Lara N, et al: Deletion of a single β-catenin allele in osteocytes abolishes the bone anabolic response to loading. *J Bone Miner Res* 2014;29(3):705-715.

63. Wiepjes CM, de Jongh RT, de Blok CJ, et al: Bone safety during the first ten years of gender-affirming hormonal treatment in transwomen and transmen. *J Bone Miner Res* 2019;34(3):447-454.

The authors dedicate this chapter to Dr. Adele Boskey in recognition of her commitment to orthopaedic research and education. She was a treasured friend and colleague. Her outstanding contributions to science have provided fundamental knowledge on the mechanisms of mineralization and on the role that the mineral phase plays in the maintenance of bone quality. Adele's early recognition of the importance of the influence of sex on musculoskeletal health has been critical to the development of this chapter. She was an invaluable mentor for scientists, engineers, physicians, and dentists, as well as orthopaedic residents, fellows, and surgeons. As the first woman president of the Orthopaedic Research Society, as a member of the American Academy of Orthopaedic Surgeons, and as an active contributor to the Orthopaedic Research Foundation, Adele showed what leadership can and should be, not only for women, but for all of us who value excellence in this field we love.

©Copyright 2021 American Academy of Orthopaedic Surgeons

25

Metabolic Bone Diseases

Se-Min Kim, MD
Michael Pazianas, MD
Tony Yuen, PhD
Roy K. Aaron, MD
Mone Zaidi, MD, PhD

Keywords: *hyperparathyroidism; osteomalacia; osteoporosis; renal osteodystrophy*

INTRODUCTION

Orthopaedic surgeons need to have a fundamental understanding of the metabolic bone diseases discussed in this chapter because these diseases compromise bone strength and increase fracture risk, including fragility fractures. A considerable number of patients treated by orthopaedic surgeons, particularly in the population older than 50 years, are at risk for a metabolic bone disease, including those patients who seek elective orthopaedic care, such as joint replacement and spine surgery. Compromised bone strength can contribute to the failure of surgical fixation and stability of the implant-bone interface. Knowledge of the diagnostic modalities and pathophysiology will help orthopaedic surgeons take an active role in the diagnosis and treatment of these diseases and the avoidance of surgical complications.

Dr. Aaron or an immediate family member has received research or institutional support from Orthofix, Inc. and an immediate family member serves as a board member, owner, officer, or committee member of the Orthopaedic Research Society. Dr. Zaidi is a member of a speakers' bureau or has made paid presentations on behalf of Diachi Sankyo, GLG, and GuidePoint; serves as a paid consultant to or is an employee of Diachi Sankyo, GLG, and GuidePoint; and serves as a board member, owner, officer, or committee member of the Alliance of Academic Internal Medicine. None of the following authors or any immediate family member has received anything of value from or has stock or stock options held in a commercial company or institution related directly or indirectly to the subject of this chapter: Dr. Kim, Dr. Pazianas, and Dr. Yuen.

SYSTEMIC CALCIUM HOMEOSTASIS

Maintenance of serum calcium concentration is a homeostatic priority because cell membrane signaling and neuromuscular signal transmission are highly sensitive to serum and extracellular calcium concentrations. Cellular responses to several hormones, excitation-contraction coupling in cardiac muscle, and skeletal muscle contraction depend upon calcium concentrations within a narrow physiologic range. To accomplish this homeostatic priority, three organ systems, gastrointestinal, renal, and skeletal, the parathyroids, parathyroid hormone (PTH), and vitamin D ($1,25(OH)_2D$), interact in an elaborate series of physiologic mechanisms to regulate serum calcium concentration.[1] Vitamin D and PTH maintain the concentrations of ionized calcium and phosphate at levels consistent with normal neuromuscular function and within safe range of the solubility product of $CaHPO_4$.

Among the organs supporting serum calcium, bone is unique in that its role as a calcium donor can compromise its structure and lead to fracture. Among the physiologic roles of bone, its role as a calcium donor can take precedence over its structural roles leading to the perspective that the primary function of bone is as the calcium reservoir for serum calcium concentration. Because of the priority to maintain serum calcium concentration, needs for serum calcium or disorders of the integrated physiologic mechanisms to support serum calcium can lead to loss of calcium from bone characterized as metabolic bone diseases, loss of bone mass, structural failure, and fracture. A type of fracture seen with decreased bone density is the fragility fracture defined as a fracture due to a fall from a standing height or with minimal trauma.

©Copyright 2021 American Academy of Orthopaedic Surgeons

CALCIUM

Serum calcium exists in serum in two general forms—ionized and protein bound, binding usually to albumin. Calcium in the ionized form is metabolically active, essential to cell membrane signal transmission. Calcium can also be bound to phosphate in serum and the resulting salts are essential for healthy bone and tooth matrix. However, phosphate binding of calcium in the gastrointestinal tract can prevent calcium absorption and phosphate binding in the serum can exceed the solubility product of calcium phosphate. Decreased serum calcium concentration, due to deficiency or the extra needs of growth, pregnancy, or lactation, stimulates a concerted response by bone, kidney, and gastrointestinal tract, modulated by PTH and vitamin D, to restore and maintain calcium concentration in its physiologic homeostatic range. Elevated vitamin D and PTH stimulate renal tubular reabsorption of calcium, phosphate diuresis, increased intestinal absorption of calcium, and osteolysis. Under these conditions, bone mineral density and mechanical strength may be sacrificed to maintain serum calcium concentration.

VITAMIN D

Vitamin D derives from two sources, calciferol, the major dietary source, and cholecalciferol which derives from 7-dehydrocholesterol. Both are irradiated in the skin which opens their sterol ring structure. Both calciferol and cholecalciferol undergo two hydroxylation steps. The first takes place in the liver and adds a hydroxyl group to the 25 carbon position to form 25(OH)D which is the storage form of vitamin D and the metabolite usually measured in serum. The second hydroxylation step takes place in the kidney at either the 1 or 24 position in the sterol ring. The 1,25(OH)D form is much more metabolically active than is the 24,25(OH)D form. Which position is hydroxylated is largely under the control of PTH and calcium that result in hydroxylation in the 1 position under a hypocalcemic stimulus. The active form of vitamin D, calcitriol (1,25(OH)$_2$D), is a steroid hormone that plays a crucial role in calcium homeostasis, in which it acts to raise serum calcium concentration. It enhances intestinal calcium and phosphate absorption and suppresses PTH secretion. In the kidney, it promotes diuresis of phosphate and stimulates tubular reabsorption of calcium. In bone, it transfers calcium to serum.

PARATHYROID HORMONE

PTH is a peptide hormone secreted by the parathyroid glands under the control of serum ionized calcium concentration. Under conditions of low ionized serum calcium, PTH is secreted and, with intact renal parenchyma, stimulates the production of 1,25(OH)D. Together, these two hormones act to raise serum ionized calcium concentration by increasing the renal tubular reabsorption of calcium, increasing calcium absorption in the small bowel, and mobilizing calcium from bone. PTH also reduces serum phosphate concentration by decreasing the tubular reabsorption of phosphate and promoting a phosphate diuresis. The consequences for bone are decreased mineral density and structural weakness to withstand physiologic stresses. Homeostatic mechanisms are less efficient in responding to hypercalcemia.[2]

KIDNEY

The kidney influences calcium homeostasis by controlling calcium and phosphate diuresis by tubular reabsorption of minerals. Diffusible calcium passes through the glomeruli and both PTH and vitamin D modulate the relative extents of tubular reabsorption of both minerals. Another important contribution of the kidney to calcium homeostasis is the second hydroxylation step of vitamin D. Under the influence of PTH, the second hydroxylation takes place at the 1 position in the sterol ring and results in the much more physiologically active 1,25(OH)D. In these ways, the kidney participates in a feedback loop that acts to raise serum calcium concentration under a hypocalcemic stimulus. Conditions that interfere with the kidney's role in calcium homeostasis can do so through (1) loss of renal parenchyma that results in a failure of the second hydroxylation of vitamin D to its active form and (2) tubular dysfunction resulting in a loss of calcium in the urine (diuresis) exerting a downward pressure on serum calcium concentration. Reductions in both active vitamin D and calcium availability stimulate secondary hyperparathyroidism that results in bone resorption and low bone mineral density.

GASTROINTESTINAL TRACT

Dietary intake of calcium varies widely. Absorption of calcium is regulated by vitamin D and PTH, both of which promote intestinal absorption to raise serum calcium. As vitamin D is fat soluble, it is dependent on intact bile salts for absorption in the proximal duodenum and proximal jejunum. Upper gastrointestinal disorders that interfere with fat digestion and absorption, notably, biliary and pancreatic disorders, can limit vitamin D absorption leading to deficiency.

BONE

Peak bone mass is attained in the third decade of life. Thereafter is a steady loss of bone mineral density (BMD) with an accelerated loss after menopause. Conditions that interfere with the attainment of peak bone mass, such as dietary deficiencies, anorexia, athletic amenorrhea, etc. can lead to age-associated osteoporosis in the later years of life. Physiologic needs for serum calcium that are unmet by other physiologic mechanisms place a downward stress on the calcium reservoir function of bone, leading to skeletal mineral depletion and reducing BMD and bone strength.

©Copyright 2021 American Academy of Orthopaedic Surgeons

Four groups of metabolic bone diseases can lead to decreased bone density—osteoporosis, osteomalacia, renal osteodystrophy, and hyperparathyroidism.[2]

FRACTURE RISK ASSESSMENT AND DIAGNOSIS OF LOW BONE DENSITY

Fractures, especially hip fractures, not only cause mortality and morbidity, but also significantly increase health care costs. In 2005, $17 billion was spent for more than two million fractures in the United States, and the cost is expected to increase.[3] As a fracture is a multifactorial event, it is imperative to assess both skeletal integrity—bone quantity and quality—and the risk of falls when estimating fracture risk. All postmenopausal women, and men aged 50 years or older, should be screened for the risk of osteoporosis. Important clinical risk factors include age ≥65 years, early menopause (age ≤45 years), prior history of fracture, history of parents having a fracture, and a history of malnutrition or eating disorder during adolescence and puberty that potentially prevents the attainment of peak bone mass. Lifestyle factors such as smoking and excessive alcohol intake can also impair bone strength. Attention has been called to the role of falls in fracture risk[4] (**Figure 1**). Many medical conditions and medications can contribute to falls particularly those resulting in visual deficits, such as glaucoma and cataracts, dehydration, postural hypotension, or loss of balance (**Table 1**).

High-risk patients for osteoporosis and fracture (eg, women ≥65 years, men ≥70 years, or younger patients with significant risk factors) should be tested for low bone density.

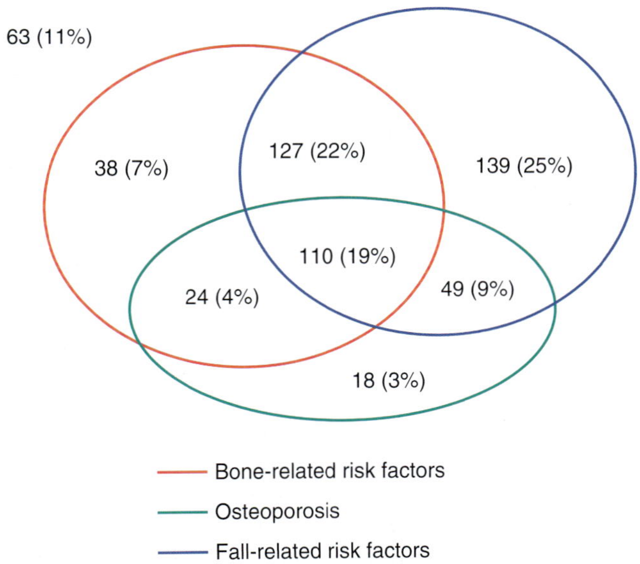

FIGURE 1 Illustration demonstrating the interactions of falls and low bone density in the fracture diathesis. Bone-related and fall-related risk factors interact with low bone density contributing to fractures. (Data from van Helden S, van Geel AC, Geusens PP, et al: Bone and fall-related fracture risks in women and men with a recent clinical fracture. *JBJS* 2008;90[2]:241-248.)

TABLE 1 Risk Factors for Fracture

Bone-Related Risk Factors	Fall-Related Risk Factors
• Fracture history	• > 1 fall last year
• Mother with fracture history	• Psychoactive drugs
• Body mass index (BMI) < 19	• Low level of activities of daily living
• Severe immobility	• Articular symptoms
• Glucocorticoids	• Impaired vision
	• Urinary incontinence
	• Parkinson Disease

Adapted from van Helden S, van Geel AC, Geusens PP, et al: Bone and fall-related fracture risks in women and men with a recent clinical fracture. *JBJS* 2008;90(2):241-248.

The most common method of assessment is dual-energy x-ray absorptiometry (DEXA) in which soft tissue is extracted from the density analysis. Bone mineral density (BMD) is expressed in g/cm^2 and is a planar rather than a volumetric measurement. BMD measured at any skeletal site is a strong predictor of hip or vertebral fracture. The Z-score compares density to an age- and sex-matched cohort; the T-score compares density to a reference group at age 20 years. The current diagnosis of low bone density and decision for treatment are often based on the T-score. Based on World Health Organization criteria, a T-score of −1.0 or above is considered normal, between −1.0 and −2.5 as osteopenia, preferably termed low bone mass, and −2.5 or below is categorized as "osteoporosis." Low BMD in the range of osteopenia or osteoporosis does not indicate a specific disease entity because DEXA does not discriminate between osteoporotic and osteomalacic bone structure. Metabolic bone histopathology can be highly characteristic and often diagnostic (**Figure 2**).

There are a number of helpful tools to assess fracture risk. Among them, the Fracture Risk Assessment Tool, or FRAX, is the most commonly used in clinical practice because it is well validated in large cohort studies and freely available (www.sheffield.ac.uk/FRAX/). FRAX predicts 10-year risks of hip fracture and major osteoporotic fractures (eg, spine, hip, proximal humerus, and distal forearm fracture) using easily accessible clinical risk factors for osteoporosis together with femoral neck bone mineral density in the FRAX calculation.

Measuring BMD using DEXA has inherent limitations because it measures areal BMD (aBMD, g/cm^2) not volumetric BMD (vBMD, g/cm^3). Patients with a smaller bone size, such as women or short individuals, can have lower aBMD despite having the same vBMD compared with age-matched counterparts. Additionally, artifacts from vertebral fractures, arthritic and degenerative changes (eg, sclerosis, osteophytes, osteochondrosis, etc), scoliosis, vascular calcification, laminectomy, and poor positioning can mislead clinicians with spuriously high or low results.

Importantly, DEXA does not assess bone quality, such as geometry, microarchitecture, trabecular connectivity, or bone turnover, which are critical determinants of bone strength. For that reason, large cohort studies have shown that skeletal health

©Copyright 2021 American Academy of Orthopaedic Surgeons

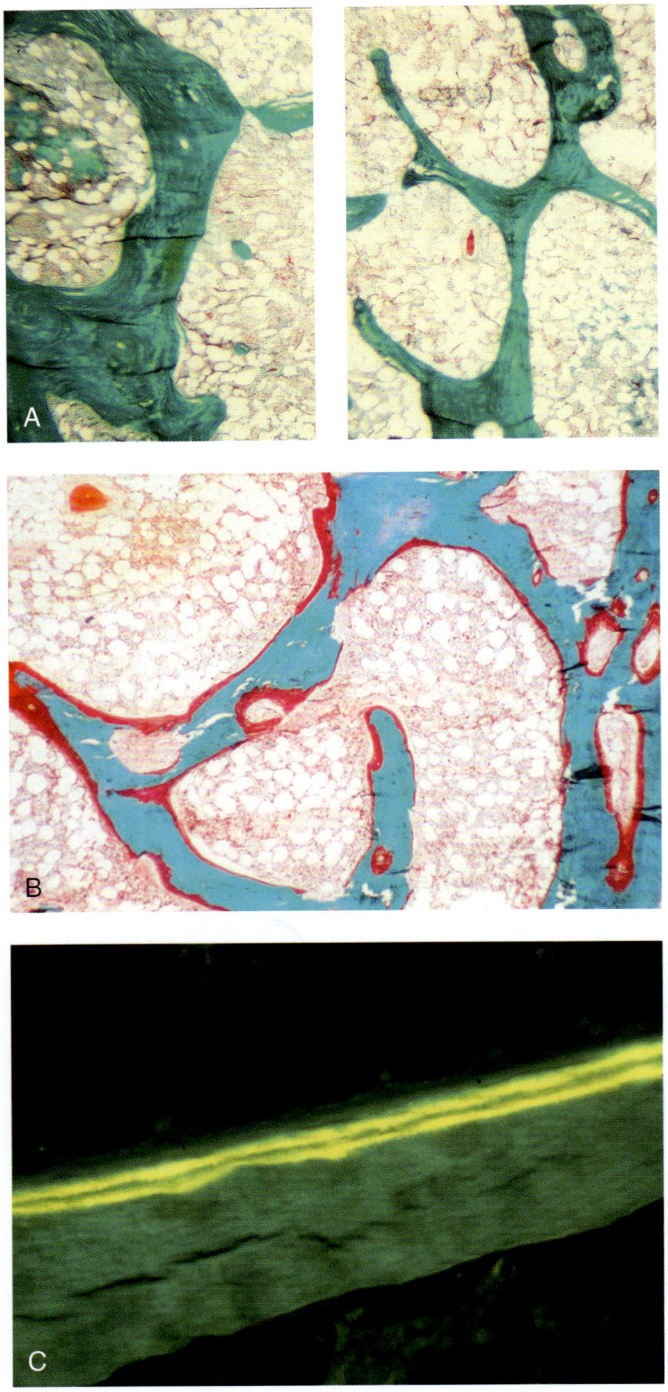

FIGURE 2 Metabolic bone histopathology. **A**, Trabecular morphology. (Left) Normal bone volume and trabecular thickness; (right) low bone volume (density) and thin discontinuous trabeculae. **B**, Osteoid borders. Trichrome stain demonstrating unmineralized osteoid (red) on trabecular surfaces. **C**, Mineralization front. Double tetracycline label is incorporated into the calcification front, fluoresces under ultraviolet light, and reveals the rate of bone formation.

assessment based on BMD alone underestimates the risk of fracture. The Manitoba Bone Density Program cohort showed that more than 60% of fractures in postmenopausal females occurred with normal BMD or low bone mass.[5] Importantly, patients with type 2 diabetes have significantly high risks of fracture despite having normal or even high BMD.[6]

MEASURING BONE QUALITY

Advances in imaging techniques and bioengineering allow the study of bone quality parameters without invasive bone biopsy (**Table 2**). Trabecular bone scoring (TBS) is an indirect measurement of trabecular bone structure. This software analyzes conventional DEXA lumbar spine images and quantifies grayscale values of each pixel. Dense trabecular structure yields high TBS scores, whereas porous trabecular bone produces a low TBS score. TBS has been validated in postmenopausal women and in older men.[7]

Quantitative ultrasonography (QUS) measures the attenuation of sound waves and the speed of sound through bone tissue and provides information on mechanical properties such as bone stiffness and elasticity. QUS of the calcaneus predicted the risk of osteoporotic fractures and discriminated between patients with or without fragility fractures.[8]

CT-based technologies are capable of assessing skeletal microarchitecture. A reconstructed three-dimensional image of femur or vertebra from low-resolution quantitative volumetric CT (QCT) provides not only vBMD but also geometry and structure. vBMD using QCT has demonstrated better predictive value than aBMD in postmenopausal women receiving long-term glucocorticoids.[9] However, measuring axial bone density using QCT is associated with significant radiation exposure compared with DEXA. High-resolution peripheral QCT (HR-pQCT) has a high spatial resolution up to ~40 μm (thickness of a single trabeculae is 100 to 150 μm and of the cortex is ~500 μm) and separately examines cortical and trabecular compartments. Trabecular connectivity and cortical porosity can be assessed.[10] Evaluating the cortical component provides

TABLE 2 Techniques for Measuring Material Properties of Bone

Techniques	Parameters
• DEXA with trabecular bone Scoring	• DEXA quantifies bone density • TBS assesses trabecular microarchitecture of the lumbar spine
• Quantitative ultrasonography	• Quantifies bone mechanics
• Quantitative CT	• Assesses bone microarchitectures
• High-resolution peripheral QCT	• Assesses microarchitecture and cortical porosity
• Indentation testing	• Measures resistance to plastic deformation

DEXA = dual energy x-ray absorptiometry, TBS = trabecular bone scoring, QCT = quantitative volumetric CT

©Copyright 2021 American Academy of Orthopaedic Surgeons

important insight in understanding the pathophysiology of secondary osteoporosis. For example, patients with type 2 diabetes have normal or high trabecular bone density, but significantly increased cortical porosity that might explain the increased risk of fracture in this group.[11] The major drawback of HR-pQCT is that it examines only peripheral appendicular bone.

Indentation testing permits studying the material properties of bone. A rigid indenter with a depth-sensing indenter tip applies a determined force into smooth and flat areas of interest (tibial midshaft). The resulting impression quantifies resistance to plastic deformation and characterizes mechanical properties with an order of individual trabeculae and osteons. With a higher spatial resolution, nanoindentation can examine bone structures as small as individual lamellae and lacunae (~1 μm).[12]

OSTEOPOROSIS

Osteoporosis is the most common cause of low bone density and is associated with low energy or, fragility, fractures. In the United States alone, 40 million adults suffer from osteoporosis or low bone density.[13] Osteoporosis is characterized by low bone volume, endosteal resorption, cortical thinning and increased porosity, and trabecular thinning and loss of connectivity (**Figure 3**). Deterioration of bone microarchitecture significantly reduces bone strength and increases the risk of fracture. Radiographically, trabecular resorption is characteristic and endosteal resorption is seen as widening of the medullary canal (**Figure 4**).

Once osteoporosis is diagnosed, possible secondary causes should be sought and treated. Vitamin D deficiency (discussed below) is very common and can be diagnosed by measuring the storage form of vitamin D, (25(OH)D). Other conditions can result in low bone density and mimic osteoporosis including prominently the endocrine disorders, hyperparathyroidism,

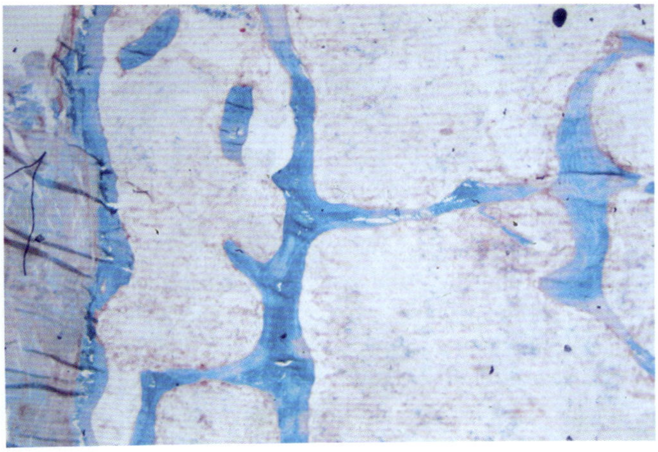

FIGURE 3 Histologic image of osteoporosis histology. Osteoporotic bone exhibits low bone volume, cortical thinning, and thin, discontinuous trabeculae.

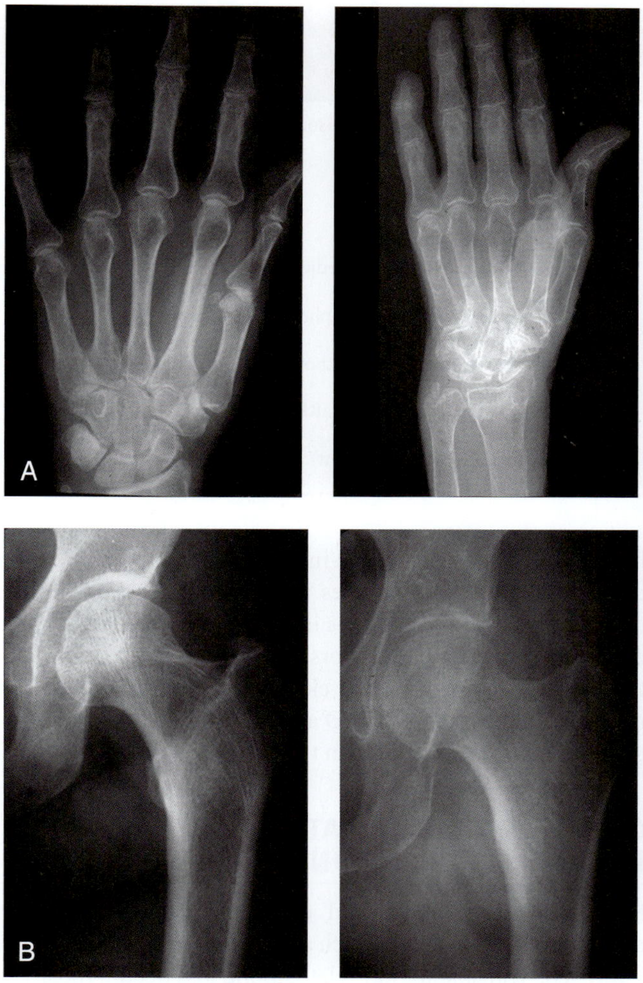

FIGURE 4 Radiographs of osteoporotic bone (**A**) Hand. In normal bone, the two cortices of the third metacarpal of should occupy about ½ the width of the bone (left). Osteoporotic bone exhibits endosteal resorption of the cortices and widening of the medullary canal (right). An incidental distal radius fracture is seen. **B**, Hip. In the normal proximal femur, thick cortices and well-defined trabeculae are seen (left). In the osteoporotic proximal femur, trabeculae are not distinct due to resorption (right).

hypercortisolism, hyperthyroidism, diabetes, and hypogonadism. A variety of other conditions including premature menopause, anorexia nervosa, athletic amenorrhea, immobilization, and alcohol abuse can also result in osteoporosis. Other, more rare conditions that include osteoporosis are discussed in Chapter 25. Medications can also contribute to osteoporosis (**Table 3**). Important conditions associated with low bone mass are hormonal therapies, organ transplantation, and immunosuppression.

HORMONAL THERAPY

Adjuvant hormonal therapy for prostate or breast cancer can significantly decrease BMD and increase the risk of fracture. Androgen deprivation treatment using gonadotropin-releasing

©Copyright 2021 American Academy of Orthopaedic Surgeons

TABLE 3 Medications Contributing to Osteoporosis

• Glucocorticoids (≥5 mg/d prednisone or equivalent for ≥3 mo)
• Proton pump inhibitors
• Heparin
• Oral hypoglycemics: thiazolidinedione, SGLT-2 inhibitors
• Anticonvulsants: phenobarbital, phenytoin, carbamazepine
• Immune-modulating agents: methotrexate, tacrolimus, cyclosporine
• Hormonal suppressive agents: GnRH, aromatase inhibitors, tamoxifen
• Thyroid hormone (over treatment)

hormone agonist/antagonists in patients with prostate cancer decreases BMD and increases fracture risk. Loss of bone is noted in multiple skeletal sites including trabecular and cortical bone.[14] Aromatase inhibitors used for breast cancer deprive the skeleton of estrogen and elevate follicle-stimulating hormone (FSH), decreasing BMD and increasing the risk of fracture compared with tamoxifen treatment.[15]

ORGAN TRANSPLANTATION AND IMMUNOSUPPRESSION

End-stage organ failure and organ transplantation-related osteoporosis have gained much attention as survival rates have improved. Transplantation related bone loss occurs mostly in the first 3 to 6 months post-transplant. A significant decline in lumbar spine BMD has been observed (6.8%) during the first 6 months after renal transplantation, which accounts for most of the bone loss (8.8%) over 18 months. BMD in the radial shaft did not show significant bone loss within 6 months,[16] suggesting that trabecular bone is more affected than is cortical bone during the initial posttransplantation period. This acute, rapid and severe bone loss after renal transplantation is caused by multiple factors, including immunosuppressant-induced bone loss, immobilization, vitamin D deficiency, preexisting osteodystrophy, and hyperparathyroidism.[17]

The pattern of acute, rapid, and severe bone loss is also notable in orthotopic liver transplantation.[18] As expected, the decrements in BMD in transplant patients pose a significant risk of fracture that is especially high in the early posttransplant period.[19]

Pretransplant BMD and duration of use of glucocorticoids are the key determinants of the high risk of fracture. Glucocorticoids reduce bone formation primarily by inhibiting osteoblast differentiation and cause apoptosis of osteocytes. Another group of commonly used immunosuppressants, calcineurin inhibitors such as cyclosporine (CsA) and tacrolimus (FK506), also negatively affect bone. They inhibit the activity of the enzyme, calcineurin, which is expressed in osteoblasts and osteoclasts and plays a key role in bone remodeling. Inhibiting calcineurin resulted in increased bone resorption and trabecular bone loss in in vivo study.[20] Patients with cyclosporine monotherapy showed increased osteoclastic activity and decreased osteoblastic bone formation based on histomorphometry.[21] The mammalian target of rapamycin (mTOR) inhibitor, rapamycin, is considered safer, as it does not show significant bone loss compared with cyclosporine.[22] Another immunosuppressant, mycophenolate mofetil (MMF), did not cause bone loss measured by histomorphometric parameters but suppressed osteocalcin levels.[23]

OSTEOPOROSIS PHARMACOTHERAPIES

In osteoporosis, the balance of bone homeostasis favors bone resorption, resulting in bone loss. Therefore, the initial goal is to slow down accelerated resorptive activity with antiresorptive agents and thus restore homeostatic balance of bone formation and resorption to prevent further bone loss. Osteoporosis, however, is characterized by microstructural damage. Therefore, repairing the structural defects is the next goal and anabolic agents, intermittent parathyroid hormone (PTH) administration and PTH-related peptide (PTH-rP) analogue, have reparative effects on bone microarchitecture.

Calcium and Vitamin D Supplements

The importance of vitamin D and calcium for bone health is well established, and deficiencies should be corrected before pharmacotherapy for osteoporosis. Although controversial, the routine use of vitamin D and calcium supplementation has recently been questioned because of a possible increased risk of cardiovascular disease with high calcium intake. Current guidelines advise 1,200 mg of calcium daily (total diet plus supplement) and 800 IU of vitamin D daily for postmenopausal women with osteoporosis.

Estrogen

Estrogens are important in maintaining skeletal homeostasis during growth and development and bone mass during adulthood. Loss of estrogens at menopause causes increased bone remodeling rates and bone loss. Indirectly, estrogens affect the differentiation of osteoclasts by reducing the actions of the receptor activator of nuclear factor-κβ (RANK) system. At menopause, the RANK-RANK ligand (RANKL) system is overactive which stimulates osteoclast development and activity and results in accelerated bone loss. It takes several years for the imbalance caused by the loss of estrogens to reach a new steady state and the rapid bone loss to subside.[24] Hormone replacement therapy had been the mainstay of therapy of postmenopausal osteoporosis for many years but the findings of the Women's Health Initiative study in 2002 marginalized their use. Estrogen with progesterone in women with an intact uterus has been associated with increased risk of breast cancer and cardiovascular events including heart attack and stroke. The use of estrogen alone in women who have had a hysterectomy showed a significantly decreased risk for breast cancer, but the

©Copyright 2021 American Academy of Orthopaedic Surgeons

risk of cardiovascular disease and venous thromboembolism (VTE) persisted. Both estrogen with progesterone and estrogen alone showed a clear reduction in fracture risk from 30% to 70% depending upon anatomic site.[25] While estrogens are effective in relieving menopausal symptoms and preventing perimenopausal bone loss, their use as first-line therapy in osteoporosis is no longer recommended from the risk-benefit perspective.[26]

Selective Estrogen Receptor Modulators

Selective estrogen receptor modulators (SERMs) are a diverse group of compounds with tissue-specific estrogen receptor agonist or antagonist activity; they are agonists to bone while being antagonists to breast. They decrease bone loss as well as the risk of breast cancer in women. The first SERM developed specifically for osteoporosis treatment was raloxifene, an estrogen agonist in bone and liver. It does not stimulate the endometrium and is a potent antagonist in the breast. In the large Multiple Outcomes of Raloxifene Evaluation (MORE) trial, eight years' follow-up of a total of 7,705 women demonstrated significant increases in BMD at the spine and hip and a significant reduction in vertebral fractures.[27] Their main drawback is perimenopausal symptoms such as hot flashes and an increased risk of VTE.

Diphosphonates

Diphosphonates are the first line of treatment for osteoporosis. Diphosphonates are analogues of pyrophosphate, bind to the surface of hydroxyapatite crystals in bone, and inhibit osteoclastic bone resorption. Their antiresorptive action results from both their affinity for bone mineral and their inhibitory effect on osteoclasts. Not all diphosphonates operate through the same mechanisms. Non-nitrogen-containing diphosphonates such as etidronate or clodronate act as metabolized cytotoxic molecules in the osteoclast that cause loss of mitochondrial membrane potential and apoptosis. Clodronate has been used mainly in the treatment of bone metastases. Nitrogen-containing diphosphonates, such as alendronate, risedronate, ibandronate, and zoledronate are currently used as the first-line treatment for osteoporosis. When internalized by the osteoclast, these compounds inhibit farnesyl diphosphonate synthase, interfering with the formation of the "ruffled border" of osteoclasts that is necessary for forming resorptive pits where bone resorption occurs.[28]

Randomized controlled trials have shown that alendronate (Fosamax), risedronate (Actonel), and zoledronate (Reclast) reduce the risk of vertebral, nonvertebral, and hip fractures, whereas ibandronate (Boniva) showed antifracture efficacy only at vertebral sites.[14,29,30] This difference arises primarily from trial design and the study population. Alendronate and risedronate are available in oral form only; zoledronate is available for intravenous use only; and ibandronate in both forms. Although diphosphonates share several common properties as a drug class, there are chemical, biochemical, and pharmacological differences among them in binding affinities for bone mineral, which may influence their distribution within bone, potency, and duration of action. These differences may be clinically relevant in terms of the onset of fracture reduction, efficacy at different skeletal sites, and the degree and duration of reduction of bone turnover. For example, diphosphonates with higher binding affinity and potential retention, such as alendronate and zoledronate, are associated with greater reduction of bone turnover with longer residual effect after discontinuation. In patients who were treated with alendronate for 5 years, bone turnover markers remained reduced, well below premenopausal levels, for up to 5 years after discontinuation. Following a single infusion of zoledronate, bone turnover markers were suppressed for three or more years. However, in patients treated with a lower binding affinity diphosphonate, such as risedronate, bone turnover markers returned to pretreatment levels within 1 year after discontinuation. No clinical trials have directly compared the clinical efficacy of individual diphosphonates with fractures as an end point.

Diphosphonates are highly effective and safe. GI intolerance (oral diphosphonates), renal impairment (IV diphosphonates), and acute-phase reactions, particularly after the first IV administration, are common. Rare events such as osteonecrosis of the jaw and atypical femur fractures (AFFs) have generated concern although a mechanistic association with diphosphonates has not been fully established. The American Society of Bone and Mineral Research (ASBMR) defined AFFs as stress fractures with specific characteristic radiographic findings. The fracture may have a localized periosteal or endosteal thickening, or an incomplete fracture, of the lateral cortex. The completed fracture is located in the femoral diaphysis, originating at the lateral cortex with a transverse orientation and is noncomminuted.[31] Although the absolute risk of AFFs with diphosphonate use is minimal, the association of prolonged diphosphonate use and an increased risk of AFFs is clear. The age-adjusted incidence rates were 1.78/100,000 per year with less than a 2-year treatment compared with rates of 113.1/100,000 per year with treatment for 8 to 9.9 years.[32] Although antifracture efficacy of the short-term (3 year) diphosphonate treatment clearly outweighs the risk of AFFs, benefit beyond 5 years of diphosphonate use is not clearly shown mainly due to limited long-term data. In 2016, the ASMBR task force offered guidance for long-term diphosphonates and "drug holiday" in terms of risk/benefit assessment. The optimal duration of treatment should be based on individualized fracture risk. The optimal duration of a "drug holiday" has not been clearly defined.[33]

Denosumab

Denosumab (Prolia) is the first drug targeting RANK/RANKL/OPG signaling pathway that controls osteoclast differentiation. Denosumab is a human monoclonal antibody that acts as a "decoy" receptor for RANKL. It blocks RANK-RANKL interaction and thereby inhibits the differentiation and activation of osteoclasts. However, it lacks the bone selectivity of the diphosphonates. In the Fracture Reduction Evaluation of Denosumab in Osteoporosis every 6 Months (FREEDOM)

©Copyright 2021 American Academy of Orthopaedic Surgeons

phase III clinical trial, including 7,808 postmenopausal women with osteoporosis, denosumab significantly reduced vertebral, nonvertebral, and hip fractures by 68%, 20%, and 40%, respectively, compared with placebo. Further studies involving over 12,000 patients have confirmed the efficacy and overall safety of denosumab out to 10 years of treatment. Denosumab also increased BMD at the total hip, femoral neck, and lumbar spine and reduced markers of bone turnover to a significantly greater extent than did oral diphosphonates in women who were naïve to diphosphonates or had switched from alendronate to denosumab.[9] However, anabolic claims for denosumab have not been confirmed in histomorphometric studies from postmenopausal women with osteoporosis treated with either denosumab or teriparatide.[34] The effects of denosumab rapidly reverse on discontinuation,[35] so that ensuring compliance is important if benefits are to be sustained.

Unlike diphosphonates that are cleared intact through the kidneys, the clearance of denosumab is not dependent on renal function. Rare cases of osteonecrosis of the jaw and AFFs have been described in patients on denosumab, although, like diphosphonates, no clear mechanism has been uncovered. In the FREEDOM study, serious infections leading to hospitalization were reported more frequently in the denosumab than in the placebo group. Serious skin infections, as well as endocarditis, and infections of the abdomen, urinary tract, and ear, were more frequent in patients treated with denosumab. It is thus prudent to avoid denosumab in patients on concomitant immunosuppressant agents or with impaired immune systems, who may themselves be at increased risk for serious infection.[9]

Calcitonin

Calcitonin is a hormone secreted by the C cells of the thyroid gland. It acts directly on the osteoclast and causes a change in its shape and structure and temporarily ceases its resorptive activity. The injectable form, initially used for the treatment of Paget disease, has been replaced by a nasal spray. The antifracture effects are weak in osteoporotic patients and its use has been superseded by more effective treatments. Recent studies with oral calcitonin have also proved disappointing.[36]

Parathyroid Hormone and Parathyroid Hormone-Related Peptide

Parathyroid hormone 1 to 34, teriparatide (Forteo) and the recently approved PTH-rP analogue, abaloparatide (Tymlos), are the only anabolic agents for osteoporosis treatment. Teriparatide is a recombinant PTH consisting of the first (N-terminus) 34 amino acids, which is the bioactive portion of the hormone. Osteoblasts and preosteoblasts express PTH1R, the receptor for PTH, which is also expressed in renal tubular cells in kidney. Intermittent daily administration of PTH stimulates bone formation at a greater rate than bone resorption, resulting in a net anabolic effect on bone. The anabolic effect of PTH leads to bone formation in cortical and trabecular compartments and reconnection of disrupted trabeculae.

Teriparatide

In osteoporotic women with a history of fractures, daily subcutaneously administered teriparatide decreased the risk of vertebral and nonvertebral fractures and increased the vertebral, femoral, and total body BMD with a median duration of 21 months of treatment. Compared with the placebo group, a 20 μg regimen increased BMD at the lumbar spine by 9% and at the femoral neck by 3%; BMD at the distal radius did not change. Significant improvements in trabecular bone microarchitecture have also been observed. The bone formation marker, N-terminal propeptide of type 1 collagen (P1NP), peaked between 6 and 12 months followed by a plateau at significantly above baseline levels up to 36 months. There was a rise in circulating carboxyl-terminal collagen cross-links (CTX) in later stages suggesting bone resorption. However, two-year histomorphometric data showed that the increase in both resorption and formation in later stage is still anabolic. The "anabolic window" (the period of time when the actions of PTH are maximally anabolic) remains open for at least 2 years.[37] The maximum recommended treatment course is 24 months because of the concern of the risk of osteosarcoma. Rats administered teriparatide at doses 60 times higher than in humans with subcutaneous doses of 20 μg developed osteosarcoma. However, with over 15 years of postmarketing experience and millions of prescriptions, there has been no evidence of an increased clinical risk. At the end of the 2-year course, the patient should be switched to an antiresorptive.

Abaloparatide

Abaloparatide, a PTH-rP analogue, was approved in 2017 by the FDA for the treatment of postmenopausal women with high-risk osteoporosis. It shares 76% amino acid sequence identity with human PTH-rP (1 to 34) and 41% with human PTH (1 to 34). Abaloparatide binds to PTH1R with high selectivity resulting in transient stimulation of the receptor.[38] This leads to greater overall anabolic effect than teriparatide. Daily subcutaneous administration of abaloparatide for 18 months significantly reduced the risk of new vertebral and nonvertebral fractures compared with placebo in a randomized controlled trial (ACTIVE trial). Treatment with abaloparatide was also associated with modestly higher BMD gains, including sites rich in cortical bone, compared with the placebo and teriparatide groups. This is likely due an increased rate of bone mineralization compared with teriparatide. The incidence of hypercalcemia was lower with abaloparatide than with teriparatide. Overall, there were no differences in serious adverse events between the treatment groups.[39] The recommended dosage is 80 μg subcutaneous injection once daily. Like teriparatide, the recommended cumulative use of abaloparatide is limited to 2 years.

Combination and Sequential Treatments

The treatment of osteoporosis is a long process, and many patients will require treatment with more than one type of drug over their lifetime. To date, no substantial evidence

©Copyright 2021 American Academy of Orthopaedic Surgeons

supports the long-term efficacy of the existing treatments. Clinical decision making, therefore, raises several considerations. Which drugs should be used first for treatment and is there any preferred sequence? Also, will any of the drugs interfere with the action of the next? Furthermore, can drugs be used concurrently? As a monotherapy, diphosphonates are the recommended first choice. Denosumab could be considered in certain circumstance such as renal impairment. Recent reports caution against transitioning patients from denosumab to teriparatide because of a notable decline in BMD at the radius and hip. By contrast, when patients on teriparatide are switched to denosumab, BMD continues to increase.[40] Following discontinuation of denosumab, administration of a diphosphonate is recommended to prevent new vertebral fractures.

In summary, diphosphonates only maintain the structure of bone including any accumulated structural or material faults. However, their bone selectivity and effectiveness in reducing the risk of fractures, together with their low cost, has established them as the first line of treatment for osteoporosis. The osteoanabolics, teriparatide and abaloparatide, increase new bone formation, but there is a combined 2-year limit in their use, and the cost remains a consideration. Based on long-term efficacy and safety profile, denosumab has become an attractive option especially for patients with renal impairment. However, compliance is crucial as the rebound risk of fracture was noted with any lapse.

Antiresorptive Drugs and Fracture Healing

There have been concerns that antiresorptive drugs might impair fracture healing, but this has not been borne out in practice. Several animal models showed no impairment of fracture healing unless very high doses of drugs were used. Furthermore, in the major clinical studies with the antiresorptive drugs, there has been no evidence of delayed fracture healing or malunion.[41] Indeed, there is no early stage in fracture healing in which antiresorptive drugs would be expected to act. It is only during the later stages of remodeling of the calcified callus that one would expect antiresorptive drugs to have an impact. In contrast to these concerns, several studies suggested that diphosphonates might enhance fracture repair by stabilizing the fracture callus.

OSTEOMALACIA AND RICKETS

Undermineralized, newly formed bone is the hallmark of both osteomalacia and rickets. On radiographs, bones appear osteopenic and stress fractures with radiodense lines adjacent to regions of radiolucency (called Looser zones or pseudofractures) appear on the concave sides of long bones[42] (**Figure 5**). Characteristic hip fractures resembling slipped femoral capital epiphyses are often present in advanced cases (**Figure 6**). On technetium bone scintigraphy, stress fractures are visible as hot spots (**Figure 7**). In cases of strong clinical suspicion of osteomalacia and negative radiological findings, bone biopsy is diagnostic. It shows widening of osteoid seams due to the lack of mineralization and smudging of tetracycline labels from the slow mineralization rate (**Figure 8**). Deficiencies in calcium or vitamin D represent the prototype of the disease. Vitamin D deficiency leads to malabsorption of calcium and phosphate, resulting in osteomalacia in adults and rickets in children. According to the National Health and Nutrition

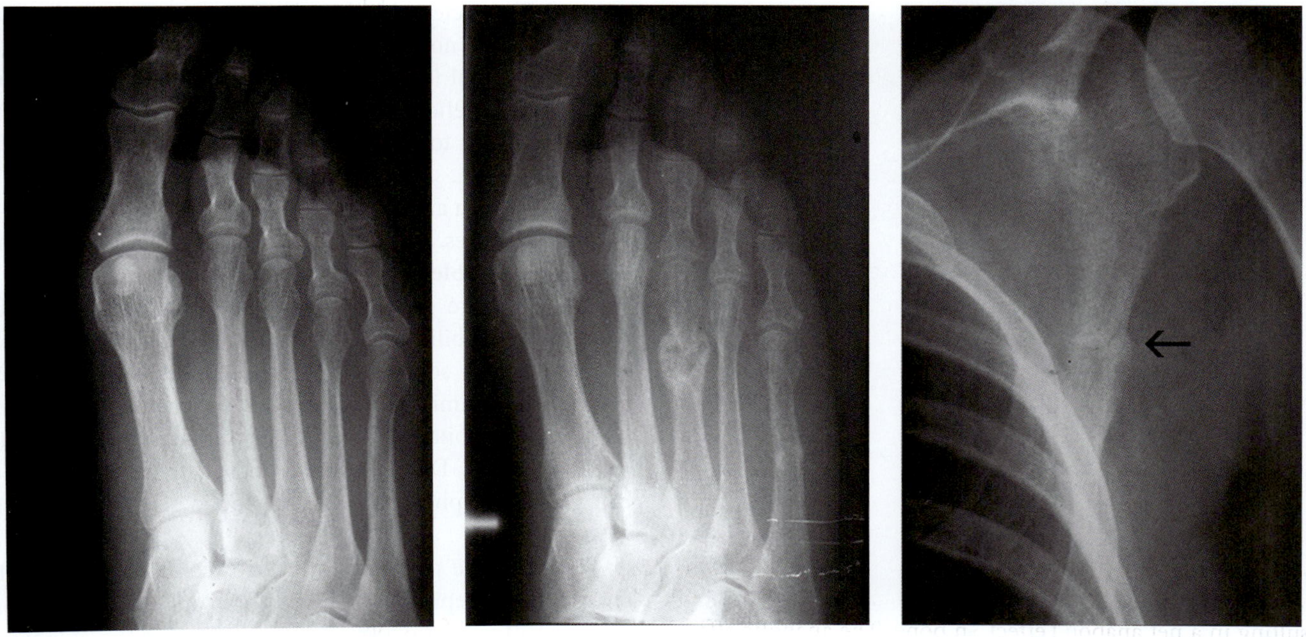

FIGURE 5 Radiographs of stress fractures in osteomalacia. Stress fractures may be seen in osteomalacia that maybe more apparent in the healing phase (left and middle) and on concave bone surfaces known as Looser lines (arrow) (right).

©Copyright 2021 American Academy of Orthopaedic Surgeons

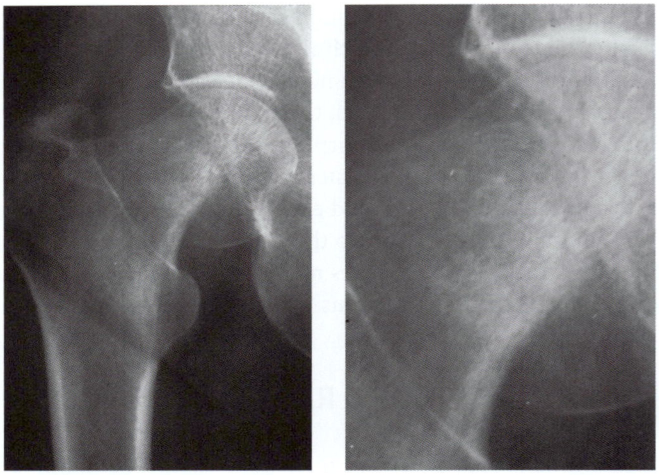

FIGURE 6 Radiographs of osteomalacic hip fractures. Hip fractures in osteomalacic bone may resemble slipped femoral capital epiphyses. They may present with chronic rather than acute bone pain, and deformity may progress over time.

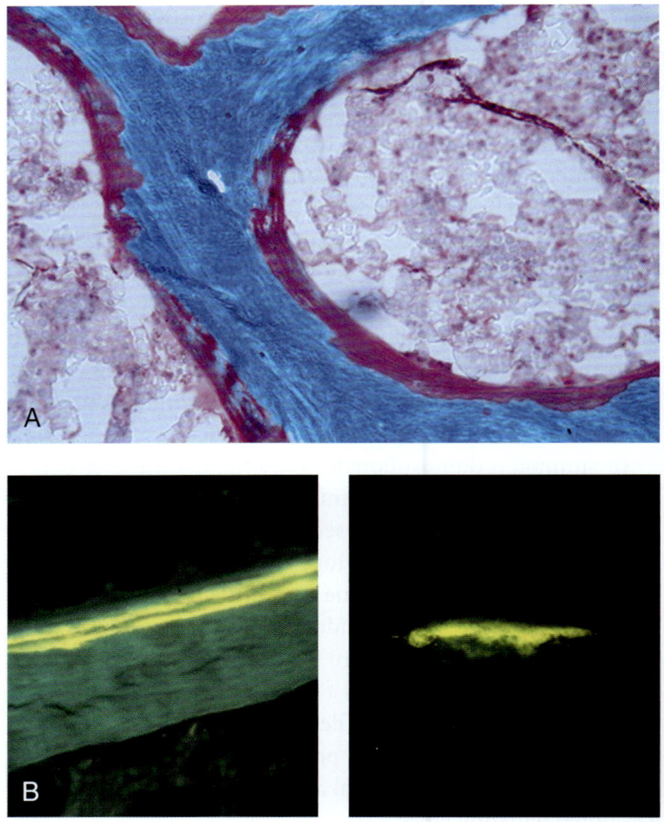

FIGURE 8 Histology and mineralization front in osteomalacia. **A**, Trichrome stain demonstrating unmineralized osteoid borders (red) rimming the length of trabeculae. **B**, In contrast to well-defined bands of double tetracycline labeling in normal bone (left), osteomalacic bone exhibits only a smudge of tetracycline uptake reflecting deficient mineralization (right).

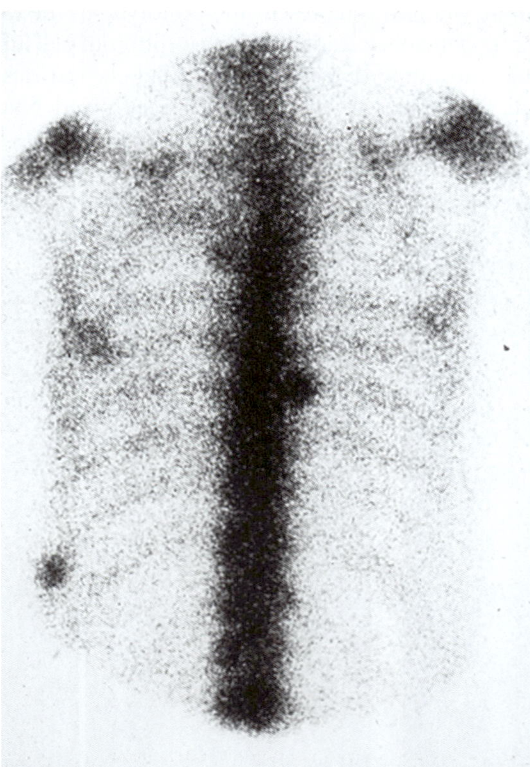

FIGURE 7 Bone scan in osteomalacia. Technetium bone scan demonstrating increased uptake at sites of multiple rib fractures in osteomalacia.

Examination Survey (NHANES) 2005 to 2006 data, the overall prevalence rate of vitamin D deficiency (defined as a serum 25-hydroxyvitamin D [25(OH)D] concentrations ≤20 ng/mL [50 nmol/L]) was 41.6%, with the highest rate seen in blacks (82.1%), followed by Hispanics (69.2%).[43] The diagnosis of vitamin D deficiency is based on measurements of serum 25(OH)D and not on the active metabolite, $1,25(OH)_2D$, which is normal (or high) in most patients. Several criteria for vitamin D deficiency have been proposed, but at this time, the consensus is to supplement vitamin D if serum values are below 30 ng/mL.

Osteomalacia and vitamin D deficiency can be induced by secondary causes. More common causes of osteomalacia are presented in **Table 4**. The most common secondary causes of osteomalacia are gastrointestinal disorders including celiac disease, hepatobiliary, and pancreatic disease, short bowel syndrome, and some bariatric procedures causing malabsorption of vitamin D; medications such as the anticonvulsants phenobarbital, phenytoin, and carbamazepine can alter hepatic vitamin D metabolism; phosphate-binding antacids can cause hypophosphatemia, metabolic acidosis, and renal osteodystrophy.

Rickets is the pediatric form of osteomalacia. In rachitic children whose epiphyseal plates are still open, defective chondrocyte differentiation and mineralization of the epiphyseal plate are pathophysiologic hallmarks. The lack of mineralization in the provisional zone of calcification results in physeal

©Copyright 2021 American Academy of Orthopaedic Surgeons

TABLE 4 Rare Causes of Osteomalacia

Deficiency	Calcium Vitamin D
Absorptive	Gastric Biliary Enteric
Renal tubular	
Renal osteodystrophy	

Adapted from Mankin HJ: Metabolic bone disease. *JBJS* 1994;76(5):760-788.

cupping and widening and metaphyseal flaring (**Figure 9**). Undermineralization of growing bones can lead to frontal skull bossing, enlarged costochondral junctions (the rachitic rosary), bowing of long bones, and delayed eruption of permanent teeth. Furthermore, in addition to increased fracture risk, bone pain in the legs with proximal muscle weakness and gait instability can be present, together with frequent falling, delayed age of standing or walking, and delayed growth. Hypocalcemic seizures and tetanic spasms in the first year of life may be the initial manifestation of rickets.[44] The diagnosis of nutritional rickets is made on the basis of history, physical examination, and biochemical testing and is confirmed by radiographs. The typical biochemical profile includes low 25(OH)D, low to low-normal serum calcium and phosphate and urinary calcium. PTH, alkaline phosphatase activity, and urine phosphate are usually elevated. However, biochemistry alone cannot differentiate whether the primary cause is vitamin D or dietary calcium deficiency because combined deficiencies are common.

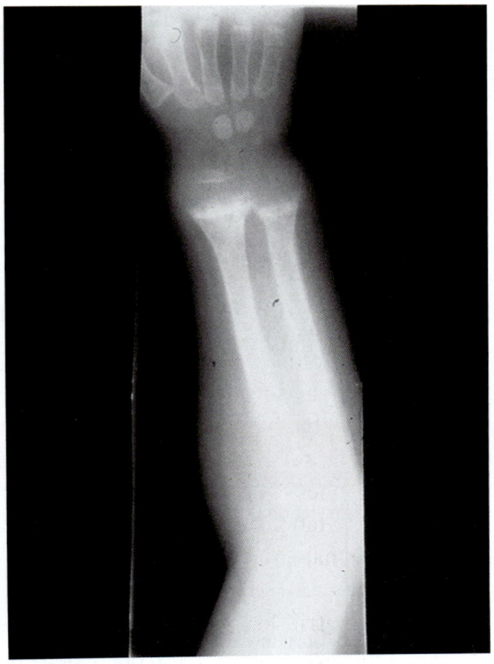

FIGURE 9 Epiphyseal plate in rickets. Radiograph of rachitic epiphyseal plate in the distal radius exhibiting cupping, flaring, and metaphyseal widening associated with deficient mineralization.

Treatment is correction of the vitamin D deficiency. In the United States, the Endocrine Society Clinical Practice Guidelines recommend the use of either vitamin D2 (ergocalciferol) or vitamin D3 (cholecalciferol) for the treatment and prevention of vitamin D deficiency. They suggest that all adults who are vitamin D deficient be treated with 50,000 IU of vitamin D2 or vitamin D3 once a week for 6 to 8 week or its equivalent of 5,000 IU of vitamin D2 or vitamin D3 daily to achieve a blood level of 25(OH)D above 30 ng/mL, followed by maintenance therapy of 1,000 to 2,000 IU/d.[45]

PRIMARY HYPERPARATHYROIDISM

Primary hyperparathyroidism is a common endocrine disorder of calcium metabolism characterized by hypercalcemia and elevated concentrations of parathyroid hormone. Most cases occur from a solitary adenoma on one of the four parathyroid glands (80% of cases) or as a multiple gland disorder (15% to 20% of cases). Typically, there are four parathyroid glands, located on the back of the thyroid gland. The presence of a fifth parathyroid gland, usually in the mediastinum, is not uncommon (2% and 6%); parathyroid cancer is rare (<1%).[46]

Elevated serum calcium found in routine biochemical testing of otherwise asymptomatic individuals is the most common presentation. More than half of patients with primary hyperparathyroidism are detected in patients older than 50 years. The disease is mostly sporadic, without a personal or family history of primary hyperparathyroidism or other endocrinopathies.[46] In primary hyperparathyroidism, elevated PTH is associated with elevated serum calcium (except the cases of normocalcaemic primary hyperparathyroidism), bone alkaline phosphatase activity, and a low or low-normal serum phosphate level. Both calcium and phosphate levels are elevated in the urine (**Table 5**). Although vitamin D deficiency is common with primary hyperparathyroidism, active $1,25(OH)_2D$ is close to the upper end of the normal range or elevated. Clinically, the identification of patients with primary hyperparathyroidism at the asymptomatic phase has changed

TABLE 5 Hyperparathyroidism

Physiology	Clinical
1,25 dihydroxy vitamin D production in kidney	
Increase in intestinal calcium absorption	↑ Serum calcium
Increase in tubular reabsorption of calcium	↓ urine calcium
Decrease in tubular reabsorption of phosphate	↑ urine phosphate
Bone resorption	↓ bone density

©Copyright 2021 American Academy of Orthopaedic Surgeons

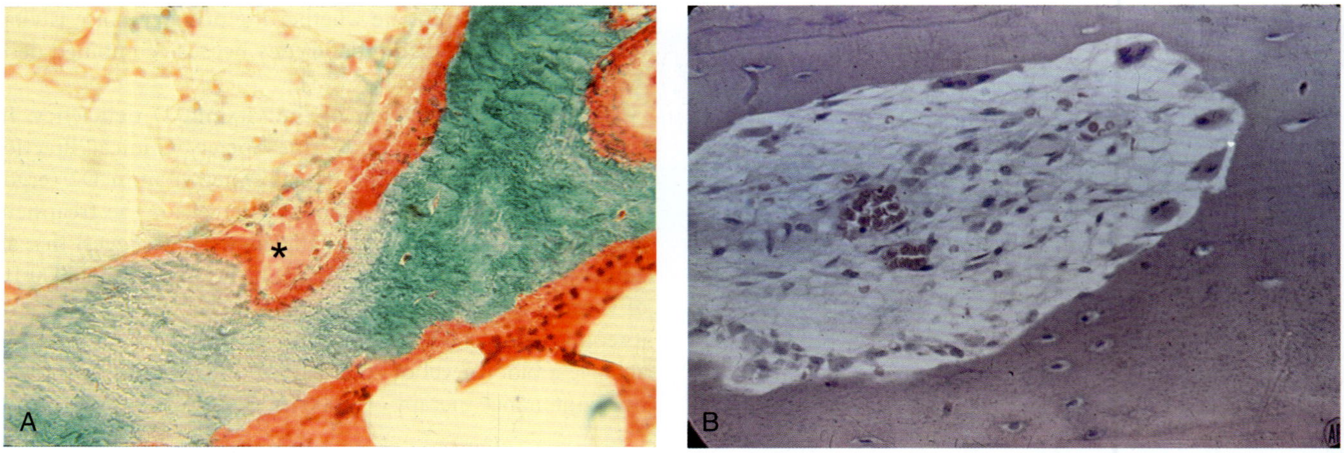

FIGURE 10 Histology of bone resorption in hyperparathyroidism. **A**, Hyperparathyroidism creates porosity in bone by indirectly stimulating osteoclastic resorption (asterisk). **B**, Osteoclastic "cutting cones" create tunneling and porosity.

the clinical phenotype of the disease, and today, fewer patients suffer from severe complications, such as nephrolithiasis or osteitis fibrosa cystica, hallmarks of the skeletal involvement, at the time of the diagnosis. When increased porosity is observed, it is the result of osteoclastic bone resorption (**Figure 10**). Demineralization of bones is mostly cortical, and the radiological features of osteitis fibrosa cystica include salt and pepper degranulation of the skull, tapering of the distal clavicle, subperiosteal resorption of the distal phalanges, bone cysts, and brown tumors. These radiological features can be associated with fractures, skeletal deformities, and bone pain.[46] In advanced cases, there is the risk of proximal muscle weakness, peptic ulcer disease, pancreatitis, hypertension, and atherosclerotic heart disease.

Treatment can be supportive only if patients are asymptomatic, vitamin D levels are within normal range, and hypercalcemia is mild without skeletal or renal involvement. For these patients, an annual assessment of serum calcium and 24-hour urine calcium/creatinine, and BMD measurements every 1 to 2 years is recommended. Symptomatic patients, however, should undergo surgical excision of the parathyroid gland with the adenoma, or excision of 3.5 glands in cases of the hyperplastic glands. After treatment, BMD gradually improves, but it can take several years for complete recovery to occur.[47]

RENAL OSTEODYSTROPHY (CHRONIC KIDNEY DISEASE–MINERAL BONE DISORDER)

Renal osteodystrophy consists of osteomalacia and secondary hyperparathyroidism and refers to alterations in bone morphology associated with chronic kidney disease. Loss of renal parenchyma leads to several physiologic changes affecting bone (**Table 6**). Loss of renal function unifies a spectrum of disparate bone disorders including secondary hyperparathyroidism or osteitis fibrosa (a high-turnover bone disease), osteomalacia (defective mineralization), mixed renal osteodystrophy (hyperparathyroid bone disease with a superimposed mineralization defect), and adynamic bone disease (diminished bone formation and resorption) (**Figure 11**).

The currently used term "Chronic Kidney Disease–Mineral and Bone Disorder (CKD–MBD)" describes the broader clinical syndrome encompassing mineral, bone, and calcific cardiovascular abnormalities that develop as a complication of chronic kidney disease. The term renal osteodystrophy has been used exclusively to define the bone pathology associated with chronic kidney disease.[48] The histologic examination is the benchmark and provides type and severity of the bone disease. However, bone biopsy is invasive and, therefore, not commonly done. Bone radiographs can be useful in demonstrating abnormal bone texture and subperiosteal resorption in the fingers, particularly in the radial side of the middle phalanx of the index and middle fingers in osteitis fibrosa cystica (**Figure 12**). Patchy osteosclerosis is also common and accounts for the classic appearance of "rugger jersey" spine (ie, horizontal bands of alternating intensity) and the "salt and pepper" appearance of the skull. However, radiologic features appear late, so individuals with quite marked secondary

TABLE 6 Renal Osteodystrophy

1. Failure of second hydroxylation (1-α hydroxylation) of vitamin D in the kidney
2. Hyperphosphatemia decreases serum calcium
3. Both decrease calcium absorption from the intestine
4. The result is hypocalcemia, hyperphosphatemia, and hypocalciuria which lead to secondary hyperparathyroidism

©Copyright 2021 American Academy of Orthopaedic Surgeons

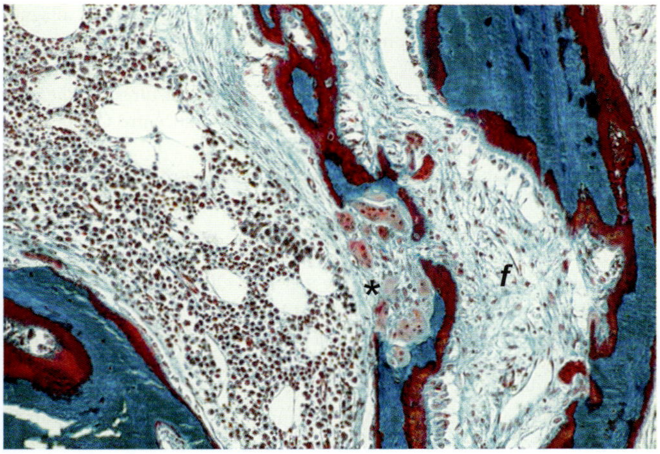

FIGURE 11 Histology in renal osteodystrophy. Osteitis fibrosa cystica comprised of (1) mineralization failure demonstrated by increased osteoid borders (red), (2) secondary hyperparathyroidism with osteoclastic resorption (asterisk), and (3) peritrabecular fibrosis ("f").

hyperparathyroidism may have normal radiographs. The most common phenotype, adynamic or "aplastic" bone disease, is characterized by reduced bone turnover. Many factors contribute to this disease: aging, underlying diabetes, phosphate binders, diphosphonates, and uremia. Aluminum-induced osteomalacia was prevalent when aluminum-containing phosphate binders were used, but currently is relatively infrequent[49] (**Figure 13**).

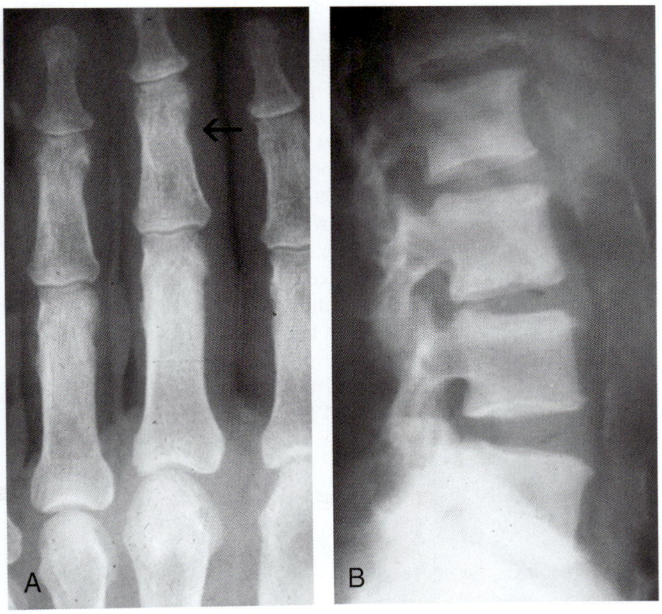

FIGURE 12 Radiographs in renal osteodystrophy. **A**, Subperiosteal resorption of the middle phalanx (arrow). **B**, Focal paradoxical sclerosis manifested by vertebral end plate density termed "rugger jersey spine."

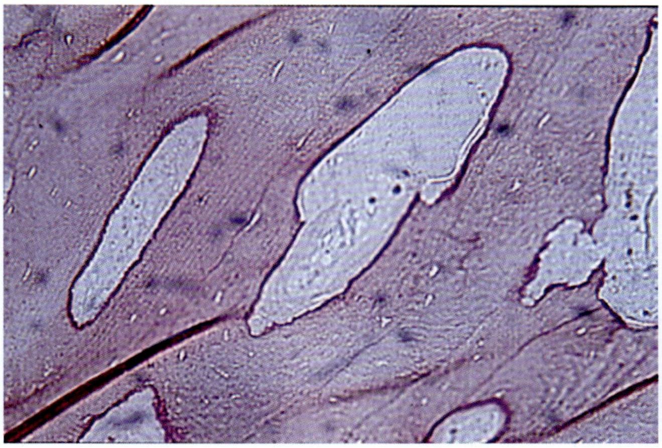

FIGURE 13 Histology of aluminum-associated osteomalacia in renal bone disease. Aluminum deposition (pink stain) at the mineralization front preventing mineralization of osteoid.

REFERENCES

1. Mankin HJ: Rickets, osteomalacia, and renal osteodystrophy. Part II. *J Bone Joint Surg Am Vol* 1974;56(2):352-386.
2. Mankin HJ: Metabolic bone disease. *JBJS* 1994;76(5):760-788.
3. Budhia S, Mikyas Y, Tang M, Badamgarav E: Osteoporotic fractures: A systematic review of U.S. Healthcare costs and resource utilization. *PharmacoEconomics* 2012;30(2):147-170.
4. van Helden S, van Geel AC, Geusens PP, et al: Bone and fall-related fracture risks in women and men with a recent clinical fracture. *JBJS* 2008;90(2):241-248.
5. Port L, Center J, Briffa NK, et al: Osteoporotic fracture: Missed opportunity for intervention. *Osteoporos Int* 2003;14(9):780-784.
6. McLellan A, Reid DM, Forbes K, et al: *Effectiveness of Strategies for the Secondary Prevention of Osteoporotic Fractures in Scotland (CEPS 99/03)*. Scotland, NHS Quality Improvement, 2004.
7. Edwards BJ, Bunta AD, Simonelli C, et al: Prior fractures are common in patients with subsequent hip fractures. *Clin Orthop Relat Res* 2007;461:226-230.
8. Black DM, Cummings SR, Karpf DB, et al: Randomised trial of effect of alendronate on risk of fracture in women with existing vertebral fractures. Fracture Intervention Trial Research Group. *Lancet* 1996;348(9041):1535-1541.
9. Cummings SR, San Martin J, McClung MR, et al: Denosumab for prevention of fractures in postmenopausal women with osteoporosis. *N Engl J Med* 2009;361(8):756-765.
10. Torgerson DJ, Bell-Syer SE: Hormone replacement therapy and prevention of nonvertebral fractures: A meta-analysis of randomized trials. *J Am Med Assoc* 2001;285(22):2891-2897.
11. Ettinger B, Black DM, Mitlak BH, et al: Reduction of vertebral fracture risk in postmenopausal women with osteoporosis treated with raloxifene: Results from a 3-year randomized clinical trial. Multiple Outcomes of Raloxifene Evaluation (MORE) Investigators. *J Am Med Assoc* 1999;282(7):637-645.
12. McClung MR, Geusens P, Miller PD, et al: Effect of risedronate on the risk of hip fracture in elderly women. Hip Intervention Program Study Group. *N Engl J Med* 2001;344(5):333-340.
13. Reginster J, Minne HW, Sorensen OH, et al: Randomized trial of the effects of risedronate on vertebral fractures in women with established postmenopausal osteoporosis. Vertebral Efficacy with Risedronate Therapy (VERT) Study Group. *Osteoporos Int* 2000;11(1):83-91.

©Copyright 2021 American Academy of Orthopaedic Surgeons

14. Harris ST, Watts NB, Genant HK, et al: Effects of risedronate treatment on vertebral and nonvertebral fractures in women with postmenopausal osteoporosis: A randomized controlled trial. Vertebral Efficacy With Risedronate Therapy (VERT) Study Group. *J Am Med Assoc* 1999;282(14):1344-1352.
15. Neer RM, Arnaud CD, Zanchetta JR, et al: Effect of parathyroid hormone (1-34) on fractures and bone mineral density in postmenopausal women with osteoporosis. *N Engl J Med* 2001;344(19):1434-1441.
16. Black DM, Delmas PD, Eastell R, et al: Once-yearly zoledronic acid for treatment of postmenopausal osteoporosis. *N Engl J Med* 2007;356(18):1809-1822.
17. Lyles KW, Colón-Emeric CS, Magaziner JS, et al: Zoledronic acid in reducing clinical fracture and mortality after hip fracture. *N Engl J Med* 2007;357:nihpa40967.
18. Khan SA, de Geus C, Holroyd B, Russell AS: Osteoporosis follow-up after wrist fractures following minor trauma. *Arch Intern Med* 2001;161(10):1309-1312.
19. Juby AG, De Geus-Wenceslau CM: Evaluation of osteoporosis treatment in seniors after hip fracture. *Osteoporos Int* 2002;13(3):205-210.
20. Meadows LM, Mrkonjic LA, O'Brien MD, Tink W: The importance of communication in secondary fragility fracture treatment and prevention. *Osteoporos Int* 2007;18(2):159-166.
21. Singh S, Foster R, Khan KM: Accident or osteoporosis?: Survey of community follow-up after low-trauma fracture. *Can Fam Physician* 2011;57(4):e128-e133.
22. Davis JC, Ashe MC, Guy P, Khan KM: Undertreatment after hip fracture: A retrospective study of osteoporosis overlooked. *J Am Geriatr Soc* 2006;54(6):1019-1020.
23. Ashe MC, McKay HA, Janssen P, Guy P, Khan KM: Improving osteoporosis management in at-risk fracture clinic patients. *J Am Geriatr Soc* 2005;53(4):727-728.
24. Byszewski A, Lemay G, Molnar F, Azad N, McMartin SE: Closing the osteoporosis care gap in hip fracture patients: An opportunity to decrease recurrent fractures and hospital admissions. *J Osteoporos* 2011;2011:404969.
25. Petrella RJ, Jones TJ: Do patients receive recommended treatment of osteoporosis following hip fracture in primary care? *BMC Fam Pract* 2006;7:31.
26. Hamel ME, Sebaldt RJ, Siminoski K, et al: Influence of fracture history and bone mineral density testing on the treatment of osteoporosis in two non-academic community centers. *Osteoporos Int* 2005;16(2):208-215.
27. Hajcsar EE, Hawker G, Bogoch ER: Investigation and treatment of osteoporosis in patients with fragility fractures. *CMAJ (Can Med Assoc J)* 2000;163(7):819-822.
28. Khandwala HM, Kolla N, Grover VK: Evaluation and treatment of osteoporosis in patients with a fragility hip fracture. *Endocr Pract* 2005;11(6):370-375.
29. International Osteoporosis Foundation: *Capture the Fracture: A Global Campaign to Break the Fragility Fracture Cycle*, Nyon, 2012.
30. Elliot-Gibson V, Bogoch ER, Jamal SA, Beaton DE: Practice patterns in the diagnosis and treatment of osteoporosis after a fragility fracture: A systematic review. *Osteoporos Int* 2004;15(10):767-778.
31. Giangregorio L, Papaioannou A, Cranney A, Zytaruk N, Adachi JD: Fragility fractures and the osteoporosis care gap: An international phenomenon. *Semin Arthritis Rheum* 2006;35(5):293-305.
32. Bessette L, Ste-Marie LG, Jean S, et al: The care gap in diagnosis and treatment of women with a fragility fracture. *Osteoporos Int* 2008;19(1):79-86.
33. Fraser LA, Ioannidis G, Adachi JD, et al: Fragility fractures and the osteoporosis care gap in women: The Canadian Multicentre Osteoporosis Study. *Osteoporos Int* 2011;22(3):789-796.
34. Leslie WD, Brennan SL, Prior HJ, et al: The post-fracture care gap among Canadian First Nations peoples: A retrospective cohort study. *Osteoporos Int* 2012;23(3):929-936.
35. Leslie WD, Giangregorio LM, Yogendran M, et al: A population-based analysis of the post-fracture care gap 1996–2008: The situation is not improving. *Osteoporos Int* 2012;23(5):1623-1629.
36. Metge CJ, Leslie WD, Manness LJ, et al: Postfracture care for older women: Gaps between optimal care and actual care. *Can Fam Physician* 2008;54(9):1270-1276.
37. Papaioannou A, Kennedy CC, Ioannidis G, et al: The osteoporosis care gap in men with fragility fractures: The Canadian Multicentre Osteoporosis Study. *Osteoporos Int* 2008;19(4):581-587.
38. Perreault S, Dragomir A, Desgagné A, et al: Trends and determinants of antiresorptive drug use for osteoporosis among elderly women. *Pharmacoepidemiol Drug Saf* 2005;14(10):685-695.
39. Vanasse A, Dagenais P, Niyonsenga T, et al: Bone mineral density measurement and osteoporosis treatment after a fragility fracture in older adults: Regional variation and determinants of use in Quebec. *BMC Musculoskelet Disord* 2005;6:33.
40. Marsh D, Akesson K, Beaton DE, et al: Coordinator-based systems for secondary prevention in fragility fracture patients. *Osteoporos Int* 2011;22(7):2051-2065.
41. Akesson K, Marsh D, Mitchell PJ, et al: Capture the fracture: A Best Practice Framework and global campaign to break the fragility fracture cycle. *Osteoporos Int* 2013;24(8):2135-2152.
42. U.S. Department of Health and Human Services: *Bone Health and Osteoporosis: A Report of the Surgeon General*. Rockville, MD, U.S. Department of Health and Human Services, Office of the Surgeon General, 2004.
43. Tosi LL, Gliklich R, Kannan K, Koval KJ: The American Orthopaedic Association's "own the bone" initiative to prevent secondary fractures. *J Bone Joint Surg Am* 2008;90(1):163-173.
44. American Orthopaedic Association: *Own the Bone Website*. 2012. Available at: http://www.ownthebone.org/. Accessed January 17, 2012.
45. American Academy of Orthopaedic Surgeons and American Association of Orthopaedic Surgeons: *Position Statement: Recommendations for Enhancing the Care of Patients With Fragility Fractures*. 2003. Available at: http://www.aaos.org/about/papers/position/1159.asp. Accessed December 10, 2012.
46. Eisman JA, Bogoch ER, Dell R, et al: Making the first fracture the last fracture: ASBMR task force report on secondary fracture prevention. *J Bone Miner Res* 2012;27(10):2039-2046.
47. National Bone Health Alliance: *NBHA Secondary Fracture Prevention Initiative*. 2013. Available at: http://www.nbha.org/projects/secondary-fracture-prevention-initiative. Accessed February 4, 2013.
48. International Society for Fracture Repair: *Osteoporotic Fracture Campaign*. 2011. Available from: http://www.fractures.com/about_ofc.html. Accessed October 28, 2011.
49. NSW Government Health: *NSW Model of Care for Osteoporotic Refracture Prevention*. Chatswood, NSW Agency for Clinical Innovation Musculoskeletal Network, 2011.

©Copyright 2021 American Academy of Orthopaedic Surgeons

26

Rare Genetic Bone Diseases of Orthopaedic Significance

Charit Taneja, MD
Tony Yuen, PhD
Jameel Iqbal, MD, PhD
Maria New, MD
Roy K. Aaron, MD
Mone Zaidi, MD, PhD
Se-Min Kim, MD

Keywords: *genetic skeletal disorder; rare bone disease; skeletal dysplasia*

INTRODUCTION

"Rare diseases" are defined by the Orphan Drug Act of 1983 as any disease or condition that affects less than 200,000 persons in the United States.[1] Of these, rare genetic skeletal diseases (or skeletal dysplasias) constitute a group of heterogeneous bone disorders arising from a defect in the complex processes of skeletal development, modeling, and remodeling. Due to the emergence of next-generation sequencing, namely whole genome sequencing, whole exome sequencing, and RNAseq, and bioinformatics, the once-undiagnosed diseases have now been characterized and better understood. The undiagnosed disease network (UDN phase 1) reported diagnoses in 35% of previously undiagnosed diseases, of which 10% presented with musculoskeletal phenotype. Seventy-four percent of diagnoses were made by newly found genetic information. Importantly, these new diagnoses led to a change in therapeutic plan in 21% of the all referred cases, and 31 new syndromes were discovered.[2]

New genetic information and careful phenotyping have together allowed genetic skeletal disorders to be organized into 42 groups based on the 2015 revision of nosology and classification of genetic skeletal disorders.[3] The broad categorization of the disease is due to heterogeneity of clinical phenotype, incomplete penetrance, and the limitation in sorting diseases based on metabolic phenotype (metabolomics). To simplify and provide practical clinical guidance, the Skeletal Rare Disease Working Group of International Osteoporosis Foundation made an effort to classify these disorders according to pathogenetic mechanism: altered osteoblast, osteoclast or osteocyte function; altered bone matrix proteins; altered bone microenvironmental regulators: and altered calciotropic hormone activity.[4]

This chapter reviews relatively common and well-studied genetic skeletal disorders that represent different phenotypes, (ie, high *vs* low bone mass) and pathogeneses (ie, skeletal development, connective tissue defects, enzyme deficiency).

OSTEOPETROSIS

Osteopetrosis is a rare genetic skeletal disorder that is characterized by failure of osteoclastic bone resorption. The clinical spectrum of osteopetrosis is broad from the severe early-onset autosomal recessive "malignant" form to

Dr. Aaron or an immediate family member has received research or institutional support from Orthofix, Inc. and serves as a board member, owner, officer, or committee member of the Orthopaedic Research Society. Dr. Zaidi is a member of a speakers' bureau or has made paid presentations on behalf of Diachi Sankyo, GLG, and GuidePoint; serves as a paid consultant to or is an employee of Diachi Sankyo, GLG, and GuidePoint; and serves as a board member, owner, officer, or committee member of the Alliance of Academic Internal Medicine. None of the following authors or any immediate family member has received anything of value from or has stock or stock options held in a commercial company or institution related directly or indirectly to the subject of this chapter: Dr. Taneja, Dr. Yuen, Dr. New, and Dr. Kim.

©Copyright 2021 American Academy of Orthopaedic Surgeons

mild adult-onset autosomal dominant "benign" form. The incidence of the autosomal dominant form is about 1 per 20,000 live births, and the autosomal recessive (infantile) "malignant" form is much rarer (1 *per* 200,000 to 250,000 live births).[5]

The patients with adult-onset osteopetrosis can be asymptomatic and have a normal life expectancy. Some, however, present with bone pain and frequent fractures accompanied by nerve compression, hearing or visual loss, and carpal tunnel syndrome. The autosomal recessive (infantile) form is lethal, presenting with pathological fractures, impaired hematopoiesis caused by bony expansion into bone marrow cavity resulting in pancytopenia with secondary hematopoiesis, immune deficiency with serious infection such as osteomyelitis, and sepsis.[5]

The defect arises from any step involved in osteoclastic bone resorption including osteoclast differentiation, resorptive pit formation (ruffled border formation), and acidification. Most genetic defects involve the acidification process, and about 70% of the autosomal recessive form is caused by mutations in *TCIRG1* (osteoclast vacuolar proton pump) and *CLCN7* (H^+-Cl^- exchange transporter 7) genes.[6] In a rare autosomal recessive type with a mutation in carbonic anhydrase II gene, patients develop renal tubular acidosis, nephrolithiasis, nephrocalcinosis, basal ganglia calcification, and cognitive dysfunction.[7]

The diagnosis of osteopetrosis is based on clinical and radiographic findings. Notable radiological features include "rugger jersey spine" (normal appearing vertebral body between dense superior and inferior endplates) and "bone-within-bone." Calvarial and basilar thickening can be seen. Cartilage "bars" or "islands" that represent calcified primary spongiosa are pathognomonic histologic findings.[8]

Treatment depends on the severity and pathogenetic mechanism underlying the osteoclast dysfunction. Calcitriol and PTH analog have been used to stimulate bone remodeling in a milder disease.[9] Hematopoietic stem cell transplant (HSCT) can repopulate normal osteoclasts and restore bone remodeling but should be used in the specific autosomal recessive form with mutations intrinsic to osteoclasts (osteoclast-poor phenotype).[8] Clinicians should be aware of potential complications of HSCT such as graft versus host disease. Although not curative, interferon-γ has been used to recover normal hematopoiesis.[5]

FIBROUS DYSPLASIA

Fibrous dysplasia is a rare skeletal disorder with tumor-like fibro-osseous lesions replacing normal skeletal tissue, which can be accompanied by nonskeletal manifestations, such as cutaneous hyperpigmentation (*café-au-lait* macules) and hyperfunctioning endocrinopathies (McCune-Albright syndrome), which includes gonadotropin-independent precocious puberty, Cushing syndrome, growth hormone excess, FGF23-mediated phosphate wasting, and hyperthyroidism.[10]

Fibrous dysplasia is a mosaic disease caused by a postzygotic activating mutation in *GNAS*, the gene encoding the alpha subunit of the stimulatory G protein (Gsα).[11] Missense mutations (R201H, R201C, R201G) have been reported.[12,13] The mutations occur in skeletal pluripotent cells in an initial developmental stage, and the mutated cells are randomly distributed to any location in the skeleton from craniofacial bones to the axial and appendicular skeleton. As a result, bone marrow stromal cells proliferate and differentiate into skeletal progenitors at the expense of adipogenesis or hematopoiesis; tumor-like fibro-osseous lesions proliferate and replace normal skeletal tissue. The histologic patterns are diverse from thin, irregular, and disconnected bony trabecular type (so-called "Chinese writing") to sclerotic pagetoid and sclerotic hypercellular patterns. Abnormal collagen in Sharpey fibers, at sites of insertion of tendons and ligaments, and retracted/stellate shaped osteoblasts are hallmarks of the diagnosis. In some cases, osteomalacic changes are noted likely due to excessive FGF23 production, which causes a lag in mineralization.[14]

The clinical spectrum ranges from none or mild symptoms to disabling deformities with chronic pain, swelling, and pathological fractures depending on the location and extent of skeletal involvement: isolated (monostotic), multiple bones (polyostotic), or the entire skeleton (panostotic). The disease affects any skeletal site, most commonly the proximal metaphysis of the femur and skull base.[15] Appendicular skeletal involvement causes limb pain and pathologic fractures (**Figure 1**). Craniofacial skeletal involvement may lead to facial deformities and cranial nerve impingement with hearing or

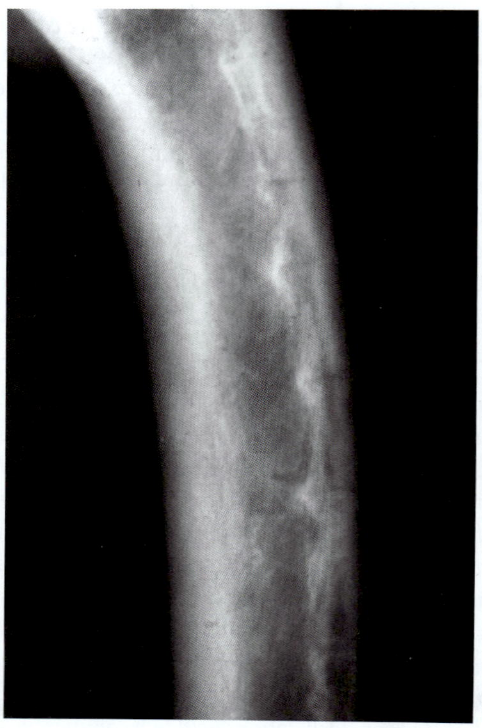

FIGURE 1 Radiograph showing fibrous dysplasia. Bowing of the femur with stress fractures on the convex side.

©Copyright 2021 American Academy of Orthopaedic Surgeons

vision impairment. Vertebral bone involvement can cause scoliosis. With aging, active proliferative lesions become sclerotic as mutant stem cells fail to self-renew and their progeny are consumed by apoptosis.[16] As a result, skeletal lesions are usually stable in adulthood, although the pain persists along with impaired mobility. The risk of malignancy is minimal; a study reported 28 cases of sarcoma among 1,122 cases of fibrous dysplasia.[17]

The diagnosis is based on the finding of two or more typical clinical features. The expansion of lesions from the medullary space with cortical thinning can be seen on radiographs. Bone scintigraphy can delineate the extent of the disease. Molecular testing is helpful in distinguishing other fibro-osseous lesions with similar clinical pictures (ie, osteofibrous dysplasia and ossifying fibromas of the mandible or maxilla).[10,14]

The goal of management is to relieve pain and prevent skeletal deformity and fracture. An open-label phase III study using diphosphonate demonstrated a decrease in the severity of bone pain.[18] An IL-6 receptor antagonist and receptor activator of nuclear factor-κ B (NFκB) ligand (RANKL) antagonist are also possible therapeutic options. Patients might need surgery to manage refractory pain at weight-bearing sites or to correct deformity. Fracture or impending fracture of the proximal femur can be stabilized with insertion of intramedullary nails.[19]

OSTEOGENESIS IMPERFECTA

Osteogenesis imperfecta (OI), or brittle bone disease, is relatively common with a prevalence of around 1 in every 20,000 births.[20] It is a collagen disorder resulting from a mutation in genes involved in collagen synthesis (COL1A1 or COL1A2). About 85% to 90% of patients who have clinical OI have abnormalities of type I collagen, the most abundant structural protein of bone, skin, and extracellular matrix.[21] Different mutations result in varying degrees of disruption in type 1 collagen synthesis, which accounts for the heterogenous phenotype in OI, ranging from perinatal death to late-onset mild osteopenia.[21] Most patients present with osteopenia/osteoporosis with fragility fractures, hearing defects, blue sclera, and dentinogenesis imperfecta (**Figure 2**).

The Sillence classification described four types of OI (I-IV) based on the clinical phenotype.[22] Type I is the mildest form of the disease. Patients usually have osteopenia with classic features of postnatal fractures, blue sclera, hearing loss, and dental imperfections. In many cases, the disease is not detected until late adulthood. Patients rarely suffer from long bone deformities and are of average height. Type II (lethal perinatal type) has high mortality in utero or in early infancy due to multiple pathological fractures, pulmonary hypoplasia, and CNS malformations. Families with this severe form benefit from genetic counseling and early prenatal screening. Type III is described as a progressively deforming type, the most severe survivable form. The patients often sustain multiple fractures in childhood, complicated with growth retardation, long bone deformities, and kyphoscoliosis, which can compromise cardiorespiratory function. Type IV is a moderate form of the disease. The classification of OI has evolved as new genes have been discovered. The 2015 revision of nosology and classification of genetic skeletal disorders added type V, which presents with calcification of the interosseous membranes and/or hypertrophic callus and distinct radiographic findings from types I-IV.[3]

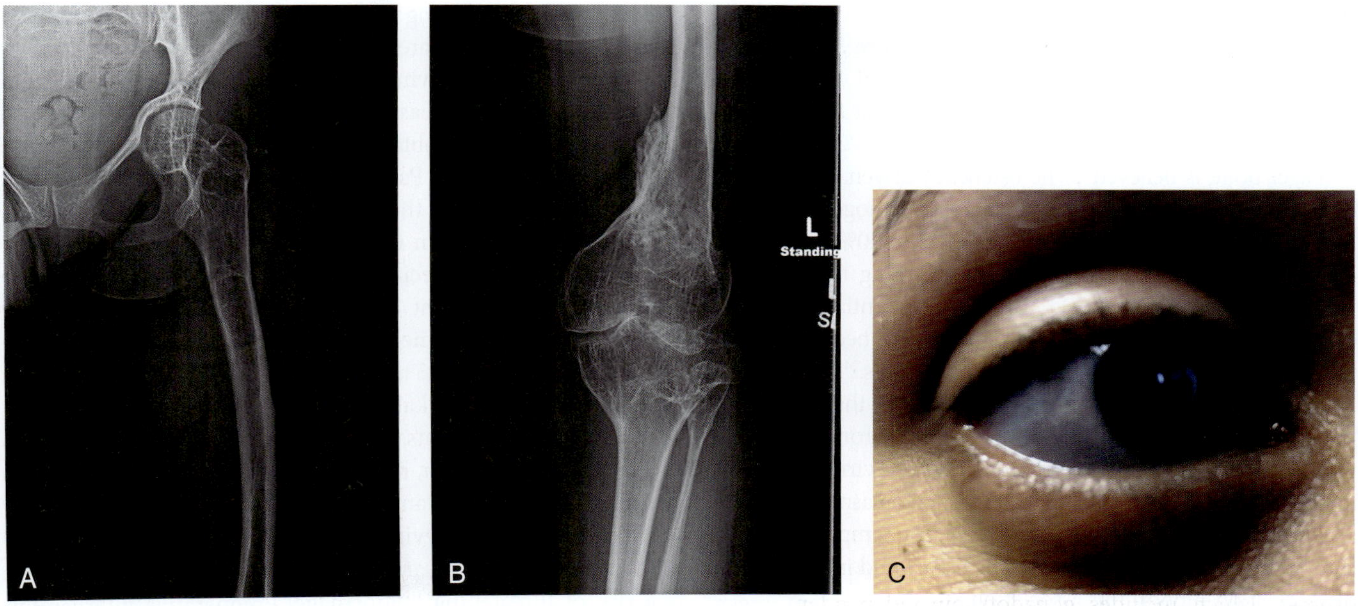

FIGURE 2 Osteogenesis imperfecta. **A** and **B**, AP radiographs. **A**, Bone deformity with severe loss of bone at the hip and bowing of the femur. **B**, Pathological fracture of the distal femur. **C**, Photograph of Blue sclera.

©Copyright 2021 American Academy of Orthopaedic Surgeons

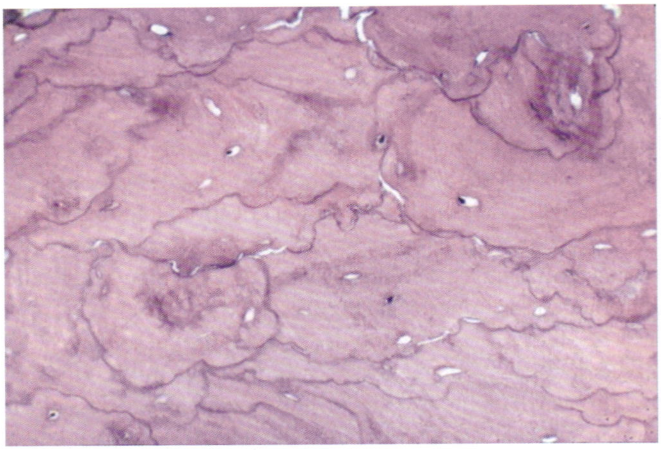

FIGURE 3 Paget disease. Histological section of Pagetic bone demonstrating mosaic pattern of cement lines undergoing uncoordinated remodeling. (Reproduced with permission from OrthoInfo © American Academy of Orthopaedic Surgeons. https://orthoinfo.aaos.org/en/diseases--conditions/pagets-disease-of-bone/. Accessed October 2019.)

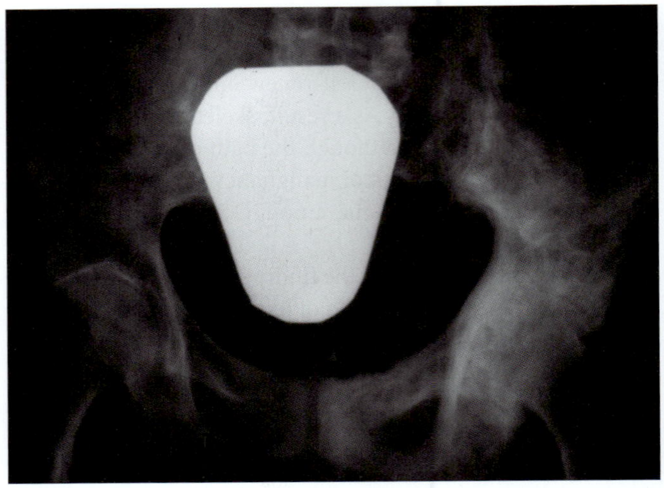

FIGURE 4 Paget disease. AP radiograph of the pelvis with sclerotic Paget disease in the left hemipelvis and severe osteoarthritis of the left hip with loss of joint space. The right hemipelvis is less involved with mixed lytic and sclerotic lesions and there may be a lytic form of Paget disease anteriorly.

The treatment is mainly supportive, focusing on physical rehabilitation. Diphosphonates are used to reduce the risk of fracture. Orthopaedic procedures using intramedullary rods can stabilize fractured bone and correct long bone deformities. Patients with severe scoliosis might need spinal fusion to prevent cardiopulmonary complications.

PAGET DISEASE OF BONE

Paget bone disease, a localized disorder of excessive and uncoordinated bone remodeling, has now become a rare disease. In affected bone, increased bone turnover caused by abnormal osteoclasts results in a disordered woven and lamellar bone often termed a "mosaic" pattern (**Figure 3**). Paget disease occurs most commonly in individuals of Anglo-Saxon descent and rarely in individuals from Asian or Scandinavian countries. It is rare below the age of 50 years.

Paget bone is believed to be osteoclast-driven. Both genetic and environmental factors contribute to the pathogenesis. Family history is positive for Paget disease in 10% to 40% of patients.[23] The mutations in the SQSTM1 gene encoding the SQSTM1/p62 protein (Sequestosome-1), which is an essential regulator of osteoclast RANK-mediated NFκB signaling, has been reported in up to 50% of familial, and some sporadic, cases.[24] Patients with *SQSTM1* mutations often have a severe form of the disease with high penetrance. A causative association with chronic paramyxoviral infection (ie, measles, respiratory syncytial virus, canine distemper virus) has been postulated since cytoplasmic inclusions are often present in affected osteoclasts. The temporal relationship of the declining incidence of the disease and increased rates of vaccination support this association.[25]

Most patients are asymptomatic and are often detected incidentally on radiographs or blood tests, namely elevated alkaline phosphatase. However, some patients develop pain, deformity, pathological fractures, and nerve compression such as hearing loss. The process tends to spread across the affected bone, causing an increase in bone size, which has both lytic and sclerotic elements on radiographs. The newly formed bone is disordered, hypervascular, and susceptible to microfracture which can result in bowing deformity. The disease can affect a single bone (monostotic) or multiple bones (polyostotic). It rarely spreads to a new location after the initial diagnosis. The most commonly affected bones are pelvis, lumbar and thoracic spine, femur, calvarium, tibia, scapula, and proximal humerus. When Paget disease affects joints, typically the hip, a secondary osteoarthritis may result, contributing to bone pain (**Figure 4**). Osteosarcoma and giant cell tumors are a rare complication (<1%).[26]

In patients with symptoms or elevated alkaline phosphatase without liver disease, a plain radiograph of the suspected area(s) should be obtained. A "cotton-wool" appearance is characteristic of a Pagetic skull, and "fissure fractures" of the convex aspect of the Pagetic bowed bones are observed. Bone scintigraphy can determine the extent of the disease.[27] Diphosphonates, especially zoledronic acid, have become the mainstay of treatment of symptomatic individuals or those with increased alkaline phosphatase activity. A single zoledronic acid infusion (5 mg IV) causes a biochemical remission in 87% of patients. Alkaline phosphatase levels have remained stable in 79% of patients throughout a follow-up period of up to 72 months.[28] However, relapses can occur anytime. Symptoms should be monitored and alkaline phosphatase checked every 1 to 2 years after achieving remission.[27] In cases where surgical intervention is necessary, especially hip replacement, there is a risk of threatening hemorrhage. Preoperative intervention with bisphosphonates or calcitonin mitigates this risk and makes surgical intervention feasible.[29]

©Copyright 2021 American Academy of Orthopaedic Surgeons

MARFAN SYNDROME

Marfan syndrome is a common heritable connective tissue disorder, with an incidence of 1 in 5,000 individuals. Most commonly, mutation in the FBN1 gene causes the disease. Several hundred mutations in the FBN1 gene have been identified in classic Marfan syndrome. FBN1 and the closely related FBN2 gene encode microfibrils, a major component of extracellular matrix structure. Therefore, Marfan syndrome often involves a variety of organs, including muscle, bone, eyes, skin, and cardiopulmonary systems.

The Ghent nosology, which categorizes Marfan syndromes based on clinical characteristics and genetic profiles, provides clinical guidance.[30] Given the excessive growth in long bones and laxity of joints, many patients develop scoliosis, and their median height is usually greater than the general population. Other skeletal manifestations include arachnodactyly, abnormal body segment ratios, kyphosis, protrusio acetabuli, pectus excavatum, and hindfoot deformities. Cardiovascular complications such as aortic root dilatation/dissection and mitral valve prolapse increase mortality. Other nonskeletal features are ectopia lentis (80% of patients), skin striae, dural ectasia, and spontaneous pneumothorax. Congenital contractural arachnodactyly, caused by a mutation in FBN2, is a Marfan-like disorder characterized by arachnodactyly, dolichostenomelia, scoliosis, and multiple congenital contractures without aortic or ocular involvement.[31]

The overall management of Marfan syndrome requires a multidisciplinary approach with a geneticist, pediatrician, orthopaedic surgeon, cardiologist, psychiatrist, and cardiovascular surgeon as the patients often suffer from the physical and emotional burden, chronic pain, limited physical activity, depression, and anxiety. Periodic musculoskeletal and cardiovascular surveillance with echocardiogram is necessary to detect complications early. Two groups of patients require strict monitoring: pregnant females and athletes given the risk of aortic dilation and rupture. Orthopaedic complications, such as scoliosis (curve >45°), severe deformities, and joint laxity may require surgical correction.

EHLERS-DANLOS SYNDROME

Ehlers-Danlos syndrome constitutes a group of rare connective tissue disorders, characterized by increased connective tissue fragility, skin hyperelasticity, joint hypermobility, easy bruising, and delayed wound healing. The latest international classification of Ehlers-Danlos syndromes describes 13 subtypes, with the hypermobile type (hEDS or type III) being the most common.[32] The disease is caused by mutations in genes responsible for collagen synthesis and processing, commonly type I, III, and V. Various mutations with distinct inheritance patterns have been described for each subtype. The genetic heterogeneity reflects a broad spectrum of clinical phenotype, and as a result, the diagnostic criteria for each subtype differ from one another. Common musculoskeletal manifestations include joint dislocations or subluxations, contractures, kyphoscoliosis, and early degenerative arthritis. The management focuses on physical rehabilitation to promote joint stability, often using braces and pads. Unfortunately, repetitive injuries may necessitate arthroscopic reconstructive procedures, best described for shoulder and patellar instability.[33]

HYPOPHOSPHATASIA

Hypophosphatasia (HPP) is a rare skeletal disorder with a decreased activity of tissue-nonspecific alkaline phosphatase. A number of mutations have been identified with different inheritance patterns, and the autosomal recessive diseases present with the most severe phenotype.[34] Alkaline phosphatase is involved in mineralization of bone and teeth, and a defect in the enzyme results in osteomalacia or rickets in children, along with dental abnormalities. The different forms of HPP include perinatal, infantile, childhood, adult, and odontohypophosphatasia. The patients often present with bone and muscle pain, fractures, poor dentition and premature loss of teeth, chondrocalcinosis, and nephrocalcinosis. The patients generally fall under four broad phenotypic groups: (1) Perinatal or in utero HPP is inevitably fatal, due to severe skeletal defects. (2) Infantile form (younger than 6 months) manifests with rickets resulting in severe demineralization of bones and premature craniosynostosis, and sometimes life-threatening respiratory complication. (3) Childhood HPP results in short stature, abnormal gait, and premature loss of teeth. (4) Adult-onset HPP is often detected after recurrent stress fractures with poor healing, bone and muscle pain, osteoarthropathy, and calcinosis. Management is mainly supportive: relieving pain, correcting fractures, and preventing respiratory complications. Recently, the FDA has approved recombinant alkaline phosphatase (asfotase alfa) for patients with perinatal, infantile, and childhood forms of the disease, as well as adult forms with a history of rickets.[35]

GAUCHER DISEASE

Gaucher disease is an autosomal recessive disorder with mutations in the glucocerebrosidase-1 gene (GBA1). It is highly prevalent in Ashkenazi Jews. The enzymatic deficiency of glucocerebrosidase (also termed beta-glucosidase) results in the accumulation of glucocerebrosides and glycolipids within lysosomes of macrophages, resulting in organomegaly and impaired hematologic function.

Skeletal manifestations, often in nonneuronopathic type 1 Gaucher disease, are associated with a high degree of morbidity and impact on activities of daily living. Skeletal manifestations include osteopenia, bone pain, osteonecrosis, and focal

©Copyright 2021 American Academy of Orthopaedic Surgeons

lytic lesions. A study using genetically modified mice with conditional deletion of Gba demonstrated decreased osteoblast viability secondary to osteotoxic sphingosine accumulation, suggesting Gba2 inhibition as a potential therapeutic target.[36]

There are three agents approved by the FDA for enzyme replacement therapy in Gaucher disease: imiglucerase, velaglucerase alfa, and taliglucerase alfa. Other therapies include substrate reduction therapy with Eliglustat, as well as splenectomy and stem cell transplantation. Diphosphonates also have been used as adjunctive therapy. As osteonecrosis and pathologic fractures are irreversible, prevention and early detection is critical.[37]

FIBRODYSPLASIA OSSIFICANS PROGRESSIVA

Fibrodysplasia ossificans progressiva (FOP) is an extremely rare skeletal disorder, with a prevalence of one in two million.[38] Typically, patients present with congenital malformation of great toes and progressive heterotopic ossification.[39] The transformation of connective tissues (ie, fascia, ligament, tendon, skeletal muscles) into bone occurs in the temporal pattern mimicking normal embryonic skeletal formation: first the dorsal, axial, cranial, proximal region followed by the ventral, appendicular, caudal, and distal regions. Interestingly, cardiac muscles, smooth muscles, and certain skeletal muscles such as diaphragm, tongue, and extraocular muscles are spared.[40]

The pathogenesis of FOP is dysregulation of the bone morphogenetic protein (BMP) signaling pathway. A highly conserved BMP pathway regulates embryogenesis and postdevelopment, including bone remodeling. Several BMPs and the types 1 and 2 BMP receptors are expressed in osteoblasts. The activating mutation in ACVR1/ALK2 gene encoding activin A receptor type I/activin-like kinase 2 (type 1 BMP receptor) causes heterotopic ossification.[41]

As low-traumatic events can trigger heterotrophic ossification, the treatment of FOP is mainly supportive and focuses on preventing flare-ups with anti-inflammatory agents such as glucocorticoids and NSAIDs.[38] Targeted therapies using an activin A antibody and a retinoid receptor agonist palovarotene are currently in clinical trials.

ACHONDROPLASIA

Achondroplasia is the most common skeletal dysplasia and is a cause of disproportionate dwarfism, which is caused by the mutations in fibroblast growth factor receptor 3 (*FGFR3*) gene. A missense mutation, (G380R), accounts for the majority of the cases. It is an autosomal dominant disorder associated with increased paternal age, with more than 80% of cases result from a de novo mutation.[42] The activating mutation in FGFR3 decelerates cartilage growth at the epiphyseal plate and impairs endochondral ossification, leading to shortened and misshapen long bones with relatively normal trunk length, facial bone hypoplasia, frontal bossing, and spinal stenosis.

Although hormonal treatments such as growth hormone therapy have been tried for achondroplasia, the response is variable, and the cost is prohibitive. A C–natriuretic peptide (CNP) agonist, BMN-111, has showed promising efficacy and safety; it increased growth rate by ~50%.[43] Both CNP agonist and meclizine, an antiemetic agent, modulate intracellular MAP kinase and inhibit constitutively active FGFR3 signaling. None of these agents corrects deformities that are already in place, and the drugs are used to prevent rather than correct deformity. Surgical procedures such as osteotomy and limb-lengthening are being widely used.

X-LINKED HYPOPHOSPHATEMIA

X-linked hypophosphatemia (XLH) is a cause of vitamin D–resistant rickets. It has been identified as a disorder in phosphate homeostasis. XLH is the prototype disorder of fibroblast growth factor 23 (FGF23)–mediated hypophosphatemia and is the most common heritable form of any phosphate wasting disorder. FGF23 decreases the expression of Na/P cotransporter and inhibits 1-alpha hydroxylase in vitamin D metabolism. The loss of function mutation in a phosphate-regulating gene with homology to endopeptidase located on the X chromosome (PHEX) is a causative mutation.[44] Other forms of hypophosphatemic rickets include autosomal dominant hypophosphatemia, autosomal recessive hypophosphatemia, and tumor-induced osteomalacia.

Clinical manifestations vary regarding severity. Most commonly, pediatric patients present with progressive bowing deformities of the legs and short stature. Metaphyseal changes of rickets and osteomalacia are observed as key radiographic findings. Dental abscesses, arthritis, and calcification of tendons and ligament with disabling pain are common skeletal complications. Patients have low serum phosphorus and low-normal 1,25 dihydroxyvitamin D levels. Measuring fasting tubular reabsorption of phosphate is helpful in diagnosis.[45]

The treatment goal in the growth phase is to achieve standard height while correcting bowing deformities. Primary treatment is calcitriol and phosphate supplements. However, normalizing phosphate levels have to be done cautiously since it can cause secondary hyperparathyroidism with resultant hypercalcemia, hypercalciuria, nephrocalcinosis, and renal impairment.[46] For an adult, the treatment for symptomatic patients targets spontaneous insufficiency fractures with orthopaedic procedures, treatment of biochemical osteomalacia, and relief of disabling skeletal pain.[47] A new anti-FGF-23 antibody has been approved by the FDA recently.

©Copyright 2021 American Academy of Orthopaedic Surgeons

SUMMARY

The rare genetic skeletal disorder field will only expand its spectrum and breadth due to developing "multiomic" analyses in clinical diagnosis. RNAseq and whole exome sequencing could serve as a starting point for the identification of disease-causing genes. Metabolomics would provide additional valuable information to understand the metabolic phenotype and pathogenesis. Detailed clinical phenotyping nonetheless must precede molecular testing and is required, given the variable expression and incomplete penetrance. Still, at the moment, the management of rare skeletal disorders is primarily targeting symptomatic relief and prevention of complications: relieving chronic pain and correcting deformities by the orthopeedic procedures. However, as we gain a better understanding of the pathogenesis of these disorders, new gene-specific treatments directed at the cause of the disease are becoming more common.

REFERENCES

1. O'Neill SC, Queally JM, Devitt BM, Doran PP, O'Byrne JM: The role of osteoblasts in peri-prosthetic osteolysis. *Bone Joint Lett J* 2013;95-B:1022-1026.
2. Splinter K, Adams DR, Bacino CA, et al: Effect of genetic diagnosis on patients with previously undiagnosed disease. *N Engl J Med* 2018;379:2131-2139.
3. Bonafe L, Cormier-Daire V, Hall C, et al: Nosology and classification of genetic skeletal disorders: 2015 revision. *Am J Med Genet* 2015;167A:2869-2892.
4. Masi L, Agnusdei D, Bilezikian J, et al: Taxonomy of rare genetic metabolic bone disorders. *Osteoporos Int* 2015;26:2529-2558.
5. Bacon S, Crowley R: Developments in rare bone diseases and mineral disorders. *Ther Adv Chronic Dis* 2018;9:51-60.
6. Sobacchi C, Schulz A, Coxon FP, Villa A, Helfrich MH: Osteopetrosis: Genetics, treatment and new insights into osteoclast function. *Nat Rev Endocrinol* 2013;9:522-536.
7. Del Fattore A, Cappariello A, Teti A: Genetics, pathogenesis and complications of osteopetrosis. *Bone* 2008;42:19-29.
8. Wu CC, Econs MJ, DiMeglio LA, et al: Diagnosis and management of osteopetrosis: Consensus guidelines from the osteopetrosis working group. *J Clin Endocrinol Metab* 2017;102:3111-3123.
9. Tolar J, Teitelbaum SL, Orchard PJ: Osteopetrosis. *N Engl J Med* 2004;351:2839-2849.
10. Boyce AM, Florenzano P, de Castro LF, Collins MT: Fibrous dysplasia/McCune-albright syndrome, in Adam MP, Ardinger HH, Pagon RA, et al, eds: *GeneReviews((R))*. Seattle, WA, 1993.
11. Weinstein LS, Shenker A, Gejman PV, Merino MJ, Friedman E, Spiegel AM: Activating mutations of the stimulatory G protein in the McCune-Albright syndrome. *N Engl J Med* 1991;325:1688-1695.
12. Bianco P, Riminucci M, Majolagbe A, et al: Mutations of the GNAS1 gene, stromal cell dysfunction, and osteomalacic changes in non-McCune-Albright fibrous dysplasia of bone. *J Bone Miner Res* 2000;15:120-128.
13. Riminucci M, Fisher LW, Majolagbe A, et al: A novel GNAS1 mutation, R201G, in McCune-albright syndrome. *J Bone Miner Res* 1999;14:1987-1989.
14. Riminucci M, Liu B, Corsi A, et al: The histopathology of fibrous dysplasia of bone in patients with activating mutations of the gs alpha gene: Site-specific patterns and recurrent histological hallmarks. *J Pathol* 1999;187:249-258.
15. Kelly MH, Brillante B, Collins MT: Pain in fibrous dysplasia of bone: Age-related changes and the anatomical distribution of skeletal lesions. *Osteoporos Int* 2008;19:57-63.
16. Kuznetsov SA, Cherman N, Riminucci M, Collins MT, Robey PG, Bianco P: Age-dependent demise of GNAS-mutated skeletal stem cells and "normalization" of fibrous dysplasia of bone. *J Bone Miner Res* 2008;23:1731-1740.
17. Ruggieri P, Sim FH, Bond JR, Unni KK: Malignancies in fibrous dysplasia. *Cancer* 1994;73:1411-1424.
18. Chapurlat RD, Delmas PD, Liens D, Meunier PJ: Long-term effects of intravenous pamidronate in fibrous dysplasia of bone. *J Bone Miner Res* 1997;12:1746-1752.
19. Stanton RP: Surgery for fibrous dysplasia. *J Bone Miner Res* 2006;21 suppl 2:P105-P109.
20. Forlino A, Marini JC: Osteogenesis imperfecta. *Lancet* 2016;387:1657-1671.
21. Marini JC, Forlino A, Bachinger HP, et al: Osteogenesis imperfecta. *Nat Rev Dis Primers* 2017;3:17052.
22. Sillence DO, Rimoin DL: Classification of osteogenesis imperfect. *Lancet* 1978;1:1041-1042.
23. Seton M, Choi HK, Hansen MF, Sebaldt RJ, Cooper C: Analysis of environmental factors in familial versus sporadic Paget's disease of bone–the New England Registry for Paget's disease of bone. *J Bone Miner Res* 2003;18:1519-1524.
24. Morissette J, Laurin N, Brown JP: Sequestosome 1: Mutation frequencies, haplotypes, and phenotypes in familial Paget's disease of bone. *J Bone Miner Res* 2006;21 suppl 2:P38-P44.
25. Albagha OM, Wani SE, Visconti MR, et al: Genome-wide association identifies three new susceptibility loci for Paget's disease of bone. *Nat Genet* 2011;43:685-689.
26. Shaker JL: Paget's disease of bone: A review of epidemiology, pathophysiology and management. *Ther Adv Musculoskelet Dis* 2009;1:107-125.
27. Singer FR, Bone HG III, Hosking DJ, et al: Paget's disease of bone: An endocrine society clinical practice guideline. *J Clin Endocrinol Metab* 2014;99:4408-4422.
28. Reid IR, Lyles K, Su G, et al: A single infusion of zoledronic acid produces sustained remissions in Paget disease: Data to 6.5 years. *J Bone Miner Res* 2011;26:2261-2270.
29. Tucci JR: Preoperative management of Paget's disease, in Aaron RK, ed: *Diagnosis and Management of Hip Disease: Biological Bases of Clinical Care*. Cham, Springer International Publishing, 2015, pp 159-184.
30. Loeys BL, Dietz HC, Braverman AC, et al: The revised Ghent nosology for the Marfan syndrome. *J Med Genet* 2010;47:476-485.
31. Putnam EA, Zhang H, Ramirez F, Milewicz DM: Fibrillin-2 (FBN2) mutations result in the Marfan-like disorder, congenital contractural arachnodactyly. *Nat Genet* 1995;11:456-458.
32. Malfait F, Francomano C, Byers P, et al: The 2017 international classification of the Ehlers-Danlos syndromes. *Am J Med Genet C Semin Med Genet* 2017;175:8-26.
33. Shirley ED, Demaio M, Bodurtha J: Ehlers-danlos syndrome in orthopaedics: Etiology, diagnosis, and treatment implications. *Sports Health* 2012;4:394-403.
34. Whyte MP: Hypophosphatasia - aetiology, nosology, pathogenesis, diagnosis and treatment. *Nat Rev Endocrinol* 2016;12:233-246.
35. Orimo H: Pathophysiology of hypophosphatasia and the potential role of asfotase alfa. *Ther Clin Risk Manag* 2016;12:777-786.
36. Mistry PK, Liu J, Sun L, et al: Glucocerebrosidase 2 gene deletion rescues type 1 Gaucher disease. *Proc Natl Acad Sci USA* 2014;111:4934-4939.
37. Mistry PK, Sadan S, Yang R, Yee J, Yang M: Consequences of diagnostic delays in type 1 gaucher disease: The need for greater awareness among hematologists-oncologists and an opportunity for early diagnosis and intervention. *Am J Hematol* 2007;82:697-701.

©Copyright 2021 American Academy of Orthopaedic Surgeons

38. Kaplan FS, Shen Q, Lounev V, et al: Skeletal metamorphosis in fibrodysplasia ossificans progressiva (FOP). *J Bone Miner Metab* 2008;26:521-530.
39. Cohen RB, Hahn GV, Tabas JA, et al: The natural history of heterotopic ossification in patients who have fibrodysplasia ossificans progressiva. A study of forty-four patients. *J Bone Joint Surg Am* 1993;75:215-219.
40. Connor JM, Evans DA: Fibrodysplasia ossificans progressiva. The clinical features and natural history of 34 patients. *J Bone Joint Surg Br* 1982;64:76-83.
41. Zaidi M, Yuen T, Sun L, Rosen CJ: Regulation of skeletal homeostasis. *Endocr Rev* 2018;39:701-718.
42. Shiang R, Thompson LM, Zhu YZ, et al: Mutations in the transmembrane domain of FGFR3 cause the most common genetic form of dwarfism, achondroplasia. *Cell* 1994;78:335-342.
43. Unger S, Bonafe L, Gouze E: Current care and investigational therapies in achondroplasia. *Curr Osteoporos Rep* 2017;15:53-60.
44. Francis F, Hennig S, Korn B, et al: A gene (PEX) with homologies to endopeptidases is mutated in patients with X-linked hypophosphatemic rickets. The HYP Consortium. *Nat Genet* 1995;11:130-136.
45. Makitie O, Doria A, Kooh SW, Cole WG, Daneman A, Sochett E: Early treatment improves growth and biochemical and radiographic outcome in X-linked hypophosphatemic rickets. *J Clin Endocrinol Metab* 2003;88:3591-3597.
46. Carpenter TO: New perspectives on the biology and treatment of X-linked hypophosphatemic rickets. *Pediatr Clin North Am* 1997;44:443-466.
47. Carpenter TO, Imel EA, Holm IA, Jan de Beur SM, Insogna KL: A clinician's guide to X-linked hypophosphatemia. *J Bone Miner Res* 2011;26:1381-1388.

©Copyright 2021 American Academy of Orthopaedic Surgeons

27

Osteonecrosis

Hiba K. Anis, MD
Nipun Sodhi, MD
Joseph O. Ehiorobo, MD
Michael A. Mont, MD

Keywords: *core decompression; hip arthroplasty; osteonecrosis of the femoral head*

INTRODUCTION

Osteonecrosis (ON) is a debilitating condition that can result in joint pain and progressive joint destruction most commonly in relatively young and active patients. In the United States, the disease is estimated to affect 10,000 to 30,000 new patients per year, who are primarily between the ages of 30 and 50 years. The prevalence of ON is increasing, and many associated risk factors have been identified. Corticosteroid use and alcohol abuse are notable modifiable risk factors associated in approximately 80% of cases.[1] Recently, alongside these acquired risk factors, there has also been interest in identifying potential genetic predispositions for this disease. Although the etiology of this condition is considered multifactorial, the fundamental cause is thought to potentially be a prolonged interruption of blood flow to the femoral head that leads to ischemia and ultimately infarction and resorption of the subchondral trabeculae followed by subchondral fracture. Subchondral fracture usually progresses to collapse and joint incongruity. The characteristic radiographic appearance of advanced ON is mixed zones of sclerosis and radiolucency, reflecting dead or repaired bone and areas of resorption, respectively.

Given the progressive nature of the disease, prompt diagnosis is critical for optimal head preservation outcomes. Detailed histories with thorough physical examinations are crucial as early stages of osteonecrosis can be difficult to detect clinically. The most common site for ON is the hip with the knee and shoulder following in prevalence. ON of the hip will be referenced here for pathophysiology and treatment. Advanced stages of hip ON are characterized by femoral head collapse often with painful arthritis, joint space narrowing, and acetabular involvement. Varying staging systems have been developed and largely rely on abnormalities seen on imaging. The importance of these staging systems lies in their guidance for treatment. According to the disease severity, several medical and surgical treatments are available to delay progression or reverse the damage. Surgical management options are further categorized depending on whether they preserve the native femoral head. Joint preservation procedures are largely reserved for patients with precollapse disease, whereas, femoral head replacement is often the only feasible option for postcollapse patients.

In this chapter, we review the current knowledge on osteonecrosis and its management. First, to get an understanding of the disease process, the associated risk factors and pathophysiology will be discussed. Next, the clinical and diagnostic

---

Dr. Mont or an immediate family member has received royalties from Microport and Stryker; serves as a paid consultant to or is an employee of Cymedica, DJ Orthopaedics, Flexion Therapeutics, Johnson & Johnson, Ongoing Care Solutions, Orthosensor, Pacira, Peerwell, Performance Dynamics, Pfizer, Skye Biologics, Stryker, and Tissue Gene; has stock or stock options held in Peerwell and USMI; has received research or institutional support from DJ Orthopaedics, Johnson & Johnson, National Institutes of Health (NIAMS & NICHD), Ongoing Care Solutions, Orthosensor, Stryker, and TissueGene; and serves as a board member, owner, officer, or committee member of the American Academy of Orthopaedic Surgeons, the American Association of Hip and Knee Surgeons, and the Knee Society. None of the following authors or any immediate family member has received anything of value from or has stock or stock options held in a commercial company or institution related directly or indirectly to the subject of this chapter: Dr. Anis, Dr. Sodhi, and Dr. Ehiorobo.

©Copyright 2021 American Academy of Orthopaedic Surgeons

features of osteonecrosis will be described including the current staging systems. In the latter part of the chapter, we will review available treatment options.

EPIDEMIOLOGY AND ETIOLOGY

Every year, approximately 20,000 to 30,000 patients are newly diagnosed with osteonecrosis of the femoral head in the United States.[2] It is the underlying condition for which approximately 10% of total hip arthroplasties (THAs) are performed and therefore places a substantial burden on healthcare cost and utilization. The disease affects people of all ages but is most common in those aged between 30 and 50 years. As the disease primarily affects young, active patients, the resulting changes and limitations to their daily and leisure activities can be drastic. The extent of disability and effect on quality of life is compounded when the contralateral hip is involved as is the case in 50% to 80% of the patients.

Associated risk factors for this disease are varied and are now believed to be multifactorial. However, associated risk factors can be broadly classified as traumatic or nontraumatic.

TRAUMATIC OSTEONECROSIS

Trauma is one broad classification of risk factors that can result in osteonecrosis due to the direct impact on the vascular supply. The vasculature of the femoral head and its compromise with trauma have been described in a recent review on skeletal circulation.[3] The femoral head is primarily supplied by three arterial systems: retinacular, foveolar, and intraosseous. The superior and inferior retinacular arteries branch off the medial circumflex artery (MCFA), and in adults, these arteries are the dominant arterial supply to the femoral head. Fractures of the femoral neck and dislocation of the hip can compromise this blood supply since the terminal branches are located in the posterior aspect of the femoral head-neck junction. Ischemia and infarction of the femoral head may be caused directly by disruption to these terminal vessels or indirectly by tamponade by intra-articular fracture hematomas.

Fractures of the femoral neck are often associated with osteonecrosis, and the risk is often determined by the fracture location and displacement, as well as patient age and the quality and timing of reduction. The retinacular arteries supplying the femoral head are most susceptible to mechanical damage in femoral head fractures, which are therefore associated with the highest incidence of osteonecrosis of up to 40%.[4-6] Due to the proximity to the MCFA and its terminal branches, medial neck fractures are more likely to interrupt the blood flow and lead to subchondral bone infarction compared with lateral neck fractures. The incidence of osteonecrosis can be 50% higher in displaced femoral neck fractures compared with nondisplaced fractures.[7,8] Similarly, patients with fractures that are malreduced with severe residual varus or valgus deformities are at an increased risk. In comparison to femoral head and neck fractures, osteonecrosis is rarely seen following intertrochanteric or femoral shaft fractures due to their distance from the MCFA.

The incidence of osteonecrosis following hip dislocation varies between 10% and 25% depending on various contributing factors.[9] The risk is far higher among those with concomitant femoral head or acetabulum fractures as there is an increased likelihood of damage to the blood vessels. Patients with posterior hip dislocations are also at a higher risk for osteonecrosis compared with those with anterior dislocations (29% vs 9%). Delays in treatment of the dislocation have also been associated with an increased incidence of osteonecrosis.

NONTRAUMATIC OSTEONECROSIS

Several nontraumatic risk factors for ON have been identified (**Table 1**). These can be broadly classified according to their contributions to the circulatory pathophysiology of ON. In addition to the vascular disruption described in traumatic ON, the blood supply to the femoral head is vulnerable to extravascular compression and intravascular occlusion.[10] There is presently no consensus regarding the relative contributions of several putative etiological risk factors for ON, most likely due to the varying methodologies, prospective and retrospective, used to determine associations in current literature.

TABLE 1 Traumatic and Nontraumatic Risk Factors for Osteonecrosis

Traumatic Risk Factors
Fracture
Hip dislocation
Nontraumatic Risk Factors
Intraosseous Extravascular Compression
Corticosteroid use
Alcohol
Gaucher disease
Intravascular Occlusion
Sickle cell disease
Coagulation disorders
Smoking
Other Etiologies
Caisson disease
Radiation
Chemotherapy
Genetic predisposition

©Copyright 2021 American Academy of Orthopaedic Surgeons

INTRAOSSEOUS EXTRAVASCULAR COMPRESSION

Microcirculatory blood flow in the femoral head is susceptible to compression by increases in extravascular pressure as the bone is thought to function as a rigid-walled chamber surrounding the vasculature.[10] When the pressure in the intraosseous extravascular compartment exceeds capillary pressure, the small vessels in the femoral head are compressed and the resulting reduction in arterial flow leads to regional ischemia. Corticosteroid use, excessive alcohol intake, and Gaucher disease are all examples of conditions that have been associated with reduced arterial supply secondary to increased intraosseous extravascular pressures.

Corticosteroid use is thought to be one of the most commonly associated risk factors of nontraumatic osteonecrosis.[9,11,12,13,14] Although this association has long been established, the exact mechanism is poorly understood. Corticosteroids can result in an increase in the number and size of adipocytes in the bone marrow resulting in venous congestion, raised intraosseous pressure, and ultimately inadequate arterial blood flow. Chronic corticosteroid use may result in further vascular dysregulation by their inhibition of vasodilatation. Additionally, corticosteroids have shown to impair bone repair processes by inducing osteoblast and osteocyte apoptosis as well as suppressing osteoblast production in the bone marrow. It is also thought that the antiangiogenic and prothrombotic effects of corticosteroids contribute to the risk of osteonecrosis through the impairment of bone repair and the interruption of intraosseous blood flow.

Excessive alcohol intake is also a major risk factor for nontraumatic osteonecrosis and is estimated to be a risk factor in 20% to 40% of all osteonecrosis cases.[15] It has been suggested that alcohol consumption leads to induced adipogenesis and decreased osteogenesis in the bone marrow which might contribute to the development of raised intraosseous extravascular pressures and subsequent reductions in arterial flow. Studies have found that the increased risk in osteonecrosis with excessive alcohol use is dose-dependent. Compared with nondrinkers, the odds of developing osteonecrosis have been found to be 2.8, 9.4, and 14.8 times higher for those drinking <320, 320 to 799, and >800 g of alcohol/week, respectively.[16] Smoking has also been implicated as a major risk factor for this disease.[16]

Raised intraosseous extravascular pressure is suggested to be the underlying mechanism for the development of osteonecrosis in patients with Gaucher disease as well. In these patients, the deficiency of beta-glucocerebrosidase leads to the accumulation of glucocerebrosides in the lysosomes of histiocytes, known as "Gaucher cells." The large collections over time of Gaucher cells in the extravascular space raises intraosseous pressures and compress the small vessels supplying the femoral head resulting in ischemia.

INTRAVASCULAR OCCLUSION

Arterial supply to the femoral head can also be compromised through intravascular obstruction. Examples of potential obstructions are sickle cell aggregates, thrombi, and lipid thrombi.

Almost half of all sickle cell disease patients develop osteonecrosis by the age of 35 years. Low oxygen tension environments are thought to polymerize abnormal hemoglobin, produced as a result of a genetic mutation, and lead to the characteristic sickling of red blood cells. These abnormal red blood cells adhere to each other and lead to intravascular occlusion. The femoral head is particularly susceptible to ischemia from intravascular obstruction by sickled red blood cells as the osseous vasculature tends to have low blood flow.[17]

Several medical conditions and hypercoagulable states are also important risk factors for intravascular occlusion and therefore nontraumatic osteonecrosis. Examples include antiphospholipid syndrome, thrombophilias, and hypofibrinolysis. The prevalence of inherited coagulation disorders have been reported to be notably higher among osteonecrosis patients. Factor V Leiden thrombophilia was reported to be almost four times more prevalent in osteonecrosis patients compared with controls (18% vs 4.6%) in a retrospective study,[18] and in another prospective study, hypofibrinolysis secondary to excess plasminogen activator inhibitor was reported to be 10 times more prevalent in osteonecrosis patients compared with controls (31% vs 3%).[19]

PATHOPHYSIOLOGY

Although there are many putative etiology associations with osteonecrosis, they are all considered to contribute to a unifying pathophysiology: ischemia and infarction of the bone (**Figure 1**). Together, compromised circulation is a final common pathway, and is a unifying concept, of many etiologies of ON. Vascular occlusion can be the result of extravascular compression from intraosseous hypertension, microcirculatory thrombi from intravascular coagulation, or mechanical interruption from trauma. In all cases, a reduction in blood flow to the femoral head leads to bone infarction and osteocyte necrosis.[20]

In the context of prolonged corticosteroid use and alcohol abuse, it is postulated that the following mechanism occurs: bone marrow stem cells convert from an osteoblastic to adipogenic lineage and differentiate into fat cells which subsequently hypertrophy, occupy the intraosseous extravascular space, and result in intraosseous hypertension, venous congestion, microvascular coagulation, and impaired arterial flow to the subchondral bone.[21,22] Intramedullary ischemia further stimulates the conversion of bone marrow stem cells to fat cells creating a vicious cycle.[23,24] A similar process is observed in Gaucher disease, whereby glucocerebrosides accumulate in the bone marrow.[25]

Several hereditary thrombophilias and hypercoagulable states put patients at risk of osteonecrosis given the particularly vulnerable vasculature of the femoral head. The lateral epiphyseal artery, which is derived from the MCFA, provides the principal blood supply to the femoral head. Vascular occlusion from microthrombi can result in ischemia at the peripheral

©Copyright 2021 American Academy of Orthopaedic Surgeons

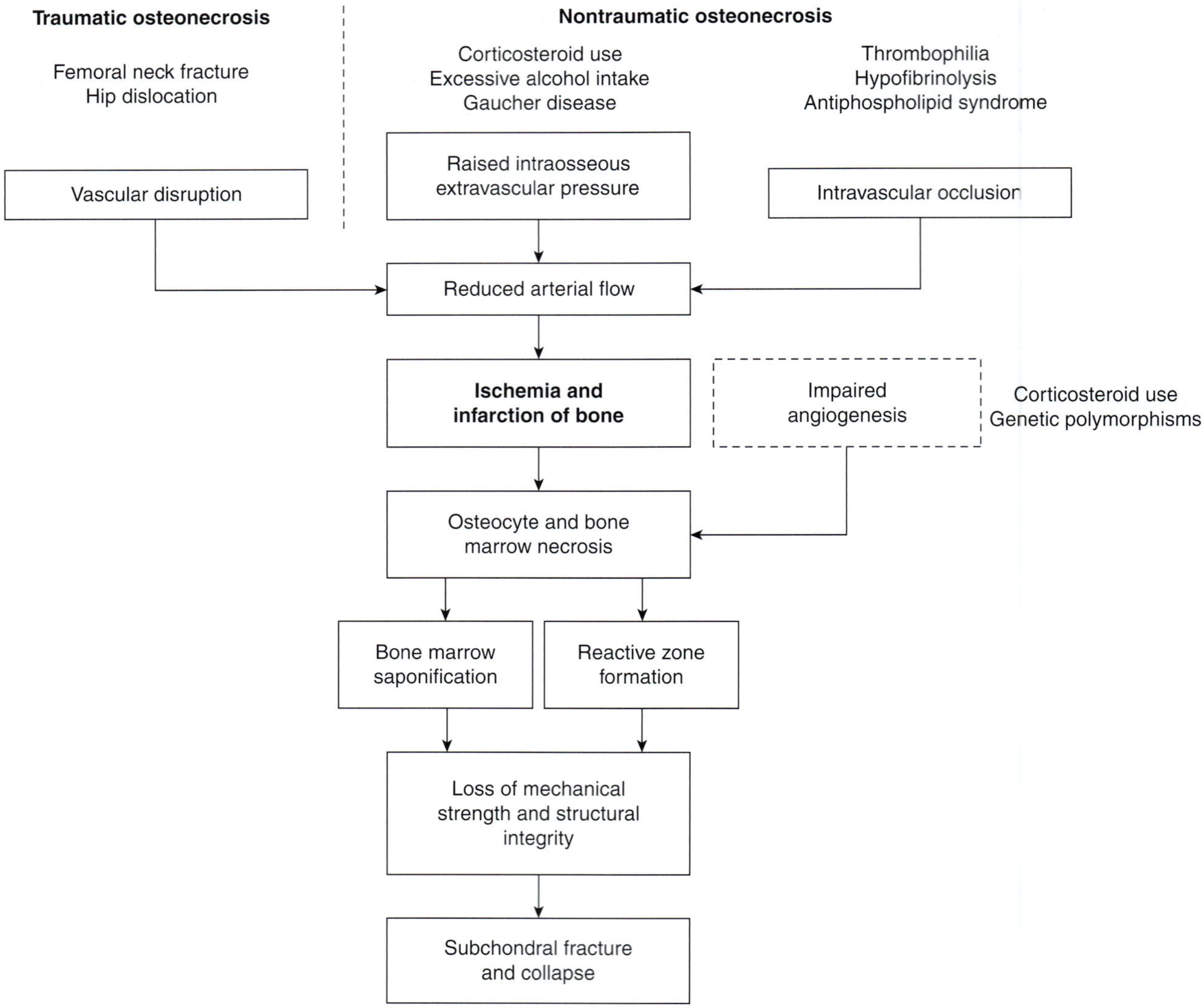

FIGURE 1 Illustration demonstrating the pathophysiology of osteonecrosis.

zone of the lateral epiphyseal artery in the subchondral bone. When the ischemia is transient, the lesion is less likely to progress to osteonecrosis, as is seen in borderline necrosis or bone marrow edema syndrome. However, prolonged ischemia with osteocyte and bone marrow necrosis leads to progression of the lesion to osteonecrosis.

An impairment of angiogenesis following bone marrow necrosis puts patients at an increased risk for osteonecrosis. It has been suggested that corticosteroid use and genetic polymorphisms suppress the reactive processes of new vessel formation.[19,26-29] Moreover, the natural reparative processes surrounding the lesion are thought to compromise the structural integrity of the femoral head. The necrotic lesion is surrounded by a fibrous capsule formed of histiocytes and giant cells, termed the reactive zone, which in itself is surrounded by bone marrow edema. Finite element modeling has demonstrated that the loss of structural integrity is due to resorption of subchondral trabeculae leading to fracture beneath the subchondral plate.[30] Additionally, the necrotic bone marrow undergoes saponification from the released fatty acids thereby losing its mechanical strength and structural integrity. At the macroscopic level, these processes lead to depression of the articular cartilage and ultimately collapse of the femoral head.[31-34]

CLINICAL FEATURES AND DIAGNOSIS

Early diagnosis leads to better outcomes as it allows the opportunity to halt disease progression, prevent subchondral collapse, and ultimately avoid the need for joint replacement. Left untreated, 80% of patients will progress to femoral head collapse within 2 years. Therefore, there should be a high index of suspicion for osteonecrosis among patients, with known risk factors presenting with anterior groin pain, a painful hip, or pain in other joints.

A detailed history is critical especially in nontraumatic osteoarthritis when the timing of insult is uncertain. In

©Copyright 2021 American Academy of Orthopaedic Surgeons

addition to elucidating potential risk factors, it is important to consider other affected joints as many patients have multiple joint involvement. It is important to note that pain rarely occurs at the onset of disease. Findings of osteonecrosis on MRI usually precede pain and studies have found that the duration of this asymptomatic period can vary between 3 months and 3 years.[35-37] Nevertheless, the most common presenting symptom in osteonecrosis of the hip is deep groin pain on movement or on weight bearing. Pain at rest or during the night occurs in some patients as well. On physical examination, patients with advanced stages of the disease may also have a limited range of motion, pain on forced internal rotation, and an antalgic gait.

IMAGING

Definitive diagnoses are made with imaging studies. MRI scans are the most sensitive and specific imaging modality for osteonecrosis; however, some features are discernible on plain radiographs, bone scans, and CT scans as well.

Plain radiographs are often used as the first imaging modality in osteonecrosis. For the hip, anterior-posterior views and frog leg lateral views are required for adequate visualization of the femoral head. The earliest radiographic sign is an increased density around the femoral head, correlating to areas of revascularization and repair, followed by sclerosis and cysts. The pathognomonic crescent sign refers to a radiolucent line along the subchondral portion of the femoral head and represents subchondral collapse. In advanced stages of the disease, joint space narrowing and degenerative changes in the acetabulum are also visible on plain radiographs. However, changes are only visible several months after disease onset, and therefore, patients with early stages of osteonecrosis often have normal plain radiographs. In the knee, tunnel views often demonstrate subchondral radiolucency of the femoral condyle in osteonecrosis. CT scans are particularly useful for delineating subchondral fractures.

Radionuclide bone scanning was previously used in patients with a high suspicion of osteonecrosis, but with negative radiographs. ^{99}Technetium bone scans identify areas of increased bone turnover surrounding the necrotic bone which is known as the "doughnut sign." However, bone scans are not as sensitive or specific for osteonecrosis as are MRI scans. Existing literature reveals that, in patients with osteonecrosis confirmed with histology or MRI, bone scans are false-negative in 25% to 45% of the cases,[38-41] so their routine diagnostic use has been superseded by MRI.

MRI is considered the standard for diagnostic imaging in osteonecrosis given that its sensitivity and specificity for osteonecrosis are reported to be 99% or greater.[9,38,40] Its ability to reveal soft-tissue abnormalities and changes of fat distribution in the bone marrow, particularly in the early stage of osteonecrosis, has meant that it is utilized to diagnose, facilitate staging, and guide treatment. T1-weighted imaging reveals low-intensity "band-like" lesions which correspond to the interface between the ischemic and normal bone. T2-weighted imaging also reveal a second high-intensity line representing the hypervascular granulation tissue thus creating the pathognomonic "double-line" sign; an outer rim of low intensity and an inner rim of high intensity. In addition, fat suppressed sequences reveal the extent of bone marrow edema that often correlates with pain and can contribute to treatment choices, especially decompression.

In a prospective cohort study by Aaron et al,[42] the authors demonstrated the value in early diagnosis with a prospective MRI screening of at-risk patients compared with a reactive strategy of MRI scanning patients who develop hip pain. In this population of patients who were all being newly treated with corticosteroids, it was found that periodic prospective MRI screening detected osteonecrosis at a much earlier stage than did reactive MRI of symptomatic patients. Prospective MRI screening enabled treatment without arthroplasty in all patients who were identified to have osteonecrosis with this strategy whereas patients who were diagnosed with osteonecrosis after reactive MRI scanning had an arthroplasty rate of 45%.

STAGING AND CLASSIFICATION SYSTEMS

Several staging systems exist for osteonecrosis to help guide treatment and assess prognosis. Mont et al[43] identified 17 major classification systems and found that the three most commonly used were the Ficat system, University of Pennsylvania system, and the Association of Research Circulation Osseous (ARCO) system (**Table 2**).

The Ficat system was the first classification system and has undergone modifications with the most current version being a five-stage system based on plain radiographic findings.[44] Stage 0 is the preclinical and preradiographic stage and often occurs in the context of bilateral osteonecrosis; the truly "silent hip." Radiographs remain normal in stage I; however, patients report groin pain and range of motion may be limited on physical examination. In stage II, some changes are visible in the femoral head such as cysts within the necrotic area or surrounding sclerosis which may be diffuse or localized. As MRI was not widely available when this staging system was first introduced, functional exploration of the bone was required for diagnosis in these early stages of osteonecrosis. Functional exploration of the bone is invasive and consists of the following three stages: measuring bone marrow pressure; intramedullary venography; and core biopsy. In comparison, diagnosis without core biopsy could be made in stage III which is characterized by subchondral collapse. A broken contour of the femoral head is visible on plain radiograph; however, joint space is preserved. In stage IV, radiographs have the appearance of osteoarthritis superimposed on a collapsed femoral head. There is progressive loss of articular cartilage and joint space as well as acetabular involvement. It is possible at this stage to incorrectly diagnose primary osteoarthritis, if there is no obvious sequestrum on the radiographs.

©Copyright 2021 American Academy of Orthopaedic Surgeons

TABLE 2 Commonly Used Staging Systems for Osteonecrosis of the Femoral Head

Stage	Ficat and Arlet Staging	Stage	University of Pennsylvania Classification	Stage	ARCO Classification
0	Normal radiograph Asymptomatic	0	Normal radiograph, bone scan, MRI	0	Normal radiograph, bone scan, MRI
I	Normal radiograph Symptomatic hip	I	Normal radiograph Abnormal bone scan or MRI	1	Normal radiograph Abnormal bone scan or MRI
			A: Mild (<15% of head affected)		A: Minimal (<15%)
			B: Moderate (15%-30%)		B: Moderate (15%-30%)
			C: Severe (>30%)		C: Extensive (>30%)
II	Diffuse osteoporosis, sclerosis, and/or cysts on radiograph	II	Femoral head radiolucency and sclerosis	2	Focal porosis, sclerosis, and/or osteolysis
			A: Mild (<15%)		A: Minimal (<15%)
			B: Moderate (15%-30%)		B: Moderate (15%-30%)
			C: Severe (>30%)		C: Extensive (>30%)
III	Subchondral collapse on radiograph ("crescent sign")	III	Subchondral collapse without femoral head flattening	3	Subchondral collapse
			A: Mild (<15% articular surface)		A: Minimal (<15% articular surface or <2 mm depression)
			B: Moderate (15%-30% articular surface)		B: Moderate (15%-30% articular surface or 2-4 mm depression)
			C: Severe (>30% articular surface)		C: Extensive (>30% articular surface or >4 mm depression)
IV	Progressive degenerative disease (secondary osteoarthritis) on radiograph	IV	Subchondral collapse with femoral head flattening	4	Acetabular changes, secondary osteoarthritis
			A: Mild (<15% articular surface or <2 mm depression)		
			B: Moderate (15%-30% articular surface or 2-4 mm depression)		
			C: Severe (>30% articular surface or >4 mm depression)		
		V	Joint space narrowing or acetabular changes		
			A: Mild		
			B: Moderate		
			C: Severe		
		VI	Advanced degenerative changes		

Data from Ficat RP: Idiopathic bone necrosis of the femoral head. Early diagnosis and treatment. *J Bone Joint Surg Br* 1985;67:3-9; Steinberg DR, Steinberg ME: *The University of Pennsylvania Classification of Osteonecrosis*. Springer, 2014, p 201-206; and Gardeniers J: A new international classification of osteonecrosis of the ARCO Committee on Terminology and Classification. *J Jpn Orthop Assoc* 1992;66:18-20.

©Copyright 2021 American Academy of Orthopaedic Surgeons

The University of Pennsylvania classification system was an important advancement in osteonecrosis staging as it incorporated both MRI findings and the extent of femoral head involvement.[45] In stage 0, radiographs, bone scans, and MRI are all normal; however, the patient is suspected to have osteonecrosis based on precipitating events. In the subsequent stages, each stage is separated into grades according to the extent of femoral head involvement: A (mild) corresponds to <15%, B (moderate) corresponds to 15% to 30%, and C (severe) corresponds to >30%. Similar to the Ficat system, radiographs are also normal in stage I; however, in the University of Pennsylvania classification, MRI and bone scans reveal abnormalities. In stage II, there are radiolucent and sclerotic changes on plain radiographs in addition to abnormalities on MRI and bone scans. The pathognomonic crescent sign is visible on plain radiographs in stage III indicating subchondral collapse without flattening of the femoral head. In stage IV, there is both femoral head collapse along with flattening. Joint space narrowing and acetabular involvement is seen in stage V. The final stage, stage VI, is characterized by advanced degenerative changes whereby the joint line is no longer visible on imaging.

Developed in the 1990s, the ARCO system stages the disease from onset to complete joint destruction from stage 0 to stage 4.[46] In stage 0, all current diagnostic studies, including MRI, are negative except for histology on core biopsy. Stages 1 to 3 are subclassified into grades according to the extent of the described abnormality: A (minimal) corresponds to <15% involvement or <2 mm depression, B (moderate) corresponds to 15% to 30% involvement or 2 to 4 mm depression, and C (extensive) corresponds to >30% involvement or >4 mm depression. A low-intensity band-like lesion is seen on MRI in stage 1, which is quantified to grade, whereas plain radiographs remain normal. In stage 2, there may be subtle signs of sclerosis or cystic changes on plain radiographs which can be used alongside the MRI to grade the stage. Subchondral collapse is evident on plain radiograph in stage 3 (crescent sign), and the percentage of surface collapse or dome depression is used to grade. In stage 4, there is destruction of the joint with acetabular changes with an appearance of osteoarthritis on plain radiographs.

The size of necrotic lesions has been correlated with the outcome and prognoses in osteonecrosis.[47,48] Kerboul et al[49] developed a method to estimate the extent of femoral head necrosis by measuring the arc of the affected femoral surface. Defined in 1974, the Kerboul angle is measured with plain radiographs but has since undergone modifications by other authors to include measurements with MRI.[50] Femoral head lesions are classified as small, medium, or large according to the Kerboul angle. Both anterior-posterior and lateral radiographs are required to calculate the angle. Once the center of the femoral head is identified, two lines are drawn from the center to either side of the lesion on the femoral surface. The Kerboul angle is calculated by taking the sum of the angles in the anterior-posterior and lateral views. Small lesions are those with a Kerboul angle of <160°, medium lesions are 160° to 200°, and large lesions are >200°.

TREATMENT

The primary factors to consider in the management of osteonecrosis are largely those discernible on imaging: stage (pre- or postcollapse), amount of head depression, size of necrotic lesion, and acetabular involvement. In addition, secondary factors such as patient age and comorbidities should also be taken into consideration.

NONSURGICAL TREATMENT

Although there is some literature evaluating pharmacological treatment options in osteonecrosis, there remains the need for large-scale randomized clinical trials to definitively determine their efficacy in delaying disease progression and preventing collapse. Diphosphonates inhibit osteoclast activity, and it is thought that this may prevent collapse in osteonecrosis. In a level IV study with 395 patients with Ficat stage I to III osteonecrosis, 92% of patients treated with alendronate had improved function and survivorship at a mean follow-up of 4 years. However, in a randomized controlled trial including 110 patients with Steinberg stage I to II osteonecrosis, there was no difference in the incidence of femoral head collapse in the alendronate group compared with the placebo group (53% vs 40%, $P = 0.251$).

Adipogenesis is considered an important contributing factor to ischemia and infarction in nontraumatic osteonecrosis. The use of lipid-lowering agents such as statins has been studied in those at risk of corticosteroid-induced osteonecrosis. However, the existing evidence is largely based on cellular or animal model studies with few low-level clinical studies. Similarly, anticoagulants may theoretically alleviate another pathophysiologic feature of osteonecrosis; vascular occlusion. However, their ability to prevent progression has only been suggested in low-level studies, and large-scale randomized controlled trials are necessary to corroborate these findings.

SURGICAL TREATMENT

The ultimate goal of joint preserving treatment is to prevent collapse and avoid replacing the native joint. Joint preservation procedures, such as core decompression, percutaneous drilling, bone grafting, or osteotomy, are feasible options in precollapse patients. However, following subchondral collapse, femoral head replacement with arthroplasty are the only options.

CORE DECOMPRESSION

Initially used by Ficat and Arlet as a diagnostic procedure to obtain specimens, core decompression has become the most common procedure to treat precollapse osteonecrosis with small lesions. This technique addresses the intraosseous hypertension that is due in part to the compartmental nature of bone

©Copyright 2021 American Academy of Orthopaedic Surgeons

and increases arterial flow by reducing microvascular compression. To illustrate the physiological role of this treatment modality and its value, Hungerford described the parallels between core decompression for osteonecrosis and decompression for compartment syndrome.[51] In both scenarios, the success of treatment depends on the magnitude of the original ischemic injury and the extent of necrosis. As with compartment syndrome, core decompression is ineffective by the time all the cells have died in the late stages of disease. However, decompression in the early stages of both osteonecrosis and compartment syndrome can lead to the reversal of the ischemic injury or at least the arrest of its progression. Thus, core decompression relieves bone marrow pressure and increases neovascularization around the core track thereby promoting the formation of new, healthy bone in the femoral head.

In traditional core decompression, an 8 to 10 mm cannulated trephine is used after which necrotic bone is removed with a burr. More recently, newer surgical techniques have been introduced which involve multiple drilling. Success rates of 71% have been reported in patients with Ficat stage I and II treated with multiple drilling procedures in which two to three core tracts with smaller 3 mm pins were utilized.[52] Mont et al[53] reviewed 42 studies including 1,206 patients treated with core decompression and found that the percentage of patients with satisfactory clinical results was almost three times greater in the core decompression group (64%) compared with the nonsurgical group (23%).

Current evidence suggests higher success rates when core decompression is combined with adjunctive procedures. Talathi et al[54] treated 43 hips in 28 ARCO classification Ia to ARCO IIc patients with autologous stem cell implantation and core decompression. The group found significant decreases in pre- to postoperative pain (8 vs 3 points; $P < 0.0001$). Additionally, 40 of the 43 hips revealed no radiographic disease progression at mean 16-months follow-up. Zhao et al[55] evaluated 76 patients with nontraumatic osteonecrosis of the femoral head who underwent core decompression with synthetic calcium-sulfate bone grafting. The group found significantly improved Harris hip and visual analog scale scores from pre- to postoperatively at 3 and 12 months ($P < 0.05$), as well as more stable image findings ($P < 0.05$).

Overall, core decompression can be a potential option for many osteonecrosis patients who exhibit no subchondral collapse, especially those with bone marrow edema. Adjunctive therapies with core decompression are promising but require further study. Due to the success, this treatment modality can likely be recommended for the majority of early stage osteonecrosis patients.

PERCUTANEOUS DRILLING

Percutaneous drilling utilizes small diameter pins compared with core decompression, and these pins are passed through the lesion multiple times.[56,57] After the patient is placed in the supine position, sedated, and appropriately prepped and draped, fluoroscopy is used to guide a Steinman pin or drill is inserted laterally, above the level of the lesser trochanter. Typically, 1 to 3 passes are made through the lesion, with larger lesions receiving more passes. Once the drill or pin has passed through the lesion, it can be removed and a simple sterile wound dressing can be placed. Patients are recommended initial 50% weight bearing for the first 6 weeks, followed by full weight bearing thereafter, and return to full sport at 1 year.

Multiple studies have identified the benefits of percutaneous drilling. Song et al[57] reviewed 136 patients (163 hips) with nontraumatic ON who underwent percutaneous drilling with 9/64-inch Steinmann pins. The group found 79% of patients with stage 1 and 77% of patients with stage 2 disease did not require additional surgery at mean 5-year follow-up. The group also found that 100% of small and 84% of medium-sized lesions had successful outcomes after percutaneous drilling, which was defined as no additional surgery, or a Harris hip score greater than 75. Another study reported on 45 patients who underwent percutaneous drilling with a 3-mm Steinman pin. The group found 71% of patients to not require any additional surgeries at mean 2-year follow-up. They also found that 80% of patients with stage 1 disease and 57% of patients with stage 2 disease had successful outcomes. Given the successful outcomes of this procedure, as well as the associated relative safety and low morbidity, percutaneous drilling can prove to be an effective option for patients with early, prefracture stage disease.

NONVASCULARIZED BONE GRAFTING

Bone grafting is an effective treatment option for medium-sized lesions in precollapse or early postcollapse osteonecrosis. Nonvascularized bone grafting provides structural support for the articular cartilage surface after the decompression and removal of necrotic bone. It also stimulates subchondral remodeling and healing with growth factors including bone morphogenetic proteins. Growth factors are known to be functionally involved with bone healing and therefore have great potential in improving bone regeneration in the setting of osteonecrosis with preserved structural integrity. Although preliminary data on the use of bone morphogenetic proteins and other growth factors are currently limited by small study populations and short-term follow-up, promising results have been reported on their adjunctive use with bone grafting.[58-60]

There are three different approaches to introduce bone graft: (1) a window in the femoral neck ("light bulb" procedure); (2) a core tract (Phemister procedure); and (3) a "trapdoor" in the femoral head.

In the light bulb procedure, a 1.0 by 1.5 cm window is made in the femoral neck with osteotomes through which the necrotic bone is removed. The resulting cavity is typically

©Copyright 2021 American Academy of Orthopaedic Surgeons

packed with harvested iliac bone, and the cortical segment is replaced and fixed. In a retrospective review of 33 patients, 80% of patients with small or medium-sized lesions and 22% with large lesions required no further surgery following the light bulb procedure.[60] The Phemister procedure is less commonly used in current practice. It involves removing an 8 to 10 mm diameter cylindrical core from the femoral neck and head which is then filled with harvested cancellous bone. When the articular cartilage is damaged, the trapdoor procedure may be an effective alternative procedure in which autogenous cortical and cancellous bone grafting is performed through an opening in the femoral head after the removal of the necrotic bone segment.[61]

VASCULARIZED BONE GRAFTING

Vascularized bone grafting restores blood supply in the femoral head in addition to structural support, and there are three different methods to do so: (1) muscle pedicle grafting; (2) free fibular vascularized grafting; and (3) vascularized iliac bone grafting. In the first method, the vasculature of four muscles and their pedicles are used to restore blood supply. Free fibular vascularized grafting entails a lengthy procedure in which the vascular pedicle of the fibula is anastomosed to the lateral circumflex artery. With vascularized iliac bone grafting, a tricortical iliac bone graft and its vascular pedicle are mobilized and fixed to the femoral neck. Although these techniques are often effective, vascularized bone grafting is seldom used in current practice due to the technical challenges and extensive resources required including a dedicated microvascular surgical center with multiple teams to harvest and place the graft.[62]

TOTAL HIP ARTHROPLASTY

For most patients presenting with advanced osteonecrosis with subchondral fracture or collapse, THA is the most effective treatment option. Johannson et al[63] conducted a meta-analysis of 67 studies, including a total of 3,277 hips, to evaluate outcomes after THA in osteonecrosis patients with a mean follow-up of 8 years. The authors reported a survival rate of 83% prior to 1990 whereas THAs performed after 1990 had a survival rate of 97%. These findings may be the result of improved second-generation cementing techniques and proximally coated femoral stems. The study also found that the underlying diagnosis was a determinant of outcomes. Patients with sickle cell disease, Gaucher disease, or renal transplants were at a higher risk of implant loosening. In contrast, those with systemic lupus erythematosus, heart transplants, or idiopathic osteonecrosis were less likely to undergo revision. Overall, THA provides excellent outcomes for patients with late-stage osteonecrosis and individualizing treatment may further improve outcomes.

SUMMARY

Osteonecrosis of the femoral head affects a young and active population who have high functional demands at diagnosis. The etiology is multifactorial, and there remain many unanswered questions regarding the pathophysiology of the disease with recent interest in potential genetic predispositions. It is a progressive disease which results in complete joint destruction and therefore early diagnosis is crucial for a satisfactory prognosis. MRI is the most sensitive and specific imaging modality and even detects the disease in the asymptomatic stages, whereas, plain radiographs may remain normal for many months after disease onset. Current staging systems incorporate findings from MRI and CT imaging to guide treatment by evaluating the following factors: whether subchondral fracture or collapse has occurred, the extent of femoral head depression, lesion size, and acetabular involvement. Nonsurgical treatment options have been suggested in current literature; however, further study is warranted to determine their efficacy. Core decompression and percutaneous drilling, with or without the addition of bone grafts or stem cells, have been shown to be effective procedures for small- or medium-sized precollapse lesions. Large-sized lesions or early postcollapse lesions can be treated with nonvascularized or vascularized bone grafts which may preserve the native joint. Arthroplasty is indicated for advanced osteonecrosis particularly for those with subchondral collapse, marked femoral head depression, and degenerative changes.

REFERENCES

1. Mont MA, Hungerford DS: Non-traumatic avascular necrosis of the femoral head. *J Bone Joint Surg Am* 1995;77:459-474.
2. Moya-Angeler J, Gianakos AL, Villa JC, Ni A, Lane JM: Current concepts on osteonecrosis of the femoral head. *World J Orthop* 2015;6:590-601. doi:10.5312/wjo.v6.i8.590.
3. Lorich DG, Lazaro LE: Fractures and bone repair, in Aaron RK, ed: *Skeletal Circulation in Clinical Practice*. Singapore, World Scientific Press, 2016, pp 185-208. doi:10.1142/9746.
4. Yeranosian M, Horneff JG, Baldwin K, Hosalkar HS: Factors affecting the outcome of fractures of the femoral neck in children and adolescents: A systematic review. *Bone Joint Lett J* 2013;95-B:135-142. doi:10.1302/0301-620X.95B1.30161.
5. Guo JJ, Tang N, Yang HL, Qin L, Leung KS: Impact of surgical approach on postoperative heterotopic ossification and avascular necrosis in femoral head fractures: A systematic review. *Int Orthop* 2010;34:319-322. doi:10.1007/s00264-009-0849-3.
6. Moon ES, Mehlman CT: Risk factors for avascular necrosis after femoral neck fractures in children: 25 Cincinnati cases and meta-analysis of 360 cases. *J Orthop Trauma* 2006;20:323-329.
7. Massie WK: Treatment of femoral neck fractures emphasizing long term follow-up observations on aseptic necrosis. *Clin Orthop Relat Res* 1973;(92):16-62.

©Copyright 2021 American Academy of Orthopaedic Surgeons

8. Cleveland M, Fielding JW: A continuing end-result study of intracapsular fracture of the neck of the femur. *J Bone Joint Surg Am* 1954;36-A:1020-1030.
9. Lieberman JR, Berry DJ, Mont MA, et al: Osteonecrosis of the hip: Management in the 21st century. *Instr Course Lect* 2003;52:337-355.
10. Shah KN, Racine J, Jones LC, Aaron RK: Pathophysiology and risk factors for osteonecrosis. *Curr Rev Musculoskelet Med* 2015;8:201-209. doi:10.1007/s12178-015-9277-8.
11. Arlet J: Nontraumatic avascular necrosis of the femoral head. Past, present, and future. *Clin Orthop Relat Res* 1992;(277):12-21.
12. Gebhard KL, Maibach HI: Relationship between systemic corticosteroids and osteonecrosis. *Am J Clin Dermatol* 2001;2:377-388. doi:10.2165/00128071-200102060-00004.
13. Vakil N, Sparberg M: Steroid-related osteonecrosis in inflammatory bowel disease. *Gastroenterology* 1989;96:62-67.
14. Felson DT, Anderson JJ: Across-study evaluation of association between steroid dose and bolus steroids and avascular necrosis of bone. *Lancet (London, England)* 1987;1:902-906. doi:10.1016/s0140-6736(87)92870-4.
15. Bradway JK, Morrey BF: The natural history of the silent hip in bilateral atraumatic osteonecrosis. *J Arthroplasty* 1993;8:383-387.
16. Hirota Y, Hirohata T, Fukuda K, et al: Association of alcohol intake, cigarette smoking, and occupational status with the risk of idiopathic osteonecrosis of the femoral head. *Am J Epidemiol* 1993;137:530-538.
17. Colin Y, Le Van Kim C, El Nemer W: Red cell adhesion in human diseases. *Curr Opin Hematol* 2014;21:186-192. doi:10.1097/MOH.0000000000000036.
18. Zalavras CG, Vartholomatos G, Dokou E, Malizos KN: Genetic background of osteonecrosis: Associated with thrombophilic mutations? *Clin Orthop Relat Res* 2004;422:251-255.
19. Glueck CJ, Freiberg RA, Boppana S, Wang P: Thrombophilia, hypofibrinolysis, the eNOS T-786C polymorphism, and multifocal osteonecrosis. *J Bone Joint Surg Am* 2008;90:2220-2229. doi:10.2106/JBJS.G.00616.
20. Aaron RK: Osteonecrosis: Etiology, pathophysiology, and diagnosis, in Callaghan J, Rosenberg A, Rubash H, eds: *Adult Hip*. Philadelphia, Lippincott Williams & Wilkins, 1998, pp 451-466.
21. Hungerford DS, Lennox DW: The importance of increased intraosseous pressure in the development of osteonecrosis of the femoral head: Implications for treatment. *Orthop Clin North Am* 1985;16:635-654.
22. Wang GJ, Sweet DE, Reger SI, Thompson RC: Fat-cell changes as a mechanism of avascular necrosis of the femoral head in cortisone-treated rabbits. *J Bone Joint Surg Am* 1977;59:729-735.
23. Kricun ME: Red-yellow marrow conversion: Its effect on the location of some solitary bone lesions. *Skeletal Radiol* 1985;14·10-19.
24. Koo KH, Dussault R, Kaplan P, et al: Age-related marrow conversion in the proximal metaphysis of the femur: Evaluation with T1-weighted MR imaging. *Radiology* 1998;206:745-748. doi:10.1148/radiology.206.3.9494495.
25. Amstutz HC, Carey EJ: Skeletal manifestations and treatment of Gaucher's disease. Review of twenty cases. *J Bone Joint Surg Am* 1966;48:670-701.
26. Koo K-H, Lee JS, Lee YJ, Kim K-J, Yoo JJ, Kim HJ: Endothelial nitric oxide synthase gene polymorphisms in patients with nontraumatic femoral head osteonecrosis. *J Orthop Res* 2006;24:1722-1728. doi:10.1002/jor.20164.
27. Kim T-H, Hong JM, Lee J-Y, et al: Promoter polymorphisms of the vascular endothelial growth factor gene is associated with an osteonecrosis of the femoral head in the Korean population. *Osteoarthr Cartil* 2008;16:287-291. doi:10.1016/j.joca.2007.06.017.
28. Lee YJ, Lee JS, Kang EH, et al: Vascular endothelial growth factor polymorphisms in patients with steroid-induced femoral head osteonecrosis. *J Orthop Res* 2012;30:21-27. doi:10.1002/jor.21492.
29. Kabata T, Matsumoto T, Yagishita S, Wakayama T, Iseki S, Tomita K: Vascular endothelial growth factor in rabbits during development of corticosteroid-induced osteonecrosis: A controlled experiment. *J Rheumatol* 2008;35:2383-2390. doi:10.3899/jrheum.070838.
30. Brown TD, Baker KJ, Brand RA: Structural consequences of subchondral bone involvement in segmental osteonecrosis of the femoral head. *J Orthop Res* 1992;10:79-87. doi:10.1002/jor.1100100110.
31. Koo KH, Ahn IO, Kim R, et al: Bone marrow edema and associated pain in early stage osteonecrosis of the femoral head: Prospective study with serial MR images. *Radiology* 1999;213:715-722. doi:10.1148/radiology.213.3.r99dc06715.
32. Glimcher MJ, Kenzora JE: Nicolas Andry award. The biology of osteonecrosis of the human femoral head and its clinical implications: 1. Tissue biology. *Clin Orthop Relat Res* 1979;(138):284-309.
33. Glimcher MJ, Kenzora JE: The biology of osteonecrosis of the human femoral head and its clinical implications: II. The pathological changes in the femoral head as an organ and in the hip joint. *Clin Orthop Relat Res* 1979;(139):283-312.
34. Glimcher MJ, Kenzora JE: The biology of osteonecrosis of the human femoral head and its clinical implications. III. Discussion of the etiology and genesis of the pathological sequelae; comments on treatment. *Clin Orthop Relat Res* 1979;(140):273-312.
35. Min B-W, Song K-S, Cho C-H, Lee S-M, Lee K-J: Untreated asymptomatic hips in patients with osteonecrosis of the femoral head. *Clin Orthop Relat Res* 2008;466:1087-1092. doi:10.1007/s11999-008-0191-x.
36. Hernigou P, Habibi A, Bachir D, Galacteros F: The natural history of asymptomatic osteonecrosis of the femoral head in adults with sickle cell disease. *J Bone Joint Surg Am* 2006;88:2565-2572. doi:10.2106/JBJS.E.01455.
37. Kopecky KK, Braunstein EM, Brandt KD, et al: Apparent avascular necrosis of the hip: Appearance and spontaneous resolution of MR findings in renal allograft recipients. *Radiology* 1991;179:523-527. doi:10.1148/radiology.179.2.2014304.
38. Mont MA, Ulrich SD, Seyler TM, et al: Bone scanning of limited value for diagnosis of symptomatic oligofocal and multifocal osteonecrosis. *J Rheumatol* 2008;35:1629-1634.
39. Mitchell DG, Rao VM, Dalinka MK, et al: Femoral head avascular necrosis: Correlation of MR imaging, radiographic staging, radionuclide imaging, and clinical findings. *Radiology* 1987;162:709-715. doi:10.1148/radiology.162.3.3809484.
40. Markisz JA, Knowles RJ, Altchek DW, Schneider R, Whalen JP, Cahill PT: Segmental patterns of avascular necrosis of the femoral heads: Early detection with MR imaging. *Radiology* 1987;162:717-720. doi:10.1148/radiology.162.3.3809485.
41. Beltran J, Herman LJ, Burk JM, et al: Femoral head avascular necrosis: MR imaging with clinical-pathologic and radionuclide correlation. *Radiology* 1988;166:215-220. doi:10.1148/radiology.166.1.3336682.
42. Aaron RK, Voisinet A, Racine J, Ali Y, Feller ER: Corticosteroid-associated avascular necrosis: Dose relationships and early diagnosis. *Ann N Y Acad Sci* 2011;1240:38-46. doi:10.1111/j.1749-6632.2011.06218.x.
43. Mont MA, Marulanda GA, Jones LC, et al: Systematic analysis of classification systems for osteonecrosis of the femoral head. *J Bone Joint Surg Am* 2006;88(suppl 3):16-26. doi:10.2106/JBJS.F.00457.
44. Ficat RP: Idiopathic bone necrosis of the femoral head. Early diagnosis and treatment. *J Bone Joint Surg Br* 1985;67:3-9.
45. Steinberg DR, Steinberg ME: The University of Pennsylvania classification of osteonecrosis, in Koo KH, Mont MA, Jones LC, eds: *Osteonecrosis*. Heidelberg, Springer, 2014, pp 201-206.
46. Gardeniers J: A new international classification of osteonecrosis of the ARCO Committee on Terminology and Classification. *J Jpn Orthop Assoc* 1992;66:18-20.
47. Lieberman JR, Engstrom SM, Meneghini RM, SooHoo NF: Which factors influence preservation of the osteonecrotic femoral head? *Clin Orthop Relat Res* 2012;470:525-534. doi:10.1007/s11999-011-2050-4.
48. Nishii T, Sugano N, Ohzono K, Sakai T, Sato Y, Yoshikawa H: Significance of lesion size and location in the prediction of collapse of osteonecrosis of the femoral head: A new three-dimensional quantification using magnetic resonance imaging. *J Orthop Res* 2002;20:130-136. doi:10.1016/S0736-0266(01)00063-8.

©Copyright 2021 American Academy of Orthopaedic Surgeons

49. Kerboul M, Thomine J, Postel M, Merle d'Aubigne R: The conservative surgical treatment of idiopathic aseptic necrosis of the femoral head. *J Bone Joint Surg Br* 1974;56:291-296.
50. Ha Y-C, Jung WH, Kim J-R, Seong NH, Kim S-Y, Koo K-H: Prediction of collapse in femoral head osteonecrosis: A modified Kerboul method with use of magnetic resonance images. *J Bone Joint Surg Am* 2006;88(suppl 3):35-40. doi:10.2106/JBJS.F.00535.
51. Hungerford DS: Response: The role of core decompression in the treatment of ischemic necrosis of the femoral head. *Arthritis Rheum* 1989;32:801-806.
52. Mont MA, Ragland PS, Etienne G: Core decompression of the femoral head for osteonecrosis using percutaneous multiple small-diameter drilling. *Clin Orthop Relat Res* 2004;(429):131-138.
53. Mont MA, Carbone JJ, Fairbank AC: Core decompression versus nonoperative management for osteonecrosis of the hip. *Clin Orthop Relat Res* 1996;(324):169-178.
54. Talathi NS, Kamath AF: Autologous stem cell implantation with core decompression for avascular necrosis of the femoral head. *J Clin Orthop Trauma* 2018;9:349-352. doi:10.1016/j.jcot.2018.05.014.
55. Zhao P, Hao J: Analysis of the long-term efficacy of core decompression with synthetic calcium-sulfate bone grafting on non-traumatic osteonecrosis of the femoral head. *Med Sci* 2018;34(Focus issue F1):43-46. doi:10.1051/medsci/201834f108.
56. Pierce TP, Jauregui JJ, Elmallah RK, Lavernia CJ, Mont MA, Nace J: A current review of core decompression in the treatment of osteonecrosis of the femoral head. *Curr Rev Musculoskelet Med* 2015;8:228-232. doi:10.1007/s12178-015-9280-0.
57. Song WS, Yoo JJ, Kim Y-M, Kim HJ: Results of multiple drilling compared with those of conventional methods of core decompression. *Clin Orthop Relat Res* 2007;454:139-146. doi:10.1097/01.blo.0000229342.96103.73.
58. Lieberman JR, Conduah A, Urist MR: Treatment of osteonecrosis of the femoral head with core decompression and human bone morphogenetic protein. *Clin Orthop Relat Res* 2004;429:139-145. doi:10.1097/01.blo.0000150312.53937.6f.
59. Mont MA, Etienne G, Ragland PS: Outcome of nonvascularized bone grafting for osteonecrosis of the femoral head. *Clin Orthop Relat Res* 2003;417:84-92. doi:10.1097/01.blo.0000096826.67494.38.
60. Seyler TM, Marker DR, Ulrich SD, Fatscher T, Mont MA: Nonvascularized bone grafting defers joint arthroplasty in hip osteonecrosis. *Clin Orthop Relat Res* 2008;466:1125-1132. doi:10.1007/s11999-008-0211-x.
61. Mont MA, Einhorn TA, Sponseller PD, Hungerford DS: The trapdoor procedure using autogenous cortical and cancellous bone grafts for osteonecrosis of the femoral head. *J Bone Joint Surg Br* 1998;80:56-62.
62. Chughtai M, Piuzzi NS, Khlopas A, Jones LC, Goodman SB, Mont MA: An evidence-based guide to the treatment of osteonecrosis of the femoral head. *Bone Joint Lett J* 2017;99-B:1267-1279. doi:10.1302/0301-620X.99B10.BJJ-2017-0233.R2.
63. Johannson HR, Zywiel MG, Marker DR, Jones LC, McGrath MS, Mont MA: Osteonecrosis is not a predictor of poor outcomes in primary total hip arthroplasty: A systematic literature review. *Int Orthop* 2011;35:465-473. doi:10.1007/s00264-010-0979-7.

©Copyright 2021 American Academy of Orthopaedic Surgeons

28

Osteoarthritis

Joel A. Block, MD

Keywords: *degenerative cartilage; osteoarthritis/pain mechanisms; osteoarthritis/pathogenesis; osteoarthritis/risk factors; osteoarthritis/therapy*

INTRODUCTION

Osteoarthritis (OA) is a heterogeneous disease characterized by pain and functional loss. It is overwhelmingly the most common form of arthritis; adults have a 40%-50% lifetime risk of developing symptomatic OA.[1,2] In addition, OA causes vast societal cost and morbidity worldwide,[1,3] consuming approximately 0.5% of the GDP of industrialized societies.[4] It represents one of the largest sources of days lost from work and is the single greatest source of functional mobility limitation among the elderly.[1,5] Finally, it predominantly affects the middle-aged and elderly and is exacerbated by obesity; hence, the societal burden is rising dramatically as the developed world ages and becomes more obese.

Dr. Block or an immediate family member has received royalties from Agios, Inc., Daiichi Sankyo, Inc., and Omeros Inc.; serves as a paid consultant to or is an employee of GlaxoSmithKline, Medivir Inc.; has stock or stock options held in Gilead, Inc.; has received research or institutional support from AstraZeneca, Novartis, and Pfizer ; and serves as a board member, owner, officer, or committee member of the American College of Rheumatology and the OsteoArthritis Research Society International.

DEFINITION

OA was formerly considered to be a disease of degenerative cartilage, and throughout the 20th century, research directed at treating or delaying disease progression was focused largely on preserving or repairing cartilage. However, cartilage degeneration alone is both painless and a normal process of aging, suggesting it alone cannot be the sole source of the painful disease that is OA. It is now clear that OA is whole organ disease of the joint and not merely of cartilage. Hence, a modern definition is:

OA is a painful degenerative process that affects all joint structures and involves the progressive deterioration of articular cartilage and reactive alterations of subchondral bone and the surrounding joint structures. OA is not a systemic inflammatory process, but local inflammation is common and is thought to be reactive rather than a primary component of OA.

EPIDEMIOLOGY

A number of large longitudinal observational studies have reported the natural history of OA and collectively have provided a great deal of insight regarding its epidemiology. As noted, its prevalence has increased dramatically as the population of the developed world has aged. Approximately 27 million Americans had physician-diagnosed OA in 2005, which was a 30% increase from a decade earlier, and this is expected to reach at least 67 million by 2030.[3] Historically, community-based epidemiology studies identified OA on the basis of radiographic disease—the presence of osteophytes, joint space narrowing, and subchondral sclerosis. Radiographic OA increases dramatically with aging, and while it is rare prior to

©Copyright 2021 American Academy of Orthopaedic Surgeons

the age of 45 years, by the seventh decade, it is virtually universal. However, this structural definition overstates the number with clinical disease. A large number of asymptomatic individuals have radiographic involvement, but only approximately 7% to 17% of those older than 44 years actually have symptomatic OA. The prevalence is higher in women than men, and in African Americans relative to Caucasian Americans.[1]

RISK FACTORS FOR OSTEOARTHRITIS

Risk factors for incident OA may be divided into those that are modifiable and those that are nonmodifiable. The strongest nonmodifiable factor is aging; this is true both for radiographic degeneration and for symptomatic OA. Other important nonmodifiable risks include genetics and female sex, especially after menopause. The most significant heritable component is for OA of the hand or hip and is estimated at between 48% and 65% for so-called "generalized OA" characterized by osteophytes of the distal interphalangeal (DIP) joints (Heberden nodes) or the proximal interphalangeal (PIP) joints (Bouchard nodes). In contrast to nonmodifiable risk factors, modifiable OA risk factors may provide potential targets for prevention. The most important of these is obesity, which alone confers approximately threefold increased risk of incident OA. Occupational and lifestyle activities that involve repeated trauma or excessive loading may be associated with increased risk of OA. These include chronic squatting, bending, and lifting such as by warehouse workers and laborers, who have increased knee involvement, and classically, pneumatic drill operators who develop OA of the wrist and elbow. Posttraumatic OA is recognized as a distinct syndrome, often with onset much earlier in life than primary OA.[6] Major knee or ankle injury, for example, is strongly associated with the subsequent development of OA in the injured joint. Finally, progressive OA has been shown to be mediated by aberrant loading of joints,[7] as well as by abnormal joint alignment.

THE JOINT IN OSTEOARTHRITIS

OA is not one disease, but rather arises from a variety of different pathogenic mechanisms that collectively encompass the degeneration of joint structures with the development of pain. Although both processes occur concomitantly, there is well-described discordance between the severity of structural degeneration and the magnitude of pain felt by patients. The mechanisms of structural degeneration have been well studied for decades, but the biology of OA pain is less well understood.

Each of the joint tissues has been discussed separately in previous chapters; however, a functional joint must operate as an integrated organ encompassing the component tissues (**Figure 1**). These include the articular cartilage, fibrocartilaginous meniscus (in some joints), synovium, ligaments, subchondral bone, periarticular musculature, and innervation. An intact synovial joint efficiently bears loads and articulates smoothly. The articular cartilage is the best studied of the tissues in OA (Chapter 12), as OA was historically considered primarily a disease of degenerative cartilage. Its biomechanical function is to bear loads during joint function and to provide virtually frictionless articulation. The former is accomplished by its compressive stiffness combined with tensile strength (see Chapter 13); these physicochemical properties are endowed by the fibrillary collagen network entrapping highly hydrophilic and anionic aggregates of the proteoglycan aggrecan. In addition to load-bearing, the articular surface helps to maintain a virtually frictionless environment through a combination of fluid-film and boundary lubrication that is provided by a variety of macromolecular components of the synovial fluid, principally hyaluronan and lubricin, respectively.[8] As a unit, the intact joint has among the lowest coefficients of friction known. The synovium is the source of the synovial fluid and is a highly vascularized structure consisting of few cell layers composed of synoviocytes which are either fibroblast- or macrophage-derived (Chapter 15). As articular cartilage is avascular, the synovial fluid provides much of the nutrition to the chondrocytes through passive diffusion. The ligaments, tendons, and periarticular musculature provide mechanical stability for the joint and of course are responsible for joint motion. Finally, whereas articular cartilage is aneural, the other joint structures are well innervated with nociceptors and a full array of somatosensory afferents, the most prominent of which are the proprioceptors. OA represents a failure of the synovial joint as an organ, and must be viewed holistically. Structurally, this includes degenerative changes in all tissues.

ARTICULAR CARTILAGE

Both aging and OA involve progressive loss of the articular cartilage. Early changes include enzymatic degradation of the extracellular matrix, now appreciated to involve the aggrecanases (principally ADAMTS-4 and -5) and the collagenases (principally MMP13), augmented by the production of catabolic cytokines, including interleukin (IL)-1 and tumor necrosis factor-α (TNF-α) (**Figure 2**). These serve to augment an imbalance between anabolic repair and catabolic degradation, further accelerating cartilage loss. Adult cartilage remains metabolically active throughout life; however, it is fundamentally a nonhealing tissue, and adult chondrocytes are unable to elaborate mechanically stable type 2 collagen fibers. Thus, early disruption of the collagen fibrillar network promotes swelling of the matrix, rendering the cartilage less able to resist compressive loads. As the degenerative process proceeds, chondrocytes themselves undergo apoptosis, which further jeopardizes the repair process.

MENISCUS

The knees and selected other joints contain fibrocartilaginous menisci that add to joint stability. These are innervated and vascularized and thus are often a source of articular pain. The

©Copyright 2021 American Academy of Orthopaedic Surgeons

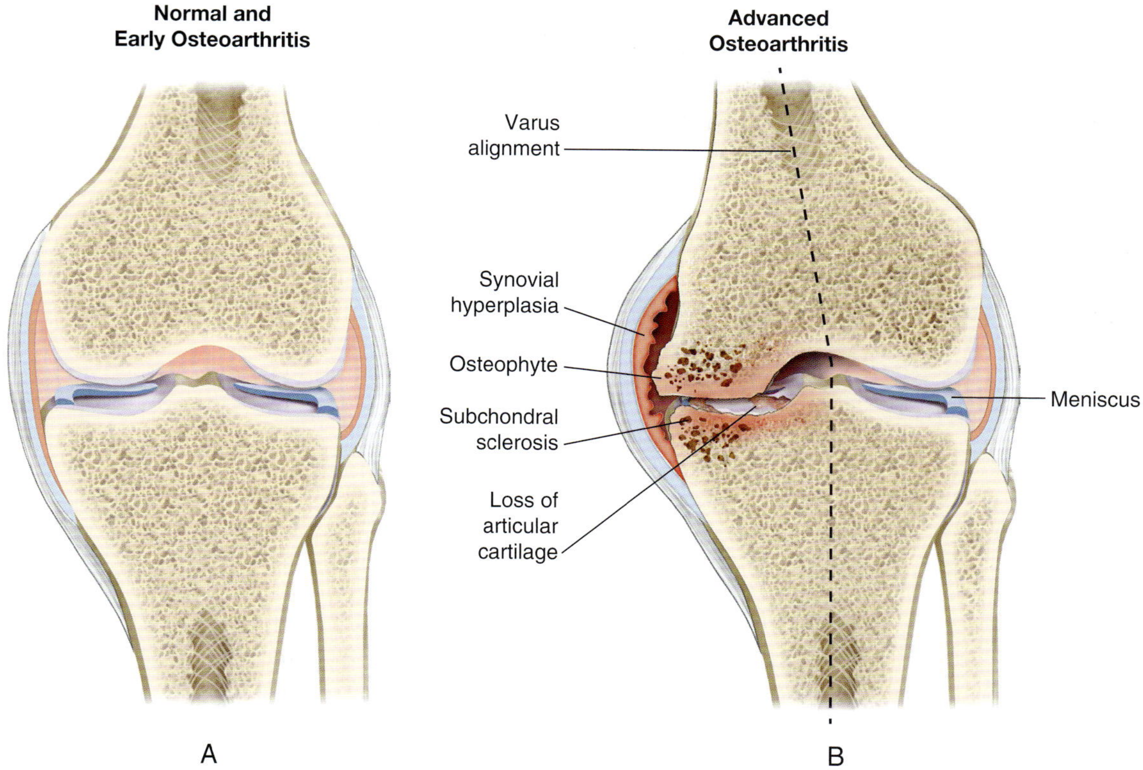

FIGURE 1 Artist's sketch of the **Degenerative changes of osteoarthritis**. A normal synovial joint integrates each of the articular tissues in a smooth and functional manner. As OA develops, the articular cartilage degenerates, resulting in significant joint space narrowing. Concomitantly, subchondral bony sclerosis develops underlying the diseased cartilage, and osteophytes form at the joint margins. Synovial hypertrophy is common, and menisci are frequently involved and displaced. Eventually, the joint becomes malaligned; varus deformity occurs when the medial compartment is most affected. **A,** A normal knee joint with intact joint structures and alignment. **B,** Advanced OA in a knee, with loss of articular cartilage, osteophyte formation, synovial hyptertrophy, and subchondral sclerosis. Because of the asymmetric cartilage loss, mainly in the medial compartment, varus alignment develops (shown by the mechanical angle outlined in black lines).

menisci are almost always degenerative in symptomatic knee OA. Moreover, degeneration and displacement of menisci represents a major source of radiographic joint space narrowing in knee OA.

BONE

The subchondral bone becomes sclerotic and develops pathological microfractures. It is controversial whether this process is a *result* of the diminished cushioning provided by degenerative cartilage, or if the bony changes *precede* and influence cartilage degeneration. In any case, these changes are matched with the degenerative processes in the overlying cartilage. The interface between the subchondral bone and the cartilage is a zone of calcified cartilage, which in OA has been shown to develop sensory neurovascular infiltration via osteochondral channels into areas that are normally poorly innervated and that connect the subchondral bone with overlying cartilage, and which may contribute to the pain of OA[9,10] (**Figure 2**). Beyond the subchondral bone, the periarticular bone undergoes OA-related changes, such as with osteophyte growth; these pathological bony formations develop from endochondral calcification at the joint margins and are cardinal manifestations of OA (**Figure 1**). Their function remains unknown, but it has been hypothesized that they may provide mechanical stability as struts supporting the joint.

SYNOVIUM

Whereas OA is primarily a degenerative rather than an inflammatory arthritis, it is frequently accompanied by local inflammation, characterized by mild synovitis. Histologically, the findings are similar to the synovitis of rheumatoid arthritis, with hyperplasia, vascularization, and infiltration of immune cells. The presence of local synovitis in OA has been associated with painful flares, and modern imaging has revealed it to be common in OA joints.[11] Synovial effusions are also common in OA and may cause pain by distension of the synovial capsule; while they are characteristically noninflammatory, with less than 2000 WBC/mm^3, they nevertheless contain a variety of inflammatory mediators, which may exacerbate both the pain and the catabolic processes of OA.

©Copyright 2021 American Academy of Orthopaedic Surgeons

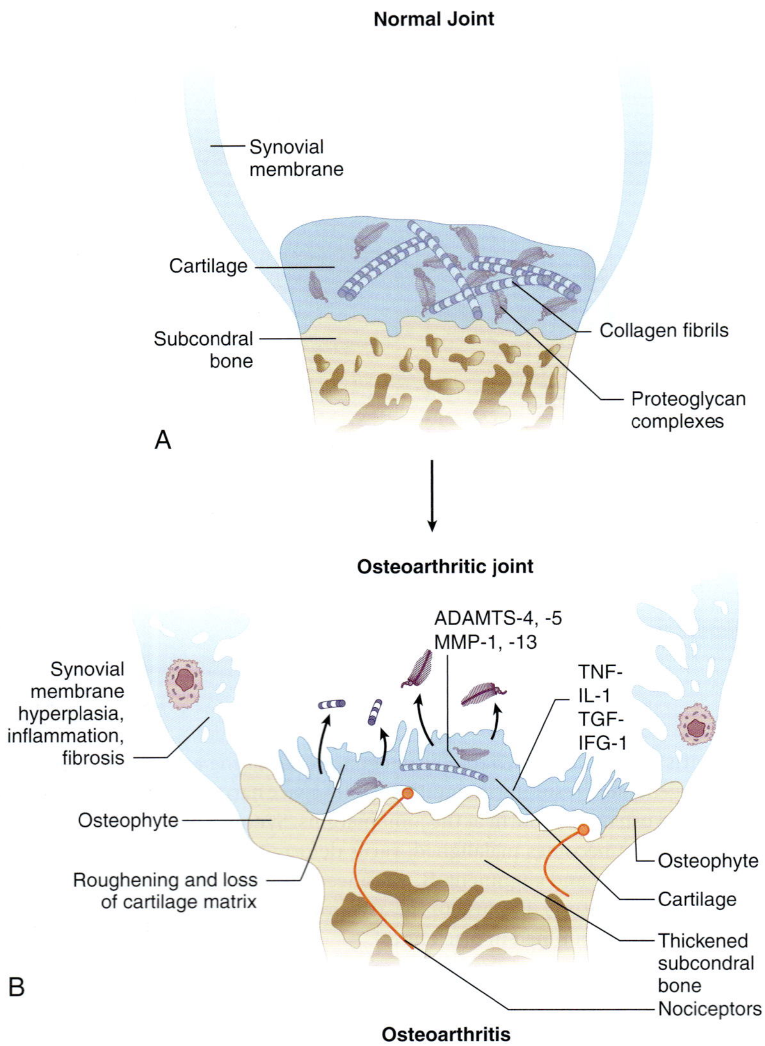

FIGURE 2 Sketch illustrating the intra-articular tissues affected by the osteoarthritis (OA) process. **A,** The intra-articular mileu of a normal joint. **B,** An osteoarthritic joint. Note the degradation of the articular cartilage, local synovitis, osteophyte formation, and the subchondral bony reaction. Nociceptors penetrate the subchondral plate via neurovascular channels and connect the subchondral bone with the overlying cartilage. (Redrawn with permission from Glyn-Jones S, Palmer AJR, Agricola R, et al: Osteoarthritis. *Lancet* 2015;386[9991]:376-387.)

PERIARTICULAR MUSCULATURE

OA patients tend to have weak periarticular musculature. Although disuse and deconditioning may explain part of this, weakness has been observed in people with structural OA who have not yet developed symptomatic disease, as well as in more distal muscles. These observations raise the question of whether weakness itself may be pathogenically important rather than a simple consequence of the disease process.[12] Moreover, there are biomechanical consequences to muscle weakness, where this may result in altered joint loading during gait and subsequent progression of OA.

INNERVATION

OA is associated with a variety of somatosensory deficits, including diminished proprioception, altered allodynia, and widespread vibratory diminution.[12-14] These are largely systemic and not restricted to the involved joint(s), suggesting that OA may be a systemic disease, even if symptomatic in only a few joints. It remains unclear whether somatosensory dysfunction antedates the onset of OA, suggesting a pathogenic role, or if it is a consequence of the degenerative structural changes in OA. In addition, peripheral and central nervous system sensitization in the form of hyperalgesia and allodynia are characteristic of OA,[13] which may have implications for the treatment of OA pain.

PATHOGENIC MECHANISMS

OA is a multifactorial syndrome that comprises multiple etiologies, many unidentified. It is typically referred to as "primary" when no underlying etiology is identifiable and "secondary" when a specific etiology is known. Multiple factors are clearly involved in OA onset and progression.

©Copyright 2021 American Academy of Orthopaedic Surgeons

AGING

Aging results in a variety of well described alterations at the molecular, cellular, and tissue levels across all parts of the joint. Many of these are normal degenerative events and are associated with the chronic low-grade inflammation of aging, termed "inflammaging,"[15] and occur in the cells of each of the connective tissues. For example, as chondrocytes senesce, they undergo a secretory phenotype associated with increased production of proinflammatory cytokines, such as IL-1 and IL-6, growth factors, including transforming growth factor-β (TGF-β), and matrix metalloproteinases, including MMP-13, which all result in altered cartilage matrix and loss of mechanical function.[16] In addition, carboxylation associated with oxidative stress occurs with advancing age and can alter protein folding, weaken tissues, and increase susceptibility to proteolytic cleavage. Finally, DNA methylation, histone acetylation and methylation, and microRNAs are important means of epigenetic regulation of changes in gene expression associated with aging in the cells of joint tissues.[17]

Independent of cellular action, advanced glycation endproducts (AGEs) accumulate in a nonenzymatic manner on all long-lasting matrix components; in the cartilage, this primarily affects the fibrillar type 2 collagen network. However, chondrocytes express AGE receptors (RAGE),[18] which, when activated by AGE binding, further stimulate release of proinflammatory cytokines such as IL-6 and IL-8. Similar changes occur in the menisci and ligaments, and these aging-related responses diminish chondrocytes' ability to respond to injury and render the joint more vulnerable to aberrant loads with diminished capacity to adapt that leads to cartilage degeneration. Nonetheless, the link between these alterations and symptomatic OA remains poorly understood.

BIOMECHANICS

It has been appreciated for decades that aberrant loading of joints mediates the evolution of structural joint degeneration and, in many cases, may contribute to the initiation of the process. For example, abnormal loading of the contralateral joints during unilateral lower extremity OA, such as with limping, has been shown to markedly increase the risk of severe OA in the overloaded joint.[19] In addition, malalignment at the knee markedly increases the likelihood of subsequent OA in that knee. Abnormal joint loading precipitated by joint instability, malalignment, trauma, or congenital or inherited connective tissue diseases may be transmitted through the cartilage matrix, pathologically activating chondrocytes as well as inducing remodeling of the subchondral bone. Similarly, abnormal neuromuscular signaling, such as in cases of deficient somatosensory perception, may result in abnormal loading that can drive the OA process.

OBESITY

Obesity has long been recognized as a major risk factor for OA, and the association of the metabolic syndrome with OA has been well documented. The risk was generally ascribed to excessive loading across weight-bearing joints (eg, Ref. 20). However, obesity and the metabolic syndrome increase the OA risk in non–weight-bearing joints as well, such as in the hands.[21,22] As the hormonal and inflammatory influences of adipose tissue have been elucidated, obesity has been appreciated to play a direct role in OA pathogenesis, independent of mechanical overloading. Obesity, with or without the metabolic syndrome, is a state of chronic low intensity inflammation; it influences the innate immune system, stimulating transition of macrophages to the proinflammatory M1 macrophage phenotype, and altering T cell populations.[23,24] The inflammatory milieu is procatabolic and antianabolic and thereby contributes to degeneration of articular cartilage and the joint tissues and may predispose them to excess damage from otherwise minor insults. In addition, adipose tissue is a rich source of adipokines (adipose-derived cytokines) which form the metabolic link between obesity and OA. The adipokines, principally leptin, adiponectin, visfatin, and resistin, stimulate production of proinflammatory cytokines such as IL-1, TNF-α, and IL-6, which in turn can augment joint damage.[23-25]

INFLAMMATION

OA is conventionally considered a degenerative rather than an inflammatory arthritis, and the local inflammatory component of synovial effusion formerly was thought to be merely an epiphenomenon. As understanding of the innate immune system has evolved, it has become clear that while OA is truly not a *systemic* inflammatory process, local inflammation may be a central component of the pain and structural degeneration inherent in the disease process.

SYNOVITIS

Cool synovial effusions are a hallmark of large joint OA. While the cell count is formally "noninflammatory" in OA, <2,000 cells/μL, the presence of the effusion and the leukocytes suggests a low-grade inflammation. Moreover, sensitive imaging techniques such as ultrasonography or MRI have demonstrated the presence of synovial hypertrophy in a large percentage of knee OA patients,[26,27] and the presence of synovitis is associated with OA pain and progression.[28] Moreover, the presence of ultrasonography- or MRI-detectable synovitis has been found to be predictive of the development of incident OA.[11,29] Pathologically, the synovitis found in OA joints appears histologically similar to rheumatoid synovitis, with infiltrating lymphocytes and macrophages, synovial lining hyperplasia, and increased vascularity.[30] Moreover, the presence of activated macrophages in the joint capsule has been associated with structural OA progression and pain, again suggesting a pathogenic role.[29]

THE INNATE IMMUNE SYSTEM

The innate immune system serves as rapid response surveillance protection and acts via activation of pattern recognition receptors present on a variety of cells. In OA, RAGE and toll-like

©Copyright 2021 American Academy of Orthopaedic Surgeons

receptors present on chondrocytes, synoviocytes, and synovial macrophages recognize a variety of so-called damage-associated molecular patterns (DAMPs), including cartilage matrix breakdown products and alarmins that are present in the degenerative joint; these in turn stimulate release of a robust cascade of proinflammatory cytokines, including IL-1β, TNF-α, IL-6, as well as chemokines, nitric oxide, and reactive oxygen species, all of which further activate the catabolic system. Thus, chondrocytes are active participants in the breakdown of cartilage matrix, and the system is amplified by the ongoing degradation. In addition, adipose tissue (itself proinflammatory, as noted above) within the joint, principally in the infrapatellar fat pad in the knee, has been implicated as an active participant in this inflammation. Ultimately, this vicious cycle of matrix degradation products activating the innate immune system and inducing further damage is widely present in OA, and there is evidence that this contributes both to OA pain and to structural progression.

GENETICS

As OA is neither a single disease nor clearly transmitted by Mendelian genetics, the contribution of genetics to OA pathogenesis is complex. Among OA phenotypes, so-called nodal OA involving osteophytes of the DIPs and the PIPs of the hand appears to have a strong familial component. Early searches for a genetic component in OA pathogenesis were candidate gene-based approaches and sought mutations in the structural proteins of the cartilage and joint tissues. However, actual single-gene defects that lead to OA-like disease, such as collagen II or lubricin gene mutations, are exceptionally uncommon and appear to be restricted to small kindreds. The widespread application of genome-wide association studies (GWAS) technology has greatly broadened the understanding of the contribution of the genome to OA in populations, and has identified more than 45 genetic loci associated with OA.[31-33] Most of these are common in the population, with allele frequencies >4%, and have small to moderate effect sizes, which is consistent with the polygenic and multifactorial etiology of OA. Nonetheless, many of the polymorphisms are in genes that regulate skeletal development and proliferation or are in structural proteins. Polymorphisms that are associated with OA pain, such as in the genes encoding PACE4 and TRPV1, have also been identified. Finally, epigenetic modifications appear to have a substantial role in regulating chondrocyte environmental responses. A variety of genome-wide methylation studies have identified multiple genes with methylation differences in OA chondrocytes related to maturation and apoptosis. Similarly, histone modifications and noncoding RNAs have been extensively evaluated in OA tissue and appear to have a pathogenic role.[17,32]

TRAUMA

Major trauma with disruption of joint structures is one of the few well-described etiologies that clearly leads to the subsequent development of OA. In addition, it provides a potential window of opportunity during which, in theory, OA could be prevented using yet-to-be defined therapeutic strategies. It also is the one form of OA for which a true baseline time point can be determined. Posttraumatic OA itself is common, accounting for at least 12% of OA cases[6] and is the primary etiology of OA in otherwise unusually affected joints such as the ankle or the elbow. Moreover, as it predominantly affects a much younger demographic than idiopathic OA, its societal morbidity is significantly amplified. The etiology of posttraumatic OA is complex and involves many of the mechanisms already described, including intra-articular inflammation and response to injury, damage to the articular cartilage, menisci, and subchondral bone, and aberrant loading both acutely due to pain and chronically due to joint pathology. The risk for development of posttraumatic OA after injury has been estimated at 20% to 50%,[34] and the time course is variable but may encompass years to decades.

PAIN IN OSTEOARTHRITIS

The pathophysiology of OA pain remains poorly understood. Articular cartilage is not innervated, and thus even historically, when OA was thought to be primarily a cartilage disease, OA pain was ascribed to other sources, including local inflammation associated with effusion, subchondral bone remodeling, and degenerative menisci. Recent investigation has yielded important new insights. Pain may be categorized as nociceptive or neuropathic, and it is now appreciated that both types are present in OA. Nociceptive pain is the classic pain sensation felt as a result of trauma or inflammation. It results from activation of the nociceptors, a group of small diameter afferent nerve fibers, by any of a variety of noxious stimuli such as tissue injury, heat, or pressure. It is conventionally felt as a sharp, aching, or throbbing pain. As it is an injury response, nociceptive pain tends to resolve with healing of the insult. In contrast, neuropathic pain tends to be chronic once it has developed. It is associated with alterations of nerve fibers, often with reorganization of pathways both in the peripheral and in the central nervous systems to perpetuate the pain sensation. In addition to altered sensitivity, neuropathic pain may intensify over time. Its symptoms are typically described as sensations of burning, tingling, electrical shock, or a heavy sensation or numbness. Neuropathic pain has increasingly been appreciated as a significant component of the pain experience in OA.[35] Systematic analyses have revealed that a large proportion of OA patients complain of neuropathic symptoms—burning, numbness, and paresthesias.[1,36] Neuropathic pain is not relieved by conventional analgesics, and its prevalence in OA may be one source of the discordance between the degree of structural degeneration observed in many patients and the magnitude of pain. Of related interest, it has become clear that OA is associated with a spectrum of somatosensory deficits, including diminished proprioception and vibratory sensation,[14,37] similarly suggesting a neuropathic component to OA pathogenesis.

©Copyright 2021 American Academy of Orthopaedic Surgeons

PAIN FROM JOINT STRUCTURES

While the cartilage is aneural, the joint is highly innervated and includes both somatosensory and nociceptive afferents.[38] There is rich innervation in the synovial capsule, ligaments, and the peripheral aspects of menisci, as well as the periosteum and subchondral bone, and each of these structures may be a source of pain.[39] In aggregate, these structures may account for the majority of the nociceptive pain in OA. Moreover, the articular cartilage and menisci undergo degradation and remodeling as part of the OA process, which involves activation of metalloproteinases and the release of inflammatory mediators and matrix degradation products, all of which may activate nociceptors and contribute to the pain response.

Local inflammation itself is another significant contributor to OA pain and may explain in part the efficacy of NSAIDs and intra-articular glucocorticoids for OA pain. As noted, many OA joints have synovitis, and this may play a prominent role in painful OA flares. In addition, even the "noninflammatory" effusions may cause pain by distending the synovial capsule and are a rich source of inflammatory mediators that also may precipitate pain.

Aberrant mechanical loading across joints is a distinct structural source of OA pain. This has been studied extensively in knee OA, where OA joints bear significantly higher loads during ambulation than normal joints, and the overloading is associated with the magnitude of pain.[7] The biomechanical function of articular cartilage is to cushion subchondral bone during articulation, and as cartilage degenerates, the subchondral bone undergoes extensive remodeling, including the development of sclerosis, bone cysts, microfractures, and osteonecrosis. These changes, each of which may produce pain, are routinely observed radiographically and may be associated with bone marrow lesions (BMLs) observed by MRI.

PAIN SENSITIZATION

Nociceptive pain may be amplified through a process termed sensitization, wherein neurons are sensitized by activation and become hyperresponsive, inducing physiologic alterations in the dorsal horns and more centrally. In OA, peripheral sensitization is thought to be mediated by constant nociceptive stimulation at the level of the joint, modulating spinal cord pathways and leading to decreased activation thresholds and increased synaptic excitability. Central sensitization arises from synaptic plasticity within the dorsal horns and may result in chronic pain even after the initial nociceptive stimulus has resolved.[39,40] Clinically assessable signs of sensitization include allodynia (the sense of pain resulting from a normally innocuous stimulus), hyperalgesia (increased painful intensity from painful stimuli), and temporal summation (repeated stimuli become increasingly painful over time). Analyses of these manifestations among OA patients have revealed a high prevalence of sensitization, which likely plays an important role in the chronic pain of OA.[13,35,41]

BIOPSYCHOSOCIAL ASPECTS OF OSTEOARTHRITIS PAIN

As it has become clear that chronic pain is an important component of OA, the biopsychosocial factors that mediate the complex interactions between noxious stimuli and peripheral and central nervous system responses have been found to be active components of the pain experience.[42,43] It is also clear that the severity and character of an individual's OA pain may depend on that individual's unique social, cultural, and personal state. Qualitative analyses of OA pain and distress have identified distinct patterns of intermittent versus background chronic pain, with negative effects on mood, sleep, and social participation.[42] In addition, fatigue, psychological distress, and social context each augment the pain perceived in OA, and individuals with poor self-efficacy or pain catastrophizing have greater pain and poorer outcomes.[44] One reason that OA pain therapy remains inadequate is this complexity, involving nociceptive, neuropathic, and biopsychosocial aspects; the contribution of each of these differs among individual patients, rendering uniform treatment guidelines less valuable than for more discrete conditions. Nonetheless, an understanding of these processes has provided insight to design novel regimens to target OA pain.[45]

CLINICAL MANIFESTATIONS

SYMPTOMS

In OA, by the time clinical symptoms appear, the pathological events underlying the disease have been ongoing for years. With clinical disease, symptoms vary dramatically over time, both in severity and in character (**Table 1**). In addition, especially early in the clinical course, patients may

TABLE 1 Clinical Features of Osteoarthritis

Symptoms	Signs
Pain and discomfort	Bony prominence at joint margins (osteophytes)
Loss of cosmesis (especially hands, feet, and knees)	Crepitus
Sensation of stiffness ("gelling" phenomenon)	Cool effusion
Reduced function	Observable deformity
Weakness	Tenderness
Grinding or clicking	Altered gait
Instability/buckling	Limitation of motion
	Ligamentous laxity

©Copyright 2021 American Academy of Orthopaedic Surgeons

experience prolonged asymptomatic periods punctuated by painful flares of joint symptoms that may last several weeks or months.

Pain

Pain is the primary symptom of OA and is typically the reason that patients seek medical attention. Movement worsens joint pain, especially loading the involved joint, as with weight bearing or stair climbing in the large joints. Conversely, the sensation of joint stiffness is often exacerbated by prolonged inactivity (eg, after sitting). With disease progression, pain tends to become more persistent, and frequently patients experience nocturnal pain which disturbs sleep. OA pain can wax and wane throughout the protracted course of the disease, though there is evidence that over time people develop a fairly stable pain level that may persist for years.[46] Some patients may be minimally symptomatic and able to function almost normally most of the time, while others with a comparable degree of structural disease experience severe pain, work limitations, and more extensive disability. The sources of this heterogeneity remain poorly understood.

Joint Stiffness

The inflammatory arthritides, such as rheumatoid arthritis, are characterized by prolonged morning stiffness, but this is explicitly not a characteristic of OA. Nonetheless, OA patients do describe feeling stiff when rising or when standing after prolonged sitting. This sensation resolves quickly (substantially less than 30 minutes) and is called a "gelling" phenomenon. Importantly, gelling tends to be restricted to affected joints and is not felt systemically.

Joint Deformity and Swelling

A common component of OA-related joint degeneration is the formation of osteophytes. These are noticeable in superficial joints as deformities. Hence, after pain, the most common presentation of hand OA is complaints of the cosmetic changes caused by osteophytes at the DIPs (Heberden nodes) or at the PIPs (Bouchard nodes) (**Figure 3**). These may have painful phases, particularly during enlargement; however, they generally are asymptomatic and troublesome largely for their appearance. Similarly, osteophytes in the knee OA may be visually evident. Joint swelling is a related finding because patients frequently conflate the bony enlargement caused by osteophytes with synovial effusions and describe both as "swelling." Nonetheless, joint swelling is distinct from bony enlargement and is a common report in OA, especially in the knees. The swelling may be warm and erythematous but is usually described as a cool effusion. Effusions may occur in any involved joints; however, the small joints of the hands do not typically develop OA effusions and the hips are too deep for patients to feel the swelling.

Mechanical Symptoms

During the course of OA involving the weight bearing joints, patients may note a sensation of instability during ambulation; in the knees, this may be felt as buckling or as "giving out" and is frequently associated with sharp pain. This is often not due to actual mechanical instability, but rather to a subjective sense that the joint cannot support weight. In addition, patients may note a grinding feeling during joint motion, which occasionally is accompanied by pain; this sensation may be the symptomatic result of crepitus. Finally, with advanced structural OA, there may be symptomatic loss of range of motion, even in the absence of synovial effusion.

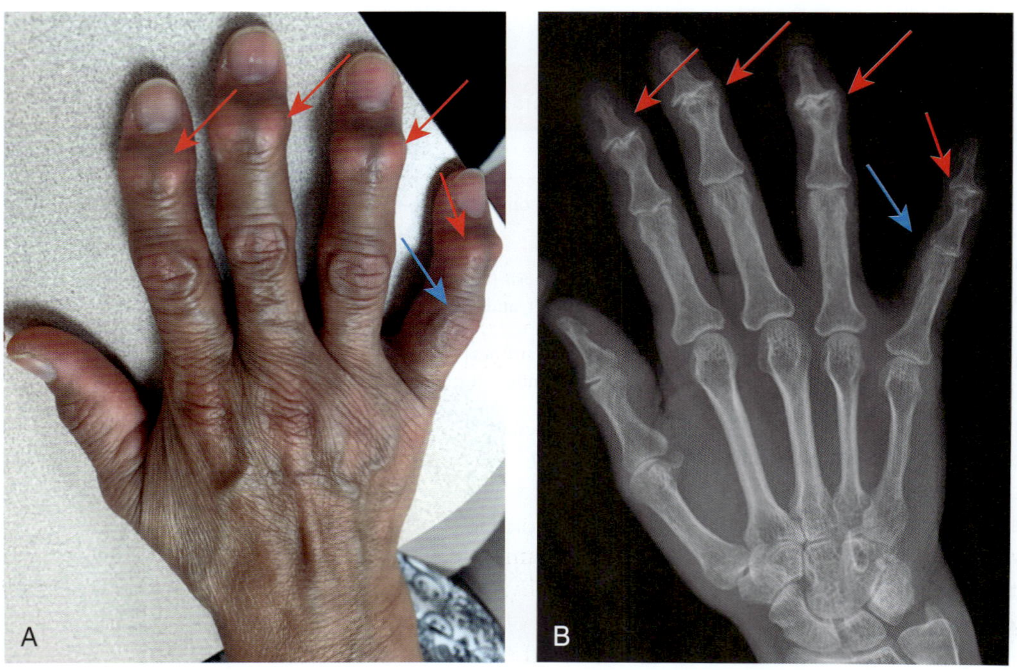

FIGURE 3 Nodal osteoarthritis (OA). Bony changes of the hand frequently involve deformities of the distal interphalangeal (DIP) and proximal interphalangeal (PIP) joints, termed Bouchard nodes and Heberden nodes, respectively. **A**, The noninflamed bony enlargement of Bouchard nodes (blue arrows) and Heberden nodes (red arrows) are evident in this photograph. **B**, Radiographic appearance of interphalangeal joint OA, with osteophytes and joint space narrowing; radiographs are obtained from a different patient. (Courtesy of Augustine Manadan, MD.)

©Copyright 2021 American Academy of Orthopaedic Surgeons

SIGNS

The signs detected by physical examination reflect the structural disease of OA, characterized by deterioration of the articular cartilage, osteophyte formation, and degenerative changes of the tendons, ligaments, muscles, and other periarticular tissue (**Table 1**). However, as OA is primarily degenerative rather than inflammatory, signs of systemic disease are absent.

Crepitus

When intact, articular hyaline cartilage provides essentially frictionless articulation. In OA, as it degenerates, the articular surface loses its smoothness, and a grinding sensation (crepitus) can be appreciated when palpating a joint in passive motion. This is pathognomonic of cartilage damage and can often be appreciated in knees prior to the development of clinical symptoms. Crepitus, which is pathologic, is distinct from the audible clicking that occasionally accompanies joint motion in normal joints and is benign.

Joint Enlargement

When superficial joints develop osteophytes, these may be palpable as joint enlargement. This enlargement is bony and is most prominent at the joint margins. These are usually asymptomatic, but occasionally can be tender. In addition, joint effusions may cause a soft ballotable swelling of the synovial capsule. As noted previously, these are usually noninflammatory and cool in OA, in contrast to the warm and erythematous infusions of the inflammatory arthritides. However, OA effusions may be warm during painful flares, denoting local inflammation.

Gait

OA in the lower extremities is associated with abnormal gait as a consequence of pain and deformities. With severe disease, this may be observable as a limp or as slowed cadence, or as is often seen with hip OA, an antalgic gait. However, overloading of the weight-bearing joints is also part of a complex gait adaptation that is pathophysiologically related to disease progression,[47] but which requires formal kinematic analyses to detect.[7]

CLINICAL PATTERNS

OA may involve any diarthrodial joint, though certain joints are commonly affected and others are only rarely involved. While OA may be monoarticular, it is typically bilateral and affects multiple joints. The pattern of involvement helps to distinguish OA from the inflammatory arthritides clinically. Whereas inflammatory arthritis, such as rheumatoid arthritis, commonly involves elbows, wrists, ankles, and the metacarpal-phalangeal (MCPs) joints, these are only rarely involved in OA except after trauma. In contrast, OA often involves the DIPs and PIPs. However, it is important to remember that as OA is such a widely prevalent disease, even unusual presentations are seen regularly by most caregivers.

Lower Extremities

The large weight-bearing joints are commonly involved. Knee OA is at least fourfold more common than hip OA and may involve any or all of the knee compartments. The majority of patients have medial compartment involvement (likely related to the fact that the medial compartment bears the majority of the knee loads) and may lead to varus deformity. Patellofemoral compartment OA has received increasing attention as it tends to be very symptomatic and more refractory to analgesia. It is characteristically exacerbated by walking stairs. Knee OA is often associated with synovial cysts and anserine or prepatellar bursitis. Hip OA may be distinguished by pain felt in the groin and radiating to the anterior thigh or to the knee. Early hip OA is characterized by restricted internal rotation and may progress to limited motion in general and to limb length discrepancy. In the foot, OA typically involves the first MTP, resulting in a bunion deformity, though midfoot pain is increasingly recognized.

Upper Extremities

The hands are the most commonly affected areas of the upper extremities. Involvement of the first CMC, at the base of the thumb, is usually symptomatic and interferes with grasping, buttoning, and turning doorknobs. Palpable osteophytes of the DIPs and of the PIPs are often the initial sign of hand OA (**Figure 3**) and may be otherwise asymptomatic though these joints may have periods of painful flares. This pattern of hand OA is termed "primary generalized OA" or "nodal OA." Erosive or inflammatory OA is a less common but distinct subset in which erosions develop in the DIPs and PIPs and are associated with repeated episodes of acute inflammatory symptoms.[48]

Spine

OA of the spine is common, but is conventionally dealt with as a separate disease encompassing degenerative disk disease. It typically involves the lumbar and cervical vertebrae, affecting the facet and uncovertebral joints.

DIAGNOSIS

The diagnosis of OA is a clinical decision. There are no laboratory tests that are sufficiently specific to be useful, and imaging provides information only about structure, which correlates only loosely with clinical symptoms. OA is not a systemic disease, and tests that assess organ function are generally normal, as are conventional markers of inflammation. The blood count, comprehensive metabolic panel, sedimentation rate, and conventional CRP should be normal. However, as OA is prevalent among the middle-aged and elderly, a demographic that has a high prevalence of comorbidities, coexisting conditions may confound the interpretation of laboratory testing. When joint effusions are present, examination of the synovial

©Copyright 2021 American Academy of Orthopaedic Surgeons

fluid should yield a noninflammatory sample. Total leukocyte counts are typically less than 1,500 to 2,000 cells/mm^3 with a predominance of lymphocytes rather than neutrophils. Incidental findings of crystals, such as calcium pyrophosphate dihydrate, or of cartilage fragments may sometimes be observed. At present, there are no clinically useful biomarkers for the diagnosis or prognostication of OA, notwithstanding a decades-long search.

IMAGING

Imaging technology provides a great deal of structural information about the joint tissues, but imaging is of only adjunctive benefit in OA, as the diagnosis is made on clinical grounds. Conventional radiography remains the primary imaging modality useful for OA in clinical practice, and quantitative assessment of radiographic joint space width still provides the only structural outcome recognized by regulatory agencies for assessing OA progression. Characteristic radiographic features of OA include narrowed joint space, osteophytes, and subchondral bone sclerosis (**Figure 4**), though not all features need to be present in any patient. There is not a clean relationship between radiographic appearance and clinical symptomatology, and it is important to remember that the radiographic changes of OA occur only after the degenerative process has been ongoing for several years. Cartilage is radiolucent and the radiographic appearance of cartilage degeneration—radiographic joint space narrowing—requires a great deal of cartilage loss before it is evident. Similarly, subchondral sclerosis and osteophyte formation occur as a response to long-standing structural processes. Thus, individuals may have symptomatic, clinically significant OA for several years prior to developing radiographically evident changes.

Advanced imaging modalities are most useful for research or for specific tasks such as planning surgery or for excluding other potential pathology such as degenerative menisci, ligamentous injuries, and unrelated diseases. Clinical MRI provides detailed images of each of the joint structures, detecting even subtle defects of articular cartilage. It also sensitively identifies subchondral bone marrow lesions that are associated with painful episodes in OA, as well as synovitis, meniscal pathology, osteophytes, and periarticular muscular lesions. A variety of methods and grading scales have been described for the quantitative and semiquantitative assessment of each of these structures, as well as for the joint as a whole, but to date, these have not had an effect on nonsurgical decision making, or on the clinical management of patients with OA.[49] More sophisticated techniques, such as compositional MR imaging and positron emission tomography CT (PET-CT) or PET-MR provide additional information about the ultrastructure and physiology of the joint, but have limited clinical applicability.[50]

Ultrasonography has been widely adopted for office-based imaging because it provides detailed information of joint structure without exposing the patient to ionizing radiation and is available at the bedside. In experienced hands, it has been shown to sensitively identify features such as occult osteophytes undetectable by standard radiography, subtle articular cartilage lesions, and mild local synovitis. In addition, it has proven useful to guide intra-articular injections, especially in deep joints such as the hip.[49]

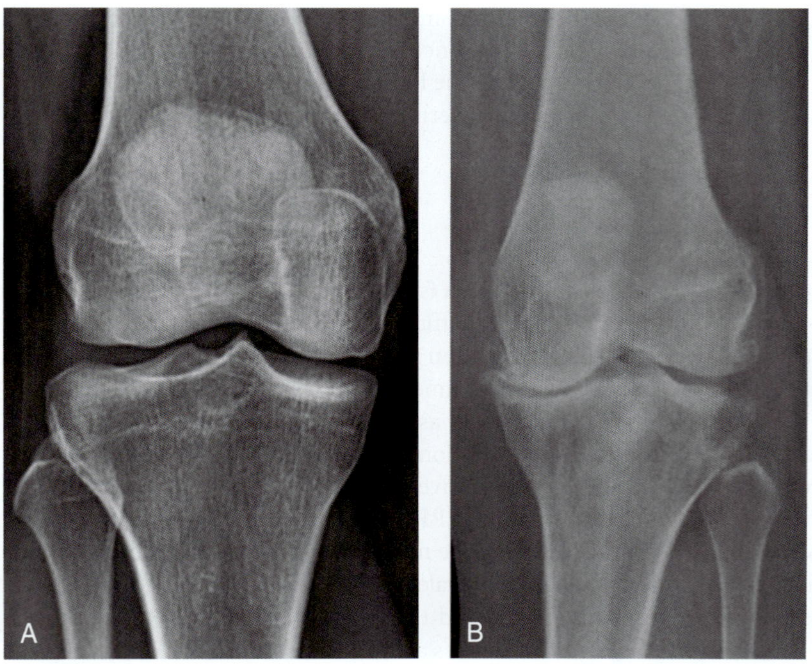

FIGURE 4 Radiographic osteoarthritis (OA) of the knee. **A**, Weight-bearing AP radiograph of a normal knee. There is abundant joint space, without bony hypertrophy or subchondral sclerosis. **B**, Weight-bearing radiograph of a knee with medial compartment advanced OA. There is loss of the radiographic joint space medially, with large osteophyte at the medial femoral condyle and the medial tibial plateau, and subchondral sclerosis, worst at the femoral condyle. (B, Courtesy of Augustine Manadan, MD.)

©Copyright 2021 American Academy of Orthopaedic Surgeons

TREATMENT

At present there are no therapeutic strategies that have been shown to retard or reverse disease progression. Ultimately, joint replacement is definitive treatment for refractory end-stage disease and is widely available for several joints. However, there are a variety of modalities that effectively relieve pain and maintain function short of surgical intervention. As with all conditions, patient education and support are critical; self-help programs alone have been shown to improve outcomes in OA. Patients should be provided thorough information about the natural course of OA, their own role in disease management, and appropriate expectations.

PHYSICAL MEASURES

Exercise, especially focusing on the periarticular muscles of affected joints, has been consistently shown to improve function and to provide significant pain palliation. Physical Therapy for appropriate strength training and to improve and maintain range of motion is almost always indicated.[51] Also, as OA pain may be mediated by aberrant biomechanical loading, ambulatory assist devices such as canes and walkers, which significantly reduce loads across the knee during gait, can reduce pain and improve stability. Unloading knee braces have been approved for knee OA for decades and may be effective, though they are cumbersome often not tolerated.

MEDICATION

With time, most patients require medication to provide adequate pain palliation. This is complicated by the fact that elderly OA patients typically have comorbidities that may circumscribe medication options. Topical NSAIDs may reduce risks of systemic adverse effects and may be as effective as oral NSAIDs;[52] in the United States, diclofenac is available as a gel, but additional NSAIDs are available in other countries. Topical capsaicin is approved for knee OA, but is only marginally effective and has a high risk of adverse effects, so it is only occasionally used.

When topical agents are insufficient, oral analgesics are often the next step. There is controversy regarding the use of acetaminophen. Whereas many organizations recommend its use in OA, there is compelling evidence that chronic use is not substantially better than placebo[53,54] and carries risks, suggesting that it is not an optimal choice. Tramadol has been shown to be effective for OA, but carries a risk of dependency, and the more potent opiates are associated with substantially increased morbidity among the elderly, especially due to the risk for traumatic falls. NSAIDs remain the category of medication that has been consistently demonstrated to be effective for OA pain and to retain efficacy for years.[55] Although there are concerns of potential toxicities, these medications remain the mainstay of OA therapy. They may not be a viable option for patients with significant renal, cardiac, or gastrointestinal conditions, though proton pump inhibitors or misoprostol can provide gastric protection in middle-aged and elderly patients and those at risk for gastrointestinal bleeding. Cyclooxygenase-2 inhibitors are an additional option; in the United States, celecoxib is the only agent available in this class. Finally, as the neuropathic component of OA has been appreciated, neuroactive agents have been employed. Duloxetine hydrochloride, a serotonin and norepinephrine reuptake inhibitor was approved by the US FDA in 2010 for the treatment of OA pain. This efficacy is widely considered to be a class effect and has led to the frequently off-label use of a variety of neuroactive medications. Moreover, inhibitors of nerve growth factor have shown potent efficacy for OA pain[56] and, notwithstanding their potential toxicity, are likely to be approved in the United States by 2020.

INTRA-ARTICULAR THERAPY

Intra-articular glucocorticoids have been used for OA painful flares for decades and have shown to be effective for short term relief.[57] In practice, injections are limited to a maximum of four times annually because of theoretical concerns of toxicity to articular cartilage. A new, extended release preparation of triamcinolone was approved for use in 2017, but has not yet been demonstrated to have superior efficacy. Hyaluronan derivatives are also available for injection to relieve OA pain, but the magnitude of relief provided beyond placebo remains controversial.[58] This modality is referred to as viscosupplementation because extrinsic hyaluronans were initially intended to supplement the viscosity of synovial fluid and thereby improve articular lubrication. However, their intra-articular residence time is too brief to have this effect and their mechanism of action in vivo is poorly understood.

COMPLEMENTARY AND ALTERNATIVE MEDICINE

As is common with chronic painful conditions for which conventional medicine has inadequate therapy, OA patients frequently use complementary modalities. Among the more popular are glucosamine, chondroitin, and acupuncture. Although none has been demonstrated to substantially retard structural progression, and independently funded trials have been consistently negative,[59] many patients derive pain relief. These results may be confounded by the substantial placebo response that is observed in any blinded study of OA pain,[60] and there is controversy regarding whether these approaches provide incremental pain relief over that obtained with placebo; nonetheless, many of these approaches can be safely utilized by individuals who feel that they benefit from them.

©Copyright 2021 American Academy of Orthopaedic Surgeons

NOVEL AGENTS UNDER DEVELOPMENT

A discussion of potential disease-modifying OA drugs (DMOADs) and the state of the pipeline for this condition is beyond the scope of this chapter. Several recent reviews thoroughly describe the active candidate molecules, however. For example, see Refs. 61 or 62.

SUMMARY

OA is the most prevalent form of arthritis and accounts for vast societal costs and morbidity. It is not a single disease, but represents a painful degenerative process of joints from a multitude of etiologies. The most important risk factors of incident disease include aging, obesity, and trauma. Pathogenesis involves an imbalance between anabolic repair and catabolic degradation of joint tissues and is mediated by local inflammation, aberrant biomechanics, aging, and genetic factors. There are at present no therapeutic strategies that have been shown to alter the natural history of the disease; however, a variety of modalities effectively relieve pain and preserve function. Ultimately, for end-stage disease with refractory pain, joint replacement in appropriate joints has been shown to be definitive.

REFERENCES

1. Neogi T: The epidemiology and impact of pain in osteoarthritis. *Osteoarthr Cartil* 2013;21(9):1145-1153.
2. Murphy L, Schwartz TA, Helmick CG, et al: Lifetime risk of symptomatic knee osteoarthritis. *Arthritis Rheum* 2008;59(9):1207-1213.
3. Lawrence RC, Felson DT, Helmick CG, et al: Estimates of the prevalence of arthritis and other rheumatic conditions in the United States. Part II. *Arthritis Rheum* 2008;58(1):26-35.
4. Puig-Junoy J, Ruiz Zamora A: Socio-economic costs of osteoarthritis: A systematic review of cost-of-illness studies. *Semin Arthritis Rheum.* 2015;44(5):531-541.
5. Hunter DJ, Guermazi A, Roemer F, Zhang Y, Neogi T: Structural correlates of pain in joints with osteoarthritis. *Osteoarthr Cartil* 2013;21(9):1170-1178.
6. Brown TD, Johnston RC, Saltzman CL, Marsh JL, Buckwalter JA: Posttraumatic osteoarthritis: A first estimate of incidence, prevalence, and burden of disease. *J Orthop Trauma* 2006;20(10):739-744.
7. Block JA, Shakoor N: Lower limb osteoarthritis: Biomechanical alterations and implications for therapy. *Curr Opin Rheumatol* 2010;22(5):544-550.
8. Jahn S, Seror J, Klein J: Lubrication of articular cartilage. *Annu Rev Biomed Eng* 2016;18:235-258.
9. Suri S, Walsh DA: Osteochondral alterations in osteoarthritis. *Bone* 2012;51(2):204-211.
10. Thakur M, Dickenson AH, Baron R: Osteoarthritis pain: Nociceptive or neuropathic? *Nat Rev Rheumatol.* 2014;10(6):374-380.
11. Scanzello CR: Role of low-grade inflammation in osteoarthritis. *Curr Opin Rheumatol* 2017;29(1):79-85.
12. Roos EM, Herzog W, Block JA, Bennell KL: Muscle weakness, afferent sensory dysfunction and exercise in knee osteoarthritis. *Nat Rev Rheumatol* 2010;7(1):57-63.
13. Dua AB, Neogi T, Mikolaitis RA, Block JA, Shakoor N: Somatosensation in OA: Exploring the relationships of pain sensitization, vibratory perception and spontaneous pain. *BMC Muscoskelet Disord* 2018;19(1):307.
14. Shakoor N, Lee KJ, Fogg LF, Block JA: Generalized vibratory deficits in osteoarthritis of the hip. *Arthritis Rheum* 2008;59(9):1237-1240. [Erratum appears in *Arthritis Rheum* 2009;61(1):142].
15. Franceschi C, Bonafe M, Valensin S, et al: Inflamm-aging. An evolutionary perspective on immunosenescence. *Ann NY Acad Sci* 2000;908:244-254.
16. Li YS, Xiao WF, Luo W: Cellular aging towards osteoarthritis. *Mech Ageing Develop* 2017;162:80-84.
17. Coutinho de Almeida R, Ramos YFM, Meulenbelt I: Involvement of epigenetics in osteoarthritis. *Baillieres Best Pract Res Clin Rheumatol* 2017;31(5):634-648.
18. Loeser RF, Yammani RR, Carlson CS, et al: Articular chondrocytes express the receptor for advanced glycation end products: Potential role in osteoarthritis. *Arthritis Rheum* 2005;52(8):2376-2385.
19. Shakoor N, Block JA, Shott S, Case JP: Nonrandom evolution of end-stage osteoarthritis of the lower limbs. *Arthritis Rheum* 2002;46(12):3185-3189.
20. Engstrom G, Gerhardsson de Verdier M, Rollof J, Nilsson PM, Lohmander LS: C-reactive protein, metabolic syndrome and incidence of severe hip and knee osteoarthritis. A population-based cohort study. *Osteoarthr Cartil* 2009;17(2):168-173.
21. Visser AW, de Mutsert R, le Cessie S, den Heijer M, Rosendaal FR, Kloppenburg M: The relative contribution of mechanical stress and systemic processes in different types of osteoarthritis: The NEO study. *Ann Rheum Dis* 2015;74(10):1842-1847.
22. Courties A, Sellam J, Berenbaum F: Metabolic syndrome-associated osteoarthritis. *Curr Opin Rheumatol* 2017;29(2):214-222.
23. Wang T, He C: Pro-inflammatory cytokines: The link between obesity and osteoarthritis. *Cytokine Growth Factor Rev* 2018;44:38-50.
24. Francisco V, Perez T, Pino J, et al: Biomechanics, obesity, and osteoarthritis. The role of adipokines: When the levee breaks. *J Orthop Res* 2017;36(2):594-604.
25. Urban H, Little CB: The role of fat and inflammation in the pathogenesis and management of osteoarthritis. *Rheumatology* 2018;57(suppl 4):iv10-iv21.
26. Roemer FW, Kassim Javaid M, Guermazi A, et al: Anatomical distribution of synovitis in knee osteoarthritis and its association with joint effusion assessed on non-enhanced and contrast-enhanced MRI. *Osteoarthr Cartil* 2010;18(10):1269-1274.
27. Sarmanova A, Hall M, Moses J, Doherty M, Zhang W: Synovial changes detected by ultrasound in people with knee osteoarthritis – A meta-analysis of observational studies. *Osteoarthr Cartil* 2016;24(8):1376-1383.
28. Sarmanova A, Hall M, Fernandes GS, et al: Association between ultrasound-detected synovitis and knee pain: A population-based case–control study with both cross-sectional and follow-up data. *Arthritis Res Ther* 2017;19(1):281.
29. Kalaitzoglou E, Griffin TM, Humphrey MB: Innate immune responses and osteoarthritis. *Curr Rheumatol Rep* 2017;19(8):45.
30. Scanzello CR: Pathologic and pathogenic processes in osteoarthritis: The effects of synovitis. *HSS J* 2012;8(1):20-22.
31. Cibrian Uhalte E, Wilkinson JM, Southam L, Zeggini E: Pathways to understanding the genomic aetiology of osteoarthritis. *Hum Mol Genet* 2017;26(R2):R193-R201.
32. Jeffries MA: Osteoarthritis year in review 2018: Genetics and epigenetics. *Osteoarthr Cartil* 2019;27(3):371-377.
33. MacArthur J, Bowler E, Cerezo M, et al: The new NHGRI-EBI Catalog of published genome-wide association studies (GWAS Catalog). *Nucleic Acids Res* 2017;45(D1):D896-D901.
34. Riordan EA, Little C, Hunter D: Pathogenesis of post-traumatic OA with a view to intervention. *Best Pract Res Clin Rheumatol* 2014;28(1):17-30.
35. French HP, Smart KM, Doyle F: Prevalence of neuropathic pain in knee or hip osteoarthritis: A systematic review and meta-analysis. *Semin Arthritis Rheum* 2017;47(1):1-8.

©Copyright 2021 American Academy of Orthopaedic Surgeons

36. Hochman JR, French MR, Bermingham SL, Hawker GA: The nerve of osteoarthritis pain. *Arthritis Care Res* 2010;62(7):1019-1023.
37. Wylde V, Palmer S, Learmonth ID, Dieppe P: Somatosensory abnormalities in knee OA. *Rheumatology* 2012;51(3):535-543.
38. Courties A, Sellam J, Berenbaum F: Role of the autonomic nervous system in osteoarthritis. *Baillieres Best Pract Res Clin Rheumatol* 2017;31(5):661-675.
39. Malfait AM, Schnitzer TJ: Towards a mechanism-based approach to pain management in osteoarthritis. *Nat Rev Rheumatol.* 2013;17:10.
40. Dimitroulas T, Duarte RV, Behura A, Kitas GD, Raphael JH: Neuropathic pain in osteoarthritis: A review of pathophysiological mechanisms and implications for treatment. *Semin Arthritis Rheum* 2014;44(2):145-154.
41. Fingleton C, Smart K, Moloney N, Fullen BM, Doody C: Pain sensitization in people with knee osteoarthritis: A systematic review and meta-analysis. *Osteoarthr Cartil* 2015;23(7):1043-1056.
42. Hawker GA: Experiencing painful osteoarthritis: What have we learned from listening? *Curr Opin Rheumatol* 2009;21(5):507-512.
43. Bennell KL, Nelligan R, Dobson F, et al: Effectiveness of an internet-delivered exercise and pain-coping skills training intervention for persons with chronic knee pain: A randomized trial. *Ann Intern Med* 2017;166(7):453-462.
44. Rayahin JE, Chmiel JS, Hayes KW, et al: Factors associated with pain experience outcome in knee osteoarthritis. *Arthritis Care Res* 2014;66(12):1828-1835.
45. Hausmann LRM, Youk A, Kwoh CK, et al: Testing a positive psychological intervention for osteoarthritis. *Pain Med* 2017;18(10):1908-1920.
46. Pan F, Tian J, Aitken D, Cicuttini F, Jones G: Predictors of pain severity trajectory in older adults: A 10.7-year follow-up study. *Osteoarthr Cartil* 2018;26(12):1619-1626.
47. Shakoor N, Hurwitz DE, Block JA, Shott S, Case JP: Asymmetric knee loading in advanced unilateral hip osteoarthritis. *Arthritis Rheum* 2003;48(6):1556-1561.
48. Gazeley DJ, Yeturi S, Patel PJ, Rosenthal AK: Erosive osteoarthritis: A systematic analysis of definitions used in the literature. *Semin Arthritis Rheum* 2017;46(4):395-403.
49. Wang X, Oo WM, Linklater JM: What is the role of imaging in the clinical diagnosis of osteoarthritis and disease management? *Rheumatology* 2018;57(suppl 4):iv51-iv60.
50. Hayashi D, Roemer FW, Guermazi A: Imaging of osteoarthritis by conventional radiography, MR imaging, PET-computed tomography, and PET-MR imaging. *Pet Clin* 2019;14(1):17-29.
51. Wellsandt E, Golightly Y: Exercise in the management of knee and hip osteoarthritis. *Curr Opin Rheumatol* 2018;30(2):151-159.
52. Derry S, Conaghan P, Da Silva JA, Wiffen PJ, Moore RA: Topical NSAIDs for chronic musculoskeletal pain in adults. *Cochrane Database Syst Rev* 2016;4:CD007400.
53. Leopoldino AO, Machado GC, Ferreira PH, et al: Paracetamol versus placebo for knee and hip osteoarthritis. *Cochrane Database Syst Rev* 2019;2:CD013273.
54. Case JP, Baliunas AJ, Block JA: Lack of efficacy of acetaminophen in treating symptomatic knee osteoarthritis: A randomized, double-blind, placebo-controlled comparison trial with diclofenac sodium. *Arch Intern Med* 2003;163(2):169-178.
55. Bannuru RR, Schmid CH, Kent DM, Vaysbrot EE, Wong JB, McAlindon TE: Comparative effectiveness of pharmacologic interventions for knee osteoarthritis: A systematic review and network meta-analysis. *Ann Intern Med.* 2015;162(1):46-54.
56. Miller RE, Block JA, Malfait AM: What is new in pain modification in osteoarthritis? *Rheumatology* 2018;57(suppl 4):iv99-iv107.
57. Juni P, Hari R, Rutjes AW, et al: Intra-articular corticosteroid for knee osteoarthritis. *Cochrane Database Syst Rev* 2015;(10):CD005328.
58. Richardson C, Plaas A, Block JA: Intra-articular Hyaluronan Therapy for Symptomatic Knee Osteoarthritis. *Rheum Dis Clin North Am* 2019;45(3):439-451.
59. Block JA, Oegema TR, Sandy JD, Plaas A: The effects of oral glucosamine on joint health: Is a change in research approach needed? *Osteoarthr Cartil* 2010;18(1):5-11.
60. Dieppe P, Goldingay S, Greville-Harris M: The power and value of placebo and nocebo in painful osteoarthritis. *Osteoarthr Cartil* 2016;24(11):1850-1857.
61. Yu SP-C, Hunter DJ: Emerging drugs for the treatment of knee osteoarthritis. *Expert Opin Emerg Drugs* 2015;20(3):361-378.
62. Huang Z, Ding C, Li T, Yu SP-C: Current status and future prospects for disease modification in osteoarthritis. *Rheumatology* 2018;57(suppl 4):iv108-iv23.

©Copyright 2021 American Academy of Orthopaedic Surgeons

29

Neuromuscular Diseases

Daniel Weltsch, MD
Keith D. Baldwin, MD, MSPT, MPH

Keywords: *motor neuron disease; muscular dystrophy; myopathy; neuromuscular junction; neuropathy*

INTRODUCTION

The nervous system in conjunction with the musculoskeletal system confers the ability to perform voluntary movements, maintain an erect posture, and perform activities of daily living. Neuromuscular diseases are pathological conditions that originate in either the musculoskeletal system, the nervous system, or the interface between the two. The clinical presentation of neuromuscular disorders may vary, as specific pathologies originate in different anatomic areas of the neuraxis, nervous system, neuromuscular junction (NMJ), or muscle tissue itself. These injuries can be progressive or static in nature. Additionally, host factors and medical treatment rendered may play a role in the phenotypical expression of the disease. There is a wide variety of neuromuscular disorders, and recent advances have been made in the understanding of the genetic basis of neuromuscular disorders. Diseases may possess congenital, developmental, or acquired etiologies. The impact on patients and families are burdensome, and as such, these conditions require an early establishment of an accurate diagnosis and multidisciplinary treatment planning. This chapter focuses on the pathological basis of these diseases (**Figure 1**) and the basic science relevant to the orthopaedic surgeon treating them.

Dr. Baldwin serves as a paid consultant to or is an employee of Pfizer and Synthes Trauma and has stock or stock options held in Pfizer. Neither Dr. Weltsch nor any immediate family member has received anything of value from or has stock or stock options held in a commercial company or institution related directly or indirectly to the subject of this chapter.

ANATOMIC CONSIDERATIONS

NERVOUS SYSTEM

The nervous system is a complex network of intercellular communications that control and regulate many processes throughout the body. In broad generality, nervous functions may be:

1. Sensory—providing data about the outside world to the central nervous system for the organism to interpret its surroundings.
2. Motor—providing action potentials to muscles to allow the organism to locomote or perform tasks on its surroundings.
3. Autonomic—providing internal regulation of bodily maintenance functions such as heart rate, blood pressure, vascular tone, and internal temperature.

The nervous system is broken up into the central nervous system (brain and spinal cord) and peripheral nervous system (peripheral nerves and effector organs). The principal cell of the nervous system is the neuron. A neuron consists of a cell body where all genetic and metabolic activity takes place at, proximal signal-recipient processes (dendrites), and a distal elongation (axon) responsible for further transmitting electrical signals to other neurons or effector organs. There are several types of neurons differentiated by size and by insulation with myelin. Electrical signals travel faster in axons that are myelinated via a process known as saltatory conduction.

©Copyright 2021 American Academy of Orthopaedic Surgeons

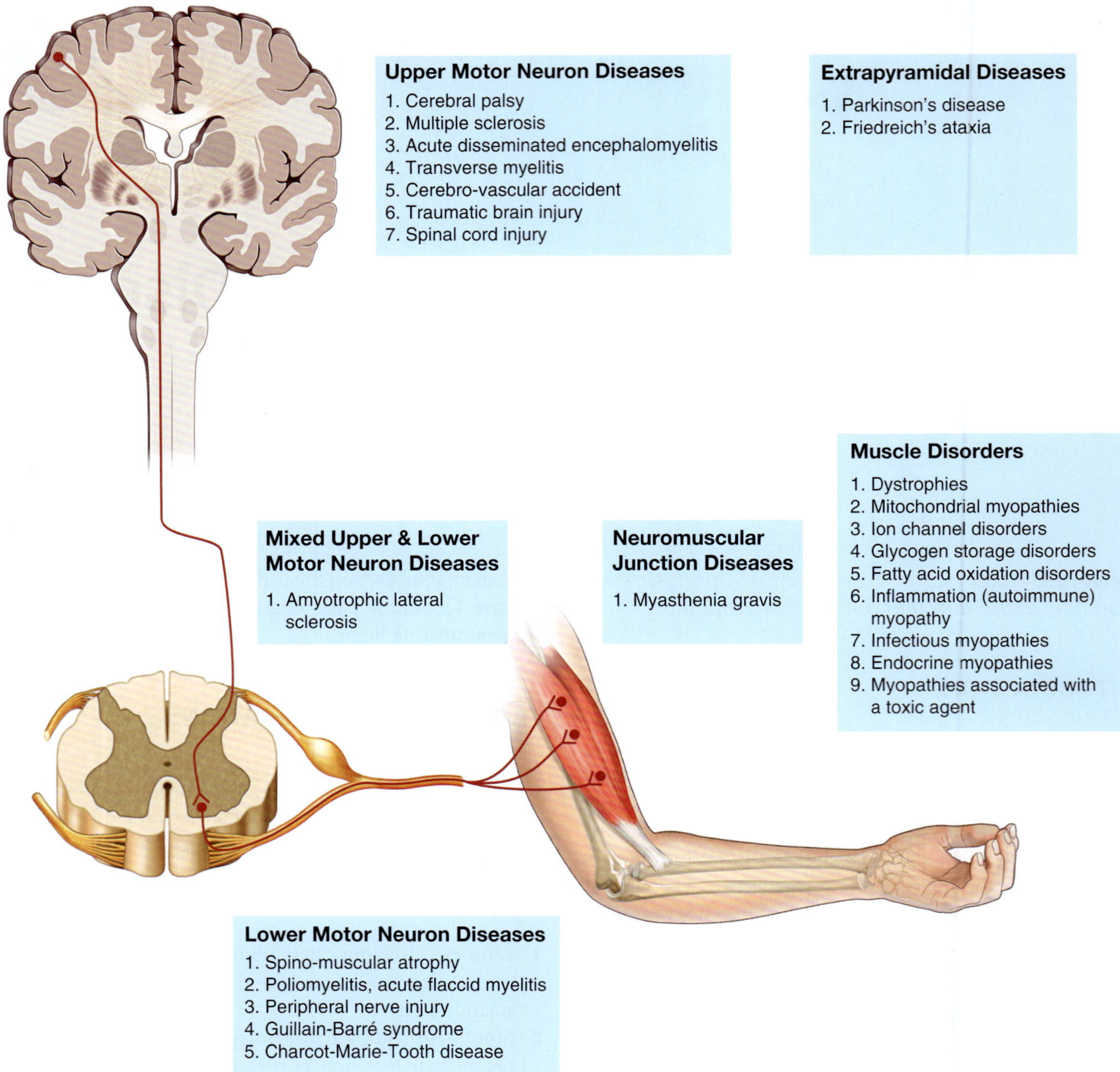

FIGURE 1 Illustration demonstrating neuromuscular diseases geographic classification.

The myelin layout on the neuron is in segments. Between two myelin segments, areas named Nodes of Ranvier are found. Only these areas provide the surface for neuronal ion exchange. This specific layout in myelinated nerves leads to a faster propagation of action potentials, as sodium gradients are efficiently conducted to the Nodes of Ranvier. It is important to note that all motor neuron bodies exist within the central nervous system, whereas generally the peripheral nervous system is occupied by the axons which relay the signals of the central nervous system to effector muscles through peripheral motor nerves. In the case of the sensory and autonomic nervous systems ganglia exist in the peripheral nervous system, which contain clusters of relay neurons. Although this chapter will primarily concern itself with motor nerves, sensory loss and autonomic dysfunction are highly essential parts of disorders of the nervous system and have a significant impact on patient function, safety, and health.

MUSCULAR SYSTEM

Muscle in the human body can be skeletal, smooth, or cardiac. Smooth muscle and cardiac muscle are primarily governed by the autonomic nervous system and will not be covered extensively here. Skeletal muscle is a specific muscle type involved in voluntary movements and activities of daily living. Skeletal muscles are innervated by axons of motor nerves, which dwell

©Copyright 2021 American Academy of Orthopaedic Surgeons

in the anterior horn of the spinal cord. Upon activation, the muscle fibers shorten across the axis of one or more joints producing motion. Nerves transmit their electrical action potential to muscles calcium-mediated chemical gates by way of the NMJ.

NEUROMUSCULAR JUNCTION

The neuromuscular junction (NMJ) is the conduit which bridges the nervous system and the muscular effector. This junction transforms an electrical impulse which can be conducted by the nerve to a chemical signal which is used by the muscle. Action potentials which propagate down a motor nerve terminate in the NMJ at the presynaptic terminal. This impulse activates calcium channels in the NMJ which in turn cause the release of acetylcholine (ACh) which binds to receptors in the cell membrane of the muscle. ACh receptor (AChR) activation results in depolarization of the muscle fibers and subsequent contraction (shortening) of the muscle.

DIAGNOSIS

HISTORY AND PHYSICAL EXAMINATION

History and physical examination are important with respect to diagnosis, treatment, and surgical planning for neuromuscular disorders. Upon presentation of a new patient with a neuromuscular finding, defining the onset of symptoms is critical. Acute weakness, facial droop, or loss of bowel or bladder function is highly concerning and warrants emergent diagnostic workup and potentially urgent or emergent intervention. Alternatively, findings or a time course that is more subacute may be worked up on a less urgent, elective outpatient schedule and time course. For concerning lesions which are slowly progressive, a neurology consult is often warranted to provide specific diagnostic and prognostic information which could be clinically useful to the orthopaedic surgeon. The pattern of "positive" (findings in addition to normal) and "negative" (missing or deficient factors from neurotypical function) symptoms along with pathologic reflexes is often helpful in localizing the lesion geographically as an upper motor neuron injury (brain and spinal cord), versus lower motor neuron (peripheral nervous system). Broadly, there are several differences (**Table 1**) between these groups. Localizing signs can additionally be used to estimate the site of the lesion and direct imaging and neurodiagnostic studies.

TABLE 1 Main Characteristics of Motor Neuron Diseases

Upper Motor Neuron	Lower Motor Neuron
Mild-moderate weakness	Severe weakness
Spastic tone	Flaccid tone
Minimal disuse atrophy	Marked muscular atrophy
Hyperreflexia	Reduced or absent reflexes
Pathological Babinski sign	No Babinski sign
Clonus may be present	No clonus
No fasciculations	Fasciculations

MUSCLE ENZYME STUDIES

Laboratory blood tests can be a clinically useful diagnostic modality in a variety of settings. Serum muscle enzyme assays are valuable indicators for muscle pathology. Serum creatinine kinase (CK) levels are elevated in the setting of muscle damage and necrosis and as such can be increased in a variety of syndromes such as rhabdomyolysis, compartment syndrome, dystrophinopathies, and even in direct trauma. CK concentrations are often more than 10 times higher than normal value in the presence of myopathies. However, in later stages as more muscle is replaced by fibrofatty infiltration, CK levels may decrease because not as much muscle tissue is available. In this setting, other enzymes may be measured but are often not as specific for muscle damage.

It is important to keep in mind that an elevated CK is highly nonspecific and indicates only that muscle has been damaged. As such it is not pathognomic for any specific condition. Contrarily, normal CK concentrations, especially in patients with decreased muscle mass or slowly progressive disease, do not rule out muscular myopathies. CK levels provide supportive data and should be considered in the context of the clinical picture and other diagnostic results.

ELECTROMYOGRAPHY AND NERVE CONDUCTION VELOCITY STUDIES

Electromyography (EMG) and Nerve conduction velocity (NCV) studies are highly useful diagnostic procedures that can help localize the site of a lesion and identify functionally working nerves and muscles from nonworking ones. Recognizing the patterns of activation and findings on EMG can assist in concluding the diagnosis.

Myopathic Diseases

Typically myopathies involve wasting of muscle and relative preservation of the nerve signal to that muscle. As such signal picked up by EMG will typically be lower amplitude, because of the lower amount of muscle available to activate. Increased frequency will be observed as well as decreased duration of signals and insertional activity. This is referred to as a "myogenic" pattern.

Neurogenic Diseases

Neurogenic diseases such as polio or amyotrophic lateral sclerosis (ALS) involve loss of motor neurons, as such muscles

©Copyright 2021 American Academy of Orthopaedic Surgeons

hypotrophy and the remaining motor units are forced to innervate a greater number of muscle fibers. Secondary to this, the amplitude of action potentials is larger with lower frequency and higher duration. Fibrillations can be detected by EMG-NCV studies and are noted in several neurogenic diseases.

EMG is also useful after trauma to assess if a nerve is damaged or severed. Typically, an EMG is obtained 3 to 6 months after a nerve injury is identified to determine if reinnervation is occurring or if nerve reconstruction or tendon transfers are warranted.

IMAGING STUDIES

Imaging studies are critically important in the assessment of neuromuscular disorders. Imaging is more commonly obtained in the setting of acute neuromuscular complaints but can also be of prognostic value for diseases such as cerebral palsy where localizing the area of damage can be helpful to guide treatment. CT is commonly used in the acute setting of a traumatic brain injury (TBI) to identify bleeding and change in the degree of hematoma in the short term to guide neurosurgical management and gauge safety of other surgical interventions. MRI has a higher resolution for soft tissues and is the work-horse of imaging of the neuraxis. Typically, MRI is employed following a physical examination or other investigations, which suggest a lesion at a particular level of the neuraxis. MRI can then characterize the lesion to assist in neurosurgical or orthopaedic management of that condition.

MUSCLE BIOPSY

Muscle biopsy is a classic method for assessing muscle tissue via various histochemical stains. It is clinically useful in the setting of muscle pathology and dystrophinopathies. In many ways, genetic testing has replaced muscle biopsy as a diagnostic modality. Occasionally, in atypical presentations, a muscle biopsy is thought to be diagnostically useful. When performed, ideally the biopsy should be performed on a muscle which still functions. The biopsy should be taken from an area where the muscle has been undisturbed (ie, not recently tested with EMG, or treated with botulinum toxin, or other intramuscular injection). The vastus lateralis is a popular location for muscle biopsy. Histochemical staining may be employed to detect abnormal proteins and discern between different types of myopathies:

Myopathic Pattern

Myopathic patterns of staining may find muscle necrosis, degeneration, and fibrofatty infiltrate. Additionally, there may be an abundance of nuclei and infiltration of connective tissue.

Neuropathic Pattern

Muscles in neuropathic disease are often atrophied, but otherwise healthy fibers will be present as well; connective tissue infiltration is typically not seen.

Inflammatory Pattern

In myositis, an abundance of inflammatory cells will be observed, along with perivascular infiltrates and edema.

GENETIC STUDIES

Genetic testing is a newer modality of diagnosis which can be clinically useful in dystrophinopathies, Charcot-Marie-Tooth, and congenital syndromes in which neuromuscular disease is a component. The process generally involves obtaining a sample of DNA from the patient and amplifying the DNA, and then testing it against known disorders using assays. These tests are best to run in consultation with neurologic specialists. Several specific DNA mutations have been identified to be associated with expression of neuromuscular diseases and conditions. These tests are considered diagnostic for some diseases but are performed at highly specialized centers, and hence results can often take significant time to return.

EXAMINATION UNDER ANESTHESIA

Examination under anesthesia before surgery (typically as part of the same surgical episode) is a critically important part of the diagnostic matrix when planning surgery. It is difficult to assess muscle length while the patient is awake in patients with hypertonia, as such the examination under anesthesia provides the ability to evaluate muscle length in the absence of tone. This can help the surgeon gauge the "dose" of surgery and finalize the surgical plan.

GAIT ANALYSIS

Gait analysis has changed the way operational decisions are made in neuromuscular diseases in ambulatory patients. This tool is important both for surgical decision making and for measuring postoperative outcomes. Gait analysis commonly starts with an observational part and includes preexamination slow motion videotaping of the gait and a standardized physical examination. The recorded video can be archived for further longitudinal comparison. The standardized physical examination evaluates skeletal deformities and fixed muscular contractures, joint range of motion, muscle force, and muscle tone. Instrumented analysis forms the basis of modern gait analytics. It combines inputs from videotaping, using body markers, EMG electrodes, and pressure sensors simultaneously. These inputs are recorded and provide detailed information including gait kinematics and kinetics, spatiotemporal, and EMG data, that is further broken down into gait cycle time, speed and length characters, plantar pressure maps, multiplanar alignment, movement arcs, joint moments, and muscle recruitment patterns including timing and intensity activation of specific muscle groups. Gait analysis allows a better understanding of the mechanics of each

©Copyright 2021 American Academy of Orthopaedic Surgeons

neuromuscular patient and assists in formulating a treatment plan to produce normal gait patterns with decreased energy expenditure.

SPECIFIC DISEASES

MUSCLE DISORDERS

BACKGROUND

A disease of muscle tissue is termed a myopathy. Individual myopathies are rare. Myopathies are commonly divided into inherited diseases and acquired conditions. Inherited myopathies include conditions such as muscular dystrophies, mitochondrial myopathies, ion channel disorders, glycogen storage disorders, and fatty acid oxidation disorders. The acquired myopathies include inflammation (autoimmune) myopathies, infectious myopathies, endocrine myopathies, and myopathies associated with a toxic agent.

Muscular dystrophies have a prevalence of 19.8 to 25.1 cases per 100,000 people.[1] These disorders are heterogeneous, and typically result in varying degrees and patterns of muscle weakness and degeneration of muscle tissue. The population, time of presentation, and severity may differ depending on the characters of the gene mutation and affected target protein (**Table 2**). The most common type of muscular dystrophies is dystrophinopathies including Duchenne and Becker's dystrophy. The genetic mutation of both diseases occurs at the same location in the dystrophin (DMD) gene. The DMD gene is the largest gene yet identified in humans, and it includes the data to form a protein called dystrophin. Dystrophin is a cytoskeletal protein located on the inner (cytoplasmic) side of the myocyte membrane. It helps to stabilize the cellular membrane and links the actin cytoskeleton to the extracellular matrix. The presence of dystrophin prevents myocyte membrane from collapsing during a muscle contraction. When dystrophin is missing, the cellular membrane becomes weakened and compromised, leading to unregulated calcium influx that eventually leads to muscle cell necrosis. Other dystrophinopathies include limb-girdle muscular dystrophies, facioscapulohumeral muscular dystrophy, and Emery-Dreifuss muscular dystrophy.

DUCHENNE MUSCULAR DYSTROPHY

Duchenne muscular dystrophy (DMD) is a rare disease; however, it is the most common form of inherited muscle disease in childhood with an incidence of 1 in 3,500 live male births[2] and prevalence of 1.7 to 4.2 cases per 100,000 people.[1]

Pathogenesis

DMD is an X-linked recessive disease, characterized by progressive deterioration of muscle mass in boys. In 70% to 80% of the cases a genetic link can be identified; the remainder of the cases are the result of "de-novo" mutation.[3] Mutations in the DMD gene (Xp21.2) are most often caused by a deletion or duplication of a promoter region which leads to frameshift-type mutation and formation of nonsense dystrophin which undergoes rapid degradation. The result of this mutation is an absence (or insufficient levels) of dystrophin protein in muscle tissue. This lack of function results in the inability to shield muscle from mechanical stress during repeated contractions. As such the cell membrane becomes disrupted leading to cell death. At the tissue level, the repeated breakdown of cellular integrity leads to prolonged inflammation process and ultimately fibrosis and fat deposition of the muscles. Dystrophin protein is also found in cardiac muscle tissue; therefore, DMD patients are at risk for dilated cardiomyopathy.

Clinical Presentation

In the first few years of life, muscle regeneration is excellent; however, as the child ages, muscle tissue degeneration outpaces their ability to replace it. This is particularly true in proximal muscles. The first symptoms usually appear between 2 and 3 years of age. The symptoms may include flat feet, delay in motor milestones including walking, pseudohypertrophy of the calves, balance issues, and clumsiness. The so-called "Gower's" sign is present when the child uses his hands to push up off the legs to aid the weak legs in standing. The plurality of patients will achieve the ability to walk; however, gait is characterized by a broad base of support, and toe walking is common. Flexion contractures of hips and knees and equinus contractures of the ankles are common as weakness progresses, eventually leading to the patient being restricted to a wheelchair. Hip flexion contractures will lead to lumbar hyperlordosis and scoliosis. Proximal muscle weakness in the upper limbs is manifested by difficulty with shoulder elevation during feeding. Cardiac and respiratory failure will ultimately lead to the patients' demise typically in the third decade of life.

Diagnosis

A high index of suspicion of DMD should arise in cases of unexplained increase in serum transaminases, a positive family history in the setting of abnormal muscle function, or a delay in walking beyond age 16 to 18 months. CK levels can serve as a screening test. The confirmation of DMD is usually made through genetic testing. The majority of cases (70%) are due to duplication or deletion in the gene that codes for dystrophin.[4] In other instances, genetic sequencing is performed to screen for less common mutations. Finally, if a diagnosis cannot be made with genetic testing, a muscle biopsy should be obtained for further testing.

Management

The general goals for the management of DMD patients are the preservation of function, maintaining bone health, and reducing contractures. The orthopaedic surgeon's role is to assist neurology and physical medicine by providing assessment and treatment of contractures, scoliosis, fractures, and optimization of bone health. Lengthening of muscles to produce braceable feet to preserve ambulatory function is critical as it can potentially decrease the rate of obesity and osteoporosis which is seen in later stage disease.

©Copyright 2021 American Academy of Orthopaedic Surgeons

TABLE 2 Dystrophies Pathogenesis Description

Disease	Transcribed Protein	Mutated Gene	Site of Mutation	Inheritance Mode
Duchenne and Becker muscular dystrophy	Dystrophin	DMD	Xq21.2	X-linked
LGMD-1A	Myotilin	MYOT	5q31.2	AD
LGMD-1B	Lamin A/C	LMNA	1q22	AD
LGMD-1C	Caveolin-3	CAV3	3p25.3	AD
LGMD-1D	DnaJ heat shock protein family (Hsp40) member B6	DNAJB6	7q36.3	AD
LGMD-1E	Desmin	DES	2q35	AD
LGMD-1F	Transportin 3	TNP03	7q32.1	AD
LGMD-1G	Heterogeneous nuclear ribonucleoprotein D like protein	HNRPDL	4q21.22	AD
LGMD-1H	Unknown	Unknown	3p23–p25	AD
LGMD-2A	Calpain-3	CAPN3	15q15.1	AR
LGMD-2B	Dysferlin	DYSF	2p13.2	AR
LGMD-2C	Gamma component (subunit) of sarcoglycan protein complex	SGCG	13q12.12	AR
LGMD-2D	Alfa component (subunit) of sarcoglycan protein complex	SGCA	17q21.33	AR
LGMD-2E	Beta component (subunit) of sarcoglycan protein complex	SGCB	4q12	AR
LGMD-2F	Delta component (subunit) of sarcoglycan protein complex	SGCD	5q33.2-q33.3	AR
LGMD-2G	Titin	TCAP	17q12	AR
LGMD-2H	Member of the tripartite motif (TRIM)	TRIM32	9q33.1	AR
LGMD-2I	Fukutin-related protein (FKRP)	FKRP	19q13.32	AR
LGMD-2J	Titin	TTN	2q31.2	AR
LGMD-2K	Member (1) of protein O-mannosyltransferase (POMT) enzyme complex	POMT1	9q34.13	AR
LGMD-2L	Anoctamin 5	ANO5	11p14.3	AR
LGMD-2M	Fukutin	FKTN	9q31.2	AR
LGMD-2N	Member (2) of protein O-mannosyltransferase (POMT) enzyme complex	POMT2	14q24.3	AR
LGMD-2O	Protein O-linked-mannose beta-1,2-N-acetylglucosaminyltransferase 1	POMGnT1	1p34.1	AR
LGMD-2P	Dystroglycan	DAG1	3p21.31	AR
LGMD-2Q	Plectin	PLEC1	8q24.3	AR
LGMD-2R	Desmin	DES	2q35	AR
LGMD-2S	Subunit of the TRAPP (transport protein particle) tethering complex	TRAPPC11	4q35.1	AR
LGMD-2T	GDP-mannose pyrophosphorylase	GMPPB	3p21.31	AR

©Copyright 2021 American Academy of Orthopaedic Surgeons

TABLE 2 Dystrophies Pathogenesis Description (Continued)

Disease	Transcribed Protein	Mutated Gene	Site of Mutation	Inheritance Mode
LGMD-2U	Isoprenoid synthase domain protein	ISPD	7p21.2	AR
LGMD-2V	Acid alpha-glucosidase (also known as acid maltase)	GAA	17q25.3	AR
LGMD-2W	PINCH2	LIMS2	2q14.3	AR
LGMD-2X	Blood vessel epicardial substance (BVES) also known as Popeye domain-containing protein 1 (POPDC1)	BVES	6q21	AR
LGMD-2Y	Torsin 1A interacting protein 1	TOR1AIP1	1q25.2	AR
FSHMD-1	Double homeobox 4	DUX4	4q35.2	AD
FSHMD-2	Structural maintenance of chromosomes flexible hinge domain containing 1	SMCHD1	18p11.32,	AD
EDMD-1	Emerin	EMD	Xq28	X-linked
EDMD-2	Lamin A/C	LMNA	1q22	AD
EDMD-3	Lamin A/C	LMNA	1q22	AR

AD = autosomal dominant, AR = autosomal recessive, EDMD = Emery-Dreifuss muscular dystrophy, FSHMD = facioscapulohumeral muscular dystrophy, LGMD = limb-girdle muscular dystrophy

Disease severity dictates treatment methods. Ambulatory patients use orthoses to facilitate walking assist during longer distances; contractures (mostly of the ankle) are addressed by surgical lengthening followed by casting and physical therapy. Administration of long-term corticosteroids has been shown to improve muscle strength, delay the loss of ambulation, preserve upper limb and respiratory functions, and decrease the need for spinal fusion for scoliosis.[5,6] In nonambulatory patients, great effort is directed at maintaining joint range of motion. Physical therapy and orthoses are used to delay the onset of contractures. Contractures of the lower limbs are addressed to maintain comfortable sitting and free movement of hip and knee joints. Scoliosis is addressed early with posterior spinal instrumented fusion to sustain an upright posture and decrease the work of breathing. In contrast to other disorders, spinal fusion is often encouraged much earlier in DMD than other disorders (as early as 20°) because of the natural history of cardiopulmonary decline shortly after scoliosis presents.

Pharmacological treatments including corticosteroids have been used in DMD patients in the last decade with great success. They have revolutionized the treatment of Duchenne's boys and prolonged their lives and in some cases their independence.[5] Theoretically, steroids may have an anti-inflammatory effect, which delays the muscle degeneration process while not explicitly addressing the underlying pathology.[3] However, these medications can exacerbate osteoporosis in these patients. Fractures are extremely common, particularly as the disease progresses. More recently with a better understanding of the genetic pathogenesis, the goal of treatment has been directed toward of mutation-specific drugs. Examples include ataluren and eteplirsen. Ataluren targets a stop codon in the mature mRNA of the dystrophin gene; it blocks the stop codon and allows mRNA translation to be completed, so a functional protein is produced. Eteplirsen specifically recognizes exon 51 in the pre-mRNA sequence (which become the stop codon on mRNA); by binding the pre-mRNA it changes the splicing process allowing mRNA-reading to become in-frame and allows a functional protein to be formed.

Cardiac and pulmonary function should be assessed in DMD patients. Cardiologists and Pulmonologists are critical members of the team particularly in its later stages where patients experience such multisystem organ decline. Consultation with these specialists is vital before surgery because of the limited pulmonary reserve. Additionally, malignant hyperthermia is associated with muscle disease, so vigilance on the part of anesthesia and the surgical team is needed.

Becker Muscular Dystrophy

Becker muscular dystrophy (BMD) is the second most common type of dystrophinopathy, and its prevalence is estimated to be 0.4 to 3.6 cases per 100,000 people.[1] It is a recessive, X-linked disease with a milder phenotypic expression than DMD. The mutation in BMD leads to a production of a shorter dystrophin protein with varying degrees of functionality. The severity of the disease depends on the quantity of functional dystrophin protein in the muscle cells. In contrast to DMD patients, BMD patients remain ambulatory until a mean of 27 years and survive into their fifth decade. Laboratory analysis shows moderately elevated CK levels, but genetic testing is the mainstay of confirmation of the disease. The goals of orthopaedic treatment are similar to DMD, but treatment is generally initiated later.

©Copyright 2021 American Academy of Orthopaedic Surgeons

Limb-Girdle Muscular Dystrophies

Limb-girdle muscular dystrophy (LGMD) refers to a group of genetic muscle disorders characterized by reduced or absent expression of specific muscle proteins (eg, sarcoglycans). The estimated prevalence of LGMD is 0.9 to 2.3 cases in 100,000 people.[1] It is common to divide the diseases based on the pattern of inheritance into autosomal dominant and autosomal recessive types. Currently, there are eight subtypes of LGMD type 1 (AD) and 26 subtypes of LGMD type 2 (AR). Type 2 variants are more common than the type 1 variants.[7]

Clinical Presentation

LGMD can be expressed in both genders. It mostly affects shoulder or pelvic girdle muscles with a phenotypic variation which depends on the type and severity of deficiency of the protein. As such the onset and the severity of disease, as well as the rate of progression, vary between different subtypes of LGMD. The disease onset is at the late first or second decade of life. Weakness and muscle wasting are the hallmark features. The upper limb muscles usually involve the trapezius, rhomboids, latissimus dorsi, serratus anterior, and the pectoralis major, whereas lower limb muscles mostly include the iliopsoas, gluteus maximus, and the quadriceps muscles.

Management

In the past, LGMD had been considered to be untreatable. Nowadays, molecular-based treatments are being developed to target genetic mutations; however, they are still in clinical trials stages. Orthopaedic management consists of supportive care with mobility aids, bracing treatment, and therapy.

Facioscapulohumeral Muscular Dystrophy

Facioscapulohumeral muscular dystrophy (FSHD) is a slowly progressive disease and is the third most common muscular dystrophy with a prevalence of 3.2 to 4.6 cases per 100,000 people.[1]

Pathogenesis

FSHD-related mutations primarily affect DNA packaging, leading to exposure of normally silenced genes and their translation into abnormal proteins that damage the muscle. FSHD type 1 (70% to 90% of cases) is autosomal dominant, and it is associated with mutations on chromosome 4. The mutations cause a reduction in the number of copies of a repeated region named D4Z4. D4Z4 has a crucial effect on silencing genes that are toxic to skeletal muscle, that is, DUX4 (double homeobox 4) retrogene. Upon alteration in the number of D4Z4 regions, DUX4 may be translated. FSHD severity usually depends on the amount of DUX4 transcribed.[8] FSHD type 2 is sporadic, and the related de novo mutations are associated with a packaging protein named SMCHD1, which lead to transcription of muscle-toxic proteins.

Clinical Presentation

Symptoms typically begin between the first and third decade. Weakness begins in the facial muscles with a typical presentation being difficulty drinking through a straw. Weakness progresses to the shoulder girdle (trapezius) and arms (biceps, triceps, pectoral). A winged scapula is a common report. Footdrop is also quite common and may be a presenting report. The Beevor sign which is an upward movement of the umbilicus with neck flexion is characteristic of FSHD. Other symptoms may include an absence of eye and forehead wrinkles, incomplete eye closure (seen mostly during sleep), transverse smile, difficulty with whistling. Extramuscular manifestations include atrial arrhythmias, sensorineural hearing loss, retinal telangiectasias, restrictive respiratory disease, and seizures. People diagnosed with FSHD usually live a normal lifespan. Diagnosis is mostly at a clinical and genetic level because CPK levels are typically normal.

Management

There are currently no pharmacological disease-modifying treatments in FSHD. Nonpharmaceutical interventions that can be offered include physiotherapy to maintain strength and range of motion of affected muscles and ankle-foot orthoses (AFO) for patients with footdrop. Surgical intervention is primarily targeted at the shoulder girdle as scapulothoracic fusion can improve the elevation of the upper extremities."

Emery-Dreifuss Muscular Dystrophy

Emery-Dreifuss muscular dystrophy (EDMD) is a rare inherited condition with a prevalence of 0.1 to 0.4 cases per 100,000 people.[1]

Pathogenesis

EDMD primarily affect the production of proteins associated with the nuclear membrane of cells in both skeletal and cardiac muscles.[9] The mutation affects the EMD gene and in turn the production of the protein called Emerin, an inner nuclear membrane protein which helps anchor the cell membrane to the cytoskeleton. Although ubiquitous, Emerin is more highly represented in skeletal and cardiac muscle. The LMNA is also associated with both the autosomal dominant and recessive types of EDMD. LMNA contains the codes for the production of lamin-A and lamin-C which are intermediate filaments in the nuclear membrane and nucleoplasm of most cells and contribute to the nuclear shape. They are essential for DNA replication and mRNA transcription.

Clinical Presentation

EDMD presents in the second decade. It is a slowly progressive disease in which contractures and weakness are prevalent and primarily affect muscles of the arms, legs, and neck. Patients usually are able to walk up until the fifth decade. Scoliosis may be seen and often characterized by slow progression of curves. Cardiac arrhythmias are common and sudden cardiac death is a frequent cause of mortality.

Management

No specific treatment exists for EDMD. Bracing treatment, physical therapy, or orthopaedic surgery can mitigate some of the effects of the contractures on walking and function.

©Copyright 2021 American Academy of Orthopaedic Surgeons

DISEASES AT THE LEVEL OF THE NMJ

MYASTHENIA GRAVIS

Myasthenia gravis (MG) is an autoimmune disorder affecting the NMJ. Prevalence is estimated between 10 to 20 cases per 100,000 population in the United States.[10]

Pathogenesis

Myasthenia gravis is caused by antibodies directed mainly against postsynaptic acetylcholine receptors (AChRs). Although ACh is released from the nerve in normal concentration, a relatively decreased concentration of AChRs present on the end plate muscle membrane (because of auto-destruction of AChRs) leads to interference of neuromuscular transmission. In about 15% of patients with myasthenia gravis, AChR antibodies are absent, and these patients may have antibodies against other NMJ proteins, such as muscle-specific kinase (MuSK), lipoprotein-related protein 4 (LRP4), or agrin in the postsynaptic membrane.[11]

Clinical Presentation

MG follows a typical bimodal age and gender pattern, with one peak in young females around age 30 and another peak in population (mostly males) at age 50, followed by a steady rise in incidence as age increases.[12] MG presentation includes painless fatigue and muscle weakness. Weakness may be fluctuating and generally gets worse with exertion and increased repetitive muscle use ("end of day weakness"). Weakness distribution may vary: about two-thirds initially present with ocular symptoms (ptosis and miosis). Bulbar fascial symptoms (dysphagia, dysarthria, reduced facial expression) and proximal muscles weakness of limbs may also occur. About 75% of patients will develop generalized weakness, mostly within the first 2 to 3 years following the initial presentation.[10] MG exacerbations are commonly triggered by an infection, increased emotional stress, sudden decrease in MG treatment (steroids), warmer environment temperature. Thymoma is associated with myasthenia gravis, 30% to 60% of thymomas are associated with myasthenia gravis, and about 10% of patients with MG have a thymic tumor.[11] Although it is more common in younger patients, all MG patients should be screened with mediastinal imaging (CT or MRI). Thymomas have slow growth pattern, but also have an increased ability to invade locally and metastasize regionally. Surgical removal is the mainstay of treatment mainly in younger patients, and adjuvant radiation is recommended for invasive thymoma.[13]

Management

Oral anticholinesterase (pyridostigmine) is the first-line treatment for symptomatic relief. Second-line treatment includes corticosteroids. It is more effective in earlier phases of the diseases and should be started as a low dose with a gradual increase by need. Azathioprine suppresses the inflammation process, but its response is slow, so it is typically used as an adjunct to steroids. Cyclosporine, methotrexate, and cyclophosphamide can be useful for those who do not respond to or cannot tolerate azathioprine.[11]

Myasthenic Crisis

Myasthenic crisis is a term describing respiratory failure caused by weakness of respiratory musculature. Forced vital capacity (FVC) is critically reduced on pulmonary function testing. The treatment is based on supportive measures including intubation and mechanical ventilation, as well as an intense immune suppression with high-dose steroids or intravenous immunoglobulin. In extreme cases, plasmapheresis may be used. Early diagnosis and treatment make this condition fully reversible.

DISEASES LEVEL OF THE LOWER MOTOR NEURON

BACKGROUND

The nervous system employs a sequence of motor neurons to carry out signals from the brain to the skeletal muscle cells. This, in turn, causes muscles to contract, which effects the movement of joints. A hierarchical description is commonly used to describe this sequence in the motor nervous system. This description is useful clinically albeit somewhat oversimplified. This system though useful ignores the neurons in the premotor area along with the delicate interplay of posture, balance, and lower brain function, which all serve to modulate motor nerve function. For the purposes of this chapter, the lower motor neuron is the second-order neuron. The body of a lower motor neuron is located in a motor nucleus in the anterior horn of the spinal cord. Upon activation, the lower motor neuron then transmits its signal via its projecting axon bundled in a peripheral nerve to its designated set of muscle fibers leading to muscle activation.

One simple method of description of neurologic disease is based on its region of origin in this hierarchical scheme. This is particularly useful in diseases caused by injury to neurologic tissue as characteristic sets of symptoms are typical given the location of the lesion. Damage to a lower motor neuron would lead to direct denervation of the muscle fibers. Involved muscles will lose the capacity of contraction (paralysis) and lead to severe muscle weakness (plegia). In addition, such injury could decrease muscle tone (flaccidity) in the affected region. The stretch reflexes would be diminished or lost. Over time the denervated muscles will exhibit muscle wasting (atrophy). In the beginning, spontaneous depolarizations of an injured muscle will lead to "fibrillations" which are usually too fine and fast to be seen by the clinician's eye. In turn, in an attempt to compensate and reinnervate the region, involuntary contractions or "fasciculations" may occur and present as muscle twitches lasting a few seconds at a time.

SPINAL MUSCULAR ATROPHY

Spinal muscular atrophy (SMA) is the leading genetic cause of infant mortality and is characterized by the degeneration of spinal cord alpha motor neurons and resultant skeletal muscles atrophy and weakness. The incidence of SMA is 1 in 10,000 to 11,000 live births with a carrier frequency of 1 in 50 to 54.[14,15]

©Copyright 2021 American Academy of Orthopaedic Surgeons

Pathogenesis

SMA is an autosomal recessive disease, caused by a defect in survival motor neuron (SMN) gene. SMN genes translate proteins essential for the vitality of the neuron. There are two types of SMN genes, SMN1(telomeric form) and SMN2 (centromeric form). SMN1 gene is the leading provider of SMN proteins. SMN2 gene is found only in humans and is nearly identical to SMN1; only it has a nucleotide change from C to T in exon 7. This nucleotide change leads to the formation of substantially less SMN proteins from SMN2 gene because of an RNA splicing error. Normally, in about 85% to 90% of the cases, exon seven is excluded during transcription, which leads to a decrease in the transcription of a full-length mRNA that can form functional proteins.[15] In more than 95% of the cases of SMA, a homozygous disruption (deletion, conversion, or mutation) occurs in exons 7 to 8 of SMN1 on chromosome 5q13.[14,15] Whenever SMN1 is disrupted, the severity of the disease depends on the ability of SMN2 to form proteins; decreased levels of SMN2 are correlated with a more severe form of SMA. A reduced amount of SMN proteins leads to selective destruction of lower motor neurons found in the anterior horn of the spinal cord and associated muscle weakness.

Clinical Presentation

The hallmark of SMA is weakness of the trunk and proximal hip muscles, which in turn lead to scoliosis deformity and hip instability. However, SMA presentation is highly variable, and the clinical features can be classified into four main phenotypes based on the age of onset and motor function:

Type 0 SMA (preterm type)—is used to describe disease onset in the first month of life (neonates), who present with severe hypotonia and weakness. In these infants, respiratory failure is severe, and mortality is in the neonatal period.

Type 1 SMA (infant type)—also known as Werdnig-Hoffman disease. It is the most severe form of SMA to survive out of the neonatal period. The onset of symptoms is in infancy before 6 months of age. Clinical manifestations include hypotonia, poor head control, tongue atrophy, pharyngeal muscle weakness with associated difficulty in swallowing and reflux, intercostal muscle weakness with breathing problems, and reduced or absent tendon reflexes. As the infant grows, they are unable to sit unassisted. Cognition is typically normal. These patients are at high risk for morbidity because of feeding problems, which can lead to recurrent aspiration events and mortality in early childhood from respiratory failure.

Type 2 SMA (intermediate type)—is the most common form of SMA. Symptom onset ranges from age 6 to 18 months. Most commonly patients will gain the ability to sit unassisted but will be unable to walk. Children present with profound weakness of the lower limbs associated with hypotonia and areflexia. Other manifestations include skeletal deformities of the spine (scoliosis) and joint contractures. Involvement of respiratory muscles may lead to complications including restrictive lung disease. Patients typically survive into their third decade.

Type 3 SMA (juvenile type)—also known as Kugelberg-Welander disease is a milder form of SMA, presenting mostly after 18 months of age. Patients will typically gain the ability to walk, and most will be able to walk unassisted. The primary clinical manifestations include weakness of the proximal muscles of the lower limb that may impact the ability to climb stairs and may lead to increased lumbar lordosis. Respiratory muscles are mostly spared. Fortunately, in most patients, the cognition and life expectancy are not markedly altered from healthy controls.

Type 4 SMA (adult onset type)—is also a mild form of the disease, and it is the least common type of SMA. Patients have similar clinical manifestations as type 3, and the onset of the disease is in adulthood years usually at the fourth decade of life.

Diagnosis

SMA should always be considered in children with developmental delays or hypotonia. Molecular genetic testing is the benchmark as it first identifies SMN1 deletions, whereas a quantitative test for SMN2 can help predict the disease severity.[16] CK serum levels are usually normal or only mildly elevated in SMA. Therefore, testing cannot be used to rule out SMA. Other diagnostic studies such as electrodiagnostic studies and muscle biopsies are mainly of historical interest in the diagnosis of SMA as typically genetic testing is used, and these tests are now reserved for when the diagnosis is in doubt.

Management

There is no cure for SMA. Efforts are being made to provide a directed genetic solution. Several candidate treatment agents are in clinical trials with promising results. In addition, over the last years, a marked advancement had been made in the supportive care of patients, with improved nutritional gastrointestinal and pulmonary care. Nusinersen is a relatively new drug that had become an integral part of clinical care in SMA patients. By modifying splicing processes of the SMN2 gene, it is able to increase the level of SMN protein and can improve motor function. It is currently delivered through repeated intrathecal injections and as such is a consideration for the orthopaedic surgeon when spinal fusion is considered.

The orthopaedic treatment is targeted mainly on maintaining function, preventing deterioration in functionality. Physiotherapy and bracing treatment are focused at opposing contractures and prevention or slowing down of skeletal deformities. Scoliosis is a common issue especially in nonambulatory individuals with SMA. If left untreated, can lead to chest cage deformities and decreased respiratory function. The vertical expandable prosthetic titanium rib (VEPTR) device is a novel solution in treating young SMA patients with severe deformities of the chest, spine, and ribs. This device has shown pulmonary functions improvements among these patients.[17] Nevertheless, bracing treatment and spinal fusion remains the mainstay of the orthopaedic treatment in scoliosis of SMA patients.[18]

©Copyright 2021 American Academy of Orthopaedic Surgeons

Poliomyelitis and Acute Flaccid Myelitis (Poliolike Syndrome)

Poliomyelitis

Acute poliomyelitis is an infectious viral disease that affects the central nervous system. It is caused by poliovirus which is transmitted by the fecal-oral route, initially presents with gastrointestinal symptoms and then accesses the CNS to attack the anterior horn cells of the spinal cord. It mostly affects children below the age of 5 and is characterized by a sudden onset of fever, muscle pain, and paralysis.

Eradication of Polio

A worldwide effort to eradicate the disease has reduced the incidence of poliomyelitis cases by more than 99% since its launch in 1988. The incidence successfully decreased from 350,000 annual cases in 125 endemic countries to 20 cases in two countries in 2017. More than 16 million people who would otherwise have been paralyzed by poliovirus infection are today walking.[19]

Postpolio Syndrome

Because of the successful public health endeavor that was the eradication of polio, in the modern era, most orthopaedic surgeons will only encounter this entity in its postpolio syndrome (PPS) form. PPS develops in survivors aged 30 to 40 after a period of stability after acute polio infection. The exact cause of PPS is unknown but appears to be related to an imbalance in the interplay between denervation and reinnervation compensation process of previously affected motor neurons.[20] The reinnervation of denervated muscle fibers through terminal axonal sprouting of new axons by nearby nerve cells results in giant motor units.[21] Common symptoms include general fatigue, muscle pain with intolerance to cold, slowly progressive weakness and atrophy of muscles, and joint pain. There is no cure for PPS. As these patients age, they may experience scoliosis, joints degradation, and progressive weakness. All of the above are the main concerns, providing a considerable challenge to the orthopaedic surgeon. One of the most significant issues with PPS is that the strategy to deal with it generally entails joint preservation and limitation of activity rather than aggressive physical therapy. As such the treatment of PPS may be counterintuitive to the general orthopaedic surgeon.

Acute Flaccid Myelitis

Acute flaccid myelitis (AFM) is described as an acute onset of flaccid limb weakness, with imaging showing spinal cord gray matter lesions suggestive of anterior myelitis.[22] It is mostly seen in children who present with paralysis of one or more limbs. In recent years, AFM has reemerged and is currently under surveillance. The CDC reported 386 confirmed cases with AFM in the period between August 2014 to September 2018 across the United States, occurring mostly in the pediatric population.

The cause of AFM remains unknown. The most recent hypothesis connects enterovirus D68 with the disease.[23] This association is made based on the detection of trends of incidence of AFM and enterovirus D68 in the United States since 2014. Interestingly outbreaks of enterovirus D68 and sequential AFM diagnosis happens every other year with a peak around the end of summer. In some reported cases the virus was isolated from respiratory specimens of AFM patients. However, no virus had been detected in cerebrospinal fluid (CSF) of the same patients. It seems that further prospective studies evaluating the epidemiological association between enterovirus D68 and AFM are needed to fully confirm this causation and perhaps search for a future vaccination.

Peripheral Nerve Injury

Peripheral nerve injury is discussed in Chapter 36 of this book.

Guillain-Barré Syndrome

Guillain-Barré syndrome (GBS) is also termed acute inflammatory demyelinating polyneuropathy. It is an immune-mediated inflammatory disorder of the peripheral nervous system that is considered to be the most common cause of acute flaccid paralysis. GBS is relatively rare; its annual incidence in the United States is 1.65 to 1.79 per 100,000 persons, and it is more frequent in males than in females.[24]

Pathogenesis

GBS typically manifests as a rapidly progressive ascending paralysis. Sensory dysesthesias are common. The disease is associated with infection and has even been associated with vaccination. *Campylobacter jejuni* is the most common bacteria associated with GBS; however, many other bacteria and viruses have been implicated, including but not limited to *Mycoplasma pneumonia*, *Haemophilus influenzae*, cytomegalovirus (CMV), Epstein-Barr virus, influenza A virus, hepatitis (A, B, and E), and Zika virus. The nerve injury is antibody mediated although both T cells and B cells appear to play a role. Cross-reacting antibodies may attack peripheral motor or sensory neurons and may lead to pure demyelination, pure axonal damage, or a mixed picture.[25]

Clinical Presentation

Onset of the disease is rapid, and progressive, and will often last 2 weeks, followed by a phase of plateau for 2 to 4 weeks, followed by a slow recovery over months to years. The presenting symptoms may include severe back pain and distal limb paresthesia with either tingling or "tight band" sensation. After a few days, symmetric weakness appears with reduced or absent deep tendon reflexes. In addition, autonomic dysfunction (dysautonomia)-related symptoms such as cardiac arrhythmias, blood pressure fluctuations, ileus, and urinary retention may also occur. Patients are at high risk for rapid onset respiratory failure because of respiratory

©Copyright 2021 American Academy of Orthopaedic Surgeons

muscle weakness, and approximately 30% of patients with GBS ultimately require mechanical ventilation.[26]

Diagnosis

The clinical picture is very suggestive of GBS; however, lumbar puncture (LP) with CSF analysis which shows elevated protein and a normal leukocyte count may provide confirmatory evidence. EMG and NCV studies may reveal slowing of nerve conduction in 80% of patients.[27] Repetitive measurements of vital capacity and negative inspiratory force are required to monitor respiratory status.

Management

Treatment of GBS is supportive; disease-modifying treatments such intravenous immunoglobulin (IVIG) or plasma exchange can be given within 4 weeks of symptoms onset, and by neutralization or removal or the circulating antigens/immune complexes they accelerate time to recovery[28] and reduce the need for mechanical ventilation.

Charcot-Marie-Tooth

Charcot-Marie-Tooth (CMT) disease is an inherited peripheral neuropathy and is the most common inherited neuromuscular disorder. Prevalence is estimated to be 10 to 40/100,000.[29]

Pathogenesis

CMT is a group of genetic disorders caused by mutations in the genes that produce proteins involved in the structure, metabolism, or function of peripheral nerve axons or the myelin sheaths. The two main resultant pathologic processes are demyelination leading to decreased conduction velocities and axon degeneration which reduces the transmission of action potentials. These processes within a peripheral nerve may lead to motor and sensory deficits.

Clinical Presentation

The typical clinical phenotype of CMT is characterized by progressive, distal limb weakness and muscle wasting with symmetric distal sensory loss. The onset of symptoms is typically in the first two decades of life but can be later in milder forms. Muscle imbalance in the hands and the feet most commonly present. In the feet, as intrinsic muscles weaken, the first ray dorsiflexes (pes cavus), and hammer toes appear. Intrinsic wasting in the hands is subtler but often presents as loss of coordination and thenar wasting[30] Distal decreases in vibratory sense as well as decreased deep tendon reflexes are noted. In time, motor impairments and loss of sensation slowly progress proximally. Pain is a common symptom in CMT, particularly in the lower limbs, and lumbar spine. Many patients will remain ambulatory throughout their life. Life expectancy is unchanged in patients with CMT.

Classification

Increase in genetic understanding of CMT diseases has led to stepwise modifications in CMT classification system, rendering it more complicated. The most common types are CMT1, CMT2, Dejerine-Sottas CMT4, and CMTX.

CMT1 is characterized by being an autosomal dominant demyelinating form of the disease. It is the most common form of CMT and has several subtypes affecting different target myelin-associated proteins. It follows the typical clinical phenotype of CMT. On conduction testing it shows slow nerve conduction velocities and the nerve biopsy may show myelin abnormalities, with pathological proliferation of Schwann cells that on histologic studies have an appearance reminiscent of an onion bulb. Later stages may show secondary axonal damage.

CMT2 is an autosomal dominant disease predominantly characterized by axonal damage. It accounts for roughly one-quarter of CMT cases. Clinically it overlaps with the typical phenotype of CMT1. EMG shows preserved or only mildly slowed nerve conduction velocities (>38 m/s). Pathological evidence of chronic axonal degeneration and regeneration are seen on nerve biopsy.

Dejerine-Sottas or CMT3 is an early-onset form of the CMT. It is considered the most severe form of demyelinating CMT. The inheritance pattern may be both AR and AD. EMG shows slow nerve conduction. CMT4 is an autosomal recessive demyelinating form of the disease. It is characterized by an earlier onset and by a more severe course than the typical presentation. Additionally, it may present with vocal cord paralysis, sensorineural deafness, and facial weakness and diaphragmatic weakness.

CMTX is a relatively rare type and accounts for approximately 1% to 2% of all CMT cases.

Management

The approach to CMT patients starts with confirmation of the diagnosis by an analysis of combined data from patient's clinical manifestations, family history and suspected mode of inheritance, nerve conduction tests, and genetic testing. Because genetic testing is available and noninvasive, nerve biopsy is reserved for cases of atypical or inconclusive genetic testing.

No effective drug therapy for CMT has been identified. Supportive treatment includes symptomatic relief and physical therapy focused on affected and neighboring muscle stamina exercise and strengthening. The Coleman's block test is often helpful to determine if the forefoot cavus is driving the hindfoot varus. If it is, often a recessed first metatarsal orthosis with a lateral hindfoot post is helpful. In more severe cases where steppage gait is observed, an ankle-foot orthosis is additionally considered to support more fluid gait. Surgical orthopaedic treatment may involve plantar fascia release, tendon transfers, osteotomies, and fusions to correct pathological posture and overcome deformities. As a rule, early treatment is advised to allow for treatment of a more flexible deformity before degenerative changes occur.[31] Rigid deformity or arthritic joints typically indicate fusion procedures. Several surgical techniques have been proposed for different CMT related scenarios[32]; however, a detailed description is beyond the scope of this chapter.

©Copyright 2021 American Academy of Orthopaedic Surgeons

DISEASES OF THE UPPER MOTOR NEURON

Background

An upper motor neuron is a first-order neuron. It transmits signals from its cell body in the motor cortex of the brain, which then enters the cortico-spinal tract (for the body) and cortico-bulbar tract (for the cranial nerves). These fibers descend along the internal capsule and then cross (decussate) in the pyramidal area of the midbrain. 90% of these fibers then proceed contralateral to their site of origination in the brain to the body of a lower motor neuron in the spinal cord.

The sequelae of such damage lead to an increased muscular tone which is often unbalanced favoring dominant muscle groups. Upper motor neurons have both excitatory and inhibitory effects on the lower motor neurons. After injury resulting in loss of an inhibitory effect, more pronounced stretch reflexes will appear. A velocity-dependent resistance to passive elongation of muscles (spasticity) could also evolve and can worsen over time. Spasticity usually becomes distinct after few weeks from the date of injury. Primitive reflex patterns are typically present. Classically positive tests are Babinski in the lower extremities (extension of the great toe upon stroking the plantar surface) or the Hoffman reflex (thumb flexion with the flicking of the middle finger DIP). Over time motor imbalance and fixed positioning may progress to muscular contractures, decreased joint motion, pain, and functional impairments.

Cerebral Palsy

Cerebral palsy (CP) is a common upper motor neuron condition in children. Notably, CP may entail disorders of motor planning, dystonia, extrapyramidal movements, and a cadre of other neurologic findings. It is effectively a static brain injury that occurs in a very young child. From an orthopaedic standpoint, the most relevant form of cerebral palsy is spastic cerebral palsy. Clinical presentation depends on which part of the brain is damaged. There is a wide variation in presentation, which ranges from hemiplegic who had a brain bleed when they were an infant to a spastic quadriplegic who had an anoxic brain injury at birth. CP is the most common cause of physical disability in childhood in developed countries with a prevalence ranging from 1.5 to 4 per 1,000 live births.[33]

Definition and Pathogenesis

A recent working group revised the definition of cerebral palsy:

> *A group of permanent disorders of the development of movement and posture, causing activity limitation, that are attributed to non-progressive disturbances that occurred in the developing fetal or infant brain. The motor disorders of cerebral palsy are often accompanied by disturbances of sensation, perception, cognition, communication, and behavior, by epilepsy, and by secondary musculoskeletal problems.*[34]

This definition occasionally produces confusion among clinicians in that the clinical presentation of children can change drastically throughout their lives. Although the primary lesion of the brain is nonprogressive, because of the secondary muscle spasticity that results, bony deformity can develop. As such the secondary issues such as spasticity contracture and bony torsion can be progressive even as the primary brain injury is not. This nonprogressive nature of the neurologic injury serves to separate CP from genetic, glycogen storage, or other neurodegenerative conditions. From a definitional perspective, the lesion involved in CP would be an upper motor (brain) injury that is nonprogressive.

If the damage occurs in a motor rich area such as the motor strip or the posterior limb of the internal capsule, one would expect the typical manifestations of upper motor neuron disease (hyperreflexia, spasticity, weakness, and increased reflexes). In a growing child, these manifestations of CP paired with longitudinal growth of the limb result in further contracture and bony torsions which may become clinically relevant as the child matures. Depending on the site of the brain injury, patients may manifest positive symptoms such as spasticity, dystonia, and dyskinetic movements, or negative symptoms such as blindness, weakness, or limited balance. The nature of the brain injury as it relates to the function of the patient is beyond the scope of this chapter, but the net effect in spastic CP is that patients suffer from progressive secondary manifestations such as muscle stiffness and contractures which impart abnormal deforming forces on an immature skeleton. Patients may then compensate for these abnormal forces by developing tertiary strategies to overcome the issues involved with the secondary deformities (ie, vaulting over a leg with an equinus contracture). Independent ambulation may be significantly impacted by these many issues and as such provides a diagnostic challenge for the orthopaedic surgeon. In addition to the motor defect, CP patients may be accompanied by disturbances of sensation, seizure disorders, movement disorders, and cognitive issues. Many patients will experience delays in motor milestones, and often milder CP will be diagnosed as a result of this.

Etiology and Risk Factors

Causes for cerebral palsy are multifactorial, but by definition involve a discrete injury to brain tissue. The hypothesis is that during brain development and growth, the brain is subjected to internal or external insult affecting gross motor function regions in the brain. Insult risk factors and etiologies may vary (**Figure 2**), and timing may be during pregnancy (prenatal period), delivery (perinatal), or up to a few years after birth (postnatal). Prematurity is a significant risk factor for CP in the developed world, with the incidence of CP being 1.5 to 2.5/1,000 live births in term babies and approximately 10 times higher in preterm infants.[35]

Clinical Presentation

The diagnosis of CP is suspected clinically though MR imaging may help reveal the pathologic basis or the nature of the

©Copyright 2021 American Academy of Orthopaedic Surgeons

Prenatal Period	Perinatal Period	Postnatal Period
• Drug or alcohol exposure • TORCH syndrome • Polyhydramnios • RH incompatibility • Breech position • Placental rupture • Umbilical cord prolapse • Chorioamnionitis	• Premature birth • Asphyxia during labor • Trauma during labor • Brain hemorrhage • Low birth weight infants (<1500 Gr) • Oxytocin augmentation	• Asphyxia • Trauma • Infections (meningitis and encephalitis) • Seizures • Brain infarcts

FIGURE 2 Categorization of suggested risk factors and etiologies for CP.

condition. MRI is recommended to rule in the diagnosis as it can visualize the area of damage in the brain. White matter and basal ganglia lesions are most common (42.5%, 12.8%), cortical or subcortical lesions (9.4%), focal infarcts (7.4%), cerebellar lesions, and diffuse lesions are also observed but in lower rates.[36] White matter damage interrupts pathways such as cerebral control of muscle tone and may clinically manifest as spasticity. The geography of the disease correlates with the severity of weakness and spasticity in the limbs affected. Movement disorders or dystonia, by contrast, can be observed with basal ganglia infarcts, however, if this damage is part of wider spread damage, a more globally involved picture may ensue. Middle cerebral artery infarcts generally produce a hemiplegic picture, whereas focal infarcts may produce isolated milder deficits. Cerebellar involvement may lead to ataxia and poor modulation of movement. Although CP is a static brain injury, secondary problems such as spasticity contracture and bony torsion can progress. Walking ability is multifactorial but often of great interest to families and caregivers.[37] A commonly used predictor for the ability to walk is an independent sitting by age 2 years. Studies show that 97.9% to 100% of patients who can sit by 24 months will be able to walk.[38,39]

Classifications

Cerebral palsy is classified in a number of different ways. A so-called "topologic" or "geographic" classification references which limbs are involved (hemiplegic—one half of the body; diplegic—both legs; quadriplegic—all four limbs). A more deficit related classifications help indicate the prominent type of deficit (spastic, dystonic, mixed, ataxic, etc.). These classifications, though useful for descriptive purposes, are not of much help in determining treatment and prognosis. The Gross Motor Function Classification System (GMFCS) was devised as a functional classification[40] and has been found to be both durable and resistant to change over time. It can provide information as to the natural history of groups of patients and may guide treatment. Although it is stratified by age, it is somewhat unreliable before the age of 2 years. The classification contains five levels and is based on functional ability. The GMFCS classification is used ubiquitously in the literature to help describe patients and as such has been helpful to group common patients.[41] Distinction between patients with spastic CP is still clinically important for orthopaedic surgeons. Many different deficits exist in CP; however, if a nonmotor pathology (movement disorder, etc) is dominant, often physiatry treatment dominates. Often orthopaedic surgeons study spastic CP as this is the form of CP which tends to develop orthopaedically relevant pathology. Nevertheless, the GMFCS has been very helpful as a "common language" by which to describe patients.

Management

Managing CP patients requires an in-depth understanding of the patho-anatomy, patho-mechanics, and variability of the natural history of the diagnosis. The approach to a patient includes patient's history, current complaints, assessment of the gross motor functional classification system level, as well as spine alignment, rotational profile of the limbs, joint range of motion, muscle strength, selective motor control, muscle tone, and observational and occasionally an instrumented gait analysis. All these data points are taken in the context of the patient's overall cognition, level of function, and social situation. An interdisciplinary, holistic treatment strategy is best suited to these types of patients. Surgeons take their place with physiatrists, neurologists, physical and occupational therapists, social workers, and caregivers as partners when decision making related to the child is considered. After providing the treatment details, a discussion of the timeline and logistics of the treatment should be made. Lastly, expectations must be set to ensure a full understanding of all participating parties, most importantly the patient and his or her family.[42]

Goals of orthopaedic treatment for cerebral palsy are to facilitate mobility, limit pain and deformity, promote painless sitting posture, and promote the most energy efficient gait for patients who are able to walk. The methods by which these goals are optimally met vary considerably as patients age and also vary with the functional level of the child in question. Nonsurgical methods by which this may be achieved in spastic patients include local treatment methods to limit tone such as botulinum toxin and phenol, or global treatments such as baclofen and other muscle relaxants. Bracing treatment is another excellent method as an adjunct to other treatments for mobility. Whereas chemical treatments assist with tone, bracing treatment can provide supplemental strength in either the coronal or sagittal planes. Axial plane control is very difficult to achieve using bracing treatment. Therapies (physical, occupational, and speech) are excellent methods of treatment for children with cerebral palsy and should be considered first line as they may allow for increased strength, increased range of motion, better function, and a sense of accomplishment for the child.

Increased muscular tone can be addressed by reversible pharmaceutical agents. The most common drug used is baclofen. It acts as an agonist on centrally located GABA receptors. Baclofen can be given either by an enteral or by an

©Copyright 2021 American Academy of Orthopaedic Surgeons

intrathecal route. In enteral delivery, baclofen is well absorbed and widely distributed throughout the body; however, increased blood concentrations hence increased dosage is needed to cross the blood-brain barrier (BBB). For intrathecal delivery, the dosage can be reduced significantly because the molecule does not need to pass the BBB. A decreased dosage of baclofen is preferred because of the decrease in unwanted side effects (ie, sedation, drooling) associated with baclofen. Additionally, the rate and timing of administration are well controlled with the pump. The downside of this method of delivery is that a pump needs to be placed surgically and occasionally refilled. Botulinum toxin is a potent neurotoxin, produced by the bacteria *Clostridium botulinum*. Commonly botulinum type A is used locally in muscles. The toxin is a competitive inhibitor of presynaptic cholinergic receptors in the NMJ. It typically remains effective for 3 to 4 months. However, long-term usage of botulinum toxin decreases the efficacy of the treatment because this toxin induces the formation of an extensive network of nerve-terminal sprouts that can overcome its effect.[43] Botulinum toxin injections should be provided in conjunction with physical therapy as it reduces tone but does not produce any new range of motion, whereas it can enable new motion through the plastic deformation of muscle and tendon tissue. Phenol is a second injectable agent against focal spasticity. Phenol causes neural damage by demyelination and a decrease in the muscle-spindle activity. It is associated with pain at the injection site, transient dysesthesias, and numbness. Phenol's therapeutic effect lasts for 4 to 12 months, longer then botulinum toxin. Nevertheless, it can be used together with botulinum toxin to allow more injection sites and larger doses per site.

Surgical treatment includes muscle lengthening, tendon transfers, bony surgeries including osteotomies, fusions, and guided growth.[44,45] The decision making for these types of surgeries is beyond the scope of this chapter.

Multiple Sclerosis

Multiple sclerosis (MS) is a challenging neurodegenerative condition which affects the myelin sheath in CNS neurons and may lead to substantial functional impairment. It is a multifocal disease somewhat heterogeneous in presentation with a prevalence of 46.3 per 100,000 people in the United States.[46]

Pathogenesis

Although a genetic factor (eg, HLA DRB1*15:01) has been described as an etiologic factor in MS development, it seems that environmental factors may play a more significant role in the pathologic manifestation of MS. Factors such as vitamin D deficiency, obesity, cigarette smoking, and Epstein-Barr virus infection have been linked with the disease. MS is characterized by an autoimmune inflammatory response confined to the CNS. The autoimmune inflammatory process appears to involve T cells, B cells, and macrophages, which are centered around the destruction of myelin.[47] The pathologic process results in demyelination of axons, as well as neuron and oligodendrocytes loss.

Clinical Presentation

Age of presentation of MS is typically later in life (50 to 60 years of age).[48] However, earlier presentation in young females is not uncommon. Clinical presentation of MS depends on the affected site of lesion and the extent of the inflammation process. Initial presentation is abrupt in onset and commonly includes unilateral optic neuritis; however, other symptoms such as weakness, paresthesia, gait and balance disturbances, muscle cramps or pain, and bowel or bladder incontinence may follow.

The timing and progression of subsequent attacks help differentiate between the different courses of the disease. Remitting-relapsing (RR) type is the most common (50%) pattern of presentation and is characterized by neurologic recovery between episodes of acute exacerbations.[47] Primary progressive type is less common and characterized by slow continuously progressing symptoms with no relapses or remissions. Secondary progressive type starts as RR, and after a period of time (mostly several years), approximately 75% to 85% of RR will become progressive. Progressive relapsing type is the least common type characterized by a steadily worsening disease state without remissions from the beginning, with acute relapses. Patients with MS are at higher risk for osteoporosis and fragility fractures.[49] This is partially due to the association with low vitamin D levels, but also due to inactivity from neurologic involvement. Repetitive steroid treatment or decreased mobilization may also affect bone mineral density. Another risk for fractures includes impaired balance and an increased tendency to falls. Mood and cognitive changes may occur at later stages in the disease course. Patients with MS have a shorter mean life expectancy of about 5 years than that of the general population. Recurrent urinary tract and respiratory infections are typical causes of mortality.

Diagnosis

The diagnosis is suspected by the clinical symptoms that are disseminated in time/space. Younger patients may also have bilateral intranuclear ophthalmoplegia, which results in double vision with a lateral gaze. This finding occurs because the medial longitudinal fasciculus is a heavily myelinated tract associated with the abducens nerve which is typically affected nerve. Confirmatory MRI exhibits hyperintense lesions of CNS white matter on T2-weighted images. An ovoid-shaped periventricular white matter lesion is another common finding in MRI. LP and CSF analysis may help support the diagnosis as 85% of patients with MS have evidence of oligoclonal bands and elevated IgG index. Opening pressure and other cerebrospinal fluid measures are typically normal.

Management

In acute exacerbations, first-line treatment includes corticosteroids as they can provide anti-inflammatory activity. In cases of steroid-resistant disease relapses plasmapheresis is offered. Several disease-modifying treatments (**Table 3**) have been approved for MS patients. These treatments target different

©Copyright 2021 American Academy of Orthopaedic Surgeons

TABLE 3 Multiple Sclerosis Disease—Modifying Treatment Description

Suggested Drug	Mechanism of Action	Common Side Effects
Interferon beta (as a group)	Reduction of antigen presentation, cytokine modulation, inhibition of T-cell activation and proliferation	Flulike symptoms, headache, injection site reactions and pain, low white blood cell count, abnormal liver function tests
Glatiramer acetate	Shifts T cells from proinflammatory Th1 T cells to regulatory Th2 T cells	Injection-site reactions, flushing, lipoatrophy
Dimethyl fumarate	Decreases absolute lymphocyte counts (most profoundly CD8+ T cells), activates nuclear factor (erythroid-derived 2)-like 2 (Nrf2), down regulates nuclear factor kappa B (Nf-κB)	Flushing, gastrointestinal symptoms (nausea, diarrhea, abdominal pain), lymphopenia
Teriflunomide	Blocking the enzyme dihydroorotate dehydrogenase (inhibit pyrimidine "de novo" synthesis and affect lymphocyte proliferation)	Hair thinning, gastrointestinal symptoms (nausea, diarrhea, abdominal pain), abnormal liver function tests
Fingolimod	Antagonist of sphingosine 1-phosphate receptors (inhibits migration of lymphocytes from lymph nodes)	Bradyarrhythmia (first dose), increased risk of infections, lymphopenia, gastrointestinal symptoms (diarrhea, abdominal pain), abnormal liver function tests, increased risk for basal cell carcinoma
Cladribine	Deoxyadenosine analogue and adenosine deaminase inhibitor (depletes B and T cells)	Lymphopenia, increased risk of infections
Alemtuzumab	Humanized monoclonal antibody against CD52 on lymphocyte and monocyte (depletes B and T cells)	Increased risk of infection, secondary autoimmunity (mainly thyroid, TTP)
Natalizumab	Humanized monoclonal antibody against α-4 integrin (prevents lymphocytes from crossing blood-brain barrier and entering the central nervous system)	Dizziness, skin rash, gastrointestinal symptoms (nausea, diarrhea, abdominal pain), increased risk of infection
Ocrelizumab	Humanized monoclonal antibody against CD20 on B cell surface (deplete B cell)	Infusion reactions increased risk of infections

Adapted from Thompson AJ, Baranzini SE, Geurts J, Hemmer B, Ciccarelli O: Multiple sclerosis. *Lancet* 2018;391(10130):1622-1636 and Dobson R, Giovannoni G: Multiple sclerosis - a review. *Eur J Neurol* 2019;26(1):27-40.

factors of the inflammatory processes and are indicated for chronic maintenance therapy in patients with relapsing-remitting disease. Spastic patients can be treated with baclofen or tizanidine; nonpharmacological measures include physical therapy and orthosis. Orthopaedic surgery focuses on treating contractures, to improve hygiene and sometimes function.

Acute Disseminated Encephalomyelitis

Acute disseminated encephalomyelitis (ADEM) is an abrupt, widespread, inflammatory demyelinating disease affecting the brain and spinal cord. ADEM clinically bears a close resemblance to MS because of its multifocal character; however, unlike MS, its course is mostly monophasic.

The incidence of ADEM has had a slight increase in the last decade and currently estimated to be 0.6 per 100,000 persons.[50]

Pathogenesis

ADEM is presumed to be preceded by a viral infection or rarely by vaccination. Viral agents include influenza, measles, mumps, rubella, varicella-zoster, Epstein-Barr virus, cytomegalovirus, and herpes simplex virus. The pathologic process consists of immune-mediated demyelination in the CNS white matter. Demyelination appears in perivenular sleeves with infiltration of a variety of immune cells.

Clinical Presentation

ADEM is more common in children but may also be seen in adults. Children younger than 12 years of age are most commonly affected; the median age of diagnosis is between 5 and 8 years.[51] Clinical presentation is acute in nature and usually includes an encephalopathic pattern with altered behavior or consciousness level in addition to polyfocal symptoms such as headaches, nausea, vomiting, muscle weakness, ataxia, fever seizures, and vision loss. The course of the disease is progressive with peak in symptoms mentioned at 5 days from onset. 80% of cases leads to full recovery within 6 months. About 20% of cases may relapse and defined as multiphasic disease. These cases are associated with seropositive anti-MOG antibodies.[52]

Diagnosis

The diagnosis is made by first ruling out more common causes such as infection or compressive disorders of the spine or brain.

©Copyright 2021 American Academy of Orthopaedic Surgeons

As such an MRI of the brain and spine are recommended. On MRI a bilateral, asymmetric multiple hyperintense lesions can be seen on T2 sequences. Lesions typically involve the white matter, basal ganglia, and cortical gray matter. On LP and CSF, analysis show increased white blood cells (lymphocytes and monocytes) and protein. No oligoclonal bands are present.

Management

Treatment with intravenous high-dose corticosteroids is first-line therapy followed by oral corticosteroids. IVIG and plasma-exchange treatments remain salvage second-line treatment in steroid-refractory cases.

Transverse Myelitis

Transverse myelitis (TM) is a rare acquired neuroimmune CNS disorder characterized by an inflammation of myelin tissue surrounding the neurons. TM is a monophasic-monofocal disease and is confined to the spinal cord. The term "transverse" refers to the hallmark bandlike pattern across the trunk of the body, with sensory changes below it. The annual incidence of TM in the United States is estimated at 1.3 to 4.6 cases per million people.[53]

Pathogenesis

TM mostly occurs as an idiopathic disease and its exact causation is unknown. It is thought to follow an autoimmune postinfectious course where molecular mimicry plays a role in the pathogenesis. In TM spinal inflammation is caused by circulating antibodies that target aquaporin 4, a protein located on distal end foot of astrocytes which provide nutrients to the spinal cord.[54] A second, less common target for antibodies is the myelin oligodendrocyte glycoprotein (MOG) found on the outer most surface of myelin sheets. Inflammation interrupts signal transmission from the CNS to the rest of the body below the level of lesion.

Clinical Presentation

Transverse myelitis can affect people of any age, gender, or race. The peak of onset is bimodal, 10 to 19 years and 30 to 39 years. Symptoms typically develop suddenly over hours or days and may include rapidly progressive weakness of the lower extremities associated with pain, sensory alterations such as partial or complete loss of sensation below a clear spinal level. Autonomic dysfunction is present in most cases and includes dysfunctional bladder, bowel, sexual, cardiovascular, and thermoregulatory processes. Physical examination can reveal muscle flaccidity and hyporeflexia at first, but over time, spasticity and hyperreflexia follow.

Diagnosis

An MRI of the entire spine as well as brain MRI are both mandatory in suspected patients. Imaging of the spine is needed first to locate the inflammatory process and secondarily to rule out mechanical compression of the spinal cord. The inflammatory process is mostly seen as a high-intensity centromedullary lesion on an MRI T2 sequence, extending over at least one vertebral segment and involving more than two-thirds of the cross-sectional area of the spinal cord.[55] LP and CSF analysis is an important tool in the diagnosis and characterized by increased protein and WBC count. Blood should be tested for autoantibodies (anti-aquaporin 4, antimyelin oligodendrocyte).

Management

There is no cure for transverse myelitis. High-dose glucocorticoids are given to help prevent or minimize permanent neurological deficits. Plasmapheresis can be offered to patients with poor or no response to steroids.

Stroke

Stroke or cerebrovascular accidents (CVA) is a leading cause of death and disability in the United States and other countries in the developed world. A stroke occurs when the cells of the brain are deprived of oxygen and nutrients, because of reduced or interrupted blood supply. The term ischemic stroke implies a clotted or a blocked blood vessel, whereas hemorrhagic stroke implies vessel rupture as a cause.

Epidemiology and risk factors

In the United States, incidence of CVA is 795,000 per year,[56] survival rate is 80% to 90%, and the majority of patients require rehabilitation.[57] As a result of improved acute care, total survivorship has increased, and the burden of care has subsequently become greater. Historically the majority of stroke patients were 50 or older, but recent evidence shows a rise in the number of younger patients (aged 18 to 50) diagnosed with stroke (10:1 ratio respectively).[58] Ischemic stroke is highly associated with atherosclerosis. As such classic risk factors include smoking, diabetes, obesity, and hypertension. In young adults, additional risk factors had been identified including illicit drug use, malignancy, pregnancy, use of oral contraceptives, autoimmune disorders (ie, antiphospholipid syndrome), arterial dissection, and patent foramen ovale (PFO).[58]

Clinical Presentation

Early presentation patients may include sudden headache; confusion; speaking difficulties; numbness or weakness of the face, arm, or leg, most of one side of the body; and loss of balance or coordination. In later stages, stroke survivors may experience residual problems in several domains. For many patients a motor deficit is most prominent; however, they may also experience deficits in mood, language, cognitive function, as well as sensory abnormalities. As in patients with TBI, poststroke patients are at increased risk for the development of heterotopic ossification, particularly with direct injuries.

Management

The acute phase of treatment for CVA is handled by emergency services, neurology, and occasionally neurosurgery.

©Copyright 2021 American Academy of Orthopaedic Surgeons

Treatment is aimed at specific pathology. Neuroimaging is crucial to understand the nature of pathology and to guide treatment. In cases where the diagnosis is made rapidly, more pathology directed treatment is possible allowing for minimal hypoxia of neurons. Tissue plasminogen activator (TPA) in the case of clots or surgical treatment of other causes is possible with a rapid diagnosis. Recent evidence shows great potential in the safety and efficacy of intra-arterial thrombolysis (IAT) of middle cerebral artery (MCA) occlusions treated within 6 hours.[59] Patients may require long-term rehabilitation after stabilization. Goals of poststroke-rehabilitation are targeted at return to independence, improve functionality, and reduction of chronic pain. Multiple services are needed. Orthopaedics is directed at preventing and correcting deformity. Equinovarus deformity, knee flexion deformity, and various upper extremity deformities are common. Neurologic ongoing treatment, fall prevention strategies, and seizure treatment are critical. Physical and occupational therapy treatment is mandatory and often ongoing.

Traumatic Brain Injury

Traumatic brain injury (TBI) is a challenging condition that can lead to severe disability or death. Severe TBI is extremely heterogeneous and a somewhat more recent clinical phenomenon as only recently have we had the technology to make the initial injuries survivable. As such the prognosis of any given injury is never clear. As orthopaedic surgeons, the most prudent course of action early in TBI is to act under the assumption that a full recovery will be made. It is sometimes difficult otherwise to overcome misguided decisions made early in patient care which can lead to malunions, nonunions, or disability later in the patient's recovery.

TBI itself is defined as a disruption of brain activity or architecture due to an external biomechanical force directing on to the head. This includes both closed-head injuries and penetrating head trauma. In penetrating trauma, the injury is typically due to direct disruption of brain tissue. In blunt trauma, damage is due to either axonal injury, pressure caused by hematoma formation, anoxia, or shear forces.

Epidemiology and Mechanism of injury

Each year in the United States, there are 2.5 million TBI-related ED visits,282,000 TBI-related hospitalizations, and 56,000 TBI-related deaths.[60] The Center for Disease Control's National Center for Injury Prevention and Control estimates that 5.3 million US citizens (2% of the population) are living with a disability as a result of a TBI. TBI affects people of all ages; however, in the United States, children aged 0 to 4 years, adolescents aged 15 to 19 years, and adults aged 75 years and older are at higher risk to have a TBI-related emergency department visit or hospitalization with TBI.[61] Patients aged 75 years and older are at greatest risk for hospitalization and death. More than half of the injuries are due to motor vehicle accidents (MVAs) followed by falls (27%) and violence associated injuries (11%).[62]

Clinical Presentation

The severity of TBI can be classified as mild, moderate, or severe from the clinical presentation of a patient's neurologic signs and symptoms. Although sports medicine physicians may commonly identify mild TBI also termed concussions through their work on the field in sporting events, more severe TBI are likely to be identified in trauma victims. Symptoms of TBI vary with severity.

The diagnosis is clinical usually with the assistance of standardized neuropsychological tests and physical examination. Patients require rest and removal from play or activity. Return to activity is based on resolution of symptomology as assessed clinically.

Moderate and severe TBI often present with altered sensorium, weakness, increased muscle tone, seizures, disability, and a myriad of other manifestations. The final common pathway of patients with TBI is similar to other patients with upper motor neuron diseases, with pathologic positive symptoms such as increased muscle tone, pathologic reflexes, and negative symptoms such as weakness and loss of balance, vision, or other senses. Orthopaedic surgeons are often called upon to manage tone and contractures, and the armamentarium is quite similar to cerebral palsy and other spastic upper motor neuron diseases. When considering a treatment plan, the orthopaedic surgeon should seek to optimize function. This may entail encouraging active function, assisting in ease of care, or promoting hygiene or improving passive function by relieving contractures in a nonfunctional limb.

Heterotopic Ossification

Heterotopic ossification (HO) is a pathological process often seen in TBI, spinal cord injury, burns, and direct trauma. In fact, when both a brain injury and direct trauma to the hip occurs, the rate of HO approaches 100%. The pathologic process is a process in which ectopic lamellar bone grows in soft tissue. On a cellular level, the process described is an osteogenic differentiation of progenitor cells in soft tissues.[63] HO is associated with traumatic injuries and neurologic issues (TBI, SCI), but can also be related to burns, surgical procedures (arthroplasty), and amputations. Despite numerous efforts to identify the exact cellular and molecular processes that lead to HO, the mechanisms of pathogenesis and the exact relationship to different scenarios mentioned remain unknown. HO mostly involves calcification of soft tissues, typically in close-proximity to joint capsules around large joints (hip, knee, shoulder, and elbow) but may also comprise more distant muscles and tendons (**Figure 3**). It may lead to different complications including chronic pain, nerve entrapment, decreased ROM, and joint ankylosis. In selected cases of functional impairment around the inflicted joint or of pain, it can be excised. Low-dose radiation and certain nonsteroidal anti-inflammatory medications namely nonselective cyclooxygenase (COX)-1 and COX-2 inhibitor (indomethacin) are

 ©Copyright 2021 American Academy of Orthopaedic Surgeons

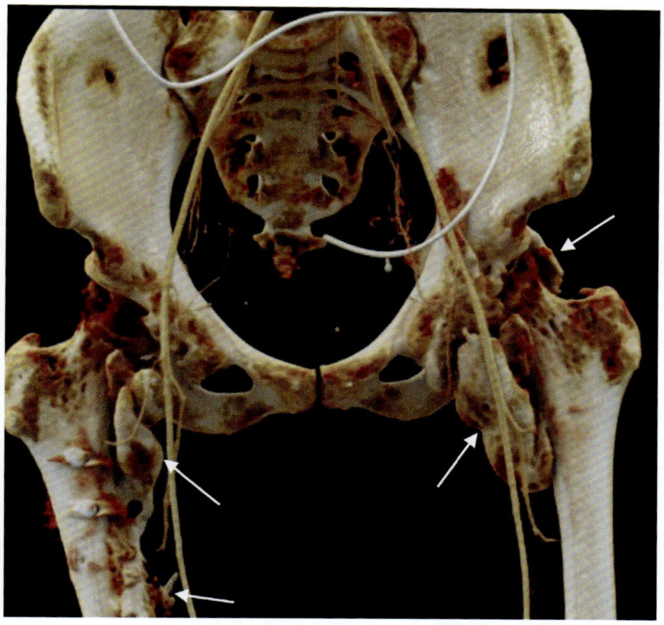

FIGURE 3 An MRI 3D visualization of a bilateral heterotopic ossification around the hip. Arrows show abnormal ossifications.

agents of prophylaxis against heterotopic ossification. The use of antiresorptive agents including diphosphonates for prophylaxis of HO remains controversial.[63]

Spinal Cord Injury

Spinal cord injury (SCI) is a devastating event that may lead to temporary or permanent impairment of motor, sensory, or autonomic functions and may have deleterious effects on survival.

Epidemiology and Mechanism of Injury

The incidence of SCI in the United States is about 17,700 new cases annually. In addition, the prevalence of SCI patients who are living in the United States is expected to be approximately 288,000 persons, with a range from 247,000 to 358,000 persons. The bimodal age distribution is related to increased high-energy trauma accidents in patients of younger age and a combined effect of either narrowed spine canal (stenosis) or an ankylosed spine with increased fracture potential and low-energy trauma in the relatively older aged patients. MVAs remain the most common mechanism of injury accounting for 38% of cases. Falls are widespread accounting for 31.6% of cases. Other common mechanisms of injury are violence (mainly gunshot wounds), sports injuries, and iatrogenic injuries.[64] Recent studies report an unappreciated toll of additional neurological damage due to improper immobilization or methodology of transportation as patients are transferred to acute care facilities (after the initial accident).

Pathogenesis

The pathogenesis of SCI includes a primary stage which occurs at the time of injury and within seconds-minutes after injury. During this period an insult to neurons in the spinal cord arises from either the direct transfer of energy and deformation of the cord itself, or from a laceration, distraction, or compressive force of the neighboring vertebra or disks onto the cord. It may also result from damage to vertebral arteries that may lead to either ischemia or a compressive effect from a hematoma. A second stage usually starts minutes after the injury and may last for weeks or months afterward. The second stage may further damage the cord neurons from indirect processes originating in nearby tissues including biochemical interactions, inflammatory responses, free radical formation, and lipid peroxidation.

Clinical Presentation

The clinical presentation may vary by anatomic location (**Figure 4**) and extent of the injury (complete or incomplete. The most commonly involved vertebral segment of the spine is the cervical spine. A higher (cervical) injury is often associated with quadriplegia, a term referring to an impaired function of both upper and lower limbs. Sensation and motor loss are below the level of the lesion. A lower spinal injury (thoracic and lumbar) may lead to paraplegia, in which the upper limbs are intact, but impairment of legs, trunk, and pelvic organs are present. In injuries that involve the upper part of the thoracic spine (above T6) autonomic dysreflexia (ADys) may occur. ADys is precipitated by different triggers (pain, urinary distention, fecal impaction) and lead to an uncontrolled autonomic response. Clinically ADys is characterized by an inappropriate response to autonomic activation with a predominant sympathetic excitation below the level of injury and a strong compensatory parasympathetic activation above the level of injury. Patients appear with severe hypertension, bradycardia, headaches, facial flushing, excessive sweating, and nasal congestion. If left untreated, this autonomic imbalance can lead to an increased risk of both intracranial hemorrhage and cardiovascular complications. Extent of the injury refers to the remainder of neurologic function retained below the injury. The American Spinal Injury Association (ASIA) classification describes the extent of the residual function below the lesion.[65] This classification (Figure 4) categorizes the neurologic (sensory and motor) function and the injury severity. Incomplete quadriplegia is most common accounting for nearly half the cases since 2015.[64] As in TBI heterotopic ossification is a common finding in SCI especially in higher levels of injuries (cervical, thoracic) and in complete injuries.

Spinal Shock

Spinal shock is a transient condition that accompanies acute SCI. It consists of a temporary combined loss of sensorimotor function and reflexes, below the level of injury, as well as autonomous dysfunction and loss of function pelvic organs. At the physiological level, at this state, neurons become hyperpolarized and are unresponsive to stimuli from the brain. One of the hallmarks of spinal shock is the temporary absence of the bulbocavernosus reflex. The reflex creates a contraction of the anal sphincter as a reaction to squeezing of glans penis

©Copyright 2021 American Academy of Orthopaedic Surgeons

ASIA — AMERICAN SPINAL INJURY ASSOCIATION

INTERNATIONAL STANDARDS FOR NEUROLOGICAL CLASSIFICATION OF SPINAL CORD INJURY (ISNCSCI)

ISCOS

Patient Name__________ Date/Time of Exam __________

Examiner Name __________ Signature __________

RIGHT — MOTOR KEY MUSCLES — SENSORY KEY SENSORY POINTS: Light Touch (LTR), Pin Prick (PPR)

C2, C3, C4

UER (Upper Extremity Right): Elbow flexors C5; Wrist extensors C6; Elbow extensors C7; Finger flexors C8; Finger abductors (little finger) T1

T2, T3, T4, T5, T6, T7, T8, T9, T10, T11, T12, L1

Comments (Non-key Muscle? Reason for NT? Pain? Non-SCI condition?):

LER (Lower Extremity Right): Hip flexors L2; Knee extensors L3; Ankle dorsiflexors L4; Long toe extensors L5; Ankle plantar flexors S1

S2, S3, S4-5

(VAC) Voluntary Anal Contraction (Yes/No)

RIGHT TOTALS (MAXIMUM) (50) (56) (56)

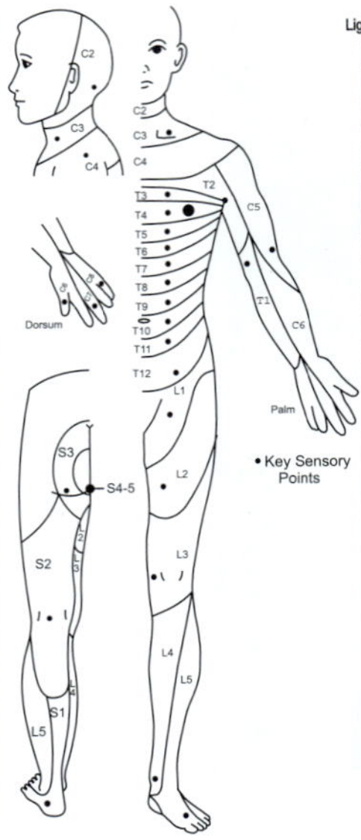

LEFT — SENSORY KEY SENSORY POINTS: Light Touch (LTL), Pin Prick (PPL) — MOTOR KEY MUSCLES

C2, C3, C4

UEL (Upper Extremity Left): C5 Elbow flexors; C6 Wrist extensors; C7 Elbow extensors; C8 Finger flexors; T1 Finger abductors (little finger)

T2, T3, T4, T5, T6, T7, T8, T9, T10, T11, T12, L1

MOTOR (SCORING ON REVERSE SIDE)

0 = Total paralysis
1 = Palpable or visible contraction
2 = Active movement, gravity eliminated
3 = Active movement, against gravity
4 = Active movement, against some resistance
5 = Active movement, against full resistance
NT = Not testable
0*, 1*, 2*, 3*, 4*, NT* = Non-SCI condition present

SENSORY (SCORING ON REVERSE SIDE)

0 = Absent; 1 = Altered; 2 = Normal; NT = Not testable; 0*, 1*, NT* = Non-SCI condition present

LEL (Lower Extremity Left): L2 Hip flexors; L3 Knee extensors; L4 Ankle dorsiflexors; L5 Long toe extensors; S1 Ankle plantar flexors

S2, S3, S4-5

(DAP) Deep Anal Pressure (Yes/No)

LEFT TOTALS (MAXIMUM) (56) (56) (50)

MOTOR SUBSCORES

UER _ + UEL _ = UEMS TOTAL _ — MAX (25) (25) (50)

LER _ + LEL _ = LEMS TOTAL _ — MAX (25) (25) (50)

SENSORY SUBSCORES

LTR _ + LTL _ = LT TOTAL _ — MAX (56) (56) (112)

PPR _ + PPL _ = PP TOTAL _ — MAX (56) (56) (112)

NEUROLOGICAL LEVELS (Steps 1-6 for classification as on reverse): 1. SENSORY R L; 2. MOTOR R L

3. NEUROLOGICAL LEVEL OF INJURY (NLI)

4. COMPLETE OR INCOMPLETE? (Incomplete = Any sensory or motor function in S4-5)

5. ASIA IMPAIRMENT SCALE (AIS)

6. ZONE OF PARTIAL PRESERVATION (In injuries with absent motor OR sensory function in S4-5 only) — Most caudal levels with any innervation: SENSORY R L; MOTOR R L

Page 1/2

This form may be copied freely but should not be altered without permission from the American Spinal Injury Association.

REV 04/19

Muscle Function Grading

0 = Total paralysis

1 = Palpable or visible contraction

2 = Active movement, full range of motion (ROM) with gravity eliminated

3 = Active movement, full ROM against gravity

4 = Active movement, full ROM against gravity and moderate resistance in a muscle specific position

5 = (Normal) active movement, full ROM against gravity and full resistance in a functional muscle position expected from an otherwise unimpaired person

NT = Not testable (i.e. due to immobilization, severe pain such that the patient cannot be graded, amputation of limb, or contracture of > 50% of the normal ROM)

0*, 1*, 2*, 3*, 4*, NT* = Non-SCI condition present [a]

Sensory Grading

0 = Absent 1 = Altered, either decreased/impaired sensation or hypersensitivity

2 = Normal NT = Not testable

0*, 1*, NT* = Non-SCI condition present [a]

[a] Note: Abnormal motor and sensory scores should be tagged with a '*' to indicate an impairment due to a non-SCI condition. The non-SCI condition should be explained in the comments box together with information about how the score is rated for classification purposes (at least normal / not normal for classification).

When to Test Non-Key Muscles:

In a patient with an apparent AIS B classification, non-key muscle functions more than 3 levels below the motor level on each side should be tested to most accurately classify the injury (differentiate between AIS B and C).

Movement	Root level
Shoulder: Flexion, extension, adduction, adduction, internal and external rotation **Elbow:** Supination	C5
Elbow: Pronation **Wrist:** Flexion	C6
Finger: Flexion at proximal joint, extension **Thumb:** Flexion, extension and abduction in plane of thumb	C7
Finger: Flexion at MCP joint **Thumb:** Opposition, adduction and abduction perpendicular to palm	C8
Finger: Abduction of the index finger	T1
Hip: Adduction	L2
Hip: External rotation	L3
Hip: Extension, abduction, internal rotation **Knee:** Flexion **Ankle:** Inversion and eversion **Toe:** MP and IP extension	L4
Hallux and Toe: DIP and PIP flexion and abduction	L5
Hallux: Adduction	S1

ASIA Impairment Scale (AIS)

A = Complete. No sensory or motor function is preserved in the sacral segments S4-5.

B = Sensory Incomplete. Sensory but not motor function is preserved below the neurological level and includes the sacral segments S4-5 (light touch or pin prick at S4-5 or deep anal pressure) AND no motor function is preserved more than three levels below the motor level on either side of the body.

C = Motor Incomplete. Motor function is preserved at the most caudal sacral segments for voluntary anal contraction (VAC) OR the patient meets the criteria for sensory incomplete status (sensory function preserved at the most caudal sacral segments S4-5 by LT, PP or DAP), and has some sparing of motor function more than three levels below the ipsilateral motor level on either side of the body. (This includes key or non-key muscle functions to determine motor incomplete status.) For AIS C – less than half of key muscle functions below the single NLI have a muscle grade ≥ 3.

D = Motor Incomplete. Motor incomplete status as defined above, with at least half (half or more) of key muscle functions below the single NLI having a muscle grade ≥ 3.

E = Normal. If sensation and motor function as tested with the ISNCSCI are graded as normal in all segments, and the patient had prior deficits, then the AIS grade is E. Someone without an initial SCI does not receive an AIS grade.

Using ND: To document the sensory, motor and NLI levels, the ASIA Impairment Scale grade, and/or the zone of partial preservation (ZPP) when they are unable to be determined based on the examination results.

ASIA — AMERICAN SPINAL INJURY ASSOCIATION

INTERNATIONAL STANDARDS FOR NEUROLOGICAL CLASSIFICATION OF SPINAL CORD INJURY

ISCOS — INTERNATIONAL SPINAL CORD SOCIETY

Page 2/2

Steps in Classification

The following order is recommended for determining the classification of individuals with SCI.

1. Determine sensory levels for right and left sides.
The sensory level is the most caudal, intact dermatome for both pin prick and light touch sensation.

2. Determine motor levels for right and left sides.
Defined by the lowest key muscle function that has a grade of at least 3 (on supine testing), providing the key muscle functions represented by segments above that level are judged to be intact (graded as a 5).
Note: in regions where there is no myotome to test, the motor level is presumed to be the same as the sensory level, if testable motor function above that level is also normal.

3. Determine the neurological level of injury (NLI).
This refers to the most caudal segment of the cord with intact sensation and antigravity (3 or more) muscle function strength, provided that there is normal (intact) sensory and motor function rostrally respectively.
The NLI is the most cephalad of the sensory and motor levels determined in steps 1 and 2.

4. Determine whether the injury is Complete or Incomplete.
(i.e. absence or presence of sacral sparing)
*If voluntary anal contraction = **No** AND all S4-5 sensory scores = **0** AND deep anal pressure = **No**, then injury is **Complete**.*
*Otherwise, injury is **Incomplete**.*

5. Determine ASIA Impairment Scale (AIS) Grade.
Is injury Complete? If YES, AIS=A

NO ↓

Is injury Motor Complete? If YES, AIS=B

NO ↓ (No=voluntary anal contraction OR motor function more than three levels below the motor level on a given side, if the patient has sensory incomplete classification)

Are at least half (half or more) of the key muscles below the neurological level of injury graded 3 or better?

NO ↓ AIS=C — **YES ↓ AIS=D**

If sensation and motor function is normal in all segments, AIS=E
Note: AIS E is used in follow-up testing when an individual with a documented SCI has recovered normal function. If at initial testing no deficits are found, the individual is neurologically intact and the ASIA Impairment Scale does not apply.

6. Determine the zone of partial preservation (ZPP).
The ZPP is used only in injuries with absent motor (no VAC) OR sensory function (no DAP, no LT and no PP sensation) in the lowest sacral segments S4-5, and refers to those dermatomes and myotomes caudal to the sensory and motor levels that remain partially innervated. With sacral sparing of sensory function, the sensory ZPP is not applicable and therefore "NA" is recorded in the block of the worksheet. Accordingly, if VAC is present, the motor ZPP is not applicable and is noted as "NA".

FIGURE 4 The American Spinal Injury Association (ASIA) International Standards for Neurological Classification of Spinal Cord Injury. (© 2011 American Spinal Injury Association. Reprinted with permission.)

©Copyright 2021 American Academy of Orthopaedic Surgeons

or clitoris. The return of bulbocavernosus reflex indicates the end of the spinal shock. Spinal shock symptoms may last hours-days; its end is marked by the return of the bulbocavernosus reflex. Emphasis should be made, as one should not be confused between spinal shock and neurologic shock. Spinal shock is distinct from neurologic shock, as the latter represents the systemic effect of blood pressure decline, bradycardia, and hypothermia due to loss of sympathetic tone as well as loss of regulated control of both vascular tone and sinoatrial activation of the heart.

Common SCI Patterns

Patterns of incomplete SCI are distinguished based on their clinical presentations and location of the injury within the spinal cord and can provide prognostic guidance.

Central cord syndrome is most common. It is caused by an insult to central gray matter of the spinal cord, often a hyperextension injury of the cervical spine. It leads to preferential upper extremity limb paralysis and loss of sensation because of the anatomic location of the nerve tracts to the upper extremities. Sacral functioning is spared. Affected patients usually manage to ambulate, but experience clumsiness, wide-based mechanical gait, and have difficulty with upper limb function. The prognosis of this disorder is better than many SCI disorders because ambulatory function is preserved, and patients have maintained bowel and bladder function.

Brown-Séquard syndrome is characterized by a complete hemi-section of the spinal cord leading to loss of motor and proprioceptive sensation at the same side (ipsilateral) of injury, combined with contralateral loss of temperature and pain sensation. The affected patients usually have a good prognosis, and ambulatory function is largely maintained.

Anterior cord syndrome is mainly caused by compression of the anterior cord or disruption to its blood supply; it is characterized by loss of motor and sensory (pain and temperature sensation) below the level of the lesion. Because posterior columns are spared, deep touch, proprioception, and vibratory sensation are mostly preserved. Affected patients have a worse prognosis for recovery, and usually cannot ambulate.

Management

A final diagnosis is made by combining the physical examination with radiographic findings. CT scan is the preferred modality for bony assessment and fracture evaluation. Surgical stabilization and urgent treatment can be guided in part by CT. An MRI is superior for soft tissue examination including ligamentous disruption, neural cord damage, disk pressure, edema formation.[66]

The first priority in the management of SCI is cardiopulmonary support to maintain blood pressure, monitor for proper ventilation and oxygenation, and prevent anemia. After the patient is stabilized and adequate diagnosis had been made, an early surgical decompression can yield better neurologic recovery and long-term results. Nonsurgical treatment such as steroid treatment remains controversial and seems to offer no significant benefit. Induced hypothermia has had mixed results, but effectiveness has not been tested in randomized clinical trials.[67] A pursuit for other novel nonsurgical operative treatments continues. The primary goals are optimizing mobility, self-care, and other daily needs. Rehabilitation methods usually include intact muscle strengthening, maintenances of joints range of motion, stabilization of posture, as well as accommodative therapies. Orthopaedic surgical treatments include HO excision and upper extremity tendon transfers to maintain or improve function.

MIXED UPPER AND LOWER MOTOR NEURON DISEASES

AMYOTROPHIC LATERAL SCLEROSIS

Amyotrophic lateral sclerosis (ALS) is a fatal, heterogenic neurodegenerative disease. The classic ALS includes involvement of both upper and lower motor neurons. Different terminologies are used for specific variants of ALS. Approximately 5,600 individuals have been diagnosed with ALS annually in the United States,[68] and its prevalence is estimated to be 5 per 100,000 population in the United States. ALS is more common in Caucasians, non-Hispanics, males, and military veterans.[69]

Pathogenesis

Most patients with ALS have the sporadic type; in these cases, the etiology, as well as the actual pathologic underpinnings of disease, is poorly understood. On the other hand, in the familial form which represents about 10% of all ALS cases, there is a somewhat better understanding of the underlying pathogenesis. The familial form is mostly inherited via an autosomal dominant pattern and has a 50% penetrance.[70] There are more than 30 different genes that had been associated with familial form of ALS. Most familial ALS patients (60% to 80%) are associated with one out of four specific genes including C9orf72 (40%), SOD1 (20%), FUS (1% to 5%), and TARBDP (1% to 5%).[70] Genetic mutations lead to pathological aggregation and accumulation of ubiquitinated proteinaceous inclusions in the affected motor neurons.[71]

Clinical Presentation

The initial clinical presentation of ALS may vary. Asymmetric muscle weakness and stiffness are common initial presentations and may involve the limbs or affect activities related to cranial nerves (dysarthria, dysphagia, facial expressions). The average age of onset in classic ALS is 65 years. The disease onset in patients with the familial disease is typically 10 to 20 years earlier. As ALS progresses, weakness usually spreads within or to more anatomic regions, and the speed of progression may also vary between individuals. Other signs and symptoms of ALS include muscle cramps and balance issues. Spasticity and hyperreflexia reflect the UMN degeneration, whereas muscle

©Copyright 2021 American Academy of Orthopaedic Surgeons

atrophy and fasciculations represent the lower motor neuron damage. In addition, cognitive and mood changes are seen in 50% of ALS patients. In 5% to 15% of ALS patients, there is an association with frontotemporal dementia characterized by shrinking of the frontal and temporal anterior lobes of the brain—leading to apathy, socially inappropriate behavior, and language fluency disturbances. Death usually results from respiratory failure because of the involvement of respiratory muscles with progression of the disease. About half of ALS patients live 3 or more years after diagnosis with a quarter living at least 5 years postdiagnosis and up to 10% living 10 years or longer.

Diagnosis

The diagnosis of ALS is made by exclusion and mainly from the clinical presentation. EMG and NCV studies may help to confirm the diagnosis. It shows characteristics of both upper and lower motor neuron disease. Imaging with MRI is used only for ruling out other differential diagnosis and is not necessary for confirmation of ALS.

Management

There is no cure for ALS. Treatment is supportive including physiotherapy, speech therapy, feeding gastrostomy tube, noninvasive ventilatory support. As of 2017, the only widely available drug is riluzole, which was found to prolong survival of patients with ALS.[72] The exact mechanism of this drug is unclear, but the current understanding holds that riluzole can block the release of glutamate from nerve cells and reduce the rate of glutamate-induced deterioration in the nerves. In 2017, the FDA approved a second drug, edaravone, a potent pyrazolone free radical scavenger and antioxidant, which is theorized to decrease the effects of oxidative stress in neurons affected by ALS.[68]

EXTRAPYRAMIDAL DISORDERS OF ORTHOPAEDIC INTEREST

Parkinson's Disease

Parkinson's disease (PD) is a progressive neurodegenerative disease that affects dopaminergic neurons in the substantia nigra region of the basal ganglia. PD prevalence among individuals over the age of 45 years is 572/100,000 persons. This prevalence increases with age,[73] and it is estimated that PD is affecting 2% to 3% of persons aged 65 years and older.

Pathogenesis

Parkinson's disease is believed to be caused by an interplay of genetics and environmental factors. Risk factors such as male gender, repeated head trauma, exposures to metals and pesticides have been associated with PD. The final common pathway, however, is the loss of dopaminergic neurons in the brain. Histologically, Lewy bodies (abnormal protein deposits) appear in the basal ganglia as concentric, eosinophilic, cytoplasmic inclusions with peripheral halos. Impairments of cellular processes, related-abnormalities in protein aggregation, intracellular protein or membrane trafficking, and protein disposal are suggested as the mechanism of neuronal damage. In addition, aberrations in synaptic structure and function of the nerves may also be related to failed signal transmission.[74]

Clinical Presentation

PD symptoms slowly develop and may usually occur 5 to 8 years after the onset of the disease. There is a broad range of symptoms. However, four cardinal movement-related symptoms are common in PD patients. These symptoms are muscular rigidity, resting tremor, bradykinesia, and postural instability. Nonmovement symptoms may also be present such as constipation, urinary incontinence, depressed mood, sleep disorders, cognitive impairment of attention, planning, language, memory, or even dementia. Other manifestations include small handwriting (micrographia), decreased facial expression (hypomimia), soft speech (hypophonia), and reduced rate of eye blinking. Orthopaedic surgeons may encounter PD patients due to spine deformities as well as increased risk for fractures in relation to postural instability.[75,76] The median survival of PD from positive symptoms onset is approximately 15 years.

Diagnosis

Clinical diagnosis depends on recognition of the early movement-related cardinal features of PD (tremor, rigidity, bradykinesia). Therapeutic improvement with dopamine agonists or levodopa provides supportive evidence. In terms of imaging, MRI is considered controversial. Striatal dopamine transporter scan (DaTSCAN) is a type of nuclear scan that uses Ioflupane (^{123}I) which has a high affinity for dopamine transporters located in the basal region of the brain. PD patients have relatively low uptake isotope in the striatal region. DaTSCAN is a reliable method to diagnose PD, particularly with atypical presentations.

Treatment

Available pharmacological therapies for Parkinson's disease can only treat symptoms of the disease. Levodopa and dopamine agonists (eg, pramipexole, bromocriptine) are typically used as the first-line treatment of PD. Levodopa is very useful in symptom control but with prolonged use can lead to several motor complications (ie, fluctuations and dyskinesia). For this reason, it is typically reserved for patients older than 65 years of age. Younger patients (age <65) are treated with a levodopa sparing strategy which mostly includes dopamine agonists. Other pharmacological treatments may include monoamine oxidase (MAO-B) inhibitors that decrease dopamine breakdown, amantadine that lead to increased dopamine release,

 ©Copyright 2021 American Academy of Orthopaedic Surgeons

anticholinergics which can decrease acetylcholine effect and catechol-O-methyl transferase (COMT) inhibitors, which can prolong levodopa's effect. Deep brain stimulation is a non-pharmacological method of treatment that can improve PD cardinal symptoms. It is often used when pharmacological treatment had failed. This device uses a specific pulse made from pulse-generator implanted in the chest, to signal a lead inserted into the targeted structure in the brain.

Friedreich's Ataxia

Friedreich's ataxia (FRDA) is the most common progressive spinocerebellar degenerative disorder. This disease is characterized by ataxia meaning an abnormal, uncoordinated motor activation and movements. The disease estimated prevalence is about 2 to 4 cases per 100,000 people.[77]

Pathogenesis

FRDA is an autosomal recessive disease generated by a mutation in the Frataxin gene, located in the long arm of chromosome 9 (9q13-q21). Pathological expansions of the guanine-adenine-adenine (GAA) triplet repeats in the first intron are inhibiting the expression of frataxin gene (FXN). Disease-causing alleles carry expanded GAA sequences ranging from 66 to 1,500 repeats. Frataxin proteins are found in mitochondria and involved in the regulation of iron metabolism and oxidative stress. The lack of frataxin protein leads to an accumulation of mitochondrial iron stores and the formation of free radicals and ultimately lead to cell death. Loss of myelin affects mainly large myelinated neuron fibers at the root ganglia and posterior columns of the spinal cord.[78]

Clinical Presentation

Symptoms begin in the first two decades of life and include generalized clumsiness, weakness of the proximal muscles, particularly the gluteus maximus, wide-based gait, scoliosis and foot deformities (pes cavus or equinovarus). The onset of the disease depends on the number of GAA repeats, the larger the number of repeats the earlier the symptoms appear.[79] At later stages, additional manifestations include nystagmus and dysarthria and eventually loss of ability to ambulate. Both knee and ankle areflexia and positive plantar response are usually found on physical examination. Diabetes mellitus and hypertrophic cardiomyopathy are also associated with the disease. Cardiomyopathy may lead to arrhythmia, congestive heart failure, and premature death by the third or fourth decade.[46]

Treatment

Currently, there is no curative treatment for FRDA, and treatment is mainly supportive. Physical therapy may help with the usage of the limbs. Other orthopaedic-related problems, that is, scoliosis or foot deformities can be corrected. Nonrigid deformities can be braced whereas rigid deformities are treated surgically.

SUMMARY

Neuromuscular disorders include a wide-ranging set of conditions. The presenting symptoms and signs may vary but may also be very familiar as many diseases may overlap at their presentation at first stages. Many of the orthopaedic treatments available treat symptoms of the disease, but it is important to be aware of the overall prognosis and natural history to devise an appropriate treatment plan. The advancement of the genetic field holds a promise in improvements of both diagnostic methods and treatments directed at modifying the course of the disease. Orthopaedic treatment strategies will likely change in the future as a result of this pharmacologic alteration of the natural history.

The orthopaedic approach to patients with neuromuscular diseases can be challenging as both surgical and supportive methods of interventions are available, and the timing of each should be chosen carefully and be placed in context of the patients' overall function and the point in time of recovery.

In general, an interdisciplinary approach with regular longitudinal follow-ups will hopefully provide patients and their family an improved day-to-day satisfaction alongside with optimal clinical outcomes.

REFERENCES

1. Theadom A, Rodrigues M, Roxburgh R, et al: Prevalence of muscular dystrophies: A systematic literature review. *Neuroepidemiology* 2014;43(3-4):259-268.
2. Emery AEH: Population frequencies of inherited neuromuscular diseases—a world survey. *Neuromuscul Disord* 1991;1:19-29.
3. Sussman M: Duchenne muscular dystrophy. *J Am Acad Orthop Surg* 2002;10(2):138-151.
4. Birnkrant DJ, Bushby K, Bann CM, et al, for the DMD Care Considerations Working Group: Diagnosis and management of Duchenne muscular dystrophy, part 2: Respiratory, cardiac, bone health, and orthopaedic management. *Review Lancet Neurol* 2018;17:251-267.
5. Birnkrant DJ, Bushby K, Bann CM, et al; DMD Care Considerations Working Group: Diagnosis and management of Duchenne muscular dystrophy, part 1: Diagnosis, and neuromuscular, rehabilitation, endocrine, and gastrointestinal and nutritional management. *Lancet Neurol* 2018;17(3):251-267.
6. Apkon SD, Alman B, Birnkrant DJ, et al: Orthopedic and surgical management of the patient with Duchenne muscular dystrophy. *Pediatrics* 2018;142(suppl 2):S82-S89.
7. Chu ML, Moran E: The limb-girdle muscular dystrophies: Is treatment on the horizon? *Neurotherapeutics* 2018;15(4):849-862.
8. Hamel J, Tawil R: Facioscapulohumeral muscular dystrophy: Update on pathogenesis and future treatments. *Neurotherapeutics* 2018;15(4):863-871.
9. Mercuri E, Muntoni F: Muscular dystrophies. *Lancet* 2013;381(9869): 845-860.

©Copyright 2021 American Academy of Orthopaedic Surgeons

10. Hehir MK, Silvestri NJ: Generalized myasthenia gravis: Classification, clinical presentation, natural history, and epidemiology. *Neurol Clin* 2018;36(2):253-260.
11. Gilhus NE, Verschuuren JJ: Myasthenia gravis: Subgroup classification and therapeutic strategies. *Lancet Neurol* 2015;14(10):1023-1036.
12. Vincent A, Palace J, Hilton-Jones D: Myasthenia gravis. *Lancet* 2001;357(9274):2122-2128.
13. Riedel RF, Burfeind WR Jr: Thymoma: Benign appearance, malignant potential. *Oncologist* 2006;11(8):887-894.
14. Kolb SJ, Kissel JT: Spinal muscular atrophy. *Neurol Clin* 2015;33(4):831-846.
15. Lunn MR, Wang CH: Spinal muscular atrophy. *Lancet* 2008;371(9630):2120-2133.
16. Mercuri E, Finkel RS, Muntoni F, et al: Diagnosis and management of spinal muscular atrophy. Part 1: Recommendations for diagnosis, rehabilitation, orthopedic and nutritional care. *Neuromuscul Disord* 2018;28(2):103-115.
17. Vitale MG, Matsumoto H, Mueller JD, et al: Improvement of pulmonary function measured by patient-reported outcomes in patients with spinal muscular atrophy after VEPTR surgery. *Spine Deformity* 2016;4(6):459.
18. Mesfin A, Sponseller PD, Leet AI: Spinal muscular atrophy: Manifestations and management. *J Am Acad Orthop Surg* 2012;20(6):393-401.
19. Zaffran M, McGovern M, Hossaini R, Martin R, Wenger J: The polio endgame: Securing a world free of all polioviruses. *Lancet* 2018;391(10115):11-13.
20. Gonzalez H, Olsson T, Borg K: Management of postpolio syndrome. *Lancet Neurol* 2010;9(6):634-642.
21. Sheth NP, Keenan MA: Orthopedic surgery considerations in post-polio syndrome. *Am J Orthop (Belle Mead NJ)* 2007;36(7):348-353.
22. Centers for Disease Control and Prevention: Notes from the field: Acute flaccid myelitis among persons aged ≤21 years- United States, August 1–November 13, 2014. *MMWR Morb Mortal Wkly Rep* 2015;63:1243-1244.
23. Messacar K, Asturias EJ, Hixon AM, et al: Enterovirus D68 and acute flaccid myelitis-evaluating the evidence for causality. *Lancet Infect Dis* 2018;18(8):e239-e247.
24. Alshekhlee A, Hussain Z, Sultan B, Katirji B: Guillain-Barré syndrome: Incidence and mortality rates in US hospitals. *Neurology* 2008;70(18):1608-1613.
25. van den Berg B, Walgaard C, Drenthen J, Fokke C, Jacobs BC, van Doorn PA: Guillain-Barré syndrome: Pathogenesis, diagnosis, treatment and prognosis. *Nat Rev Neurol* 2014;10(8):469-482.
26. Willison HJ, Jacobs BC, van Doorn PA: Guillain-Barré syndrome. *Lancet* 2016;388(10045):717-727.
27. Goodfellow JA, Willison HJ: Guillain-Barré syndrome: A century of progress. *Nat Rev Neurol* 2016;12(12):723-731.
28. Chen EY, Stratton C, Mercer B, Hohler A, Tannoury TY, Tannoury C: Guillain-Barré syndrome after elective spinal surgery. 2017;25(8):587-593.
29. Barreto LC, Oliveira FS, Nunes PS, et al: Epidemiologic study of Charcot-Marie-Tooth disease: A systematic review. *Neuroepidemiology* 2016;46:157-165.
30. Pareyson D, Marchesi C: Diagnosis, natural history, and management of Charcot-Marie-Tooth disease. *Lancet Neurol* 2009;8(7):654-667.
31. Faldini C, Traina F, Nanni M, et al: Surgical treatment of cavus foot in Charcot-Marie-Tooth disease: A review of twenty-four cases: AAOS exhibit selection. *J Bone Joint Surg Am* 2015;97(6):e30.
32. Georgiadis AG, Spiegel DA, Baldwin KD: The Cavovarus foot in Hereditary motor and sensory neuropathies. *JBJS Rev* 2015;3(12). pii:01874474-201512000-00003. doi:10.2106/JBJS.RVW.O.00024.
33. Stavsky M, Mor O, Mastrolia SA, Greenbaum S, Than NG, Erez O: Cerebral palsy—trends in epidemiology and recent development in prenatal mechanisms of disease, treatment, and prevention. *Front Pediatr* 2017;5:21.
34. Rosenbaum P, Paneth N, Leviton A, et al: A report: The definition and classification of cerebral palsy April 2006. *Med Child Neurol* 2007;49(suppl 109):8-14.
35. Panteh N, Hong T, Korzeniewski S: The descriptive epidemiology of cerebral palsy *Clin Perinatol* 2006;33:251-267.
36. Bax M, Tydeman C, Flodmark O: Clinical and MRI correlates of cerebral palsy: The European Cerebral Palsy Study. *J Am Med Assoc* 2006;296(13):1602-1608.
37. Givon U: Gait research in cerebral palsy: Should we zoom in or zoom out? *Dev Med Child Neurol* 2018;60(8):738-739. doi:10.1111/dmcn.13742.
38. Watt JM, Robertson CM, Grace MG: Early prognosis for ambulation of neonatal intensive care survivors with cerebral palsy. *Dev Med Child Neurol* 1989;31(6):766-773.
39. da Paz Ju´nior AC, Burnett SM, Braga LW: Walking prognosis in cerebral palsy: A 22-year retrospective analysis. *Dev Med Child Neurol* 1994;36(2):130-134.
40. Palisano R, Rosenbaum P, Walter S, Russell D, Wood E, Galuppi B: Development and reliability of a system to classify gross motor function in children with cerebral palsy. *Dev Med Child Neurol* 1997;39(4):214-223.
41. Davids JR: Management of neuromuscular hip dysplasia in children with cerebral palsy: Lessons and challenges. *J Pediatr Orthop* 2018;38(suppl 1):S21-S27.
42. Georgiadis AG, Schwartz MH, Walt K, Ward ME, Kim PD, Novacheck TF: Team approach: Single-event multilevel surgery in ambulatory patients with cerebral palsy. *JBJS Rev* 2017;5(8):e10.
43. Pamphlett R: Early terminal and nodal sprouting of motor axons after botulinum toxin. 1989;92(2-3):181-192.
44. Winterton MT, Baldwin KD: The neuro-orthopaedic approach. *Phys Med Rehabil Clin N Am* 2018;29(3):567-591.
45. Chan G, Miller F: Assessment and treatment of children with cerebral palsy. *Orthop Clin North Am* 2014;45(3):313-325. doi:10.1016/j.ocl.2014.03.003.
46. Dilokthornsakul P, Valuck RJ, Nair KV, Corboy JR, Allen RR, Campbell JD: Multiple sclerosis prevalence in the United States commercially insured population. *Neurology* 2016;86(11):1014-1021.
47. Thompson AJ, Baranzini SE, Geurts J, Hemmer B, Ciccarelli O: Multiple sclerosis. *Lancet* 2018;391(10130):1622-1636.
48. Pidgeon TS, Borenstein T, Daniels Alan H, Murali J, Hayda RA: Understanding multiple sclerosis: Essentials for the orthopaedic surgeon. *JBJS Rev* 2014;2(7):1-9.
49. Bhatt P, Bray L, Raju S, et al: Temporal trends of pediatric hospitalizations with acute disseminated encephalomyelitis in the United States: An analysis from 2006 to 2014 using National Inpatient Sample. *J Pediatr* 2019;206:26-32.e1.
50. Pohl D, Alper G, Van Haren K, et al: Acute disseminated encephalomyelitis: Updates on an inflammatory CNS syndrome. *Neurology* 2016;87(9 suppl 2):S38-S45.
51. Young NP, Weinshenker BG, Lucchinetti CF: Acute disseminated encephalomyelitis: Current understanding and controversies. *Semin Neurol* 2008;28(1):84-94.
52. West TW: Transverse myelitis–a review of the presentation, diagnosis, and initial management. *Discov Med* 2013;16(88):167-177.
53. Absoud M, Greenberg BM, Lim M, Lotze T, Thomas T, Deiva K: Pediatric transverse myelitis. *Neurology* 2016;87(9 suppl 2):S46-S52.
54. Beh SC, Greenberg BM, Frohman T, Frohman EM: Transverse myelitis. *Neurol Clin* 2013;31(1):79-138.
55. Mozaffarian D, Benjamin EJ, Go AS, et al; American Heart Association Statistics Committee and Stroke Statistics Subcommittee: Heart disease and stroke statistics-2016 update: A report from the American Heart Association [published correction appears in Circulation. 2016;133(15):e599]. *Circulation* 2016;133(4):e38-e360.
56. Broderick J, Brott T, Kothari R, et al: The Greater Cincinnati/Northern Kentucky Stroke Study: Preliminary first-ever and total incidence rates of stroke among blacks. *Stroke* 1998;29:415-421.
57. Ekker MS, Boot EM, Singhal AB, et al: Epidemiology, etiology, and management of ischemic stroke in young adults. *Lancet Neurol* 2018;17(9):790-801.

©Copyright 2021 American Academy of Orthopaedic Surgeons

58. Fields JD, Khatri P, Nesbit GM, et al: Meta-analysis of randomized intra-arterial thrombolytic trials for the treatment of acute stroke due to middle cerebral artery occlusion. *J Neurointerv Surg* 2011;3(2):151-155.
59. Taylor CA, Bell JM, Breiding MJ, Xu L: Traumatic brain injury-related emergency department visits, hospitalizations, and deaths - United States, 2007 and 2013. *MMWR Surveill Summ* 2017;66(9):1-16.
60. Faul M, Xu L, Wald MM, Coronado V, Dellinger AM: Traumatic brain injury in the United States: National estimates of prevalence and incidence, 2002-2006. *Inj Prev* 2010;16:A268.
61. National Database: 2018 Profile of People within the Traumatic Brain Injury Model Systems.
62. Ranganathan K, Loder S, Agarwal S, et al: Heterotopic ossification: Basic-science principles and clinical correlates. *J Bone Joint Surg Am* 2015;97(13):1101-1111.
63. White N-H: *Spinal Cord Injury Facts and Figures at a Glance.* National Spinal Cord Injury Statistical Center. Birmingham, Alabama, 2018.
64. Roberts TT, Leonard GR, Cepela DJ: Classifications in brief: American Spinal Injury Association (ASIA) impairment scale. *Clin Orthop Relat Res* 2017;475(5):1499-1504.
65. Schouten R, Albert T, Kwon BK: The spine-injured patient: Initial assessment and emergency treatment. *J Am Acad Orthop Surg* 2012;20(6):336-346. doi:10.5435/JAAOS-20-06-336.
66. Haller J, Bice M, Lawrence B: Mediating the secondary effects of spinal cord injury through optimization of key physiologic parameters. *J Am Acad Orthop Surg* 2016;24(3):160-171.
67. Cruz MP: Edaravone (Radicava): A novel neuroprotective agent for the treatment of amyotrophic lateral sclerosis. *P & T* 2018;43(1):25-28.
68. Mehta P, Kaye W, Raymond J, et al: Prevalence of amyotrophic lateral sclerosis — United States, 2014. *MMWR Morb Mortal Wkly Rep* 2018;67:216-218.
69. Renton AE, Chio A, Traynor BJ: State of play in amyotrophic lateral sclerosis genetics. *Nat Neurosci* 2014;17:17-23.
70. Hardiman O, Al-Chalabi A, Chio A, et al: Amyotrophic lateral sclerosis. *Nat Rev Dis Primers* 2017;3:17071.
71. Van Es MA, Hardiman O, Chio A, et al: Amyotrophic lateral sclerosis. *Lancet* 2017;390(10107):2084-2098.
72. Dharmadasa T, Kiernan MC: Riluzole, disease stage and survival in ALS. *Lancet Neurol* 2018;17(5):385-386. doi:10.1016/S1474-4422(18)30091-7.
73. Marras C, Beck JC, Bower JH, et al: Prevalence of Parkinson's disease across North America. *NPJ Parkinsons Dis* 2018;4:21.
74. Kalia LV, Lang AE: Parkinson's disease. *Lancet* 2015;386(9996):896-912. doi:10.1016/S0140-6736(14)61393-3.
75. Baker JF, McClelland S III, Hart RA, Bess RS: Management of spinal conditions in patients with Parkinson disease. *J Am Acad Orthop Surg* 2017;25(8):e157-e165.
76. Zuckerman LM: Parkinson's disease and the orthopaedic patient. *J Am Acad Orthop Surg* 2009;17(1):48-55.
77. De Michele G, Filla A: Movement disorders: Friedreich ataxia today—preparing for the final battle. *Nat Rev Neurol* 2015;11(4):188-190.
78. Tsirikos AI, Smith G: Scoliosis in patients with Friedreich's ataxia. *J Bone Joint Surg Br* 2012;94(5):684-689.
79. Bürk K: Friedreich ataxia: Current status and future prospects. *Cerebellum Ataxias* 2017;4:4.

©Copyright 2021 American Academy of Orthopaedic Surgeons

30

Lumbar Spondylosis, Degenerative Disk Disease, and Radiculopathy

Brad A. Webb, DO
Jeffrey S. Fischgrund, MD
Jad G. Khalil, MD

Keywords: *intervertebral disk degeneration; lumbar facet joint osteoarthritis; spinal nerve compression*

INTRODUCTION

Low back pain (LBP) is a complicated disorder and is a leading cause of disability worldwide. The causes of LBP include an extensive differential diagnoses, of which degenerative changes within the lumbar bony anatomy and intervertebral disks play a significant role. Lumbar spine spondylosis can be an associated cause of LBP and is a common condition with an estimated prevalence ranging from 40% to 85%.[1] Lumbar spondylosis is due to a degenerative cascade that has an association with intervertebral disk degeneration (IDD) (**Figure 1**). Mechanical progression and associated disk space narrowing leads to adjacent level pedicle approximation with narrowing of the superior-inferior dimensions of the intervertebral foraminal canal. Laxity of the associated ligaments and vertebral column translate into altered loading mechanics and an altered pressure relationship on the vertebral bone and joint surfaces, which is believed to influence both osteophyte formation and facet joint hypertrophy.[2] IDD is a complicated multifactorial process characterized by altered biomechanics of loading, an imbalance of extracellular matrix synthesis and degradation, increased secretion of proinflammatory cytokines, and increased apoptosis and senescence in the nucleus pulposus (NP) cells.[3,4] These altered biomechanics lead to further degenerative changes and osteophyte formation. This has the potential to cause lumbar central and foraminal stenosis leading to symptomatic nerve compression and radiculopathy.

LUMBAR DEGENERATIVE DISK

The human spine possesses 23 intervertebral disks that separate the vertebrae and provide flexibility. They account for about 20% to 30% of the length of the spine and increase in size from the cervical to the lumbar regions.[5] The disk contains two regions, a more central region—the gelatinous NP, which is surrounded by a fibrous ring, the anulus fibrosus (AF) (**Figure 2**). Each vertebral body has cartilage end plates,

---

Dr. Webb or an immediate family member has received nonincome support (such as equipment or services), commercially derived honoraria, or other non-research-related funding (such as paid travel) from DePuy, A Johnson & Johnson Company and Stryker. Dr. Fischgrund or an immediate family member serves as a paid consultant to or is an employee of FzioMed, Relievant, and Stryker; has stock or stock options held in Understand.com; has received research or institutional support from Smith & Nephew and Stryker; and serves as a board member, owner, officer, or committee member of the Cervical Spine Research Society, and the Lumbar Spine Research Society. Dr. Khalil or an immediate family member is a member of a speakers' bureau or has made paid presentations on behalf of Johnson & Johnson, Spinewave, and Stryker; serves as a paid consultant to or is an employee of Camber Spine, Innovasis, Johnson & Johnson, and Stryker; has stock or stock options held in Johnson & Johnson, and Medtronic; has received research or institutional support from Centinel Spine, Innovative surgical designs, Johnson & Johnson, Limiflex, Medtronic, and Relievant; and serves as a board member, owner, officer, or committee member of the American Academy of Orthopaedic Surgeons.

©Copyright 2021 American Academy of Orthopaedic Surgeons

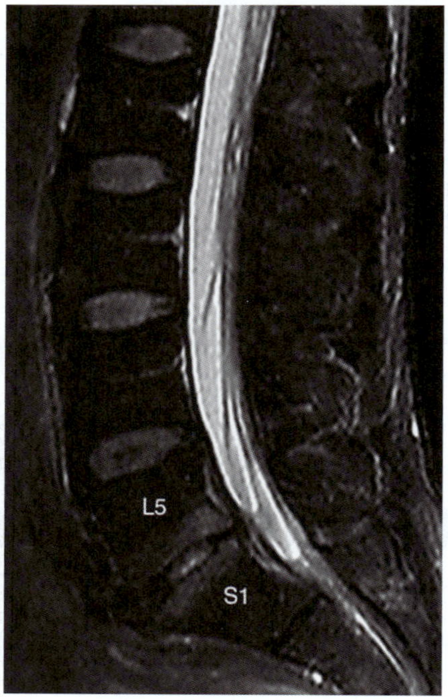

FIGURE 1 Lumbar sagittal T2-weighted MRI demonstrating lumbar degenerative disk and end plate (Modic) changes at the L5-S1 interspace. (Reproduced with permission from Madigan L, Vaccaro AR, Spector LR, Milam AR: Management of symptomatic lumbar degenerative disk disease. *J Am Acad Orthop Surg* 2009;17[2]:102-111.)

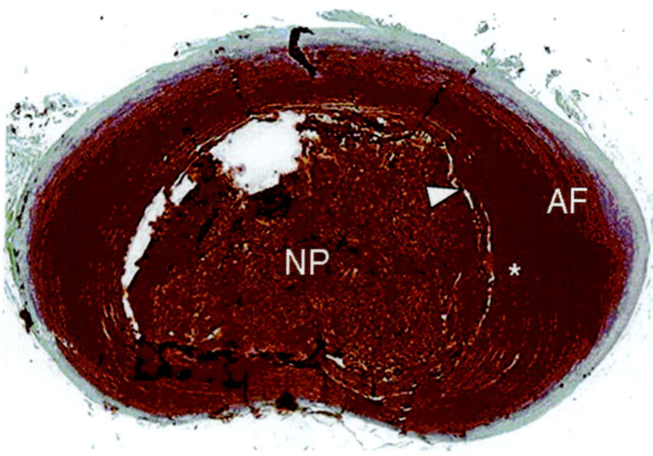

FIGURE 2 Photomicrograph of a rabbit intervertebral disk showing the four regions of the disk: outer anulus fibrosus (AF), inner AF (*), transition zone (arrowhead), and nucleus pulposus (NP). (Reproduced with permission from Kepler CK, Anderson GD, Tannoury C, Ponnappan RK: Intervertebral disk degeneration and emerging biologic treatments. *J Am Acad Orthop Surg* 2011;19[9]:543-553 and Originally adapted with permission from Walker MH, Anderson DG: Molecular basis of intervertebral disc degeneration. *Spine J* 2004;4[6 suppl]:158S-166S.)

which are a thin layer of hyaline cartilage tissue that separate the adjacent vertebrae. The composition of the two intervertebral disk regions differs in their cellular types. The NP consists mainly of a high concentration of proteoglycans and water, which are surrounded by a loose type II collagen network. In the NP, the collagen fibrils assume a random orientation and are interspersed in the matrix, which is rich in proteoglycans and water; this is an ideal organization for resisting compressive forces induced with axial loading of the spine.[5,6] The AF has a low proteoglycan and water content and a high concentration of type I collagens as well as a small concentration of type II collagens, organized into concentric lamellae.[5,6] The AF is described as possessing 20 to 25 lamellae, which are rich in collagen fibrils arranged in a parallel fashion (**Figure 3**). In each adjacent lamella, the collagen fibrils along the axis are fashioned in the opposite direction as to create an alternating pattern between the lamellae. This arrangement is best suited for resisting the tensile forces seen in both bending and twisting of the spine.[7] There are also a set of cells within the disk that help maintain the homeostasis by producing and maintaining proteoglycans, collagen, and matrix cells.

The composition of the intervertebral disk varies not only by location, but also with age. The content of water and the proteoglycan concentration within the disk increases when progressing from the AF to the NP. In contrast, the content of collagen within the disk decreases from the outer anulus to the nucleus. With increasing age the proteoglycan and water content of the nucleus decrease. In relation to the level of the spine, the composition of the disk will also vary, with the collagen content of the nucleus being the highest in the cervical disks and lowest in the lumbar disks. There is an opposite trend when evaluating the proteoglycan content.[8,9]

DISK MATRIX AND CELLULAR CHANGES

The extracellular matrix of the NP contains a high concentration of proteoglycans, with aggrecan the most abundant. In a mature disk, aggrecan possesses both chondroitin sulfate and keratin sulfate chains bound to the same core protein. The synthesized aggrecan interacts with hyaluronan to form the proteoglycan aggregates.[10] In healthy disks, the proteoglycans produce a negative charge, which generates an osmotic potential; this potential is converted into biomechanical hydrostatic pressure through the attraction of water.[11] The water content of the disk is dependent on both the concentration of proteoglycan and collagen contents. Proteoglycans provide the swelling pressure required to increase the water content and the collagen providing the resistance to swelling.[11,12] The functional ability related to the proteoglycan and collagen content has been shown to decline with age. Other proteoglycan aggregate components, such as hyaluronan and matrix proteins, also display concentration and structural changes with age. Hyaluronan is found throughout the disk and its concentration increases with age, but the exact mechanism for the resultant accumulation is not entirely understood.[13] Link

©Copyright 2021 American Academy of Orthopaedic Surgeons

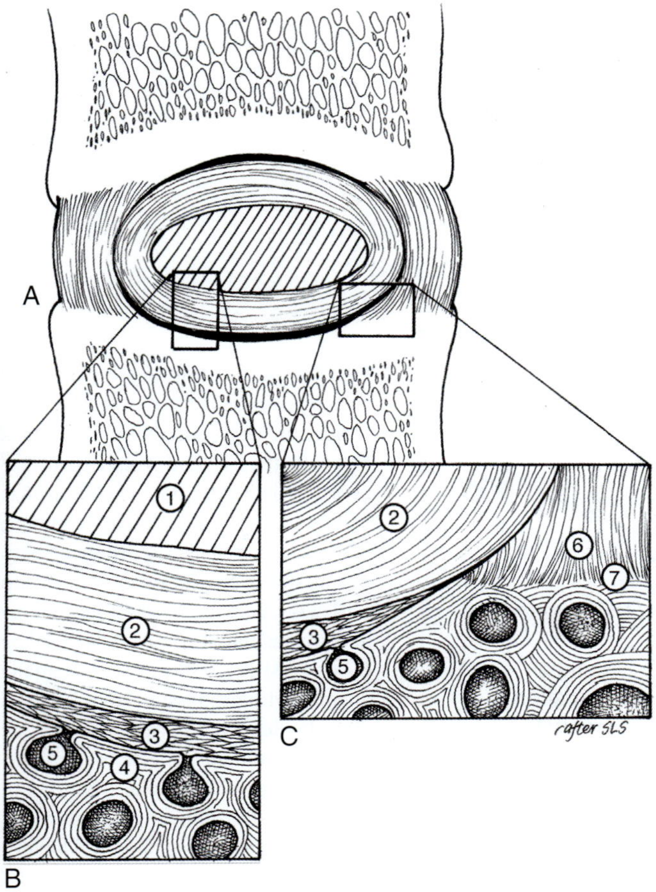

FIGURE 3 Illustrations demonstrating the arrangement of the fibrocartilaginous fibers of the anulus fibrosus. **A**, Fibers are arranged in a concentric lamellar fashion. **B**, Magnified view of the central part of the disk. 1 = Nucleus pulposus, 2 = anulus fibrosus, 3 = horizontal disposition of the collagen fibers of the cartilaginous end plate, 4 = bony end plate, 5 = vascular channel in direct contact with the cartilaginous end plate. **C**, Fiber arrangement of the peripheral part of the disk. 6 = Outer fibers of the anulus fibrosus, 7 = anchoring of the fibers to the bony end plate (Sharpey-type fibers). (Reproduced with permission from Biyani A, Andersson GBJ: Low back pain: Pathophysiology and management. *J Am Acad Orthop Surg* 2004;12(2):106-115 and Originally adapted with permission from Dupuis PR: The anatomy of the lumbosacral spine, in Kirkaldy-Willis WH, Burton CV, eds: *Managing Low Back Pain*, ed 3. New York, NY, Churchill Livingstone, 1992, pp 10-27.)

proteins are also present throughout the disk, but it is found that their concentration decreases with age in contrast to that of hyaluronan. Along with this, the proteolytic process of the link proteins increases with aging and degeneration.[14]

Further evaluation of the population of matrix proteins contains a group of both fibrous and cartilaginous connective tissue proteins whose function is similar as found in other sites outside of the vertebral disks. Two main proteins of note are fibronectin and elastin. Little has been reported on the exact function or cause from the degradation of these two proteins. It has been determined that fibronectin increases as we age and will exhibit an increase in degradation fragmentation, with these fragments thought to cause an increase in the catabolic events of disk degeneration.[15] Elastin is found in the elastic fibers within the intervertebral disk. Elastin constitutes only about 2% of the dry weight of the anulus; however, it contributes greatly to the overall functioning of the normal healthy disk. The orientation and structure have been evaluated, but it is not clear how degradation of the intervertebral disk influences the structure and function of elastin as well as the overall affect elastin has on the degeneration process of the disk.[16]

Intervertebral disks are believed to undergo a degenerative cascade, which is proposed to initiate with the introduction of proinflammatory mediators, degenerative enzymes, and a decrease in nutritional support, with genetic and biomechanical influences. This leads to the development of painful tears of the outer disk anulus with end plate separation, leading to a potential compromise in disk nutrition and waste removal. Small annular tears coalesce to form larger radial tears that potentiate disk protrusion and impact the ability of the intervertebral disk to maintain water, leading to subsequent disk desiccation and reduced disk height.[17] The loss of disk height leads to mechanical integrity loss, which potentiates progressive disk changes in resorption, and internal disruption.[18]

Intervertebral disk degeneration results from degradation of matrix macromolecules leading to early features of proteoglycan loss in the regulation of disk hydration and load-bearing properties. Proteoglycan biochemistry, which helps to determine disk osmolarity and hyaluronan content and support proteoglycan aggregation, is important to normal disk function.[19]

Within the degenerating intervertebral disk, there is a progressive increase in the expression of inflammatory cytokines like interleukin-1 (IL-1) and tumor necrosis factor-α (TNF-α).[20,21] It has been shown that TNF-α induces multiple cellular responses in relation to the proinflammatory cascade, which includes the decrease expression of both aggrecan and type II collagen genes. This leads to a decreased accumulation and overall synthesis of aggrecan and collagen, with an increased expression of MMPs and ADAMTS (A Disintegrin and Metalloproteinase with Thrombospondin Motifs) enzymes. Together these cellular responses lead to a loss of extracellular matrix and proteoglycan content within the NP.[4]

It has been evaluated that proteolysis is considered a major component of the degenerative processes that takes place in the disk. It has been proposed that matrix metalloproteinases (MMPs) play a significant role in the extracellular matrix degeneration, and an imbalance between their activation and inhibition leads to a probable cause of disk degeneration.[22] The family of MMPs account for much of the degradation of collagen, aggrecan, and link proteins. The ADAMTS family of metalloproteinases, particularly ADAMTS-4 and ADAMTS-5, has a high affinity for aggrecan and are considered aggrecanases[23,24] (**Figure 4**).

©Copyright 2021 American Academy of Orthopaedic Surgeons

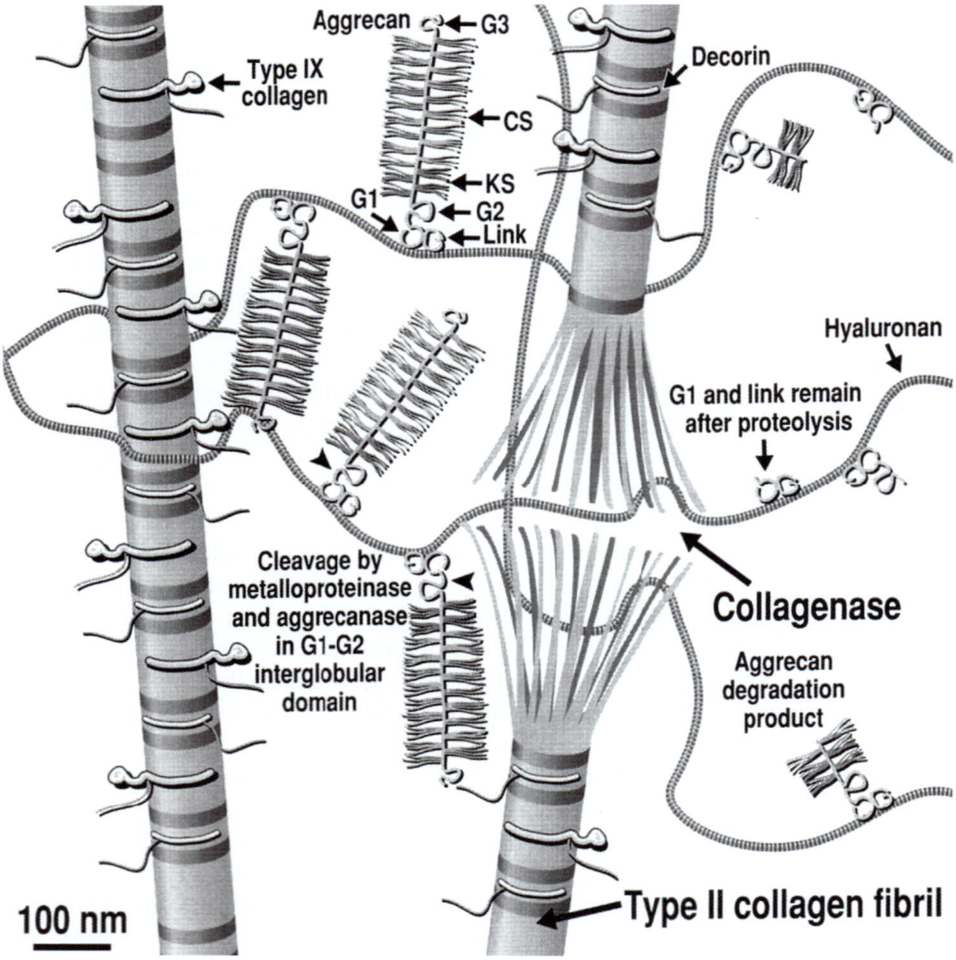

FIGURE 4 Illustration showing the structure of collagen and the proteoglycan aggrecan. Sites of attack by collagenase and other proteinases (arrowheads). CS = chondroitin sulfate, G1-G3 = globular domains, KS = keratin sulfate. (Reproduced with permission from Biyani A, Andersson GBJ: Low back pain: Pathophysiology and management. *J Am Acad Orthop Surg* 2004;12[2]:106-115. Originally adapted with permission from Recklies AD, Poole AR, Banerjee S, et al: Pathophysiologic aspects of inflammation in diarthrodial joints, in Buckwalter JA, Einhorn TA, Simon SR, eds: *Orthopaedic Basic Science: Biology and Biomechanics of the Musculoskeletal System*, ed 2. Rosemont, IL, American Academy of Orthopaedic Surgeons, 2000, pp 489-530.)

ETIOLOGY OF INTERVERTEBRAL DISK DEGENERATION

A factor that leads to the progression of disk degeneration is the decrease in nutrient supply, which leads to the loss of cell viability and failure to synthesize macromolecules.[25] The supply of nutrients is mainly provided by the blood vessels at the disk-end plate interface where the blood vessels penetrate the subchondral space at the level of the vertebral end plate. The nutrients diffuse from the blood vessels, through the cartilaginous end plate and the extracellular matrix of the adjoining disk to provide nutrition to the associated cells.[25,26] Declining nutritional transport appears to be a critical event responsible for the changes of the NP cellular matrix. As an intervertebral disk undergoes disk degeneration, the blood supply to the periphery of the disk declines. This leads to a decrease in waste product removal and accumulation of degraded matrix macromolecules, which in turn decreases water content within the central disk[27,28] (**Table 1**).

Abnormal mechanical loads are also thought to provide a pathway to disk degeneration. There have been some evaluations of biomechanical and loading forces that influence intervertebral disk cell and matrix vitality. Studies have shown that intervertebral disks which under go prolonged underloading, overloading, or static loading forces are more susceptible to unfavorable matrix changes and disk degeneration.[29-31]

Several studies suggest that the factors that lead to disk degeneration may have important genetic components. Several studies suggest that factors contributing to disk degeneration may have important genetic components.[32] Aggrecan can be more susceptible to disk degeneration as a result of changes to its functional composition, particularly the chondroitin sulfate content. It has been postulated that gene polymorphism within the aggrecan gene, specifically short alleles for chondroitin sulfate, contributes to early disk degeneration.[33]

LUMBAR SPONDYLOSIS

Osteoarthritis is the outcome of a disease process that results in structural and functional failure of synovial joints. This process has been characterized by damage to articular cartilage, subchondral bone alterations, synovial inflammatory response, and an overgrowth of bone and cartilage.[34] In the spine, both the presence of intervertebral disk degeneration

©Copyright 2021 American Academy of Orthopaedic Surgeons

TABLE 1 Pathophysiology of Intervertebral Disk Aging and Degeneration

Process	Effects
Diminished cellular responses	Senescence (alteration in gene expression and transcription factors) Apoptosis (programmed cell death)
Biochemical processes	Imbalance between catabolic and anabolic activity: Posttranslational protein modification Increased collagen cross-linking through nonenzymatic glycation, lipid peroxidation Loss of proteoglycans Altered diffusion of nutrients Impaired assembly of newly synthesized molecules
End plate changes	Diminished vascularity and decreased porosity because of end plate calcification ↓ Elevated lactate levels and reduced pH ↓ Cell apoptosis ↓ Thinning or microfracture of the end plate ↓ Increased permeability and altered hydraulic property ↓ Nonuniform load transference and increased focal shear stresses ↓ Disk degeneration and annular damage

Reproduced with permission from Biyani A, Andersson GBJ: Low back pain: Pathophysiology and management. *J Am Acad Orthop Surg* 2004;12(2):106-115.

and osteophyte formation at the same vertebral level has been used to describe lumbar spine osteoarthritis, also known as spondylosis. Similar to other synovial joints, degenerative changes of the facet joints occur in the form of degeneration of joint cartilage, remodeling of subchondral bones, osteosclerosis, and bone spur formation. These changes are similar to those in other load-bearing joints. Alignment abnormalities cause dynamic loads to be unbalanced on the facet joints.[35]

FACET JOINT ARTHRITIS AND OSTEOPHYTE FORMATION

The facet joints of the posterior spine are true synovial joints, which are anatomically and functionally different than the fibrocartilaginous articulation of the intervertebral disk. The combination of these three anatomical structures (one disk and two facet joints) is termed the three-joint complex or spinal motion segment. The spine is a structure composed of multiple motion segments connected in series with the total motion being a combination of each individual segment.[35,36] The orientation of the facet joints varies by location and relates to the principal planes of motion and forces seen at each spinal level. Within the lumbar spine, the facet joints are inclined to a nearly vertical orientation. This sagittal orientation reduces rotation and the risk of forward displacement of the vertebral bodies on one another.[36] It is thought that joint alignment and load distributions are major factors in the development and progression of facet joint arthritis and spondylosis. Pathology of the facet joints accounts for 5% to 15% of chronic axial low back pain.[37] It is hypothesized that the pain arises from any component of the structure of the facet joint, including the fibrous capsule, synovial membrane, hyaline cartilage, or bone. The degeneration is thought to be a result of repetitive stresses and cumulative low-level trauma and degeneration. This can lead to inflammation causing the facet joints to develop an effusion and stretching of the joint capsule, further aggravating the inflammatory response.[38]

The loss of disk structure and biomechanical properties can lead to altered loading and alignment of the vertebral bodies, facet joints, spinal ligaments, and muscles. This can decrease the ability of the motion segments to absorb and distribute loads applied to them. Altering the biomechanical function of the spine and alignment of the facet joints may initiate or accelerate development of osteoarthritis of the facet joints and lumbar spine.[38,39] This combination associated with increased facet degeneration may induce subluxation and instability. Instability and associated altered disk mechanics leads to continued fibrosis and the formation of osteophytes.[39] However, the presence of facet joint osteoarthritis has been found to be present even in the absence of intervertebral disk degeneration.[40]

Early changes of facet joint osteoarthritis involve the articular cartilage, synovium, and the capsule with later changes involving the subchondral bone and bone capsule margins.[41] Early changes in the cartilage involve fibrillation and pitting that affects the cartilage surface, progressing to deeper fibrillation and fissuring, and eventually erosion down to subchondral bone. Clustering of the chondrocytes is seen in early cartilage lesions, with the presence of fibrocartilage suggesting attempts at cartilage repair.[42]

Studies evaluating osteophyte formation demonstrate that osteophyte lipping originates from the periosteum through the proliferation of articular cartilage by way of endochondral ossification.[43,44] Proposed mediators of the osteophyte formation are mesenchymal stem cells of the synovium or periosteum and associated synovial macrophages via growth factors and extracellular matrix molecules.[44] Osteophyte formation in the vertebral column has been shown to be a general indicator of age, but osteophytes have also been found in healthy joints.[45] However, there is a strong correlation between the presence of disk space narrowing and osteophyte formation.[34] During the lumbar degenerative cascade, the presence of anterior lumbar vertebral osteophytes were speculated to be toward the end of the cascade and is postulated the formation is to help stabilize and unstable spinal column.[46]

©Copyright 2021 American Academy of Orthopaedic Surgeons

PROINFLAMMATORY RESPONSE WITH VERTEBRAL OSTEOARTHRITIS

Chemical factors may play a role in radiculopathy caused by lumbar disk herniation.[41] Inflammatory cytokines produced from the cartilage, ventral capsule, and synovial tissue of the facet joints are linked to the advancement of osteoarthritis and generation of pain. TNF-α, interleukin-1β (IL-1β), and interleukin-6 (IL-6) can be found in the facet joint tissues in degenerative lumbar disorders.[44] IL-6 from the synovium and cartilage of the facet joints is elevated mainly in lumbar spinal canal stenosis and related degenerative conditions.[47] IL-1β is present in higher concentrations with lumbar spinal stenosis and degenerative changes compared with lumbar herniated disks.

This higher expression of IL-1β was found to have a higher association with leg pain and declining quality of life in lumbar degenerative patients when compared with other inflammatory cytokines.[48] IL-1β simulates the production of MMPs through activation signaling pathways (**Table 2**). Typically, IL-1β and MMPs are markedly increased in degenerative facets, leading to further proteoglycan degeneration and destruction of the cartilage and joint.[49]

The relationship of facet joint osteoarthritis with adiponectin, an adipocyte factor secreted from fat cells, has also been evaluated. Adiponectin has a multimeric (several protein chain subunits) structure and circulates in the blood as low-molecular-weight (LMW) and high-molecular-weight (HMW) complexes. HMW adiponectin has a proinflammatory response whereas the (LMW) isoform has an anti-inflammatory function.[50,51] Identified in different metabolic and cardiovascular diseases, adiponectin was found to interact with proinflammatory cytokines.[52] Adiponectin has the potential to be catabolic mediator of osteoarthritis by increasing several MMPs and inducible nitric oxide synthase (iNOS).[53] In one study, it was shown that adiponectin was identified in the process of facet joint osteoarthritis and was shown to have greater expression for facet joint osteoarthritis when compared with IL-1β and TNF-α.[52]

TABLE 2 Common Chemical Substances and Their Functions

Chemical Substance	Function
Phospholipase A_2	Mediates mechanical hyperalgesia
Nitric oxide	Inhibits mechanical hyperalgesia and produces thermal hyperalgesia
MMP-2 (gelatinase A) and MMP-9 (gelatinase)	Degrade gelatin (denatured fibrillar collagens) and other matrix molecules Act synergistically with MMP-1
MMP-1 (collagenase-1)	MMP-1 degrades collagen
MMP-3 (stromelysin-1)	Both MMP-1 and MMP-2 may play a role in spontaneous regression of the herniated disk
IL-1, TNF-α, prostaglandin E_2	Promote matrix degradation Enhance production of MMPs
CGRP, glutamate, substance P (neurotransmitters)	Modulate dorsal root ganglion responses
IL-6	Induces synthesis of TIMP-1
TIMP-1	Inhibits MMPs
TGF-β superfamily	Blocks synthesis of MMPs
IGF-I, PDGF	Have an antiapoptotic effect

CGRP = calcitonin gene–related peptide, IGF = insulinlike growth factor, IL = interleukin, MMP = matrix metalloproteinase, PDGF = platelet-derived growth factor, TGF = transforming growth factor, TIMP = tissue inhibitor of metalloproteinase

Reproduced with permission from Biyani A, Andersson GBJ: Low back pain: Pathophysiology and management. *J Am Acad Orthop Surg* 2004;12(2):106-115.

LUMBAR RADICULOPATHY

Compression of the nerve roots can be related to facet joint deformation and osteophyte formation. The consequences of nerve root injury and radiculopathy can be understood in terms of motor weakness and sensory abnormalities that can express as numbness, paresthesia, and burning pain. The prevalence of lumbar radiculopathy ranges from 2% to 43%.[54] The causes of radiculopathy can vary and include metabolic and vascular dysfunction due to a mechanical and chemical response. The inflammatory mediators from the ventral capsule of a degenerative facet joint in lumbar stenosis may be partially responsible for the neuropathic and radicular symptoms an individual would experience with degenerative spinal conditions.[48] In terms of spinal degenerative changes, mechanical compression of the nerve root can occur from disk herniations, thickened ligamentum flavum, osteoarthritic facet joints, and/or osteophyte formation. Nerve root compression can lead to diminished nerve conduction and blood supply to the nerve and may even lead to structural nerve damage.[55]

MECHANICAL COMPRESSION

The lumbosacral nerve roots are often involved in disease processes and injuries, including pathological conditions of the spine, that can lead to the creation of radiculopathy. Spinal nerve roots are more susceptible to compression than peripheral nerves. The dorsal root ganglia are highly sensitive to mechanical compression and hypoxia, resulting in the abnormal sensations and pain of radiculopathy.[56] Mechanical compression can also lead to a series of intraneural tissue reactions, including intraneural edema formation, demyelination, and fibrosis.[57,58] There have been several published studies, which have evaluated the series of events after experimentally

©Copyright 2021 American Academy of Orthopaedic Surgeons

applied nerve compression. They have described the physiologic and morphologic changes in connection with acute[59-61] and chronic[58,62] nerve root compression. Intraneural edema can be a consequence of increased vascular permeability initiated from nerve compression,[63] and vascular permeability is more pronounced for rapid, rather than the slow onset of compression.[64]

The associated intraneural edema and decreased microvascular flow affects the nutrition to the nerve root.[65] Following continued mechanical nerve root compression, the nerve fibers undergo marked demyelination as the process of Wallerian degeneration of the nerve root occurs from disruption of the axonal continuity.[58,66] Macrophages have been found in connection with removal of foreign material, similar to the macrophages within the spinal cord and nerve roots. Macrophages are seen in increased numbers in regions of the nerve root undergoing Wallerian degeneration and are thought to enter the nerve roots as a result of a breakdown of the blood-nerve barrier in acutely injured nerve roots.[66] Macrophages are labeled as the principal cells that initiate and potentiate inflammatory neuritis. Inflammatory mediators activated by macrophages are involved in the inflammatory process by enhancing vascular permeability, providing chemotactic signals, and modulating inflammatory cells.

BIOCHEMICAL AFFECTS OF RADICULOPATHY

The concept of chemical radiculitis is an inflammatory condition of the nerve root. Inflammation of the spinal nerve root may be initiated from cytokines found from the degenerative disk or from the facet joint arthritis. The cycle of inflammatory cell recruitment is partly directed by macrophages in respect to degeneration of nerves and production of cytokines.[67] The inflammatory physiologic state associated with neuropathy can include those induced by lowered pH, bradykinin, histamine, or prostaglandin release. Extrinsic factors can cause the inflammatory cascade responsible for radiculopathy. Thus, nerve root injury from either mechanical or chemical responses can give rise to an upregulation of proinflammatory cytokines such as TNF-α.[68] The upregulation of TNF-α has the ability to upregulate and work together with other cytokines such as IL-1β and IL-6.[67,69] This upregulation of proinflammatory cytokines occurs in dorsal root ganglion, Schwann cells, perineurial cells, and endothelial cells.[70,71] Clinical and experimental studies have shown that cartilage and synovial tissue of the facet joint contain inflammatory cytokines, which come into contact with a nerve root. Once in contact, pathologic changes can occur to the nerve tissue, and then neurologic deficits may be seen.[72,73] These findings suggest that the biochemical inflammatory factors such as IL-1B and MMPs released from a degenerative facet joint can induce radicular symptoms. There are significant expressions of both proinflammatory

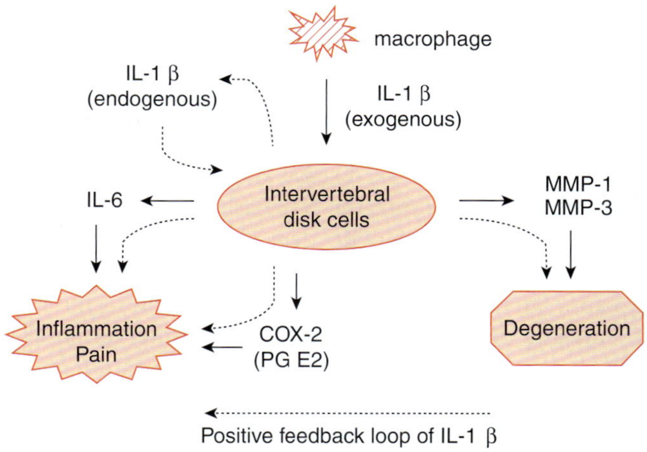

FIGURE 5 Schematic illustration of a positive feedback loop of interleukin (IL)-1β in intervertebral disk herniation (IDH) cells. Endogenous IL-1β was produced from the IDH cells in response to exogenous IL-1β, which affected the cells of IDH in a way similar to exogenous IL-1β. This positive feedback loop of IL-1β upregulated the production of IL-6, cyclooxygenase (COX)-2, and matrix metalloproteinase (MMP)-1 and MMP-3, resulting in inflammation, neurologic pain, and disk degeneration. PG E2 = prostaglandin E2. (Reproduced with permission from Kepler CK, Anderson GD, Tannoury C, Ponnappan RK: Intervertebral disk degeneration and emerging biologic treatments. *J Am Acad Orthop Surg* 2011;19[9]:543-553. Originally adapted with permission from Jimbo K, Park JS, Yokosuka K, Sato K, Nagata K: Positive feedback loop of interleukin-1beta upregulating production of inflammatory mediators in human intervertebral disc cells in vitro. *J Neurosurg Spine* 2005;2[5]:589-595.)

cytokines as well as MMPs from degenerative and herniated disk tissue[33,74] (**Figure 5**), and the relationships between the two interact in a way to modulate an environment, which escalates inflammation and nerve tissue changes.

SUMMARY

Lumbar spondylosis is predominantly a radiographic diagnosis that refers to the degenerative changes of the intervertebral disks, vertebral bodies, and paired zygapophysial facet joints of the lumbar spine. The etiology of lumbar spondylosis remains relatively unclear, but is characterized as osteoarthritis of the spine. It results from increased stresses, with repetitive microtrauma leading to an imbalance in the synthesis and degradation of cartilage, combined with an increased stress placed on the bones and ligaments leading to osteophyte formation. Some investigators believe the process of lumbar spondylosis is due partly to a proinflammatory degenerative cascade, thought to be initiated by intervertebral disk and

©Copyright 2021 American Academy of Orthopaedic Surgeons

facet degeneration. TNF-α is one of the main catalyzers of the proinflammatory cytokine response to lumbar spondylosis.

The most important physiological change of lumbar degenerative disk disease starts with the extracellular matrix within the NP. Early changes include the increased proteolytic degradation of aggrecan, coupled with an accumulation of degraded proteoglycans. This can further impair the diffusion of nutrients and oxygen throughout the disk. Intervertebral disk degeneration also results in disorganization and destruction of the collagen network. Increased levels of proinflammatory cytokines leads to an increase production of proteinases such as MMPs and ADAMTS families that lead to a breakdown of the intervertebral disk collagens. As disk hydration decreases, the disk height decreases with solidification of the NP. The combined effects of aging, unfavorable genetics, altered nutrition and metabolite transport, and excessive or repetitive loading all have been implicated in contributing to the process of intervertebral disk degeneration.

Lumbar radiculopathy is a complex disease, which involves multiple processes that cause nerve dysfunction such as ischemic, inflammatory, mechanical, and biochemical. Mechanical compression on the nerve roots and dorsal root ganglions can reduce blood flow and cause ischemic change. The ischemia further triggers increased nerve damage. The continued nerve damage induces the release of chemical factors and accentuates the inflammatory cascade. Chemical insults to the nerve are predominately induced by an inflammatory response that surrounds the spinal nerve roots and dorsal root ganglion. The inflammatory and pain response is accentuated by a subsequent increase in inflammatory mediators. It is important to recognize the role of cytokines such as TNF-α and MMPs in the role of neural inflammation and radicular pain. Furthermore, spinal nerve roots already sensitized to inflammatory mediators and now with associated mechanical compression and injury exacerbate the neural immune insult, causing macrophage-mediated degeneration with a further increase in TNF concentrations.

REFERENCES

1. Goode A, Carey T, Jordan J: Low back pain and lumbar spine osteoarthritis: How are they related? *Curr Rheumatol Rep* 2013;15(2):305.
2. Schneck CD: The anatomy of the lumbar spondylosis. *Clin Orthop Rlat Res* 1985;193:20-36.
3. Kim KW, Chung HN, Ha KY, Lee JS, Kim YY: Senescence mechanisms of nucleus pulposus chondrocytes in human intervertebral discs. *Spine J* 2009;9(8):658-666.
4. Sequin CA, Pilliar RN, Roughley PJ, Kandel RA: Tumor necrosis factor-alpha modulates matrix production and catabolism in nucleus pulposus tissue. *Spine* 2005;30(17):1940-1948.
5. Chan CW, Sze KL, Samartzis D, Leung YL, Chan D: Structure and biology of the intervertebral disk in health and disease. *Orthop Clin North Am* 2011;42:447-464.
6. Roberts S, Evans H, Trivedi J, Menage J: Histology and pathology of the human intervertebral disc. *J Bone Joint Surg Am* 2006;88(2):10-14.
7. Vergroesen P, Kingma I, Emanuel K, et al: Mechanics and biology in intervertebral disc degeneration: A vicious circle. *Osteo and Cartilage* 2015;23:1057-1070.
8. Buckwalter JA: Aging and degeneration of the human intervertebral disc. *Spine* 1995;20:1307-1314.
9. Boos N, Weissback S, Rohrhack H, Weiler C, Spratt K, Nerlich A: Classification of age-related changes in lumbar intervertebral discs. Volvo Award in basic science. *Spine* 2002;27:2631-2644.
10. Taylor J, Scott J, Cribb A, Bosworth T: Human intervertebral disc acid glycosaminoglycans. *J Anat* 1992;180:137-141.
11. Urban JP, McMullin JF: Swelling pressure of the lumbar intervertebral discs: Influence of age, spinal level, composition, and degeneration. *Spine* 1988;13(2):179-187.
12. Nachemson A: The load on lumbar disks in different positions of the body. *Clin Orthop Relat Res* 1966;45:107-122.
13. Scott J, Bosworth T, Cribb A, Taylor J: The chemical morphology of age-related changes in human intervertebral disc glycosaminoglycans from cervical, thoracic, and lumbar nucleus pulposus and annulus fibrosus. *J Anat* 1994;184:73-82.
14. Pearce R, Mathieson J, Mort J, Roughley P: Effect of age on the abundance and fragmentation of link proteins of the human intervertebral disc. *J Orthop Res* 1989;7:861-867.
15. Oegema T, Johnson S, Aguiar D, Ogilvie J: Fibronectin and its fragments increase with degeneration in the human intervertebral disc. *Spine* 2000;25:2742-2747.
16. Yu J: Elastic tissues of the intervertebral disc. *Biochem Soc Trans* 2002;30:848-852.
17. Choi Y: Pathophysiology of degenerative disc disease. *Asian Spine J* 2009;3(1):39-44.
18. Kirkaldy-Willis WH, Wedge JH, Yong-Hing K, et al: Pathology and pathogenesis of lumbar spondylosis and stenosis. *Spine* 1978;3:319-328.
19. Roughley PJ: Biology of intervertebral disc aging and degeneration: Involvement of the extracellular matrix. *Spine* 2004;29:2691-2699.
20. Purmessur D, Walter B, Roughley P, Laudier D, Hecht A, Iatridis J: A role for TNFα in intervertebral disc degeneration: A non-recoverable catabolic shift. *Biochem Biophys Res Commun* 2013;433(1):151-156.
21. Le Maitre C, Freemont A, Hoyland J: The role of interleukin-1 in the pathogenesis of human intervertebral disc degeneration. *Arthritis Res Ther* 2005;7(4):732-745.
22. Goupille P, Jayson M, Valat J, Freemont A: Matrix metalloproteinases: The clue to intervertebral disc degeneration? *Spine* 1998;23:1612-1626.
23. Roberts S, Caterson B, Menage J, Evans E, Jaffray D, Eisenstein S: Matrix metalloproteinases and aggrecanase: Their role in disorders of the human intervertebral disc. *Spine* 2000;25:3005-3013.
24. Tang B: Adamts: A novel family of extracellular matrix proteases. *Int J Biochem Cell Biol* 2001;33:33-44.
25. Maroudas a, Stockwell RA, Nachemson a, Urban J: Factors involved in the nutrition of the human lumbar intervertebral disc: Cellularity and diffusion of glucose in vitro. *J Anat* 1975;120:113-130.
26. Benneker LM, Heini PF, Alini M, Anderson SE, Ito K: 2004 Young Investigator Award Winner: Vertebral endplate marrow contact channel occlusions and intervertebral disc degeneration. *Spine* 2005;30:167-173.
27. Urban JP, Holm S, Maroudas A, Nachemson A: Nutrition of the intervertebral disk. An in vivo study of solute transport. *Clin Orthop Relat Res* 1977:101-114.
28. Boubriak Oa, Watson N, Sivan SS, Stubbens N, Urban JPG: Factors regulating viable cell density in the intervertebral disc: Blood supply in relation to disc height. *J Anat* 2013;222:341-348.

 ©Copyright 2021 American Academy of Orthopaedic Surgeons

29. Lotz J, Chin J: Intervertebral disc cell death is dependent on the magnitude and duration of spinal loading. *Spine* 2000;25:1477-1482.
30. MacLean J, Lee C, Grad S, Ito K, Alini M, Iatridis J: Effects of immobilization and dynamic compression on intervertebral disc cell gene expression in vivo. *Spine* 2003;28:973-981.
31. Walsh A, Lotz J: Biological response of the intervertebral disc to dynamic loading. *J Biomech* 2004;37:329-337.
32. Ala-Kokko L: Genetic risk factors for lumbar disc disease. *Ann Med* 2002;34:42-47.
33. Kawaguchi Y, Osada R, Kanamori M, et al: Association between an aggrecan gene polymorphism and lumbar disc degeneration. *Spine* 1999;24:2456-2460.
34. de Schepper El, Damen J, van Meurs J, et al: The association between lumbar disc degeneration and low back pain: The influence of age, gender, and individual radiographic features. *Spine* 2010;35(5):531-536.
35. Tischer T, Aktas T, Milz S, Putz R: Detailed pathological changes of human lumbar facet joints L1-L5 in elderly individuals. *Eur Spine J* 2005;15:308-315.
36. Adams M, Hutton W: The mechanical function of the lumbar apophyseal joints. *Spine* 1983;8:327-330.
37. Manchikanti L, Boswell M, Singh V, Pampati V, Damron K, Beyer C: Prevalence of facet joint pain in chronic spinal pain of cervical, thoracic, and lumbar regions. *BMC Musculoskelet Disord* 2004;5:15.
38. Yang K, King A: Mechanism of facet load transmission as a hypothesis for low back pain. *Spine* 1984;9:557-565.
39. Gellhorn A, Katz J, Pradeep S: Osteoarthritis of the spine: The facet joints. *Nat Rev Rheumatol* 2013;9(4):216-224.
40. Grobler L, Robertson P, Novotny J, Pope M: Etiology of spondylolisthesis. Assessment of the role played by the lumbar facet joint morphology. *Spine* 1993;18:80-91.
41. Eisenstein S, Parry C: The lumbar facet arthrosis syndrome. Clinical presentation and articular surface changes. *J Bone Joint Surg Br* 1987;69:3-7.
42. Menkes CJ, Lane NE: Are osteophytes good or bad? *Osteo Cartilage* 2004;12(suppl A):S53-S54.
43. Blom AB, Van Lent PL, holfhuysen AE, et al: Synovial lining macrophages mediate osteophyte formation during experimental osteoarthritis. *Osteo Cartilage* 2004;12(8):627-635.
44. Igarashi A, Kikuchi S, Konno S, Olmarker K: Inflammatory cytokines released from the facet joint tissue in degenerative lumbar spinal disorders. *Spine* 2004;29(19):2091-2095.
45. Klaassen Z, Tubbs R, Apaydin N, Hage R, Jordan R, Loukas M: Vertebral spinal osteophytes. *Anat Sci Int* 2011;86(1):1-9.
46. Pate D, Goobar J, Resnick D, Haghighi P, Sartoris D, Pathria M: Traction osteophytes of the lumbar spine: Radiographic-pathologic correlation. *Radiology* 1988;166:843-846.
47. Dionne C, Dunn K, Croft P, et al: A consensus approach toward the standardization of back pain definitions for use in prevalence studies. *Spine* 2008;33(1):95-103.
48. Igarashi A, Kikuchi S, Konno S: Correlation between inflammatory cytokines released from lumbar facet joint tissues and symptoms in degenerative lumbar spinal disorders. *J Orthop Sci* 2007;12:154-160.
49. Xu D, Sun Y, Bao G, et al: MMP-1 overexpression induced by IL-1β: Possible mechanism for inflammation in degenerative lumbar facet joint. *J Orthop Sci* 2013;18:1012-1019.
50. Song H, Chan J, Rovin B: Induction of chemokine expression by adiponectin in vitro is isoform dependent. *Transl Res* 2009;154:18-26.
51. Neumeier M, Weigert J, Schaffler A, et al: Different effects of adiponectin isoforms in human monocytic cells. *J Leukoc Biol* 2006;79:803-808.
52. Lai Q, Liu Y, Huang L et al: Expression of adiponectin in the subchondral bone of lumbar facet joints with different degrees of degeneration. *BMC Muscoskelet Disord* 2017;18:427-435.
53. Kang E, Lee Y, Kim T, et al: Adiponectin is a potential catabolic mediator in osteoarthritis cartilage. *Arthritis Res Ther* 2010;12(6):231-242.
54. Valat J, Genevay S, Marty M, Rozenberg S, Koes B: Sciatica. *Best Pract Res Clin Rheumatol* 2010;24(2):241-252.
55. Sommer C, Galbraith J, Heckman H, Myers R: Pathology of experimental compression neuropathy producing hyperesthesia. *J Neuropathol Exp Neurol* 1993;52(3):223-233.
56. Sugawara O, Atsuta Y, Iwahara T, Muramoto T, Watakabe M, Takemitsu Y: The effects of mechanical compression and hypoxia on nerve root and dorsal root ganglia. An analysis of ectopic firing using and in vitro model. *Spine* 1996;21(18):2089-2094.
57. Rydevik B, Brown M, Lundberg G: Pathoanatomy and pathophysiology of nerve root compression. *Spine* 1984;9:7-17.
58. Yoshizawa H, Kobayashi S, Morita T: Chronic nerve root compression: Pathophysiologic mechanism of nerve root dysfunction. *Spine* 1995;20:397-407.
59. Delamarter R, Bohlman H, Dodge L, Boro C: Experimental lumbar spinal stenosis; analysis of the cortical evoked potential, micro-vasculature, and histopathology. *J Bone Joint Surg Am* 1990;72:110-120.
60. Rydevik B, Pedowtiz R, Hargens A, Swenson M, Myers R, Garfin S: Effects of acute graded compression on spinal nerve root function and structure; an experimental study of the pig cauda equina. *Spine* 1991;16:487-493.
61. Sato K, Konno S, Yabuki S, Mao G, Olmarker K, Kikuchi S: A model for acute, chronic, and delayed graded compression of the dog cauda equina. Neurophysiologic and histologic changes induced by acute, graded compression. *Spine* 1995;20(22):2389-2391.
62. Iwamoto H, Kuwahaea H, Matsuda H, Noriage A, Yamano Y: Production of chronic compression of the cauda equina in rats for use in studies of lumbar spinal canal stenosis. *Spine* 1995;20:2750-2757.
63. Rydevik B, Lundborg G: Permeability of intraneural microvessels and perineurium following acute, graded experimental nerve compression. *Scand J Plast Reconstr Surg* 1977;11:179-187.
64. Olmarker K: Spinal nerve root compression. Nutrition and function of the porcine cauda equina compressed in vivo. *Acta Orthop Scand Suppl* 1991;242:1-27.
65. Myers R, Murakami H, Powell H: Reduced nerve blood flow in edematous neuropathies: A biomechanical mechanism. *Microvasc Res* 1986;32:145-151.
66. Kobayashi S, Yoshizawa H, Yamada S: Pathology of lumbar nerve root compression Part 1: Intraradicular inflammatory changes induced by mechanical compression. *Journal of Orthop Res* 2004;22:170-179.
67. Myers R, Rydevik B, Olmarker K, Kikucki S: Nerve root pain in disc herniation and spinal stenosis: A basic science review, in Garfin S, Eismont F, Bell G, Fischgrund J, Bono C, eds: *Rothman-Simeone and Herkowitz's The Spine*, ed 7. Philadelphia, PA, Elsevier-Saunders, 2018, pp 119-131.
68. Olmarker K, Larsson K: Tumor necrosis factor alpha and nucleus-pulposus-induced nerve root injury. *Spine* 1998;23:2538-2544.
69. McGee D, Bamberg T, Vitkus S, McGhee J: A synergistic relationship between TNF-alpha, IL-1 beta, and TGF-beta 1 on IL-6 secretion by the IEC-6 intestinal epithelial cell line. *Immunology* 1995;86:6-11.
70. Watts M, Arnold S, Chaplin D: Changes in coagulation and permeability properties of human endothelial cells in vitro induced by TNF-alpha or 5,6 MeXAA. *Br J Cancer* 1996;74(suppl 27):S164-S167.
71. Sorkin L, Xiao W, Wagner R, et al: Tumor necrosis factor-alpha induces ectopic activity in nociceptive primary afferent fibers. *Neuroscience* 1997;81:255-262.
72. Cohen S, Raja S: Pathogenesis, diagnosis, and treatment of lumbar zygapophysial (facet) joint pain. *Anesthesiology* 2007;106:591-614.
73. Ng L, Chaudhary N, Sell P: The efficacy of corticosteroids in periradicular infiltration for chronic radicular pain: A randomized, double-blind, controlled trail. *Spine* 2005;30:857-862.
74. Bachmeier B, Nerlich A, Mittermaier N, et al: Matrix metalloproteinase expression levels suggest distinct enzyme roles during lumbar disc herniation and degeneration. *Eur Spine J* 2009;18(11):1573-1586.

©Copyright 2021 American Academy of Orthopaedic Surgeons

4

REPAIR AND REGENERATION

SECTION EDITORS

Robert L. Sah, MD, ScD
Barbara D. Boyan, PhD

31

Fracture Repair

Hamish Simpson, BM, BCh, DM (Oxon), MA (Cantab), FRCS (Eng & Ed)
James Ryaby, PhD

Keywords: *fracture healing, fracture nonunion, osteoblast*

INTRODUCTION

The WHO recognized trauma as a major healthcare epidemic with over 16,000 people dying each day and injury accounting for 16% of the global burden of disease.[1] In the United States, approximately 60 million fractures occur each year.[2] People in low-income settings are far more likely to suffer complications from traumatic injury than those in high-income settings.[3] For every death linked to trauma there are many more injured, which causes considerable suffering. In addition, fractures often occur in patients of working age, and this can cause substantial economic hardship. Thus, fractures are one of the major causes of morbidity and create a significant drain on a country's resources.

Fragility fractures in the older population create an additional layer of morbidity as they result in sustained loss of independence, and many patients are fearful that they may never regain their independence. As a consequence of this, 80% of patients suffering a fracture have stated that they would rather die than sustain a hip fracture.[4]

There is therefore a pressing need to ensure that patients' fractures of all ages heal uneventfully in a timely manner. However, up to 9% of fractures fail to unite[5] and cause considerable additional hardship. To minimize the rate of nonunion, it is essential to understand the principles of fracture repair.

However, bone healing is a complex process involving the activation of thousands of genes and the release of multiple growth factors and cytokines coupled with the proliferation and differentiation of progenitor cells,[6] which all has to occur in a favorable mechanical environment.

FRACTURE PREVENTION AND REPAIR MECHANISMS

The skeleton is vital for a diverse range of mechanical activities essential for the existence of the human, such as respiration, mastication, locomotion, and protection of vital structures such as the brain; as well as biological functions such as calcium homeostasis and hematopoiesis. There are therefore a number of features of bone that maintain its integrity. These include both fracture prevention and fracture repair mechanisms. The basic processes that are relevant for fracture repair can be considered under the following categories:

1. Fracture prevention
2. Bone homeostasis
3. Bone maintenance
4. Wound healing

Dr. Simpson is a member of a speakers' bureau or has made paid presentations on behalf of Orthofix, Inc.; has received research or institutional support from Biocomposites, DePuy, A Johnson & Johnson Company, Orthofix, Inc., Smith & Nephew, and Stryker; and serves as a board member, owner, officer, or committee member of the British Orthopaedic Association, the British Orthopaedic Research Society, the Combined Service Orthopaedic Society, and the Orthopaedic Trauma Care Foundation Global Research Committee. Dr. Ryaby serves as a paid consultant to or is an employee of Orthofix, Inc.; has stock or stock options held in Orthofix, Inc.; and has received research or institutional support from Orthofix, Inc.

©Copyright 2021 American Academy of Orthopaedic Surgeons

FRACTURE PREVENTION

Materials such as glass are brittle materials. A small crack in one region can propagate across the structure resulting in failure. Composite materials such as fiberglass and carbon fiber have numerous boundaries within the structure that prevent a crack from propagating across the material. Bone has such a composite structure with the organic component (primarily collagen) and the mineral component (primarily calcium hydroxyapatite). However, cracks can occur in the composite structure and, although they will not propagate instantaneously, they can accumulate in the material, and if they are not removed (see bone maintenance below), they can eventually result in catastrophic failure.

BONE HOMEOSTASIS

It has long been recognized that bone adapts to the loads to which it is subjected. This was encapsulated in Wolff's Law[7] in 1892. The original title was the law of transformation of the bone in which Wolff described the relationship between bone geometry and the mechanical influences on bone. Subsequently, Harold Frost proposed an updated concept—he coined the term, *mechanostat* to encapsulate the homeostatic concept of bone suggesting that bone growth and bone loss were stimulated by the local mechanical elastic deformation of bone. If a local region of bone experienced too high a strain in response to an applied load, then bone formation would be stimulated. Conversely, if no strain was experienced in response to an applied load then bone resorption would occur (Frost HN[8]). It is now generally considered that microscopic fluid movement within the lacunar-canalicular system is the major physical stimulus that osteocytes within bone sense.[9,10]

In a landmark paper by Rubin and Lanyon, the frequency of application of load rather than its magnitude was explored.[11] Remarkably they demonstrated that only four consecutive cycles per day of external loading was sufficient to prevent disuse remodelling and maintain the bone mass. If there were fewer than this, disuse osteoporosis occurred. Thirty six cycles per day at 0.5 Hz resulted in considerable periosteal and endosteal new bone formation. Importantly, neither the size nor the character of the bone changes were affected by any additional increase in the number of loading cycles after 36 cycles. A possible mechanism for this daily memory was suggested by Skerry et al,[12] who reported that the matrix became aligned with loading and maintained this structure for approximately 24 hours.

CLINICAL NOTE During fracture repair, a gradually increasing load would be expected to result in a stronger callus but maximum stimulus of the callus would be expected to be achieved after approximately 40 cycles of loading. Significantly, more cycles of loading beyond this would not be expected to provide any additional repair stimulus, but may put the callus at risk of mechanical breakdown and hypertrophic nonunion. This suggests that, in the early stages of fracture repair, progressively increasing the load patients take through the fractured limb but limiting the number of loading cycles may be most appropriate.

BONE MAINTENANCE

During regular activity, small amounts of subclinical damage occur to the bone in the form of microcracks. These microcracks are the structural manifestation of cyclical loading-dependent failure at the microscopic level. The extent of microdamage has been shown to be higher in individuals of older than 40 years.[13] Bone has a remarkable system of removing these microcracks. Bone is thought to perceive and react to this through an osteocyte-mediated mechanism. The formation of linear microcracks leads to regulated (apoptotic) death of osteocytes in the region of the crack. Dying osteocytes trigger expression of receptor activator of nuclear factor-κ B ligand (RANKL) by neighboring surviving osteocytes, which results in osteoclast formation and bone resorption. If, however, the rate at which the cracks are accumulating exceeds the rate at which they are removed, then a fracture line will slowly propagate across the whole bone and result in a stress fracture. This is classically seen in the metatarsals of new recruits to the army but can also be seen in individuals with less intense physical activity, whose repair mechanisms are slowed. The removal of these microcracks requires osteoclasts to tunnel to the site of the microcracks and resorb bone. The exposed surfaces of the wall of the tunnel, behind the osteoclasts, are covered in osteoblasts that lay down layers of new lamellar bone. This whole structure is referred to as a cutting cone. These cutting cones are responsible for remodelling.

CLINICAL NOTE

- Agents such as diphosphonates and denosumab block the maturation of osteoclasts and prevent the formation of cutting cones. Prolonged usage of these agents results in accumulation of the microcracks and eventually to atypical fractures.
- Primary bone healing utilizes the process of remodelling and, therefore, may be inhibited by diphosphonates and denosumab.[14]

©Copyright 2021 American Academy of Orthopaedic Surgeons

WOUND HEALING

The body's standard response to injury is an acute inflammation response. This involves an initial stage of hematoma formation, followed by a phase of inflammation and demolition, and finally a phase of ingrowth of granulation into the tissue. In the inflammatory phase, the fibrin exudate and neutrophil polymorph infiltrate are replaced with a mononuclear cell infiltrate, and this indicates the onset of the demolition phase in which macrophages engulf fibrin and cellular infiltrate. Following this, granulation tissue is formed by the proliferation and migration of the surrounding connective tissue elements consisting of capillary loops and fibroblastic cells. This process of healing is used in a specialized way in secondary bone repair.

TYPES OF FRACTURE REPAIR

PRIMARY BONE HEALING (DIRECT OR OSTEONAL BONE REPAIR)

Primary bone healing occurs when accurate reduction and rigid internal fixation has been performed. The central components of primary bone healing are "cutting cones" which consist of a spearhead of osteoclasts that cut a space in bone. Within this space, there is a central blood vessel and the walls of the cavity behind the osteoclasts are lined with osteoblasts, which lay down new bone. Multiple cutting cones traverse the fracture gap perceiving it to be a "giant microcrack." Eventually, the fracture line is obliterated as it is removed and is replaced with new bone by the osteoblasts (**Figure 1**).

In order for a fracture to heal by primary bone healing, the fracture needs to be fixed rigidly (ie, the strain of the facture surface needs to be less than 2%) and there needs to be no significant gap between the bone surfaces (ie, less than ~ 0.1 mm). This process does not have an inflammatory phase but does require active osteoclasts and may, therefore, be impaired by agents that inhibit osteoclasts such as diphosphonates.

GAP HEALING

Gap healing is a modified form of primary bone repair. This occurs if a fracture has been rigidly fixed but the gap at the fracture site is in the order of a few hundred microns. In this situation, immature bone is initially laid down along the fracture surface of each bone end so that the gap now becomes small enough to allow cutting cones to traverse the fracture as in primary bone healing.

SECONDARY BONE REPAIR

The majority of fractures heal by secondary bone repair which is a form of wound healing. It can be considered to consist of five stages—ie, (1) hematoma, (2) inflammation, (3) soft callus, (4) hard callus, and (5) remodeling; however, in practice, there is a continuum and many of these phases overlap (**Figure 2**).

HEMATOMA

Immediately after a fracture, bleeding from the bone surfaces and from the surrounding soft tissue occurs. This blood clot is rich in a number of factors such as VEGF (vascular endothelial growth factor). These factors are important in initiating the inflammatory response and recruiting cells and blood vessels to the site of injury. It has been shown that removal of the

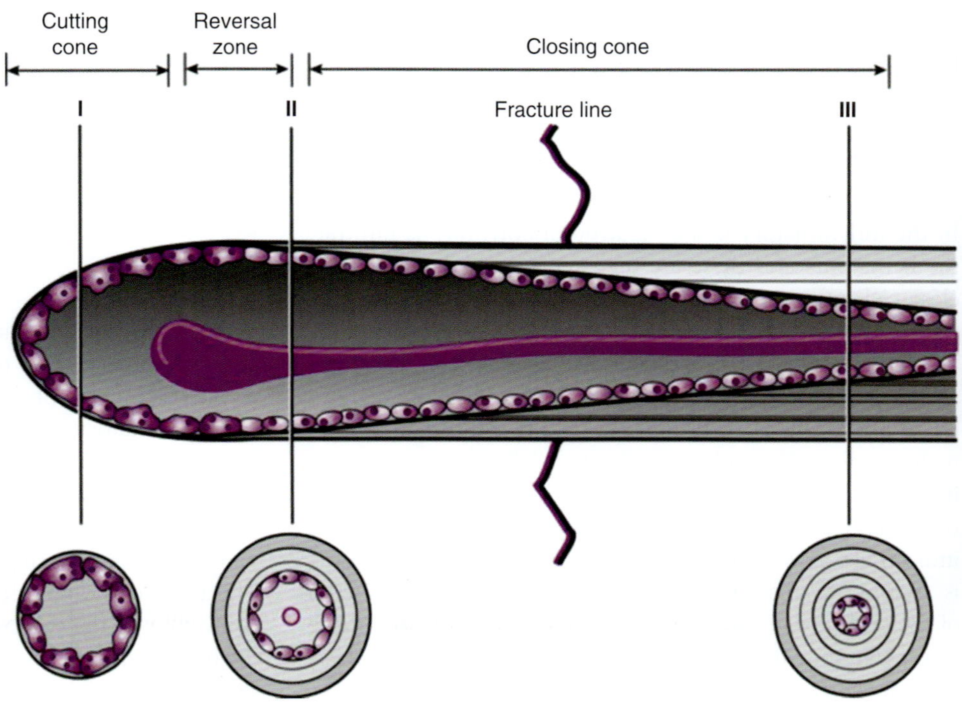

FIGURE 1 Illustration showing direct fracture repair. Cutting cones consisting of osteoclasts burrowing their way across the fracture line, creating a cavity with a blood vessel in its middle and osteoblasts on the walls of cavity laying down bone. (Reproduced with permission from Court-Brown C, Heckman JD, McKee M, McQueen MM, Ricci W, Tornetta P: *Rockwood and Green's Fractures in Adults*. Philadelphia: Wolters Kluwer, 2014.)

4: Repair and Regeneration

©Copyright 2021 American Academy of Orthopaedic Surgeons

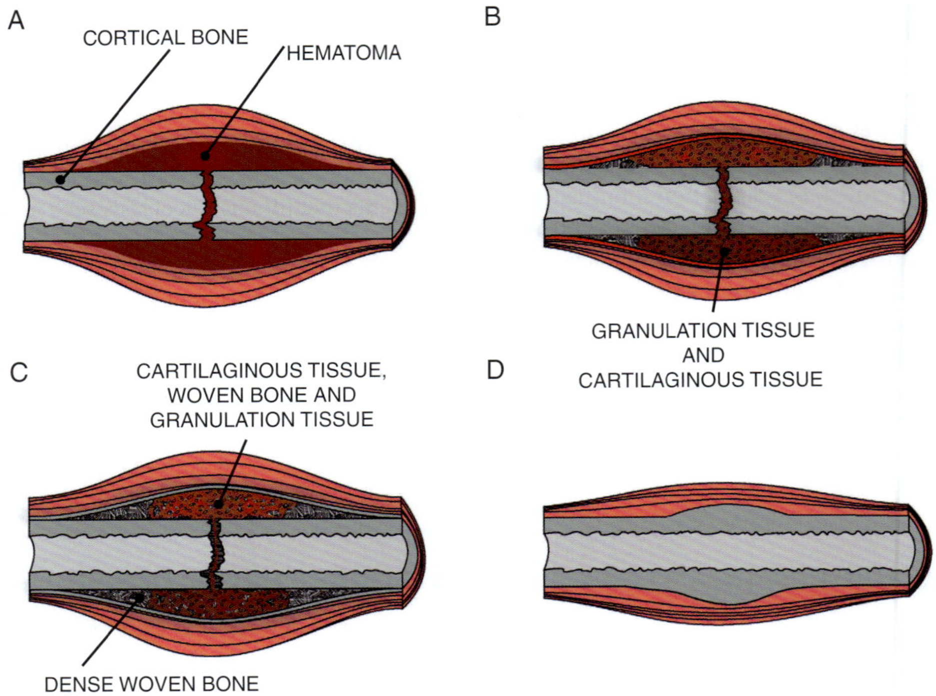

FIGURE 2 Illustrations showing indirect fracture repair. Indirect fracture repair occurs in fractures that have not been rigidly fixed. The repair process can be considered to follow five stages; however, in real life, these stages are not distinct, but overlap. **A**, Stages 1 and 2—Stage 1 (Day 0): Hematoma formation, which is rich in important growth factors such as vascular endothelial growth factor (VEGF) and platelet-derived growth factor (PDGF). Stage 2 (Days 1-10): Inflammation. In this phase, there is an invasion of inflammatory cells; firstly neutrophils, then macrophages, which phagocytose debris and necrotic tissues. Osteoclasts are recruited that start to resorb the necrotic bone ends. **B**, Stage 3 (week 1-8): In this phase, organization of the blood clot occurs with invasion of capillaries and fibroblasts. Fibroblasts and chondrocytes lay down a fibrocartilaginous matrix between the fracture ends. The muscle and the deep cambial layer of the periosteum contribute to the external callus. The medullary tissue and the bone ends contribute to the internal callus. **C**, Stage 4 (Months 2-6): Hard Callus formation. In this phase the matrix becomes mineralised. **D**, Stage 5 (Months 3-24): Remodeling. In the final phase of fracture repair, the woven bone is gradually remodelled and replaced by lamellar bone with Haversian canals. There can also be reconstitution of the medullary canal. (Reproduced with permission from Casanova M, Schindeler A, Little D, Müller R, Schneider P: Quantitative phenotyping of bone fracture repair: A review. *Bonekey Rep* 2014;3:550. doi:10.1038/bonekey.2014.45.)

hematoma results in delayed fracture healing and the absence of the hematoma in open fractures is likely to contribute to the impaired healing in these patients.[15]

Inflammatory Phase

In the inflammatory phase, neutrophil polymorphs infiltrate the hematoma and these are then replaced with a mononuclear cell infiltrate of macrophages, which engulf fibrin and red cells. In addition, other inflammatory cells such as T-cells, B-cells, and mast cells also play a role. Inflammatory cytokines such as tumor necrosis factor-alpha (TNF-α), the interleukins (ILs), specifically IL-1, IL-6, IL-11, and IL-18, recruit inflammatory cells and stimulate angiogenesis.[16] TNF-α acts through its receptors TNFR1 and TNFR2, which are expressed on osteoblasts and osteoclasts. TNFR2 is only present after injury, indicating it may have a particular role in fracture repair. IL-1 is secreted by macrophages, which regulates the expression of the cyclo-oxygenase enzymes (Cox1 and Cox2) that make prostaglandins at the fracture site.[17] NSAIDS inhibit these enzymes and may inhibit the repair process. In addition, IL-1 induces osteoblasts to produce IL-6 and stimulates angiogenesis at the fracture site. IL-6 also stimulates angiogenesis and in addition stimulates the differentiation of osteoblasts and osteoclasts.[18] Factors in the complement cascade also have a role in fracture repair; however, at present this is poorly defined.[19,20]

Soft Callus

In this phase, organization of the blood clot occurs with invasion of capillaries and fibroblasts. The macrophages, present at the fracture site, begin to change their phenotype from a proinflammatory one induced by toll-like receptors (TLR) to an anti-inflammatory phenotype.

Fibroblasts and chondrocytes lay down a fibrocartilaginous matrix between the fracture ends. A bridge of soft callus forms where the tissue is being subjected to a strain of less than 20%. The muscle and the deep cambial layer of the periosteum contribute to the external callus. The medullary tissue and the bone ends contribute to the internal callus. Mesenchymal stem cells (MSCs) are derived from these tissues, and recent

 ©Copyright 2021 American Academy of Orthopaedic Surgeons

evidence indicates that they are recruited from the circulation (Granero-Molto et al[21] and Kitaori et al[22]). Stromal cell derived factor-1 and its receptor CXCR-4 appear to be crucial for the homing of appropriate MSCs to the fracture site.[21-23] However, lineage tracing work indicates that most of the cells are derived from the periosteum, endosteum and bone marrow.[24]

TNF-α also has a key role in recruiting osteoprogenitor stem cells, stimulating apoptosis of hypertrophic chondrocytes and enhancing the recruitment of osteoclasts to the calcified cartilage callus.[25]

Hard Callus

In some respects, adult fracture repair recapitulates embryonic endochondral ossification (**Figure 3**). In both processes, MSCs condense at the sites of bone formation. The process involves activation of transcription factors such as Hoxa 4, Cart 1, CBFA 1, and Sox 9 as well as growth factors such as those of the transforming growth factor beta (TGF-β) superfamily (including the bone morphogenic proteins [BMPs]).[26]

In addition members of the Wnt family of molecules, which are known to have a major role in development, have also been shown to contribute to fracture repair and to regulate the differentiation of MSCs.[27]

As the recruited MSCs differentiate into chondroblasts and osteoblasts, they are stimulated to form type 2 and type 1 collagen, by members of the TGF-beta superfamily, such as BMP-2 which is important for the initiation of healing. BMP-5 and BMP-6 are important for intramembranous ossification and TGF-β2 and growth/differentiation factor-5 (GDF-5) for chondrogenesis during endochondral ossification.[28]

In this phase, the matrix becomes mineralized; calcium-containing granules are accumulated in the cytoplasm and then transported to the extracellular matrix where they combine with phosphate and precipitate and become the nidus for apatite crystal formation.[29]

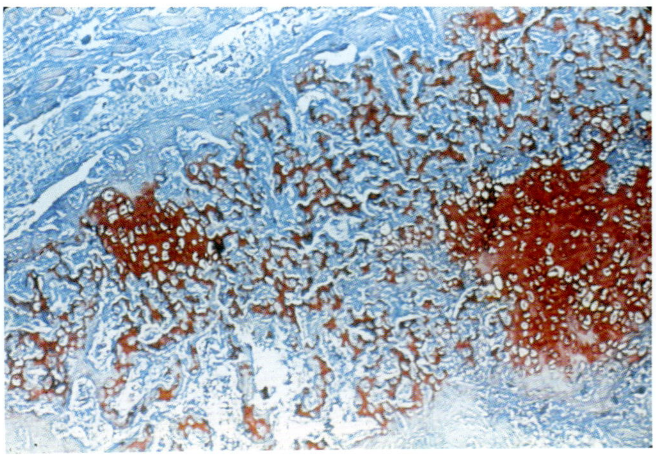

FIGURE 3 Histologic image of endochondral ossification: cartilage extracellular matrix (staining red) is being replaced by bone (staining blue) mediated by chondroclasts and osteoblasts and resulting in stable fracture callus.

As the soft callus becomes stiffer, the tissue strains reach a level where bone can form and osteoblasts are able to ossify the tissue. Provided there are regions where the callus is now under the breaking strain of bone (ie, approximately 2%), a bridge of hard callus is able to form. If there is excessive movement at this stage and there are no zones where the strain is under 2%, then a hypertrophic nonunion will occur. The hard callus initially consists of a "repair" form of bone (ie, woven bone) which consists of type 3 as well as type 1 collagen.

Remodelling

Once the bone ends have been joined together by a solid bridge of woven bone, this tissue is gradually replaced with lamellar bone by a cutting cone process called remodeling. This new bone is laid down along the lines of stress in response to the mechanical requirements of the bone. The process of secondary bone healing is remarkable in that the bone regenerates without a scar and reforms healthy new bone.

MECHANICS OF FRACTURE REPAIR

OPTIMAL MECHANICAL ENVIRONMENT FOR FRACTURE REPAIR

The optimum mechanical environment of healing depends upon the treatment modality used. (1) For primary bone healing, the strain at the fracture site should be less than 2% at all times. (2) For secondary fracture healing, a degree of movement is necessary to stimulate the repair process, but excess movement/instability will inhibit fracture repair (**Figure 4**).

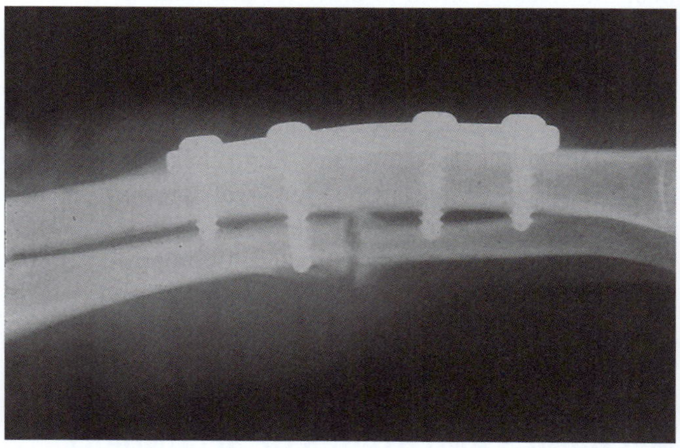

FIGURE 4 Lateral radiograph illustrating fracture healing in two different mechanical environments: the fracture fixed with a rigid plate experiences minimal mechanical strain and heals by direct osteonal repair. The fracture subject to micromotion is healing by endochondral ossification. In both cases, extracellular matrix is being regulated by the biophysical environment. (Reproduced with permission from Aaron RK, Bolander ME: *Physical Regulation of Skeletal Repair*. American Academy of Orthopaedic Surgeons, 2005.)

©Copyright 2021 American Academy of Orthopaedic Surgeons

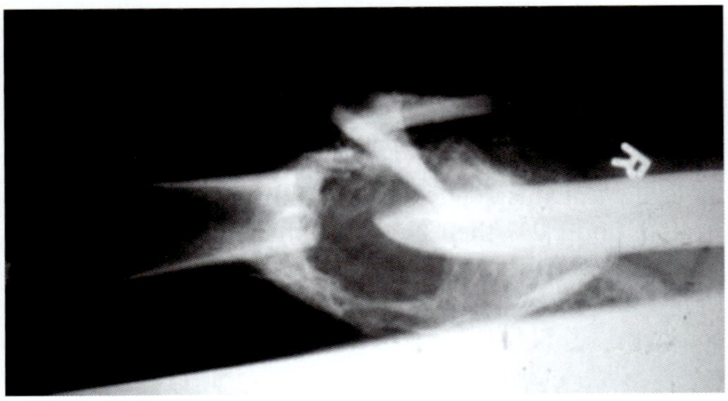

FIGURE 5 Lateral radiograph showing a femoral fracture treated by skeletal traction. New bone is formed where the strain on the tissue is under 2%. Initially this is at the periphery of the fracture callus, but as callus stiffens and the strain on the tissue close to the bone ends is reduced, bone is laid down progressively closer to the bone ends.

Locking plates can provide too rigid an environment and inhibit secondary fracture repair.[30] In contrast, hybrid external fixators stabilizing metaphyseal fractures applied with the diaphyseal fixation block too far from the metaphysis results in excess shear movement and predispose the patient to hypertrophic nonunion.

PERREN STRAIN THEORY

The amount of deformation that a tissue can tolerate and still function varies from intact bone, which has a breaking strain of 2%, to granulation tissue that can withstand 100% strain before breaking. Fibrocartilage has an intermediate breaking strain in the order of 10%. The amount of movement of the fracture ends has to result in a strain on the material lower than the breaking strain in order for that material to bridge across the fracture gap[31] (**Figure 5**).

MICROMOVEMENT

In a sheep study, it was shown that 1 mm of axial micromovement (ie, displacement) applied for 17 minutes per day to a 3 mm osteotomy gap resulted in improved healing compared with rigid external fixation.[32] Subsequently, improved healing was also shown in patients, who received micromovement in a prospective randomized control trial of 85 tibial fractures treated with external fixation.[33]

MECHANICS AND STAGES OF SECONDARY FRACTURE REPAIR

As the callus matures, it becomes stiffer, reducing the interfragmentary movement sufficiently so that bridging or hard bony callus can occur. By expanding the volume of callus and laying down material at a distance away from the center of the fracture, the body is able progressively to decrease the strain experienced by the tissue in the fracture gap.

Fracture Repair and Aging

Children's fractures are known to heal faster than adults, which has been attributed to their thicker periosteum and because they form a larger subperiosteal hematoma, resulting in more rapid callus formation.[34] As some of the fracture healing and limb development pathways overlap, some of the bone formation processes will already be active in the immature skeleton and this may also contribute to the faster healing in children.

With aging, slower fracture healing is thought to be multifactorial. There are changes in the function of inflammatory cells which slow the early phase of fracture repair. Delayed periosteal cell differentiation, delayed periosteal bone formation, prolonged endochondral phase, and blood vessel invasion into the cartilage have been reported in experimental fracture healing.[35] Delayed healing has also been attributed to reduced expression of key growth factors (Naik et al[35]).

Metaphyseal Fracture Healing

In metaphyseal fractures, there is a broader surface area of cancellous bone and there is no medullary canal. The bone is well vascularized, and it is likely that in patients with these fractures, there is less death of the bone ends, possibly because the thinner trabecular elements fail without causing as much damage to the blood vessels. Union is able to occur without external callus, provided that the strains at the fracture surface are under 2%. Woven bone forms directly from mesenchymal cells by the faster intramembranous ossification route. The woven bone subsequently remodels into lamellar bone. Lamellar bone formation has also been reported to occur directly on the surface of preexisting trabeculae.[36,37]

INHIBITION OF FRACTURE HEALING

HOST FACTORS ASSOCIATED WITH DELAYED FRACTURE HEALING AND NONUNION

Diabetes

In patients with diabetes, there is a reduced cell proliferation in the early phase associated with reduced levels of a variety of growth factors (including insulin-like growth factor [IGF1], VEGF, TGF-β).[38] Clinical studies have demonstrated a significantly higher incidence of delayed union, nonunion, and a doubling of the time to healing of fractures in diabetics compared with non-diabetics.[39] This can be minimized by optimizing the control of blood glucose levels.[40]

Anemia

Iron deficient anemic rats have been shown to have had impaired bone healing which has been attributed to the poor oxygen levels and a deficiency of iron, which is required for the electron transport system within the cell and for hydroxylation of proline in collagen.[41] The impairment in bone repair is primarily due to hypovolaemia associated with anemia as normovolemic anemic

©Copyright 2021 American Academy of Orthopaedic Surgeons

animals healed satisfactorily. This suggests that in patients, early correction of hypovolemia after trauma is beneficial for fracture healing and after the acute phase, correction of iron deficiency will reduce the rate of non-union.

Hypothyroidism

Hypothyroidism inhibits endochondral ossification. Treatment with thyroxine overcomes this inhibition. It is important therefore to consider hypothyroidism especially in the elderly, in whom it is often undiagnosed.

Malnutrition

Metabolic requirements increased during fracture repair and nutritional deficiencies are associated with impaired fracture healing. In particular, low albumin and low levels of vitamins B, C, and D have been associated with a reduced chance of returning to their prefracture level of independence and impaired fracture healing.

Peripheral Vascular Disease

Impaired blood flow to the limb will reduce the delivery of oxygen, inflammatory cells, and nutrients to the fracture site and result in an increase in carbon dioxide and other metabolites resulting in a local acidic environment.

PRESCRIBED MEDICATIONS

Nonsteroidal Anti-inflammatory Drugs

The effect of NSAIDs on fracture healing may be biphasic. Both Cox 1 and Cox 2, inhibitors have been shown to inhibit bone repair in animal models. However, a short course of nonsteroidals (less than 72 hours) may not be detrimental for fracture healing perhaps because the inflammatory phase is not at its peak at this period. An increased rate of nonunion was observed in the associated limb fractures in patients taking indomethacin as part of a randomized controlled trial to evaluate the role of indomethacin in preventing heterotopic ossification post acetabular fracture fixation.[42] Thus, the use of NSAIDs after the first few days of injury should be carefully considered.

Corticosteroids

Corticosteroids are immunosuppressive and anti-inflammatory. Short-term administration of corticosteroids does not appear to be detrimental but prolonged administration of corticosteroids does inhibit fracture repair. If patients have to be on steroids during fracture repair, they should be warned that their healing time is likely to be longer and a method of stabilisation should be chosen to allow for a prolonged healing time.

Anticoagulants

Agents such as heparin and warfarin may be prescribed to reduce the risk of deep vein thrombosis and pulmonary embolism after certain types of fracture. There is a small amount of animal work that reports that these agents may impair fracture repair. It is possible that the hematoma phase of fracture repair is particularly sensitive to these agents.

Antibiotics

Infection is associated with impaired fracture healing. However certain antibiotics (eg, the fluoroquinolones) have been reported in animal models to also impair fracture healing. Cell culture studies have demonstrated that a range of antibiotics including aminoglycosides and rifampicin inhibit osteoblasts in cell culture, and it is possible therefore that high doses of these antibiotics may impair fracture repair. However, this needs to be explored further in clinical studies.

NONPRESCRIBED MEDICATIONS

Smoking

Smoking is associated with impaired fracture healing.[43,44] This has been postulated to be due to (1) a reduced blood supply, (2) high levels reaction oxygen intermediates, (3) low concentrations of antioxidant vitamins, and (4) the effects of nicotine on arterial endothelial receptors. In one study, a tobacco extract not containing nicotine significantly reduced the mechanical strength of healing femoral fractures while nicotine alone did not affect the mechanical properties.[45] A prospective clinical study of open tibial fractures demonstrated that smokers were 37% more likely to develop nonunion and twice and likely to develop infection.[46]

Alcohol

Individuals consuming excessive alcohol are prone to delayed fracture healing. There appears to be a dose-dependent toxic effect of alcohol on osteoblasts. In addition, alcohol decreases the synthesis of the extracellular matrix and ossification.

FRACTURE NONUNION

Nonunions result in prolonged pain, inability to work, and a considerable impairment of the quality of life such that patients refer to their life being "on hold" until their nonunion is healed. They also place a considerable burden on the healthcare system with median treatment costs for nonunions being over double that of uncomplicated healing fractures.[47] The overall incidence of fracture nonunion is 20 per 100,000 population and peaks in the fourth decade of life;[5,48] therefore, there are likely to be ~100,000 nonunions every year in the United States. The causes of nonunion can be considered to be due to infection, mechanical, or biological factors. The latter can be further subdivided into local and systemic biological causes. Whatever the cause, there is a pressing need for urgent identification and treatment to prevent the prolonged morbidity these patients suffer.

EPIDEMIOLOGY OF FRACTURE NONUNION

In a study of almost 5,000 symptomatic nonunions, the overall rate of nonunion was 1.9% per fracture. However, for specific groups, the rate was over 5%. In the 35- to 44-year age

©Copyright 2021 American Academy of Orthopaedic Surgeons

group with clavicle/scapula fractures, the rate of nonunion was 8.1% and, with tibial fractures, the rate of nonunion was 9.2% (**Figure 4**).

Although the number of fractures increased with age, the number of nonunions per fracture did not. The nonunion rate per fracture was highest in the 30 to 44 year age group, 20 times greater than that in the 0- to 14-year-olds and 2.5 times higher than that in those aged ≥75 years.

When the pattern of acute fracture incidence, nonunion incidence, and nonunion per fracture incidence according to age and sex were compared, the patterns were markedly different. The overall fracture incidence in men and women was similar (11.6 per 1,000 population per year), but with an age distribution that was bimodal in males and unimodal in females. In contrast, the nonunion incidence was unimodal peaking in the 35- to 44-year age group in both sexes with a gradual decline thereafter (**Figure 6**).

The risk factors for nonunion are multifactorial, with host factors, mechanical factors, and biological bone factors all playing a role.[49] However, the risk of fracture nonunion does not increase with age-related loss of bone density. After case-control matching (1:2), one study concluded that osteoporosis was not a risk factor for fracture nonunion. This prospective study of 1498 acute fracture patients older than 50 years who all underwent screening for osteoporosis and of whom 40 developed nonunion.[50]

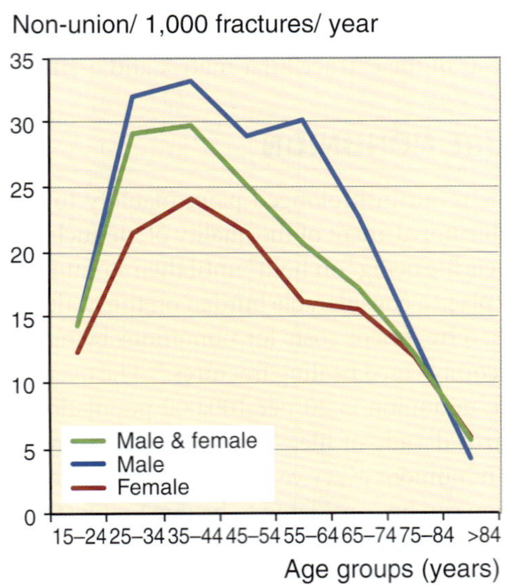

FIGURE 6 Line graph shows that the risk of nonunion per fracture is highest in the 30- to 45-year age band, who are still sustaining high-energy injuries, but in whom the healing potential is likely to be less than the 15- to 29-year age band. (Reproduced with permission from Mills LA, Aitken SA, Simpson AHRW: The risk of non-union per fracture: current myths and revised figures from a population of over 4 million adults. *Acta Orthop* 2017;88(4):434-439.)

High-energy and open fractures are at increased risk of disturbed fracture healing[51-54]. The average age for sustaining a fracture from a fall down a step or from standing height is in the sixth and seventh decade, whereas fractures caused by an higher-energy mode such as from sport, a direct blow, or a motor vehicle accident occur in the younger adult population (25 to 39 years of age on average).[54,55]

PRINCIPLES OF MANAGEMENT OF FRACTURE NONUNIONS

When treating a patient with a nonunion, it is important to consider (1) whether there is bone loss (ie, a gap), (2) whether infection is present, (3) whether the mechanical environment is conducive to healing, and (4) what the biology is of the nonunion.

Gap Versus No Gap

The presence and size of a bone gap has major implications for the reconstruction options. A small to moderate gap can often be treated with bone graft or osteoinductive substances. A large bone gap poses major treatment challenges, which in some patients may mean that attempts at healing the nonunion are abandoned and the defect is treated with amputation or endoprosthetic replacement. The bone ends may have sclerotic caps, which are associated with atrophic nonunions.

Infection Versus Aseptic

Infection is a known aetiological factor for impaired bone healing. It has been reported to be present in 38% of cases presenting to a nonunion clinic.[50] In 5% of cases, there are no features in the history (such as open fracture, early wound infection) to suggest infection, and the patients present with a failure of bone healing analogous to infected joint replacements presenting with loosening rather than systemic sepsis. Low virulence organisms (such as *Propionibacterium acnes, Staphylococcus epidermis*) should be suspected in these cases and it is essential to send multiple samples for microbiological analysis as well as tissue for histology. Histological examination has been shown to be of diagnostic use in nonunions as well as infected arthroplasties.[56]

Mechanical Environment

As described earlier, for a fracture to heal, at each stage of fracture healing the mechanical environment must be conducive for healing and in particular the prevailing strains at the fracture site must be lower than the failure strain of the tissue present at that stage of healing. For example, in the later stages of repair, when tissue such as hard callus/woven bone with a failure strain of ~2% is present at the fracture site, if the prevailing strains at the fracture site exceed 2%, then a hypertrophic nonunion will develop.

©Copyright 2021 American Academy of Orthopaedic Surgeons

Biological Activity of the Nonunion

Although by definition, all nonunions have the loss of mechanical integrity in common, they differ greatly in their biology, and this has major implications for the treatment options for the patient. Several different ways of classifying of nonunions have been described. Most surgeons use either the Weber and Čech[57] or AO classification.[58] Both classifications suggest nonunions have viable and nonviable types; those in the viable group are considered to have the biological ability to heal but are prevented by underlying mechanical/instability issues, whereas the nonviable group consists of comminuted devascularized fractures that do not have the blood supply to heal. These classifications divide patients on the basis of their radiological appearance and x-rays are used to infer the biological viability at the nonunion site. With hypertrophic nonunions the radiograph may be a reasonable indicator of the biology (vascular and active), however, nonunions with an atrophic appearance on radiograph have very variable biology. In particular, the allocation of the atrophic and oligotrophic subtype to their categories is very subjective and challenging.

Therefore, the common approach of inferring the biological activity of a nonunion by using plain x-rays is unreliable. Weber and Cech in their classic descriptions of nonunions were fully aware that some nonunions with poor callus formation were still active and referred to these as oligotrophic. However, in practice, atrophic/oligotrophic radiographic pattern does not distinguish those nonunions that are biologically nonactive from those that are not; reinforcing the fact that the lack of radio density of the nonunion tissue does not indicate lack of biological activity (**Figure 7**).

Appearance of Nonunions at Surgery

Macroscopic appearance: In septic cases, there may be a sinus and visible pus but as noted above there may be no visible signs of infection. In aseptic cases, there may be (1) abundant vascular-dense gritty callus, (2) vascular "fibrous" tissue between the bone ends with or without a small amount of callus, or (3) a fibrous false capsule containing fluid with a synovial-like lining. The Ilizarov description of nonunions as stiff or mobile reflects the different tissue connecting the bone ends with those connected by "fibrous" tissue and the hypertrophic ones being stiff while those with a false capsule and fluid between the bone ends being mobile.

Microscopic appearance: The nonunion consists of connective tissue of varying density containing primarily fibroblast-like mononuclear cells. There can also be regions of fibrocartilage and woven bone, which are most common in hypertrophic nonunions. High levels of collagen III can be visible in the nonunions. This is consistent with the findings of Lawton et al.

Vascularity of Nonunions

In a series of patients undergoing treatment at the same time, tissues were obtained from the fracture site in patients with stiff "atrophic/oligotrophic" nonunions, hypertrophic nonunions, and fractures undergoing normal healing. Importantly, the vascularity of patients with "atrophic/oligotrophic" nonunions was the same as those with hypertrophic nonunions and, in fact, both had similar blood vessel numbers to normal healing fractures.[59] Therefore, a lack of vascularity at the nonunion stage was not the cause of the failure of healing.

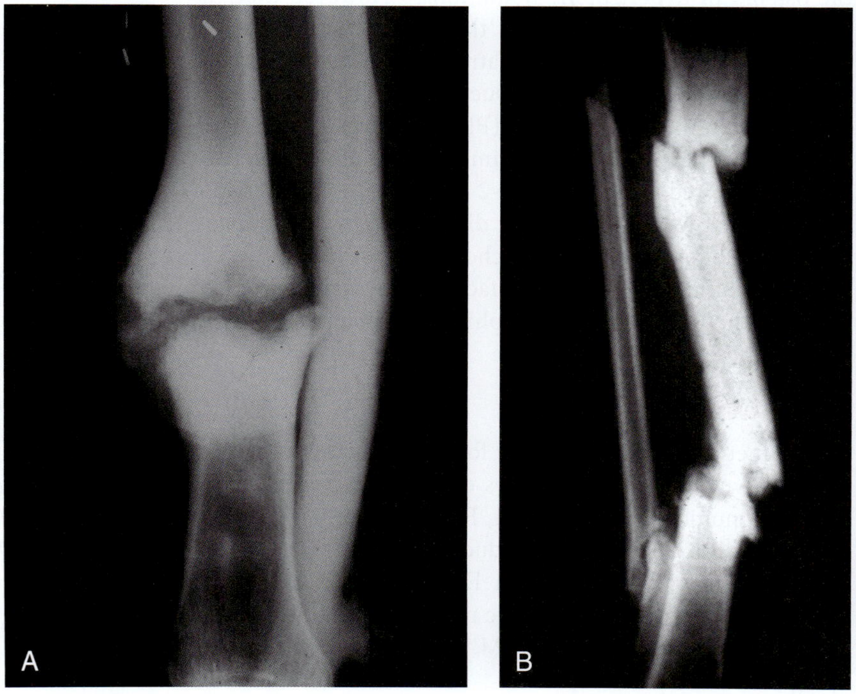

FIGURE 7 **A**, Lateral radiograph of distal tibia. A hypertrophic nonunion. The nonunion tissue is vascular and has osteoblastic potential as it will heal if the correct mechanical environment is applied. **B**, AP radiograph of tibial shaft. A segmental tibial fracture that has an oligotrophic/atrophic radiographic appearance. At surgery, fluid was found between the bone ends at both proximal and distal fracture sites, which lacked any healing potential. (**A**, Photo courtesy of Roy Aaron, MD.)

©Copyright 2021 American Academy of Orthopaedic Surgeons

TABLE 1 The Radiographic Appearance is Not a Good Indicator of the Biological Potential of the Tissue at the Nonunion Site (Except for Hypertrophic Nonunions)

	Hypertrophic	Oligotrophic	Atrophic
Osteoblastic	✓	—	—
Pluripotent	—	?	?
Apotent	—	?	?

Cellular Components

Cells with a fibroblastic appearance, phagocytes, and chondrocytes are present in nonunions. In hypertrophic nonunions, MSCs are present.[60] In atrophic/oligotrophic nonunions, the tissue has been found to be pluripotential but the individual cells less so.[61] Bajada et al[62] also reported some biologically active cells that were positive for the MSC marker CD105, but negative for the haematopoietic markers CD34 and CD45. However, they also found that a higher proportion of the cells were senescent and that the cells had a reduced capacity for osteogenic differentiation and mineralization in vitro. These cells were deficient when compared with bone marrow cells, which have elevated levels of Dickkopf-1 (Dkk-1) which inhibits Wnt signalling during osteogenesis.

Growth Factors

Bone morphogenetic proteins are part of the TGFβ superfamily; they have a major role in the control of cell proliferation and differentiation. BMP-2, BMP-4, and BMP-7 as well as BMP receptors have been found in the osteoblasts lining the osteoid of hypertrophic nonunions.[63] However, there is some disagreement concerning the presence of BMP-7.[64] Conversely, in an established atrophic/oligotrophic nonunion model, the cells in the tissue were negative for TGFβ, platelet-derived growth factor (PDGF), fibroblast growth factor (FGF)-β, and BMP 2/4.[65] Similarly, in human material, a significant reduction in BMP-2 and BMP-14 expression was observed with no statistical differences in the endogenous expression of noggin and chordin (BMP inhibitors).[66] Thus, the difference in growth factor expression may play a role in the persistence of atrophic nonunions but further work in this area is needed.

Gene Expression

Hoffman et al[67] reported that the following genes are significantly down regulated in cultures of osteoblast from hypertrophic nonunions: IGF-2, FGF-1, FGF-receptor 2 (FGF-R2), BMP-4, TGF-b2, PDGF, Wnt-induced proteins (WISP2 and 3), b-catenin and prostaglandin E2 receptor EP4. Fajardo et al[64] also examined hypertrophic nonunions and found that the BMP antagonist genes (DRM, follistatin, noggin) were upregulated.

SUMMARY

The biology of the tissue at fracture nonunion sites is very diverse ranging from acellular fluid to vascular "fibrous" tissue. Growth factor expression ranges from low to relatively high in vascular mineralized tissue. The potential of nonunions to heal varies greatly, and therefore, it is important to consider the nature of the tissue between the bone ends. This can be described as (1) osteoblastic, (2) pluripotent, or (3) apotent. Importantly, it is vital to note that the ability of bone to heal is not indicated by radiograph appearance (**Table 1**). The osteoblastic tissue of a nonunion has the potential to heal with the provision of a suitable mechanical environment. The pluripotent tissue would be expected to be a receptive target for biological, pharmacological, and biophysical stimuli such as electrical, electromagnetic, and ultrasonography. The apotent material will not respond to these interventions and may require bone grafting, application of growth factors, or osteoinductive agents.

REFERENCES

1. Mock C, Lormand JD, Goosen J, et al: *Guidelines for Essential Trauma Care*. Geneva: World Health Organization, 2004.
2. Hadjiargyrou M, O'Keefe RJ: The convergence of fracture repair and stem cells: Interplay of genes, aging, environmental factors and disease. *J Bone Miner Res* 2014;29(11):2307-2322. doi:10.1002/jbmr.2373.
3. Mock CN, Adzotor KE, Conklin E, et al: Trauma outcomes in the rural developing world: Comparison with an urban level I trauma center. *J Trauma* 1993;35:518-523.
4. Salkeld G, Cameron ID, Cumming RG, et al: Quality of life related to fear of falling and hip fracture in older women: A time trade off study. *Br Med J* 2000;320:241-246.
5. Mills LA, Aitken SA, Simpson AHRW: The risk of non-union per fracture: Current myths and revised figures from a population of over 4 million adults. *Acta Orthop* 2017;88(4):434-439. doi:10.1080/17453674.2017.1321351.
6. Hadjiargyrou M, Lombardo F, Zhao S, et al: Transcriptional profiling of bone regeneration Insight into the molecular complexity of wound repair. *J Biol Chem* 2002;277(33):30177-30182.

 ©Copyright 2021 American Academy of Orthopaedic Surgeons

7. Wolff J: *The Law of Bone Remodeling*. Berlin, Heidelberg, New York: Springer, 1986 (translation of the German 1892 edition).
8. Frost HN: Defining osteopenias and osteoporosis: Another view (with insights from a new paradigm). *Bone* 1997;20(5):385-391.
9. Fritton SP, Weinbaum S: Fluid and solute transport in bone: Flow induced mechanotransduction. *Annu Rev Fluid Mech* 2009;41:347-374.
10. Schaffler MB, Kennedy OD: Osteocyte signalling in bone. *Curr Osteoporos Rep* 2012;10(2):118-125.
11. Rubin CT, Lanyon LE: Regulation of bone formation by applied dynamic loads. *J Bone Joint Surg Am* 1984;66(3):397-402.
12. Skerry TM, Bitensky L, Chayen J, Lanyon LE: Loading-related reorientation of bone proteoglycan in vivo. Strain memory in bone tissue? *J Orthop Res* 1988;6(4):547-551.
13. Schaffler MB, Choi K, Milgrom C: Aging and matrix microdamage accumulation in human compact bone. *Bone* 1995;17(6):521-525.
14. Savaridas T, Wallace RJ, Salter DM, Simpson AH: Do bisphosphonates inhibit direct fracture healing?: A laboratory investigation using an animal model. *Bone Joint J* 2013;95-B(9):1263-1268. doi:10.1302/0301-620X.95B9.31562.
15. Park SH, Silva M, Bahk WJ, McKellop H, Lieberman JR: Effect of repeated irrigation and debridement on fracture healing in an animal model. *J Orthop Res* 2002;20(6):1197-1204.
16. Gerstenfeld LC, Cullinane DM, Barnes GL, et al: Fracture healing as a post-natal developmental process: Molecular, spatial, and temporal aspects of its regulation. *J Cell Biochem* 2003;88(5):873-884.
17. Bankers-Fulbright JL, Kalli KR, McKean DJ: Interleukin-1 signal transduction. *Life Sci* 1996;59:61-83.
18. Yang X, Ricciardi BF, Hernandez-Soria A, et al: Callus mineralization and maturation are delayed during fracture healing in interleukin-6 knockout mice. *Bone* 2007;41(6):928-936.
19. Ehrnthaller C, Huber-Lang M, Nilsson P, et al: Complement C3 and C5 deficiency affects fracture healing. *PLoS One* 2013;8:e81341.
20. Kovtun A, Bergdolt S, Hagele Y, et al: Complement receptors C5aR1 and C5aR2 act differentially during the early immune response after bone fracture but are similarly involved in bone repair. *Sci Rep* 2017; 7:14061.
21. Granero-Molto F, Weis JA, Miga MI, et al: Regenerative effects of transplanted mesenchymal stem cells in fracture healing. *Stem Cells* 2009;27(8):1887-1898.
22. Kitaori T, Ito H, Schwarz EM, et al: Stromal cell-derived factor 1/CXCR4 signaling is critical for the recruitment of mesenchymal stem cells to the fracture site during skeletal repair in a mouse model. *Arthritis Rheum* 2009;60(3):813-823.
23. Ma J, Ge J, Zhang S, et al: Time course of myocardial stromal cell-derived factor 1 expression and beneficial effects of intravenously administered bone marrow stem cells in rats with experimental myocardial infarction. *Basic Res Cardiol* 2005;100(3):217-223.
24. Colnot C: Skeletal cell fate decisions within periosteum and bone marrow during bone regeneration. *J Bone Miner Res* 2008;24:274-282.
25. Gerstenfeld LC, Cho TJ, Kon T, et al: Impaired intramembranous bone formation during bone repair in the absence of tumor necrosis factor-alpha signaling. *Cells Tissues Organs* 2001;169(3):285-294.
26. Ferguson C, Alpern E, Miclau T, Helms J: Does adult fracture repair recapitulate embryonic skeletal formation? *Mech Dev* 1999;87: 57-66.
27. Chen Y, Alman BA: Wnt pathway, an essential role in bone regeneration. *J Cell Biochem* 2009;106(3):353-362.
28. Marsell R, Einhorn TA: The role of endogenous bone morphogenetic proteins in normal skeletal repair. *Injury* 2009;40(suppl 3):S4-S7.
29. Ketenjian AY, Arsenis C: Morphological and biochemical studies during differentiation and calcification of fracture callus cartilage. *Clin Orthop Relat Res* 1975;107:266-273.
30. MacLeod AR, Pankaj P: Pre-operative planning for fracture fixation using locking plates: Device configuration and other considerations. *Injury* 2018;49(suppl 1):S12-S18. doi:10.1016/S0020-1383(18)30296-1.
31. Perren SM: Evolution of the internal fixation of long bone fractures. The scientific basis of biological internal fixation: Choosing a new balance between stability and biology. *J Bone Joint Surg* 2002;84-B:1093-1110.
32. Goodship AE, Kenwright J: The influence of induced micromovement on the healing of experimental tibial fractures. *J Bone Joint Surg Br* 1985;67-B:650-655.
33. Kenwright J, Richardson JB, Cunningham JL, et al: Axial movement and tibial fractures. A controlled randomised trial of treatment. *J Bone Joint Surg Br* 1991;73(4):654-659.
34. Lindaman LM: Bone healing in children. *Clin Podiatr Med Surg* 2001;18(1):97-108.
35. Naik AA, Xie C, Zuscik MJ, et al: Reduced COX-2 expression in aged mice is associated with impaired fracture healing. *J Bone Miner Res* 2009;24(2):251-264.
36. Aspenberg P, Sandberg O: Distal radial fracture heal by direct woven bone formation. *Acta Orthop* 2013;84:297-300.
37. Chen WT, Han da C, Zhang PX, et al: A special healing pattern in stable metaphyseal fractures. *Acta Orthop* 2015;86(2):238-242.
38. Gandhi A, Doumas C, O'Connor JP, Parsons JR, Lin SS: The effects of local platelet rich plasma delivery on diabetic fracture healing. *Bone* 2006;38:540-546.
39. Loder RT: The influence of diabetes mellitus on the healing of closed fractures. *Clin Orthop* 1988;232:210-216.
40. Bibbo C, Lin SS, Beam HA, Behrens FF: Complications of ankle fractures in diabetic patients. *Orthop Clin North Am* 2001;32:113-133.
41. Rothman RH, Klemek JS, Toton JJ: The effect of iron deficiency anemia on fracture healing. *Clin Orthop* 1971;77:276-283.
42. Burd TA, Hughes MS, Anglen JO: Heterotopic ossification prophylaxis with indomethacin increases the risk of long-bone nonunion. *J Bone Joint Surg Br* 2003;85-B:700-705.
43. Patel RA, Wilson RF, Patel PA, Palmer RM: The effect of smoking on bone healing. *Bone Joint Res* 2013;2(6):102-111.
44. Hernigou J, Schuind F: Tobacco, bone and fractures: A review of the facts and issues that every orthopaedic surgeon should know. *Bone Joint Res* 2019;8(6):255-265.
45. Skott M, Andreassen TT, Ulrich-Vinther M, et al: Tobacco extract but not nicotine impairs the mechanical strength of fracture healing in rats. *J Orthop Res* 2006;24:1472-1479.
46. Castillo RC, Bosse MJ, MacKenzie EJ, Patterson BM, LEAP Study Group: Impact of smoking on fracture healing and risk of complications in limb-threatening open tibia fractures. *J Orthop Trauma* 2005;19:151-157.
47. Antonova E, Le TK, Burge R, Mershon J: Tibia shaft fractures: Costly burden of nonunions. *BMC Muscoskelet Disord* 2013;14:42.
48. Mills LA, Simpson AHRW: The relative incidence of fracture non-union in the Scottish population (5.17 million): A 5-year epidemiological study. *BMJ Open* 2013;3:e002276.
49. Mills L, Tsang J, Hopper G, Keenan G, Simpson AHRW: The multifactorial aetiology of fracture non-union and the importance of searching for latent infection. *Bone Joint Res* 2016;5(10):512-519.
50. van Wunnik BP, Weijers PH, van Helden SH, Brink PR, Poeze M: Osteoporosis is not a risk factor for the development of nonunion: A cohort nested case-control study. *Injury* 2011;42(12):1491-1494.
51. Robinson CM: Fractures of the clavicle in the adult. Epidemiology and classification. *J Bone Joint Surg Br* 1998;80(3):476-484.
52. Bhandari M, Tornetta P III, Sprague S, et al: Predictors of reoperation following operative management of fractures of the tibial shaft. *J Orthop Trauma* 2003;17(5):353-361.
53. Court-Brown C, Aitken SA, Forward D, O'Toole R: The epidemiology of adult fractures, in Bucholz RW, Court-Brown C, Heckman JD, Tornetta P, eds: *Rockwood and Green's Fractures in Adults*. Philadelphia, Lippincott Williams & Wilkins, 2009, pp. 53-84.
54. Schemitsch EH, Bhandari M, Guyatt G, et al: Study to prospectively evaluate reamed intramedullary nails in patients with tibial fractures (SPRINT) investigators. Prognostic factors for predicting outcomes after intramedullary nailing of the tibia. *J Bone Joint Surg Am* 2012;94(19):1786-1793.

©Copyright 2021 American Academy of Orthopaedic Surgeons

55. Enninghorst N, McDougall D, Evans JA, Sisak K, Balogh ZJ: Population based epidemiology of femur shaft fractures. *J Trauma Acute Care Surg* 2013;74(6):1516-1520.
56. Simpson AH, Wood MK, Athanasou NA: Histological assessment of the presence or absence of infection in fracture non-union. *Injury* 2002;33(2):151-155.
57. Weber BG, Cech O, Konstam P: *Pseudarthrosis: Pathophysiology, Biomechanics, Therapy, Results.* New York, London: Grune and Stratton, 1976.
58. McKee M: Aseptic nonunion, in Ruedi T, Murphy W, eds: *AO-Principles of Fracture Management.* Stuttgart, New York: Georg Thieme Verlag, 2000, pp 748-762.
59. Reed AA, Joyner CJ, Brownlow HC, Simpson AH: Human atrophic fracture non-unions are not avascular. *J Orthop Res* 2002;20(3):593-599.
60. Iwakura T, Miwa M, Sakai Y, et al: Human hypertrophic nonunion tissue contains mesenchymal progenitor cells with multilineage capacity in vitro. *J Orthop Res* 2009;27(2):208-215. doi:10.1002/jor.20739.
61. Tawonsawatruk T, Kelly M, Simpson H: Evaluation of native mesenchymal stem cells from bone marrow and local tissue in an atrophic nonunion model. *Tissue Eng C Methods* 2014;20(6):524-532. doi:10.1089/ten.TEC.2013.0465.
62. Bajada S, Marshall MJ, Wright KT, Richardson JB, Johnson WE: Decreased osteogenesis, increased cell senescence and elevated Dickkopf-1 secretion in human fracture non union stromal cells. *Bone* 2009;45(4):726-735. doi:10.1016/j.bone.2009.06.015.
63. Kloen P, Doty SB, Gordon E, Rubel IF, Goumans MJ, Helfet DL: Expression and activation of the BMP-signaling components in human fracture nonunions. *J Bone Joint Surg Am* 2002;84(11):1909-1918.
64. Fajardo M, Liu CJ, Egol K: Levels of expression for BMP-7 and several BMP antagonists may play an integral role in a fracture nonunion: A pilot study. *Clin Orthop Relat Res* 2009;467(12):3071-3078. doi:10.1007/s11999-009-0981-9.
65. Brownlow HC, Reed A, Simpson AH: Growth factor expression during the development of atrophic non-union. *Injury* 2001;32(7):519-524.
66. Kwong FN, Hoyland JA, Freemont AJ, Evans CH: Altered relative expression of BMPs and BMP inhibitors in cartilaginous areas of human fractures progressing towards nonunion. *J Orthop Res* 2009;27(6):752-757. doi:10.1002/jor.20794.
67. Hofmann A, Ritz U, Hessmann MH, et al: Cell viability, osteoblast differentiation, and gene expression are altered in human osteoblasts from hypertrophic fracture non-unions. *Bone* 2008;42(5):894-906. doi:10.1016/j.bone.2008.01.013.

©Copyright 2021 American Academy of Orthopaedic Surgeons

32

Contemporary Concepts in Soft-Tissue Wound Management

Andrew R. Evans, MD, FACS
Roman A. Hayda, MD, COL(Ret.)

Keywords: *healing; management; soft tissue; wound*

INTRODUCTION

Musculoskeletal soft-tissue injury refers to mechanical, thermal, or chemical injury of skin, subcutaneous tissue, muscle, ligament, tendon, vascular, lymphatic, or periosteal tissues of the body (**Figure 1**). Due to their highly specialized structure and repair mechanisms, injury of tissues such as ligaments and tendons will be discussed in separate dedicated chapters of this book.

Skin tissue consists of stratified squamous (keratinized) epithelium, made up of an outer keratin layer, a series of layers transitioning from flattened squamous epithelial cells to cuboidal epithelial cells situated adjacent to a basal/basement membrane/lamina. Epithelium is avascular and is supplied nutrients and oxygen through diffusion from capillaries in the underlying basal lamina.

Dr. Evans or an immediate family member is a member of a speakers' bureau or has made paid presentations on behalf of Synthes; serves as a paid consultant to or is an employee of Zimmer; and serves as a board member, owner, officer, or committee member of the Center for Orthopedic Trauma Advancement (COTA) - BOD and the Orthopaedic Trauma Association. Dr. Hayda or an immediate family member is a member of a speakers' bureau or has made paid presentations on behalf of AONA and Synthes; serves as an unpaid consultant to BioIntraface; and serves as a board member, owner, officer, or committee member of the American Academy of Orthopaedic Surgeons, METRC, and the Orthopaedic Trauma Association.

The primary function of skin tissue is to provide a water-impermeable barrier that resists mechanical abrasion/laceration and microbial invasion. When the epidermis is injured, the dermis and other underlying tissues are no longer contained in their native physical and chemical milieu and are therefore no longer protected from dessication, infection, and exposure to other cytotoxic conditions and/or chemicals.

Tissues underlying skin consist of a variety of connective tissues derived from undifferentiated mesenchymal stem cells. These tissue/cell types include adipose (adipocytes), fascia (fibroblasts), muscle (myoblasts/myocytes), vascular (endothelial cells), cartilage (chondrocytes), and bone (osteoblasts/osteocytes). This discussion of normal and injured soft tissues will focus primarily on the soft-tissue components including adipose, fascia, muscle, and vascular tissue. Obviously, these soft tissues do not live isolated from bone and cartilage, and we will discuss how the soft tissues are affected by the integrity and mechanical stability afforded by the underlying skeleton.

The structure of skeletal muscle consists of several hundred myoblasts lined up and fused end-to-end to form myotubes. Myotubes are filled with myofibrils consisting of myofilament arrays, the protein units responsible for the contractile function of skeletal muscle. Skeletal muscle fibers are arranged in parallel with intervening continuous capillaries, with individual myotubes contained in endomysium, muscle fascicles contained in perimysium, and entire muscles contained in epimysium. The microscopic structure and function of skeletal muscle will be described in further detail in other chapters. However, a facile understanding of this structure and function is required to understand the mechanisms for healing of skeletal muscle and its potential for regeneration. Skeletal muscle cells do not have mitotic capability, but skeletal muscle tissue does have regenerative capability due to the presence of

©Copyright 2021 American Academy of Orthopaedic Surgeons

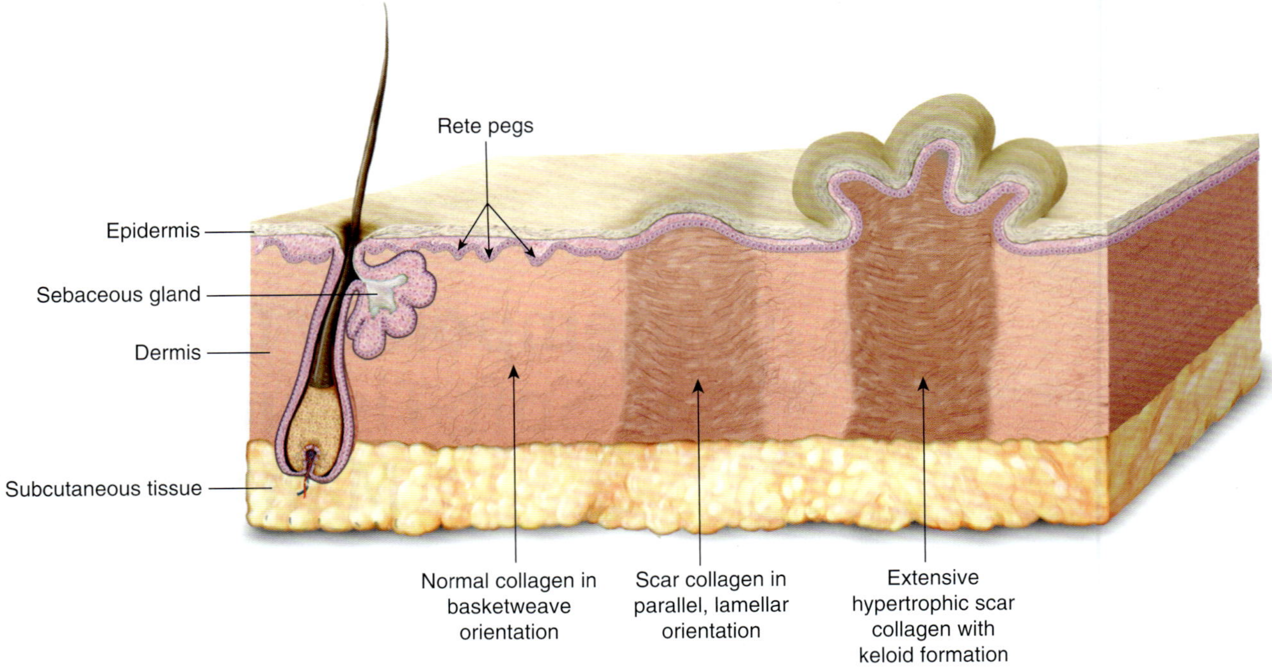

FIGURE 1 Illustration demonstrating the comparison of normal skin and scarred skin.

satellite, or mesenchymal stem cells. As a result, skeletal muscle is capable of undergoing hyperplasia (cell multiplication) and hypertrophy (cell fusion and spatial growth); however, the specificity and reliability of regenerating myoneural junctions is less well controlled or understood in response to injury.

CELLULAR AND MOLECULAR MECHANISMS OF SOFT-TISSUE HEALING

Healing of skin, subcutaneous, fascial/connective, and muscle tissues often occurs through scar formation[1] (**Figure 1**). Although each of these tissues has some potential for regeneration with "scarless" healing through stem cells, most wounds that result from trauma rely on scar tissue formation and even wound contracture. Advanced stem cell therapies that are being developed in the translational arena will be discussed in other parts of this chapter and textbook.

Soft-tissue wound healing occurs along a spectrum, with "scarless" tissue regeneration on one end, normal scar tissue formation in the center, and hypertrophic scar or even keloid formation on the other end (**Figure 2**). Wound healing classically occurs in three overlapping stages: inflammation, proliferation, and remodeling (**Figure 3**). The inflammatory phase of cellular recruitment to injury through autocrine and paracrine mechanisms typically lasts 48 to 72 hours following injury. The proliferative phase, where cell-mediated wound débridement occurs, granulation tissue forms, and vascularity proliferates, evolves over a period of at least 2 to 3 weeks, depending upon wound size and conditions. Once sufficient wound débridement has occurred to establish a well-vascularized wound bed, then the process of reepithelialization can occur, and eventually collagen fibrils are laid down, initially in a disorganized proliferative fashion, but are later gradually remodeled into a more organized collagen structure that never reaches the full tensile strength of normal tissue, but restores sufficient tissue integrity to reestablish the local biological environment.

Following the destruction or laceration of soft tissue, a hematoma containing fibrin and platelets forms. This hematoma facilitates hemostasis and also initiates a cellular and molecular cascade of events that result in the induction of an inflammatory response. That inflammatory response consists of degranulating platelets that release several inflammatory mediators (eg, platelet-derived growth factor [PDGF]) and cytokines (eg, interleukin-8 [IL-8]). Resident mast cells in the local tissues also release mediators including thrombin, complement factors, and others that increase blood flow through vasodilation and enhanced vascular permeability. The chemoattractants generated by this process recruit neutrophils and macrophages into the wound to phagocytose cellular debris, foreign debris, and bacteria. In response, neutrophils amplify the inflammatory reaction through release of inflammatory cytokines including IL-1, IL-6, and tumor necrosis factor (TNF)-α. These, along with transforming growth factor (TGF)-β, monocyte chemoattractant protein-1 (MCP-1), and various extracellular matrix (ECM) proteins further attract monocytes to the wound and stimulate differentiation into macrophages, which become the dominant cell type in the wound during the latter portions of the inflammatory phase, and subsequent transition to the proliferative phase of healing. This transition is mediated in large

©Copyright 2021 American Academy of Orthopaedic Surgeons

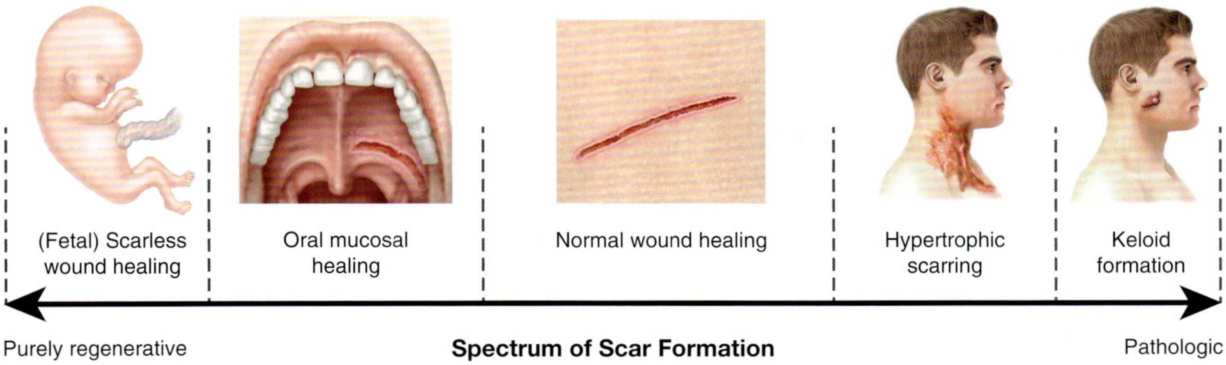

FIGURE 2 Illustration showing the spectrum of scar formation. On one end is scarless wound healing which occurs in fetal cutaneous tissue, then normal wound healing, and linear scar formation. On the pathologic end of the spectrum is hypertrophic scarring, such as that following a burn, and keloid formation, for which there appears to be some genetic predisposition.

part by macrophage-mediated release of chemicals including PDGF and vascular endothelial growth factor (VEGF), fibroblast growth factor (FGF), nerve growth factor (NGF), TGF-β, connective tissue growth factor (CTGF), and cysteine-rich 61 (Cyr-61), which promote the formation of proliferative granulation tissue. T-lymphocytes, fibrocytes, and eosinophils also participate in the inflammatory phase.

The proliferative phase of wound healing, when granulation tissue is formed, is dominated from a cellular perspective by fibroblasts which form extracellular matrix (ECM), and endothelial cells which form blood vessels. Fibroblasts are stimulated to migrate in large part by PDGF, and upon arrival at the wound, many differentiate into myofibroblasts. Myofibroblasts are able to upregulate myocardin-related transcription factor-A, which facilitates expression of smooth muscle actin and causes wound contraction. Fibroblasts that remain travel along connective tissue fibers, aided by interactions between cell-surface integrins and ECM components

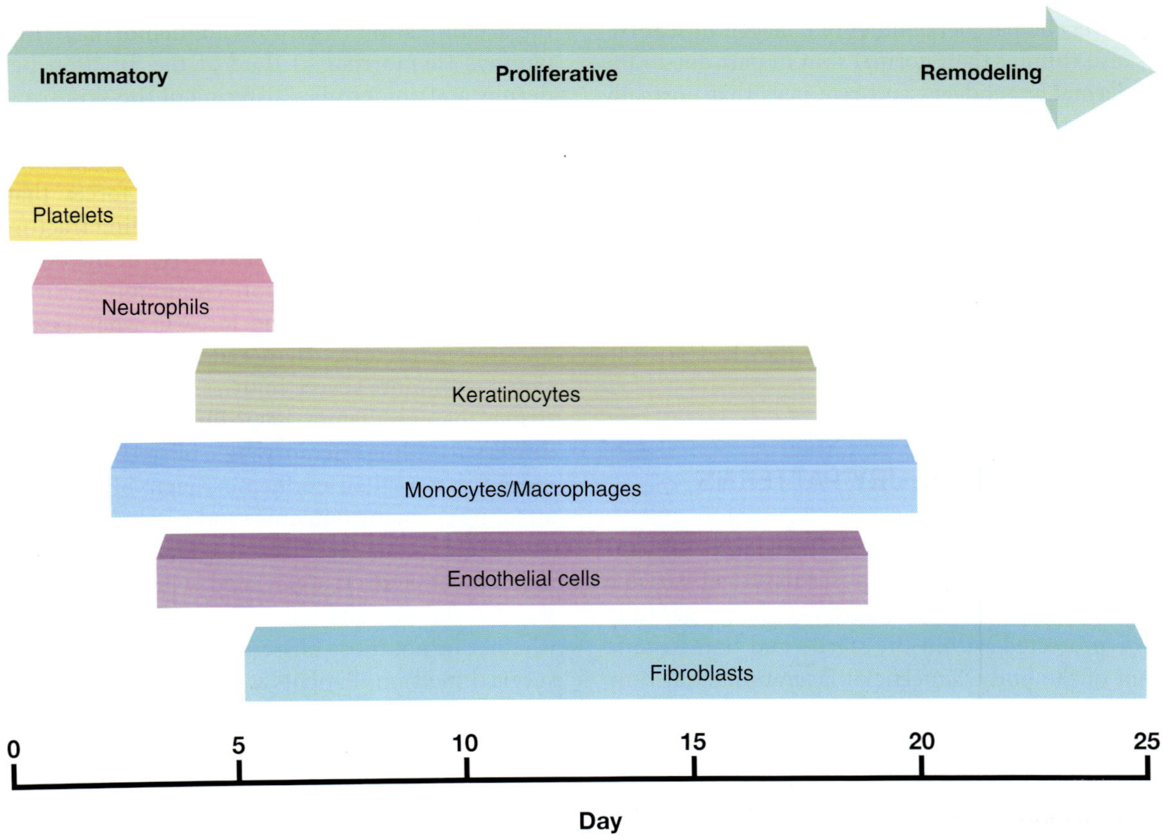

FIGURE 3 Illustration showing the three phases of soft-tissue healing and scar formation.

©Copyright 2021 American Academy of Orthopaedic Surgeons

including fibrin, fibronectin, vitronectin, and hyaluronic acid. They clear pathways within wounded tissue to move through secretion of matrix metalloproteinases (MMPs) that not only break down ECM components to facilitate fibroblast migration, but also to facilitate new blood vessel ingrowth. Local endothelial cells break down the basement membranes of the capillaries they line to enhance vascular permeability and form tubules that eventually become new capillaries. Angiogenesis is promoted by secretion of VEGF, FGF, angiopoietin, TGF-β, as well as local hypoxia with lactic acid. As granulation tissue proliferates to cover the injured tissue/wound bed, the fibroblasts secrete cytokines such as Neu differentiation factor (NDF), which promotes keratinocyte migration from the wound edge and nearby hair follicles, thereby facilitating the process of epithelialization.

Once a wound is epithelialized, the scar tissue formed over this wound largely consists of disorganized type III collagen fibrils and ECM without any dermal appendages (eg, hair follicles, sweat glands), and epithelium. Many of the cells involved in the repair process, including fibroblasts, macrophages, and endothelial cells, go on to apoptosis. As the type III collagen fibrils are remodeled and reorganized into type I collagen, the strength of the wound repair improves to approximately 70% of its original tensile strength, and the scar becomes more flat, firm, and less vascular. A mature scar is made up of 80% to 90% type I collagen arranged in parallel bundles, the rest type III collagen. Collagen in normal skin is present in a basketweave orientation, improving its tensile strength over the parallel bundles of collagen in scar tissue. Scar is also thinner than normal skin in part due to the absence of dermal appendages and rete pegs that normally penetrate the dermis, as well as a lack of stem cells that typically inhabit these structures. The ECM of scar tissue also contains less elastin than normal skin, thereby reducing its elasticity, and when coupled with scar contracture mediated by fibroblasts and myofibroblasts, and significantly restrict the mobility of the injured soft tissues to the point where normal surrounding tissues such as muscles, tendons, and even joints no longer retain the mobility they had prior to the injury.

ACUTE SOFT-TISSUE INJURY PATTERNS

Laceration of soft-tissues refers to the incision or disruption of soft tissues in a way that exposes tissues at variable levels to the environment. Those tissues are no longer fully contained or protected within the sterile and homeostatic environment of the body. Superficial lacerations may only involve skin or subcutaneous tissues, whereas deeper lacerations can potentially involve all soft-tissue layers including muscle, fascia, ligaments, tendons, periosteum, and even bone in the case of open fractures. The tissue layers involved are disrupted at the cellular level, where cells are directly damaged and caused to undergo apoptosis and/or senescence. The mechanical environment in which the tissues typically live is disrupted through wound gaping or even flap formation. More profound alteration of the mechanical environment occurs when the underlying fascial, or even bony structures are disrupted, in which case ongoing mechanical injury to the tissues can occur until those tissues can be stabilized mechanically through skeletal fixation and suture repair. In addition to mechanical disruption and direct injury at the cellular level, lacerated tissues also experience disruption of their blood supply, thereby depriving variable tissue regions of nutrients and oxygen delivery. This lack of blood supply leads to a disruption of the normal respiratory process at the cellular level, resulting in ischemia and tissue necrosis unless that blood supply can be restored in a timely fashion.

Blood supply to and from tissues at all layers depend upon the integrity of the arterial, venous, and capillary networks that exist throughout the body. Laceration and most other forms of soft-tissue injury result in injury or compromise of those important vascular structures to some extent. Superficial tissues such as skin and subcutaneous tissue depend upon perforator vessels and capillary networks for their perfusion, and when those networks are damaged without sufficient collateral flow to compensate, skin necrosis occurs.

Most superficially, blisters of the skin can occur due to thermal, chemical, or mechanical injury at the interface of the epidermis and dermis. Injury at this level results in the accumulation of serous (nonhemorrhagic) or serosanguinous (hemorrhagic) fluid at the junction between the dermis and epidermis. Blistering of the skin from mechanical causes results from shearing forces being applied to the skin, whether it is superficial shearing forces coming from outside the body or shearing forces that emanate from deeper tissue disruptions, including fracture blisters.[2] Blisters can occur in almost any area of the body; however, they occur significantly more commonly in the dorsal foot, ankle, lower leg, wrist, and forearm when associated with underlying fractures. Hemorrhagic blisters tend to be associated with more severe injuries of the skin and underlying tissues than nonhemorrhagic blisters, although this is not a universal finding. Hemorrhagic blisters are associated with more scarring than nonhemorrhagic blisters, significantly affecting cosmetic outcomes and patient satisfaction scores. The presence of fracture blisters, either hemorrhagic or nonhemorrhagic, is associated with an increased risk of skin breakdown and subsequent infection, irrespective of whether or not those blistered areas are incorporated into a surgical incision. Patients with diabetes mellitus and other conditions associated with peripheral vascular disease are at particularly high risk of soft-tissue complications and infection in blistered areas.

The Morel-Lavallee lesion (MLL), a traumatic separation of the hypodermis and underlying deep fascia resulting in

©Copyright 2021 American Academy of Orthopaedic Surgeons

the development of a potential space that fills with blood, serosanguinous fluid, and necrotic fat, was first described by Victor-Auguste-Morel-Lavallee in 1863.[3] The disruption of perforating vascular and lymphatic structures results in the formation of a hemolymphatic fluid collection containing blood clot, fibrin, as well as normal and necrotic fat—an environment at elevated potential risk of infection. Initially, when the shearing injury occurs between the superficial and deep tissue layers, a potential space is created that fills with blood, lymph, and fatty debris, much of which becomes necrotic due to the concomitant injury to tissue blood supply[4] (**Figure 4**). Gradually, as this mixture of fluids is replaced by serosanguinous fluid, the volume of the collection typically increases, and eventually a pseudocapsule forms around it.[5] Morel-Lavallee lesions have been described to occur in one of six patterns, based primarily on MRI imaging characteristics, as described by Mellado and Bencardino.[6] Type 1 is a simple seroma, type 2 is a subacute hematoma, type 3 is a mature organized hematoma, type 4 is a closed fatty laceration complicated by perifascial dissection, type 5 is a perifascial nodular lesion, and type 6 is an infected lesion with sinus tract, septations, and capsular formation (**Figure 5**). If sufficient pressure is exerted on the overlying skin, the skin can experience necrosis, which ultimately leads to bacterial exposure and infection if débridement is not performed prior to recognition of this problem. Due to the necrotic and static nature of this fluid collection, it is often considered to be at risk of infection, even when overlying skin breakdown does not occur, and some studies have demonstrated that up to almost 50% of these lesions are culture positive when aspirated. Lesions treated with surgical débridement are at higher risk of infection than standard surgical wounds. Surgical indications, as well as techniques for management, remain controversial.[7] Lesions treated with aspiration or surgical débridement are not only at higher risk of infection, but are also highly likely to recur with fluid reaccumulation. If closed lesions are treated nonsurgicallyy, and do not develop infection, the fluid pocket typically persists for months, and sometimes years. Typically the fluid will eventually resorb, and changes to the overlying skin will persist, including

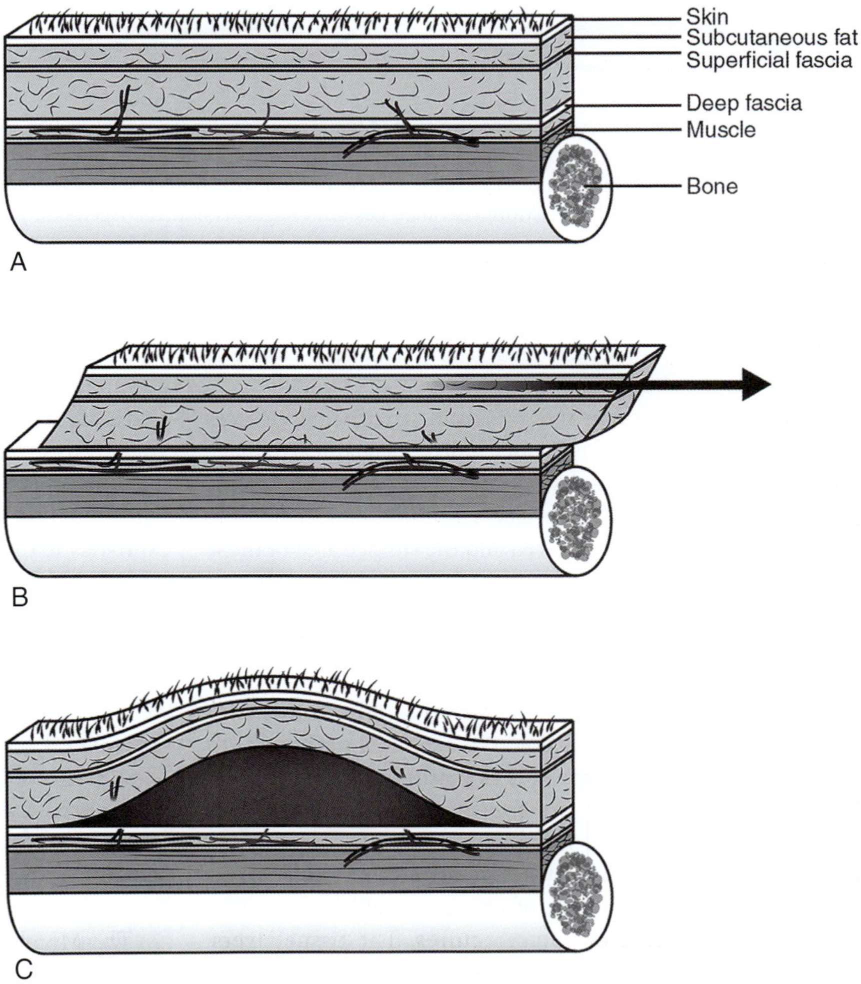

FIGURE 4 Cross-sectional illustration of how a Morel-Lavalee lesion occurs through traumatic shear injury. Normal skin and soft-tissues overlying bone (**A**), when subjected to shear forces (**B**), subsequently accumulate serosanguinous fluid and necrotic tissue between the subcutaneous tissue layer and deep fascia (**C**). (Reproduced from Scolaro JA, Chao T, Zamorano DP: The Morel-Lavallée Lesion: Diagnosis and management. *J Am Acad Orthop Surg* 2016;24(10):667. doi:10.5435/JAAOS-D-15-00181.)

©Copyright 2021 American Academy of Orthopaedic Surgeons

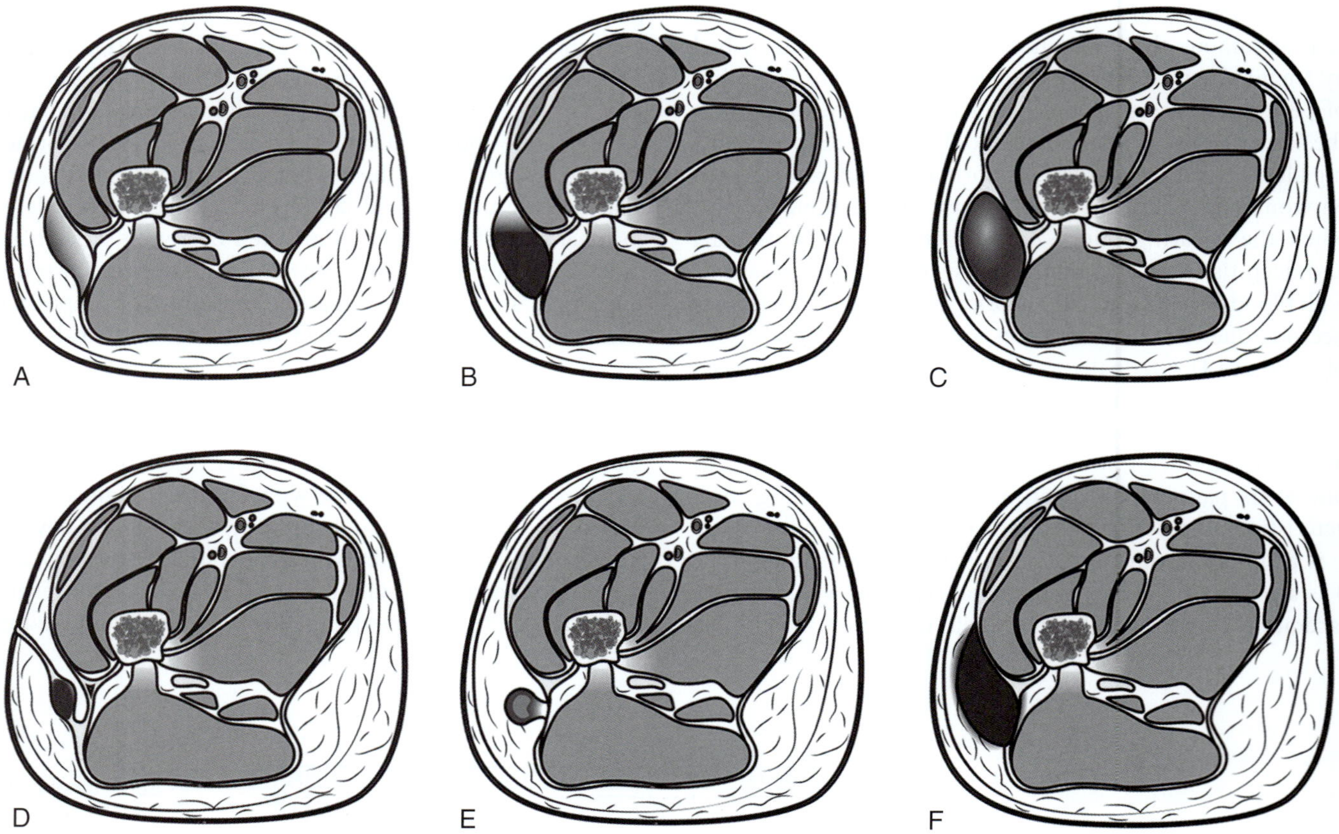

FIGURE 5 Illustration showing the classification of the Morel-Lavallee lesion by Mellado and Bencardino. **A**, Type 1, simple seroma. **B**, Type 2, subacute hematoma. **C**, Type 3, mature organized hematoma. **D**, Type 4, closed fatty laceration complicated by perifascial dissection. **E**, Type 5, perifascial nodular lesion. **F**, Type 6, infected lesion with sinus tract, septations, and capsular formation. (Reproduced from Scolaro JA, Chao T, Zamorano DP: The Morel-Lavallée Lesion: Diagnosis and management. *J Am Acad Orthop Surg* 2016;24(10):667. doi:10.5435/JAAOS-D-15-00181.)

thinning of the skin, which results in permanent cosmetic deformity at the site.

Direct pressure on skin and soft tissues, if sufficiently forceful or prolonged, induced ischemia and/or mechanical damage to that soft tissue that results in pressure-induced skin necrosis, or ulcer formation. These ulcers/wounds vary depending upon the depth of tissue involved and the surface area of those affected tissues. Pressure sores/ulcers are a significant source of morbidity and mortality, particularly in patients with impaired mobility, increased age, and with comorbidities that impair the normal wound healing process.

Ballistic injuries are a unique form of injury to the skin and soft tissues because of the area of injury peripheral to the primary site of injury. This is commonly seen in bullet wounds, where there is direct laceration or disruption of the tissues through which the bullet passes, but there is also a variable area of injury surrounding that bullet tract, caused by a traumatic wave of energy capable of disrupting the viability of tissues surrounding that area. Higher velocity firearms, larger bullet sizes and postimpact shapes (ie, flattening of hollow-tipped bullets), and closer range injury all lead to higher levels tissue damage, including ballistic injury of tissues surrounding the primary point(s) of penetration. Blast effects, resulting from explosions, occur in similar fashion to ballistic injuries described above, but on a much larger scale, potentially resulting in catastrophic soft-tissue injury or even amputation.

Thermal and chemical burns are additional forms of soft-tissue injury that can range from superficial to deep. They can affect all layers of soft tissues, and typically result in necrosis of the layers they affect.[8] There is typically a focus of injury where the primary injury occurs, and a peripheral area of lesser injury until reaching tissues that are unaffected. Patients who experience thermal or chemical burns are often left with scarring, often severe, and therefore can experience contractures that prohibit normal motion of the affected skin and soft tissues. When burns occur in areas overlying joints, contractures often develop in ways that inhibit normal joint motion, and can require contracture releases.

©Copyright 2021 American Academy of Orthopaedic Surgeons

Lacerations resulting in the exposure of underlying osseous fractures are referred to as open or compound fractures. The presence of the underlying fracture creates a unique clinical situation in which the soft tissues, extending down to and including the bone, are at elevated risk of infection. The underlying skeletal instability is harmful to the overlying soft tissues, thereby creating an area of variably compromised soft-tissue viability at all layers, further enhancing the risk of infection to this area. Open fractures typically require timely surgical débridement and skeletal stabilization to minimize the risk of infection, or even amputation. The severity of open fractures has been graded and classified many ways over the last several decades; however, the two most prominent classifications currently in use include the Gustilo and Anderson classification, and the Orthopaedic Trauma Association (OTA) Open Fracture Classification (OFC).[9,10] The Gustilo and Anderson classification rates the severity of injury based upon the size and depth of soft-tissue injury, the extent of fracture comminution and instability of the fracture pattern, and the nature and degree of contamination at the site of injury. The Gustilo and Anderson classification, although arguably the most commonly used classification in clinical practice among orthopaedic and nonorthopaedic specialties, suffers from a well-documented lack of interobserver reliability. As a result, the OTA OFC was created using methods that clearly demonstrate significantly enhanced interobserver reliability over Gustilo and Anderson. It also helps to stratify injury severity using a distinct nomenclature and scoring system, aids in the development of treatment strategies, and also possesses the capability to predict or anticipate outcomes for patients who sustain open fractures. The OTA OFC incorporates into its nomenclature and structure, injury severity stratifications for skin, muscle, and bone, as well as accounts for whether any associated arterial injury creates limb ischemia, and how extensive any wound contamination is around the open fracture. This classification helps to predict whether certain injury patterns, or levels of severity, will require multiple surgical debridements, benefit from use of modalities such as negative pressure wound therapy (NPWT) vacuum-assisted closure (VAC) devices or antibiotic-impregnated poly methyl methacrylate (AIPMMA) beads, and what levels of injury severity are likely to lead to the need for amputation.

NORMAL WOUND HEALING

Soft-tissue injuries heal through the variety of cellular and molecular mechanisms that are described above. This typically involves the formation of scar tissue in a way that restores the integrity of the soft-tissue envelope of the body, thereby restoring its function as a barrier to infection and facilitating the restoration of biomechanics and kinetics. Certain mechanisms, which typically involve pluripotent mesenchymal stem cells and the inhibition of a normal inflammatory reaction, produce "scarless" healing through tissue regeneration. The technology to create conditions that will facilitate "scarless" tissue regeneration, as opposed to scar formation, is a major subject of active research. The incorporation of stem cells in many techniques for treatment of soft-tissue injuries is also rapidly becoming an enormous industry, due in part to the perceived, and in many cases, real benefits seen when tissues are capable of regeneration rather than scar formation. Scar formation never fully restores the mechanical strength and flexibility of tissues it replaces. When scar formation becomes pathologic, hyperplastic scars, or even keloids form, which are functionally and cosmetically problematic.

FACTORS THAT PROMOTE WOUND HEALING

Normal wound healing is promoted through the optimization of numerous factors including nutrition, oxygen delivery, and provision of mechanical support to soft tissues. Optimizing nutrition through normal dietary intake mechanisms, or through supplementation, has been shown to significantly improve the quality and efficiency of soft-tissue wound healing. Low bodily levels of protein (eg, albumin, prealbumin) have been shown to be associated with prolonged wound healing times and, as a result, higher rates of infection and subsequent wound breakdown/nonhealing.

Impaired oxygen delivery to injured soft tissues also leads to prolonged wound healing times, and higher rates of infection. Impaired oxygen delivery can occur as the result of many different circumstances or comorbidities, including impaired perfusion from direct tissue/vascular damage, impaired circulation due to peripheral large vessel or small vessel disease (eg, peripheral vascular disease [PVD], diabetes, smoking, etc), and impaired oxygen intake due to comorbidities that impair normal lung function (eg, chronic obstructive pulmonary disease [COPD], reactive airway disease [asthma], etc). Improvement of oxygen delivery through restoration of tissue perfusion (eg, suture repair, skeletal stabilization), enhancement of local blood flow (eg, angioplasty, stenting, vascular bypass, etc), optimization of pulmonary function, and even provision of oxygen from exogenous sources (ie, hyperbaric oxygen therapy (HBOT), have all been shown to have positive effects on the ability of soft-tissue wounds to heal.[11]

Mechanical support and management of soft-tissue gapping through laceration repair and soft-tissue approximation will reduce the volume of wounds and thereby significantly decrease the time and quantity of metabolic resources needed to achieve wound healing. This can be achieved through many avenues including fracture reduction and deformity minimization, as well as

©Copyright 2021 American Academy of Orthopaedic Surgeons

suture-mediated or adhesive-mediated wound closure/approximation.[12] For wounds that cannot close primarily, supplementing the local injured tissue or granulation tissue with cellular or acellular matrices and scaffoldings can further accelerate wound healing and improve the ability of those tissues to fight infection.[13,14] There is a large emerging market of these matrices, some of which include cellular components and some that do not. The use of stem cells is also becoming very popular, despite its enormous expense, and in some cases, unproven benefits.[15,16] Early coverage of soft-tissue defects with exposed tendon or bone with rotational or free tissue transfers provides enhanced vascularity to injured tissues and can help to reduced susceptibility of those tissues to infection.[17]

FACTORS THAT NEGATIVELY AFFECT SOFT-TISSUE HEALING

Normal soft-tissue healing can be impaired by a wide variety of factors, including medical comorbidities, age, medication and/or chemical exposures, and, most certainly, by infection. Comorbidities such as diabetes mellitus, connective tissue disorders (eg, scleroderma, Sjogren syndrome), autoimmune disorders (RA, lupus), and immune deficiencies can all cause significant disruption of normal wound healing pathways. This can be due to alterations in local biochemistry, impaired metabolism, structural abnormalities in collagen manufacture, impaired immune response, and overactive immune responses that become deleterious to already injured tissues. Many of these types of conditions can be treated to lessen and, in some cases, even eliminate the negative impacts that the comorbid disease process has on wound healing. Immune deficiencies, such as HIV/AIDS, or patients on immune suppression therapy due to transplants or other autoimmune phenomena exhibit impaired wound healing. Nutritional deficiencies caused by poor dietary habits, as well as malnutrition from starvation, cancer, or other problems negatively impacts wound healing. Exposure to chemicals such as nicotine, which influences peripheral blood flow, smoke toxins, and other substances, impairs wound healing capacity. The use of exogenous steroids also impairs normal wound healing, both through impaired mechanisms for scar tissue formation, as well as impaired ability to fight infection.

Wound healing capacity general diminishes with age. “Scarless” wound healing has been shown to occur normally in the fetus, up to approximately 24 weeks of age. Thereafter, scar formation is a normal part of wound healing, but one’s ability to form scar tissue, and the quality of the collagen being incorporated into those scars, decreases gradually over the course of a lifetime. This is likely due to a number of factors ranging from control of the immune response to an injury, to concentration and number of progenitor/stem cells available to contribute to the healing process, and diminishing quality of cellular function/efficiency over time. This is not only seen with aging, but also with radiation exposures that include sun exposure, as well as therapeutic radiation exposure used to treat cancer or other amenable ailments.

EFFECTS OF MICROBIAL INFECTION ON SOFT-TISSUE HEALING

The disruptive role of infection in healing of all tissue types is well known and will be discussed in greater detail in other chapters of this book. However, the influence of infection on the capability of soft tissues to heal also cannot be understated. All treatment strategies for management of soft-tissue injuries are aimed, in one way or another, at limiting the ability of pathogens to achieve infection of a compromised soft-tissue envelope. Wounds can be colonized with pathogens without actually being infected; however, this occurs when pathogen concentrations/effects are insufficient to generate a meaningful immune response. As soon as the threshold of pathogen concentration is reached that a sufficient immune response is generated, a wound is considered infected. The treatment of wound colonization or infection is an enormous topic that extends beyond the scope of this chapter. However, the role of interventions that include antibiotics and surgical débridement must be considered to eliminate infection and facilitate a return to a more normal state of wound healing, as has been described above.

Colonization and infection of soft-tissue wounds interferes with the normal wound healing process and, if left unchecked, produces further tissue necrosis and will prevent wounds from healing altogether. Surgical débridement helps to eliminate areas of compromised or necrotic tissue that have no defense mechanisms to fight infection. Areas of compromised or necrotic tissue lack access to the body’s immune system and are compromised in their ability to receive systemically administered antibiotics carried in the bloodstream. Antibiotics can be administered systemically (oral, intramuscular, intravenous) and/or locally (AIPMMA beads or spacers, direct antibiotic powder application, etc) to fight pathogens and restore the body’s ability to advance wound healing. Appropriate surgical débridement and judicious selection of antibiotics are critically important tools needed to fight infection and promote wound healing.

INTERVENTIONS

Fortunately, most surgical and traumatic wounds heal uneventfully and rapidly. However, disturbed healing does occur in predictable and sometimes unpredictable settings as described previously. Healing in these situations can be facilitated by certain techniques and interventions.

©Copyright 2021 American Academy of Orthopaedic Surgeons

Tissue handling during surgery and closure limits soft-tissue damage and can promote healing. Specific suturing technique notable the Donati-Allgower vertical buried mattress technique has been shown to maintain the best perfusion to the skin edges and is therefore felt to set optimal conditions to healing.[18]

Limiting subcutaneous dead space through suturing and use of drains is felt to be an important adjunct. Drains are routinely utilized in some types of surgery to decrease the accumulation of fluid subcutaneously. However, drains have also been associated with infection and with inadvertent retention upon attempted removal. There is no consensus on the optimal use of drains.

NEGATIVE PRESSURE WOUND THERAPY

Negative pressure wound therapy has become a widely adopted technique to assist with wound healing both for closed and open wounds.[19,20] In its standard form, an open cell foam is applied to the wound with an occlusive dressing. Subatmospheric pressure between 75 and 125 mm Hg is generated with a pump on an intermittent or continuous basis. Several advantages have been reported with the use of this technique. In addition to sealing the wound providing a barrier to outside contaminants, the pressure gradient withdraws fluids and may decrease interstitial edema.[21-23] Studies have shown an improvement of tissue oxygenation which promotes wound healing and reduces risk of infection.[24] The effects on edema control have been harder to quantify. Clinical series in procedures at risk for wound failure and infection such as pilon, calcaneus, and bicondylar plateau fractures have shown a reduction in wound complications.[25] Similar use in obese patients with acetabular surgery and total hip replacement have shown positive effects.[26-28]

The foundational work for this technique was performed in pigs. In a series of four experiments, Morykwas demonstrated at a pressure of 125 mm Hg (1) blood flow to the wound and surrounding tissue was increased by a factor of 4, (2) granulation tissue was improved with both continuous and intermittent flow (63% and 103% respectively), (3) bacterial clearance was improved in contaminated wounds after dressing removal in 4 days, and (4) random flap survival improved by 21%.[24] Further work is being done to elucidate efficacy in specific clinical scenarios and method of action.[23]

At the cellular level work has shown that under subatmospheric pressure cytokines become modulated to an anti-inflammatory profile with mechanoreceptor and chemoreceptors signaling for vascular growth and generation of extracellular matrix. These effects ultimately promote granulation tissue growth and wound healing.[29] More specifically, TNF is downregulated while VEGF, FGF-2, TGF-β, and PDGF were increased. Interestingly, differences were noted in acute versus chronic wounds; IL-1β was reduced in acute wounds only confirming somewhat different effects in wound types.

OPEN WOUNDS

Wounds that have dehisced or where there is insufficient tissue for skin closure present an altogether different problem. Whether they are acute or chronic, these wounds can be colonized with bacteria or frankly infected. In these settings, healing depends on creating conditions that promote endothelial growth while limiting bacterial proliferation. Healing can be attained by secondary intention with progressive epithelialization and contracture or through delayed primary closure, skin grafting, or flap coverage. No firm criteria exist in regard to the level of colonization acceptable to proceed with closure although in the presence of infection wounds should not be closed.

Chronic wounds have been shown to have an elevated inflammatory state which inhibits healing.[30] Chronic wounds have elevated inflammatory cytokines[31-33] with a prolonged and hyperactive neutrophil response sometimes 100 greater than that seen in acute wounds.[34] The impaired healing is felt to be due to degraded growth factors and impaired cellular adhesion fostered by this inflammatory milieu.[32] Therefore therapies directed at control of this inflammation may promote healing.

Early work demonstrated that a moist environment favored epithelization both in pigs[35] and humans.[36] Other investigators have shown that the moist environment of an occlusive dressing similarly promotes epithelial growth in skin grafts accelerating it by as much as 40%.[37]

Other dressings have been developed to modulate the wound bed by controlling the exudates or directly addressing infection. Collagen forms a key component of extracellular matrix. In its application to wounds as an exogenous product from various sources (bovine, porcine, etc), it can stabilize the wound bed allowing a structure for platelet as well as fibroblast, macrophage, and granulocyte aggregation allowing for hemostasis and healing.[30,38] Bilayer constructs combining collagen with a temporary silastic cover allow for generation of a granulation tissue layer even over limited areas of exposed tendon or bone, which are subsequently skin grafted, as shown in **Figure 6**.[30,39]

A variety of antimicrobials and antiseptic materials have also been used to control bacterial colonization and infection. However, a balance must be maintained between antibacterial efficacy as opposed to toxicity to the regenerating cells lines for healing. Dakin solution, a buffered sodium hypochlorite solution, gained wide use during World War I with continued interest with its ability to control various bacterial infections to include *Staphylococcus aureus*, *Pseudomonas*, *Enterococcus* and *Escherichia coli*.[40] A recent in vitro study has demonstrated the most favorable response at a concentration of 0.00025% in controlling four different mold species with limited cytotoxicity specifically for human keratinocytes, osteoblasts and fibroblasts when compared with amphotericin and mafenide.[41] Various iodine compounds have also been advocated and is commonly used in skin

©Copyright 2021 American Academy of Orthopaedic Surgeons

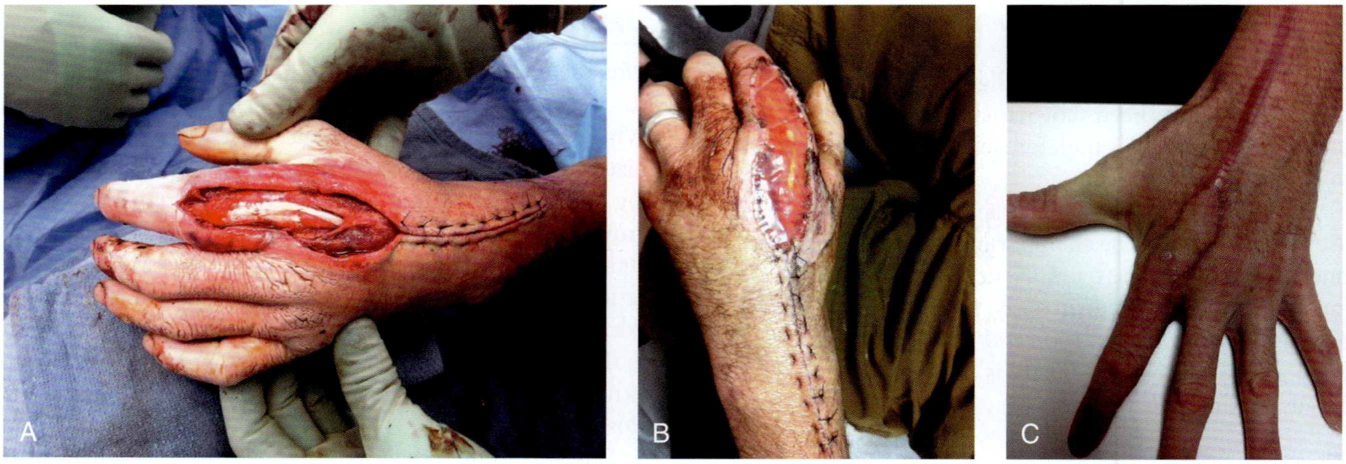

FIGURE 6 Photographs showing hand wound with exposed tendon treated with bilayer silastic/collagen implant—(**A**) wound following débridement, (**B**) applied bilayer implant following granulation tissue ingrowth, and (**C**) healed split-thickness skin graft. (Courtesy of Christopher Got, MD.)

preparation due to its wide spectrum of antibacterial action. However, high iodine concentrations have similarly noted to be cytotoxic. Recent work has shown povidone-iodine is cytotoxic to human skin fibroblasts.[42] At a concentration of 0.01%, growth was retarded, while it was completely arrested at 0.1% (**Table 1**).

Hydrogen peroxide application to wounds is a more complex topic, as it is known to play a role in various cellular functions to include phagocytosis. However, it is thought to be a contributor to chronic wounds when present in higher concentrations. Therefore, its role as an additive in wound treatment has not been fully clarified. Recent work in a rat model demonstrated a delay in wound healing with topical application at 166 mM which is equivalent to clinical use of 0.5% solution. However, by day 8 to 10, no difference was seen compared with controls when looking at wound size.[43] The investigators felt that peroxide increased the proteolytic environment and collagen formation but ultimately did not impair wound healing in this model.

Given the conflicting information on the various topical antimicrobial solutions regarding potential toxicity, it is not possible to provide a firm recommendation which a clinician should use. However, careful clinical observation should direct continued therapy.

TABLE 1 Antiseptic and Antimicrobial Solutions With Concentrations, Mode of Action, and Toxicity

Antiseptic/Antimicrobial/ Antifungal Solution	Concentration Used in Clinical Practice	Mode of Action	Toxicity
Dakin solution (buffered sodium hypochlorite)	0.125%-0.5% ("quarter to full strength")	Germicidal bleaching agent	Decreased neutrophil viability and migration 0.025%-0.00025%[40] Human fibroblast death at 0.5% visibility at 0.005%[40] Mouse fibroblast @0.25%[40]
Iodine solution	1%-10%	Microbicidal against microbial protein and DNA	Fibroblast growth progressively retarded @ 0.01%-0.025%; totally inhibited by 0.1%-1% povidone-iodine solutions[42]
Hydrogen peroxide	<3%	Oxidative	0.5% reduced connective tissue formation[43]
Mafenide (Sulfamylon)	5%	Bacteriostatic, mechanism unknown	50% fibroblast death with 2% solution[41]
Amphotericin	2-20 mg/mL	Binds with fungus cell wall and disrupts it	50% fibroblast death with >30 min exposure to 2 mg/mL[41]

Reproduced with permission from Orthopaedic Trauma Association: Open Fracture Study Group: A new classification scheme for open fractures. *J Orthop Trauma* 2010;24(8):457-464.

©Copyright 2021 American Academy of Orthopaedic Surgeons

SUMMARY

Soft-tissue injuries occur in many different forms, ranging from simple lacerations, to chemical or thermal burns, to degloving and devascularizing lesions such as Morel-Lavallee lesions. Soft-tissue injuries most commonly heal through scar tissue formation, although regeneration can occur to a limited extent, and scarring can occur pathologically with hypertrophic scar and even keloid formation. Wound healing typically occurs in 3 phases: inflammatory, proliferative, and remodeling phases. Each of these phases contributes to the progressive organization of collagen in a manner that restores the integrity of the soft-tissue envelope to the point where it can resume its function as a barrier to microbial infection. An intricate cellular and molecular cascade of events is triggered by trauma to the soft tissues that recruits appropriate cell types to the area of injury that can débride nonviable tissue, reestablish vascularity to the wound bed, gradually build scar tissue, and, in some cases, regenerate the original tissue that was injured. The resultant scar tissue typically does not reach the full tensile strength of the native tissue and often retains an altered appearance.

Efficient and effective soft-tissue healing can be facilitated by surgical débridement, wound edge approximation/repair, and, if necessary, provision of extracellular matrix to facilitate/guide the scar formation process. Many host factors can positively and negatively affect a patient's capacity for soft-tissue healing, ranging from nutritional and metabolic factors that facilitate tissue repair, to autoimmune disorders or immune deficiencies that inhibit healing and promote susceptibility to microbial infection. Techniques ranging from optimal intraoperative soft-tissue handling and suture techniques, to the use of negative pressure wound therapy devices/dressings, and selective use of antimicrobial chemicals and antibiotics can help to optimize conditions for wound healing.

REFERENCES

1. Marshall CD, Hu MS, Leavitt T, Barnes LA, Lorenz HP, Longaker MT: Cutaneous scarring: Basic science, current treatments, and future directions. *Adv Wound Care* 2018;7(2):29-45.
2. Strauss EJ, Petrucelli G, Bong M, Koval KJ, Egol KA: Blisters associated with lower extremity fracture: Results of a prospective treatment protocol. *J Orthop Trauma* 2006;20(9):618-622.
3. Morel-Lavallee VAL: Decollments tramatiques de la peau et des couches sous jacentes. *Archives of General Medicine* 1863;1:20-38, 172-200, 300-332.
4. Scolaro JA, Chao T, Zamorano DP: The morel-lavallee lesion: Diagnosis and management. *JAAOS* 2016;24(10):667-672.
5. Diviti S, Gupta N, Hooda K, Sharma K, Lawrence L: Morel-lavallee lesions – review of pathophysiology, clinical findings, imaging findings, and management. *J Clin Diagn Res* 2017;11(4):1-4.
6. Mellado JM, Bencardino JT: Morel-lavalee lesion: Review with emphasis on MR imaging. *Magn Recon Imaging Clin N Am* 2005;13(4):775-782.
7. Greenhill D, Haydel C, Rehman S: Management of the morel-lavallee lesion. *Orthop Clin N Am* 2016;47:115-125.
8. Yousuf Y, Jeschke MG, Shah A, et al: The response of muscle progenitor cells to cutaneous thermal injury. *Stem Cell Res Ther* 2017;8(234):1-12.
9. Orthopaedic Trauma Association: Open Fracture Study Group: A new classification scheme for open fractures. *J Orthop Trauma* 2010;24(8):457-465.
10. Gustilo RB, Anderson JT: Prevention of infection in the treatment of one thousand and twenty-five open fractures of long bones. *JBJS-Am* 1976;58:453-458.
11. Mathieu D, Marroni A, Kot J: Tenth European Consensus Conference on Hyperbaric Medicine: Recommendations for accepted and non-accepted clinical indications and practice of hyperbaric oxygen treatment. *Diving and Hyperbaric Medicine* 2017;47(1):24-32.
12. Buchanan PJ, Kung TA, Cederna PS: Evidence-based medicine: Wound closure. *Plast Reconstr Surg* 2016;138(3S):257S-270S.
13. Rosenbaum AJ, Banerjee S, Rezak KM, Uhl RL: Advances in wound management. *JAAOS* 2018;26(23):833-843.
14. Hughes OB, Rakosi A, Nacquhae F, Herskovitz I, Fox JD, Kirsner RS: A review of cellular and acellular matrix products: Indications, techniques, and outcomes. *Plast Reconstr Surg* 2016;138(3S):138S-147S.
15. Lee D, Ayoub N, Agrawal DK: Mesenchymal stem cells and cutaneous wound healing: Novel methods to increase cell delivery and therapeutic efficacy. *Stem Cell Res Ther* 2016;7(37):1-8.
16. Balaji S, Kewsani SG, Crombleholme TM: The role of mesenchymal stem cells in the regenerative wound healing phenotype. *Adv Wound Care* 2012;1(4):159-165.
17. Levin LS: Principles of definitive soft tissue coverage with flaps. *J Orthop Trauma* 2008;22(10):S161-S166.
18. Sagi HC, Papp S, Dipasquale T: The effect of suture pattern and tension on cutaneous blood flow as assessed by laser Doppler flowmetry in a pig model. *J Orthop Trauma* 2008;22(3):171-175.
19. Liu DSH, Sofiadellis F, Ashton M, MacGill K, Webb A: Early soft tissue coverage an negative pressure wound therapy optimises patient outcomes in lower limb trauma. *Injury* 2012;43:772-778.
20. Green T, Kavros S, Springer S, Drez D Jr, McCabe M, Gremillion J: Team Approach: Complex dermal wound-healing utilizing negative-pressure wound therapy (NPWT) in orthopaedic trauma. *JBJS Reviews* 2018;6(1):1-8.
21. Wood BC, Molnar JA: Subatmospheric ppressure therapy: Basic science review. *J Surg Orthop Adv* 2011;20(3):168-175.
22. Murphey GC, Macias BR, Hargens AR: Depth of penetration of negative pressure wound therapy into underlying tissues. *Wound Repair Regen* 2009;17(1):113-117.
23. Morykwas MJ, Simpson J, Punger K, Argenta A, Kremers L, Argenta J: Vacuum-assisted closure: State of basic research and physiologic foundation. *Plast Reconstr Surg* 2006;117(7 Suppl):121S-6S.
24. Morykwas MJ, Argenta LC, Shelton-Brown EI, McGuirt W: Vacuum-assisted closure: A new method for wound control and treatment:animal studies and basic foundation. *Ann Plast Surg* 1997;38(6):553-562.
25. Stannard JP, Volgas DA, McGwin G III, et al: Incisional negative pressure wound therapy after high-risk lower extremity fractures. *J Orthop Trauma* 2012;26:37-42.
26. Hansen E, Durinka JB, Costanzo JA, et al: Negative pressure wound therapy is associated with resolution of incisional drainage in most wounds after hip arthroplasty. *Clin Orthop Relat Res* 2013;471:3230-3236.
27. Pachowsky M, Gusinde J, Klein A, et al: Negative pressure wound therapy to prevent seromas and treat surgical incisions after total hip arthroplasty. *Int Orthop* 2012;36:719-722.
28. Reddix RN Jr, Tyler HK, Kulp B, et al: Incisional vacuum-assisted wound closure in morbidly obese patients undergoing acetabular fracture surgery. *Am J Orthop (Belle Mead NJ)* 2009;38:446-449.
29. Glass GE, Murphy GF, Esmaeili A, Lai LM, Nanchahal J: Systematic review of molecular mechanism of action of negative-pressure wound therapy. *Br J Surg* 2014;101(13):1627-1636.

©Copyright 2021 American Academy of Orthopaedic Surgeons

30. Fan K, Tang J, Escandon J, Kirsner RS: State of the art in topical wound-healing products. *Plast Reconstr Surg* 2011;127(suppl 1):44S-59S.
31. Wang XJ, Han G, Owens P, Siddiqui Y, Li AG: Role of TGF beta-mediated inflammation in cutaneous wound healing. *Investig Dermatol Symp Proc* 2006;11:112-117.
32. Trengove NJ, Bielefeldt-Ohmann H, Stacey MC: Mitogenic activity and cytokine levels in non-healing and healing chronic leg ulcers. *Wound Repair Regen* 2000;8:13-25.
33. Wetzler C, Kampfer H, Stallmeyer B, Pfeilschifter J, Frank S: Large and sustained induction of chemokines during impaired wound healing in the genetically diabetic mouse: Prolonged persistence of neutrophils and macrophages during the late phase of repair. *J Invest Dermatol* 2000;115:245-253.
34. Tarnuzzer RW, Schultz GS: Biochemical analysis of acute and chronic wound environments. *Wound Repair Regen* 1996;4:321-325.
35. Winter GD: Formation of the scab and the rate of epithelization of superficial wounds in the skin of the young domestic pig. *Nature* 1962;193:293-294.
36. Hinman CD, Miabach H: Effect of air exposure and occlusion on experimental human skin wounds. *Nature* 1963;200:377-378.
37. Eaglstein WH, Mertz PM: New methods for assessing epidermal wound healing: The effects of triamcinolone acetonide and polyethelene film occlusion. *J Invest Dermatol* 1978;71:382-384.
38. Chattopadhyay S, Raines RT: Collagen-based biomaterials for wound healing. *Biopolymers* 2014;101(8):821-833.
39. Wilkins LM, Watson SR, Prosky SJ, Meunier SF, Parenteau NL: Development of a bilayered living skin construct for clinical applications. *Biotechnol Bioeng* 1994;43:747-756.
40. McCullough M, CarlsonG W: Dakin's solution historical perspective and current practice. *Ann Plast Surg* 2014;73:254-256.
41. Barsoumian A, Sanchez CJ, Mende K, et al: In vitro toxicity and activity of Dakin's solution, mafenide acetate, and amphotericin B on filamentous fungi and human cells. *J Orthop Trauma* 2013;27:428-436.
42. Balin AK, Pratt L: Dilute povidone iodine solution inhibit human skin fibroblast growth. *Dermatol Surg* 2002;28:210-214.
43. Loo AEK, Wong YT, Ho R, et al: Effects of hydrogen peroxide on wound healing in mice in relation to oxidative damage. *PLoS One* 2012;7(11):e49215. doi:10.1371/journal.pone.0049215.

©Copyright 2021 American Academy of Orthopaedic Surgeons

Articular Cartilage Repair: Augmentation, Regeneration, Replacement, and Substitution

Erica G. Gacasan, MS
Robert L. Sah, MD, ScD

Keywords: *autologous chondrocyte implantation; biochemical signals; cartilage; cells; focal defects; joint replacement; microfracture; osteoarthritis; osteochondral; osteochondral grafting; repair; scaffolds*

INTRODUCTION

Throughout adult life, the articular cartilage normally functions as a key component of diarthrodial joints, withstanding years of repetitive loading and facilitating pain-free motion. However, with injury and aging, this cartilage is often damaged. Unfortunately, damaged adult articular cartilage exhibits a limited intrinsic repair response and often deteriorates.[1] Thus, damaged articular cartilage is an attractive candidate for reparative interventions.[2] In general, cartilage repair strategies aim to augment, regenerate, replace, or substitute the damaged or missing tissue. Augmentation strategies seek to generate a tissue, often fibrous and not identical to the articular cartilage, but one that reduces pain and restores some function. In contrast, regenerative strategies aim to elicit a biological response that reforms normal adult articular cartilage. Both strategies use cells, scaffolds, and signals as components which induce or facilitate biological responses, including those that recapitulate development and growth. Repair by tissue replacement entails placement of a tissue graft containing articular cartilage (eg, autograft or allograft). Finally, repair by substitution involves placement of a nonliving prosthetic structure (eg, total joint replacement).

This chapter begins with a brief overview of normal articular cartilage and its poor intrinsic healing response, and then addresses restorative components for damaged cartilage, how they are delivered, the focal defect and osteoarthritic cartilage that are targeted for repair, and strategies for assessing repair. It then summarizes the established surgical procedures for cartilage repair, beginning with the bone marrow stimulation by standard and enhanced microfracture, then covering autologous chondrocyte implantation as it has evolved over multiple generations, and concluding with osteochondral grafts, both autogenic and allogeneic. It then reviews current and emerging strategies for cartilage augmentation, regeneration, or replacement. Emphasized throughout are the biological and biomechanical processes involved in repair within a synovial joint, and how resultant changes lead to measurable structural and functional outcomes.

Dr. Sah or an immediate family member has stock or stock options held in GlaxoSmithKline, Johnson & Johnson, and Medtronic. Neither Ms. Gacasan nor any immediate family member has received anything of value from or has stock or stock options held in a commercial company or institution related directly or indirectly to the subject of this chapter.

©Copyright 2021 American Academy of Orthopaedic Surgeons

KEY POINTS

- Damaged adult articular cartilage does not typically mount an effective repair response.
- The type of cartilage damage targeted for repair is of two main types: focal defects and osteoarthritis.
- The types of cartilage repair that target regeneration and replacement aim to restore the damaged region to normal articular cartilage, mimicking native structural, biochemical, and biomechanical properties; in contrast, cartilage repair by augmentation does not aim to necessarily restore normal tissue, and cartilage repair by substitution inserts a classic inert biomaterial.
- Cartilage repair via augmentation, regeneration, or replacement all use one or more of the following components: cells, chemical and physical signals, and scaffolds.
- Cartilage repair strategies can be classified by their primary therapeutic modality as biomechanical or biological.
- Cartilage repair strategies can also be classified according to their mode of delivery, systemic, local, or surgical.
- Treatments for cartilage damage are used when symptoms persist despite pharmacologic and nonpharmacologic physical interventions.
- Treatment of focal defects by either microfracture, autologous chondrocyte implantation, or osteochondral autograft or allograft is based on the size and location of the defect, quality of the surrounding cartilage, as well as patient age, lifestyle, and presence of comorbidities such as obesity, joint malalignment, and ligamentous instability.
- Experimental studies are underway to develop more effective or readily available treatments for focal cartilage defects, and also to create effective treatments for damaged or eroded cartilage in OA.

ARTICULAR CARTILAGE FUNCTION, STRUCTURE, AND LIMITATIONS OF INTRINSIC REPAIR

Articular cartilage is a hyaline cartilage covering the subchondral bone in diarthrodial joints. This cartilage provides a load-bearing, low-permeability, low-friction, and wear-resistant surface for pain-free joint movement. Regional, site, and depth-dependent variation in tissue organization is critical to normal function under complex loading.[3,4] Healthy adult articular cartilage is composed of resident chondrocytes (~2% v/v), extracellular matrix (~20% to 40% w/w), and water (~60% to 80% w/w).[5] The extracellular matrix is largely comprised of collagen type II (~200 mg/g wet weight) and proteoglycan (~25 mg/g wet weight).[5] The chondrocytes produce and maintain the cartilage matrix, balancing its synthesis and degradation. The collagen network contributes to overall tissue integrity and the resistance of cartilage to tension. Negatively charged proteoglycans, mainly aggrecan, are entrapped within the collagen network and contribute to compressive resistance, providing a high osmotic pressure within the tissue. The relatively high density, charged nature, and binding sites within the extracellular matrix affects storage, partitioning, and transport of solutes, including regulatory factors, nutrients, and waste products through and within the tissue.[6,7] Different types of mechanical stimuli, static and dynamic, compressive and shear, distinctly regulate indwelling cells and matrix turnover. Additionally, the synovial joint, including the articular cartilage, subchondral bone, synovium, and synovial fluid, acts as an interactive organ system. Each joint organ can change with time and interact with the more traditional organ systems. Just as abnormalities of system components cause joint degeneration, repair of components may restore the homeostatic function of joint systems.

Unfortunately, adult articular cartilage exhibits limited intrinsic repair as demonstrated by experimental studies in animal models and supported by clinical observations. Mature articular cartilage is mostly avascular and receives nutrients primarily by diffusion from the synovial fluid. Thus, when lacerated, articular cartilage does not bleed or undergo the classic wound-healing response. The resultant wound repair response is ineffective, with only proliferation of some nearby cells, possibly driven by release of matrix-bound FGF-2.[8] In addition, resident chondrocytes are largely immobilized within the dense extracellular matrix and exhibit limited migration to injured sites. Finally, damaged tissue does not normally secrete sufficient chemotactic factors to attract reparative cells.

Thus, long-standing approaches to stimulating a biologic response to repair cartilage defects involve surgical penetration of the subchondral plate to initiate a cascade of events occurring in particular locations with characteristic times[9] (**Figure 1**). Initially, there is an influx of blood and marrow elements including stem cells and growth factors from the subchondral marrow and vasculature. During and following clot formation, the repair cells undergo the regulated fate processes of differentiation, proliferation, and apoptosis. Subsequently, the repair cells gradually form and maintain the extracellular matrix, ideally to create bulk cartilage tissue with appropriate site-specific and depth-dependent biological and biomechanical properties. Additionally, such cartilaginous tissue should form the appropriate interfaces with the surrounding tissues for the various types of defect repair (**Figure 2**), integrating with adjacent cartilage, transitioning to subchondral bone, and maintaining a lubricated articular surface. Unfortunately, although such stimulated repair exhibits many regenerative features, it does not result in reliable formation of

©Copyright 2021 American Academy of Orthopaedic Surgeons

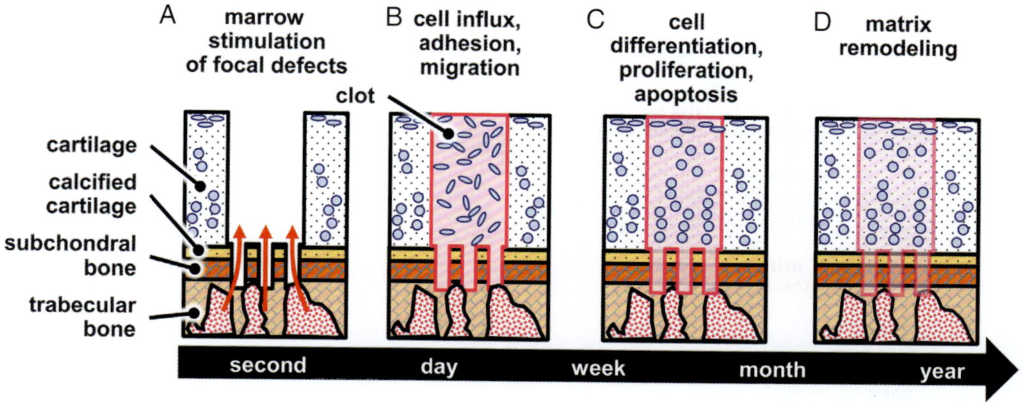

FIGURE 1 Characteristic time frames of focal defect repair by bone marrow stimulation. In microfracture, (**A**) penetration of the subchondral bone plate leads to (**B**) formation of a clot containing cells, growth factors, and matrix molecules. Over time, (**C**) cells remain at the defect site, differentiate, and (**D**) form and maintain the repair tissue.

stable hyaline articular cartilage, but rather a fibrocartilage or inadequate articular-like cartilage that does not fully fill the defect and/or deteriorates in the ensuing months.

COMPONENTS FOR, AND APPROACHES TO, CARTILAGE AUGMENTATION, REGENERATION, AND REPLACEMENT

The goal of many cartilage treatment strategies is to deliver or attract cells, effective in repair and regeneration, within and adjacent to the defect site, to ultimately regenerate normal articular cartilage. Interventions which aim to augment, replace, or regenerate injured tissues often use a variety of components which can be classified as cells, signals, or scaffolds, which enable a biological response (**Figure 3**). Cartilage repair strategies can be classified according to (1) their primary mode of therapeutic action, biomechanical or biological, and (2) their mode of delivery, systemic, local, or surgical (**Table 1**).

Mechanically directed treatment strategies aim to correct abnormal joint loading and joint malalignment or provide mechanically functional (ie, load bearing) tissues or tissue substitutes. Changes in normal loading due to injury, joint laxity, neuromuscular changes, obesity, and varus-valgus malalignment may initiate degenerative pathways leading to cartilage deterioration and osteoarthritis.[10] If identified early, abnormal joint mechanics leading to cartilage deterioration may be ameliorated by improving joint alignment.[11] Surgical interventions such as osteotomy and joint distraction aim to enable intrinsic cartilage repair by either restoring normal joint alignment or decreasing mechanical loading on compromised portions of the joint. Other nonsurgical interventions include orthotics and unloader braces. Conversely, implantation of fully functional tissue, or tissue substitutes, may use autologous or allogeneic grafts, or synthetic implants such as metal and plastic protheses, to resurface joints with widespread deterioration.

Many cartilage regenerative therapies enable a biological response which aim to regenerate the tissue, restore normal structure and function, and may involve cells, scaffolds, and

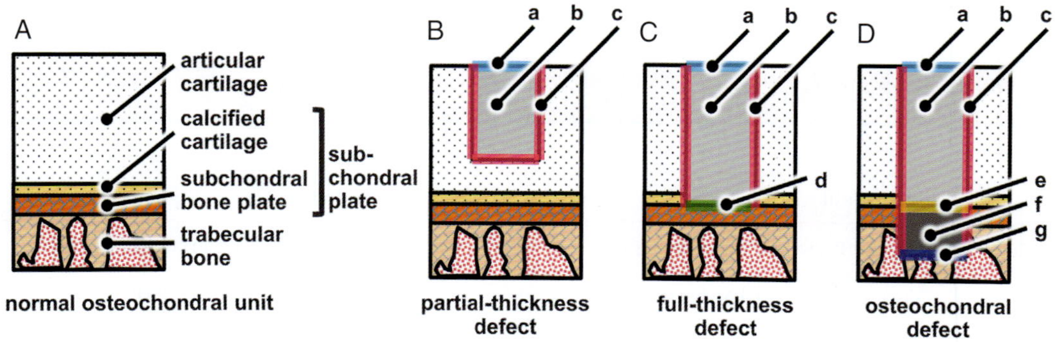

FIGURE 2 Normal osteochondral unit and spatial aspects of repair of cartilage defects. **A**, Normal osteochondral unit. Defects that are (**B**) partial-thickness, (**C**) full-thickness, and (**D**) osteochondral and spatial aspects of repair strategies. Specialized surfaces, tissues, and interfaces include the (a) articular surface, (b) bulk cartilage, (c) interface of repair with host cartilage, (d) interface of repair cartilage with subchondral plate, (e) formation of a bone-cartilage interface, (f) repair of trabecular bone, and (g) interface of repair with host bone.

©Copyright 2021 American Academy of Orthopaedic Surgeons

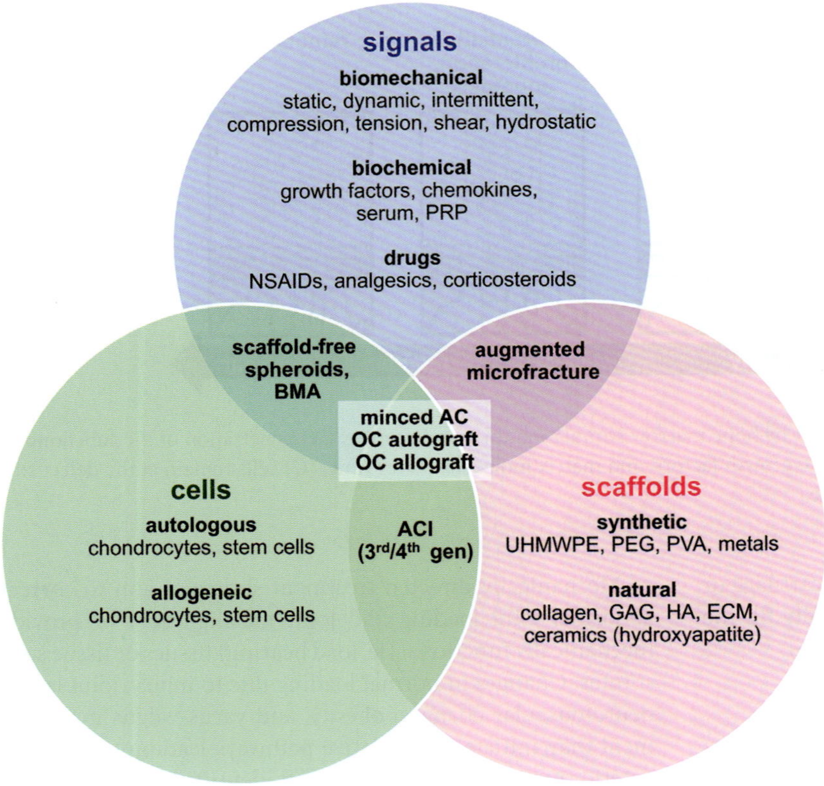

FIGURE 3 Engineered tissue components. Signals, cells, and scaffolds are the major elements of pharmacologic and tissue engineering approaches to cartilage repair. These elements may be used separately, or in combination, to treat symptomology or affect regeneration or restoration of tissue function.

small molecules, individually and in combination. Perforation of the subchondral bone to release a milieu of mesenchymal stem cells and growth factors via bone marrow stimulation techniques is commonly used to incite formation of fibrocartilage repair tissue at the defect site. Similarly, use of platelet-rich plasma (PRP), containing a mixture of platelets, leukocytes, growth factors, and cytokines depending on the formulation, alone or to augment repair, has shown promise, although more clinical studies are necessary.[12] Autologous chondrocyte implantation (ACI), in which autologous chondrocytes are harvested, expanded, and implanted to the defect site, initially developed in the 1990s, has since undergone several generations of development and is a promising cell-based treatment for cartilage lesions.

Combination strategies, which attempt to acutely, mechanically restore function to the tissue as well as enable a long-term functional biological repair, have also been developed. For instance, cell-free osteochondral scaffolds have robust mechanical properties which rapidly restore mechanical function but also contain osteoconductive scaffolding, which allows for bone growth and integration of the implant with host tissue.

Depending on the biological components used, human cells, tissues, and cellular-based products (HCT/Ps) may be designated as "minimally manipulated" by the United States FDA. Minimally manipulated products are those that have not altered the original relevant characteristics of the tissue or cell-type relating to its utilization for homologous reconstruction,

TABLE 1 Repair Strategies to Treat (osteo)chondral Lesions

Mode of delivery	Therapy: Mechanical	Therapy: Biological
Systemic	Exercise/PT, weight loss, orthotics	NSAIDs, analgesics, nutritional supplements
Local	Viscosupplements, CPM, braces	Corticosteroids, stem cells, PRP
Surgical	Osteotomy, allografts, autografts, total/partial joint replacement	Bone marrow stimulation, ACI, minced cartilage, joint distraction

Repair strategies can be classified according to their primary therapeutic mode of action, biomechanical or biological, and also by mode of delivery (systemic, local, or surgical). ACI = autologous chondrocyte implantation, CPM = continuous passive motion, PRP = platelet-rich plasma , PT = physical therapy

©Copyright 2021 American Academy of Orthopaedic Surgeons

TABLE 2 Acellular Scaffold-based Therapies to Treat (osteo)chondral Lesions

Product	Company	Material	Procedure	Market Status
Agili-C	Cartiheal (Kfar Saba, Israel)	Hyaluronan, aragonite	Cell-free osteochondral scaffold	✔(Europe), clinical trials (USA)
BioCartilage	Arthrex (Naples, FL, USA)	Allogeneic cartilage matrix	Augmented microfracture	✔
BioPoly RS	BioPoly (Fort Wayne, IN, USA)	Ultra-high-molecular-weight polyethylene	Focal defect repair	✔ (Europe), clinical trials (USA)
BST-CarGel	Smith & Nephew (London, UK)	Chitosan	Augmented microfracture	✔ (Canada, Europe)
Cartifill	Sewon Cellontech (Seoul, South Korea)	Collagen	Augmented microfracture	Withdrawn
Cartilage allograft matrix	MTF Biologics (Edison, NJ, USA)	Allogeneic cartilage matrix	Augmented microfracture	✔
Cartiva	Cartiva (Alpharetta, GA, USA)	Polyvinyl alcohol	Metatarsophalangeal joint replacement	✔
Chondrofix	Zimmer Biomet (Warsaw, IN, USA)	Devitalized osteochondral allograft	Osteochondral allograft	✔
GelrinC	Regentis Biomaterials (Haifa, Israel)	Poly(ethylene glycol)–modified fibrinogen	Augmented microfracture	✔ (Europe), clinical trials (USA)
HemiCap Classic	Arthrosurface (Franklin, MA, USA)	Metal	Focal defect repair	✔
Hyalofast	Anika Therapeutics (Bedford, MA, USA)	Hyaluronan	Augmented microfracture	✔ (Europe), clinical trials (USA)
Maioregen	Fin-ceramica (Faenza, Italy)	Collagen I, hydroxyapatite	Cell-free osteochondral scaffold	✔ (Europe)
Trufit CB	Smith& Nephew (London, UK)	Poly(glycolic acid), poly(lactic-co-glycolic acid), calcium sulfate	Cell-free osteochondral scaffold	Withdrawn

repair, or replacement and do not require premarket approval by the FDA.[13] If a HCT/P does not qualify as minimally manipulated, it may be classified as a drug, device, or biologic material and are subjected to the requisite regulations. Many acellular (**Table 2**) and cellular (**Table 3**) products targeting cartilage repair have been developed, are currently marketed, or are in development.

FOCAL DEFECTS AND OSTEOARTHRITIC DEGENERATION AS TARGETS FOR ARTICULAR CARTILAGE REPAIR

FOCAL DEFECTS

The current articular cartilage repair strategies address focal defects, some of which are large. Of the six types of synovial joints, hinge (eg, knee, ankle, finger) and spherical joints (eg, hip, shoulder) are currently targets for biological intervention.[14-18] Other synovial joints include pivot, saddle, plane, and condyloid joints. Joint motion, either translation or rotation, is constrained by joint geometry and surrounding tissue structures. The incidence of joint pathologies is in part dependent on joint type and motion, age, anatomic location, as well as other risk factors including genetics, joint malalignment, and ligamentous instability. Joint pathologies including articular cartilage encompass osteoarthritis, focal chondral defects, chondromalacia patellae, osteochondritis dissecans, acetabular impingement, joint malalignment, and other types.[19]

Focal chondral and osteochondral defects are injuries or areas of degeneration which are limited to a defined focal area. Focal defects may occur because of acute traumatic injury causing compression, shear, or both, disorders of the bone or cartilage, including subchondral osteonecrosis, or may be idiopathic. Defects can present as (1) partial-thickness chondral defects where damage is restricted to the chondral layer and where resurfacing of the articular cartilage may be helpful, (2) full-thickness chondral defects extending completely to the calcified cartilage or subchondral bone, and (3) osteochondral defects which affect both the cartilage and underlying bone where repair may

©Copyright 2021 American Academy of Orthopaedic Surgeons

TABLE 3 Cell-based Therapies to Treat (osteo)chondral Lesions

Product	Company	Cells	Material	3D Culture Conditions	Procedure	Market Status
CAIS	DePuy Mitek (Raynham, MA, USA)	Autologous chondrocytes	Minced autologous cartilage product	–	–	Withdrawn
CaReS	Arthrokinetics (Esslingen, Germany)	Autologous chondrocytes	Collagen I scaffold	10-13 d in autologous serum	Autologous chondrocyte implantation (third generation)	Withdrawn
Carticel	Genzyme Biosurgery (Cambridge, MA, USA)	Autologous chondrocytes	–	–	Autologous chondrocyte implantation (first generation)	Withdrawn
Cartiform	Arthrex (Naples, FL, USA)	Allogeneic chondrocytes	Osteochondral allograft	–	–	✔
CartiLife	Biosolution (Seoul, South Korea)	Autologous chondrocytes	Autologous ECM	–	Autologous chondrocyte implantation (fourth generation)	Phase 2 clinical trials (USA)
CartiMax	MTF Biologics (Edison, NJ, USA)	Allogeneic chondrocytes	Cartilage allograft matrix	–	–	✔
Cartistem	Medipost (Seoul, South Korea)	Allogeneic umbilical cord MSCs	–	–	Subchondral drilling	Phase 2 clinical trials (USA), approved in Korea
ChondroCelect	Tigenix (Haasrode, Belgium)	Autologous chondrocytes	–	–	Autologous chondrocyte implantation (first generation)	Withdrawn
Chondrosphere/ Spherox	Co.Don AG (Teltow, Germany)	Autologous chondrocytes (2×10^5 cells/ spheroid; 10-70 spheroids/cm^2)	Autologous ECM	14 d as cell spheroids	Autologous chondrocyte implantation (fourth generation)	✔ (Europe)
DeNovo NT	Zimmer Biomet (Warsaw, IN, USA)	Allogeneic chondrocytes	Minced allogeneic cartilage product	–	–	✔
Hyalograft-C	Anika Therapeutics (Bedford, MA, USA)	Autologous chondrocytes (1×10^6 cells/cm^2)	Hyaluronic acid ester scaffold (HYAFF-11S)	14 d	Autologous chondrocyte implantation (third generation)	Withdrawn
MACI	Genzyme Biosurgery (Cambridge, MA, USA)	Autologous chondrocytes ($0.5\text{-}1.0 \times 10^6$ cells/cm^2)	Collagen I/III scaffold	3 d in autologous serum	Autologous chondrocyte implantation (third generation)	✔
NeoCart	Histogenics (Waltham, MA, USA)	Autologous chondrocytes	Honeycomb collagen I scaffold	7 d in bioreactor culture (high pressure, oxygen concentration, perfusion), 3D static culture for 2-4 wk	Autologous chondrocyte implantation (fourth generation)	Phase 3 clinical trials (USA)

 ©Copyright 2021 American Academy of Orthopaedic Surgeons

TABLE 3 Cell-based Therapies to Treat (osteo)chondral Lesions (Continued)

Product	Company	Cells	Material	3D Culture Conditions	Procedure	Market Status
Novocart	TETEC GmbH (Reutlingen, Germany)	Autologous chondrocytes	–	–	Autologous chondrocyte implantation (first generation)	Withdrawn
Novocart 3D	TETEC GmbH (Reutlingen, Germany)	Autologous chondrocytes ($0.5\text{-}3.0 \times 10^6$ cells/cm^2)	Biphasic collagen scaffold with chondroitin sulfate	2 d in autologous serum	Autologous chondrocyte implantation (third generation)	Phase 3 clinical trials (USA)
ProChondrix	Allosource (Centennial, CO, USA)	Allogeneic chondrocytes	Osteochondral allograft	–	–	✔
Tissue Gene-C/ Invossa	Kolon TissueGene (Rockville, MD, USA)	Allogeneic chondrocytes (18×10^6 cells/3.5 mL, virally transduced to express TGF-β)	–	–	IA injection	Phase 3 clinical trials (USA)

ECM = extracellular matrix, MSC = mesenchymal stem cell

involve interaction with, or penetration of, the subchondral plate (**Figure 2**). Defects may present as softened or partially eroded tissue and are classified according to size and geometry.[19]

Decision-making algorithms to treat cartilage injury include size of the defect and quality of the surrounding cartilage as well as patient age, lifestyle, and presence of comorbidities such as obesity, joint malalignment, and ligamentous instability. In conjunction with specific patient characteristics, treatment options for cartilage defects are generally categorized according to "small" (<2 to 4 cm^2) and "large" (>2 to 4 cm^2) lesions[17] (**Figure 4**). In addition to defect size, interventional algorithms may consider patient age and lifestyle or may require correction of comorbidities.

Surgical management of cartilage defects can be accomplished by minimally invasive arthroscopic procedures or by traditional open approaches to enable cartilage repair by bone marrow stimulation or by providing a scaffold or graft which is capable of coordinating repair. Microfracture, biopsies, and delivery of small tissue grafts can be accomplished

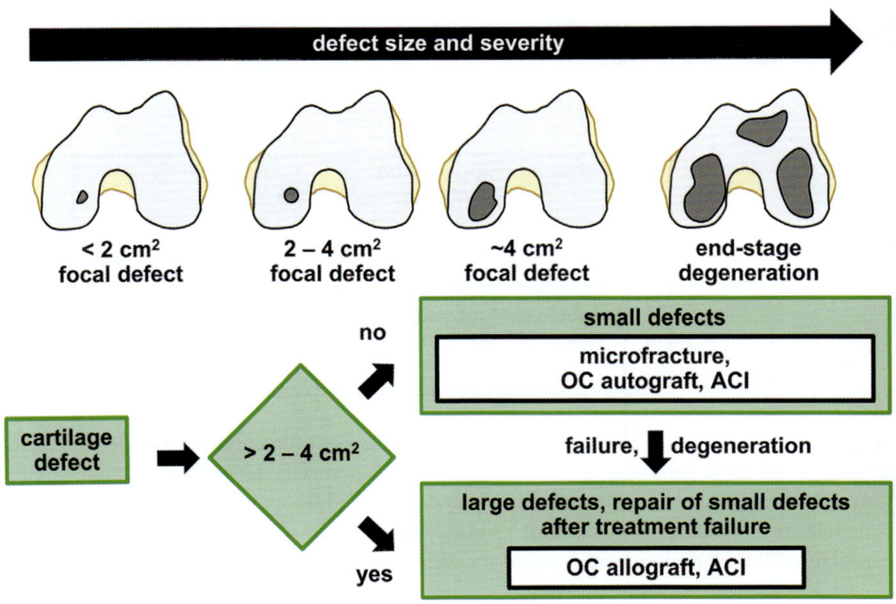

FIGURE 4 Severity and management of focal defects. Small focal defects may degenerate, extend, and coalesce into larger lesions. The type of surgical treatment for symptomatic of cartilage defects is chosen according to lesion size and previous treatments.

©Copyright 2021 American Academy of Orthopaedic Surgeons

via arthroscopy. Other arthroplasty techniques such as large auto- or allografts, partial or total joint replacement, and ACI implantation procedures can be accomplished by (mini-) arthrotomy. Open surgeries can also be used to enhance joint alignment by osteotomy or joint distraction.

OSTEOARTHRITIS

Osteoarthritis (OA) is characterized by joint degeneration due to progressive loss of articular cartilage and pathophysiologic remodeling including fibrocartilage formation, sclerosis of subchondral bone, and osteophyte formation and is diagnosed based on clinical and radiological features, as well as arthroscopic findings[20,21] (**Figure 5**). Accordingly, there are a variety of grading systems which categorize OA extent,[22] and describe function.[23] The prevalence of OA increases with age and tends to affect more women than men. Of adults 55 years or older, 67% of women and 55% of men had radiographic OA of the hand, and in people older than 80 years, 53% of women and 33% of men had radiographic osteoarthritis of the knee.[21] The natural history of OA appears to involve an interaction between cartilage, bone, and synovial tissue. In early OA, chondrocyte efforts to repair damaged tissue are countered by increased matrix metalloproteinases and aggrecanases, as well as chondrocyte senescence and apoptosis.[21,24] In addition, subchondral bone changes, including sclerosis, cyst formation, bone attrition, bone marrow lesions, and osteophyte formation, often occur before and during late-stage cartilage degeneration. Changes in cartilage and bone are accompanied by synovial inflammation and production of catabolic and proinflammatory mediators that can regulate chondrocyte-mediated repair. Such biological barriers to repair are compounded by normal loading of the joint.

Treatment of OA may be useful over the continuum of disease but is typically initiated when symptoms persist despite escalating conservative measures (**Figure 5**). Initial treatment for OA is with pharmacologic (oral analgesics) and nonpharmacologic physical (weight loss, physical therapy, use of devices including braces and aids) interventions. For patients with medial compartment OA of the knee, osteotomy may be performed.[25] End-stage OA is typically managed by joint replacement,[18] whereas joint distraction has shown promise as a salvage procedure, inducing functional tissue repair.[11]

Nonsurgical pharmacologic and nonpharmacologic treatment guidelines for OA have been published by professional organizations including the American College of Rheumatology[26] and the American Academy of Orthopaedic Surgeons.[27] Although the guidelines are generally similar, some recommendations vary between organizations.[28] Pharmacological management of OA may

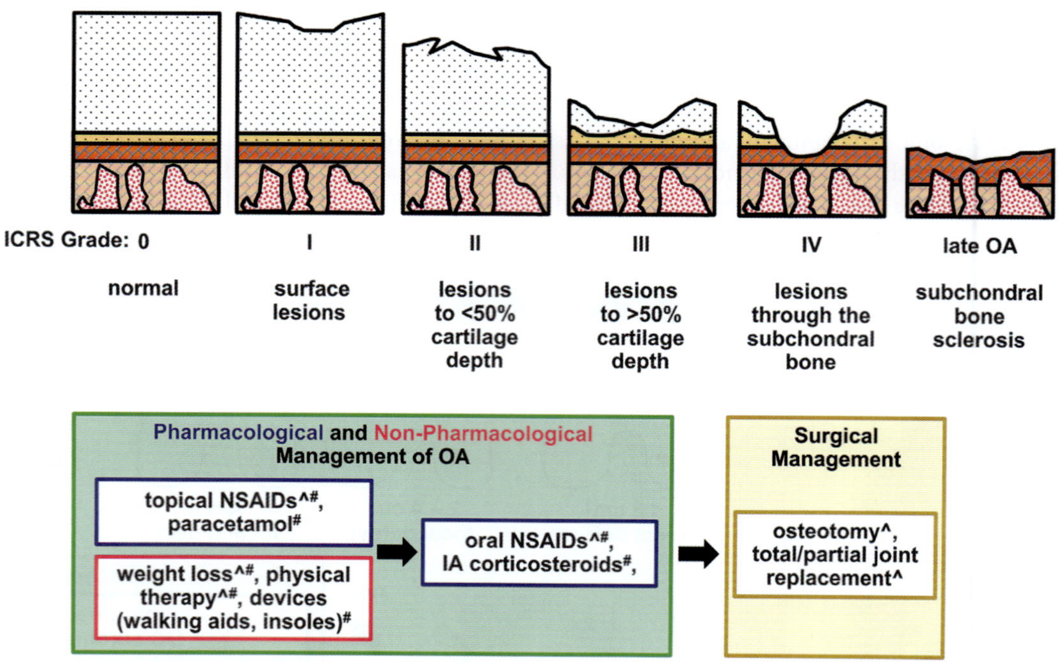

FIGURE 5 Stages of articular cartilage degeneration and management of osteoarthritis. The ICRS grading system of chondral lesions in osteoarthritis is based on arthroscopic appearance of the cartilage surface as (grade 0) normal, (grade 1) nearly normal, (grade 2) abnormal, and (grade 3, 4) severely abnormal as determined by lesion depth. In addition, late-stage OA is characterized by complete loss of cartilage and subchondral bone sclerosis. Symptomology of OA is primarily managed by a combination of pharmacological and nonpharmacological interventions until partial or total joint replacement is necessary, although clinical guidelines may vary. ^ Ref. 27. # Ref. 26.

©Copyright 2021 American Academy of Orthopaedic Surgeons

be delivered by oral or intravenous systemic administration of pharmacological agents. Currently, oral and topical agents are limited to palliative treatments which manage symptomatic inflammation (NSAIDs) and pain (analgesics) but do not modify the damaged cartilage Additionally, although improved joint health has been attributed to the use of oral nutritional supplements, including glucosamine and chondroitin, long-term human clinical studies show limited effects.[29]

Therapeutic agents, such as cell-therapies, viscosupplements, and medications, may be administered directly to the joint by intra-articular (IA) injection. Symptomatic knee OA may be managed by IA injection of viscosupplements and corticosteroids. However, joint-space residence is limited by permeability of the synovium, which increases substantially after injury and with active disease, including OA.[7] Therefore, although viscosupplementation of the joint with hyaluronic acid is widely used to improve joint lubrication and shock absorption for patients with knee OA, there is limited clinical evidence supporting enhanced function.[30] Similarly, the effect of IA injection of long-acting glucocorticoids has been shown to diminish after 1 week.[21] Investigational studies involving IA injection of biological products such as stem cells or other cell types, and PRP which may augment existing repair strategies are also limited.

STRATEGIES FOR ASSESSING CARTILAGE REPAIR

Accompanying the development of strategies for cartilage repair are an array of metrics and methodologies to assess repair mechanisms, treatment effectiveness, and overall joint health (**Figure 6**; **Table 4**). Commonly used patient-reported measures of joint function can be performed before and after an intervention and may include dimensions to assess pain, function, health-related quality of life, and activity level.[23] Conversely, although measures of knee function are useful in determination of patient satisfaction, they do not assess the quality of repair tissue. Evaluation of the repair-site by imaging modalities such as MRI and CT, with and without contrast, and ultrasonography are useful noninvasive methods of determining tissue structure and composition and to assess mechanisms of cartilage repair and joint homeostasis.[31] In addition, biochemical analysis of fluids, including urine, blood, and synovial fluid, may be used to identify byproducts of joint degeneration and assess the metabolic state of the body or joint. Arthroscopic technologies which evaluate biochemical composition and load-bearing properties of cartilage are also in development.

Histological examination of repair tissue biopsies, in addition to macroscopic, biochemical, and biomechanical

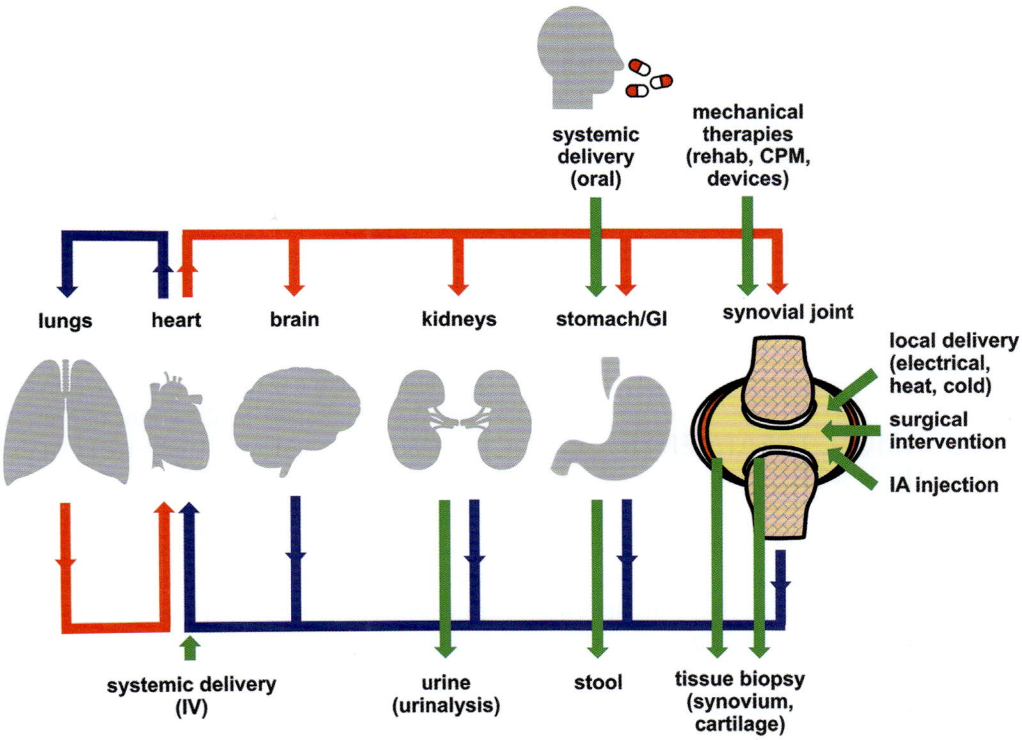

FIGURE 6 Organ system and whole-body model of transport to, and from, synovial joints. Different metrics and methodologies can be used to assess cartilage and overall joint health, before and after therapeutic interventions. Monitoring and sampling can facilitate evaluation of the general state of the body as well as the condition of specific sites within the joint or repair tissue.

©Copyright 2021 American Academy of Orthopaedic Surgeons

TABLE 4 Assessment of Cartilage Repair Therapies

Method of Evaluation	Invasive (−/+)	Destructive (−/+)	Mechanical Function	Structure	Composition/ Metabolites
Patient-reported measures of knee function (pain, function, quality of life, activity level)	−	−	✔		
Gait analysis	−	−	✔		
MRI (+contrast)	−	−		✔	(✔)
CT (+contrast)	−	−		✔	(✔)
Ultrasonography	−	−		✔	
Clinical urine/blood tests	−	−			✔
Arthrocentesis	+	−			✔
Tissue indentation (arthroscopic)	+	−	✔	✔	
Tissue biopsy	+	+		✔	✔

Evaluation methods include clinical outcome measures, imaging, and sampling of tissues and fluids. Such methods may be invasive or destructive and reflect mechanical function, tissue structure, composition, and metabolism.

analysis, is an integral component of in vivo preclinical animal studies for cartilage regeneration and occasionally used in clinical studies. Such analysis helps to elucidate the nature and underlying mechanisms of neo-tissue formation. In the clinical setting, if biopsied tissues are available, histological grading systems which assess tissue fill, structure, and cellularity of the repair are useful for determining the structure and composition of specific sites within repair tissue.[22] The interpretation of biopsy results is naturally limited by the method of sampling and in situ variability of repair within the repair site. Histological examination of tissues which represent the general state of the joint (ie, the synovium), or analysis of metabolites by fluid (ie, synovial fluid, blood, urine) analysis, may be more helpful in assessing global effects of a repair or therapeutic on joint inflammation and degradation.

ESTABLISHED SURGICAL TREATMENTS FOR DAMAGED CARTILAGE

A variety of surgical treatments are available, and many enhanced recently, to address chondral and osteochondral lesions associated with focal defects and osteoarthritis. Augmentation techniques include microfracture and other bone marrow stimulation techniques which bolster degenerated tissue but do not recreate the normal structure of articular cartilage. Regenerative techniques, which elicit a biological response to enable repair and intend to recapitulate the normal cartilage structure, include autologous chondrocyte transplantation as well as many of the next-generation strategies in development. In addition, osteochondral replacement and substitution strategies, including auto- and allografting techniques as well as prosthetic joint replacement, have been used extensively.

BONE MARROW STIMULATION

For symptomatic defects of small size (<2 cm^2), bone marrow stimulation by breach of the subchondral bone through various methods including microfracture microdrilling, and other methods, is typically a first-line treatment because of the relatively low cost and straightforward technique compared with other surgical interventions. Marrow stimulation leverages the intrinsic cartilage repair response after subchondral bone penetration.[22,32]

Microfracture, developed by Steadman et al in the 1980s, involves débridement at the defect site and then perforation of subchondral bone with an awl to create an array of small holes spaced ~3 mm apart to allow flow of bone marrow elements and blood into the defect[32,33] (**Figure 1**). At the defect, the marrow clots and provides a structural framework upon which repair can occur. However, lack of control on the differentiation process often leads to variable suboptimal fibrocartilage repair tissue with inferior biochemical and biomechanical properties having a higher proportion of type I collagen than hyaline cartilage. In a long-term follow-up study of microfracture of patients younger than 45 years with traumatic full-thickness chondral defects without accompanying ligament or meniscal injuries, Steadman et al reported that patients had improvement in clinical outcome measures including decreased pain and swelling and increased function after 7 years.[33] However, in a study of 85 consecutive patients undergoing microfracture, patients older than 40 years had worse cartilage repair

©Copyright 2021 American Academy of Orthopaedic Surgeons

scores (ICRS scoring system, modified Cincinnati score) compared with patients younger than 40 years, with evidence of tissue deterioration over time.[34] Factors affecting outcome of microfracture procedures include age, duration of symptoms, lesion size, body mass index, pre- and postoperative activity level, pervious surgery, and repair cartilage volume.[32]

Advances in microfracture involve augmentation with biomaterial scaffolds which help stabilize clot formation and promote chondrogenesis and formation of hyaline cartilage. Augmented microfracture products, which have undergone clinical trials in the United States and internationally, include micronized allogeneic cartilage (BioCartilage; Arthrex), as well as chitosan (BST-CarGel; Smith & Nephew), collagen (CartiFill; SewonCellontech), hyaluronan scaffold (Hyalofast; Anika Therapeutics), and mixed natural/synthetic products (GelrinC; Regentis Biomaterials). These products are used in a single-step procedure sometimes called autologous matrix-induced chondrogenesis (AMIC). AMIC combines microfracture with placement of a biomaterial scaffold to enable blood and marrow elements to infiltrate and clot within scaffold. In a 12-month randomized control trial comparing AMIC with BST-CarGel and microfracture alone, BST-CarGel significantly improved imaging results and clinical outcomes.[35]

AUTOLOGOUS CHONDROCYTE IMPLANTATION

Autologous chondrocyte implantation (ACI), or autologous chondrocyte transplantation, was the first commercially marketed cell-based therapy for cartilage regeneration. ACI is a two-stage procedure involving arthroscopic biopsy of cartilage from a non–load-bearing area, isolation and in vitro expansion of chondrocytes, and implantation of the cartilage suspension into the defect site (**Figure 7**). Indications for ACI are mixed and may be used for treatment of full-thickness injuries (>2 cm^2) as a primary intervention or in patients who have failed another primary intervention.[36] Cartilage (200 to 300 mg) is harvested from healthy tissue, and the sample is sent to a commercial GMP (cGMP) facility to isolate and expand chondrocytes in vitro. The final product is a liquid suspension of cells, 5 × 10^6 cells in 100 μL/vial with one or two vials used/defect,[37] or cell-laden scaffold, ~2 × 10^6 cells/cm^2,[38] which is extensively tested for chondrocyte morphology, sterility, viability, and endotoxins before it is shipped for implantation in the second stage.

First developed in the 1990s by Brittberg et al,[37] ACI evolved from successful preclinical studies in a rabbit model.[39] ACI has undergone several generations of

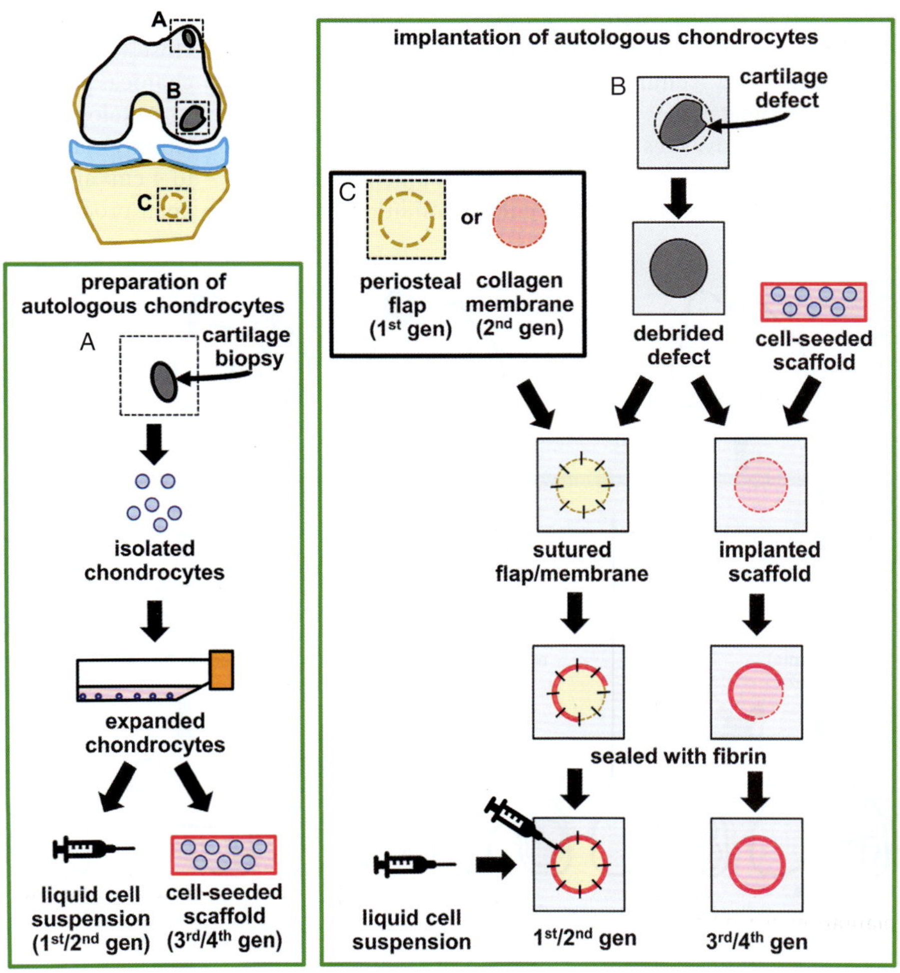

FIGURE 7 Preparation and implantation of autologous chondrocytes in first- to fourth-generation therapies. ACI techniques involve a two-stage process involving (1) isolation and preparation of autologous chondrocytes and (2) subsequent implantation. Initially, (**A**) cartilage is harvested, and the chondrocytes are isolated, expanded, and prepared either as a liquid cell suspension (for first- or second-generation ACI) or cell-seeded scaffold (for third- or fourth-generation ACI). Implantation of first- or second-generation ACI involves (**B**) preparation of the defect, (**C**) periosteal harvest (for first-generation ACI), suturing of the periosteum or collagen membrane over the defect, application of fibrin glue, and implantation of chondrocytes as a liquid cell suspension. Implantation of third- or fourth-generation ACI involves placement of a cell-seeded scaffold, adherence with fibrin (without membrane coverage).

©Copyright 2021 American Academy of Orthopaedic Surgeons

development wherein the method of in vitro expansion and anchorage to the defect site during the secondary procedure has varied.[36] In its inception, ACI involved suturing of harvested periosteum from the distal femur or proximal tibia over the defect, and implantation of chondrocytes by syringe through the periosteal flap. Proprietary first-generation products include, but are not limited to, Carticel (Genzyme Biosurgery), ChondroCelect (Tigenix), and Novocart (Tetec) which differ in their expansion and preparation of the autologous chondrocyte suspension. However, to reduce complexity and potential complications, second-generation ACI procedures employed purpose-designed collagen membranes such as Chondro-Gide (Geistlich Biomaterials) instead of periosteum.

Third-generation ACI techniques progressed from liquid-suspension preparations of autologous chondrocytes and instead expanded chondrocytes are seeded onto biomaterial scaffolds. Matrix-assisted chondrocyte transplantation (MACT) allows for culture of chondrocytes in a more physiologically relevant environment and facilitates a simpler, more rapid, and less morbid operation by removing the need for periosteal harvest or membrane suturing. During the procedure, the cellular scaffold is trimmed to size and fixed into the defect site with fibrin glue or sutures. Third-generation ACI procedures include MACI (Genzyme Biosurgery), Hyalograft C (Anika Therapeutics), CaReS (Arthrokinetics), and Novocart 3D (Tetec), among others, which differ in their preparation and culture of autologous chondrocytes and choice of biomaterial.

Additional advances in bioreactor design and cell-culture methodologies have resulted in the development of fourth-generation ACI techniques where culture conditions facilitate extracellular matrix production and preservation of chondrogenic phenotype. For instance, Neocart (Histogenics) comprises a collagen scaffold seeded with expanded autologous chondrocytes which are cultured in a biomimetic bioreactor, involving hydrostatic pressure, perfusion, and hypoxia to increase cell proliferation and matrix production, for 1 week in addition to a 2- to 4-week static culture period.[38] Also, cell-spheroid–based ACI techniques (Chondrosphere, Co.Don; CartiLife, Biosolution), where autologous chondrocytes are cultivated into spheroids containing cell aggregates and autologous cartilage-like extracellular matrix, have been developed.[38] Although third- and fourth-generation products have shown significant improvements, limitations of all ACI methodologies include high cost due to in vitro cell expansion in a cGMP facility and fragility of the initial repair tissue.

OSTEOCHONDRAL GRAFTING

Osteochondral grafting involves transfer of intact osteochondral units from either autologous sources or allogeneic cadaver sources to full-thickness cartilage defects to replace damaged tissue and restore normal load-bearing function (**Figure 8**). Osteochondral grafts consist of full-thickness articular cartilage and a layer of attached subchondral bone. Such grafting of intact hyaline cartilage closely replaces the lost tissue and restores normal biomechanical properties.

Autologous grafts, either by single or multiple (mosaicplasty) plugs, is generally used to resurface focal defects 1 to 4 cm^2 and can be accomplished arthroscopically, or as an open procedure. Osteochondral autografting has been used

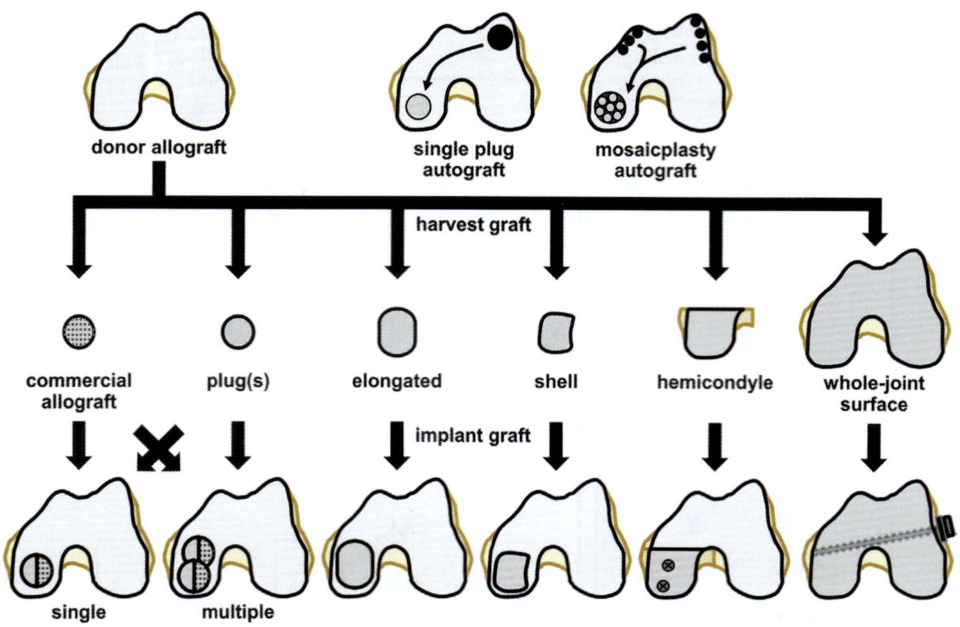

FIGURE 8 Osteochondral grafting techniques. Depending on the size of the defect, osteochondral lesions may be treated with osteochondral autografts or osteochondral allografts. Autologous grafts, consisting of single or multiple (mosaicplasty) plugs, are generally used to resurface focal defects 1 to 4 cm^2. Osteochondral allograft transplantation involves the transfer of size-matched tissue from a cadaveric donor, into defects >2 cm^2, where the type of allograft depends on lesion size and severity.

©Copyright 2021 American Academy of Orthopaedic Surgeons

to treat lesions of the femoral condyles, patellofemoral joint, talus, humeral capitular, and femoral head.[40] However, treatment size is limited by donor-site availability. Histological evaluation of transplanted tissue indicates survival of hyaline cartilage after transplantation, formation of a hyaline-to-fibrocartilage transition area between grafts, deep matrix integration of the transplanted cartilage with surrounding tissues, and at the donor site, voids become filled with cancellous bone and capped with fibrocartilage repair tissue by 8 weeks.[40] Although donor-site morbidity and lack of lateral mechanical support of the grafts remains a concern, a systematic review of osteochondral autograft transplantation indicated that of nine studies with 607 patients, patients undergoing autograft transplantation had better clinical results, with faster return to sport and lower failure rates, compared with microfracture.[41]

Osteochondral allograft transplantation involves the transfer of size-matched allograft tissue from a cadaveric donor, into chondral and osteochondral defects (>2 cm^2) which are not suitable for marrow stimulation or autograft procedures. Allografts have been used to treat lesions on the knee including of the femoral condyles, femoral trochlea, patella, and tibial plateau as well as other joints including the femoral head, glenoid, and talus due to trauma, tumor, osteoarthritis, osteonecrosis, avascular necrosis, and other conditions and restore both the hyaline cartilage as well as associated bone abnormalities.[42] To ensure fit, the lesion location, size, and the overall shape and contour of the joint are assessed such that a size-matched graft can be harvested from the donor. Depending on defect size and severity, allograft morphology may range from a single osteochondral plug to massive osteoarticular allografts (**Figure 8**). Historically, free-hand shell allografts have been used for cartilage resurfacing; however, this technique has become superseded by instrumentation and techniques which accommodate larger graft sizes. For instance, the BioUni System (Arthrex) enables harvesting large elongated grafts rather than using multiple overlapping osteochondral plugs.[43]

During allograft transplantation, donor tissue is commonly prepared by storage of the tissue for up to 28 days before implantation and removal of bone marrow elements by lavage.[42,44] Once implanted, the hyaline cartilage is expected to survive transplantation, while the osseous portion acts as an osteoconductive scaffold supporting replacement of graft bone with host bone, through a process known as "creeping substitution." A systematic review of osteochondral allograft transplantation in the knee found that good clinical outcomes with high patient satisfaction rate (86%) and low short-term complications (2.4%) were reported after 5 years with more favorable outcomes associated with younger patients, traumatic and idiopathic etiologies, and unipolar treatment.[42] Despite positive outcomes, widespread application of allografts is limited because of allograft cost, availability, and possibility of disease transmission. To increase availability, nonorthotopic sites (lateral femoral condyle for medial femoral condyle defect sites)[45] and enhanced media to extend storage (by inclusion of dexamethasone)[46] have been recently introduced.

For all grafting techniques, proper graft placement and maintenance of chondrocyte viability is necessary to successful outcomes. Development of abnormal stresses between the graft surface, adjacent grafts and tissues, and opposing articulating surfaces may inhibit healing and lead to graft failure and joint deterioration.[47,48] In addition, conservation of chondrocyte viability during graft storage, in the case of allografts, and graft insertion is necessary for success. It has been demonstrated that with prolonged storage and freezing, cartilage may fissure, delaminate, and cause chondrocyte death,[44] and that successive impact insertion of grafts negatively affects viability.[49]

ALTERING JOINT BIOMECHANICS

Osteotomy

Unloading of a localized area of the joint, as in osteotomy, aims to induce structural changes to the cartilage and bone to improve function and reduce disease progression. Joint malalignment leading to abnormal joint mechanics has been shown to lead to cartilage deterioration. For patients with isolated medial OA, high tibial osteotomy (HTO) aims to reduce supraphysiologic loads on the medial compartment of the knee by improving joint alignment. Long-term survivorship of HTO, of studies reported between 1999 and 2008, ranges from 50% to 95% after 10 years with failure associated with increased age and advanced bone attrition at time of surgery.[25]

Joint Distraction

In patients with OA, distraction of the affected synovial joint can induce functional tissue repair. Joint distraction utilizes an external fixation frame to reduce stress and prevent further wear on the articular cartilage for up to 12 weeks, and has been applied to the hip, ankle, and knee for a variety of chondral and osteochondral pathologies.[50] Distraction relieves stresses on the peri-articular bone leading to osteopenia. However, although overall density of subchondral bone decreases, an increase in bone density of low-density cystic lesions and resurfacing of bony joint contours with hyaline-like cartilage has been reported after distraction of the ankle.[50,51] Normalization of subchondral bone density between cystic and sclerotic areas has been related to clinical improvement (decreased pain and functional deficit) after joint distraction. Potential adverse events occur mainly because of use of an external fixation frame including pin tract infections, thrombosis, and neurapraxia.

©Copyright 2021 American Academy of Orthopaedic Surgeons

TISSUE SUBSTITUTION AND JOINT REPLACEMENT

Substitution of some, or all, of the osteochondral unit with nonliving metal and plastic prothesis has been used for a range of defect sizes. In the case of knee replacements, patients may undergo total knee arthroplasty or partial replacement of the medial, lateral, or patella-femoral compartments of the knee, depending on the size and severity of the lesion (**Figure 9**). For focal lesions, implants made of synthetic polymer (BioPoly RS, BioPoly) and metal (HemiCap Classic, Arthrosurface) have been developed. After failure of conservative treatment methods, total joint replacement is considered an effective and cost-effective treatment for end-stage symptomatic arthritis, which is not relieved by nonoperative treatments.[52] It is estimated that the prevalence of total hip replacements (THA) and total knee replacements (TKA) in 2010 was 2.5 and 4.7 million individuals, respectively, with prevalence increasing with age and higher among women.[53]

Clinical benefits have been reported up to 21 years follow-up with improvements in disease-specific (WOMAC, KSS scores) and general health-related quality of life (pain, function) metrics versus preoperative levels after knee replacement.[54] Adverse events leading to revision surgery include aseptic loosening of the implant, infection, as well as pain, instability, and stiffness after surgery which may be due to implant design as well as preoperative diagnosis, patient factors, surgical technique and experience, and postoperative care with the risk of revision inversely related to age at the primary procedure.[52] Although joint replacement surgeries have resulted in substantial quality-of-life gains for people with end-stage arthritis, future treatment strategies should avoid the need for major surgery.

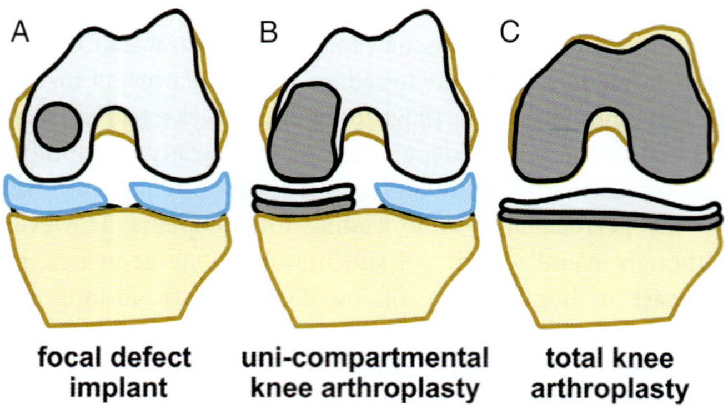

FIGURE 9 Types of (knee) joint replacement. Depending on the size and severity of the lesion, metal and plastic prothesis can be used to treat focal defects, degeneration restricted to a single compartment, or end-stage degeneration affecting multiple compartments. **A**, Focal defect implants. **B**, Unicompartmental knee arthroplasty. **C**, Total knee arthroplasty.

EMERGING STRATEGIES FOR IMPROVED CARTILAGE TREATMENT

Future directions for improved cartilage regeneration may build upon the fundamental basis of existing interventions by providing cells, signals, and structurally functional matrix to reconstitute the damaged tissue.

ALTERNATIVE CELL SOURCES

Current cell-based therapies, as in the case of ACI, are limited to autologous chondrocytes. There is increasing attention on autologous mesenchymal stem cells (MSCs) and other multipotent cell types (induced pluripotent stem cells, embryonic stem cells) that can be obtained from bone marrow aspirate and other tissues, and differentiated into both cartilage and bone depending on the nature of biomechanical and biochemical cues.[55] Alternative cell sources may be used as a stand-alone drug or biologic (ie, by IA injection), in ACI-like procedures, or as a component of future interventions along with purpose-designed scaffolds and biochemical signaling.

MSCs have been extensively studied in vitro and in vivo and are most commonly derived from autologous bone marrow or adipose tissue or from allogeneic sources. However, although there is a wide body of evidence supporting the use of MSC-based treatments of cartilage injury in animal models, there are limited large-scale clinical data.[56,57] Pilot studies in cartilage lesions indicate that IA injection of MSCs, as well as implantation of MSCs supported by scaffolds, results in improvement in pain and function, and formation of hyaline-like cartilage up to 2 years postoperation.[57] However, as of 2018, there are no MSC-based therapies authorized to market in the United States or Europe.

In Korea, there are several clinical trials investigating Cartistem (Medipost), an allogeneic product of umbilical cord MSCs which are cultured in vitro and mixed with sodium hyaluronate before arthroscopic administration into drill holes created within an articular cartilage defect >2 cm^2 in the knee. Early clinical studies have been registered for Cartistem treatment of osteochondral lesions of the knee (NCT01041001, NCT01626677, NCT01733186) and talus (NCT02338375) as well as of the ACL (NCT02755376). In an early phase I/II clinical trial of seven patients treated with Cartistem, there was evidence of hyaline-like repair tissue and improvement of pain (VAS score) and function (IKDC score) that was maintained up to 7 years, although this study was not controlled.[58] Challenges to adoption of MSC-based interventions include difficulties optimizing chondrogenic differentiation and maintaining phenotypic stability in vitro or in vivo, especially long term.

Owing to the scarcity of autologous cell populations and risk of donor-site morbidity, exogenous cell sources would be beneficial for future off-the-shelf cell therapies. Possible allogeneic

©Copyright 2021 American Academy of Orthopaedic Surgeons

cell populations for cartilage repair include chondrocytes, MSCs, induced pluripotent stem cells, and embryonic stem cells. However, there are few clinical trials of allogeneic cell-therapies other than for MSCs. In a phase II randomized study, IA injection of TissueGene-C (Kolon TissueGene, Inc.), a biologic containing genetically engineered chondrocytes virally transduced with TGF-β1 (NCT01221441), has been shown to decrease pain and improve IKDC scores versus saline.[59]

Future treatments may develop in the form of IA injection, or seeding, of cells onto structural scaffolds for implantation facilitated with advances in cell-based therapeutics. Several strategies have been developed to maximize the therapeutic benefit and safety as well as minimize production costs of stem cells including transgenic approaches and in vitro preconditioning of cells to express relevant proteins and development of homing strategies to target specific tissues.[60] However, hurdles to widespread use of cell-based therapies include determination of the number of cells, or number of injections, required to promote cartilage regeneration and long-term safety of the technique and of multipotent stem cells in general.

BIOCHEMICAL SIGNALING

Defined growth factor or small molecule treatments have been proposed as disease-modifying osteoarthritis drugs (DMOADs) to enable endogenous repair mechanisms and prevent degeneration within the joint or to direct cellular behavior within an implanted construct. Chondrogenic differentiation of multipotent cells and maintenance of chondrogenic phenotype can be directed via biochemical stimuli including those in the transforming growth factor-beta (TGF-β), fibroblast growth factor (FGF), bone morphogenetic protein (BMP), and insulinlike growth factor (IGF) families, many of which are contained within PRP, although contrasting results may occur with specific dosage, combinations, culture conditions, and mechanical cues.[6,50,57,61]

Proteases and cytokine blockers have also been proposed as targets to prevent further degeneration. For instance, after acute injury of the knee, interleukin-1 (IL-1) levels become elevated and are correlated with chondral damage. A small randomized phase I/II clinical study (NCT00332254) of administration of anakinra, an interleukin-1 receptor antagonist (IL-1ra), after acute knee injury found that IL-1ra treatment reduced pain and improved function after 2 weeks postinjury compared with placebo, although longer term results and evidence of cartilage degradation health were not assessed.[62]

Penetration of therapeutic molecules to the cartilage remains a challenge because of the great density and charged nature of the matrix. Future drug delivery strategies may leverage electrostatic interactions within and dynamic loading of the cartilage to increase solute penetration and residence time within the tissue.[6,7]

SCAFFOLDS

To enable rapid restoration of cartilage function, tissue engineering approaches are being developed to engineer cartilage tissue in vitro to withstand physiological loading soon after implantation in vivo and recapitulate the native mechanical, transport, and boundary properties of the tissue. Scaffolds for (osteo)chondral-engineering encompass synthetic materials including synthetic polymers, ceramics, and bioactive glasses as well as natural materials, including collagen, proteoglycan, and hyaluronan to recapitulate either the soft tissue (cartilage) or multiple tissues (cartilage, bone, vasculature) in an integrated construct with the appropriate cellular populations, interfaces, and integration with surrounding tissues.[63]

MINCED AND PARTICULATE CARTILAGE

Single-stage cell-based cartilage repair procedures using fresh minced cartilage products have been developed. The implanted tissue acts as a source for donor chondrocytes and reservoir of growth factors and other bioactive molecules which may help to promote formation of functional repair tissue. During the procedure, the defect is débrided, and a foil template of the defect site is created. Minced cartilage products using either fresh or cryopreserved allogeneic cartilage, such as DeNovo NT (Zimmer Biomet) and CartiMax (MTF Biologics), or autologous cartilage, as in the Cartilage Autologous Implantation System (CAIS, DePuy Mitek), are transferred onto the foil template and coated with fibrin glue. Conversely, dried particulate cartilage products act as an acellular scaffold and provide biochemical signals which may help to recruit and direct endogenous cells to the defect site and promote repair.

OSTEOCHONDRAL IMPLANTS

Engineered allogeneic osteochondral implants have become available including decellularized or cell-free osteochondral allografts and scaffolds as well as fresh cryopreserved allografts. Cell-free osteochondral implants including decellularized allografts (Chondrofix, Zimmer Biomet) and cell-free osteochondral scaffolds (Trufit CB, Smith & Nephew; Maioregen, Fin-Ceramica; Agili-C, Cartiheal) have robust mechanical properties and are composed of distinct cartilage and bone phases. The bone phase is osteoconductive and designed to promote osteointegration; however, results are mixed and further clinical studies are needed to assess efficacy.[64] Fresh cryopreserved osteochondral allografts with etched surface topographies (Cartiform, Arthrex; ProChondrix, AlloSource) to improve graft flexibility and allow for bone healing have also been produced.

Whole joint resurfacing, especially of large and diffuse cartilage lesions and end-stage OA, remains an unmet need and should be a target for development of future therapies and

©Copyright 2021 American Academy of Orthopaedic Surgeons

TABLE 5 Types of Synovial Joints Commonly Repaired

Joint	Joint Type	Geometry and Motion	Biological Therapy			Mechanical Therapy		
			Bone Marrow Stimulation	(M) ACI	Joint Distraction	Osteotomy	Tissue Grafts (Auto/Allo)	Total/ Partial Joint Arthroplasty
Knee	Modified hinge	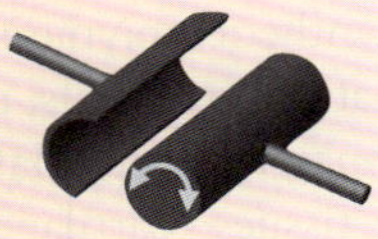	✔	✔	✔	HTO	✔	✔
Talocrural	Hinge		✔	✔	✔		✔	✔
Proximal interphalangeal	Hinge						✔	✔
Hip	Spheroidal	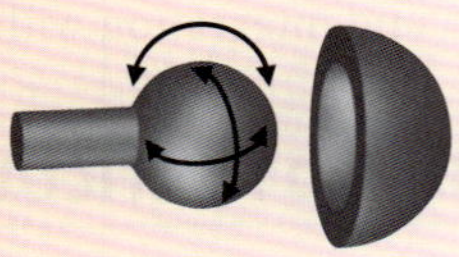	✔	✔	✔	PAO	✔	✔
Shoulder	Spheroidal		✔	✔			✔	✔

Chondral and osteochondral injuries to hinge joints (knee, ankle, fingers) and spherical joints (hip, shoulder) are common targets for treatment.
HTO = high tibial osteotomy, PAO = periacetabular osteotomy

techniques. Tissue engineering of whole joints is limited by the need for unique tissue-specific environments, integration between tissue interfaces, and lubrication that is controllable at the multiple scales.[65] Although there is significant work in the design of multiphasic scaffolds for focal osteochondral lesions, extension of these platforms to joint-scale constructs will be necessary. Such technologies may eliminate the need for joint arthroplasty with metal and plastic prothesis.

SUMMARY

Repair of cartilage injuries, including focal cartilage defects and OA, may be delivered systemically, locally by IA injection, or surgically, and may affect repair according to mechanical or biological modes of action (**Table 5**) and may intend to augment, regenerate, replace, or substitute damaged tissues. Although there are several interventions, including bone marrow stimulation, osteochondral grafting, and joint arthroplasty, which have been studied extensively, long-term high-level clinical studies of emerging paradigms, including augmented microfracture, next-generation ACI techniques, and minced cartilage, are required to establish efficacy versus conventional strategies. In addition, strategies which alter joint loading to induce structural changes to the cartilage and subchondral bone reveal critical relationships between cartilage and bone which may be leveraged to develop future therapies. Future directions for improved cartilage repair include the use of alternative cell sources, signaling molecules, and scaffolds which allow for rapid restoration of cartilage function and prevent or slow joint degeneration.

REFERENCES

1. Hunter W: Of the structure and disease of articulating cartilages. *Philos Trans R Soc London* 1743;42:514-521.
2. Mankin HJ: Chondrocyte transplantation–one answer to an old question. *N Engl J Med* 1994;331:940-941.
3. Hunziker E, Quinn T, Shimaoka E, Hauselmann H: Quantitative structural organization of the normal adult human articular cartilage. *Trans Orthop Res Soc* 2002;27:357.
4. Poole AR, Kojima T, Yasuda T, Mwale F, Kobayashi M, Laverty S: Composition and structure of articular cartilage: A template for tissue repair. *Clin Orthop Relat Res* 2001;(391 suppl):S26-S33.
5. Temple MM, Bae WC, Chen MQ, et al: Age- and site-associated biomechanical weakening of human articular cartilage of the femoral condyle. *Osteoarthr Cartil* 2007;15:1042-1052.
6. Bajpayee AG, Grodzinsky AJ: Cartilage-targeting drug delivery: Can electrostatic interactions help? *Nat Rev Rheumatol* 2017;13:183-193.
7. DiDomenico CD, Lintz M, Bonassar LJ: Molecular transport in articular cartilage – what have we learned from the past 50 years? *Nat Rev Rheumatol* 2018;14:393-403.
8. Vincent T, Hermansson M, Bolton M, Wait R, Saklatvala J: Basic FGF mediates an immediate response of articular cartilage to injury. *Proc Natl Acad Sci U S A* 2002;99:8259-8264.
9. Sah RL, Klein TJ, Schmidt TA, et al: *Articular cartilage repair, regeneration, and replacement. Arthritis and Allied Conditions: A Textbook of Rheumatology*. Philadelphia, PA, Lippincott Williams & Wilkins, 2005, pp 2277-2301.
10. Andriacchi TP, Koo S, Scanlan SF: Gait mechanics influence healthy cartilage morphology and osteoarthritis of the knee. *J Bone Joint Surg Am* 2009;91(suppl 1):95-101.
11. Lafeber FP, Intema F, Van Roermund PM, Marijnissen AC: Unloading joints to treat osteoarthritis, including joint distraction. *Curr Opin Rheumatol* 2006;18:519-525.
12. Bedi A, Feeley BT, Williams RJ III: Management of articular cartilage defects of the knee. *J Bone Joint Surg Am* 2010;92:994-1009.
13. U.S. Food and Drug Administration, FDA. Regulatory considerations for human cells, tissues, and cellular and tissue-based products: Minimal manipulation and homologous use. Guidance for Industry and Food and Drug Administration Staff. 2017.

 ©Copyright 2021 American Academy of Orthopaedic Surgeons

14. Depalma AA, Gruson KI: Management of cartilage defects in the shoulder. *Curr Rev Musculoskelet Med* 2012;5:254-262.
15. El Bitar YF, Lindner D, Jackson TJ, Domb BG: Joint-preserving surgical options for management of chondral injuries of the hip. *J Am Acad Orthop Surg* 2014;22:46-56.
16. Baums MH, Schultz W, Kostuj T, Klinger HM: Cartilage repair techniques of the talus: An update. *World J Orthop* 2014;5:171-179.
17. Tetteh ES, Bajaj S, Ghodadra NS: Basic science and surgical treatment options for articular cartilage injuries of the knee. *J Orthop Sports Phys Ther* 2012;42:243-253.
18. Bruyere O, Cooper C, Pelletier JP, et al: An algorithm recommendation for the management of knee osteoarthritis in Europe and internationally: A report from a task force of the European Society for clinical and Economic aspects of Osteoporosis and osteoarthritis (ESCEO). *Semin Arthritis Rheum* 2014;44:253-263.
19. Hjelle K, Solheim E, Strand T, Muri R, Brittberg M: Articular cartilage defects in 1,000 knee arthroscopies. *Arthroscopy* 2002;18:730-734.
20. Buckwalter JA, Saltzman C, Brown T: The impact of osteoarthritis: Implications for research. *Clin Orthop Relat Res* 2004;(427 suppl):S6-S15.
21. Bijlsma JW, Berenbaum F, Lafeber FP: Osteoarthritis: An update with relevance for clinical practice. *Lancet* 2011;377:2115-2126.
22. Rutgers M, van Pelt MJ, Dhert WJ, Creemers LB, Saris DB: Evaluation of histological scoring systems for tissue-engineered, repaired and osteoarthritic cartilage. *Osteoarthr Cartil* 2010;18:12-23.
23. Collins NJ, Misra D, Felson DT, Crossley KM, Roos EM: Measures of knee function: International Knee Documentation Committee (IKDC) Subjective Knee Evaluation Form, Knee Injury and Osteoarthritis Outcome Score (KOOS), Knee Injury and Osteoarthritis Outcome Score Physical Function Short Form (KOOS-PS), Knee Outcome Survey Activities of Daily Living Scale (KOS-ADL), Lysholm Knee Scoring Scale, Oxford Knee Score (OKS), Western Ontario and McMaster Universities Osteoarthritis Index (WOMAC), Activity Rating Scale (ARS), and Tegner Activity Score (TAS). *Arthritis Care Res* 2011;63 suppl 11:S208-S228.
24. Lotz M, Loeser RF: Effects of aging on articular cartilage homeostasis. *Bone* 2012;51:241-248.
25. Amendola A, Bonasia DE: Results of high tibial osteotomy: Review of the literature. *Int Orthop* 2010;34:155-160.
26. Hochberg MC, Altman RD, April KT, et al, American College of Rheumatology: American College of Rheumatology 2012 recommendations for the use of nonpharmacologic and pharmacologic therapies in osteoarthritis of the hand, hip, and knee. *Arthritis Care Res* 2012;64:465-474.
27. Jevsevar DS, Brown GA, Jones DL, et al, American Academy of Orthopaedic Surgeons: The American Academy of Orthopaedic Surgeons evidence-based guideline on: Treatment of osteoarthritis of the knee, 2nd edition. *J Bone Joint Surg Am* 2013;95:1885-1886.
28. Nelson AE, Allen KD, Golightly YM, Goode AP, Jordan JM: A systematic review of recommendations and guidelines for the management of osteoarthritis: The chronic osteoarthritis management initiative of the U.S. bone and joint initiative. *Semin Arthritis Rheum* 2014;43:701-712.
29. Steinmeyer J, Konttinen YT: Oral treatment options for degenerative joint disease–presence and future. *Adv Drug Deliv Rev* 2006;58:168-211.
30. McAlindon TE, Bannuru RR, Sullivan MC, et al: OARSI guidelines for the non-surgical management of knee osteoarthritis. *Osteoarthr Cartil* 2014;22:363-388.
31. Marlovits S, Singer P, Zeller P, Mandl I, Haller J, Trattnig S: Magnetic resonance observation of cartilage repair tissue (MOCART) for the evaluation of autologous chondrocyte transplantation: Determination of interobserver variability and correlation to clinical outcome after 2 years. *Eur J Radiol* 2006;57:16-23.
32. Mithoefer K, McAdams T, Williams RJ, Kreuz PC, Mandelbaum BR: Clinical efficacy of the microfracture technique for articular cartilage repair in the knee: An evidence-based systematic analysis. *Am J Sports Med* 2009;37:2053-2063.
33. Steadman JR, Briggs KK, Rodrigo JJ, Kocher MS, Gill TJ, Rodkey WG: Outcomes of microfracture for traumatic chondral defects of the knee: Average 11-year follow-up. *Arthroscopy* 2003;19:477-484.
34. Kreuz PC, Erggelet C, Steinwachs MR, et al: Is microfracture of chondral defects in the knee associated with different results in patients aged 40 years or younger? *Arthroscopy* 2006;22:1180-1186.
35. Smith BD, Grande DA: The current state of scaffolds for musculoskeletal regenerative applications. *Nat Rev Rheumatol* 2015;11:213-222.
36. Krill M, Early N, Everhart JS, Flanigan DC: Autologous chondrocyte implantation (ACI) for knee cartilage defects: A review of indications, technique, and outcomes. *JBJS reviews* 2018;6:e5.
37. Brittberg M, Lindahl A, Nilsson A, Ohlsson C, Isaksson O, Peterson L: Treatment of deep cartilage defects in the knee with autologous chondrocyte transplantation. *N Engl J Med* 1994;331:889-895.
38. Huang BJ, Hu JC, Athanasiou KA: Cell-based tissue engineering strategies used in the clinical repair of articular cartilage. *Biomaterials* 2016;98:1-22.
39. Grande DA, Pitman MI, Peterson L, Menche D, Klein M: The repair of experimentally produced defects in rabbit articular cartilage by autologous chondrocyte transplantation. *J Orthop Res* 1989;7:208-218.
40. Hangody L, Fules P: Autologous osteochondral mosaicplasty for the treatment of full-thickness defects of weight-bearing joints. Ten years of experimental and clinical experience. *J Bone Joint Surg Am* 2003;85-A suppl:25-32.
41. Lynch TS, Patel RM, Benedick A, Amin NH, Jones MH, Miniaci A: Systematic review of autogenous osteochondral transplant outcomes. *Arthroscopy* 2015;31:746-754.
42. Chahal J, Gross AE, Gross C, et al: Outcomes of osteochondral allograft transplantation in the knee. *Arthroscopy* 2013;29:575-588.
43. Jones KJ, Cash BM, Arshi A, Williams RJ: Fresh osteochondral allograft transplantation for uncontained, elongated osteochondritis dissecans lesions of the medial femoral condyle. *Arthrosc Tech* 2019;8:e267-e73.
44. Bugbee WD, Pallante-Kichura AL, Görtz S, Amiel D, Sah R: Osteochondral allograft transplantation in cartilage repair: Graft storage paradigm, translational models, and clinical applications. *J Orthop Res* 2016;34:31-38.
45. Wang D, Jones KJ, Eliasberg CD, Pais MD, Rodeo SA, Williams RJ III: Condyle-specific matching does not Improve midterm clinical outcomes of osteochondral allograft transplantation in the knee. *J Bone Joint Surg Am* 2017;99:1614-1620.
46. Bian L, Stoker AM, Marberry KM, Ateshian GA, Cook JL, Hung CT: Effects of dexamethasone on the functional properties of cartilage explants during long-term culture. *Am J Sports Med* 2010;38:78-85.
47. Wu JZ, Herzog W, Hasler EM: Inadequate placement of osteochondral plugs may induce abnormal stress-strain distributions in articular cartilage –finite element simulations. *Med Eng Phys* 2002;24:85-97.
48. Du PZ, Markolf KL, Lama CJ, McAllister DR, Jones KJ: Contact forces acting on large femoral osteochondral allografts during forced knee extension. *Am J Sports Med* 2017;45:2804-2811.
49. Su AW, Chen Y, Wailes DH, et al: Impact insertion of osteochondral grafts: Interference fit and central graft reduction affect biomechanics and cartilage damage. *J Orthop Res* 2018;36:377-386.
50. Mastbergen SC, Saris DB, Lafeber FP: Functional articular cartilage repair: Here, near, or is the best approach not yet clear? *Nat Rev Rheumatol* 2013;9:277-290.
51. Intema F, Thomas TP, Anderson DD, et al: Subchondral bone remodeling is related to clinical improvement after joint distraction in the treatment of ankle osteoarthritis. *Osteoarthr Cartil* 2011;19:668-675.
52. Carr AJ, Robertsson O, Graves S, et al: Knee replacement. *Lancet* 2012;379:1331-1340.
53. Maradit Kremers H, Larson DR, Crowson CS, et al: Prevalence of total hip and knee replacement in the United States. *J Bone Joint Surg Am* 2015;97:1386-1397.
54. Shan L, Shan B, Suzuki A, Nouh F, Saxena A: Intermediate and long-term quality of life after total knee replacement: A systematic review and meta-analysis. *J Bone Joint Surg Am* 2015;97:156-168.

©Copyright 2021 American Academy of Orthopaedic Surgeons

55. Makris EA, Gomoll AH, Malizos KN, Hu JC, Athanasiou KA: Repair and tissue engineering techniques for articular cartilage. *Nat Rev Rheumatol* 2015;11:21-34.
56. Noth U, Steinert AF, Tuan RS: Technology insight: Adult mesenchymal stem cells for osteoarthritis therapy. *Nat Clin Pract Rheumatol* 2008;4:371-380.
57. Confalonieri D, Schwab A, Walles H, Ehlicke F: Advanced therapy medicinal products: A guide for bone marrow-derived MSC application in bone and cartilage engineering. *Tissue Eng Part B Rev* 2018;24:155-169.
58. Park YB, Ha CW, Lee CH, Yoon YC, Park YG: Cartilage regeneration in osteoarthritic patients by a composite of allogeneic umbilical cord blood-derived mesenchymal stem cells and hyaluronate hydrogel: Results from a clinical trial for safety and proof-of-concept with 7 years of extended follow-up. *Stem Cells Transl Med* 2017;6:613-621.
59. Cherian JJ, Parvizi J, Bramlet D, Lee KH, Romness DW, Mont MA: Preliminary results of a phase II randomized study to determine the efficacy and safety of genetically engineered allogeneic human chondrocytes expressing TGF-beta1 in patients with grade 3 chronic degenerative joint disease of the knee. *Osteoarthr Cartil* 2015;23:2109-2118.
60. Wagner J, Kean T, Young R, Dennis JE, Caplan AI: Optimizing mesenchymal stem cell-based therapeutics. *Curr Opin Biotechnol* 2009;20:531-536.
61. Daher RJ, Chahine NO, Greenberg AS, Sgaglione NA, Grande DA: New methods to diagnose and treat cartilage degeneration. *Nat Rev Rheumatol* 2009;5:599-607.
62. Kraus VB, Birmingham J, Stabler TV, et al: Effects of intraarticular IL1-Ra for acute anterior cruciate ligament knee injury: A randomized controlled pilot trial (NCT00332254). *Osteoarthr Cartil* 2012;20:271-278.
63. Yousefi AM, Hoque ME, Prasad RG, Uth N: Current strategies in multiphasic scaffold design for osteochondral tissue engineering: A review. *J Biomed Mater Res A* 2015;103:2460-2481.
64. Kon E, Filardo G, Perdisa F, Venieri G, Marcacci M: Clinical results of multilayered biomaterials for osteochondral regeneration. *J Exp Orthop* 2014;1:10.
65. Williams GM, Chan EF, Temple-Wong MM, et al: Shape, loading, and motion in the bioengineering design, fabrication, and testing of personalized synovial joints. *J Biomech* 2010;43:156-165.

 ©Copyright 2021 American Academy of Orthopaedic Surgeons

34

Tendon and Ligament Healing

Kenneth M. Lin, MD
Scott A. Rodeo, MD

Keywords: *anterior cruciate ligament; enthesis; fibrocartilage; ligament; rotator cuff; tendon*

INTRODUCTION

Tendon and ligament injuries are common and lead to significant pain, disability, and work hours missed.[1,2] These injuries are very diverse in terms of etiology, pathogenesis, and prognosis and affect the general population, regardless of age. The spectrum of disease includes acute traumatic injuries, sports-related injuries, and chronic tendinopathy due to repetitive overuse. Injury and tissue failure may occur at the midsubstance of ligament or tendon or at the junction to bone (enthesis). There are intra- and extra-articular ligaments and tendons, as well as extra-articular but intrasynovial tendons such as the flexor tendons of the hand. It is accepted that the microstructure and composition of tendon and ligament are not reconstituted following injury or rupture, as these tissues heal by formation of scar tissue with material properties that are inferior to native healthy tissue. Various surgical and nonsurgical treatment strategies exist, with recent interest in biologic augmentation of healing. This chapter will review basic factors related to tendon and ligament healing, using rotator cuff repair and anterior cruciate ligament (ACL) reconstruction as clinical examples of each to highlight important concepts. We will conclude by summarizing the evidence for various strategies of biological augmentation of tendon and ligament healing.

Dr. Rodeo or an immediate family member serves as a paid consultant to or is an employee of Flexion Therapeutics and has stock or stock options held in Ortho RTI. Neither Dr. Lin nor any immediate family member has received anything of value from or has stock or stock options held in a commercial company or institution related directly or indirectly to the subject of this chapter.

BASIC PRINCIPLES OF TENDON HEALING

BIOLOGICAL PATHWAY OF TENDON HEALING

Tendon healing generally occurs through three overlapping biological phases: inflammatory, proliferative, and remodeling.[2] The inflammatory phase lasts about a week, during which vascular permeability increases and inflammatory cells (neutrophils, monocytes, lymphocytes, and macrophages) enter the injured area to remove necrotic material. A concomitant increase in the local concentration of cytokines and inflammatory mediators activates tendon fibroblasts, which begin to synthesize type III collagen.

The proliferative phase begins several days after initial injury and lasts for several weeks depending on the tendon involved. Fibroblasts proliferate and initiate new matrix synthesis, beginning with production of type III collagen. Increased proliferative activity correlates with accumulation of growth factors such as transforming growth factor-β (TGF-β), insulinlike growth factor (IGF-1), platelet-derived growth factor (PDGF), vascular endothelial growth factor (VEGF), and basic fibroblast growth factor (bFGF).[3] Relative blood flow, VEGF activity, and microvessel density peak at around 1 week and remain elevated for approximately 4 weeks.[4] The torn tendon hematoma becomes replaced by granulation tissue followed by immature, poorly organized collagen.

The remodeling phase follows, starting at approximately 6 weeks and lasting for many months. This phase can be divided into the consolidation and maturation stages. During consolidation, repair tissue becomes less cellular and more densely fibrous, as tenocytes and collagen fibers align based on the direction of tensile mechanical load. Collagen synthesis shifts from type III to predominantly type I.[5] During

©Copyright 2021 American Academy of Orthopaedic Surgeons

the maturation stage, cellular metabolism and overall tendon vascularity decrease concomitant with progressive matrix remodeling.

On a cellular level, there are many important mediators in tendon healing. Tenoblasts and tenocytes are present in both epitenon and endotenon, and it is also known that tendons contain a niche of intrinsic resident progenitor cells.[6] Animal studies have shown that tendon healing is initiated by proliferation of cells from the epitenon, followed later by proliferation and matrix synthesis by endotenon cells.[6] Intrinsic tenocytes derived from the endotenon secrete larger and more mature collagen fibers compared with epitenon cells and are thought to begin synthesizing collagen later in the repair process. Matrix metalloproteinases (MMPs) play an important role in collagen remodeling. Animal studies have demonstrated that MMP-9 and MMP-13 participate in collagen degradation, whereas MMP-2, 3, and 14 participate in both degradation and remodeling.[7] Additionally, chemokines, cytokines, and growth factors, initially secreted by platelets, neutrophils, and monocytes play a role in neovascularization and migration and activation of tenocytes.

The tendon healing process relies on a complex interplay of intrinsic basic cell biologic activity (cell proliferation, matrix synthesis, and remodeling), tissue vascularity, the inflammatory response to injury, and exogenous factors (cytokines and biomechanical loads).

ANATOMIC CONSIDERATIONS IN TENDON HEALING

There are several important distinctions related to tendon and ligament healing. Tendons can be intrasynovial or extrasynovial. Intrasynovial tendons (such as the flexor tendons of the hand) have a synovial sheath which allows for decreased friction, abrasion, and greater excursion; the presence of the synovial sheath also has biological implications for healing and repair strategies. All tendon healing occurs through two general pathways: Intrinsic healing occurs through proliferation of cells in the tissue itself, such as epitenon and endotenon tenocytes, while extrinsic healing occurs via invasion of cells, generally from the surrounding sheath or synovium.[8] Intrinsic tendon healing results in improved biomechanics and fewer complications, most notably better gliding mechanics, and is generally the goal of treatment; extrinsic healing tends to lead to scar formation and is the predominant mode of healing in tendon ruptures seen clinically.

Another important distinction is that between intra- and extra-articular tendons and ligaments. In general, intra-articular tendons and ligaments have poor intrinsic healing capacity and usually require surgical repair in the event of complete rupture, such as the rotator cuff and ACL. It is hypothesized that the presence of synovial fluid, matrix-degrading proteases, and other intra-articular mediators have an adverse effect on healing of intra-articular tissues. One fundamental reason for poor healing of intra-articular issues is the failure of a fibrin clot to form and serve as a provisional scaffold for healing. The presence of fibrinolysates in the injured joint prevents formation of a stable fibrin clot. Furthermore, the levels of inflammatory cytokines needed for effective healing, including PDGF, TGF-β, and FGF, may be inadequate following intra-articular ligament rupture.[9] In contrast, some extra-articular tendons and ligaments, such as the Achilles tendon and the medial collateral ligament (MCL) have been shown to heal with good outcomes following nonsurgical management, although there are exceptions such as the patellar tendon, which is almost universally treated with surgical repair. In all cases, the healed tendon tissue is composed of scar tissue, with a greater content of collagen III, smaller diameter collagen fibrils, and abnormal collagen cross-links in comparison to native tendon tissue.

MIDSUBSTANCE VERSUS TENDON-BONE HEALING

Due to material, mechanical, and biological properties of bone and the bone-tendon interface, bone-to-tendon healing differs from midsubstance tendon-to-tendon healing. Direct insertions, such as the rotator cuff (**Figure 1**) and ACL (**Figure 2**) insertions to bone, have a tendon-bone interface mediated by fibrocartilage, through four zones: tendon, unmineralized fibrocartilage, mineralized fibrocartilage, and bone. In contrast to bone-to-bone healing, spontaneous healing with restoration of the microstructure and composition of the native enthesis does not typically occur at the bone-tendon junction after injury. Failure of healing may be due to numerous factors, including the relative avascularity of the fibrocartilage region, pathological changes in the bone, the complex mechanical loading environment, and gap formation between tendon and bone at the site of injury. Animal models and limited analysis of clinical specimens have shown that tendon-bone healing occurs through fibrovascular scar tissue rather than regeneration of the native fibrocartilaginous transition zone.[1] Even at late time points following tendon rupture and healing, the structural and mechanical properties of a healed tendon to its bony insertion do not return to normal. In contrast, in midsubstance tendon or ligament healing, generation of well-aligned collagen fibers can lead to good return of function.

While tissue at a repaired enthesis is biologically inferior to native insertion site tissue, a further challenge to adequate healing is pathological change at the bone attachment site. Bone loss and focal reduction in bone mineral density has been reported after tendon rupture and repair. In a canine model of flexor tendon repair as well as a rat model of rotator cuff repair, decreased bone mineral density is seen at the insertion site even at late times following repair, suggesting that bone resorption may contribute to the clinically observed delay in tendon-bone healing, such as the inferior healing rates seen in rotator cuff repairs treated with early or excessive mechanical loading.[5]

©Copyright 2021 American Academy of Orthopaedic Surgeons

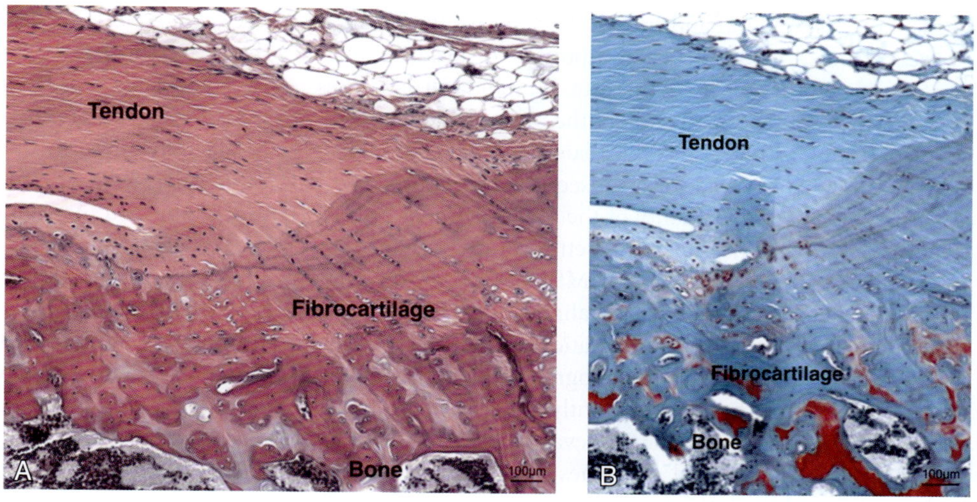

FIGURE 1 Light microscopy images of native rotator cuff insertion, 20× magnification. A, Hematoxylin and eosin (H&E) staining showing native tendon-bone interface with distinct transition zones from tendon to fibrocartilage and bone. **B**, Safranin-O staining, with proteoglycan content in the fibrocartilaginous transition zone appearing red.

CHRONIC TENDINOPATHY VERSUS ACUTE INJURY

The exact underlying cellular and molecular mechanism(s) that predispose to tendon injury are unknown, and thought to be multifactorial.[9] Many intrinsic and extrinsic factors may predispose to tendon injury, such as age, sex, disease comorbidities (diabetes, rheumatoid arthritis), medication use, sports activity, and limb alignment.[10] When categorizing tendon injuries into acute versus chronic types, acute ruptures are thought of as occurring in relatively normal tissue, although it has been demonstrated that some degree of preexisting tendinopathy is usually present for a tendon to spontaneously rupture.[11] In chronic tendinopathy, however, there is accumulation of microscopic matrix damage that occurs over time, weakening the tendon and altering the innate biological healing capacity. Degeneration is hypothesized to involve hypoxia, ischemic damage, oxidative stress, nonuniform mechanical loading, and production of inflammatory cytokines.[10] It has become increasingly clear that inflammatory mediators play an important role in the initiation of the pathological tendon changes. For example, it has been shown that administration of the inflammatory mediators prostaglandin E2 and IL-6 induce histologic changes consistent with tendinopathy.[12]

Acute injuries have a better prognosis for healing compared with chronic injuries,[13] as treatment with surgical repair is relatively straightforward. In chronic injuries, there is an inferior innate biological healing capacity, resulting in the high failure rates reported in surgical repairs of ruptured tendinopathic tendons, particularly in large rotator cuff tears.[14] Given these biological limitations, research efforts have focused on strategies to augment the biology of tendon healing, especially in chronic tendinopathy.[3]

CLINICAL ASSESSMENT OF TENDON AND LIGAMENT HEALING

In the clinical setting, objective evaluation of the quality of tendon or ligament healing is difficult. While various clinical scores and physical examination maneuvers allow assessment

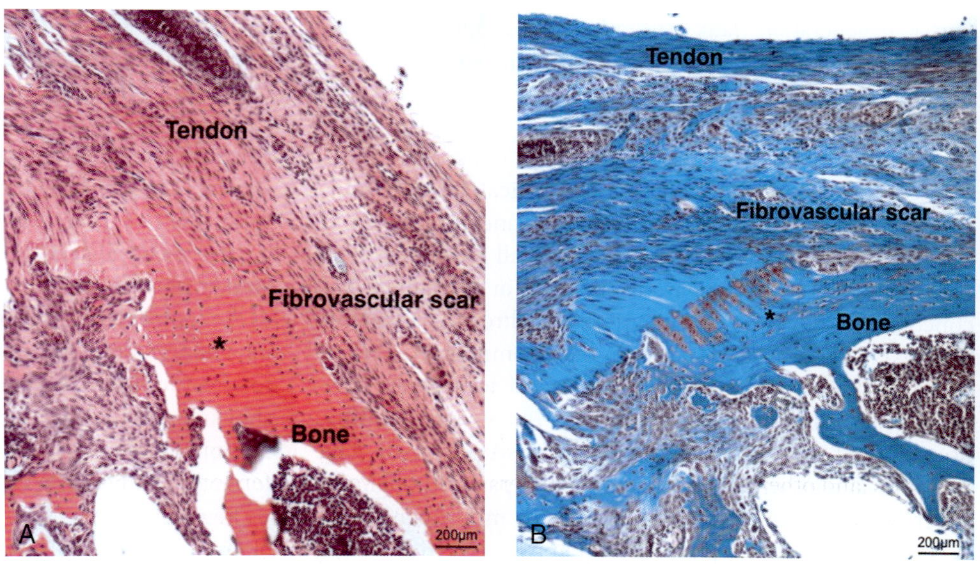

FIGURE 2 Light microscopy images of repaired rotator cuff tendon insertion, 10× magnification. Hematoxylin and eosin (**A**) and safranin-O (**B**) staining show transition from tendon to bone mediated by fibrovascular scar tissue. In the center of the images, there is a small area of fibrocartilage (asterisk), representing a portion of the native footprint that was left intact during repair.

©Copyright 2021 American Academy of Orthopaedic Surgeons

of the patient's function and the overall status of the repaired or reconstructed tendon (such as a positive or negative anterior drawer test for the ACL), there are no standardized scores for assessment of tendon healing in the postoperative patient. As second-look arthroscopy and tissue sampling is only possible in patients indicated for a subsequent procedure, direct assessment of the tissue quality of the graft is limited to MRI or ultrasonography imaging. In the setting of ACL reconstruction, oblique coronal and sagittal MRI have been used for postoperative evaluation of graft healing, and several authors have proposed scores for quantification.[15,16] When assessing graft maturity of autografts and allografts at 2 years, Li et al found that allografts had a significantly higher signal to noise quotient, suggesting a lower rate of revascularization and integration.[17] However, clinical outcomes were similar between both groups, and the lack of association between graft maturity on MRI with clinical scores has been reported from other studies as well,[18,19] suggesting that graft maturity and incorporation assessed by current noninvasive imaging techniques should not be an objective criteria for determining timing of return to sport.

CLINICAL EXAMPLE: ROTATOR CUFF REPAIR

Rotator cuff pathology is common, with symptomatic rotator cuff injuries affecting up to 30% of the population[20]; among the aging population, the prevalence of full-thickness tears is estimated to be as high as 30%.[21] Depending on injury factors, activity level, functional status, and occupation, surgical repair or reconstruction is generally the treatment of choice for injuries of the rotator cuff. The rotator cuff presents special challenges for tendon healing: its tendons are intra-articular and thus intrasynovial, there is a complex mechanical loading environment, the native fibrocartilaginous insertion to the greater tuberosity is not reconstituted, and there is almost always an element of chronic tendinopathy leading to impaired biological healing capacity on both the tendon and bone side. Factors known to be associated with failure of rotator cuff repair include muscle degeneration (fatty infiltration and atrophy), tear size, chronicity, advanced age, and other environmental factors.[22]

Treatment Techniques

Treatment of rotator cuff tears begins with nonsurgical measures such as activity modification, physical therapy, nonsteroidal anti-inflammatory medications, and corticosteroid injection. Oftentimes, however, patients will require surgical management. When tears are irreparable, or the patient has concomitant advanced glenohumeral arthrosis, alternative options such as arthroplasty can be recommended. When repair is indicated, many approaches and techniques have been described, including traditional open repairs, mini-open deltoid split approaches, and arthroscopic repair. The current standard of care is arthroscopic repair, although the superiority of arthroscopic versus open or mini-open repair is still somewhat controversial. Arthroscopic repair has been shown to have similar outcomes and failure rates, with decreased short-term pain and more rapid return to activity.[23]

The rotator cuff tends to fail at or near the tendon-bone junction, and the goal of repair is to restore the tendon to its anatomic footprint to encourage healing.[23] Historically, transosseous tunnels were used in open rotator cuff repair, with sutures placed and tied through bone tunnels from the cuff footprint to the lateral aspect of the tuberosity. Arthroscopically, repair is performed with suture anchors in various configurations—single-row, double-row, and transosseous-equivalent repair technique. Controlled laboratory studies have generally shown superiority of double-row techniques over single-row in terms of initial and ultimate failure strength, decreased gap formation, decreased strain and suture cut-through, and improved vascularity in transosseous-equivalent double-row repair.[24]

Biology of Rotator Cuff Footprint Healing

It is well-established that the anatomic structure of the rotator cuff insertion site is not regenerated after tendon-to-bone repair.[25] Repair of the rotator cuff leads to formation of a fibrovascular scar at the healing tendon-bone interface that never attains the gross, histological, or mechanical properties of native tendon[1] (**Figure 3**). Clinically, it has been shown that repair failure occurs at the tendon attachment site, with the tendon pulling through the sutures.[26] This suggests that the tendon-bone interface is slow to heal due to the formation of scar tissue with inferior material properties at the attachment site. Biologic factors that adversely affect healing include poor vascularity, the presence of excessive inflammatory mediators and matrix metalloproteinases, and the presence of chronic tendinopathic change. Furthermore, the concentration of biomechanical load on the suture-tendon interface may further impair healing. The presence of chronic tendinopathic change is almost ubiquitous in patients requiring rotator cuff repair and is associated with poor outcomes; in a controlled laboratory study in rats, repair of rotator cuff tendon with chronic degenerative change led to inferior healing, with decreased bone mineral density at the footprint, abnormal trabecular structure, and weaker biomechanical strength at the repair site.[27]

Clinical and research emphasis has been placed on footprint and tendon edge preparation in an effort to understand and manipulate healing potential. Studies in rat models comparing various techniques of footprint preparation have shown that leaving the footprint untreated (and preserving what is left of native fibrocartilage) or microfracture leads to greater mean load to failure, thicker collagen bundles, and greater fibrocartilage formation than radiofrequency ablation of the footprint or excavation of the footprint down to cancellous bone.[28] Overall bone health has also been hypothesized to affect footprint healing, as vitamin D deficiency has been shown to significantly decrease load to failure in a rat model of rotator cuff repair, with histological analysis showing less bone formation and inferior collagen fiber organization.[29]

Regarding tendon edge preparation, a clinical study using biopsy samples of cuff tissue at various distances from the

©Copyright 2021 American Academy of Orthopaedic Surgeons

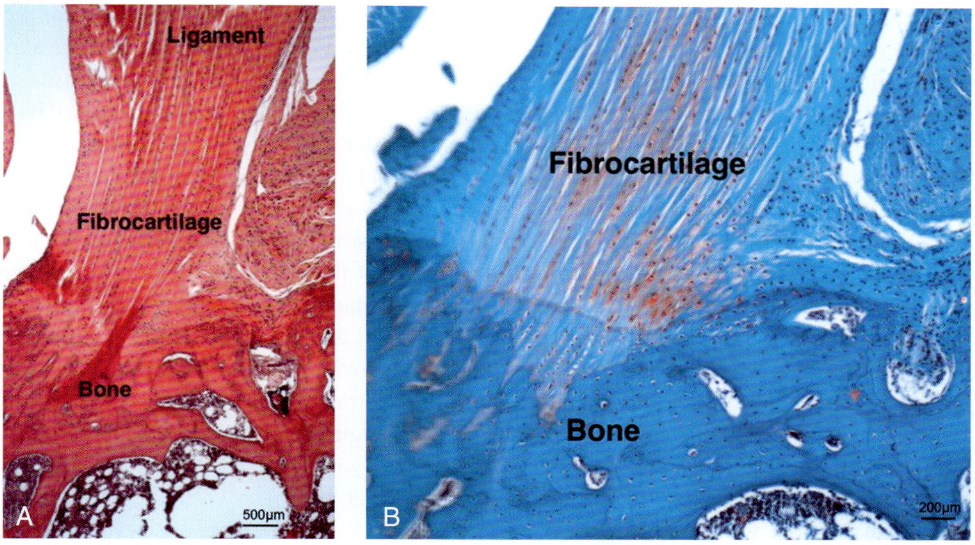

FIGURE 3 Light microscopy images of the native tibial anterior cruciate ligament (ACL) insertion. A, Hematoxylin and eosin staining at 4× magnification showing a direct insertion with a fibrocartilaginous transition zone. **B**, Safranin-O staining at 10× magnification demonstrating proteoglycan content (red) within the fibrocartilage zone.

edge of the tear from patients during arthroscopic rotator cuff repair showed increased expression of proapoptotic mediators, including caspases 3, 8, and 9, BAX (Bcl-2 associated X protein), and TNF-α closer to the tendon edge compared with a more proximal biopsy site.[30] Moving distal to proximal from the torn tendon edge, there was an increased expression of antiapoptotic Bcl-2 and anti-inflammatory IL-10. A separate analysis of the same specimens showed decreased expression of type I collagen and increasing expression of proinflammatory IL-1β and interferon gamma moving from proximal to distal, closer to the torn tendon edge.[31] The exact role of the inflammatory response remains unclear, but it is known that inflammatory mediator expression is associated with increased expression and activity of matrix metalloproteinases, and it is hypothesized that a balance must be achieved between pro- and anti-inflammatory signals.[32] In a rat model of rotator cuff repair, use of both indomethacin, a nonselective NSAID, and celecoxib, a COX-2-specific inhibitor, had negative effects on healing, with significantly lower load to failure and inferior collagen organization compared with controls in both groups.[33]

Effect of Biomechanical Load

Mechanical loads at the healing tendon-to-bone attachment site have a critical effect on healing. Cells in both tendon and bone respond to mechanical loads, and stress shielding can lead to adverse changes in these tissues.[34] However, excessive mechanical load in the early postoperative period impairs healing,[35] which may be due in part to failure of resolution of the postoperative inflammatory response. Proper tendon healing requires re-establishment of collagen fiber continuity between tendon and bone, and collagen fibrils become organized and aligned in response to biomechanical load. Biomechanical load on the healing tendon attachment site also leads to enhanced cell proliferation, and selective enhanced expression of tenocyte-related genes such as tenomodulin, but not genes related to other cell lineages such as chondrocytes or osteocytes.[36]

Despite the physiologic role of load in tendon development and homeostasis, loads applied too early to a repaired tendon can inhibit healing. Biomechanical studies in animal models of tendon healing have shown that after repair, a period of initial immobilization results in a stronger tendon-bone complex with improved collagen organization with less scar formation than immediate loading.[37] It should be noted, however, that prolonged immobilization, in both repaired and native tendons, has been shown to significantly weaken the bone-tendon complex, with a corresponding increase in MMP-13 activity.[35] A certain level of biomechanical stress is required for tendon homeostasis and repair, and this is reflected in laboratory studies of tendon development: injection of botulinum toxin A at birth into the supraspinatus showed reduction in muscle volume, fibrocartilage development, and bone mineralization, showing that a baseline level of muscle loading is required for normal development, and likely healing as well.[38] Beyond simply overstressing the repair mechanically, there are direct biological consequences of changing load on a repaired rotator cuff, such as activation of various MMPs. Further research is required to elucidate the cellular pathways involved in mechanotransduction.

While the exact pathogenesis of rotator cuff tendinopathy, rupture, and healing remains incompletely understood, knowledge of the intrinsic and extrinsic pathways and their influence on the cellular and molecular mechanisms involved in degeneration and healing provides insight into possible therapeutic targets to improve healing.

BASIC PRINCIPLES OF LIGAMENT HEALING

Ligament healing is comparable to tendon healing with similar biological principles as described above. Ligaments can be generally divided into intra-articular (such as the ACL) and extra-articular ligaments (such as the MCL), which have

©Copyright 2021 American Academy of Orthopaedic Surgeons

different healing properties, as intra-articular ligaments are known to have slower and more limited healing. Clinically, extra-articular ligaments such as the MCL can be treated conservatively, with good clinical outcomes despite persistently abnormal mechanical and histological properties.[39] Similar to tendon healing, ligament healing has been described to have distinct phases including inflammation, proliferation, and remodeling. An "epiligamentous regeneration" phase lasting 8 to 12 weeks has also been described in the response of the ACL to injury. Notable differences in intra-articular ligament healing compared with injury in other connective tissues are formation of an α-smooth muscle actin-expressing synovial layer over the surface of the ruptured ends that leads to retraction of the torn ligament stump and lack of tissue bridging at the repair site.[9] Perhaps the most studied ligament with regard to the biology of healing is the ACL, and using it as a clinical example we will summarize the current preclinical understanding of ligament healing with a focus on ACL reconstruction.

CLINICAL EXAMPLE: ANTERIOR CRUCIATE LIGAMENT RECONSTRUCTION

ACL injuries cause knee instability and dysfunction in athletes and are often treated with reconstruction. Historically, primary repair after traumatic rupture was considered an option; however, outcomes studies showed up to a 94% rate of instability at 5-year follow-up after primary suture and drill hole repair.[40] Use of more complex suture constructs improved failure rates; however, most authors have still advocated for abandonment of primary repair in favor of reconstruction which has produced more predictable outcomes.[9] Various graft options exist for reconstruction, but the most commonly used and studied are allograft and autograft using either combined semitendinosus and gracilis ("hamstrings") or patella bone-tendon-bone (BTB). A purely soft-tissue graft (hamstrings and allograft tibialis tendon or Achilles tendon) rely on tendon-bone healing inside a bone tunnel, while BTB relies on bone-to-bone healing in addition to tendon-bone healing at the apertures. Following ACL reconstruction, regardless of graft type, the structure, composition, and organization of the native ACL insertion site are not reproduced (**Figure 4**); rather, there is generation of a transitional zone of vascularized, highly cellular granulation tissue between the graft and tunnel wall which eventually leads to formation of Sharpey-like fibers bridging tendon and bone.[9]

Tendon-Bone Tunnel Healing

There are several challenges to tendon healing in a bone tunnel in the setting of ACL reconstruction. The first is the inability to truly regenerate native ACL insertion tissue; this is likely due several factors including the presence of inflammatory cells and associated inflammatory mediators and MMPs, insufficient number of progenitor cells at the healing site, and improper coordination of gene-signaling cascades leading to scar tissue formation rather than regeneration of a native enthesis. Developmental biology experiments have shown a paradigm of "scar-less healing" which is present in the embryo and early fetus prior to the development of a functioning immune system; this type of healing is possible in the absence of an acute inflammatory response.[1] The robust inflammatory response in adults, and especially at the graft-tendon junction following ACL reconstruction, contributes to healing by fibrovascular scar tissue rather than regeneration

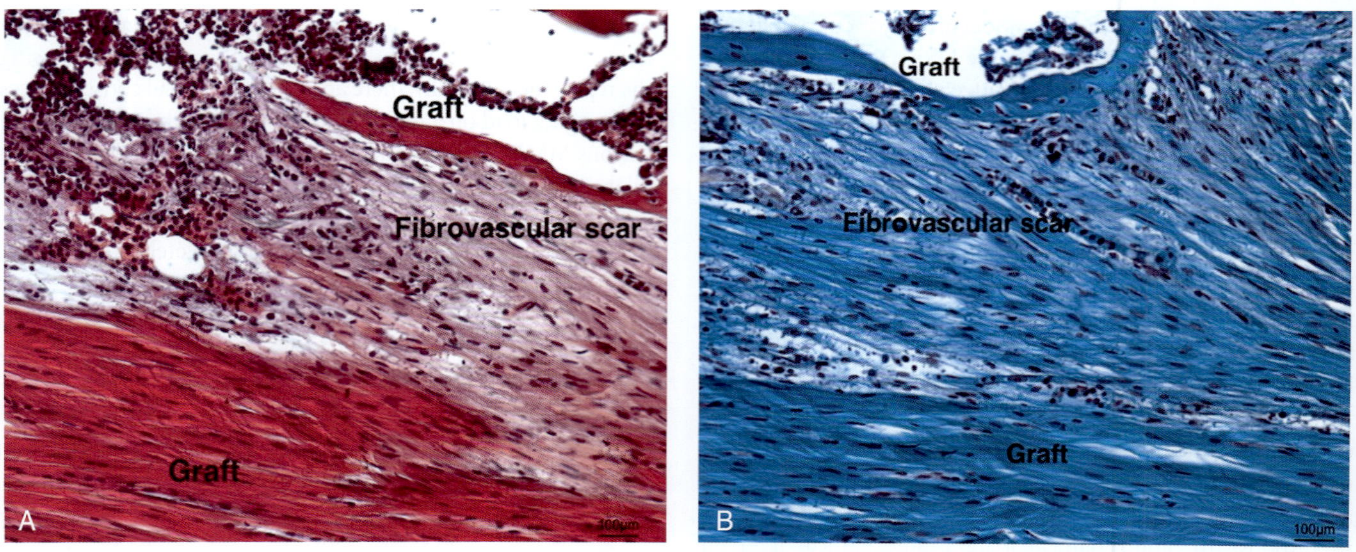

FIGURE 4 Light microscopy images of tendon-bone healing in an anterior cruciate ligament (ACL) bone tunnel following reconstruction, 20× magnification. Hematoxylin and eosin (**A**) and safranin-O (**B**) staining demonstrate a reconstructed graft-bone interface with fibrovascular scar tissue rather than regeneration of the native fibrocartilage transition zone. Note the absence of proteoglycan content on safranin-O staining.

©Copyright 2021 American Academy of Orthopaedic Surgeons

of the native insertion. Similar to the general tendon healing pathway described above, initial healing begins with a fibrin clot which releases cytokines, including TGF-β and PDGF which recruit neutrophils and then macrophages to the graft site. Increased expression of VEGF and FGF leads to influx of macrophages and fibroblasts which begin synthesizing type III collagen fibers which are then remodeled under the influence of MMPs. Endochondral new bone formation occurs with chondroid cells accumulating along the walls of the bone tunnel and depositing type II collagen. Sharpey-like type III collagen fibers are then seen bridging the grafted tendon to bone. The duration of this process has been variably reported in the literature, ranging from 8 to 30 weeks based on animal studies.[9]

Animal studies of the temporal and spatial pattern of hematopoietic lineage cell accumulation during the early tendon-bone healing process of a tendon graft in a bone tunnel (ACL reconstruction model) show that neutrophils and macrophages accumulate sequentially in the tendon-bone interface and then the outer tendon. There is little apparent contribution from proliferation of intrinsic tendon cells, suggesting that infiltrating inflammatory cells initiate the healing process.[41] Within the macrophage lineage, ED1 + proinflammatory macrophages dominate the early response (rat model), followed by accumulation of ED2 + proregenerative macrophages which promote new matrix formation by fibroblasts via TGF-β and other macrophage-derived cytokines. In a rat model, macrophage depletion led to superior healing, as demonstrated by a significantly narrower fibrous tissue interface between tendon and bone, significantly greater osteoid formation and mineral apposition rates, as well as significantly greater load to failure and stiffness of the femur-ACL graft-tibia construct.[42]

Inflammatory mediators produced during the early healing process are likely to drive scar-mediated healing and to inhibit regeneration of the native ACL insertion. At the same time, animal models of rotator cuff and patellar tendon ruptures have shown that administration of selective and nonselective nonsteroidal anti-inflammatory medications lead to histologically and biomechanically inferior tendon-bone interface.[33] This apparent disconnect can be explained by the recognition that healing in the postnatal organism is fundamentally initiated and regulated by inflammation. Although this inflammatory process leads to healing by scar tissue with inferior material properties, this is the only way that dense fibrous connective tissues heal, and thus, inhibition of inflammation negatively affects healing. Future research is warranted to identify methods to modulate the inflammatory response to decrease scar tissue formation and to optimize graft interface healing and remodeling.

Mechanical Factors

Surgical techniques for graft and tunnel preparation should largely focus on maximizing the surface area of the tendon-bone interface. Laboratory studies have shown that increasing bone tunnel length is correlated with improved quality and strength of the reconstructed tendon. Minimizing graft-tunnel size mismatch improves healing; specifically achieving a press-fit is thought to be superior. Maximizing circumferential contact area of the graft and tunnel are thought to improve healing; this must be balanced with construct stiffness; however, while use of an interference screw for aperture fixation provides increased stiffness and less relative motion by decreasing fixation-to-fixation construct length, it may decrease contact area of the graft and tunnel.[9]

The presence of graft-tunnel micromotion may delay or impair healing of the grafted tendon. In clinical studies, it has been shown that overly aggressive rehabilitation protocols after ACL reconstruction with quadrupled hamstring grafts leads to significantly greater tunnel widening, thought to be due to graft-tunnel micromotion.[9] In animal studies, initial immobilization after ACL reconstruction improved load to failure and resulted in closer bone-tendon apposition with less fibrovascular scar tissue at the healing graft-bone interface.[43] Laboratory quantification of graft-tunnel motion has been performed in a rabbit model using micro-CT, showing that motion is greatest at the tunnel apertures and least at tunnel exits, adjacent to graft fixation.[44] Healing in this model is correspondingly poorest at the apertures with a wider fibrovascular scar tissue interface interposed between the tendon and bone. Additionally, osteoclasts are seen in higher concentration at the tunnel aperture, suggesting osteoclast-mediated bone resorption as the mechanism of secondary tunnel widening.

Bone-to-Bone Healing

Healing of a bone plug to the osseous tunnel walls in ACL reconstruction using BTB autograft relies on bone-to-bone healing. The temporal biological healing process has been described in a canine model,[45] showing that bone plugs undergo ischemic necrosis and replacement by creeping substitution. By 6 weeks, there is plug incorporation with bridging cancellous bone. When compared with a soft-tissue graft, pull-out strength was greater at 3 weeks in the BTB group, and no difference at 6 weeks. By 6 weeks, the point of failure was no longer the bone tunnel interface but rather the tendon-bone plug interface. Similar to the tendon-bone tunnel interface, healing in a bone-bone tunnel interface occurs most rapidly at points farthest away from the joint, with slowest and sometimes incomplete healing at the tunnel apertures,[9] where there is typically still tendon-bone tunnel overlap. These findings suggest that there are biological or mechanical factors at the tunnel aperture, including a possibly inhibitory effect of synovial fluid (which contains high quantities of MMPs and other proteolytic enzymes) on healing, as well as the integral concept of graft micromotion. It is important to recognize that the typical length of the tendon portion of a patellar tendon BTB graft usually exceeds native ACL length, necessitating that the bone plug is recessed in the bone tunnel such that the aperture zone of the graft will be a tendon-bone interface and will rely on the principles of tendon-bone healing described above.

©Copyright 2021 American Academy of Orthopaedic Surgeons

BIOLOGICAL AUGMENTATION

Interest in the use of "biologics" to improve healing in various orthopaedic conditions has drastically increased in recent years,[39] as our preclinical understanding of injury, healing, and the limitations of native tissue regeneration continue to develop. Specific to the field of tendon and ligament healing, biological augmentation holds great promise; however, despite the increasing use and reported successes, there remain many fundamental unanswered questions. There is still no clear algorithm for the use of biologics with regard to indications, the optimal agent for different tissues and pathologies (eg, acute tendon injury vs chronic tendinopathy), and specific delivery method or surgical technique. We summarize here several important biological augmentation strategies that have been commonly reported in the recent literature (**Table 1**), acknowledging that much of the data are mixed and that new methods for augmentation are continually being developed.

TABLE 1 Factors Reported to Affect Tendon and Ligament Healing in Human and Animal Studies

Biological Factors Affecting Tendon and Ligament Healing	
Stimulatory	
BMP[25,55,56]	Bone morphogenetic protein
TGF[25]	Transforming growth factor
FGF[25]	Fibroblast growth factor
PDGF[3,9,25,39]	Platelet-derived growth factor
BMAC[46-50]	Bone marrow aspirate concentrate
PRP[25,51-54]	Platelet-rich plasma
Teriparatide[57,61,62]	Parathyroid hormone 1-34
Extracellular matrix patch[63-66]	Acellular allo- or xenogeneic scaffold
Inhibitory	
Intrinsic patient comorbidities	Diabetes, thyroid disease, renal disease, osteoporosis
Extrinsic factors[32,33]	Smoking, NSAIDs, quinolone antibiotics
MMPs[7,35,38]	Matrix metalloproteinases
TNF-α[30]	Tumor necrosis factor-α
IL-17[74]	Interleukin-17

BONE MARROW ASPIRATE CONCENTRATE

Autologous therapies such as bone marrow aspirate concentrate (BMAC) and platelet-rich plasma (PRP) have gained popularity in the field of tendon and ligament repair and reconstruction. While its benefits in the setting of ligament and tendon repair are not completely understood, BMAC has been shown to improve bone healing in the setting of fractures and nonunions.[46] BMAC is typically harvested from the iliac crest, but may also be obtained from the distal femur, proximal tibia, proximal humerus, or other long bones. Raw aspirate is mixed with a solution containing anticoagulant and centrifuged to isolate mononuclear cells. There is significant variability and lack of standardization among preparation protocols and proprietary systems. Aspiration at various locations using a small (10 mL) syringe maximizes progenitor cell concentrations.[47] The concentration of stem cells based on formal criteria in BMAC is relatively low, with reports showing 0.001% to 0.01% yield; however, in addition to progenitor cells, numerous growth factors are present and include PDGF, TGF-β, and BMP-2 and BMP-7.[48]

Preclinical data from a rabbit model of rotator cuff repair suggests increased bone formation at the rotator cuff footprint following local delivery of BMAC at the time of repair,[49] although there is minimal correlative clinical data. In a study using a rabbit model of bilateral ACL reconstructions, grafts coated with mesenchymal progenitor cells demonstrated cartilage at the tendon-bone interface, while contralateral control limbs demonstrated only fibrous tissue.[50] Clinical studies are limited; furthermore, given that all current methods of reconstruction necessitate the creation of bone tunnels, which generates an influx of bone marrow cells and factors, the additional utility of BMAC in the setting of procedures such as ACL reconstruction is unclear.

PLATELET-RICH PLASMA

PRP has been used clinically in the treatment of rotator cuff tears, elbow ulnar collateral ligament tears, lateral epicondylitis, hamstring injuries, and even osteoarthritis of the knee. Platelets are known to contain a large number of cytokines that are involved in modulating the inflammatory response and the early tendon and ligament healing response, including basic FGF, TGF-β, insulinlike growth factors, VEGF, and PDGF.[25] PRP is obtained after centrifuging autologous blood and isolating the upper buffy coat layer, which has the highest concentration of platelets. Various formulations of PRP exist, including leukocyte-rich or leukocyte-poor preparations and liquid versus semisolid forms, with very little rigorous data comparing the various formulations. Early data suggest that different formulations will be optimal for different tissues and pathologies (eg, acute vs chronic injury). In our current understanding of tendon and ligament healing, the fibroblast is the primary cell involved in new matrix synthesis. Several factors

©Copyright 2021 American Academy of Orthopaedic Surgeons

known to be present in PRP, including PDGF and TGF-β are known to stimulate fibroblast growth, migration, and biosynthetic activity.[39] In addition to the presence of cytokines that can stimulate cell proliferation and matrix synthesis, PRP also has an anti-inflammatory and immunomodulatory action.

Both preclinical and clinical studies of PRP have yielded largely equivocal results. Preclinical studies have suggested that PRP may enhance ACL graft remodeling, especially in the early stages of healing. A study using a dog model of ACL reconstruction showed improved vascularity as well as increased expression of genes thought to be involved in graft reinnervation, in the PRP-treated group compared with controls.[51] Clinical studies of PRP augmentation of ACL reconstruction have produced conflicting results. A prospective study showed earlier achievement of intra-articular graft homogeneity on MRI following reconstruction with PRP gel augmentation compared with controls (179 vs 369 days), although clinical outcomes were not reported.[52] A randomized controlled study with longer term follow-up showed no difference in subjective outcome, biomechanical performance, or graft integration at 2 years following ACL reconstruction with BTB autograft augmented with PRP gel compared with controls.[53] In the setting of rotator cuff repair, clinical studies have shown variable results with PRP augmentation. While a few studies have demonstrated a positive effect on clinical outcomes, there are very little data suggesting improved structural outcomes based on follow-up imaging with ultrasonography or MRI. A randomized controlled study of platelet-rich fibrin matrix applied to the tendon-bone interface at the time of rotator cuff repair reported no demonstrable effect on tendon healing, vascularity, strength, or clinical outcome scores and was actually shown to be correlated with a tendon defect at week 12 with an odds ratio of 5.8.[54] Similarly, studies in lateral epicondylitis and ulnar collateral ligament rupture in the elbow have yielded conflicting results.

OSTEOINDUCTIVE GROWTH FACTORS

Osteoinductive growth factors are hypothesized to improve tendon healing to bone by encouraging greater bony ingrowth into the fibrovascular scar region of a healing or repaired tendon. Research in this area has been largely limited to animal models of rotator cuff repair. A study in a sheep model demonstrated that an osteoinductive protein extract derived from bovine cortical bone (including BMPs 2-7, TGF-β1-3, and fibroblast growth factor) led to greater bone formation at the bone-tendon interface, greater reparative scar tissue cross-sectional area, and a larger fibrocartilage zone between bone and tendon.[25] However, the mechanical strength normalized by cross-sectional area of the repaired tendon was unchanged compared with controls that did not receive growth factors, suggesting that addition of these osteoinductive factors led to greater formation of new tissue with material properties still inferior to normal tendon. BMP-12 and BMP-13 are more recently described molecules that are expressed at tendon insertion sites during embryonic development and are thought to be functionally distinct from the osteoinductive BMP's (2, 4, and 7), inducing formation of tendon and fibrocartilage rather than bone.[55] In a sheep model of rotator cuff repair, delivery of recombinant human BMP-12 (rhBMP-12) in a collagen or hyaluronan sponge led to increased load to failure and increased re-establishment of collagen fiber continuity at the bone-fibrovascular scar interface at earlier time points.[56]

Particularly in rotator cuff repair, local or generalized decrease in bone mineral density is known to affect the strength and integrity of repair.[57] Anabolic agents such as teriparatide (an engineered analogue of parathyroid hormone consisting of the first 34 N-terminus amino acids) have been shown to improve bone mineral density as well as healing of fragility fractures in osteoporotic patients.[58,59] Teriparatide induces bone healing through preferential activation of osteoblasts with intermittent (typically once daily) exposure to PTH.[60] It has been shown in animal experiments to improve not only biomechanical strength of repair, but also histological appearance with increased collagen deposition at the repair site in both rotator cuff and flexor tendon repair models.[61,62]

STRUCTURAL AUGMENTATION

In rotator cuff repair and less so in ACL reconstruction, structural augmentation using various forms of tissue scaffolds has been described. In the rotator cuff, tissue patches, consisting of autogenous, allogeneic, xenogeneic, or synthetic materials have been used for massive or irreparable rotator cuff tears in either an augmentation (overlaying the repaired tissue) or a bridging construct (with native tendon and patch in series connecting to bone).[63] In the literature, autograft use has largely been limited to biceps and fascia lata. Xenograft, allograft, and synthetic patches have been shown in small series to have relatively high structural healing rates, ranging from 60% to 100%.[63] Currently in the clinical setting, the most commonly used graft is typically acellular dermis (essentially a collagen matrix patch), which has been shown to improve pain, function, strength, and motion, with high rate of intact repairs seen on imaging at 50 months post-op.[64,65] In animal studies, the use of an acellular dermal patch has been shown to produce a repaired construct with similar biomechanical strength to native tendon by 12 weeks and somewhat similar appearance to native tendon on gross and histologic examination with evidence of native cell infiltration.[66] The mechanism of healing following augmentation with various types of matrix patches has been shown to be via macrophage infiltration within the first 2 months followed by integration via fibrovascular scar formation at 2 years.[67]

In the ACL, there have been reports of periosteal patch augmentation for enhanced graft-bone healing in animal models. In vitro studies have shown that collagen patches mixed with mesenchymal cells show improved differentiation potential toward tenocytes, with enhanced adherence to the matrix and metabolic

©Copyright 2021 American Academy of Orthopaedic Surgeons

activity.[68] In addition to patch augmentation, structural augmentation using biologically inert materials, such as suture tape, has been described. This technique, also referred to as internal bracing treatment, has been described in primary ACL repair, Achilles repair, patellar tendon repair, and lateral ankle stabilization.[69-72] In the setting of ACL repair, internal bracing treatment has been used to strengthen the overall construct and protect the graft from excessive loading during rehabilitation[71,73]; however, theoretical disadvantages include possible overconstraint of the joint and excessive stress-shielding of the graft, with a resultant adverse effect on graft maturation and remodeling. Internal bracing treatment with repair has been shown to be biomechanically superior to repair alone,[70] although the literature is limited and consists only of small series thus far.

SUMMARY

This chapter summarizes the basic principles of tendon and ligament healing and reviews the rotator cuff, Achilles tendon, and ACL as distinct clinical examples. Direct insertions, such as the ACL and rotator cuff, consist of a fibrocartilage transition between bone and tendon and do not regenerate when injured; healing following repair or reconstruction instead produces a fibrovascular scar tissue bridge. Tendons and ligaments both heal through a similar process, consisting of the inflammatory, proliferative, and remodeling phases. Tendons and ligaments contain native fibroblasts which are the active cell during healing, in addition to numerous factors and recruited inflammatory and progenitor cells. Recent studies demonstrate that inflammatory cells and their mediators play an important role in the basic biology of both tendinopathy and tendon healing. Biologic augmentation of surgical repair is becoming increasingly widespread and includes many techniques, of which the most commonly used are BMAC, PRP, and growth factors. Continued research is required to further our growing understanding of the complex mechanisms of tendon and ligament healing and also to discover and develop novel strategies for manipulating the various cellular, molecular, chemical, and biomechanical mediators of the healing pathway to improve clinical outcomes.

REFERENCES

1. Galatz LM, Gerstenfeld L, Heber-Katz E, Rodeo SA: Tendon regeneration and scar formation: The concept of scarless healing. *J Orthop Res* 2015;33(6):823-831. doi:10.1002/jor.22853.
2. Thomopoulos S, Parks WC, Rifkin DB, Derwin KA: Mechanisms of tendon injury and repair. *J Orthop Res* 2015;33(6):832-839. doi:10.1002/jor.22806.
3. Molloy T, Wang Y, Murrell G: The roles of growth factors in tendon and ligament healing. *Sport Med* 2003;33(5):381-394. doi:10.2165/00007256-200333050-00004.
4. Stange R, Sahin H, Wieskotter B, et al: In vivo monitoring of angiogenesis during tendon repair: A novel MRI-based technique in a rat patellar tendon model. *Knee Surg Sports Traumatol Arthrosc* 2015;23(8):2433-2439. doi:10.1007/s00167-014-2897-5.
5. Lin TW, Cardenas L, Soslowsky LJ: Biomechanics of tendon injury and repair. *J Biomech* 2004;37(6):865-877. doi:10.1016/j.jbiomech.2003.11.005.
6. Bi Y, Ehirchiou D, Kilts TM, et al: Identification of tendon stem/progenitor cells and the role of the extracellular matrix in their niche. *Nat Med* 2007;13(10):1219-1227. doi:10.1038/nm1630.
7. Oshiro W, Lou J, Xing X, Tu Y, Manske PR: Flexor tendon healing in the rat: A histologic and gene expression study. *J Hand Surg Am* 2003;28(5):814-823.
8. Sharma P, Maffulli N: Tendon injury and tendinopathy: Healing and repair. *J Bone Joint Surg Am* 2005;87(1):187-202. doi:10.2106/jbjs.d.01850.
9. Grawe B, Sugiguchi F, Bedi A, Rodeo S: Biology of anterior cruciate ligament graft healing, in Noyes FR, Barber-Westin SD, eds: *Noyes' Knee Disorders: Surgery, Rehabilitation, Clinical Outcomes*. Philadelphia, PA, Elsevier Health Science, 2017.
10. Lipman K, Wang C, Ting K, Soo C, Zheng Z: Tendinopathy: Injury, repair, and current exploration. *Drug Des Dev Ther* 2018;12:591-603. doi:10.2147/DDDT.S154660.
11. Astrom M, Rausing A: Chronic Achilles tendinopathy. A survey of surgical and histopathologic findings. *Clin Orthop Relat Res* 1995;(316):151-164.
12. Stone D, Green C, Rao U, et al: Cytokine-induced tendinitis: A preliminary study in rabbits. *J Orthop Res* 1999;17(2):168-177. doi:10.1002/jor.1100170204.
13. Bassett RW, Cofield RH: Acute tears of the rotator cuff. The timing of surgical repair. *Clin Orthop Relat Res* 1983;(175):18-24.
14. Galatz LM, Ball CM, Teefey SA, Middleton WD, Yamaguchi K: The outcome and repair integrity of completely arthroscopically repaired large and massive rotator cuff tears. *J Bone Joint Surg Am* 2004;86-a(2):219-224.
15. Kim SI, Park HJ, Lee SY, et al: Usefulness of oblique coronal and sagittal MR images of the knee after double-bundle and selective anterior cruciate ligament reconstructions. *Acta Radiol* 2015;56(3):312-321. doi:10.1177/0284185114525952.
16. Moon SG, Hong SH, Choi JY, et al: Grading anterior cruciate ligament graft injury after ligament reconstruction surgery: Diagnostic efficacy of oblique coronal MR imaging of the knee. *Korean J Radiol* 2008;9(2):155-161. doi:10.3348/kjr.2008.9.2.155.
17. Li H, Tao H, Cho S, Chen S, Yao Z, Chen S: Difference in graft maturity of the reconstructed anterior cruciate ligament 2 years postoperatively: A comparison between autografts and allografts in young men using clinical and 3.0-T magnetic resonance imaging evaluation. *Am J Sports Med* 2012;40(7):1519-1526. doi:10.1177/0363546512443050.
18. Li H, Chen J, Li H, Wu Z, Chen S: MRI-based ACL graft maturity does not predict clinical and functional outcomes during the first year after ACL reconstruction. *Knee Surg Sports Traumatol Arthrosc* 2017;25(10):3171-3178. doi:10.1007/s00167-016-4252-5.
19. Hofbauer M, Soldati F, Szomolanyi P, et al: Hamstring tendon autografts do not show complete graft maturity 6 months postoperatively after anterior cruciate ligament reconstruction. *Knee Surg Sports Traumatol Arthrosc* 2019;27(1):130-136. doi:10.1007/s00167-018-5033-0.
20. Atesok K, Fu FH, Wolf MR, et al: Augmentation of tendon-to-bone healing. *J Bone Joint Surg Am* 2014;96(6):513-521. doi:10.2106/jbjs.m.00009.
21. Moosmayer S, Smith HJ, Tariq R, Larmo A: Prevalence and characteristics of asymptomatic tears of the rotator cuff: An ultrasonographic and clinical study. *J Bone Joint Surg Br* 2009;91(2):196-200.
22. Naranja RJ, Iannotti JP, Gartsman GM: *Orthopaedic Knowledge Update: Shoulder and Elbow*. Rosemont, IL, American Academy of Orthopaedic Surgeons, 1994, pp 157-166.

©Copyright 2021 American Academy of Orthopaedic Surgeons

23. Depres-Tremblay G, Chevrier A, Snow M, Hurtig MB, Rodeo S, Buschmann MD: Rotator cuff repair: A review of surgical techniques, animal models, and new technologies under development. *J Shoulder Elbow Surg* 2016;25(12):2078-2085. doi:10.1016/j.jse.2016.06.009.
24. Barber FA, Drew OR: A biomechanical comparison of tendon-bone interface motion and cyclic loading between single-row, triple-loaded cuff repairs and double-row, suture-tape cuff repairs using biocomposite anchors. *Arthroscopy* 2012;28(9):1197-1205. doi:10.1016/j.arthro.2012.02.015.
25. Rodeo SA: Biologic augmentation of rotator cuff tendon repair. *J Shoulder Elbow Surg* 2007;16(5 suppl):S191-S197. doi:10.1016/j.jse.2007.03.012.
26. Cummins CA, Murrell GA: Mode of failure for rotator cuff repair with suture anchors identified at revision surgery. *J Shoulder Elbow Surg* 2003;12(2):128-133. doi:10.1067/mse.2003.21.
27. Killian ML, Cavinatto LM, Ward SR, Havlioglu N, Thomopoulos S, Galatz LM: Chronic degeneration leads to poor healing of repaired massive rotator cuff tears in rats. *Am J Sports Med* 2015;43(10):2401-2410. doi:10.1177/0363546515596408.
28. Nakagawa H, Morihara T, Fujiwara H, et al: Effect of footprint preparation on tendon-to-bone healing: A histologic and biomechanical study in a rat rotator cuff repair model. *Arthroscopy* 2017;33(8):1482-1492. doi:10.1016/j.arthro.2017.03.031.
29. Angeline ME, Ma R, Pascual-Garrido C, et al: Effect of diet-induced vitamin D deficiency on rotator cuff healing in a rat model. *Am J Sports Med* 2014;42(1):27-34. doi:10.1177/0363546513505421.
30. Fabis J, Szemraj J, Strek M, Fabis A, Dutkiewicz Z, Zwierzchowski TJ: Is resection of the tendon edge necessary to enhance the healing process? An evaluation of the homeostasis of apoptotic and inflammatory processes in the distal 1 cm of a torn supraspinatus tendon: Part I. *J Shoulder Elbow Surg* 2014;23(12):1772-1778. doi:10.1016/j.jse.2014.03.018.
31. Fabis J, Szemraj J, Strek M, Fabis A, Dutkiewicz Z, Zwierzchowski TJ: Is resection of the tendon edge necessary to enhance the healing process? An evaluation of the expression of collagen type I, IL-1beta, IFN-gamma, IL-4, and IL-13 in the distal 1 cm of a torn supraspinatus tendon: Part II. *J Shoulder Elbow Surg* 2014;23(12):1779-1785. doi:10.1016/j.jse.2014.08.023.
32. Arnoczky SP, Lavagnino M, Egerbacher M, Caballero O, Gardner K: Matrix metalloproteinase inhibitors prevent a decrease in the mechanical properties of stress-deprived tendons: An in vitro experimental study. *Am J Sports Med* 2007;35(5):763-769. doi:10.1177/0363546506296043.
33. Cohen DB, Kawamura S, Ehteshami JR, Rodeo SA: Indomethacin and celecoxib impair rotator cuff tendon-to-bone healing. *Am J Sports Med* 2006;34(3):362-369. doi:10.1177/0363546505280428.
34. Rodeo SA, Arnoczky SP, Torzilli PA, Hidaka C, Warren RF: Tendon-healing in a bone tunnel. A biomechanical and histological study in the dog. *J Bone Joint Surg Am* 1993;75(12):1795-1803.
35. Hettrich CM, Gasinu S, Beamer BS, et al: The effect of immobilization on the native and repaired tendon-to-bone interface. *J Bone Joint Surg Am* 2013;95(10):925-930. doi:10.2106/jbjs.k.01329.
36. Zhang J, Wang JH: The effects of mechanical loading on tendons–an in vivo and in vitro model study. *PLoS One* 2013;8(8):e71740. doi:10.1371/journal.pone.0071740.
37. Hettrich CM, Gasinu S, Beamer BS, et al: The effect of mechanical load on tendon-to-bone healing in a rat model. *Am J Sports Med* 2014;42(5):1233-1241. doi:10.1177/0363546514526138.
38. Thomopoulos S, Kim HM, Rothermich SY, Biederstadt C, Das R, Galatz LM: Decreased muscle loading delays maturation of the tendon enthesis during postnatal development. *J Orthop Res* 2007;25(9):1154-1163. doi:10.1002/jor.20418.
39. Chahla J, Kennedy MI, Aman ZS, LaPrade RF: Ortho-biologics for ligament repair and reconstruction. *Clin Sports Med* 2019;38(1):97-107. doi:10.1016/j.csm.2018.08.003.
40. Raines BT, Naclerio E, Sherman SL: Management of anterior cruciate ligament injury: What's in and what's out? *Indian J Orthop* 2017;51(5):563-575. doi:10.4103/ortho.IJOrtho_245_17.
41. Kawamura S, Ying L, Kim HJ, Dynybil C, Rodeo SA: Macrophages accumulate in the early phase of tendon-bone healing. *J Orthop Res* 2005;23(6):1425-1432. doi:10.1016/j.orthres.2005.01.014.1100230627.
42. Hays PL, Kawamura S, Deng XH, et al: The role of macrophages in early healing of a tendon graft in a bone tunnel. *J Bone Joint Surg Am* 2008;90(3):565-579. doi:10.2106/jbjs.f.00531.
43. Sakai H, Fukui N, Kawakami A, Kurosawa H: Biological fixation of the graft within bone after anterior cruciate ligament reconstruction in rabbits: Effects of the duration of postoperative immobilization. *J Orthop Sci* 2000;5(1):43-51.
44. Rodeo SA, Kawamura S, Kim HJ, Dynybil C, Ying L: Tendon healing in a bone tunnel differs at the tunnel entrance versus the tunnel exit: An effect of graft-tunnel motion? *Am J Sports Med* 2006;34(11):1790-1800. doi:10.1177/0363546506290059.
45. Tomita F, Yasuda K, Mikami S, Sakai T, Yamazaki S, Tohyama H: Comparisons of intraosseous graft healing between the doubled flexor tendon graft and the bone-patellar tendon-bone graft in anterior cruciate ligament reconstruction. *Arthroscopy* 2001;17(5):461-476. doi:10.1053/jars.2001.24059.
46. Lin K, VandenBerg J, Putnam SM, et al: Bone marrow aspirate concentrate with cancellous allograft versus iliac crest bone graft in the treatment of long bone nonunions. *OTA Int* 2019;2(1):e012. doi:10.1097/oi9.0000000000000012.
47. Hernigou P, Homma Y, Flouzat Lachaniette CH, et al: Benefits of small volume and small syringe for bone marrow aspirations of mesenchymal stem cells. *Int Orthop* 2013;37(11):2279-2287. doi:10.1007/s00264-013-2017-z.
48. Pittenger MF, Mackay AM, Beck SC, et al: Multilineage potential of adult human mesenchymal stem cells. *Science* 1999;284(5411):143-147.
49. Liu XN, Yang CJ, Kim JE, et al: Enhanced tendon-to-bone healing of chronic rotator cuff tears by bone marrow aspirate concentrate in a rabbit model. *Clin Orthop Surg* 2018;10(1):99-110. doi:10.4055/cios.2018.10.1.99.
50. Lim JK, Hui J, Li L, Thambyah A, Goh J, Lee EH: Enhancement of tendon graft osteointegration using mesenchymal stem cells in a rabbit model of anterior cruciate ligament reconstruction. *Arthroscopy* 2004;20(9):899-910. doi:10.1016/j.arthro.2004.06.035.
51. Xie X, Zhao S, Wu H, et al: Platelet-rich plasma enhances autograft revascularization and reinnervation in a dog model of anterior cruciate ligament reconstruction. *J Surg Res* 2013;183(1):214-222. doi:10.1016/j.jss.2013.01.020.
52. Radice F, Yanez R, Gutierrez V, Rosales J, Pinedo M, Coda S: Comparison of magnetic resonance imaging findings in anterior cruciate ligament grafts with and without autologous platelet-derived growth factors. *Arthroscopy* 2010;26(1):50-57. doi:10.1016/j.arthro.2009.06.030.
53. Nin JR, Gasque GM, Azcarate AV, Beola JD, Gonzalez MH: Has platelet-rich plasma any role in anterior cruciate ligament allograft healing? *Arthroscopy* 2009;25(11):1206-1213. doi:10.1016/j.arthro.2009.06.002.
54. Rodeo SA, Delos D, Williams RJ, Adler RS, Pearle A, Warren RF: The effect of platelet-rich fibrin matrix on rotator cuff tendon healing: A prospective, randomized clinical study. *Am J Sports Med* 2012;40(6):1234-1241. doi:10.1177/0363546512442924.
55. Wolfman NM, Hattersley G, Cox K, et al: Ectopic induction of tendon and ligament in rats by growth and differentiation factors 5, 6, and 7, members of the TGF-beta gene family. *J Clin Invest* 1997;100(2):321-330. doi:10.1172/jci119537.
56. Seeherman HJ, Archambault JM, Rodeo SA, et al: rhBMP-12 accelerates healing of rotator cuff repairs in a sheep model. *J Bone Joint Surg Am* 2008;90(10):2206-2219. doi:10.2106/jbjs.g.00742.
57. Cadet ER, Hsu JW, Levine WN, Bigliani LU, Ahmad CS: The relationship between greater tuberosity osteopenia and the chronicity of rotator cuff tears. *J Shoulder Elbow Surg* 2008;17(1):73-77. doi:10.1016/j.jse.2007.04.017.
58. Yeh WL, Su CY, Chang CW, et al: Surgical outcome of atypical subtrochanteric and femoral fracture related to bisphosphonates use in osteoporotic patients with or without teriparatide treatment. *BMC Musculoskelet Disord* 2017;18(1):527. doi:10.1186/s12891-017-1878-5.

4: Repair and Regeneration

©Copyright 2021 American Academy of Orthopaedic Surgeons

59. Collinge C, Favela J: Use of teriparatide in osteoporotic fracture patients. *Injury* 2016;47 suppl 1:S36-S38. doi:10.1016/s0020-1383(16)30009-2.

60. Rubin MR, Cosman F, Lindsay R, Bilezikian JP: The anabolic effects of parathyroid hormone. *Osteoporos Int* 2002;13(4):267-277. doi:10.1007/s001980200026.

61. Lee DJ, Southgate RD, Farhat YM, et al: Parathyroid hormone 1-34 enhances extracellular matrix deposition and organization during flexor tendon repair. *J Orthop Res* 2015;33(1):17-24. doi:10.1002/jor.22735.

62. Chen X, Giambini H, Ben-Abraham E, An KN, Nassr A, Zhao C: Effect of bone mineral density on rotator cuff tear: An osteoporotic rabbit model. *PLoS One* 2015;10(10):e0139384. doi:10.1371/journal.pone.0139384.

63. Frank RM, Cvetanovich G, Savin D, Romeo AA: Superior capsular reconstruction: Indications, techniques, and clinical outcomes. *JBJS Rev* 2018;6(7):e10. doi:10.2106/jbjs.rvw.17.00141.

64. Neumann JA, Zgonis MH, Rickert KD, et al: Interposition dermal matrix xenografts: A successful alternative to traditional treatment of massive rotator cuff tears. *Am J Sports Med* 2017;45(6):1261-1268. doi:10.1177/0363546516683945.

65. Badhe SP, Lawrence TM, Smith FD, Lunn PG: An assessment of porcine dermal xenograft as an augmentation graft in the treatment of extensive rotator cuff tears. *J Shoulder Elbow Surg* 2008;17(1 suppl):35s-39s. doi:10.1016/j.jse.2007.08.005.

66. Adams JE, Zobitz ME, Reach JS Jr, An KN, Steinmann SP: Rotator cuff repair using an acellular dermal matrix graft: An in vivo study in a canine model. *Arthroscopy* 2006;22(7):700-709. doi:10.1016/j.arthro.2006.03.016.

67. Nicholson GP, Breur GJ, Van Sickle D, Yao JQ, Kim J, Blanchard CR: Evaluation of a cross-linked acellular porcine dermal patch for rotator cuff repair augmentation in an ovine model. *J Shoulder Elbow Surg* 2007;16(5 suppl):S184-S190. doi:10.1016/j.jse.2007.03.010.

68. Gantenbein B, Gadhari N, Chan SC, Kohl S, Ahmad SS: Mesenchymal stem cells and collagen patches for anterior cruciate ligament repair. *World J Stem Cells* 2015;7(2):521-534. doi:10.4252/wjsc.v7.i2.521.

69. McWilliam JR, Mackay G: The internal brace for midsubstance achilles ruptures. *Foot Ankle Int* 2016;37(7):794-800. doi:10.1177/1071100716653373.

70. Rothfeld A, Pawlak A, Liebler SAH, Morris M, Paci JM: Patellar tendon repair augmentation with a knotless suture anchor internal brace: A biomechanical cadaveric study. *Am J Sports Med* 2018;46(5):1199-1204. doi:10.1177/0363546517751916.

71. van Eck CF, Limpisvasti O, ElAttrache NS: Is there a role for internal bracing and repair of the anterior cruciate ligament? A systematic literature review. *Am J Sports Med* 2018;46(9):2291-2298. doi:10.1177/0363546517717956.

72. Yoo JS, Yang EA: Clinical results of an arthroscopic modified Brostrom operation with and without an internal brace. *J Orthop Traumatol* 2016;17(4):353-360. doi:10.1007/s10195-016-0406-y.

73. Smith PA, Bley JA: Allograft anterior cruciate ligament reconstruction utilizing internal brace augmentation. *Arthrosc Tech* 2016;5(5):e1143-e1147. doi:10.1016/j.eats.2016.06.007.

74. Millar NL, Akbar M, Campbell AL, et al: IL-17A mediates inflammatory and tissue remodelling events in early human tendinopathy. *Sci Rep* 2016;6:27149. doi:10.1038/srep27149.

©Copyright 2021 American Academy of Orthopaedic Surgeons

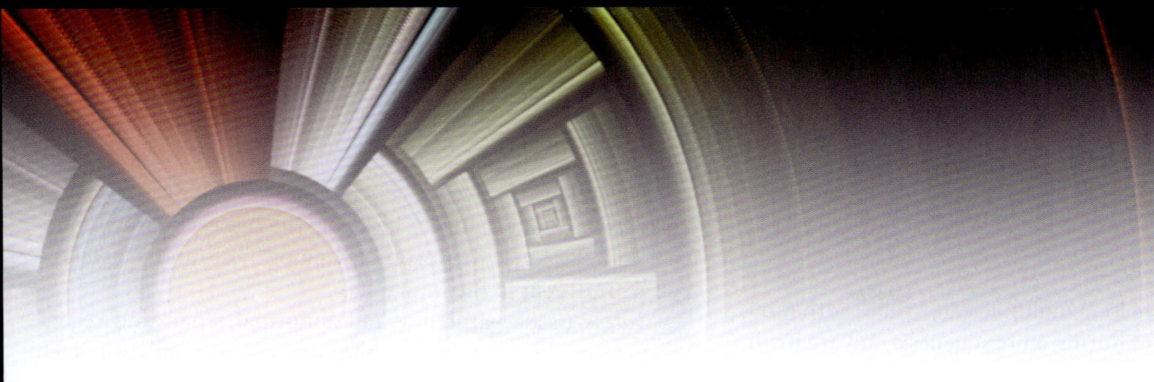

35

Skeletal Muscle Repair and Regeneration

Michael J. McClure, PhD
George J. Christ, PhD
Jonathan E. Isaacs, MD

Keywords: *atrophy; muscle injuries; regeneration; repair; skeletal muscle*

INTRODUCTION

Skeletal muscle is highly organized and one of the largest organs in the body, comprising over 40% of total body mass. The primary function of skeletal muscle contraction is to enable motor tasks ranging from respiration to locomotion. The complexity of such a wide range of motor tasks is coordinated via neural control of both sensory and motor nerves, though it is the latter that are the focus of this report. In this scenario, multiple muscle fibers that belong to a given motor unit are innervated by a single motor neuron. Each motor unit is associated with one muscle fiber type pertaining to either slow twitch oxidative (type I), fast twitch fatigable (type IIb), or fast twitch fatigue resistant (type IIa). Thus, groups of motor units innervate a heterogeneous distribution of fiber types in each large muscle group and can vary depending on the activity and genetics of the individual. This distribution of motor units in association with innate genetics plays a key role in determining the endogenous regenerative capacity of skeletal muscle.[1]

At the cellular level, bundles of striated multinucleated myofibers derive their appearance from the characteristic longitudinal sarcomeric repeats, which, in turn, are surrounded by an intricate extracellular matrix and complex neurovascular networks. Although skeletal muscle has a relatively robust regenerative capacity, traumatic injuries and surgical excision, as well as a diversity of congenital and acquired disorders/diseases, result in simultaneous destruction and/or absence of muscle fibers as well as all the critical surrounding tissue components (nerve, vessel, matrix, and the muscle stem cell niche).[2] Such injuries/conditions result in permanent functional and cosmetic deficits and are collectively referred to as volumetric muscle loss (VML) or VML-like injuries. By definition, the magnitude of tissue loss in VML and VML-like injuries exceeds the endogenous regenerative capacity of skeletal muscle.

The goal of this chapter is to illuminate the complex interplay among the vasculature, nervous system, and muscle satellite cells, and the resulting impact on muscle repair and regeneration in commonly occurring muscle disorders. To this end, we start with a brief review of normal muscle repair and regeneration, and then proceed to describe how this process is abrogated in various muscle conditions. Finally, we describe the current status and limitations of clinical care for muscle disorders, and moreover, highlight the potentially revolutionary impact that tissue engineering/regenerative medicine (TE/RM) technologies could have for improved functional outcomes.

Dr. McClure has received research or institutional support from MTF Biologics. Dr. Isaacs or an immediate family member is a member of a speakers' bureau or has made paid presentations on behalf of Trimed; serves as an unpaid consultant to AxoGen, Inc.; has received research or institutional support from AxoGen, Cook Biotech, and Polyganics, Inc.; and serves as a board member, owner, officer, or committee member of the Hand Surgery Endowment Board of Governors. Neither Dr. Christ nor any immediate family member has received anything of value from or has stock or stock options held in a commercial company or institution related directly or indirectly to the subject of this chapter.

©Copyright 2021 American Academy of Orthopaedic Surgeons

SUCCESSFUL MUSCLE REPAIR AND REGENERATION

Skeletal muscle fibers are long multinucleated tubes with thousands of nuclei that form during embryogenesis and are maintained during postnatal development. These fibers are sensitive to mechanical, electrical, and chemical stimuli and respond rapidly following damage. In situations where the fibers are mildly damaged (such as during exercise), a process of repair and regeneration occurs via necrosis, inflammation, and regeneration. Furthermore, repair and regeneration are two distinguishable processes where we define repair as the preparation of an injured site through inflammation, cellular proliferation, and synthesis of new extracellular matrix to stabilize and preserve the tissue to form either newly regenerated tissue or scar. Regeneration is defined as the reestablishment of intact functional tissue that has histologic, biochemical, and mechanical properties similar to that of native skeletal muscle, following tissue repair. These processes are described in more detail below.

INFLAMMATION

The inflammatory response plays a critical role in muscle repair and regeneration after injury. Of the major constituents of the inflammatory response, macrophage participation is considered critical and is highly regulated. Successful regeneration relies on a delicate balance of phagocytic and nonphagocytic macrophages that secrete factors into the local microenvironment to activate regenerative pathways. For instance, acute injuries result in a predictable series of events in which neutrophils and macrophages play important roles in preparing the optimal local microenvironment for regeneration. More specifically, neutrophils release myeloperoxidase, inducing membrane damage that initiates macrophage phagocytosis and efferocytosis.[3] This prompts the formation of distinct macrophage subpopulations that infiltrate the area to clear debris and promote regeneration. The first subpopulation to arrive is phagocytic CD68+ macrophages (M1), which clear debris and secrete pro-inflammatory cytokines such as interleukin-6 (IL-6). The second subpopulation of macrophages is a nonphagocytic CD163+/CD206+ phenotype (M2), which produces cytokines and growth factors regulating tissue regeneration. This shift in macrophage phenotype (polarity) is accompanied by increased release of pro-resolving and angiogenic milieu such as interleukin-10 (IL-10), vascular endothelial growth factor (VEGF), and transforming growth factor-β1 (TGF-β1) while simultaneously reducing pro-inflammatory signals like IL-6, IL-1β, and tumor necrosis factor-α (TNF-α).[4-6]

In this scenario, any imbalance may lead to impaired regeneration and favor fibrosis. For example, when the balance of phagocytic and nonphagocytic macrophages is disrupted, fibrosis can ensue through elevated numbers of M1 or M2 macrophages, shifting the scale in favor of one or the other. In fact, studies that ablated either M1 or M2 subpopulations demonstrated impaired regeneration by blocking removal of cell debris, or alternatively, blocking the release of growth factors and cytokines that promote angiogenesis and progenitor cell recruitment to the injury site.[7]

Muscle tissue pathology and abnormal repair and regeneration are closely linked to immune system regulation such as macrophage polarization following injury.[8] Severe soft-tissue injuries caused by lacerations to the muscle belly, blast, crush, or tumor resection can alter this immune response cascade and create a microenvironment rich in TGF-β1 and IL-6 that permits fibrosis.[9] In these types of injuries, the wound environment is mostly dictated by the first subpopulation of phagocytic M1 macrophages, while the second subpopulation of M2 macrophages are suppressed, limiting production of pro-regenerative factors and shifting the balance toward fibrosis.[10] Furthermore, muscle atrophy caused by denervation or disuse upregulates signaling pathways such as TNF-α, which can have deleterious effects and permit aberrant synthesis of collagen.[11] Lastly, prolonged muscular dystrophy causes enhanced fibrosis through continued breakdown and regeneration of muscle fibers, which leads to relentless M1 and M2 macrophage turnover and a slow buildup of fibrosis.[9]

REGENERATION

The generation of muscle fibers stems from a process termed, myogenesis, which occurs during both embryo development and adult regeneration in two phases, primary and secondary myogenesis. During primary myogenesis, mononucleated myogenic progenitor cells differentiate and fuse together to form long, syncytial multinucleated tubes. Multinucleated tubes grow in length and width during secondary myogenesis as more progenitor cells continue to fuse and myotubes fuse with each other. Three sources of muscle progenitors have been identified, including those that reside adjacent to myofibers (satellite cell), perivascular cells from the interstitial connective tissue, and some nonlocal cells derived from circulation such as mesenchymal stem cells.

Mesenchymal stem cells were shown to contribute to muscle regeneration following acute injuries, and specialized subpopulations that express PDGFR-a, CD34, and stem cell antigen-1 are considered to be more potent than other types.[12] In particular, it was shown that these MSCs rapidly divide and then disappear following muscle injury, interacting with satellite cells to promote regeneration. In addition, it appears these cells boost the regenerative response by regulating inflammation through production of pro-inflammatory signals to recruit phagocytic macrophages during the first phase of inflammation followed by a change to anti-inflammatory factors to aid with regeneration.[13]

The role of perivascular cells (pericytes) has been studied in both prenatal and postnatal myogenesis. In postnatal tissue, these cells encircle the endothelium of microvessels, regulating blood vessel growth, permeability, and homeostasis. In muscle, two subpopulations were identified by their myogenic capacity where cells that stained for tissue nonspecific alkaline phosphatase and

©Copyright 2021 American Academy of Orthopaedic Surgeons

CD146 possessed a stronger myogenic potential.[14] Indeed, studies that extracted CD146+ cells from muscle reported positive expression muscle-specific transcription factors. More interestingly, a recent study demonstrated that prenatal pericytes directly contributed to the postnatal satellite cell pool.[15]

The most widely accepted putative muscle progenitor cells are satellite cells. Satellite cells are found within the basal lamina of mature muscle fibers, reside as quiescent mononucleated cells within a specific niche, and are identified by their expression of Pax7, an important regulator of myogenic phenotype and cell maturation.[16] Following mild injury or exercise, satellite cells are activated, exiting their quiescent state and entering mitosis to generate progeny that will go through several rounds of proliferation and then migrate to the injury site. During this proliferative state, a large percentage of daughter cells migrate, undergo differentiation, and fuse to form new myofibers. However, not all satellite cell progeny are involved in de novo fiber formation. In contrast, a smaller percentage of progeny will self-renew to replenish the muscle satellite stem cell population following full regeneration, entering back into quiescence.[17] Although three cell types have been identified and discussed in brief, the focus of this chapter will emphasize the most prominently studied cell, the satellite cell.

SATELLITE CELL REGULATION

Satellite cells respond to environmental signals, including physical cues and regulatory factors that affect regeneration. This creates an extraordinarily complex microenvironment with diverse signaling patterns. Satellite cells are often located near capillaries, a source of endocrine signals, and are approximated to fibroblasts and immune cells, creating a source of paracrine signals which can influence satellite cell activation, proliferation, and differentiation. Neural inputs that depolarize the muscle fiber are also capable of influencing satellite cells through electrical activity, or by the chemical signals released following contraction or injury during exercise.[18]

Transforming growth factor-β (TGF-β) is a cytokine released by inflammatory cells following injury, stimulating resident fibroblasts to synthesize collagen and fibronectin. When levels of TGF-β are high, fibroblasts synthesize excessive amounts of extracellular matrix leading to fibrosis. This is observed in muscular dystrophy where dystrophic tissue has elevated levels of collagen compared with normal tissue. Furthermore, TGF-β promotes a fibrogenic phenotype in cultured myoblasts, indicating its dominant effect to promote fibrosis. In addition, recent evidence suggests that lower levels of TGF-β are required for effective regeneration, demonstrating a specific therapeutic window.[19] In contrast, insulinlike growth factor-1 (IGF-1) is associated with increased muscle mass and enhanced regeneration in mice. IGF-1 functions in a dual manner, initially increasing proliferation in cultured myoblasts followed by enhanced differentiation and fusion.[20] Hepatocyte growth factor (HGF) spikes in the early phase of regeneration. This protein is sequestered in extracellular matrix and released following injury, where it binds to the c-met receptor to activate satellite cells.[21] Moreover, fibroblast growth factors (FGFs) were shown to induce myoblast proliferation and suppress differentiation. Like HGF, FGF-2 is sequestered in muscle ECM and promotes satellite cell proliferation during the early phase of regeneration.[22]

Aside from growth factor sequestration, ECM proteins play a critical role in regulation of satellite cell proliferation and differentiation. Satellite cells reside in a niche where they adhere to a basement membrane that contains a specific concentration of collagens, laminins, fibronectin, and proteoglycans. It is widely accepted that ECM influences satellite cell proliferation, migration, and differentiation.[23] For instance, laminin and collagen are reciprocally regulated by fibronectin during muscle regeneration. In addition, fibronectin inhibits differentiation of cultured progenitor cells whereas laminin promotes it. Collectively, these diverse extracellular signals underscore the complexity of the satellite cell microenvironment and highlight factors that are capable of influencing muscle regeneration.

CONDITIONS WITH ALTERED MUSCLE REPAIR AND REGENERATION

As mentioned, skeletal muscle has the ability to fully regenerate following mild injuries by initiating a series of events. This ability is closely linked to the status of the muscle, where associated comorbidities should be considered as major determinants of regeneration. Changes muscle homeostasis ("status quo") are capable of disrupting those regenerative and reparative processes by adversely affecting satellite cell pools via loss of neural control, disuse, trauma, or other dystrophic disorders (**Figure 1**). Below we provide some salient examples.

MUSCLE ATROPHY

Skeletal muscle is a highly adaptable tissue, changing its size, structure, and function in response to changing environmental stimuli. Part of this response involves a balance between catabolic (protein degradation) and anabolic (protein synthesis) pathways that either reduce or increase the size and mass of muscle fibers. When the catabolic pathways supersede anabolic, the balance shifts toward protein degradation and muscle atrophy. Atrophy occurs through multiple mechanisms including those induced by denervation, aging, and disuse. Although atrophy is not causing a direct injury to the muscle, it does impact satellite cell activity which can have detrimental effects on an individual's ability to regenerate new muscle. Furthermore, each atrophic mechanism imposes a different effect on satellite cells.

DENERVATION ATROPHY

When muscle is denervated because of injury to the motor neurons through laceration, crush, or avulsion, the innervated muscle groups are paralyzed distal to the defect, creating a flaccid tissue with rapid atrophy and reduction in muscle mass

©Copyright 2021 American Academy of Orthopaedic Surgeons

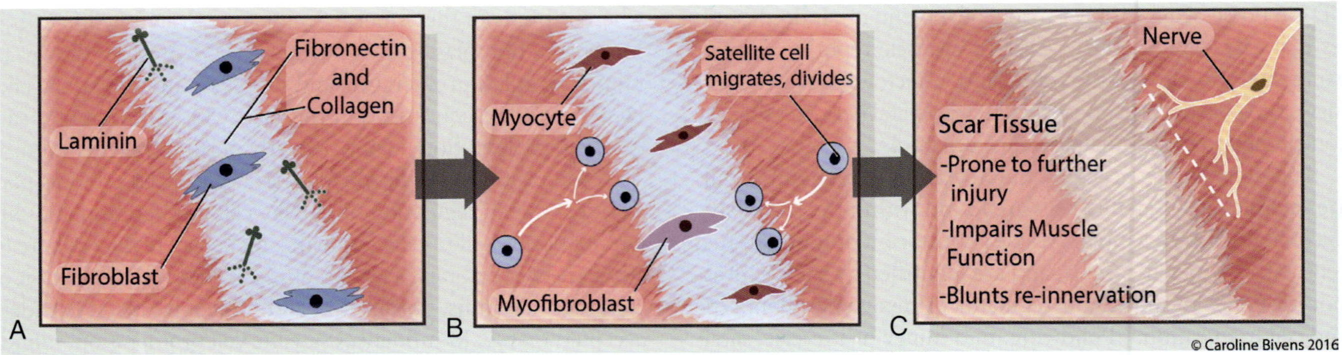

FIGURE 1 Regeneration of muscle injuries is adversely effected by the development of fibrosis (**A**), which is the aberrant synthesis of extracellular matrix in an effort to stabilize the wound. Fibrosis can reduce the number of myoblasts and myocytes that develop in the defect (**B**) by negatively impacting satellite cell motility and blunting reinnervation (**C**) due to an unfavorable cell-matrix interface. (Image courtesy of Caroline Bivens.)

and function. Depending on the degree of denervation and length of time without neural stimulation (months or years), changes in muscle can be mild or severe. Short-term changes following denervation are characterized by progressive atrophy and functional deterioration (**Figure 2**). This can be observed at the muscle fiber level where ultrastructural changes become more prominent including disruptions of the Z-line and loss of actin and myosin filaments. Blood flow to muscles is also impacted with a reduced capillary bed density following the first week of denervation, compounding the effects of injury.[24]

Denervated muscles are incapable of function without exogenous stimulation and, if spontaneous nerve regeneration does not occur, require surgery to reinnervate the muscle and reestablish neural connections.[25] In cases involving a nerve laceration or avulsion, a proximal axonal stump remains, whereas the distal portion begins to degenerate. This pathological condition is known as Wallerian degeneration. Wallerian degeneration is initiated by the absence of a survival signal from cell bodies or a pro-degenerative signal at the injury site. Following loss of core survival signals like nicotinamide mononucleotide acetyltransferases (NMNATs), SARM1, and PHR1, axonal breakdown and fragmentation are activated.[26] Furthermore, muscle and nerve attempt to preserve each other following injury and denervation. During the initiation phase of Wallerian degeneration, axons retain the ability to generate spontaneous miniature end plate potentials (MEPP) and end plate potentials (EPP) that can summate to evoke small muscle contractions. In addition, before full fragmentation, damaged axons release chemical factors that sensitize muscle to acetylcholine.[24] Because muscle relies on neural stimulation to preserve muscle fiber integrity and vice versa, targets such as those mentioned could also help prevent the degenerative events that follow Wallerian degeneration in muscle. If reinnervation cannot be achieved within a certain time frame (~18 months), the potential for recovery of muscle contraction and volume becomes less achievable.

Motor nerve injuries also cause changes in muscle fiber signaling patterns and membrane potentials. Following denervation, signaling favors the ubiquitin-proteasome pathway, where NF-κB activation causes release of several pro-inflammatory factors such as TNF-α and a variety of interleukins that collectively promote downstream pathways to degrade proteins.[24] Activation of these pathways also causes increased production and localization of ion channels, hemichannels formed by connexins (39, 43, and 45), and pannexin channels via positive feedback, heightening membrane sensitivity to changes in electric potential, and producing a more permeable membrane for ion exchange.[27] Altered sensitivity of muscle membranes via connexins increased the likelihood of continued atrophy. In support of this hypothesis a recent study demonstrated that absence of connexin 43 and 45 reduced the degree of atrophy,[27] but more study is needed to determine whether targeting connexins is useful for denervation because these changes to the membrane occur in the short-term.

Increased abundance of channels in muscle membranes produced simultaneous increases in ion currents. Membrane depolarization is associated with changes in ion currents and membrane permeability. During the initial phase of denervation, an increase in intracellular Na^+ and Ca^{2+} occurs alongside a reduction in K^+. In addition, the sarcolemma becomes more permeable to Na^+ and less permeable to K^+, allowing for massive influx of Na^+ to depolarize the membrane and create MEPPs to evoke miniature muscle contractions.[28]

SATELLITE CELL ACTIVATION FOLLOWING DENERVATION ATROPHY

Collectively, promotion of the ubiquitin-proteasome pathway and increased membrane permeability via gap junctions have a significant effect on satellite cell response. Increased inflammatory mediators and concomitant increased calcium flux activate satellite cell pools, sending progeny to repair damaged/denervated muscle. Satellite cell activity following short-term denervation increases dramatically with activation of the satellite cell pool and robust proliferation within the first 2 months (figure from our data). This is related to a general activation of the myogenic program following denervation with upregulation of early myogenic regulatory factors during

©Copyright 2021 American Academy of Orthopaedic Surgeons

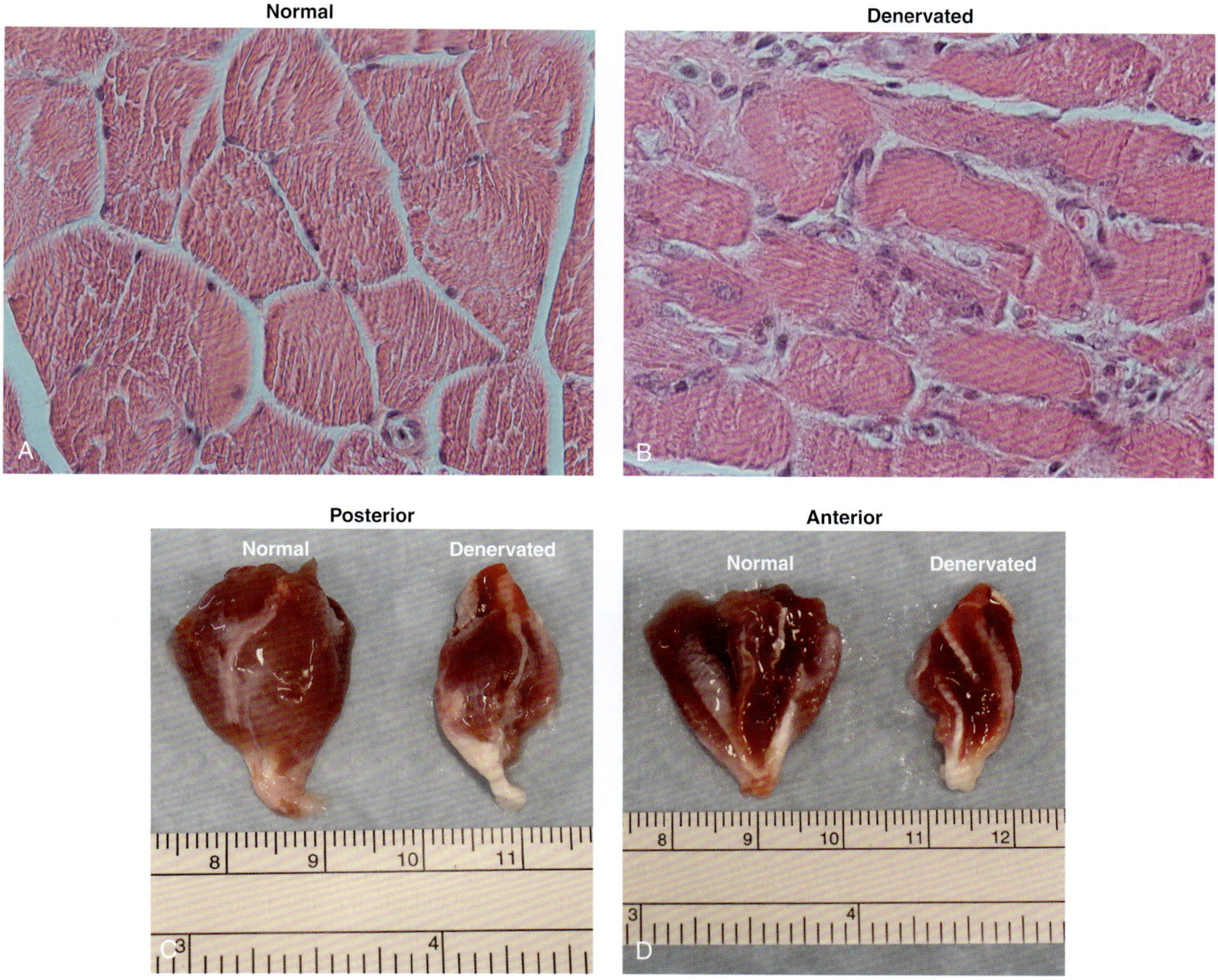

FIGURE 2 Denervation muscle atrophy results in increased number of nuclei in the muscle when normal (**A**) and denervated (**B**) muscles are compared. This also results in drastically reduced muscle mass as shown by gross morphological images of the posterior (**C**) and anterior (**D**) sides of the gastrocnemius following sciatic nerve ligation.

this early period. In contrast, long-term denervation encourages continued atrophy and degeneration of the original muscle fibers. Capillary loss becomes ever more prominent in the later stages of denervation with a 90% reduction 18 months postinjury.[29] This occurs in conjunction with a replacement of muscle mass with noncontractile connective tissue. At this stage, there is no hope for recovery despite further efforts by satellite cells to regenerate new muscle fibers. Without innervated muscle and intact neuromuscular junctions, muscle deteriorates beyond repair.

DISUSE ATROPHY

During a period of immobilization, bed rest, or change in gravitational environment, muscle remains unloaded and unused. In these situations, a reduction in muscle and strength is observed in the affected sites despite neuromuscular junctions remaining intact. Owing to low strength, individuals with disuse atrophy are at risk for other injuries. Furthermore, there is a progressive loss of mass and strength over time that, if allowed to continue, leads to an exacerbated effect. For instance, 2 weeks of bed rest resulted in an 8% and 6% reduction in muscle mass and maximum force, respectively. When the individuals were immobilized for 5 weeks, they lost 16% of their muscle mass and 18% of their maximum muscle force.[30] Furthermore, disuse atrophy due to limb immobilization is more susceptible to muscle damage during reloading or reambulation. Indeed, patients were tested for muscle injury following eccentric and concentric contractions using loads less than 65% of the maximum load initially tested before immobilization, and those loads showed increased edema in magnetic resonance imaging scans.[31]

©Copyright 2021 American Academy of Orthopaedic Surgeons

SATELLITE CELL RESPONSE TO DISUSE ATROPHY

Drastic changes in muscle size, structure, and composition are capable of influencing satellite cells, but evidence poses more questions than answers. Human studies indicate no change in myonuclear numbers with atrophy during 2 and 4 weeks immobilization, suggesting that satellite cells were unaffected by disuse.[18] Other human studies suggest that satellite cell numbers dwindle during more prolonged disuse. To more effectively study the effect of disuse on satellite cells, hindlimb suspension models were employed and it was determined that satellite cell numbers diminished over time, but that the regenerative capacity of muscle once loaded again remains unchanged.[18] These data suggest that mechanisms which influence satellite cells following disuse are different than those involving denervation. Thus, treatments that might target satellite cells in either condition would require a different approach.

AGING-INDUCED ATROPHY

A major characteristic of aging is the gradual loss of skeletal muscle mass that begins around the age of 50. This age-related muscle atrophy is a slow reduction in muscle mass and strength and results in impaired functional capacity and increased incidence of injury, costing the United States $18.5 billion in related healthcare expenses every year.[32] Age-associated mechanisms are responsible for the changes that occur in muscle leading to reduced fiber size, a shift in fiber type, a change in the number of motor units, and a reduction in innervation. Indeed, age-related muscle wasting was suggested to be similar to the events that occur following denervation, owing to a slow degeneration of neural synapses as aging progresses. To emphasize this point, Carlson and colleagues performed preclinical studies in rat and demonstrated age-related muscle fiber denervation by documenting parallel changes in myogenin and nicotinic acetylcholine receptor RNA levels when they compared aged muscle versus denervated muscle.[33] As muscle continues to age, it is accompanied by a progressive loss of type II alpha-motor neurons and expansion of type I neurons to replace denervated sites, leading to a net gain of slow oxidative muscle fibers.[34] This process draws parallels to conditions such as denervation and strengthens the importance to understanding the muscle-nerve relationship and is especially important to describe muscle's regenerative capacity. Cumulative changes such as those that occur during aging are accompanied by changes in satellite cell and affect regenerative outcomes.

EFFECT OF AGING ON SATELLITE CELLS

As aging progresses, stem cell numbers dwindle and the same is true for satellite cells. Humans and animals share a similar quantitative pattern of satellite cells over the course of a lifespan. In rats, satellite cells decline rapidly in the first month after birth and remain relatively constant until old age. When a rat exceeds the human equivalent of 50 years, satellite cells decline yet again. These age-related changes are thought to be due to intrinsic and extrinsic features that influence satellite cell proliferation and self-renewal. One of the most widely documented changes in muscle is an increase in collagen I and reduction in key basement membrane components such as laminin, proteoglycans, and collagen IV. Increased collagen I demonstrated a negative impact on satellite cell self-renewal both in vitro and in vivo, resulting in fewer satellite cells and a lower regenerative capacity. Interestingly, studies demonstrated that when satellite cells derived from older animals were implanted into young animals, their ability to regenerate and self-renew was restored,[35] underscoring the hypothesis that environmental factors like ECM play a significant role in satellite cell regulation and muscle's regenerative capacity.

MUSCLE TRAUMA

Extremity soft-tissue trauma, in particular, VML injury, results in permanent loss of skeletal muscle mass, posing a significant clinical challenge. Treatments for these devastating injuries are to first stabilize the wound. This can be achieved by allowing fibrosis to occur within the wound site. In addition, an autologous muscle can be engrafted after scar has formed. Although some autologous grafts can support limb salvage, functional recovery rates are often low (8%).[36,37] As a consequence, these grafts typically remodel into noncontractile tissue after a long healing and reparative process.[38,39] Despite postoperative efforts to rehabilitate the muscle deficit using physical therapy, patients continue to experience functional losses. In total, these surgeries and rehabilitation cost the United States $600 billion (2016 data) each year[2,37] (**Figure 3**).

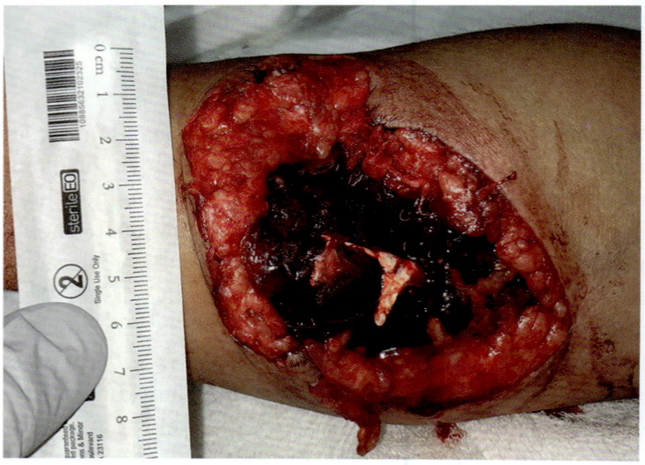

FIGURE 3 Acute volumetric muscle loss injury in the lower limb. This image also depicts injuries to the skin, fat, muscle, and bone as part of this collective injury, indicating its complexity. Note, dark appearance of the muscle indicating severe bruising and possible necrosis.

©Copyright 2021 American Academy of Orthopaedic Surgeons

The rapid degeneration of muscle fibers following traumatic muscle injury seems to be related to disuse and loss of trophic support and feedback normally provided by intact axons. Unlike most cells in the body, muscle fibers function as a syncytium of fused nucleated cells. In cases of muscle trauma, these multinucleated muscle fibers are lost in the injured area. Initially, muscle injury activates a pool of quiescent, regenerative satellite cells that migrate to the injured site, differentiate into myoblasts, and fuse with existing myofibers to bolster their reduced size. However, lack of muscle regeneration and reinnervation in the traumatized area subsequently negates these temporary mechanisms, leaving muscle to promote reparative features like fibrosis. With time, degeneration occurs, and fibrosis develops in the traumatized area. In addition, distally affected muscle fibers lose the intramuscular connections that are important in motor unit recruitment during contraction. Fibrosis, denervation, and lack of muscle regeneration collectively contribute to muscle weakness. Eventually, the injured muscle is completely replaced with fibrotic adipose tissue with no hope of recovery.

Reduced motor function is directly associated with the development of noncontractile tissue (mainly fibrosis) in the muscle injury area. This suboptimal reparative state can be ascribed to a combination of inflammatory mediators, overactive connective tissue cells, dysfunctional regenerative processes, and denervation both in the zone of injury and distal to the defect that limit de novo regeneration. As such, achieving functional gains will require treatment modalities that favor de novo muscle regeneration over fibrosis.

CURRENT CLINICAL TREATMENT OF MUSCLE DAMAGE

Clinical muscle injury can be related to a variety of traumatic and atraumatic etiologies. Clinicians must appreciate the natural history of the injury spectrum and recognize where and when intervention can favorably alter the prognosis. The spectrum of traumatic injuries includes contusions, strains, lacerations, and avulsing injuries resulting in VML (see above). However, muscles can be damaged by infection, ischemia, and toxins as well, and further, even denervation (which permanently alters the muscle structure and function) can be considered a form of injury.

The most common muscle injuries are related to athletics and typically involve contusions and muscle strains. Contusions are a result of blunt trauma and in addition to the local muscle fiber cell damage, can be associated with intramuscular hematoma (especially when associated with pathologic or medically induced coagulopathy) and swelling. Muscle "strain" is analogous to muscle "tear" and occurs from excessive stretch during muscle contraction. Strain severity ranges from minor damage (first-degree tear) to complete disruption of the muscle belly (third-degree tear). First-degree tears do not result in substantial loss of function, whereas second-degree injuries result in temporary loss of strength and mobility.[40] Almost all of these types of injuries are treated conservatively with temporary relative immobilization, ice, rest, and compression. Protecting the muscle can avoid further tearing, and cryotherapy has been shown to decrease intramuscular bleeding and inflammation.[41] After a few days (3 to 7), gentle passive range of motion is initiated often in conjunction with heat to help relax the painful and often spastic muscle. Mobilization has been shown to improve regeneration of myofibers and accelerate tissue healing, whereas early active range of motion can actually worsen the injury and increase scar formation.[42] As a full range of motion is restored typically over several weeks, gradual strengthening can be initiated.

Rarely, in the presence of severe swelling, soft-tissue imaging modalities such as ultrasonography or MRI can be used primarily to assess for focal blood collections. Some benefit has been proposed with percutaneous drainage when a well-contained, focal hematoma is identified.[43] These same imaging modalities may be indicated if active motion is not achieved and a full-thickness tear is suspected (third degree). In these cases, surgical repair may improve the final recovery though it is controversial. Complications of contusions and muscle strains are rare but include the formation of scar tissue,[44] heterotopic ossification (myositis ossificans),[45] and prolonged discomfort and loss of function.[46] Reinjury is not uncommon because function may return to "normal" despite incomplete muscle healing, and healing time can be somewhat hard to predict depending on muscle involvement and the extent of injury.

Muscle lacerations are typically related to penetrating trauma from a knife or sharp object. Partial lacerations, in which the general muscle tissue tension is maintained, will behave much like a muscle strain and have a good prognosis for spontaneous recovery with conservative treatment. The muscle belly stumps, however, will separate and retract with complete lacerations. Though scar tissue can form in the intervening space to offer some stability, the resting tension of the muscle fibers is never restored. Additionally, intramuscular nerve fibers are unable to grow across the fibrotic plane, and the muscle tissue distal to the zone of injury remains denervated.[47] These muscles suffer permanent weakness and dysfunction. Surgical repair can restore the muscle continuity more effectively and create an environment more conducive to intramuscular neural regeneration. Muscle tissue, however, does not hold sutures well, and in the absence of fascial coatings (seen at the muscle-tendon junction) midsubstance muscle repair can be likened to sewing soft white bread together. Grasping sutures incorporating the epimysium have been shown to provide the best, albeit still not great, holding strength. By convention, repaired muscles are protected with immobilization for 3 weeks before initiating gentle range of motion.

More extensive injuries as can be seen with avulsion mechanisms, open fractures, and gunshot wounds result in

©Copyright 2021 American Academy of Orthopaedic Surgeons

larger zones of injury and greater degrees of muscle damage and loss. This pattern, again, referred to as VML injury, is not directly repairable for all of the reasons enumerated above. Though the defect is stabilized by scar tissue, the remaining functional muscle tissue is weak and fibrotic and, similar to other muscle lacerations, the distal muscle is usually denervated.[48] Large zones of injury can also be seen from pressure necrosis due to crush injuries, severe soft-tissue infection and abscess formation, and ischemia due to vessel injury or undertreated compartment syndrome. Pressure severity seems to correlate with ischemia and subsequent tissue loss.[49]

The most common treatment strategy for VML injury is replacement of the missing anatomic structure with pedicled and free vascularized muscle transfer or substitution for the missing function with tendon transfer. The latissimus dorsi, for example, can be transferred as a pedicled muscle flap to create a "new" biceps, triceps, or even deltoid muscle if these muscles are irreversibly damaged and nonfunctional.[50] The thoracodorsal artery, vein, and nerve are mobilized along with the muscle so that the muscle can either be rotated to a new insertional target or completely lifted up and inset with a new origin and insertion. The gracilis is more commonly transferred as a free tissue transfer when a local option (such as the latissimus) is not available to restore elbow flexion or finger flexion. This surgery is much more complex and while the motor nerve to the gracilis and the vascular pedicle are harvested and transferred with the muscle, donor blood vessels and nerves must be identified to reestablish tissue perfusion and innervation. These surgeries suffer high complication rates (including loss of the transfer muscle) and often still restore only marginally useful muscle strength.[51,52] There are many more tendon transfer options depending on what function is lost and which muscles are available (ie, not affected by the injury). General principles of tendon transfer include identifying a redundant or functionally insignificant donor with similar strength and excursion of the muscle being replaced, preserving a straight line of pull after the transfer, and using donor and recipient synergy. Transferring the flexor carpi radialis to the extensor digitorum longus tendons for loss or chronic denervation of the extensor digitorum longus muscle is an example of a synergistic transfer. Wrist flexion is normally coupled with finger extension, so minimal functional retraining is necessary, and the patient intuitively incorporates the transfer into normal activities. Though finger extension requires much more excursion than the wrist flexor is able to provide, wrist motion compensates via a relative tenodesis effect, resulting in a highly predictable and useful tendon transfer. For all of these muscle and tendon transfers, the surgeon must adjust the resting tension of the donor muscle to optimize myofilament overlap (as based on the Blix curve[53]). When reasonable contractile function is preserved but contraction results in an inadequate arc of motion, the healed and scarred muscle belly can be released from surrounding tissue and allowed to "slide" distally. Though this maneuver can relieve contraction and shift the arc of motion to a more "useful" range, the excursion and resting tension of the muscle are not reestablished and the net range of motion does not increase and muscle force does not return to normal.[54]

With prolonged periods of denervation due to delayed nerve reconstruction, missed injuries, and most commonly, long regeneration lengths, muscle recovery can be extremely compromised. The neurotrophic environment in the chronically denervated distal nerve stump is compromised so that an insufficient number of axons reach the target muscle.[55] At least in animal models, this axon loss can be partially compensated for by enlarging motor units.[56,57] However, many of the muscle fibers suffer apoptosis and those that remain are smaller and weaker than normal.[58,59] Many reinnervated muscles are able to contract but are incapable of generating functionally useful power.

FUTURE THERAPIES

As noted above, the distinct inflammation, repair, and remodeling phases of skeletal muscle injury following blunt trauma, contusions, and lacerations are well documented. Moreover, although clinical treatment of blunt trauma, contusions, and lacerations varies, most injuries, if given sufficient time, rest, and physical rehabilitation, will repair themselves.[44] Nonetheless, despite the rather well-documented capacity of skeletal muscle to repair, regenerate, and remodel following injury, more severe traumatic injuries, such as those involving the loss of a substantial portion of muscle tissue, as characteristic of VML injuries, are not capable of full regeneration on their own. That is, such injuries involve a degree of muscle tissue loss that exceeds the endogenous regenerative capacity of muscle. VML injuries result in permanent cosmetic and functional deficits of either the injured muscle or the muscle unit (ie, in the presence of synergists). As reviewed in the previous section, current treatment for VML injury is often associated with poor engraftment and donor site morbidity. Not surprisingly, this unmet medical need has stimulated research efforts to develop new technologies for treatment of VML injuries.

Tissue engineering/regenerative medicine (TE/RM) technologies hold great promise for treating any disease, disorder, or condition associated with a loss of viable cells or tissue, especially for an unmet medical need such as VML injury. Thus, it is not surprising that a variety of such therapeutic strategies are under development for the repair of VML to craniofacial and extremity muscles, as well as similar injury conditions (eg, abdominal wall repair). The overall strategies for treatment of VML injury can be divided into two general categories, those pursuing implantation of a biological (ie, decellularized) or synthetic scaffold (**Figure 4**), and those using a scaffold in combination with cells.[60] Some of these approaches are sufficient to promote robust primary myogenesis and functionally significant neofiber formation within a

©Copyright 2021 American Academy of Orthopaedic Surgeons

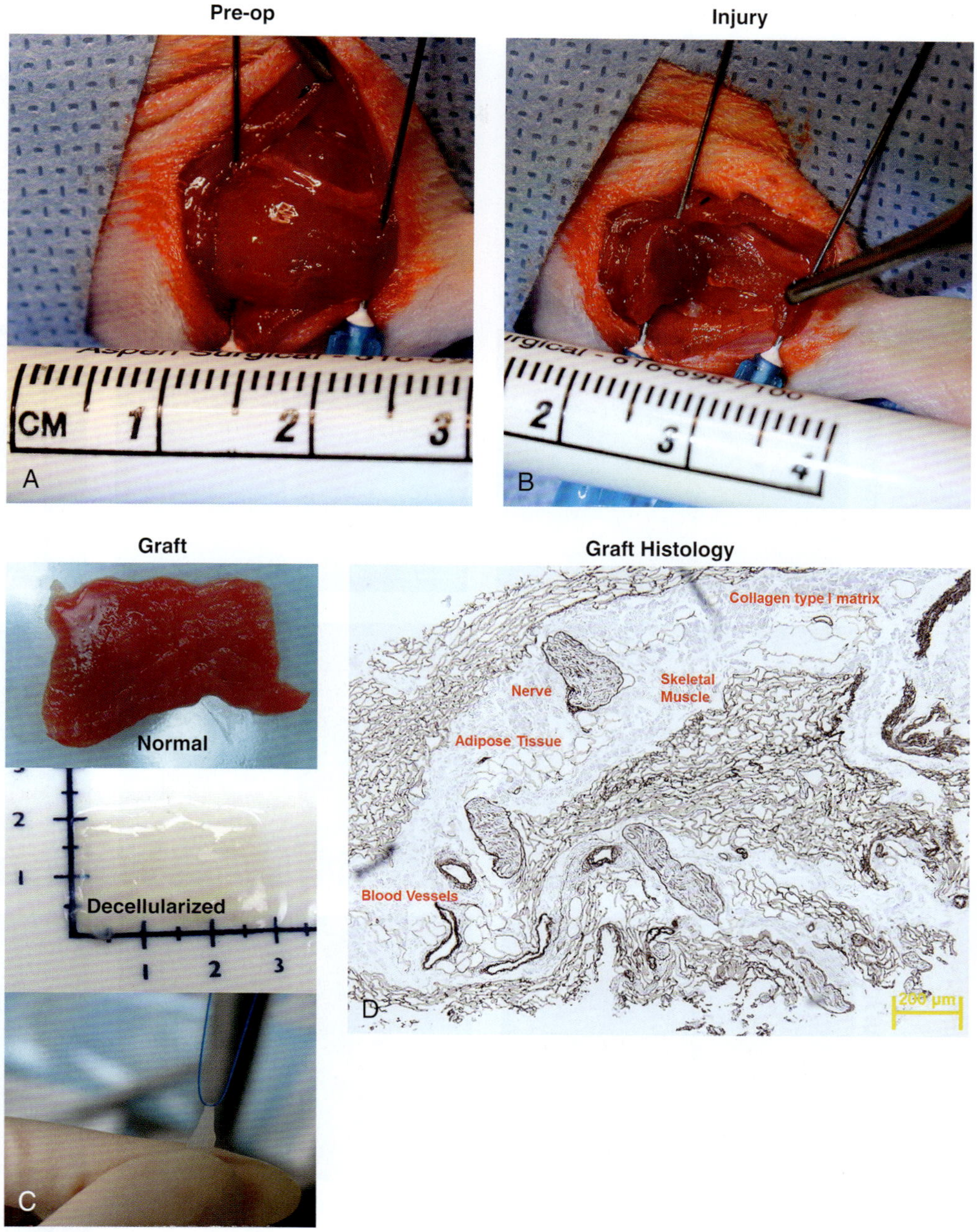

FIGURE 4 Preclinical volumetric muscle loss surgical model using the gastrocnemius. **A**, demonstrates the site of the lateral head before and after injury is made (**B**). These types of injury models allow scientists to test various products such as biologics and synthetics. In (**C**), we demonstrate use of decellularized muscle grafts derived from a human vastus lateralis, where the native components and architecture of the extracellular matrix are retained (**D**).

few millimeters of the native tissue interface. Such preclinical findings are encouraging and likely scalable to the smaller muscles of the face, hand, and shoulders. However, to treat the most devastating VML injuries will require vastly larger surgical products that positively stimulate regeneration and enhance the regenerative capacity of the site, and this need can be best observed through recent clinical studies that tested decellularized small intestinal submucosa in muscle defects[61] (**Figure 5**). Results from these studies show that while islands of muscle fibers are present, fibrosis dominates the tissue. Enhancement of these devastating injuries can be classified by noting primary and secondary myogenesis develop in the site as well as continued muscle growth and hypertrophy. Moreover, continued evolution of TE/RM technologies to explore the potential of combination therapeutics for more complete repair of VML injuries is necessary. Combination therapies include the addition of exogenous growth factors and/or progenitor cells in implantable skeletal muscle tissue engineering technologies.[60,62,63]

In summary, despite robust preclinical activity, there are currently only a few published clinical reports that use biological matrices for muscle tissue repair in patients. In these reports the investigators describe the use of an acellular matrix (porcine intestinal submucosa) for the treatment of leg muscles with VML injury.[64] Although these initial findings are encouraging for the overall tissue engineering

©Copyright 2021 American Academy of Orthopaedic Surgeons

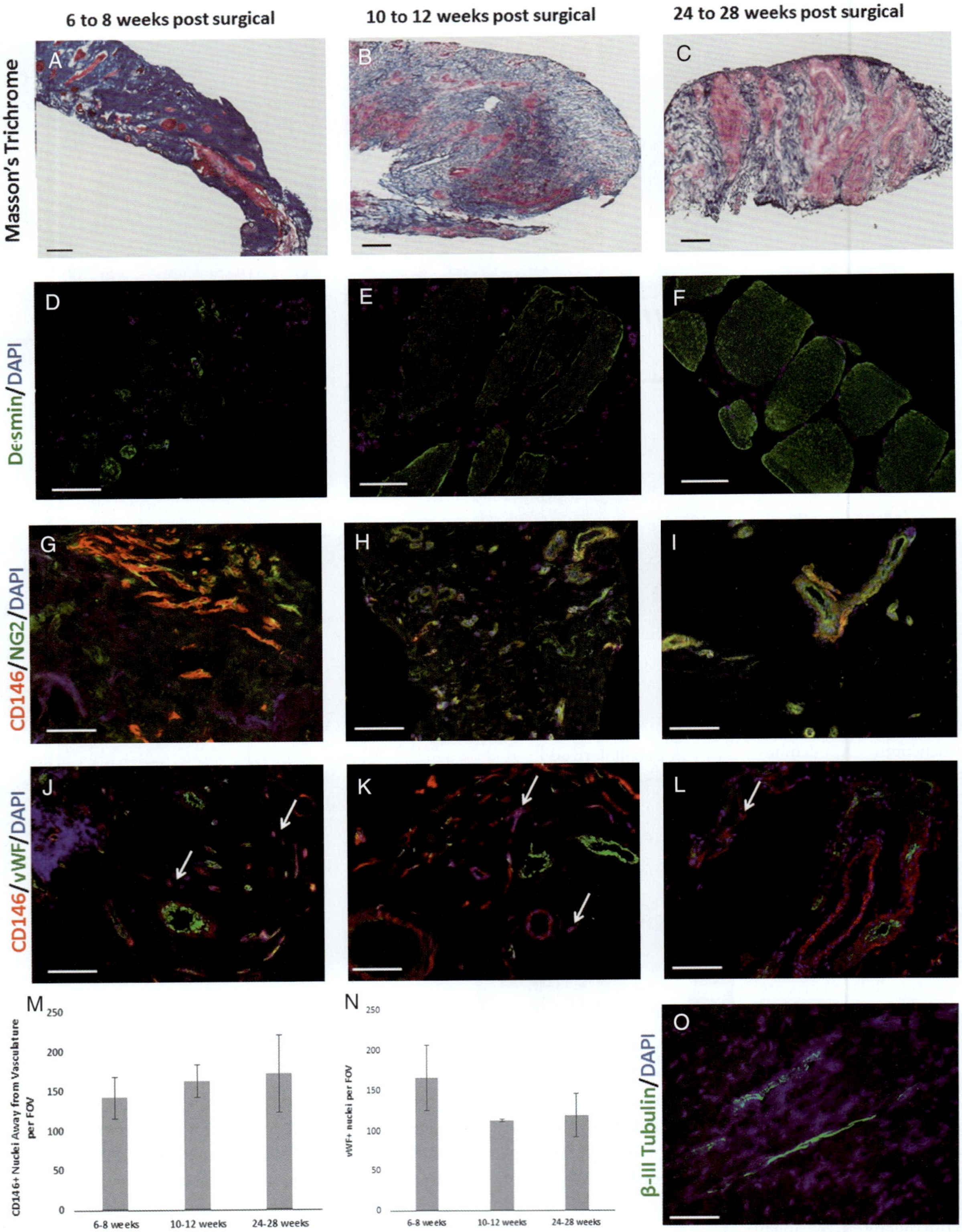

FIGURE 5 Clinical evaluation of volumetric muscle loss treatments. Biopsies of site-appropriate tissue remodeling following implantation of small intestinal submucosa (Cook Biotech) into human muscle defects. Masson's trichrome staining shows islands of muscle fibers present following surgery up to 28 weeks (**A** to **C**). Desmin staining of human muscle biopsies showed positive expression (**D** to **F**), indicating the presence of intermediate filaments proteins that connect the sarcomere and costamere. Perivascular stem cells, a subset of muscle stem cells (see Successful Muscle Repair and Regeneration), were stained using CD146+ NG2+ markers and were associated with tissue repair (**G** to **I**). In addition, those perivascular cells were stained away from the vasculature indicating their activity within the implant area (**J** to **O**). (From Dziki J, Badylak S, Yabroudi M, et al: An acellular biologic scaffold treatment for volumetric muscle loss: results of a 13-patient cohort study. *NPJ Regen Med* 2016;1:16008. Reproduced under Creative Commons Attribution License 4.0, http://creativecommons.org/licenses/by/4.0/.)

 ©Copyright 2021 American Academy of Orthopaedic Surgeons

paradigm, clearly there is still room for significant therapeutic improvement, particularly in light of the relatively modest amount of muscle regeneration and functional recovery that are currently possible.[64,65] Without question, progress to date with TE/RM approaches to VML bode well for future marked improvements, where we will need to continue to evolve our technologies to incorporate bone, neural and vascular tissue components before the achievement of durable, functional products.

SUMMARY

The mechanisms responsible for muscle repair and regeneration are tightly regulated by a series of timely events that first prepare the injury site for wound healing by clearing necrotic debris and synthesizing extracellular matrix to be populated by migrating muscle stem cells (eg, satellite cells). Those cells then undergo a process of fusion, primary tube formation, tube elongation, and hypertrophy to form mature fibers that become innervated. When any portion of these events is disrupted by severe injury or disease, the results can detrimentally impact muscle regeneration, maturity, and homeostasis. Moreover, the ability of muscle to regenerate is largely dependent on the preexisting status of the muscle at the time of injury or disease onset. Current treatments for injuries and diseases that result in permanent cosmetic and functional deficits are able to mitigate some of these negative effects but are largely ineffective to fully regenerate skeletal muscle form and function. Future therapeutics, such as tissue engineering and regenerative medicine technologies, hold promise to enhance the repair and regenerative mechanisms and are described in this chapter.

CLINICAL NOTE

Basic Science Pearls

- Regenerative capacity of the muscle is dependent on its preexisting status and whether the muscle is healthy or an additional comorbidity exists.
- Satellite cells are affected by intrinsic and extrinsic features of the muscle including local and systemic growth factors, cytokines, and local extracellular matrix. Moreover, factors that influence satellite cells are directly affected by comorbidities.
- Treatments for muscle disorders are mostly used in preclinical models, focusing on biologics, synthetics, and incorporation of various stem cells.

Clinical Pearls

- Almost all muscle strains can be treated conservatively with temporary relative immobilization, ice, rest, and, compression.
- More severe injuries such as avulsions and VML often heal with extensive fibrosis.
- Conventional treatment options for VML are limited to tendon and muscle transfers to substitute for the functional loss.

REFERENCES

1. Roberts MD, Haun CT, Mobley CB, et al: Physiological differences between low versus high skeletal muscle hypertrophic responders to resistance exercise training: Current perspectives and future research directions. *Front Physiol* 2018;9:834.
2. Grogan BF, Hsu JR: Volumetric muscle loss. *J Am Acad Orthop Surg* 2011;19(suppl 1):S35-S37.
3. Winterbourn CC, Kettle AJ, Hampton MB: Reactive oxygen species and neutrophil function. *Annu Rev Biochem* 2016;85:765-792.
4. Sunderkotter C, Steinbrink K, Goebeler M, Bhardwaj R, Sorg C: Macrophages and angiogenesis. *J Leukoc Biol* 1994;55(3):410-422.
5. Rostoker R, Yaseen H, Schif-Zuck S, Lichtenstein RG, Rabinovich GA, Ariel A: Galectin-1 induces 12/15-lipoxygenase expression in murine macrophages and favors their conversion toward a pro-resolving phenotype. *Prostaglandins Other Lipid Mediat* 2013;107:85-94.
6. Rao KM: MAP kinase activation in macrophages. *J Leukoc Biol* 2001;69(1):3-10.
7. Arnold L, Henry A, Poron F, et al: Inflammatory monocytes recruited after skeletal muscle injury switch into antiinflammatory macrophages to support myogenesis. *J Exp Med* 2007;204(5):1057-1069.
8. Wang H, Melton DW, Porter L, Sarwar ZU, McManus LM, Shireman PK: Altered macrophage phenotype transition impairs skeletal muscle regeneration. *Am J Pathol* 2014;184(4):1167-1184.
9. Klingler W, Jurkat-Rott K, Lehmann-Horn F, Schleip R: The role of fibrosis in Duchenne muscular dystrophy. *Acta Myol* 2012;31(3):184-195.
10. Hurtgen BJ, Ward CL, Garg K, et al: Severe muscle trauma triggers heightened and prolonged local musculoskeletal inflammation and impairs adjacent tibia fracture healing. *J Musculoskelet Neuronal Interact* 2016;16(2):122-134.
11. Costamagna D, Costelli P, Sampaolesi M, Penna F: Role of inflammation in muscle homeostasis and myogenesis. *Mediat Inflamm* 2015;2015:805172.
12. Joe AW, Yi L, Natarajan A, et al: Muscle injury activates resident fibro/adipogenic progenitors that facilitate myogenesis. *Nat Cell Biol* 2010;12(2):153-163.
13. Villalta SA, Nguyen HX, Deng B, Gotoh T, Tidball JG: Shifts in macrophage phenotypes and macrophage competition for arginine metabolism affect the severity of muscle pathology in muscular dystrophy. *Hum Mol Genet* 2009;18(3):482-496.
14. Cappellari O, Cossu G: Pericytes in development and pathology of skeletal muscle. *Circ Res* 2013;113(3):341-347.
15. Dellavalle A, Maroli G, Covarello D, et al: Pericytes resident in postnatal skeletal muscle differentiate into muscle fibres and generate satellite cells. *Nat Commun* 2011;2:499.
16. von Maltzahn J, Jones AE, Parks RJ, Rudnicki MA: Pax7 is critical for the normal function of satellite cells in adult skeletal muscle. *Proc Natl Acad Sci U S A* 2013;110(41):16474-16479.

©Copyright 2021 American Academy of Orthopaedic Surgeons

17. Bentzinger CF, von Maltzahn J, Rudnicki MA: Extrinsic regulation of satellite cell specification. *Stem Cell Res Ther* 2010;1.
18. Brooks NE, Myburgh KH: Skeletal muscle wasting with disuse atrophy is multi-dimensional: The response and interaction of myonuclei, satellite cells and signaling pathways. *Front Physiol* 2014;5:99.
19. Carlson ME, Conboy MJ, Hsu M, et al: Relative roles of TGF-beta1 and Wnt in the systemic regulation and aging of satellite cell responses. *Aging Cell* 2009;8(6):676-689.
20. Allen RE, Boxhorn LK: Regulation of skeletal muscle satellite cell proliferation and differentiation by transforming growth factor-beta, insulin-like growth factor I, and fibroblast growth factor. *J Cell Physiol* 1989;138(2):311-315.
21. Karalaki M, Fili S, Philippou A, Koutsilieris M: Muscle regeneration: Cellular and molecular events. *In Vivo* 2009;23(5):779-796.
22. Allen RE, Dodson MV, Luiten LS: Regulation of skeletal muscle satellite cell proliferation by bovine pituitary fibroblast growth factor. *Exp Cell Res* 1984;152(1):154-160.
23. Calve S, Odelberg SJ, Simon HG: A transitional extracellular matrix instructs cell behavior during muscle regeneration. *Dev Biol* 2010;344(1):259-271.
24. Dumitru A, Radu BM, Radu M, Cretoiu SM: Muscle changes during atrophy. *Adv Exp Med Biol* 2018;1088:73-92.
25. Isaacs J: Major peripheral nerve injuries. *Hand Clin* 2013;29(3):371-382.
26. Conforti L, Gilley J, Coleman MP: Wallerian degeneration: An emerging axon death pathway linking injury and disease. *Nat Rev Neurosci* 2014;15(6):394-409.
27. Cea LA, Cisterna BA, Puebla C, et al: De novo expression of connexin hemichannels in denervated fast skeletal muscles leads to atrophy. *Proc Natl Acad Sci U S A* 2013;110(40):16229-16234.
28. Cisterna BA, Cardozo C, Saez JC: Neuronal involvement in muscular atrophy. *Front Cell Neurosci* 2014;8:405.
29. Carlson BM: The biology of long-term denervated skeletal muscle. *Eur J Transl Myol* 2014;24(1):3293.
30. Gordon BS, Kelleher AR, Kimball SR: Regulation of muscle protein synthesis and the effects of catabolic states. *Int J Biochem Cell Biol* 2013;45(10):2147-2157.
31. Ploutz-Snyder LL, Tesch PA, Hather BM, Dudley GA: Vulnerability to dysfunction and muscle injury after unloading. *Arch Phys Med Rehabil* 1996;77(8):773-777.
32. Janssen I, Shepard DS, Katzmarzyk PT, Roubenoff R: The healthcare costs of sarcopenia in the United States. *J Am Geriatr Soc* 2004;52(1):80-85.
33. Kostrominova TY, Macpherson PC, Carlson BM, Goldman D: Regulation of myogenin protein expression in denervated muscles from young and old rats. *Am J Physiol Regul Integr Comp Physiol* 2000;279(1):R179-R188.
34. Carlson BM: Factors influencing the repair and adaptation of muscles in aged individuals: Satellite cells and innervation. *J Gerontol A Biol Sci Med Sci* 1995;50 Spec No:96-100.
35. Carosio S, Berardinelli MG, Aucello M, Musaro A: Impact of ageing on muscle cell regeneration. *Ageing Res Rev* 2011;10(1):35-42.
36. Fischer JP, Elliott RM, Kozin SH, Levin LS: Free function muscle transfers for upper extremity reconstruction: A review of indications, techniques, and outcomes. *J Hand Surg Am* 2013;38(12):2485-2490.
37. Corona BT, Rivera JC, Owens JG, Wenke JC, Rathbone CR: Volumetric muscle loss leads to permanent disability following extremity trauma. *J Rehabil Res Dev* 2015;52(7):785-792.
38. DePalma RG, Burris DG, Champion HR, Hodgson MJ: Blast injuries. *N Engl J Med* 2005;352(13):1335-1342.
39. Baechler MF, Groth AT, Nesti LJ, Martin BD: Soft tissue management of war wounds to the foot and ankle. *Foot Ankle Clin* 2010;15(1):113-138.
40. Grassi A, Quaglia A, Canata GL, Zaffagnini S: An update on the grading of muscle injuries: A narrative review from clinical to comprehensive systems. *Joints* 2016;4(1):39-46.
41. Deal DN, Tipton J, Rosencrance E, Curl WW, Smith TL: Ice reduces edema. A study of microvascular permeability in rats. *J Bone Joint Surg Am* 2002;84-A(9):1573-1578.
42. Jarvinen M: Healing of a crush injury in rat striated muscle. 2. a histological study of the effect of early mobilization and immobilization on the repair processes. *Acta Pathol Microbiol Scand* 1975;83(3):269-282.
43. Jarvinen TA, Jarvinen TL, Kaariainen M, et al: Muscle injuries: Optimising recovery. *Best Pract Res Clin Rheumatol* 2007;21(2):317-331.
44. Jarvinen TA, Jarvinen TL, Kaariainen M, Kalimo H, Jarvinen M: Muscle injuries: Biology and treatment. *Am J Sports Med* 2005;33(5):745-764.
45. Beiner JM, Jokl P: Muscle contusion injury and myositis ossificans traumatica. *Clin Orthop Relat Res* 2002;(403 suppl):S110-S119.
46. Huard J, Lu A, Mu X, Guo P, Li Y: Muscle injuries and repair: What's new on the Horizon! *Cells Tissues Organs* 2016;202(3-4):227-236.
47. Kaariainen M, Kaariainen J, Jarvinen TL, Sievanen H, Kalimo H, Jarvinen M: Correlation between biomechanical and structural changes during the regeneration of skeletal muscle after laceration injury. *J Orthop Res* 1998;16(2):197-206.
48. Corona BT, Wenke JC, Ward CL: Pathophysiology of volumetric muscle loss injury. *Cells Tissues Organs* 2016;202(3-4):180-188.
49. Criswell TL, Corona BT, Ward CL, et al: Compression-induced muscle injury in rats that mimics compartment syndrome in humans. *Am J Pathol* 2012;180(2):787-797.
50. Stevanovic MV, Cuellar VG, Ghiassi A, Sharpe F: Single-stage reconstruction of elbow flexion associated with massive soft-tissue defect using the latissimus dorsi muscle bipolar rotational transfer. *Plast Reconstr Surg Glob Open* 2016;4(9):e1066.
51. Maldonado AA, Kircher MF, Spinner RJ, Bishop AT, Shin AY: Free functioning gracilis muscle transfer with and without simultaneous intercostal nerve transfer to musculocutaneous nerve for restoration of elbow flexion after traumatic adult brachial pan-plexus injury. *J Hand Surg Am* 2017;42(4):293 e291-293 e297.
52. Lin CH, Lin YT, Yeh JT, Chen CT: Free functioning muscle transfer for lower extremity posttraumatic composite structure and functional defect. *Plast Reconstr Surg* 2007;119(7):2118-2126.
53. Blix M: Die lange und die spannung des Muskels. *Skand Arch Physiol* 1895;(5):22.
54. Sharma P, Swamy MK: Results of the Max Page muscle sliding operation for the treatment of Volkmann's ischemic contracture of the forearm. *J Orthop Traumatol* 2012;13(4):189-196.
55. Fu SY, Gordon T: Contributing factors to poor functional recovery after delayed nerve repair: Prolonged denervation. *J Neurosci* 1995;15(5 pt 2):3886-3895.
56. Luff AR, Hatcher DD, Torkko K: Enlarged motor units resulting from partial denervation of cat hindlimb muscles. *J Neurophysiol* 1988;59(5):1377-1394.
57. Gordon T, Yang JF, Ayer K, Stein RB, Tyreman N: Recovery potential of muscle after partial denervation: A comparison between rats and humans. *Brain Res Bull* 1993;30(3-4):477-482.
58. Anzil AP, Wernig A: Muscle fibre loss and reinnervation after long-term denervation. *J Neurocytol* 1989;18(6):833-845.
59. Kobayashi J, Mackinnon SE, Watanabe O, et al: The effect of duration of muscle denervation on functional recovery in the rat model. *Muscle Nerve* 1997;20(7):858-866.
60. Passipieri JA, Christ GJ: The potential of combination therapeutics for more complete repair of volumetric muscle loss injuries: The role of exogenous growth factors and/or progenitor cells in implantable skeletal muscle tissue engineering technologies. *Cells Tissues Organs* 2016;202(3-4):202-213.
61. Dziki J, Badylak S, Yabroudi M, et al: An acellular biologic scaffold treatment for volumetric muscle loss: Results of a 13-patient cohort study. *NPJ Regen Med* 2016;1:16008.

©Copyright 2021 American Academy of Orthopaedic Surgeons

62. Baker HB, Passipieri JA, Siriwardane M, et al: Cell and growth factor-loaded keratin hydrogels for treatment of volumetric muscle loss in a mouse model. *Tissue Eng Part A* 2017;23(11-12):572-584.
63. Passipieri JA, Baker HB, Siriwardane M, et al: Keratin hydrogel enhances in vivo skeletal muscle function in a rat model of volumetric muscle loss. *Tissue Eng Part A* 2017;23(11-12):556-571.
64. Mase VJ Jr, Hsu JR, Wolf SE, et al: Clinical application of an acellular biologic scaffold for surgical repair of a large, traumatic quadriceps femoris muscle defect. *Orthopedics* 2010;33(7):511.
65. Han N, Yabroudi MA, Stearns-Reider K, et al: Electrodiagnostic evaluation of individuals implanted with extracellular matrix for the treatment of volumetric muscle injury: Case series. *Phys Ther* 2016;96(4):540-549.

©Copyright 2021 American Academy of Orthopaedic Surgeons

36

Diagnosis and Repair of Peripheral Nerve Injuries

Sameer K. Puri, MD
Margaret E. Cooke, MD
Steve K. Lee, MD

Keywords: *peripheral nerve; nerve injury; nerve repair*

INTRODUCTION

Peripheral nerve injuries present challenges to surgeons in diagnosis and characterization of the injury; prognostication of outcomes with surgical and nonsurgical intervention; and choosing optimal treatment options when intervention is chosen. Suboptimal treatment can leave devastating consequences due to pain and dysfunction. Over one million people worldwide present with a peripheral nerve injury every year. These injuries affect the quality of daily life; 24% to 41% of patients with a major peripheral nerve injury are unable to return to their previous line of work.[1] Despite this, there remains a lack of consensus on optimal treatment strategies for many clinical scenarios.

The authors will attempt to present an up-to-date approach to diagnosis and management of peripheral nerve injuries, with reliance on the best available evidence when available. The goals for treating surgeons should be to (1) accurately describe the injury, (2) make a best available assessment as to the likelihood of improvement without intervention, and (3) choose the optimal intervention at the earliest time point when clarity is available. Clarity is not always obtainable, and intervention in the form of exploration may at times be indicated. Options for treatment of peripheral nerve injuries include direct repair, single or cabled autografts, allografts, conduit-assisted repairs, nerve transfers, and tendon- and muscle-based salvage options.

Dr. Lee or an immediate family member has received royalties from Arthrex, Inc.; is a member of a speakers' bureau or has made paid presentations on behalf of Axogen; serves as a paid consultant to or is an employee of Axogen, Checkpoint, Synthes, and Zimmer; serves as an unpaid consultant to HQRB; has received research or institutional support from Arthrex, Inc. and Axogen, Checkpoint, Integra, and Toyoba; has received nonincome support (such as equipment or services), commercially derived honoraria, or other non-research-related funding (such as paid travel) from Cartiva; and serves as a board member, owner, officer, or committee member of the American Society for Surgery of the Hand. Neither of the following authors nor any immediate family member has received anything of value from or has stock or stock options held in a commercial company or institution related directly or indirectly to the subject of this chapter: Dr. Puri and Dr. Cooke.

CLASSIFICATION OF NERVE INJURIES

Seddon described three types of nerve injury based on the histologic structure of nerves—neurapraxia, axonotmesis, and neurotmesis. Neurapraxia describes a conduction block of an otherwise intact nerve.[2] Axonotmesis describes an injury involving axonal discontinuity. These injures will lead to a degenerative pathway, with variable potential for regeneration, but the macroscopic structure of the visible nerve sheath remains intact. The final category, neurotmesis, describes a complete transection of all neural elements.

SUNDERLAND CLASSIFICATION

Sunderland introduced a classification of peripheral nerve injury in 1989, expanding on Seddon's classification from 1942, which has been widely accepted and is used to categorize nerve injuries (**Table 1**). The classification is based on the histologic structure of peripheral nerves, progressing in increasing severity based on the amount of damaged neural elements. When applied accurately, it can help surgeons to accurately prognosticate and make the clinical choice on whether or not to intervene.

©Copyright 2021 American Academy of Orthopaedic Surgeons

TABLE 1 Sunderland Classification of Nerve Injuries With Description of Pathoanatomy and Expected Clinical Course Without Surgical Intervention

Sunderland Grade (and Seddon Classification)	Description and Damaged Elements	Anticipated Clinical Course
1 (Neurapraxia)	A temporary conduction block. Axonal continuity remains; there is damage to the myelin sheath preventing complete or effective conduction.	There may be some sensory, and less commonly motor, sparing. As the myelin sheath repairs, clinical recovery is anticipated.
2 (Axonotmesis)	Stretch or contusion has led to axonal discontinuity and damage to the myelin sheath. The perineurium containing fascicles and endoneurium surrounding axons remain intact.	Due to axonal continuity, a degenerative process distal to the lesion will occur. With the neural structure remaining largely intact, nerve regeneration and spontaneous healing is anticipated.
3 (Axonotmesis)	As above, but with additional damage and scarring of the endoneurium within the fascicles.	Variable chance of recovery based on the amount of endoneurial scarring, and difficult to prognosticate.
4 (Axonotmesis)	Additional damage to the perineurial structure of the individual fascicles. Epineurium remains intact, with the nerve visibly in continuity from a macroscopic perspective.	With all internal neural elements damaged, there is low likelihood of regeneration. Commonly referred to as "neuroma in continuity."
5 (Neurotmesis)	Complete transection of all neural elements.	Low likelihood of spontaneous regeneration.

PHYSIOLOGIC EFFECTS OF NERVE INJURY

Understanding the physiologic effects of nerve injury helps to form the basis of clinical decision making (**Table 2**). Axonotmetic nerve injuries lead to predictable changes to the nerve stump proximal to the lesion, the cut nerve distal to the lesion, and in the target muscles and target sensory end organs that the nerve innervates. All of these factors play into clinical decision making, and the treatment choice requires a basic understanding of the physiology of nerve healing.

NERVE PROXIMAL TO THE INJURY

Proximal to axonal injury, both the nerve and the cell body undergo histologic and transcriptional changes to switch the nerve from transmission to growth mode.[2] Macrophages are recruited to the cell bodies and mediate changes in the nuclear transcriptional activity of the cell.[3-6] In the ganglia, a group of regeneration-associated genes (RAGs) are upregulated, increasing transcription of neurotrophic factors, their receptors, and structural components necessary for growth such as tubulin and actin.[7-12] These RAGs are upregulated initially after nerve injury and decline over time.[13,14] However, if an injured nerve is repaired or reaches a target, it is exposed to growth factors from the target which help to maintain the regenerative growth response.[15,16]

NERVE DISTAL TO THE INJURY

Distal to axonal injury, the nerve undergoes a process known as Wallerian degeneration. Negative connotations of the word notwithstanding, Wallerian degeneration refers to a process by which the transected nerve actively becomes more receptive to regrowth. After transection, the distal stump continues to transmit signals for hours to days, likely due to lag time from the slow pace of anterograde axoplasmic transport.[17-19] Quiescent Schwann cells dedifferentiate, upregulate expression of RAGs, recruit additional macrophages, and together phagocytose the preexisting myelin and axonal tissue.[20-24] The dedifferentiated Schwann cells line up along the basal lamina of the distal transected nerve in bands of Bungner, which help to guide and target regrowing axons.[25-28] Schwann cells continue to play an important role in keeping the nerve alive as well, which will eventually cease in the absence of neurotrophic factors.

NERVE INJURY EFFECTS ON TARGET ORGANS

Target muscle and sensory organs undergo changes when they lose neural input. The neuromuscular junction—made up of terminal Schwann cells and motor axons in the nerve and the motor end plate with its acetylcholine receptors in the muscle fiber—will degenerate and disperse acetylcholine receptors as it loses the neurotrophic factors from the efferent axon.[29,30] Atrophy of the muscle and collagen infiltration begins within weeks of denervation, but the architecture can remain intact for up to a year. By two years, fibrosis and degeneration of the muscle is likely irreversible, leading to the generally accepted guideline that a muscle must be reinnervated by 12 to 18 months from injury to hope for functional recovery.[31,32] Sensory organs are more resistant and may remain reinnervatable for 2 to 3 years.[33]

©Copyright 2021 American Academy of Orthopaedic Surgeons

TABLE 2 Important Growth Factors, Pathways, and Proteins Associated With Nerve Injury and Regeneration

Growth Factors	Effect
Vascular endothelial growth factor (VEGF)	Secreted by macrophages in response to hypoxia at the injury/repair site, stimulates angiogenesis
CCL2	Released in response to nerve injury, recruits macrophages to injury site, an essential step in promoting regeneration-associated genes (RAGs)
CSF1	Secreted by fibroblasts, recruits macrophages to dedifferentiated Schwann cells
ERK signalling pathway	Pathway for dedifferentiation of Schwann cells, driving their transition to role in postinjury state
LIF/STAT3 pathway	Utilized by macrophages to upregulate RAGs in the cell body of an injured nerve
Sox11	Transcription factor upregulated after injury, promotes neurite branching, elongation, and myelination
EphB2	Receptor upregulated by Schwann cells in distal nerve, responds to Ephrin B secreted by fibroblasts, relocalizing N-cadherin to cell surface. This drives attraction between cells, and aids in formation of bands of Bungner in distal nerve during Wallerian degeneration
N-cadherin, NCAM	Adhesion molecules upregulated by Schwann cells that may aid in migratory behavior, both for formation of bands of Bungner and to drive directionality of regrowth of axons
Chondroitin sulfate glycoproteins	Along with other breakdown products and debris, can play inhibitory role in axon regrowth and migration
Choline acetyltransferase, acetylcholine esterase	Transmission-related genes that are downregulated as RAGs become upregulated
Tubulin, actin	Cytoskeleton proteins upregulated by RAGs essential for growth cone extension from the proximal stump
BDNF, GDNF	RAG-associated neurotrophic factors
GAP-43, CAP-23, SGC-10	Growth-associated proteins upregulated by RAGs, correlated with regeneration capacity of injured neurons
IL-1, IL-6	Schwann cells upregulate production of cytokines that recruit macrophages across blood nerve barrier

BDNF = Brain-derived neurotrophic factor, GDNF = Glial derived neurotrophic factor, NCAM = Neural cell adhesion molecule

NERVE HEALING

The space between the proximal and distal stump of nerve is initially characterized by a macrophage-rich inflammatory response.[34] Local hypoxia drives migration of regional dedifferentiated Schwann cells and, with them, their neurotrophic factors and factors of angiogenesis. At the distal aspect of the nerve proximal to the injury, growth cones are formed which respond to and are led by neurotrophic factors primarily derived from the Schwann cells in the bridge between proximal and distal nerve.[35] Schwann cells progressively organize into cords that can lead regenerating axons across the gap from the proximal to distal nerve stump.[36,37] This process, especially initially, is imperfect with staggering of the crossing axons and frequent misdirection.[36,38] Upon reaching the distal stump, axons are guided by the bands of Bungner along the path of the distal nerve toward the target organ. While initially random, over time, neurotrophic factors sort the fibers appropriately toward motor and sensory end organs.[39]

MODALITIES OF DIAGNOSIS

The goals of diagnosis are to understand the location, level, and extent of the zone of a nerve injury and to understand the severity of nerve injury. When these features are known, the surgeon can make a hypothesis as to whether the patient will recover function with or without intervention. History and physical examination, along with knowledge of the patient's clinical progression since the injury, provide a groundwork for understanding the injury. Electrodiagnostic studies can be invaluable in confirming a diagnosis, assessing severity, and tracking recovery. Increasingly, imaging modalities are utilized that may aid in clinical decision making.

HISTORY

The mechanism of injury and the time when the injury occurred are paramount to the history. Peripheral nerve injuries occur from trauma and can be open from sharp laceration,

©Copyright 2021 American Academy of Orthopaedic Surgeons

crush, gunshot wounds, blast, or closed traction injuries. Injuries can also be iatrogenic from direct laceration, compression by plates or suture, and stretch. When the injury occurred is particularly important to motor nerve injuries because distal nerve, motor end plates, and target muscle degenerate and are not reinnervatable 12 to 18 months after injury.

Three essential pieces of information must be taken from history.

1. What was the mechanism of injury? Nerve deficit after sharp laceration implies high likelihood of complete neurotmesis with minimal surrounding zone of injury, and should lead to a low threshold for surgical intervention based on history alone. Open injury due to crush, gunshot, or blast mechanisms can have highly variable clinical progressions. These injuries can cause neurapraxia due to concussive trauma to the nerve, or transfer more significant amounts of energy to the nerve resulting in a degenerative pathway with a wide zone of injury. The energy imparted from the mechanism of injury is a clear prognostic factor, with worse outcomes seen in higher energy injuries.[40,41]
2. When did the injury occur? The timing of presentation relative to injury is key. As detailed above, there is a physiologic window with regard to potential for nerve regeneration. For motor recovery, the reinnervated nerve must reach its target before 12 to 18 months, likely closer to 12 months, especially in patients older than 40 years. However, outcomes are optimized with early intervention when possible depending on clinical circumstances.
3. What has the clinical course been since injury? A conduction block or neurapraxia should be expected to improve by 6 to 12 weeks from injury. Nerve regeneration after axonotmesis should be expected to progress along its anatomic course at approximately 1 mm/d after an initial latent period of 2 to 4 weeks. While there is likely variability in this rate between nerves, individual patients, and at different time points over the course of a single nerve's recovery, this estimate can be useful in evaluating likelihood of recovery without further intervention.[42]

PHYSICAL EXAMINATION

In cases of laceration, open wound, or surgical incision, the area of skin scar is palpated and percussed to attempt to elicit painful Tinel. Tenderness and positive severely painful Tinel at the site of previous open injury is a sign of neuroma and nerve injury. A Tinel sign that advances away from the site of injury or repair is a sign of nerve regeneration.

The patient's active range of motion should be compared with their contralateral extremity, and their motor strength for all pertinent muscles should be assessed. The British Medical Research Council (BMRC) method of motor grading is usually used. The sensory examination performed differs depending on the body part examined. For hand examination and digits, static two-point discrimination, a measure of innervation density, is useful.[43] Normal values are <6 mm, and protective sensation is defined as <15 mm, but typically a lacerated nerve will lead to sensation being indeterminate <10 mm.[44] For other body parts, usually light touch is used and graded by the patient reporting if the sensibility is normal, altered (paresthesia, hyperesthesia, hypoesthesia), or none (anesthetic).

Detailed knowledge of innervation patterns from root to terminal branch can help the surgeon focus the examination. Based on preserved function, identified deficits, and location of Tinel sign, the nerve and level of injury can often be identified.

ELECTRODIAGNOSTIC STUDIES

Nerve conduction testing is performed by stimulating nerves and recording their response and tests only the large, myelinated fibers of a nerve. Sensory nerves are recorded directly, whereas motor nerves are recorded in the innervated target muscle of the tested nerve. Compound muscle action potentials (CMAPs) provide a summation of the motor response to stimulation and represent the number of conducting axons. Because it is measured as a muscle response, CMAPs have larger amplitude than sensory nerve action potentials (SNAPs), which are smaller and more prone to error. Both sensory and motor nerves can be tested for their latency (time from stimulus to response) and conduction velocity (distance/time). Normative values vary by laboratory, age of patient, and environmental factors including temperature of the room.

In the setting of nerve injury, a transected nerve, or nerve fibers distal to a site of axonotmesis, will continue to conduct for, sometimes, several days after injury, prior to the onset of Wallerian degeneration. CMAPs must be recorded in an anterograde fashion and will be absent distal to axonotmesis or decreased in amplitude if there is a decrease in efferent axon count. SNAPs can be recorded antero- or retrograde. SNAPs will also be absent across the site of axonotmesis, but in the setting of preganglionic avulsion, they will be preserved in an anesthetic limb because the nerve is still in continuity with its cell body, despite being disconnected from the brain.[45] Conduction velocity and latency slowing is likely due to inefficient conduction due to demyelination or ongoing compression. Severe conduction block can lead to dispersion of the individual axonal transmission, mimicking loss of axons by decreasing the amplitude of the signal.

Needle electromyography (EMG) measures the electrical signal directly in a muscle. There is both an involuntary and voluntary portion of the test. A needle is inserted into muscle and elicits insertional activity—usually a short burst followed by silence. In the setting of muscle denervation, there is increased insertional activity followed by spontaneous fibrillations and positive sharp waves. Voluntary recruitment on needle electromyography demonstrates presence or absence of functioning motor axons and relies on patient effort and compliance. EMG recruitment categories (in order of ascending activity) are graded as none, low discrete (1-2 motor units on maximum recruitment), high discrete (3+ motor units on maximum recruitment), decreased, and full.[46] (**Figure 1**). Motor unit configuration patterns

 ©Copyright 2021 American Academy of Orthopaedic Surgeons

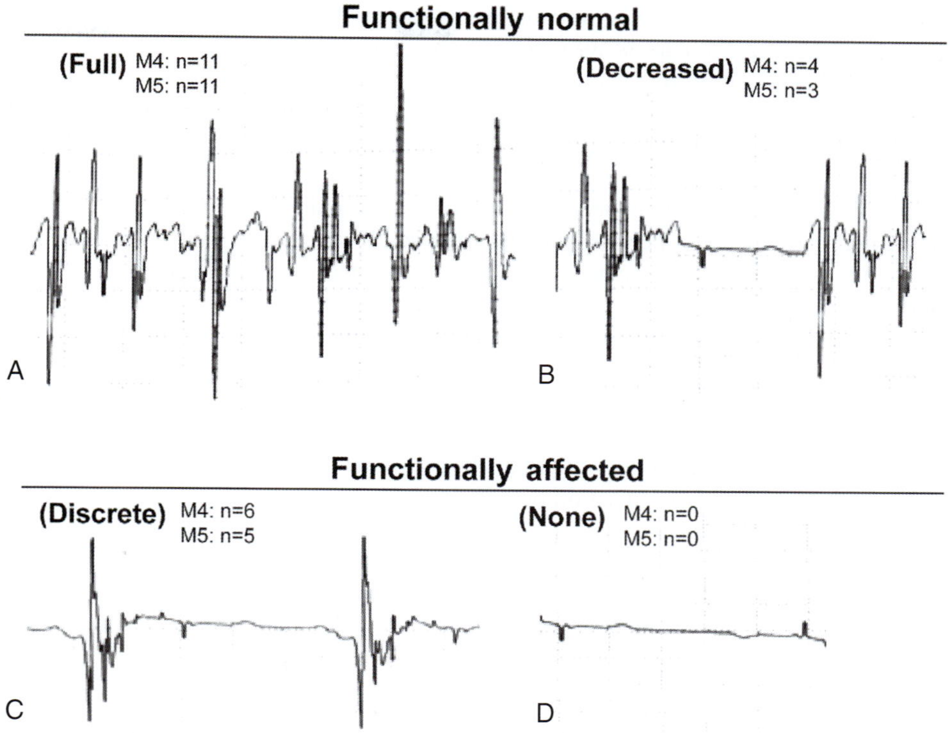

FIGURE 1 Electromyographic (EMG) recruitment grading is categorized as (**A**) full when there is there is complete voluntary activation and filling of the EMG screen, (**B**) decreased when there is less complete filling, but individual motor units are not discernible, (**C**) discrete when individual motor units can be distinguished, and (**D**) none when no motor units are activated despite full voluntary effort. (Reproduced with permission from Schreiber JJ, Feinberg JH, Byun DJ, Lee SK, Wolfe SW: Preoperative donor nerve electromyography as a predictor of nerve transfer outcomes. *J Hand Surg Am* 2014;39(1):42-49.)

categories included none, nascents, increased polyphasics, and di-/triphasics. Nascent wave configurations can be thought of as immature waves with capacity to mature to di-/triphasic waves.[47]

ULTRASONOGRAPHY

Ultrasonography (USG) is gaining popularity as a cost-effective modality to evaluate peripheral nerve injuries. USG has the ability to evaluate for fascicular continuity, areas of compression or kinking, focal areas of nerve enlargement, and complete nerve discontinuity with end neuroma formation.[48] It is particularly useful for visualization of neuromas. High rates of clinical correlation between USG and intraoperative findings have been reported.[49]

Ultrasonography-guided local anesthetic injections are a very useful diagnostic tool to confirm pain relief of a neuroma or scar-tethered nerve. Ultrasonography is limited if the nerve is very deep or underneath bone or under devices such as metal plates.

MRI

Magnetic resonance neurography (MRN) is useful to determine continuity of nerves and presence of neuroma and examine for neuritis. Features that can be seen include in evaluating nerve continuity, nerve caliber, signal intensity, perineural edema, and enhancement. An examination of the regional anatomy can aid in clinical decision making, for example, by showing the absence or presence of signs of denervation atrophy in target muscles.[50] T1, turbo spin echo T2-weighted, and diffusion tensor imaging have all been utilized and found to be useful, with higher level magnets (3T) likely yielding more useful information.[51,52] Diffusion tensor imaging (DTI) has been previously used for brain imaging and is showing promising results in visualizing neuronal microstructure.[53]

INTRAOPERATIVE ASSESSMENT

The surgical approach to injured nerves can be challenging due to abundant scar. Extensile incisions should be used to gain adequate exposure. The nerve should be dissected proximally and distally using the mantra of dissecting first in normal tissue, then moving to abnormal tissue. If there is some motor function in the nerve, an intraoperative nerve stimulator can be helpful to locate a nerve in scar. Once the nerve is located, use of small vessel loops around the nerve can be helpful to mobilize and place gentle traction on the nerve to dissect it free of adhesions, which can be very dense.

Once the nerve is isolated, it is then inspected visually and by palpation. Visual inspection under loupe magnification and headlamp light amplification is performed. Operating microscope can also be used for visual inspection. Fascicles can often be seen through the epineurium in normal healthy nerve. In the area of injury, fascicles are attempted to be identified. The nerve is palpated and should have a soft rubbery consistency, not a hard nodular feeling.

By a combination of preoperative workup and intraoperative assessment that there is discontinuity of nerve and resultant neuroma formation, the neuroma is resected to healthy appearing nerve on the proximal and distal ends. There should be pouting fascicles from the nerve ends and intrafascicular

4: Repair and Regeneration

©Copyright 2021 American Academy of Orthopaedic Surgeons

bleeding. This axotomy exposes the proximal axons for unimpaired growth and stimulates RAG expression in the proximal nerve and nerve cell body.[13] If uncertain and the institution has the capability, intraoperative histopathology can be performed to assess for axonal integrity.[54] Intraoperative somatosensory evoked potentials can also be detected from a nerve stump in electrodes placed on the scalp, confirming continuity of the peripheral nerve or nerve root being assessed.[55]

In the case of a partial nerve injury, the decision to leave the nerve in continuity or resect and repair the gap can be difficult. Intraoperative nerve stimulation can be helpful to determine the motor deficits of the partial nerve injury. Intraoperative nerve stimulation is also helpful in identifying the level of the lesion and in identifying donor nerves for nerve transfers.[56] Intraoperative nerve conduction studies can be used as a useful adjunct by attempting to send action potentials across an area with unknown level of injury severity, confirming absence or presence of conducting axons, and localizing the level of loss of conduction.[57]

DIRECT NERVE REPAIR

Direct nerve repair is the goal when tension-free repair is possible.[58] Tension at the repair site inhibits nerve regeneration.[59-61] The location of nerve injury, zone of injury in the nerve, and chronicity of the lesion may all decrease likelihood of a tension-free direct repair. Nerves in some locations—for example, the ulnar nerve at the elbow—can be mobilized to decrease the resultant gap after injury. However, excessive mobilization can devitalize the proximal and distal nerve stumps at the level of injury and should only be carried out within reason. A wide zone of injury requiring resection of scar tissue and neuroma will often preclude direct repair. Similarly, nerves that are repaired in a delayed fashion may be scarred into place, limiting mobility, and requiring resection of a larger resultant neuroma than a freshly approached nerve injury.

SUTURE TECHNIQUE

Much has been written about the advantages and disadvantages of epineurial or perineurial repair techniques, and no clear advantage to either approach has been established. Proponents of perineurial grouped fascicular repair techniques cite the ability to accurately realign fascicles and increased strength of repair as the primary advantages.[62-64] However, no meaningful clinical or animal data exist to establish the superiority of this technique, and disadvantages include surgical time and possible induction of increased scarring and fibrosis.[65-67] Our practice is to take care to align the nerve properly and perform epineurial repair when possible, sometimes with connector assist as described below (**Figure 2**). Nerve tissue should be delicately handled to avoid inadvertent damage to the nerve and subsequent scar tissue or neuroma formation. If excessive

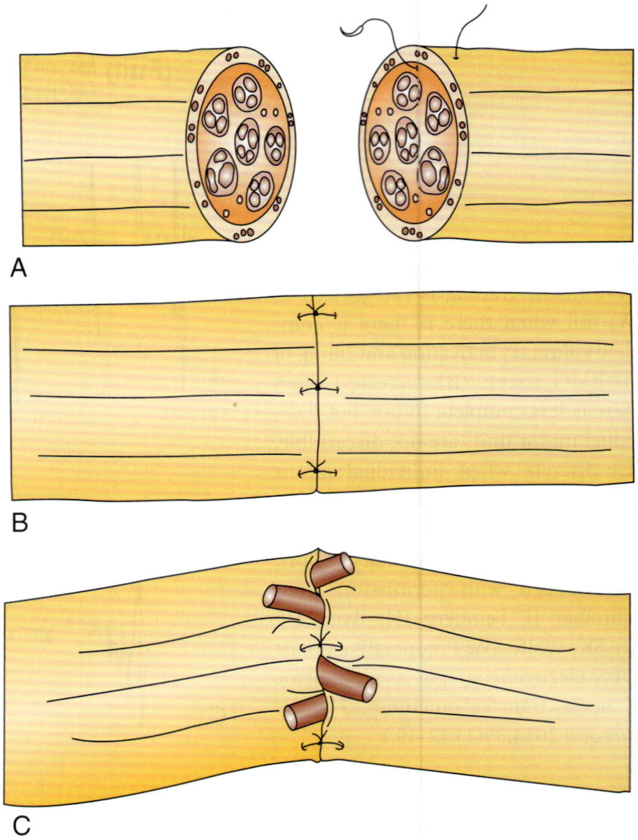

FIGURE 2 **A**, Epineurial repair is carried out with care taken to properly align fascicles. Epineurial vasculature may guide alignment. **B**, Sutures are tied to close the gap. **C**, Overtensioning the repair can lead to axonal escape ("past pointing"), preventing regeneration or leading to neuroma formation. (Adapted with permission from Trehan SK, Model Z, Lee SK: Nerve repair and nerve grafting. *Hand Clin* 2016;32(2):119-125.)

tension is required to achieve direct coaptation, an alternative to direct coaptation is used. A single 8-0 or 9-0 epineurial suture is a commonly used threshold for acceptable tension.[68]

CONNECTOR-ASSISTED REPAIR

Tension at the repair site can be present at rest, or induced by motion. A technique of using a conduit or connector to offset tension at the site of a direct coaptation has been shown to improve functional and electrophysiological results in animal models.[61] In this technique, a tube is slid over a stump of the nerve prior to direct coaptation. Direct epineurial repair is performed with a minimum of sutures, sometimes only two sutures at 180° to align the nerve. It is paramount that the nerve ends barely touch; if the nerve ends are crammed together, the fascicles may past point and nerve regeneration will not occur, but rather a neuroma will. The tube is then slid over the repair site. It is sutured to the epineurium proximal and distal to the suture line using epineurial horizontal-mattress sutures (de-tensioning sutures). Two sutures at either site of the tube have been shown

©Copyright 2021 American Academy of Orthopaedic Surgeons

to be as strong as a four-strand epineurial repair in digital nerve repair.[69] It is important that the nerve tube is not tight and allows for nerve swelling postoperatively. Alternatively a nerve protector with a slit can be used and loosely closed over with sutures or microclips (**Figure 3**). Other theoretical benefits include protection from inflammatory factors in the wound bed, reduced soft-tissue handling, and ease of repair.[70,71]

NERVE GLUE

Commercially available sealants can function as a nerve glue—on their own, in addition to direct coaptation, and in addition to connector-assisted repair—and may be a useful adjunct to protect the repair site from inflammation and add strength.[72,73] Tisseel (Baxter, Deerfield, IL) was the first commercially available fibrin sealant and is commonly available in most hospitals. Its application in nerve repair remains off-label, but commonly performed and well-studied in the literature.[74] The strength effect is likely temporary, given the maximum 4 week resorption time of commercially available sealants.[75] In addition, they are likely more valuable in resisting initial gapping, as opposed to increasing ultimate tensile strength.[75]

Several studies have shown the benefits of using fibrin glue compared with microsuturing histologically, likely by protecting the coaptation site around the time of the inflammatory cascade of wound healing, and minimizing the foreign body effect of suture.[76,77]

INDIRECT NERVE REPAIR

AUTOGRAFT

For gaps greater than 7 cm, nerve autograft must be used. For gaps less than 7 cm, it is controversial whether to use nerve autograft or nerve allograft. Until more data are available, a

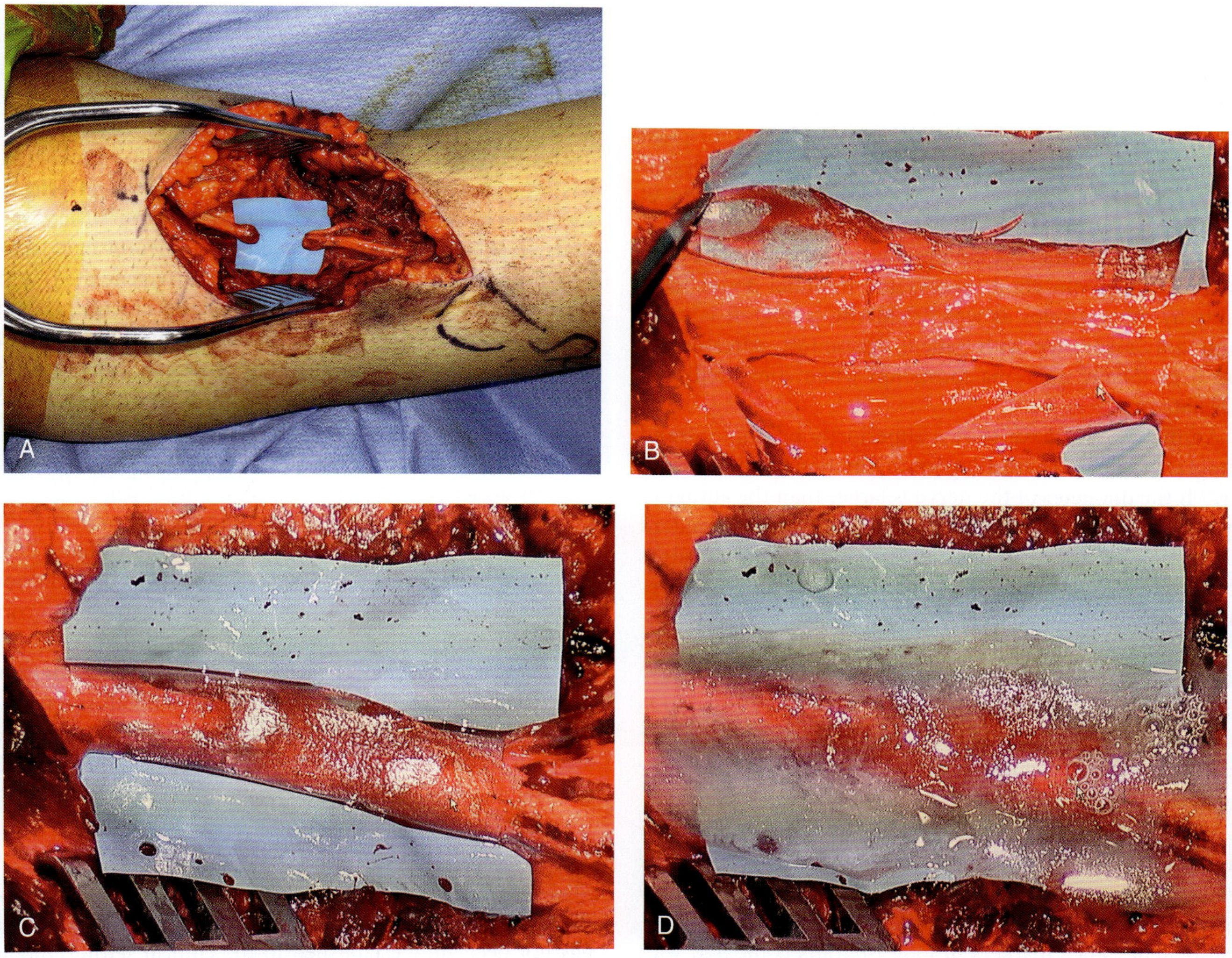

FIGURE 3 **A** to **D**, Intraoperative photographs. **A**, A surgically identified peroneal nerve laceration. **B**, After resection of damaged ends and mobilization of the proximal and distal stumps, a primary epineurial repair was performed. **C**, A previously placed nerve protector was laid over the top of the repair and closed over the repair site. De-tensioning sutures were placed proximally and distally to minimize tension at the repair site. **D**, The repair was reinforced with fibrin glue. (Courtesy of Steve K. Lee, MD, Ithaca, NY.)

4: Repair and Regeneration

©Copyright 2021 American Academy of Orthopaedic Surgeons

common practice pattern among peripheral nerve surgeons is to use nerve autograft for motor nerves and critical sensory nerves. For noncritical sensory nerves and surgical care of neuromas, nerve allograft has an increasingly indisputable role.

The longest commercially available decellularized allograft is 7 cm. For this reason, most favor use of autograft in gaps of this length or greater. For patients with preference against autograft harvest, or where donor site morbidity is deemed to be unacceptable, multiple allografts can be placed in series.[78] Yan et al showed in an animal model that there was minimal loss of axons across an additional suture line using this approach, though autografts performed better than allograft.

The sural nerve is the most common peripheral nerve graft donor. However, harvesting sural nerve for autograft does have significant donor site morbidity; 20% to 30% of patients experience pain at the donor site, cold sensitivity, or functional impairment.[79] Alternative options for autograft include the medial antebrachial cutaneous nerve (MABC), third web space branch of median, lateral antebrachial cutaneous nerve (LABC), palmar cutaneous, dorsal cutaneous branch of the ulnar nerve, and posterior interosseous nerve (PIN).[80] The selection of the donor nerve should take into consideration the ability to limit additional incisions, donor and recipient nerve caliber, and length required as well as the expected donor site morbidity. The LABC was shown by Higgins et al to be a good match in terms of size and axon counts for digital nerves distal to the common bifurcation and has been used clinically with good success and minimal donor morbidity by other groups as well.[81,82] MABC autograft is more commonly associated with patient discomfort, paresthesias, and occasionally neuroma formation when compared with PIN autograft.[83]

Animal studies have shown superiority of single-strand autograft compared with allograft in functional motor recovery.[84] If the diameter of the nerve is larger than the autograft available, cabled nerve autografting is the current standard for treating patients when tension-free direct nerve repair is not possible (**Figure 4**). The orientation of the donor nerves should be placed in reverse to avoid loss of axonal regeneration through any donor nerve branches—a theoretical advantage that has not been established in the literature.[85] Fibrin glue can be used to secure the donor nerves in a cable formation.[86] Animal studies have not shown a clear benefit of cabled autograft when compared with allograft in motor nerve recovery.[87]

While nerve autograft is helpful in bridging larger nerve gaps, the efficiency of axon regeneration decreases as the bridge gap increases. A rodent model evaluating 2 versus 6 cm nerve gaps in the sciatic nerve revealed greater expression of senescence markers in long isografts compared with the short isografts.[88] Long and large caliber nerve grafts lead to prolonged ischemia-related oxidative stress and prolonged denervation which results in arrest of proliferation and altered gene expression toward senescence.[89-91]

ALLOGRAFT

Processed allograft nerve is decellularized nerve tissue that retains the three-dimensional microstructural scaffolding and protein composition characteristic of nerve tissue. There is only one commercially available decellularized nerve allograft, Avance (AxoGen, Alachua, FL), and its maximum available length is 7 cm. There are several studies establishing sensory recovery through allograft reconstruction.[92-97] There are favorable outcomes reported on motor and mixed nerves as well, but comparative data with autograft reconstruction in the clinical setting are lacking.[94,98-100]

Given the ease of application, lack of donor site morbidity, and theoretical advantages, use of nerve allograft has become an appealing choice for surgeons.[101] The major drawbacks remain the cost and lack of comparative data with regard to motor and mixed nerves.[102]

CONDUITS

Conduits can be used to bridge short nerve gaps or as a tool to aid direct nerve repairs to place fewer sutures at the injured nerve ends. Autologous vein grafts or synthetic conduits avoid the donor site morbidity from nerve autograft.

The concept of bridging a nerve gap with a hollow tube has been described as early as 1880 when Gluck investigated the use of decalcified bone to bridge nerve gaps.[103] Nerve conduits serve to align the nerve and contain neurotropic factors beneficial to nerve regeneration in a matrix generated by the proximal and distal nerve ends. If the conduit chamber is maintained with a sufficient volume of matrix, sprouting axons can be led across the gap as in the traditional nerve healing model. However, as the matrix is dependent on volume of output proximally and distally, if the gap is large, the matrix will thin out at the center, with classic "hourglass" appearance, and limitation of crossing axons at the narrowest point in the gap.[104-107]

There are several options for commercially available conduits manufactured with collagen, polycaprolactone (PCL), porcine submucosa, and polyglycolic acid (PGA). Autogenous options such as vein grafts have compared favorably to commercially available tubes in clinical studies.[108] Early reports of conduit reconstruction of nerve deficit showed, at the time, promising results. Recent comparisons of allograft reconstruction compared with the historical results of conduit repair favor allograft reconstruction.[97,109-111] Conduit repair should likely be reserved for small nerve sensory gaps of less than 10 mm.[112,113]

ADJUNCTIVE TREATMENTS

A clear role for enhancement of the nerve healing response has not been fully established in the clinical setting, though several potential targets have been identified.

Growth factors delivered in a scaffolding tube have shown in animal models to increase axons compared with autograft.[114,115] Limitations of half life and delivery method may

©Copyright 2021 American Academy of Orthopaedic Surgeons

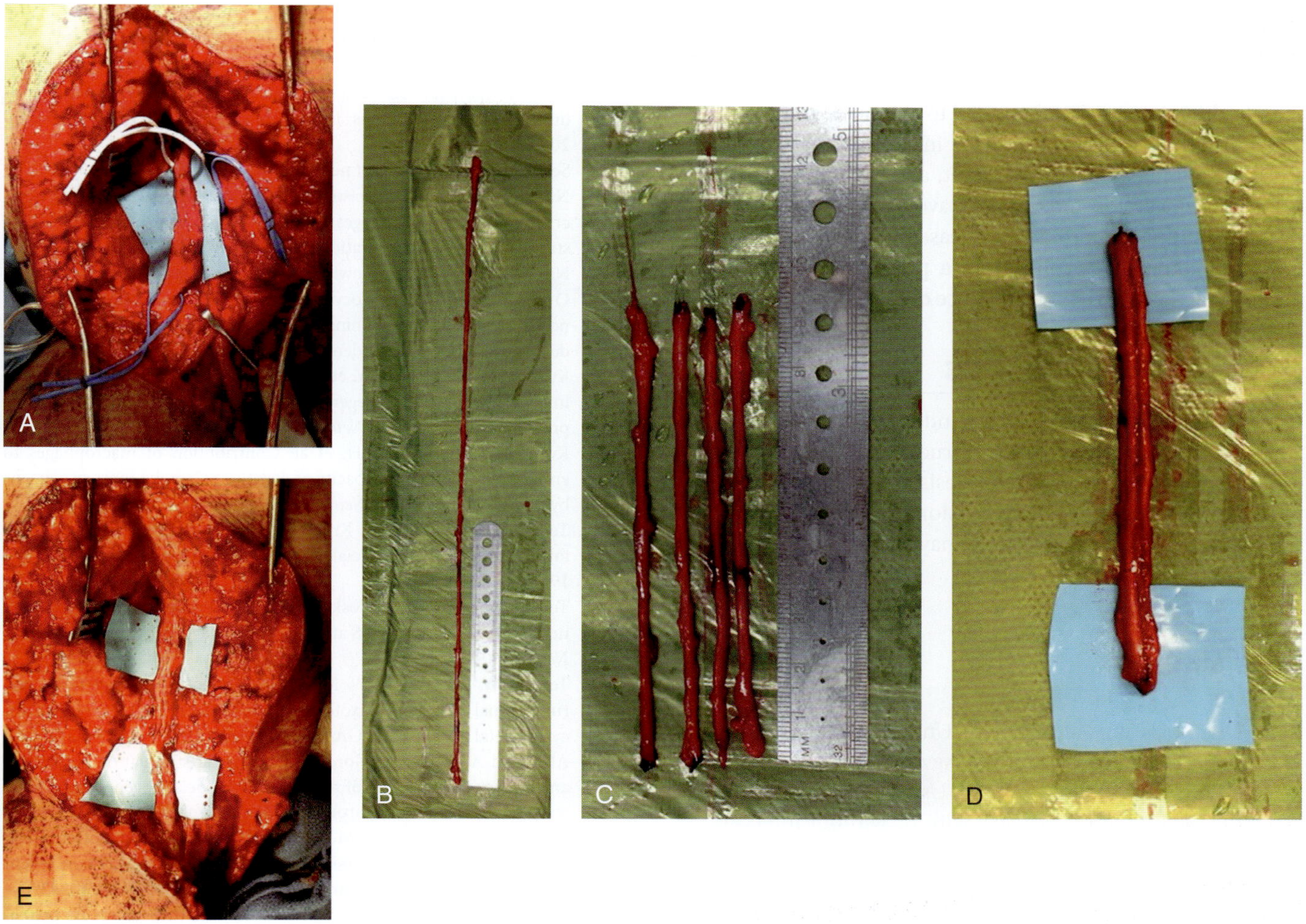

FIGURE 4 **A** and **B**, Intraoperative photographs. **A**, A peroneal nerve lesion requiring excision and grafting is exposed. **B**, Maximum sural nerve graft length is harvested. **C**, The nerve graft is cut into segments measuring 20% larger than the identified nerve defect. The segments are all reversed to prevent axonal escape during regeneration through antegrade branches. **D**, The graft segments are grouped into a size match for the target and assembled together with fibrin glue. **E**, The cabled graft in a fibrin glue tube is sutured tension-free into place to span the defect. (Reproduced with permission from Trehan SK, Model Z, Lee SK: Nerve repair and nerve grafting. *Hand Clin* 2016;32(2):119-125.)

limit application for longer grafts. Supplementation of tube or graft with betamethasone,[116] vitamin E,[117] erythropoietin,[118] rapamycin,[119] and FK506[120] have all shown some potential benefits in animal models.

Schwann cells drive much of the regenerative response and represent an attractive target for augmentation of the nerve healing response. Their use has been evaluated to augment nerve grafts and conduits in animal models.[121,122] Levi et al reported a case of clinical use of autologous harvested Schwann cells to supplement sural nerve autograft reconstruction of a 7.5 cm sural nerve defect, demonstrating clinical feasibility.[123]

Stem cells remain a potential source of augmentation due to their ability to dedifferentiate into several key cells along the regenerative pathway. Sources for stem cells include human embryo, induced pluripotent stem cells, adipose tissue, neural crest cells, and bone marrow.[124] Source, differentiation of cells, and delivery methods are all under investigation for potential future use.

ALTERNATIVES TO NERVE REPAIR OR RECONSTRUCTION

Alternatives to nerve repair or reconstruction may be advisable due to time from injury, distance of injury to target, zone of injury, severity of regional trauma, anticipated length of recovery, patient morbidity, or patient desires.

NERVE TRANSFER

With knowledge of the level of injury, when the injury occurred, and anticipating approximately 1 mm/d of axonal regeneration, the likelihood of a motor nerve reaching its target muscle within the 12 to 18 month window for reinnervation can be estimated. In situations where spontaneous recovery or nerve repair is unlikely to result in meaningful functional recovery, nerve transfer can be a preferred

©Copyright 2021 American Academy of Orthopaedic Surgeons

approach. Other indications include wide zone of injury requiring very long grafts or compromising the soft-tissue bed with dense scarring.[125]

A healthy donor nerve is coapted to a distal denervated nerve target. Advantages of this technique include decreasing the distance for reinnervation to the target, ability to use pure motor nerve to reinnervate a motor target, avoidance of a zone of scarring, lack of donor morbidity, and ease of reeducation. In addition, the donor axons come from a previously healthy nerve, minimizing the chance for senescence of the proximal nerve.

OTHER SALVAGE OPTIONS

If target muscle is outside the window for reinnervation, a goal-oriented approach to reconstruction may include splint or prosthetic use, selective arthrodesis, tendon transfer, or free functioning muscle transfer. Decisions to take this approach should be made with care and may vary largely based on patients' individual needs.

SUMMARY

- Diagnosis is goal-oriented: Understand the injured structure, understand the severity of injury, and understand the time course. Using this information, the likelihood of recovery with or without intervention can be determined.
- History and physical examination can be significantly augmented by electrodiagnostic studies and selective use of advanced imaging modalities.
- Nerve injuries can be categorized into injuries that will likely recover in the short term (conduction block), in the long term (axonotmesis with preserved neural elements), or not likely to recover (higher grade axonotmesis or neurotmesis).
- Nerves that have sustained axonal discontinuity will undergo predictable degenerative and regenerative changes at the cell body, proximal nerve stump, distal nerve stump, and target end organ.
- Tension at a nerve repair site is detrimental to healing, and direct repair should only be carried out if tension can be avoided.
- Small nerve gaps (<5 to 10 mm) can be treated with autograft, allograft, or conduit.
- Larger nerve gaps benefit from autograft or allograft reconstruction, with little comparative data available.
- Autograft is likely superior to allograft in long nerve gaps (>7 cm).
- Nerve transfers are useful when direct or indirect repair is not feasible.
- Tendon transfers and selective arthrodesis are alternatives when nerve repair or reconstruction is unlikely to succeed.

REFERENCES

1. Rebowe R, Rogers A, Yang X, et al: Nerve repair with nerve conduits: Problems, solutions and future directions. *J Hand Microsurg* 2018;10:61-65.
2. Seddon JH: Three types of nerve injury. *Brain* 1943;66:237-288.
3. Niemi JP, DeFrancesco-Lisowitz A, Roldan-Hernandez L, et al: A critical role for macrophages near axotomized neuronal cell bodies in stimulating nerve regeneration. *J Neurosci* 2013;33:16236-16248.
4. Niemi JP, DeFrancesco-Lisowitz A, Cregg JM, Howarth M, Zigmond RE: Overexpression of the monocyte chemokine CCL2 in dorsal root ganglion neurons causes a conditioning- like increase in neurite outgrowth and does so via a STAT3 dependent mechanism. *Exp Neurol* 2016;275:25-37.
5. Kwon MJ, Shin HY, Cui Y, et al: CCL2 mediates neuron-macrophage interactions to drive proregenerative macrophage activation following preconditioning injury. *J Neurosci* 2015;35:15934-15947.
6. Kwon MJ, Kim J, Shin H, et al: Contribution of macrophages to enhanced regenerative capacity of dorsal root ganglia sensory neurons by conditioning injury. *J Neurosci* 2013;33:15095-15108.
7. Tetzlaff W, Bisby MA, Kreutzberg GW: Changes in cytoskeletal proteins in the rat facial nucleus following axotomy. *J Neurosci* 1988;8:3181-3189.
8. Tetzlaff W, Bisby MA: Cytoskeletal protein synthesis and regulation of nerve regeneration in PNS and CNS neurons of the rat. *Restor Neurol Neurosci* 1990;1:189-196.
9. Tetzlaff W, Alexander SW, Miller FD, et al: Response of facial and rubrospinal neurons to axotomy: Changes in mRNA expression for cytoskeletal proteins and GAP-43. *J Neurosci* 1991;11:2528-2544.
10. Al-Majed AA, Tam SL, Gordon T: Electrical stimulation accelerates and enhances expression of regeneration-associated genes in regenerating rat femoral motoneurons. *Cell Mol Neurobiol* 2004;24:379-402.
11. Al-Majed AA, Brushart TM, Gordon T: Electrical stimulation accelerates and increases expression of BDNF and trkB mRNA in regenerating rat femoral motoneurons. *Eur J Neurosci* 2000;12:4381-4390.
12. Boyd JG, Gordon T: Neurotrophic factors and their receptors in axonal regeneration and functional recovery after peripheral nerve injury. *Mol Neurobiol* 2003;27:277-324.
13. Gordon T, You S, Cassar SL, et al: Reduced expression of regeneration associated genes in chronically axotomized facial motoneurons. *Exp Neurol* 2015;264:26-32.
14. Gordon T, Tetzlaff W: Regeneration-associated genes decline in chronically injured rat sciatic motoneurons. *Eur J Neurosci* 2015;42(10):2783-2791.
15. Funakoshi H, Belluardo N, Arenas E, et al: Muscle derived neurotrophin-4 as an activity-dependent trophic signal for adult motor neurons. *Science* 1995;268:1495-1499.
16. Funakoshi H, Frisen J, Barbany G, et al: Differential expression of mRNAs for neurotrophins and their receptors after axotomy of the sciatic nerve. *J Cell Biol* 1993;123:455-465.
17. Lubinska L: Early course of Wallerian degeneration in myelinated fibres of the rat phrenic nerve. *Brain Res* 1977;130:47-63.
18. Miledi R, Slater CR: On the degeneration of rat neuromuscular junctions after nerve section. *J Physiol* 1970;207:507-528.
19. Mackenzie SJ, Smirnov I, Calancie B: Cauda equina repair in the rat: Part 2. Time course of ventral root conduction failure. *J Neurotrauma* 2012;29:1683-1690.
20. Harrisingh MC, Perez-Nadales E, Parkinson DB, et al: The Ras/Raf/ERK signalling pathway drives Schwann cell dedifferentiation. *EMBO J* 2004;23:3061-3071.
21. Napoli I, Noon LA, Ribeiro S, et al: A central role for the ERK-signaling pathway in controlling Schwann cell plasticity and peripheral nerve regeneration in vivo. *Neuron* 2012;73:729-742.
22. Gomez-Sanchez JA, Carty L, Iruarrizaga-Lejarreta M, et al: Schwann cell autophagy, myelinophagy, initiates myelin clearance from injured nerves. *J Cell Biol* 2015;210:153-168.

©Copyright 2021 American Academy of Orthopaedic Surgeons

23. Beuche W, Friede RL: The role of non-resident cells in Wallerian degeneration. *J Neurocytol* 1984;13:767-796.
24. Scheidt P, Friede RL: Myelin phagocytosis in Wallerian degeneration. Properties of millipore diffusion chambers and immunohistochemical identification of cell populations. *Acta Neuropathol* 1987;75:77-84.
25. Fu SY, Gordon T: The cellular and molecular basis of peripheral nerve regeneration. *Mol Neurobiol* 1997;14:67-116.
26. Gonzalez-Perez F, Udina E, Navarro X: Extracellular matrix components in peripheral nerve regeneration. *Int Rev Neurobiol* 2013;108:257-275.
27. Arthur-Farraj PJ, Latouche M, Wilton DK, et al: c-Jun reprograms Schwann cells of injured nerves to generate a repair cell essential for regeneration. *Neuron* 2012;75:633-647.
28. Fontana X, Hristova M, Da Costa C, et al: c-Jun in Schwann cells promotes axonal regeneration and motoneuron survival via paracrine signaling. *J Cell Biol* 2012;198:127-141.
29. Reist NE, Werle MJ, McMahan UJ: Agrin released by motor neurons induces the aggregation of acetylcholine receptors at neuromuscular junctions. *Neuron* 1992;8(5):865-868.
30. Gautam M, Noakes PG, Moscoso L, et al: Defective neuromuscular synaptogenesis in agrin-deficient mutant mice. *Cell* 1996;85(4):525-535.
31. Dahlin LB: Nerve injury and repair: From molecule to man, in Slutsky DJ, Hentz VR, ed: *Peripheral Nerve Surgery: Practical Applications in the Upper Extremity.* Philadelphia, Churchill Livingston, Elsevier, 2006, 1-22.
32. Noaman HH, Shiha AE, Bahm J: Oberlin's ulnar nerve transfer to the biceps motor nerve in obstetric brachial plexus palsy: Indications, and good and bad results. *Microsurgery* 2004;24(3):182-187.
33. Tsao B, Boulis N, Bethoux F, et al: *Trauma of the nervous system, peripheral nerve trauma*, in *Bradley's Neurology in Clinical Practice*, ed 6. 2012, pp 984-1001.
34. Cattin AL, Burden JJ, Van Emmenis L, et al: Macrophage-induced blood vessels guide Schwann cell-mediated regeneration of peripheral nerves. *Cell* 2015;162:1127-1139.
35. Menorca RMG, Fussell T, Elfar JC: Peripheral nerve trauma: Mechanisms of injury and recovery. *Hand Clin* 2013;29(3):317-330.
36. Witzel C, Rohde C, Brushart TM: Pathway sampling by regenerating peripheral axons. *J Comp Neurol* 2005;485:183-190.
37. Parrinello S, Napoli I, Ribeiro S, et al: EphB signaling directs peripheral nerve regeneration through Sox2-dependent Schwann cell sorting. *Cell* 2010;143:145-155.
38. Gordon T: Nerve regeneration: Understanding biology and its influence on return of function after nerve transfers. *Hand Clin* 2016;32(2):103-117.
39. Brushart TM: Motor axons preferentially reinnervate motor pathways. *J Neurosci* 1993;13:2730-2738.
40. Shergill G, Bonney G, Munshi P, Birch R: The radial and posterior interosseous nerves. *JBJS (Br)* 2001;83-B:646-649.
41. Rochkind S, Strauss I, Shlitner Z, et al: Clinical aspects of ballistic peripheral nerve injury: Shrapnel versus gunshot. *Acta Neurochir* 2014;156(8):1567-1575.
42. Seddon HJ, Medawar PB, Smith H: Rate of regeneration of peripheral nerves in man. *J Physiol* 1943;102(2):191-215.
43. Moberg E: Objective methods for determining the functional value of sensibility in the hand. *J Bone Joint Surg* 1958;40B:454.
44. Callahan AD: Sensibility assessment for nerve lesions-in-continuity and nerve lacerations, In Skirven T, Osterman LA, Fedorczyk JM, et al, ed: *Rehabilitation of the Hand and Upper Extremity*, ed 6. Elsevier, 2011.
45. Bonney G, Gilliatt RW: Sensory nerve conduction after traction lesion of the brachial plexus. *Proc R Coll Med* 1958;51:365-367.
46. Schreiber JJ, Feinberg JH, Byun DJ, et al: Preoperative donor nerve electromyography as a predictor of nerve transfer outcomes. *J Hand Surg* 2014;39(1):42-49.
47. Feinberg JH, Nguyen ET, Boachie-Adjei K, et al: The electrodiagnostic natural history of parsonage-turner syndrome. *Muscle Nerve* 2017;56(4), 737-743.
48. Smith JK, Miller ME, Caroll CG, et al: High-resolution ultrasound in combat-related peripheral nerve injuries. *Muscle Nerve* 2016;54(6):1139-1144.
49. Hollister AM, Simoncini A, Sciuk A, Jordan J: High frequency ultrasound evaluation of traumatic peripheral nerve injuries. *Neurol Res* 2012;34(1):98-103.
50. Ahlawat S, Wadhwa V, Belzberg AJ, Batra K, Chhabra A: Spectrum of suprascapular nerve lesions: Normal and abnormal neuromuscular imaging appearances on 3-T MR neurography. *AJR Am J Roentgenol* 2015;204(3):589-601.
51. Aggarwal A, Srivastava DN, Jana M, et al: Comparison of different sequences of magnetic resonance imaging and ultrasonography with nerve conduction studies in peripheral neuropathies. *World Neurosurg* 2017;108:185-200.
52. Crim J, Ingalls K: Accuracy of MR neurography in the diagnosis of brachial plexopathy. *Eur J Radiol* 2017;95:24-27.
53. Andreisek G, White LM, Kassner A, Sussman MS: Evaluation of diffusion tensor imaging and fiber tractography of the median nerve: Preliminary results on intrasubject variability and precision of measurements. *AJR Am J Roentgenol* 2010;194(1):W65-W72.
54. Wolfe SW, Johnsen PH, Lee SK, Feinberg JH: Long-nerve grafts and nerve transfers demonstrate comparable outcomes for axillary nerve injuries. *J Hand Surg Am* 2014;39(7):1351-1357.
55. Landi A, Copeland SA, Wynn Parry CB, et al: The role of somatosensory evoked potentials and nerve conduction studies in the surgical management of brachial plexus injuries. *J Bone Joint Surg Br* 1980;62:492-496.
56. Noland SS, Krauss EM, Felder JM, Mackinnon SE: Surgical and clinical decision making in isolated long thoracic nerve palsy. *Hand (N Y)* 2018 13(6):689-694.
57. Kline DG, Hudson AR: *Operative care and techniques*, In *Nerve Injuries*. Philadelphia, WB Saunders, 1995, pp 118-145.
58. Goldberg SH, Jobin CM, Hayes AG, et al: Biomechanics and histology of intact and repaired digital nerves: An in vitro study. *J Hand Surg Am* 2007, 32:474-482.
59. Terzis J, Faibisoff B, Williams B: The nerve gap: Suture under tension vs. graft. *Plast Reconstr Surg* 1975;56(2):166-170.
60. Clark WL, Trumble TE, Swiontowski MF, et al: Nerve tension and blood flow in a model of immediate and delayed repairs. *J Hand Surg Am* 1992;17:677-687.
61. Schmidhammer R, Zandieh S, Hopf R, et al: Alleviated tension at the repair site enhances functional regeneration: The effect of full range of motion mobilization on the regeneration of peripheral nerves–histologic, electrophysiologic, and functional results in a rat model. *J Trauma* 2004;56(3):571-584.
62. Liu G, Zhang Q, Jin Y, Gao Z: Stress and strain analysis on the anastomosis site sutured with either epineurial or perineurial sutures after simulation of sciatic nerve injury. *Neural Regen Res* 2012;7(29):2299-2304.
63. Orgel MG, Terzis JK: Epineurial vs. perineurial repair. *Plast Reconstr Surg* 1977;60(1):80-91.
64. Spinner RJ: Operative care and technique, in: Kim DH, Midha R, Murovic JA, eds: *Kline and Hudson's Nerve Injuries*, ed 2. Philadelphia, WB Saunders, 2008, pp 87-106.
65. Tupper JW, Crick JC, Matteck LR: Fascicular nerve repairs. A comparative study of epineurial and fascicular (perineurial) techniques. *Orthop Clin North Am* 1988;19(1):57-69.
66. Bora FW Jr, Pleasure DE, Didizian NA: A study of nerve regeneration and neuroma formation after nerve suture by various techniques. *J Hand Surg Am* 1976;1(2):138-143.
67. Cabaud HE, Rodkey WG, McCarroll HR Jr, et al: Epineurial and perineurial fascicular nerve repairs: A critical comparison. *J Hand Surg Am* 1976;1(2):131-137.
68. Smetana BS, Cao J, Merrell GA, Greenberg JA: Testing of direct neurorrhaphy strain. *J Hand Surg Am* 2019;44(7):615.e1-615.e6.
69. Tang P, Schimoler PJ, Kim H, et al: The optimal number and location of sutures in conduit-assisted primary digital nerve repair. *J Hand Surg Eur* 2018;43(6):621-625.

©Copyright 2021 American Academy of Orthopaedic Surgeons

70. Ducic I, Safa B, DeVinney E: Refinements of nerve repair with connector-assisted coaptation. *Microsurgery* 2017;37(3):256-263.
71. Isaacs J, Safa B, Evans PJ, Greenberg J: Technical assessment of connector-assisted nerve repair. *J Hand Surg Am* 2016;41(7):760-766.
72. Owusu A, Mayeda B, Isaacs J: Surgeon perspectives on alternative nerve repair techniques. *Hand (N Y)* 2014;9(1):29-35.
73. Childe JR, Regal S, Schimoler P, et al: Fibrin glue increases the tensile strength of conduit-assisted primary digital nerve repair. *Hand (N Y)* 2018;13(1):45-49.
74. Sameem M, Wood TJ, Bain JR: A systematic review on the use of fibrin glue for peripheral nerve repair. *Plast Reconstr Surg* 2011;127(6):2381-2390.
75. Isaacs JE, McDaniel CO, Owen JR, Wayne JS: Comparative analysis of biomechanical performance of available "nerve glues". *J Hand Surg Am* 2008;33(6):893-899.
76. Ornelas L, Padilla L, Di Silvio M, et al: Fibrin glue: An alternative technique for nerve coaptation-Part II. Nerve regeneration and histomorphometric assessment. *J Reconstr Microsurg* 2006;22(2):123-128.
77. Martins RS, Siqueira MG, Da Silva CF, Plese JP: Overall assessment of regeneration in peripheral nerve lesion repair using fibrin glue, suture, or a combination of the 2 techniques in a rat model. Which is the ideal choice? *Surg Neurol* 2005;64:S10-S16.
78. Yan Y, Wood MD, Huntder DA, et al: The effect of short nerve grafts in series on axonal regeneration across isografts or acellular nerve allografts. *J Hand Surg Am* 2016;41(6):e113-e121.
79. Ijpma FA, Nicolai J-PA, Meek MF: Sural nerve donor-site morbidity: Thirty-four years of follow-up. *Ann Plast Surg* 2006;57:391-395.
80. Poppler LH, Davidge K, Lu JC, et al: Alternatives to sural nerve grafts in the upper extremity. *Hand (N Y)* 2015;10(1):68-75.
81. Higgins JP, Fisher S, Serletti JM, et al: Assessment of nerve graft donor sites used for reconstruction of traumatic digital nerve defects. *J Hand Surg Am* 2002;27:286-292.
82. Pilanci O, Ozel A, Basaran K, et al: Is there a profit to use the lateral antebrachial cutaneous nerve as a graft source in digital nerve reconstruction? *Microsurgery* 2014;34:367-371.
83. Stang F, Stollwerck P, Prommersberger KJ, van Schoonhoven J: Posterior interosseus nerve vs. medial cutaneous nerve of the forearm: Differences in digital nerve reconstruction. *Arch Orthop Trauma Surg* 2013;133(6):875-880.
84. Giusti G, Willems WF, Kremer T, et al: Return of motor function after segmental nerve loss in a rat model: Comparison of autogenous nerve graft, collagen conduit, and processed allograft (AxoGen). *J Bone Joint Surg Am* 2012;94(5):410-417.
85. Roberts SE, Thibaudeau S, Burrell JC, et al: To reverse or not to reverse? A systematic review of autograft polarity on functional outcomes following peripheral nerve repair surgery. *Microsurgery* 2017;37(2):169-174.
86. Draeger RW, Bynum DK Jr, Patterson JMM: Simplified cable nerve grafting with nerve-cutting guides and fibrin glue. *J Hand Microsurg* 2017;9(3):167-169.
87. Tang P, Kilic A, Konopka G, et al: Histologic and functional outcomes of nerve defects treated with acellular allograft versus cabled autograft in a rat model. *Microsurgery* 2013;33(6):460-467.
88. Hoben GM, Ee X, Schellhardt L, et al: Increasing nerve autograft length increases senescence and reduces regeneration. *Plast Reconstr Surg* 2018;142:952-996.
89. Saheb-Al-Zamani M, Yan Y, Farber SJ, et al: Limited regeneration in long acellular nerve allografts is associated with increased Schwann cell senescence. *Exp Neurol* 2013;247C:165-177.
90. Tojo T, Ushio-Fukai M, Yamaoka-Tojo M, et al: Role of gp91phox (Nox2)-containing NAD(P)H oxidase in angiogenesis in response to hindlimb ischemia. *Circulation* 2005;111:2347-2355.
91. Whitlock EL, Myckatyn TM, Tong AY, et al: Dynamic quantification of host Schwann cell migration into peripheral nerve allografts. *Exp Neurol* 2010;225:310-319.
92. Means KR Jr, Rinker BD, Higgins JP, et al: A multicenter, prospective randomized pilot study of outcomes for digital nerve repair in the hand using hollow conduit compared with processed allograft nerve. *Hand (N Y)* 2016;11(2):144-151.
93. Karabekmez FE, Duymaz A, Moran SL: Early clinical outcomes with the use of decellularized nerve allograft for repair of sensory defects within the hand. *Hand (N Y)* 2009;4:245-249.
94. Cho MS, Rinker BD, Weber RF, et al: Functional outcome following nerve repair in the upper extremity using processed nerve allograft. *J Hand Surg Am* 2012;38:2340-2349.
95. Guo Y, Chen G, Tian G, et al: Sensory recovery following decellularized nerve allograft transplantation for digital nerve repair. *J Plast Surg Hand Surg* 2013;47:451-453.
96. Zuniga JR: Sensory outcomes after reconstruction of lingual and inferior alveolar nerve discontinuities using processed nerve allograft-a case series. *J Oral Maxillofac Surg* 2015;73:734-744.
97. Taras JS, Amin N, Patel N, et al: Allograft reconstruction for digital nerve loss. *J Hand Surg Am* 2013;38:1965-1971.
98. Squintani G, Bonetti B, Paolin A, et al: Nerve regeneration across cryopreserved allografts from cadaveric donors: A novel approach for peripheral nerve reconstruction. *J Neurosurg* 2013;119:907-913.
99. Brooks DN, Weber RV, Chao JD, et al: Processed nerve allografts for peripheral nerve reconstruction: A multicenter study of utilization and outcomes in sensory, mixed and motor nerve reconstructions. *Microsurgery* 2012;32(1):1-14.
100. Isaacs J, Safa BA: Preliminary assessment of the utility of large-caliber processed nerve allografts for the repair of upper extremity nerve injuries. *Hand (N Y)* 2017;12(1):55-59.
101. Azouz SM, Lucas HD, Mahabir RC, Noland SS: A survey of the prevalence and practice patterns of human acellular nerve allograft use. *Plast Reconstr Surg Glob Open* 2018;6(8):e1803.
102. Rbia N, Shin AY: The role of nerve graft substitutes in motor and mixed motor/sensory peripheral nerve injuries. *J Hand Surg Am* 2017;42(5):367-377.
103. Gluck T: Uber Neuroplastik auf dem Wege der Transplantation. *Arch Klin Chir* 1880;25:606-616.
104. Dahlin LB, Lundborg G: Use of tubes in peripheral nerve repair. *Neurosurg Clin North Am* 2001;12:341-352.
105. Moore AM, Kasukurthi R, Magill CK, et al: Limitations of conduits in peripheral nerve repairs. *Hand (N Y)* 2009;4:180-186.
106. Isaacs J, Mallu S, Yan W, et al: Consequences of oversizing: Nerve-to-nerve tube diameter mismatch. *J Bone Joint Surg Am* 2014;96:1461-1467.
107. Liodaki E, Bos I, Lohmeyer JA, et al: Removal of collagen nerve conduits (NeuraGen) after unsuccessful implantation: Focus on histological findings. *J Reconstr Microsurg* 2013;29:517-522.
108. Rinker B, Liau J: A prospective randomized study comparing woven polyglycolic acid and autogenous vein conduits for reconstruction of digital nerve gaps. *JHS* 2011;36A:775-781.
109. Rinker BD, Ingari JV, Greenberg JA, et al: Outcomes of short-gap sensory nerve injuries reconstructed with processed nerve allografts from a multicenter registry study. *J Reconstr Microsurg* 2015;31:384-390.
110. He B, Zhu Q, Chai Y, et al: Safety and efficacy evaluation of a human acellular nerve graft as a digital nerve scaffold: A prospective multicenter controlled clinical trial. *J Tissue Eng Regen Med* 2015;9:286-295.
111. Voegelin E, Juan B: Nerve allografts and vein grafts in nerve reconstructions, in Dahlin LB, Leblebicioglu G, eds: *Current Treatment of Nerve Injuries and Disorders*. Zurich, Switzerland, Palme Publications, 2013.
112. Schmauss D, Finck T, Liodaki E, et al: Is nerve regeneration after reconstruction with collagen nerve conduits terminated after 12 months? The long-term follow-up of two prospective clinical studies. *J Reconstr Microsurg* 2014;30:561-568.

 ©Copyright 2021 American Academy of Orthopaedic Surgeons

113. Lohmeyer JA, Kern Y, Schmauss D, et al: Prospective clinical study on digital nerve repair with collagen nerve conduits and review of literature. *J Reconstr Microsurg* 2014;30:227-234.

114. Hirakawa CK, Grecco MA, Leite VM, et al: Fibroblasts growth factor and nerve fragment effect on tibial nerve regeneration in rats: A comparative study. *Acta Ortop Bras* 2007;15:114-117.

115. Marquardt LM, Ee X, Iyer N, et al: Finely tuned temporal and spatial delivery of GDNF promotes enhanced nerve regeneration in a long nerve defect model. *Tissue Eng Part A* 2015;21:2852-2864.

116. Mohammadi R, Amini K, Eskafian H: Betamethasone-enhanced vein graft conduit accelerates functional recovery in the rat sciatic nerve gap. *J Oral Maxillofac Surg* 2013, 71:786-792.

117. Azizi A, Azizi S, Heshmatian B, Amini K: Improvement of functional recovery of transected peripheral nerve by means of chitosan grafts filled with vitamin E, pyrroloquinoline quinone and their combination. *Int J Surg* 2014;12:76-82.

118. Elfar JC, Jacobson JA, Puzas JE, et al: Erythropoietin accelerates functional recovery after peripheral nerve injury. *J Bone Jt Surg Am* 2008;90:1644-1653.

119. Ding T, Zhu C, Yin JB, et al: Slow-releasing rapamycin-coated bionic peripheral nerve scaffold promotes the regeneration of rat sciatic nerve after injury. *Life Sci* 2015;122:92-99.

120. Shahraki M, Mohammadi R, Najafpour A: Influence of tacrolimus (FK506) on nerve regeneration using allografts: A rat sciatic nerve model. *J Oral Maxillofac Surg* 2015;73:1438.e1-1438.e9.

121. Hoben G, Yan Y, Iyer N, et al: Comparison of acellular nerve allograft modification with Schwann cells or VEGF. *Hand* 2015;10:396-402.

122. Strauch B, Rodriguez DM, Diaz J, et al: Autologous Schwann cells drive regeneration through a 6-cm autogenous venous nerve conduit. *J Reconstr Microsurg* 2001;17:589-598.

123. Levi AD, Burks SS, Anderson KD, et al: The use of autologous schwann cells to supplement sciatic nerve repair with a large gap—first in human experience. *Cell Transplant* 2016;25:1395-1403.

124. Jones S, Eisenberg HM, Jia X: Advances and future applications of augmented peripheral nerve regeneration. *Int J Mol Sci* 2016;17:1494.

125. Lee SK, Wolfe SW: Nerve transfers for the upper extremity: New horizons in nerve reconstruction. *J Am Acad Orthop Surg* 2012;20(8):506-517.

©Copyright 2021 American Academy of Orthopaedic Surgeons

37

Cells and Materials for Soft-Tissue Repair and Regeneration

Robert L. Mauck, PhD

Keywords: *biomaterials; cells; connective tissue repair; tissue engineering*

INTRODUCTION

Loss of function in musculoskeletal tissues initiates from either a failure of the cells that produce and maintain the extracellular matrix (ECM) or as a consequence of material failure of the ECM itself. To address these degenerative processes, the last three decades have witnessed marked advances in the identification of candidate therapeutic cell populations (to replace tissue formation capacity) and the development of new biomaterials (to restore or direct the restoration of damaged ECM). These agents can be applied alone or in combination to promote healing that alters the trajectory of disease or, potentially replace an entire tissue when damage has progressed to later stages. This chapter will provide an overview of the categories of ***cells*** and ***materials*** that are in use or in development for the treatment (and potential treatment) of damaged or diseased musculoskeletal tissues, highlighting their strengths and weaknesses, and ongoing developments to speed their reduction to clinical practice. Finally, this chapter closes with several illustrative examples of how the combination of cells and materials are being (or soon will be) used to address soft-tissue repair in humans.

Neither Dr. Mauck nor any immediate family member has received anything of value from or has stock or stock options held in a commercial company or institution related directly or indirectly to the subject of this chapter.

CELLS FOR SOFT-TISSUE REPAIR

The materials comprising the ECM of musculoskeletal tissues arise from the metabolic activity of cells within those tissues. During development, endogenous cells produce ECM that defines the mechanical properties of these tissues and allows them to carry out their role in musculoskeletal function. When endogenous cells are compromised, cell delivery may be considered. Three different types of cells are currently used in repair and regeneration scenarios: **primary cells**, **multipotent mesenchymal stem/progenitor cells**, and **pluripotent stem cells** (**Table 1**).

PRIMARY CELLS

DEFINITIONS AND APPLICATIONS

All musculoskeletal tissues contain living cells situated within a dense ECM. The phenotype of these cells is, by definition, appropriate for the generation of the ECM that defines the specialized function of the host tissue—this is their primary role. Given this, these are the most ideal source of regenerative cells after injury. Indeed, in several current clinical applications, endogenous cells are the therapeutic cell type of choice. These **primary cells** are removed from the native tissue, expanded in culture, coupled with a delivery system (in some cases), and then applied to the defect site.[1] For example, several FDA-approved cartilage repair procedures rely on the isolation of primary cells, wherein morsels of cartilage from a non–load-bearing region of the affected joint are removed (using an arthroscopic procedure), followed by extraction of living chondrocytes from these native tissue segments, and expansion in an in vitro setting. These cells are then either delivered directly or are seeded onto a provisional delivery

©Copyright 2021 American Academy of Orthopaedic Surgeons

TABLE 1 Cell Types for Musculoskeletal Regeneration and Repair

	Primary Cells	Mesenchymal Stem/Progenitor Cells	Pluripotent Stem Cells
Strengths	• Have the appropriate phenotype • Can be used in an autologous fashion	• Can be harvested in an autologous manner from multiple locations • Can differentiate towards relevant musculoskeletal lineages • Have an established safety profile for clinical use	• Can differentiate to any cell in the body • Show marked expansion capacity • Can be derived (for iPSC) in an autologous fashion
Weaknesses	• Limited in number upon isolation • Loss of phenotype with expansion • Replicative senescence with expansion • Limited potential with age/disease of donor	• Differentiation does not always match native cell phenotype • Evidence for phenotypic instability • Heterogeneity between donors and within populations • Replicative senescence with expansion	• Ethical concerns and limited number of source cells (for ESCs) • Need for reprogramming vectors (for iPSCs) • Issues of heterogeneity and phenotypic instability
Clinical progress	• In current use in procedures such as ACI and MACI	• In current clinical use, though without strong evidence to support efficacy • Large number of current clinical trials evaluating efficacy	• Limited clinical use to date, especially for musculoskeletal applications

ACI = autologous chondrocyte implantation; ESC = embryonic stem cell; iPSC = induced pluripotent stem cell; MACI = matrix-assisted autologous chondrocyte implantation

material and then reimplanted into a focal defect in the same joint. The recent approval of the matrix-assisted autologous chondrocyte implantation (MACI) procedure represents the first "tissue engineered" produce in clinical use in the musculoskeletal system.[2]

Limitations and Other Considerations

While primary cell-based therapeutics are already impacting clinical practice, several limitations do exist in this approach. Unlike most tissues in the body, the density of primary cells within adult musculoskeletal tissues is quite low, on the order of 10% of the volume or less.[3] This is due to both the primarily mechanical roles of these tissues as well as the relatively limited anabolic requirements of an already established musculoskeletal tissue. Once growth and development is complete, the role of endogenous cells is to replace the ECM in localized areas to address tissue damage. This occurs at a slow rate, however, and wholesale replacement of the ECM on a regular basis does not occur. Recent studies using carbon isotope analysis, taking advantage of the above-ground nuclear testing of the 1950s and 1960s, showed that the majority of the collagen in soft tissues that is present at the time of skeletal maturity remains present for the rest of life.[4] This suggests that, in healthy tissues in adults, cells operate at a low level of activity, and expansion in cell number is rare.

As there are so few cells, and those that are present operate mostly to maintain homeostasis, the application of these cells to in a regenerative context raises some issues. First, to populate large defects, primary cells must be dramatically expanded in number. The conditions under which this expansion occurs can impact the ultimate therapeutic efficacy of these primary cells. When primary cells undergo a high number of population doublings in vitro, typically on rigid tissue culture surfaces, cellular exhaustion (senescence) rapidly emerges. This results in the cessation of replicative capacity and the loss of cellular metabolic function.[5] Moreover, when primary cells are isolated from individuals of an advanced age, this in vitro senescence emerges more rapidly or may limit the number of population doublings that these cells can undergo. Even if expansion does not instigate senescence, the phenotype of primary cells is often lost through the expansion process. This is particularly true for chondrocytes that, within a few cell divisions, undergo a reversion to a fibroblast-like phenotype and cease production of proteoglycans and type II collagen (two essential components of the cartilage ECM).[6] Given that these cells must, de novo, generate new ECM at a rapid rate post implantation, this may compromise in vivo function of the regenerate tissue.

Current Advances

The use of primary cells has already impacted orthopaedic clinical practice. Current advances are focusing on overcoming the limitations that currently exist to make the process more efficient and cost-effective and to widen the indications for these cells. For example, work is being done to define the most optimal set of biological factors (growth factors, cytokines, etc.) and culture environments (material framework, see below) that can improve expansion efficiency while preserving phenotype. The delivery systems for these primary cells has also become more sophisticated, with newer autologous treatments for cartilage using biomaterials as a carrier to improve targeting of primary cells to the defect site and to decrease surgical complexity.[7] Likewise, advances in drug delivery have made it possible for these primary cells to be delivered along with agents that release factors to increase retention and anabolic activity post implantation. Others have explored coculture systems where, for example, primary chondrocytes are mixed with progenitor cells (described below) to take advantage of the need for fewer cells at the time of implantation,[8] allowing for these to become

©Copyright 2021 American Academy of Orthopaedic Surgeons

one-stage procedures.[9] Finally, with this and other approaches, methods are being developed to select the most efficient cartilage forming cells, including from alternative sources (such as nasal cartilage),[10] as well as to remove from the population those showing senescent or other aberrant phenotypes.[11]

MULTIPOTENT STEM/PROGENITOR CELLS

DEFINITIONS AND APPLICATIONS

While primary cells, by definition, possess the appropriate phenotype for tissue repair, in many instances the isolation of these cells is not feasible, or the isolation and expansion process may not be compatible with retention of phenotype and clinical application. To overcome this limitation, work over the last two decades has focused on the identification and application of stem cell or stem cell-like populations for musculoskeletal tissue repair. A stem cell is a cell that can replicate indefinitely to produce progeny that both maintain the original stem cell pool and/or can be induced to differentiate into a phenotype resembling the primary cells in the target tissue of interest. When the spectrum of fates is limited, these cells are called multipotent, to indicate the limited set of phenotypes that can be achieved, and are referred to most appropriately as progenitor cells (rather than stem cells).

Most popular among these cells are bone marrow-derived **mesenchymal stem/progenitor cells**, colloquially termed MSCs. These cells, first identified in the 1960s and 1970s,[12,13] can undergo lineage specification into cells resembling bone, fat, and cartilage cells, among others.[14,15] Lineage specification of these cells is generally directed using specific soluble factors in combination with culture environments permissive of a given lineage—for instance, the cartilage phenotype is best promoted when these cells are cultured in high-density micromass or pellet cultures or in a suitable three dimensional (3D) environment that can promote the rounded cell shape of a chondrocyte.[16] With appropriate induction, these progenitor cells can generate a cartilage-like matrix that increases in mechanical properties over time, resembling native tissue in terms of composition, mechanics, and molecular profile.[17,18]

Although the bone marrow is by far the most common location for sourcing of these progenitor cells, this is not the only location in the body from which multipotent cells can originate. In the early 2000s[19,20] it was found that lipoaspirate contained a population of mesenchymal-like progenitors as well, with similar differentiation capacity as those isolated from bone marrow. Since then, nearly every tissue in the musculoskeletal system has been shown to harbor a population of so called "endogenous stem cells" that can differentiate into cartilage, fat, and bone and are speculated to play a role in endogenous repair of these native tissues. For this reason, these cells are widely used as a starting source for many repair applications.

LIMITATIONS AND OTHER CONSIDERATIONS

Mesenchymal progenitors show great promise as a cellular therapeutic and for growing new tissues ex vivo for reimplantation. Given that bone marrow and adipose tissue scan be readily harvested in a relatively noninvasive manner, they also serve as a clinically relevant source of autologous starting cells. Moreover, clinical trials have shown the safety of joint injections of allogeneic MSCs in humans,[21] with recent trials showing some evidence of efficacy in some patients, though comprehensive and well-regulated trials are limited.[22]

However, limitations in this cell type do exist. First, these cells are by definition only multipotent with fixed lineage potential, not totipotent, and so can only differentiate along specific lineages and may not be able to address all tissues in the musculoskeletal system. Additionally, the extent to which they take on the appropriate primary cell phenotype is often limited, where incomplete commitment to the differentiated lineage being a common outcome. For example, if a cell becomes an "inefficient" chondrocyte, production of matrix will only occur under ideal situations, and so in vivo production and survival in the demanding environment of the joint may be compromised.[23] Also, because commitment may be incomplete, this raises the potential for subsequent transition in phenotype after implantation. For example, it has been well documented that MSCs that have undergone in vitro chondrogenesis can transition to an osteogenic phenotype after in vivo implantation.[24] This is compounded by the variation seen in these cell populations both within a single donor, and between individual donors. As every MSC population initiates from a number of different individual cells (that expand into "clones") and each of these starting cells can have a different potential, the population is by definition heterogeneous.[25] Likewise, between donors, marked variability exists, based on age of donor and other systemic comorbidities that impact the number of resident stem cells. Finally, like primary cells, mesenchymal progenitors are not "true" stem cells and so undergo replicative senescence and loss of potentiality with extended culture expansion.[26]

CURRENT ADVANCES

As with primary cells, a number of technological advances are being used to improve the therapeutic efficacy of mesenchymal progenitor cell populations. High-depth and single-cell transcriptomic analysis has uncovered patterns of expression across populations of progenitor cells that may improve selection criteria of cells with the "best" phenotype.[27,28] Likewise, material substrates have been introduced that can maintain the "stemness" of these progenitor cells during culture expansion, potentially improving their long-term function.[29] Others have used biomaterial cues (more below) and drug and gene delivery methods to help to control the phenotype of these cells, both during in vitro differentiation and after in vivo implantation. Also, as with primary cells, coculture of mesenchymal progenitors with a very small fraction of primary cells appears to improve phenotypic specialization by the progenitors as well as the retention of this specialized phenotype.[8] Finally, as the cells are typically expanded in vitro prior to being delivered back into a repair environment, they can

©Copyright 2021 American Academy of Orthopaedic Surgeons

be engineered to express a number of factors, including those that promote their own differentiation or factors that improve the host environment to increase retention/survivability after implantation.[30] This could improve their functional role, but it should be noted that any cell type that is more than "minimally manipulated" will face a more stringent review by the FDA prior to approval for clinical use.

PLURIPOTENT STEM CELLS

Definitions and Applications

The final category of cells now in development for musculoskeletal applications is **pluripotent stem cells** (PSCs). These cells can undergo lineage specification to any cell type and can reconstitute an entire organism when integrated into the germline of a developing embryo. As such, these cells represent the greatest potential for repair across the musculoskeletal system.[31] Multiple sources of PSCs now exist. The original PSCs were derived from the inner cell mass of developing mouse and human embryos and were termed embryonic stem cells (ESCs). After expansion on a feeder layer, and with careful and sequential exposure to developmentally relevant morphogens, ESCs can differentiate along all relevant lineages of the musculoskeletal system. Indeed, there are now multiple published protocols for pushing ESCs toward a cartilage-like phenotype.[32-38] In addition to ESCs, the discovery of somatic cell "reprogramming" has enabled production of PSCs from nearly any cell in the body in adult sources. These induced pluripotent stem cells (or iPSCs) are generated (typically from skin fibroblasts) by transfecting with four critical transcription factors (the so called "Yamanaka factors," based on the originator of this process).[39] This reprogramming step resets the epigenome of these cells (marks and histone organization that helps to instill differentiation) to a more primitive state, enabling their subsequent differentiation into any cell type via carefully staged induction processes that are similar to those used to direct lineage specification in ESCs. Indeed, a host of recent studies have reported on the efficient production of chondrocyte-like cells from iPSCs and have begun to show the potential of these cells in a number of regenerative scenarios.[40,41]

Limitations and Other Considerations

Limitations in the use of PSCs are consistent with (and perhaps more apparent than) those in multipotent progenitor cell sources. This includes population heterogeneity, variation in differentiation potential based on source, and stability of phenotype after differentiation. Because PSCs have a greater potential for differentiation, emergence of alternative lineages may be more difficult to control. In addition, few ESC lines are available for federally funded use, and the clinical relevance of these cells remains limited. iPSCs offer a potentially autologous alternative, though the processes for reprogramming, expansion, and induction of a stable phenotype present a number of challenges in terms of reduction to clinical practice, despite considerable research activity in this area.

Current Advances

Advances in PSCs for soft-tissue applications are focused on improvements in differentiation methods and vehicles for gene delivery for reprogramming, methods for selection of optimally differentiated cells, and the reduction of this to practice in preclinical models. While much work remains to be done for these cells to reach widespread clinical applicability, the promise of a fully autologous cell-based therapeutic for soft-tissue repair motivates continued innovation in this area.

MATERIALS FOR SOFT-TISSUE REPAIR

While cells are essential for repair, these processes cannot occur without a template on which to form new tissue. In many applications, biomaterials serve as this template, facilitating the delivery of cells to a defect site and/or capturing and organizing the ECM produced by cells. Biomaterials may also be implanted in an acellular format (lacking cells), where they are designed to engage with and recruit neighboring endogenous cell populations to improve repair. This section will review basic terminology in biomaterials and highlight advances in biomaterial design to promote exogenous and endogenous cell-mediated repair activities (**Table 2**).

CLASSES OF MATERIALS IN CLINICAL AND PRECLINICAL USE

There are a number of materials in preclinical and clinical use for the restoration of soft tissues of the musculoskeletal system. These fall into two broad classes: **natural** and **synthetic**.

Natural materials are those that can be extracted from native tissues and other organisms, purified, and then delivered to promote repair.[42,43] Examples of natural materials isolated from tissues include collagens (of various types), fibrin, and hyaluronic acid, among others. It is also important to note that the source for natural materials need not be a mammalian system. For example, many natural extracts from plants and other life forms have been used in tissue engineering and repair applications. These include agarose, alginate, and chitosan, with the former being extracts from seaweed and algae and the latter being an extract from the exoskeleton of crustaceans. Natural materials have the benefit of being comprised of materials that cells normally experience in their microenvironment, and many times contain proteins to which cells and/or released factors can bind. One drawback of natural materials, however, is that they are prone to lose their biologic features during crosslinking and stabilization of formed constructs. Another drawback of biologic materials is the potential for presence of immunogenic epitopes, particularly if the material is sourced from a different mammalian system. That said, a number of naturally derived materials are already used in clinical practice in humans. Small intestinal submucosa (SIS) has been used in a number of soft-tissue repair

©Copyright 2021 American Academy of Orthopaedic Surgeons

TABLE 2 Materials for Musculoskeletal Regeneration and Repair

	Natural Materials	Synthetic Materials
Strengths	• Sourced from animal and humans tissues • Can be used in an autologous fashion • Contain appropriate biochemical constituents and binding epitopes	• Constituents are well defined and characterized • Can be readily processed into multiple forms with defined mechanical attributes • Can be easily modified to include controlled degradation as well as binding domains for cells and growth factors
Weaknesses	• Can be immunogenic if sourced from animals • May require extensive processing and crosslinking for stabilization • Constituents may not be fully characterized and may vary based on source	• Do not endogenously contain cell-binding motifs and may elicit foreign body response • May require extensive modification for a given application, raising additional regulatory concerns
Clinical progress	• In current clinical use for procedures such as ACI and MACI	• Used commercially in multiple applications, ranging from implants to biodegradable sutures

ACI = autologous chondrocyte implantation; MACI = matrix-assisted autologous chondrocyte implantation

scenarios.[44-46] Likewise, processed membranes composed of porcine type 1/type III collagen (which were originally used to cover defects in preparation for autologous chondrocyte implantation [ACI])[47,48] are now being used a vehicle for chondrocyte delivery in the newer MACI procedures. Newer methods, involving decellularization (removal of living cells and cell debris) of native tissues have created a host of "tissue-specific" ECM formulations that are now being processed into biomaterials and applied in defined regenerative scenarios.[49-52]

Synthetic materials for soft-tissue repair, on the other hand, include a broad range of man-made nondegradable and degradable polymers.[42,43] These polymers can form networks through physical entanglement or by ionic or covalent interactions between polymers. One strength of synthetic materials is that one can design in attributes, including material properties and degradation rate. One prototypical synthetic material is polyethylene glycol (PEG). PEG is a relatively inert nondegradable polymer that can be formed into a polymeric network by modifying its end groups to enable covalent crosslinking. PEG has also undergone multiple design modifications over the years to expand its versatility in forming networks, including the generation of complex multiarm formulations to nucleate crosslinking. As PEG does not contain any endogenous biologic motifs, cell adhesion to the base material is poor. To address this, PEG can be modified to include matrix-mimicking peptides to increase adhesion of cells as well as degradable crosslinks to enable cell-mediated remodeling. Other commonly used synthetics include biodegradable polyesters, such as polylactic acid, polyglycolic acid, and copolymers of the two. These synthetic polymers undergo hydrolytic degradation in aqueous environments, with their rate of degradation controlled by the specific composition and polymer molecular weight. This material is found in degradable sutures and similar clinically used items and has been extended for use as a biomaterial scaffold for regenerative applications.

MATERIAL STRUCTURES

Beyond polymer composition, there is also considerable flexibility in the structural form that a scaffold may take. For musculoskeletal applications, the two most common forms are **hydrogels** and **porous scaffolds**. These are described below.

Hydrogels

Hydrogels are water-swollen networks composed of polymers that interact through physical, ionic, or covalent crosslinks. Hydrogels can be composed of either natural or synthetic polymers, or a combination of the two.[53] From a clinical use perspective, hydrogels have a long history of application in the delivery of bone morphogenetic protein from collagen gels that are applied during spinal fusion surgery. Because of their aqueous formulation, hydrogels can serve as a depot for the release of biologic agents (such as growth factors and other pharmaceuticals), with release defined by the diffusive characteristics of the material. Hydrogels can also serve as physical housing for encapsulated cells. Given their high water content, hydrogels can support cell viability and nutrient exchange. As the pore size of these materials can be tuned to small length scales (based on the polymer density and crosslinking), these networks can also capture large macromolecules and ECM components produced by embedded cells. Toward cartilage regeneration, a number of hydrogels have been used to encapsulate chondrocytes and chondrogenically differentiated progenitor cells to generate living cartilage constructs for implantation.[54]

Porous Scaffolds

Porous scaffolds are comprised of a solid polymeric component with void spaces that enable penetration of cells, in vitro or in vivo.[55] As with hydrogels, these porous materials can be formed from either natural or synthetic polymers, or a combination of the two. In its simplest manifestation, a porous polymeric material is produced by mixing a polymer solution with

©Copyright 2021 American Academy of Orthopaedic Surgeons

a porogen, evaporating the solvent to solidify the polymer, and then removing the porogen to create the final structure. In specialized versions, the polymer of interest may be extruded into micron-scale fibers, which can then be wrapped, braided, or woven to create a three-dimensional material.[56] For example, recent studies have used three-dimensional weaving of biodegradable filaments to produce a porous, fibrous material with mechanical properties matching that of native articular cartilage.[57] Other specialized fabrication methods, such as electrospinning, can be used to generate fibrous porous scaffolds that have fiber length scales that match that of native ECM molecules, providing topographic cues to cells that encounter these materials.[58] These materials can likewise be generated with organization in differing directions and through the depth to mimic native tissue structure/function relationships.

ADVANCES IN MATERIAL DESIGN

Upon these base material formulations, marked advances and innovations have occurred in the last two decades. Principally, this focus has been in the area of making synthetic material systems more "biologic," and in making natural material systems more "synthetic." Toward the former, it would be ideal to have the versatility of a synthetic backbone though which to control the overall properties of the material, while at the same time imparting biologic cues to direct cell behavior. As noted above, simple PEG hydrogels have been further developed[59] to include moieties that enable cell adhesion (such at RGD, a motif in fibronectin) and GFOGER (a collagen mimic)[60] as well as numerous growth factors through covalent and noncovalent mechanisms. These modifications enable presentation of cues that are normally present in the microenvironment, in a controlled manner. Likewise, synthetic aspects have been added to biologic molecules. One example of this is hyaluronic acid (HA)—a natural polysaccharide component of the cartilage ECM. Chondrocytes and chondro-progenitors can interact directly with HA through cell surface receptors. Moreover, this molecule has long been injected into joints as a lubricant and anti-inflammatory molecule. With respect to material modifications, HA has been engineered to introduce additional functionality. This includes addition of cell-binding motifs (as previously mentioned for PEG), modification to enable UV and visible light-mediated crosslinking, modification with crosslinkers that are susceptible to MMP-mediated cleavage, and modifications that promote viscoelastic material properties in formed hydrogels.[61,62] These synthetic modifications of a natural material provide enhanced functionality and can improve biologic function when cells interact with these advanced materials.

ADVANCES IN SCAFFOLD FABRICATION

The past two decades have witnessed marked advances in three-dimensional (3D) printing and rapid prototyping[63] that have enabled production of anatomic, 3D tissue engineered constructs.[63,64] Rapid prototyping relies on information garnered through advanced imaging modalities, such as MRI and microcomputed tomography (μCT), and *in silico* models generated through computer-assisted drawing (CAD) programs, which render 3D shapes into a series of 2D cross sections.[65] Rapid prototyping techniques have gained popularity because they allow for precise control of pore size and distribution[66,67] and enable scaffold fabrication in any desired shape along with components tailored to promote tissue formation and cell differentiation.[68] Image-guided tissue engineering is ideal for musculoskeletal applications, as it allows for precise size-matching for each patient. Early work in this area has shown promising results.[69-71] For example, Chang and colleagues developed molds for facial implants that were filled by injection molding with cell-seeded alginate hydrogels.[72] This work was recently extended to fashion anatomic meniscus implants.[64,73] These techniques have also been applied to articular cartilage, via stainless steel molds that generate replicas of the retro-patellar cartilage based on chondrocyte-seeded hydrogels.[69] More recently, Hollister and others have developed direct fabrication methods (3D printing) of solid porous materials with controlled geometry and pore spacing.[74] These and similar methods have likewise been implemented by Mao and colleagues to develop fully anatomic replacements for the humeral head in a rabbit model.[70] Since this early and seminal work in this arena, numerous other studies have deployed similar technologies to fashion 3D, living, engineered cartilage constructs.[49,75,76] This technology, coupled with advances in our ability to grow functional cartilage tissue in vitro using patient-derived MSCs,[77] make it now possible to advance these technologies toward clinical application.

REDUCTION TO PRACTICE: ILLUSTRATIVE EXAMPLES

As these technologies and the preclinical testing of cells and materials have advanced, the opportunity for clinical translation has also increased. Indeed, these advances have increasingly been combined and evaluated in clinically relevant models and translated to humans to improve soft-tissue repair.[78] In this final section, we review the current state of the art in cells, materials, and their combination via illustrative examples that are now in or at the cusp of clinical implementation.

CELL DELIVERY TO PROMOTE CARTILAGE REPAIR

Since the mid 1990s, it has been well appreciated that the delivery of chondrocytes to focal cartilage defects can improve long term repair outcomes.[1] This procedure, termed autologous chondrocyte implantation (ACI), underwent significant modifications as clinical experience and outcomes developed over time and has recently been further refined. This new approach, termed MACI follows a similar course as ACI but improves clinical practicality and long-term outcomes

©Copyright 2021 American Academy of Orthopaedic Surgeons

by focusing the initial cell delivery using a biomaterial support.[2] For this, patient cells are isolated from donor tissue and expanded as in ACI. However, at this stage, cells are then cultured onto a type I/type II collagen sponge for several days prior to implantation. This new method, recently approved by the FDA, is noteworthy in that it is the first real application of "tissue engineering" in the field of orthopaedics. Even more noteworthy is the untapped potential to further improve upon this procedure. Already, new developments have reduced this approach to a single-stage procedure, where isolated MSCs and chondrocytes are combined together, in coculture, for reimplantation.[9] In addition, the material used in these first MACI approvals was quite simple, a repurposing of an already accepted material used in similar procedures, but here reapplied as a cell carrier. Innovations in biomaterials are poised to generate the next generation of cell carriers that can not only efficiently deliver cells to the defect site, but also direct their fate by material design and deliver bioactive factors that expedite repair and regeneration of the cartilage.[79]

ACELLULAR MATERIALS TO PROMOTE MENISCUS REPAIR

Materials can also be instrumented to interact with endogenous primary and stem cells to promote repair, obviating the need for cell delivery. For example, in early meniscus repair scaffolds composed of both synthetic and natural materials, repair was improved by delivering a scaffold that could support invasion by cells from the remaining meniscus and the synovium.[80,81] These original formulations have been further refined via custom weaving methods that address the direction dependent properties in the meniscus.[82] While these scaffolds show promise in preclinical models and human clinical trials, advancing the rate of cell colonization and the formation of matrix may improve outcomes. To that end, Mao and colleagues 3D printed a fibrous scaffold composed of a slowly degrading synthetic material, and coupled this with biodegradable microspheres designed to deliver active factors[83] (**Figure 1**). These factors were released sequentially, and chosen for their

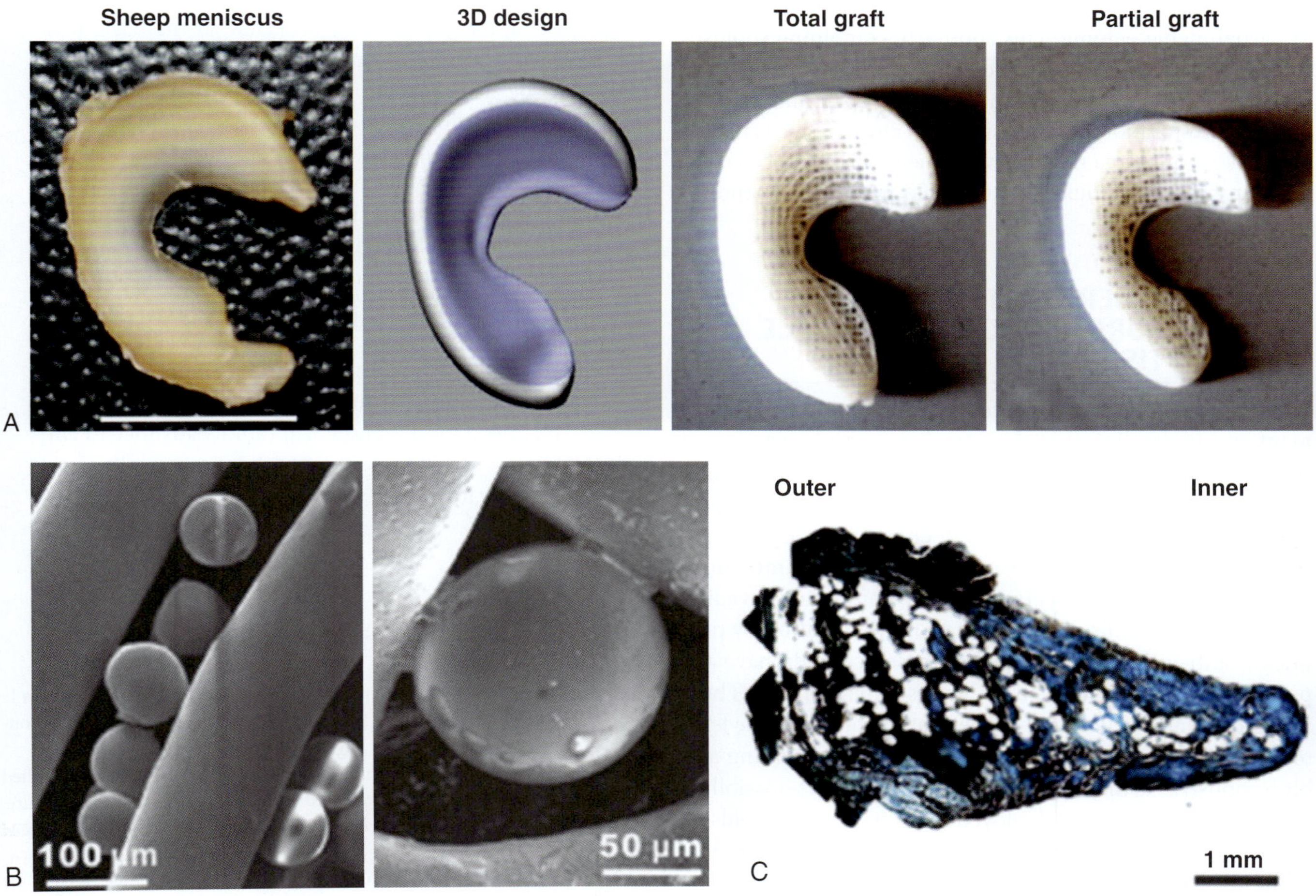

FIGURE 1 Engineering the knee meniscus via acellular 3D-printed scaffolds and drug delivery. **A**, Imaging and 3D printing of a sheep-sized meniscus. **B**, Scanning electron micrograph showing fibers and drug-delivering microspheres. **C**, Alcian blue staining of regenerated meniscus based on implanted engineered implant. (Reproduced with permission from Lee CH, Rodeo SA, Fortier LA, Lu C, Erisken C, Mao JJ: Protein-releasing polymeric scaffolds induce fibrochondrocytic differentiation of endogenous cells for knee meniscus regeneration in sheep. *Sci Transl Med* 2014;6(266):266ra171.)

©Copyright 2021 American Academy of Orthopaedic Surgeons

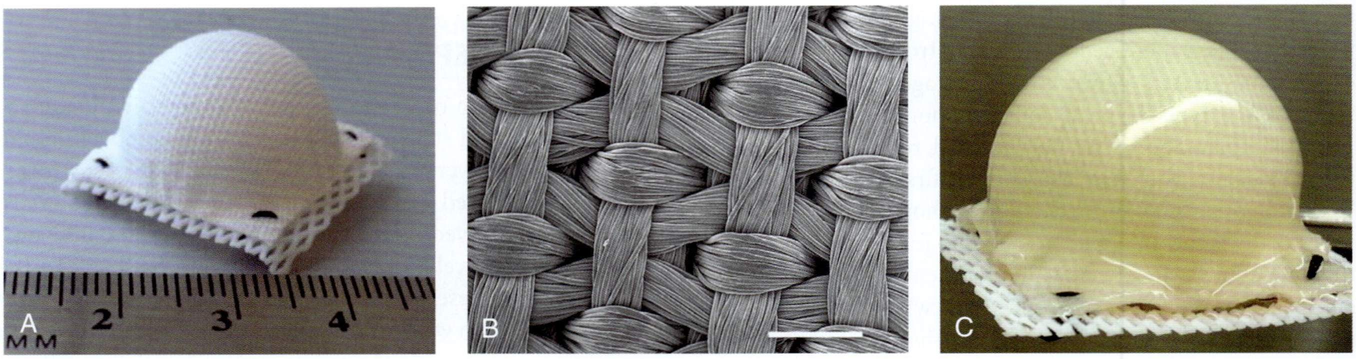

FIGURE 2 Macroscale (**A**) and microscale scanning electron micrograph (**B**) images of large anatomically shaped cartilage tissue constructs formed from a woven scaffold instrumented to deliver gene vectors that make colonizing cells resistant to inflammatory challenge. Hemispherical 3D-woven scaffold and (**C**) construct seeded with stem cells and cultured for 38 days in vitro. Scale bar = 0.5 mm. (Reproduced with permission from Moutos FT, Glass KA, Compton SA, et al: Anatomically shaped tissue-engineered cartilage with tunable and inducible anticytokine delivery for biological joint resurfacing. *Proc Natl Acad Sci U S A* 2016;113(31):E4513-E4522.)

capacity to first promote colonization of the scaffold and then cartilaginous matrix deposition. These advanced biomaterials improved the rate and quality of repair in a large animal model of partial meniscectomy. This approach, combining sophisticated 3D printing methods and tunable release of biofactors may overcome endogenous limitations to repair and improve meniscus restoration. If successful, such an approach is readily adaptable to multiple repair environments in which cell colonization by endogenous cells and rapid matrix production is required.

COMBINED THERAPEUTICS—CELLS/MATERIAL FORMULATIONS TO REPLACE DAMAGED TISSUES

Even more sophisticated scaffolds are now under development and in preclinical evaluation. For example, one recent scaffold formulation (based on woven slowly degrading polymer fibers) that mimicked native cartilage properties was instrumented with viral constructs designed to reprogram invading cells to be resistant to inflammation-mediated degradation[84] (**Figure 2**). By converting invading cells into "smart cells" that respond to inflammation by producing anti-inflammatory agents, these scaffolds have the potential to permanently alter the host environment. These scaffolds were also woven into the anatomic form of the femoral head, making the possibility of a fully conforming and bioresponsive cartilage repair construct a distinct possibility. Such scaffolds could be deployed after seeding scaffolds in vitro or could be deployed in an acellular fashion to reprogram invading cells in vivo.[30] This reprogramming may one day be extended to the reprogramming of any invading cell to a pluripotent state, followed by careful instruction toward differentiation to the intended lineage and resistance to ongoing inflammatory processes.

SUMMARY

This chapter provided an overview of the basic principles and recent advances in cells and materials that could be used for the treatment of damaged or diseased musculoskeletal tissues. Each cell type has inherent strengths and weaknesses. That said, current clinical practice relies on these cells to improve repair, and additional research and evaluation of emerging cell types (including pluripotent stem cells) may revolutionize cell therapies with autologous sourcing. Similarly, developments in materials have resulted in sophisticated synthetic and natural templates that can match native tissue properties and promote cell phenotype and function. As these developments are validated in preclinical models, they will rapidly advance to clinical trials and will undoubtedly change clinical practice in the years to come.

REFERENCES

1. Brittberg M, Lindahl A, Nilsson A, Ohlsson C, Isaksson O, Peterson L: Treatment of deep cartilage defects in the knee with autologous chondrocyte transplantation. *N Engl J Med* 1994;331(14):889-895.
2. Brittberg M, Recker D, Ilgenfritz J, Saris DBF, Group SES: Matrix-applied characterized autologous cultured chondrocytes versus microfracture: Five-year follow-up of a prospective randomized trial. *Am J Sports Med* 2018;46(6):1343-1351.
3. Jadin KD, Bae WC, Schumacher BL, Sah RL: Three-dimensional (3-D) imaging of chondrocytes in articular cartilage: Growth-associated changes in cell organization. *Biomaterials* 2007;28(2):230-239.
4. Heinemeier KM, Schjerling P, Heinemeier J, et al: Radiocarbon dating reveals minimal collagen turnover in both healthy and osteoarthritic human cartilage. *Sci Transl Med* 2016;8(346):346ra90.

©Copyright 2021 American Academy of Orthopaedic Surgeons

5. Barbero A, Grogan S, Schafer D, Heberer M, Mainil-Varlet P, Martin I: Age related changes in human articular chondrocyte yield, proliferation and post-expansion chondrogenic capacity. *Osteoarthr Cartil* 2004;12(6):476-484.
6. Ma B, Leijten JC, Wu L, et al: Gene expression profiling of dedifferentiated human articular chondrocytes in monolayer culture. *Osteoarthr Cartil* 2013;21(4):599-603.
7. Saris D, Price A, Widuchowski W, et al: Matrix-applied characterized autologous cultured chondrocytes versus microfracture: Two-year follow-up of a prospective randomized trial. *Am J Sports Med* 2014;42(6):1384-1394.
8. Kim M, Steinberg DR, Burdick JA, Mauck RL: Extracellular vesicles mediate improved functional outcomes in engineered cartilage produced from MSC/chondrocyte cocultures. *Proc Natl Acad Sci U S A* 2019;116(5):1569-1578.
9. de Windt TS, Vonk LA, Slaper-Cortenbach IC, et al: Allogeneic mesenchymal stem cells stimulate cartilage regeneration and are safe for single-stage cartilage repair in humans upon mixture with recycled autologous chondrons. *Stem Cells* 2017;35(1):256-264.
10. Mumme M, Barbero A, Miot S, et al: Nasal chondrocyte-based engineered autologous cartilage tissue for repair of articular cartilage defects: An observational first-in-human trial. *Lancet* 2016;388(10055):1985-1994.
11. Jeon OH, Kim C, Laberge RM, et al: Local clearance of senescent cells attenuates the development of post-traumatic osteoarthritis and creates a pro-regenerative environment. *Nat Med* 2017;23(6):775-781.
12. Friedenstein AJ, Deriglasova UF, Kulagina NN, et al: Precursors for fibroblasts in different populations of hematopoietic cells as detected by the in vitro colony assay method. *Exp Hematol* 1974;2(2):83-92.
13. Caplan AI: Mesenchymal stem cells. *J Orthop Res* 1991;9(5):641-650.
14. Prockop DJ: Marrow stromal cells as stem cells for nonhematopoietic tissues. *Science* 1997;276(5309):71-74.
15. Pittenger MF, Mackay AM, Beck SC, et al: Multilineage potential of adult human mesenchymal stem cells. *Science* 1999;284:143-147.
16. Johnstone B, Hering TM, Caplan AI, Goldberg VM, Yoo JU: In vitro chondrogenesis of bone marrow-derived mesenchymal progenitor cells. *Exp Cell Res* 1998;238:265-272.
17. Erickson IE, Kestle SR, Zellars KH, et al: High mesenchymal stem cell seeding densities in hyaluronic acid hydrogels produce engineered cartilage with native tissue properties. *Acta Biomater* 2012;8(8):3027-3034.
18. Bhumiratana S, Eton RE, Oungoulian SR, Wan LQ, Ateshian GA, Vunjak-Novakovic G: Large, stratified, and mechanically functional human cartilage grown in vitro by mesenchymal condensation. *Proc Natl Acad Sci U S A* 2014;111(19):6940-6945.
19. Zuk PA, Zhu M, Mizuno H, et al: Multilineage cells from human adipose tissue: Implications for cell-based therapies. *Tissue Eng* 2001;7(2):211-228.
20. Erickson GR, Gimble JM, Franklin DM, Rice HE, Awad H, Guilak F: Chondrogenic potential of adipose tissue-derived stromal cells in vitro and in vivo. *Biochem Biophys Res Commun* 2002;290(2):763-769.
21. Vangsness CT Jr, Farr J II, Boyd J, Dellaero DT, Mills CR, LeRoux-Williams M: Adult human mesenchymal stem cells delivered via intra-articular injection to the knee following partial medial meniscectomy: A randomized, double-blind, controlled study. *J Bone Joint Surg Am* 2014;96(2):90-98.
22. Iijima H, Isho T, Kuroki H, Takahashi M, Aoyama T: Effectiveness of mesenchymal stem cells for treating patients with knee osteoarthritis: A meta-analysis toward the establishment of effective regenerative rehabilitation. *NPJ Regen Med* 2018;3:15.
23. Farrell MJ, Shin JI, Smith LJ, Mauck RL: Functional consequences of glucose and oxygen deprivation on engineered mesenchymal stem cell-based cartilage constructs. *Osteoarthr Cartil* 2015;23(1):134-142.
24. Pelttari K, Winter A, Steck E, et al: Premature induction of hypertrophy during in vitro chondrogenesis of human mesenchymal stem cells correlates with calcification and vascular invasion after ectopic transplantation in SCID mice. *Arthritis Rheum* 2006;54(10):3254-3266.
25. McLeod CM, Mauck RL: On the origin and impact of mesenchymal stem cell heterogeneity: New insights and emerging tools for single cell analysis. *Eur Cell Mater* 2017;34:217-231.
26. Wagner W, Horn P, Castoldi M, et al: Replicative senescence of mesenchymal stem cells: A continuous and organized process. *PLoS One* 2008;3(5):e2213.
27. Huynh NPT, Zhang B, Guilak F: High-depth transcriptomic profiling reveals the temporal gene signature of human mesenchymal stem cells during chondrogenesis. *FASEB J* 2019;33(1):358-372.
28. Liu S, Stroncek DF, Zhao Y, et al: Single cell sequencing reveals gene expression signatures associated with bone marrow stromal cell subpopulations and time in culture. *J Transl Med* 2019;17(1):23.
29. Heo SJ, Szczesny SE, Kim DH, Saleh KS, Mauck RL: Expansion of mesenchymal stem cells on electrospun scaffolds maintains stemness, mechano-responsivity, and differentiation potential. *J Orthop Res* 2018;36(2):808-815.
30. Guilak F, Pferdehirt L, Ross AK, et al: Designer stem cells: Genome engineering and the next generation of cell-based therapies. *J Orthop Res* 2019;37(6):1287-1293.
31. Castro-Vinuelas R, Sanjurjo-Rodriguez C, Pineiro-Ramil M, et al: Induced pluripotent stem cells for cartilage repair: Current status and future perspectives. *Eur Cell Mater* 2018;36:96-109.
32. Hwang NS, Varghese S, Lee HJ, et al: In vivo commitment and functional tissue regeneration using human embryonic stem cell-derived mesenchymal cells. *Proc Natl Acad Sci U S A* 2008;105(52):20641-20646.
33. Kramer J, Hegert C, Guan K, Wobus AM, Muller PK, Rohwedel J: Embryonic stem cell-derived chondrogenic differentiation in vitro: Activation by BMP-2 and BMP-4. *Mech Dev* 2000;92(2):193-205.
34. Toh WS, Lee EH, Richards M, Cao T: In vitro derivation of chondrogenic cells from human embryonic stem cells. *Methods Mol Biol* 2010;584:317-331.
35. Gibson JD, O'Sullivan MB, Alaee F, et al: Regeneration of articular cartilage by human ESC-derived mesenchymal progenitors treated sequentially with BMP-2 and Wnt5a. *Stem Cells Transl Med* 2017;6(1):40-50.
36. Craft AM, Ahmed N, Rockel JS, et al: Specification of chondrocytes and cartilage tissues from embryonic stem cells. *Development* 2013;140(12):2597-2610.
37. Craft AM, Rockel JS, Nartiss Y, Kandel RA, Alman BA, Keller GM: Generation of articular chondrocytes from human pluripotent stem cells. *Nat Biotechnol* 2015;33(6):638-645.
38. Koay EJ, Hoben GM, Athanasiou KA: Tissue engineering with chondrogenically differentiated human embryonic stem cells. *Stem Cells* 2007;25(9):2183-2190.
39. Takahashi K, Tanabe K, Ohnuki M, et al: Induction of pluripotent stem cells from adult human fibroblasts by defined factors. *Cell* 2007;131(5):861-872.
40. Diekman BO, Christoforou N, Willard VP, et al: Cartilage tissue engineering using differentiated and purified induced pluripotent stem cells. *Proc Natl Acad Sci U S A* 2012;109(47):19172-19177.
41. Diekman BO, Guilak F: Stem cell-based therapies for osteoarthritis: Challenges and opportunities. *Curr Opin Rheumatol* 2013;25(1):119-126.
42. Liu M, Zeng X, Ma C, et al: Injectable hydrogels for cartilage and bone tissue engineering. *Bone Res* 2017;5:17014.
43. Duarte Campos DF, Drescher W, Rath B, Tingart M, Fischer H: Supporting biomaterials for articular cartilage repair. *Cartilage* 2012;3(3):205-221.
44. Badylak S, Arnoczky S, Plouhar P, et al: Naturally occurring extracellular matrix as a scaffold for musculoskeletal repair. *Clin Orthop* 1999;(367 suppl):S333-S343.
45. Cook JL, Tomlinson JL, Fox D, et al: Tissue-engineered meniscal replacment in dogs using small intestinal submucosa: Phase 2, addition of autogenous fibrin clot and biomechanical protection. *Trans Orthop Res Soc* 2001;26:599.
46. Dejardin LM, Arnoczky SP, Ewers BJ, Haut RC, Clarke RB: Tissue-engineered rotator cuff tendon using porcine small intestine submucosa. Histologic and mechanical evaluation in dogs. *Am J Sports Med* 2001;29(2):175-184.

©Copyright 2021 American Academy of Orthopaedic Surgeons

47. Haddo O, Mahroof S, Higgs D, et al: The use of chondrogide membrane in autologous chondrocyte implantation. *Knee* 2004;11(1):51-55.
48. Niemeyer P, Pestka JM, Kreuz PC, et al: Characteristic complications after autologous chondrocyte implantation for cartilage defects of the knee joint. *Am J Sports Med* 2008;36(11):2091-2099.
49. Rowland CR, Colucci LA, Guilak F: Fabrication of anatomically-shaped cartilage constructs using decellularized cartilage-derived matrix scaffolds. *Biomaterials* 2016;91:57-72.
50. Yuan X, Wei Y, Villasante A, et al: Stem cell delivery in tissue-specific hydrogel enabled meniscal repair in an orthotopic rat model. *Biomaterials* 2017;132:59-71.
51. Spang MT, Christman KL: Extracellular matrix hydrogel therapies: In vivo applications and development. *Acta Biomater* 2018;68:1-14.
52. Cunniffe GM, Diaz-Payno PJ, Sheehy EJ, et al: Tissue-specific extracellular matrix scaffolds for the regeneration of spatially complex musculoskeletal tissues. *Biomaterials* 2019;188:63-73.
53. Spiller KL, Maher SA, Lowman AM: Hydrogels for the repair of articular cartilage defects. *Tissue Eng Part B Rev* 2011;17(4):281-299.
54. Johnstone B, Alini M, Cucchiarini M, et al: Tissue engineering for articular cartilage repair–the state of the art. *Eur Cell Mater* 2013;25:248-267.
55. Matsiko A, Levingstone TJ, O'Brien FJ: Advanced strategies for articular cartilage defect repair. *Materials* 2013;6(2):637-668.
56. Cooper JA Jr, Sahota JS, Gorum WJ II, Carter J, Doty SB, Laurencin CT: Biomimetic tissue-engineered anterior cruciate ligament replacement. *Proc Natl Acad Sci U S A* 2007;104(9):3049-3054.
57. Moutos FT, Freed LE, Guilak F: A biomimetic three-dimensional woven composite scaffold for functional tissue engineering of cartilage. *Nat Mater* 2007;6(2):162-167.
58. Li WJ, Mauck RL, Tuan RS: Electrospun nanofibrous scaffolds: Production, characterization, and applications for tissue engineering and drug delivery. *J Biomed Nanotech* 2005;1(3):259-275.
59. Zhu J: Bioactive modification of poly(ethylene glycol) hydrogels for tissue engineering. *Biomaterials* 2010;31(17):4639-4656.
60. Mhanna R, Ozturk E, Vallmajo-Martin Q, Millan C, Muller M, Zenobi-Wong M: GFOGER-modified MMP-sensitive polyethylene glycol hydrogels induce chondrogenic differentiation of human mesenchymal stem cells. *Tissue Eng Part A* 2014;20(7-8):1165-1174.
61. Bian L, Guvendiren M, Mauck RL, Burdick JA: Hydrogels that mimic developmentally relevant matrix and N-cadherin interactions enhance MSC chondrogenesis. *Proc Natl Acad Sci U S A* 2013;110(25):10117-10122.
62. Loebel C, Burdick JA: Engineering stem and stromal cell therapies for musculoskeletal tissue repair. *Cell Stem Cell* 2018;22(3):325-339.
63. Mouser VHM, Levato R, Bonassar LJ, et al: Three-dimensional bioprinting and its potential in the field of articular cartilage regeneration. *Cartilage* 2017;8(4):327-340.
64. Ballyns JJ, Gleghorn JP, Niebrzydowski V, et al: Image-guided tissue engineering of anatomically shaped implants via MRI and micro-CT using injection molding. *Tissue Eng Part A* 2008;14(7):1195-1202.
65. Rengier F, Mehndiratta A, von Tengg-Kobligk H, et al: 3D printing based on imaging data: Review of medical applications. *Int J Comput Assist Radiol Surg* 2010;5(4):335-341.
66. Feinberg SE, Hollister SJ, Halloran JW, Chu TM, Krebsbach PH: Image-based biomimetic approach to reconstruction of the temporomandibular joint. *Cells Tissue Organs* 2001;169(3):309-321.
67. Hollister SJ: Porous scaffold design for tissue engineering. *Nat Mater* 2005;4(7):518-524.
68. Gonzalez-Fernandez T, Rathan S, Hobbs C, et al: Pore-forming bioinks to enable spatio-temporally defined gene delivery in bioprinted tissues. *J Control Release* 2019;301:13-27.
69. Hung CT, Lima EG, Mauck RL, et al: Anatomically shaped osteochondral constructs for articular cartilage repair. *J Biomech* 2003;36(12):1853-1864.
70. Lee CH, Cook JL, Mendelson A, Moioli EK, Yao H, Mao JJ: Regeneration of the articular surface of the rabbit synovial joint by cell homing: A proof of concept study. *Lancet* 2010;376(9739):440-448.
71. Ding C, Qiao Z, Jiang W, et al: Regeneration of a goat femoral head using a tissue-specific, biphasic scaffold fabricated with CAD/CAM technology. *Biomaterials* 2013;34(28):6706.
72. Chang SC, Rowley JA, Tobias G, et al: Injection molding of chondrocyte/alginate constructs in the shape of facial implants. *J Biomed Mater Res* 2001;55(4):503-511.
73. Ballyns JJ, Cohen DL, Malone E, et al: An optical method for evaluation of geometric fidelity for anatomically shaped tissue-engineered constructs. *Tissue Eng Part C Methods* 2010;16(4):693-703.
74. Schek RM, Taboas JM, Segvich SJ, Hollister SJ, Krebsbach PH: Engineered osteochondral grafts using biphasic composite solid free-form fabricated scaffolds. *Tissue Eng* 2004;10(9-10):1376-1385.
75. Mesallati T, Sheehy EJ, Vinardell T, Buckley CT, Kelly DJ: Tissue engineering scaled-up, anatomically shaped osteochondral constructs for joint resurfacing. *Eur Cell Mater* 2015;30:163-185; discussion 185-6.
76. Rhee S, Puetzer JL, Mason BN, Reinhart-King CA, Bonassar LJ: 3D bioprinting of spatially heterogeneous collagen constructs for cartilage tissue engineering. *ACS Biomater Sci Eng* 2016;2(10):1800-1805.
77. Martin AR, Patel JM, Zlotnick HM, Carey JL, Mauck RL: Regenerating the "red knee": Emerging therapies for cartilage repair in currently excluded populations. *NPJ Regen Med*, in press.
78. Pfeifer CG, Fisher MB, Carey JL, Mauck RL: Impact of guidance documents on translational large animal studies of cartilage repair. *Sci Transl Med* 2015;7(310):310re9.
79. Patel JM, Saleh KS, Burdick JA, Mauck RL: Bioactive factors for cartilage repair and regeneration: Improving delivery, retention, and activity. *Acta Biomater* 2019;93:222-238.
80. Rodkey WG, DeHaven KE, Montgomery WH III, et al: Comparison of the collagen meniscus implant with partial meniscectomy. A prospective randomized trial. *J Bone Joint Surg Am* 2008;90(7):1413-1426.
81. Verdonk P, Beaufils P, Bellemans J, et al: Successful treatment of painful irreparable partial meniscal defects with a polyurethane scaffold: Two-year safety and clinical outcomes. *Am J Sports Med* 2012;40(4):844-853.
82. Patel JM, Ghodbane SA, Brzezinski A, Gatt CJ Jr, Dunn MG: Tissue-engineered total meniscus replacement with a fiber-reinforced scaffold in a 2-year ovine model. *Am J Sports Med* 2018;46(8):1844-1856.
83. Lee CH, Rodeo SA, Fortier LA, Lu C, Erisken C, Mao JJ: Protein-releasing polymeric scaffolds induce fibrochondrocytic differentiation of endogenous cells for knee meniscus regeneration in sheep. *Sci Transl Med* 2014;6(266):266ra171.
84. Moutos FT, Glass KA, Compton SA, et al: Anatomically shaped tissue-engineered cartilage with tunable and inducible anticytokine delivery for biological joint resurfacing. *Proc Natl Acad Sci U S A* 2016;113(31):E4513-E4522.

©Copyright 2021 American Academy of Orthopaedic Surgeons

5

PRINCIPLES OF CLINICAL INFORMATION

SECTION EDITORS

Kurt P. Spindler, MD
Patricia D. Franklin, MD, MBA, MPH

Ethics of Clinical Practice in Orthopaedic Surgery

Christian A. Pean, MD, MS
Arthur L. Caplan, PhD

Keywords: *ethics; healthcare disparities; orthopaedic surgery; shared-decision making; value-based care*

INTRODUCTION

Ethical principles are ideas upon which norms, rules, and behavior are based.[1] The rigorous application of ethics is imperative for the clinical practice of orthopaedic surgery and an essential component of the medical profession. The repeated ethical transgressions by members of the medical profession throughout history are evidence of the need to continuously acknowledge and reinforce the role of morality in providing just and beneficent medical care.[2] This is increasingly apparent as advances in research and clinical surgery have changed the practice of orthopaedic surgery drastically and sparked the emergence of new challenging subjects such as value-based care, robotic surgery, and the use of biologics. Beyond the application of ethical principles during individual patient encounters, orthopaedic surgeons should also be cognizant of the ethical challenges that may present to them at a systems level and be conscientious practitioners of preventive ethics. Ethical dilemmas present frequently in the clinical practice of orthopaedic surgery, and the ability to anticipate and prevent ethical challenges is a critical skill orthopaedic surgeons should develop to provide the highest standard of care to their patients. This chapter will highlight the application of ethics to orthopaedic surgery from individual patient encounters to considerations at the broader level of the healthcare system and provide guidelines for orthopaedic surgeons to consider in providing ethical surgical care.

Neither of the following authors nor any immediate family member has received anything of value from or has stock or stock options held in a commercial company or institution related directly or indirectly to the subject of this chapter: Dr. Pean and Dr. Caplan.

PRINCIPLES AND A BRIEF HISTORY OF SURGICAL ETHICS

HISTORICAL CONTEXT

Surgeons and medical practitioners throughout history and across cultures have utilized ethical codes and moral guidelines to govern their profession. The origins of the ethics of clinical practice in orthopaedic surgery are varied in nature and have evolved gradually over time. Most physicians and surgeons will hearken to the Hippocratic Oath established in the fifth century BCE in their recall of the ethical principles that guide the medical profession.[3] The philosophical aspects of the Hippocratic Oath often cited in reference to the modern code of medical ethics derive from the famous doctrine of *primum non nocere*: "first, do no harm." The role of the surgeon is paradoxical to this oft-quoted maxim of nonmaleficence in that a surgical intervention *must* in some degree cause harm or pain to the patient via surgical instrumentation in an effort to ultimately cure or alleviate suffering. This aspect of the surgical profession creates a unique paradigm for the patient-physician relationship. The present-day healthcare system prioritizes evidence-based, informed, uncoerced treatment that places primacy on the patient's well-being and autonomy and frowns upon paternalism. However, ethical norms of the medical profession have changed substantially over the course of recent history.

Just how drastically ethics of patient care have changed is illustrated by a quote attributed to Henri de Mondeville, a French surgeon in medieval times who said, "If the patient is defiant, seldom will the result be successful."[4]

©Copyright 2021 American Academy of Orthopaedic Surgeons

The expectation of patient docility and the theme of paternalism are far removed from the modern emphasis on patient autonomy in clinical care. Codes of conduct for surgeons in Western medicine are traced back to 1745 when the Company of Surgeons was established. Until this time in Western society, the surgical vocation was seldom recognized in the same professional vein as other medical disciplines. As surgeons organized into a more regulated profession, individuals emerged who would begin to define the ethical foundations of modern surgery.[5] Scottish physician John Gregory (1724-1773) implored physicians and surgeons to develop sympathy defined as the "sensibility of heart which makes us feel for the distresses of our fellow-creatures…" He further believed that the physician's relationship to the patient required patients to be capable of understanding a physician's treatment recommendations and able to comply with them. These early notions of patient autonomy were more akin to the modern standard of informed consent in surgical ethics.

The American Medical Association (AMA) Code of Ethics was established in 1847 based on the idea of professional responsibility toward patients; however, surgery is mentioned in this code only in prohibiting physicians from holding patents for surgical instruments and mentioning "unusual fatigue" of the surgical cases.[6] The American College of Surgeons (ACS) was founded later in 1913. The Fellowship Pledge of the ACS was established the same year and contained elements of a foundation for a surgical ethical framework. The pledge exalted the merits of teaching and the patient's welfare above all else. Furthermore, the pledge emphasized the surgeon's obligation to scrupulous and honest financial dealings with respect to their craft, binding the surgeon to "shun dishonest money-seeking and commercialism as disgraceful to our profession."[4]

Ethical guidelines more specific to the orthopaedic surgeon were established by the American Academy of Orthopaedic Surgeons (AAOS). The AAOS was established in 1933 and is the largest medical association of musculoskeletal specialists. The AAOS established a code of professionalism and ethics specifically geared toward orthopaedic surgeons that continues to aid in the recommended behavior of those in the profession.

ETHICAL PRINCIPLES

Recently, surgeon and bioethicist Mile Little more clearly delineated the unique aspects of the surgeon-patient relationship.[7] He proposed five characteristics that made the patient-surgeon relationship distinct from other medical specialties:

1. The surgeon's power to rescue patients;
2. The intimate proximity of surgeons and their patients, especially in the operating room;
3. The ordeal that patients endure before, during, and after surgery;
4. The aftermath, both physical and emotional, of surgery; and
5. The patient's desire for the surgeon's presence throughout the experience.

As this chapter will demonstrate, it is indeed such characteristics of the surgical profession—and of orthopaedic surgery in particular—that necessitate special ethical consideration.

There are four basic principles of ethics that have prevailed in modern medicine and surgery.[1] They are listed and briefly defined below:

1. Justice: Prioritizes distributive fairness to produce societal good and emphasizes equal patient rights as well as adequate patient access at a population level.
2. Autonomy: Responsibility of the surgeon to elevate the patient's right to make well-informed decisions for themselves consistent with their own values.
3. Beneficence: Physician obligation to promote the greatest good for the patient.
4. Nonmaleficence: Often equated with *primum non nocere: "first do no harm."* Physician responsibility to inflict the least harm in working toward a positive clinical outcome.

THE SURGEON-PATIENT RELATIONSHIP

SHARED DECISION-MAKING

The foundation of orthopaedic surgical ethics begins and ends with the therapeutic relationship between the surgeon and the patient. In this regard, the ethical doctrines that govern orthopaedic surgeons are quite similar to those applicable in general medical ethics. General principles such as the necessity to disclose conflicts of interest to patients, placing the patient's benefit above other considerations in treatment, and abiding by the principle of nonmaleficence remain steadfast components of the orthopaedic surgeon's ethical framework. Romantic relationships with patients are regarded as unethical due to the asymmetric power relationship between a physician and their patient and should be avoided. As in other medical fields, confidentiality is an integral component of the relationship between a patient and their orthopaedic surgeon. The Health Insurance Portability and Accountability Act of 1996 (HIPAA) established clear guidelines and legal stipulations to protect confidentiality.[8]

Orthopaedic surgeons are tasked with using surgical means to correct physical form, facilitate function, and improve mobility. Furthermore, orthopaedic procedures are undertaken to elevate a patient's quality of life but require rehabilitation on the part of the patient to ensure a positive outcome. The ultimate success or failure of many orthopaedic surgical interventions is contingent upon a patient's willingness and ability to engage in rehabilitation properly after surgery.

©Copyright 2021 American Academy of Orthopaedic Surgeons

This aspect of orthopaedic surgery requires added effort on the part of the surgeon to properly explicate the risks and benefits of proposed treatment and describe the expected patient effort in the postoperative period. This understanding ought to be part and parcel of informed consent, an ethical principle requiring patients comprehend the risks, benefits, and alternative options to treatment proposed before moving forward with given procedure.[9] A patient may indeed have debilitating and painful knee osteoarthritis, but if they also have serious medical comorbidities that confer unreasonable surgical risk or portend a low likelihood of being able to recover after surgery, a total knee arthroplasty may not be an ethically sound course of action. The orthopaedic surgeon must be able to accurately judge when surgery is not the best option and also help a patient understand why this is the case. Ensuring a commitment to compliance and availability for follow-up are core elements in the initial consent as well.

This overall emphasis on autonomy and informed consent has led to an increased prevalence of the "shared decision-making" model of patient care in medicine.[10] The elective nature of many orthopaedic procedures dictates that this approach has considerable merit to ensure patient satisfaction with the decision to undergo surgery or elect instead for nonsurgical management. Regional variation in surgical procedure volume for total knee and total hip arthroplasty is significant, with some areas seeing up to a tenfold difference in rates of surgical procedure from demographically similar regions.[11,12] These figures suggest shared decision-making model may not be sufficiently utilized by orthopaedic surgeons.

Shared decision-making (SDM) has been defined as "an approach where clinicians and patients share the best available evidence when faced with the task of making decisions, and where patients are supported to consider options, to achieve informed preferences."[13] Over 80 randomized trials have demonstrated patients using SDM had increased involvement in treatment decisions, more confidence in decisions, and a tendency to elect for more treatment options.[14] One study indicated that introducing standardized patient decision aid tools consistent with SDM was associated with 26% fewer hip replacement surgeries and 38% fewer total knee replacements during the same period of time.[15]

Shared decision-making is a linear fluid process. It consists of "choice talk" explicitly making the patient aware of agency in the decision-making process, "option talk" narrowing discussion to available treatments for the patient to choose from, and moving to "decision talk" in which the patient and physician elect the most suitable course of action (**Figure 1**). This method of engagement with patients is useful for orthopaedic surgeons and should be used to encourage fulfillment of the principles of informed consent and patient autonomy.

DISCLOSURE OF SURGICAL ERRORS

Imagine a scenario in which during surgical fixation of a proximal humerus fracture an orthopaedic surgeon injures the axillary nerve resulting in a deltoid palsy. The patient will undoubtedly notice the new weakness and inquire about the deficit. The ethical surgeon must disclose the complication and would be hard-pressed not to do so in the face of the obvious sequelae. However, consider an alternate scenario in which the orthopaedic surgeon inadvertently injures a portion of the axillary artery during the same surgery. Though more bleeding than expected occurs, a vascular repair is completed without further complication and there are no significant sequelae from the error. Is disclosure required in both circumstances?

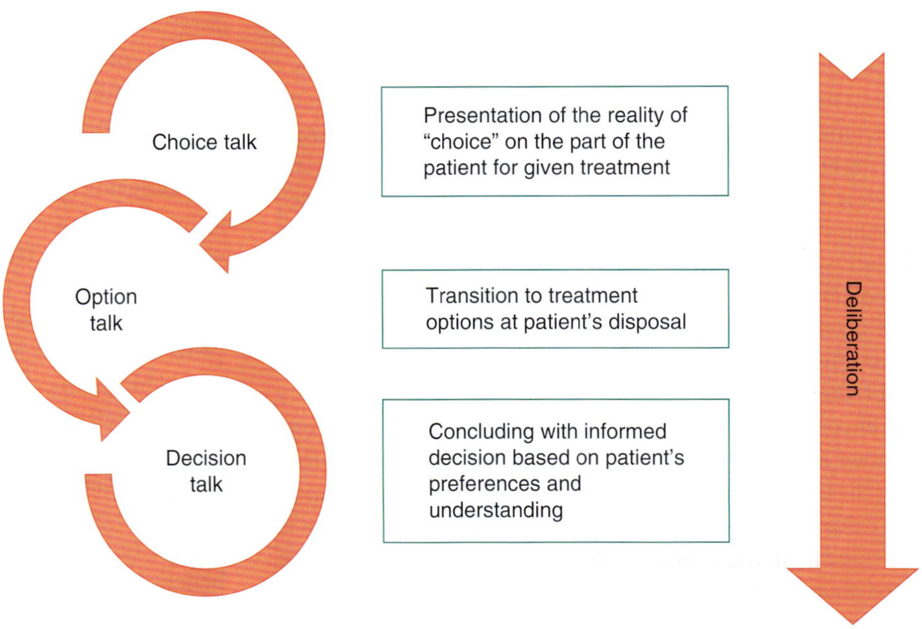

FIGURE 1 A diagram of shared decision-making.

©Copyright 2021 American Academy of Orthopaedic Surgeons

A "medical error" is defined by the Institute of Medicine as the failure of a planned action to be completed as intended or the use of a wrong plan to achieve an aim.[16] The process for disclosure of a surgical error begins before the surgery itself, during the process of informed consent. A surgeon must make their patient aware of "all" risks of the procedure explicitly. The temptation to make promises of a complication-free procedure or painless postoperative course to temporarily comfort an anxious patient should be avoided. Furthermore, when errors that result from a series of mistakes or systemic missteps happen, disclosure for all members of the healthcare team contributing to the harm is the most ethical course of action. Disclosure demonstrates respect for persons and supports patient autonomy by allowing patients to make educated decisions regarding further care after a medical error.[17]

There are multiple barriers that may impede honest and transparent disclosure of surgical errors. Fear of instigating grounds for litigation can complicate a surgeon's effort to discuss an error with a patient. The malpractice environment in the United States has created difficulties for surgeons wishing to apologize to patients. The relationship between errors and medical malpractice claims is mismatched and "lopsided" leading to a particular vulnerability for surgeons in the face of otherwise high-quality care. Fear of litigation, professional loyalty, hierarchy, and fear of retaliation have also been reported as strong deterrent to surgeons disclosing problems in care to patients. Future legislative and policy solutions to accommodate the ethical and honest disclosure of medical and surgical errors may include explicit allowances for apologies that are not admissible in court, similar to legislation passed in California and other states.[18]

Ultimately, disclosure of errors is an emotionally challenging and logistically onerous component of a surgical career. However, it is also a necessary skill for an orthopaedic surgeon to develop and practice. In one study, a communication and resolution program in which a structured response to adverse events was formulated yielded a decreased trend of new claims and legal defense costs, but no changes in other outcomes.[19] This strategy consisted of the physician and healthcare institution communicating with patients about adverse events; investigating and explaining what happened; and, when appropriate, allowing for an apology, taking responsibility, and proactively offering compensation. Another team-based model includes a "disclosure timeout" in which all involved healthcare workers collaboratively plan for communication with the patient. This occurs during a brief period set aside in the operating room after an adverse event. This permits for discrepancies about the event to be reconciled, facilitated accountability, and encourages system-wide corrective change.[20] The recommended time for communication with the patient or family is after the timeout as well as consultation with risk management or a disclosure coach. Such strategies uphold the principles of informed consent, professionalism, as well as nonmaleficence, given that undisclosed errors may lead to future individual and systemic dangers for patients.

CONSIDERATIONS OF COST AND JUSTICE

Cost considerations have not traditionally been an integral component of the patient-physician relationship. However, in the face of increasingly burdensome healthcare costs in the United States, a surgeon should consider the financial implications of their treatment for their individual patients as well as society at large. There is potential for conflict between the principles of beneficence for the individual patient and justice for the sake of society. Judgments are often made in the healthcare system that sacrifice marginal benefit for an individual patient to benefit the broader community. It may benefit a patient to spend a full uninterrupted hour with their orthopaedic surgeon in the clinic; however, this hinders the surgeon's ability to see more patients and provide access to care for a larger group of people.

According to the American College of Physicians Ethics Manual, "Physicians have a responsibility to practice effective and efficient healthcare and to use healthcare resources responsibly."[21] This is also consistent with John Stuart Mills'[22] theory of utilitarianism—espousing actions that should promote the greatest happiness for the overall benefits of society. There are many individual choices surgeons make daily that have implications for the cost burden healthcare expenditures.

Judicious use of radiologic studies is one manner of addressing costs in the field of orthopaedic surgery. Patients may demand expensive and unnecessary tests. Suppose a patient presents to the clinic with an obvious simple contusion or hematoma to the elbow, no fracture on radiographs, and no signs of instability or deformity on examination. They adamantly request an MRI study. The orthopaedic surgeon will use his clinical judgment to discern that an MRI will not yield any clinically significant findings or change in treatment, but it can be challenging to appease a demanding patient fixated on a particular test or treatment. It is the responsibility of the surgeon to explain the lack of benefit for such procedures and forge a therapeutic alliance with the patient to best move forward. Close follow-up and reevaluation at a time in the near future should be offered as an alternative to redundant imaging or unnecessary invasive procedures.

A fee-for-service model of health care may incentivize recommending patients for treatment to increase procedural volume and reimbursement rather than for reasons of clinical appropriateness. This model creates inherent financial conflicts in which the physician may have a pecuniary interest in prolonging a patient's illness or performing unnecessary procedures for financial gain. Such a clinical practice pattern would be unethical for obvious reasons. Policy proposals shifting health care to value-based care may allay these concerns, but orthopaedic surgeons must continue to diligently advocate for price transparency for their patients.[23,24] Orthopaedic surgeons also must seek evidence-based treatment and minimize the use of expensive resources that do not add demonstrable benefit to clinical care.[25] The costs of health care are becoming increasingly unsustainable in the United States. Orthopaedic

©Copyright 2021 American Academy of Orthopaedic Surgeons

surgeons have a moral obligation to steward their patients through injury and disease in a manner that satisfies the principle of beneficence and avoids burdening patients with "financial toxicity" while simultaneously upholding the principle of justice.

ETHICS OF ORTHOPAEDIC TRAUMA

Whereas many disciplines in orthopaedic surgery focus on procedures of an elective nature, orthopaedic trauma requires unique ethical considerations given the urgency and fluidity of the clinical scenarios in which an orthopaedic traumatologist operates. Patients undergoing elective orthopaedic procedures have time to contemplate their options for treatment and make informed decisions. By contrast, in orthopaedic trauma, there are many instances in which informed consent is not possible for a procedure or the patient is unable to express their wishes due to injury or duress. In these scenarios, the duty to rescue, defined as a moral obligation to prevent serious harm when one has the capacity to do so, may come at odds with the principle of informed consent. There are some patients who may express the opinion that they would rather die than live with bilateral below the knee amputations. An orthopaedic traumatologist consulted to manage two mangled lower extremities in a patient at risk of imminent death from hemorrhagic shock would question the soundness of such an expressed opinion,[26] but would also have no means to learn the basis of this preference from a patient in the midst of an emergent trauma. Surgeons will generally be steadfast in their duty to save life over limb. However, the approach to managing mangled extremities is ethically nuanced. Indeed, even the semantic bias of using the term "limb salvage" has been questioned from an ethical perspective.[27] Presentation of all treatment options and possible outcomes must be revisited by the treating surgeon at different time points after provisional initial stabilization. Orthopaedic traumatologists must forge therapeutic alliances with family members, fully elucidate informed consent when possible, consult bioethicists as needed, and pay particular attention to available data on functional outcomes to give patients a realistic expectation of their path to recovery. Such an approach is required in limb salvage, management of polytrauma patients, dealing with patients nonadherent to treatment, and many other scenarios unique to orthopaedic trauma.[28]

Elderly patients susceptible to fragility fractures present varied ethical concerns. There is substantial study on the optimal method of fixation for a hip fracture dependent on fracture morphology and patient factors.[29,30] These decisions are made using clinical data but also require ethical considerations. Orthopaedic surgery that is performed with the objective of improving a patient's mobility may seem futile if the patient in question had limited functional mobility prior to their injury. Some orthopaedic interventions are also of questionable benefit in the face of surgical risks. Recognition of extraordinary measures and deciding when not to operate on an ill patient with a poor prognosis is a skill a traumatologist must develop to uphold their moral obligations to their patients and society. If a 94-year-old wheelchair-bound woman sustains a distal femur fracture during a transfer, the goal of treatment will be comfort rather than mobility.

Cognitive deficits in the elderly population can hinder the ability to facilitate autonomy and support a patient's self-determination. Preventive ethical measures include encouraging patients to file advance directives and assign surrogate decision makers prior to onset of any debilitating conditions such as dementia. The principles of beneficence as well as justice play distinct roles in discerning the optimal treatment for these patients. Orthopaedic traumatologists will often need to rely on other consulting services such as internal medicine, general surgery, and palliative care to manage patient expectations and choose the best option of treatment.

ETHICAL CONSIDERATIONS IN PEDIATRIC ORTHOPAEDIC SURGERY

Most orthopaedic surgeons will care for pediatric patients in some capacity during their training or professional career. A firm grasp of ethical reasoning required for common dilemmas of care for children is critical. Pediatric orthopaedic surgery presents several special ethical considerations due to the fact that most children lack fully developed autonomy. An individual must traditionally display four key characteristics to have moral autonomy: (1) ability to understand information, (2) capacity to communicate a given choice, (3) ability to use information in a process of reasoning and deliberation, and (4) capacity to compare consequences of alternative courses of action to the proposed choice. Younger children typically do not meet all these criteria, and the practice of pediatric orthopaedic surgery is further complicated by the need to treat patients who are cognitively or physically impaired.

CONSENT VERSUS ASSENT

Consent is the legally binding permission that allows for treatment in health care provided by a person of legal age. For children, consent is typically provided by a parent or guardian whereas an expression of approval or agreement "assent" is often required from the child.[31] The involvement of numerous agents in the surgical decision making for a child presents several possible scenarios for ethical conflict. There are scenarios in which a parent may not opt for the course of action that is of maximal benefit for their child.

One such scenario would be an adolescent patient who has sustained several fractures necessitating surgical fixation and subsequently a blood transfusion due to postoperative anemia. If, for example, the parents of the child refuse blood transfusion and further treatment due to religious reasons, emotional distress, or a lack of understanding regarding the necessity for further treatment, this presents a conflict between the principles of informed consent and beneficence for the orthopaedic surgeon. One can imagine a scenario further complicated

©Copyright 2021 American Academy of Orthopaedic Surgeons

by the child expressing a differing opinion from their parents and wishing to move forward with the blood transfusion. An orthopaedic surgeon is required to recall the prerequisites for moral autonomy and assess whether the child possesses these qualities. If a child possesses the characteristics necessary for moral autonomy and articulates the risks and benefits of a particular procedure, the requisite for consent becomes a legal matter as well as an ethical one. Additionally, pediatric orthopaedic surgeons will treat many patients with some degree of physical or cognitive impairment secondary to genetic disease or conditions such as cerebral palsy. The degree to which an orthopaedic surgeon will be capable of sorting such complicated moral matters may be limited. Ultimately, the surgeon must advocate for the course of action that produces the maximal benefit for the patient. A low threshold to seek formal ethical consultation from a bioethicist or legal advice from the institution's risk management team is encouraged.[32]

TABLE 1 Value-Based Care Ethical Issues

Ethical Issue	Relevant Principles
Cost-reduction strategies	Justice Autonomy Conflicts of interest
Implant pricing and regulation	Autonomy Nonmaleficence Conflicts of interest Informed consent
Alternative payment models and bundled care	Justice Autonomy
Healthcare disparities	Bias Solidarity Justice

ETHICS OF VALUE-BASED CARE AND COST-CONTAINMENT STRATEGIES IN ORTHOPAEDIC SURGERY

Estimates of healthcare costs in the United States indicate $3.2 trillion USD were spent on health care in 2015, representing 18% of the country's gross domestic product.[33] Gradually, shifts from fee-for-service health care to value-based models are being implemented to counter rising healthcare costs. Initiatives such as the Medicare Payment Reform Act (MACRA) and bundled care payments are reflective of broader changes in American health care that have profound implications for orthopaedic surgeons.[34]

Ethical issues regarding healthcare financial reform can be divided into considerations for three groups: the surgeon and hospital, the patient and society, and the orthopaedic device industry. As the structure of healthcare reimbursements increasingly relies on outcome measures, new incentive schemes in patient selection are expected to emerge with implications for each of these groups. A summary of relevant values and considerations in value-based orthopaedic care is included in **Table 1**.

PATIENT RISK MODIFICATION

The ethics of patient risk factor modification have been described in the literature from several vantage points. The example of a prospective patient who uses tobacco products presents clear-cut ethical dilemmas for the orthopaedic surgeon. Numerous studies have established that smokers have higher rates of wound complications, worse functional outcomes, and prolonged hospitalization after orthopaedic procedures.[35] A surgeon performing a procedure on a patient who uses tobacco products knowingly exposes this patient to those increased risks. Most surgeons will instruct patients to undertake a tobacco cessation program to decrease this risk. If a patient acknowledges the risks of undergoing surgery and is unwilling to discontinue their tobacco use, can the surgeon comfortably proceed with an elective procedure knowing the elevated chance of complications? To do so would likely be at odds with the principle of nonmaleficence.

A patient's unwillingness to engage in a tobacco cessation program at a surgeon's recommendation may also not bode well for adherence for a postsurgical rehabilitation program. A surgeon must establish their own threshold for acceptable risk and consult with their institution for guidelines and protocols to mitigate these risks. Many centers have implemented tobacco cessation programs and have strict guidelines prohibiting patients above a certain body mass index (BMI) from undergoing elective procedures. The increased risk of complications has consequences for costs that may be passed onto other patients, and the use of such guidelines upholds the principles of justice for society as well as nonmaleficence in consideration for the patient.

PROVIDER RISK MODIFICATION

Studies have demonstrated improved outcomes among high-volume institutions compared with hospitals that perform fewer surgical procedures for intertrochanteric hip fractures, musculoskeletal tumors, as well as fusion for scoliosis.[36] The question of whether a surgeon is obligated to refer patients to their more seasoned colleagues or whether it is morally precarious to permit a patient to have surgery at a facility with poorer outcomes than an alternative center is controversial. Each orthopaedic surgeon must acknowledge their individual limitations, accept their level of expertise, and readily refer patients to more experienced colleagues when necessary.

It may be argued that systematically referring patients to higher-volume regional orthopaedic centers with lower overall complication rates is consistent with the principles of beneficence and nonmaleficence. However, this would potentially infringe on patient autonomy by limiting a patient's options

©Copyright 2021 American Academy of Orthopaedic Surgeons

to choose a provider based on a preexisting relationship or proximity to a surgeon or hospital center. Furthermore, such provider risk modification could limit access to care by discouraging the provision of orthopaedic care in rural, less populated areas. Studies have indicated that underserved minorities and disenfranchised populations are more likely to receive care from low-volume clinical facilities.[37] This is likely in part due to the difficulty in finding transport to distant sites and an inclination for patients to seek care at facilities in close proximity to their place of residence. Thus, requiring referral to high-volume centers may inadvertently restrict access to care for these patients. The solution may be to encourage thresholds for patient care volume at a given center and create standardized protocols to improve patient outcomes.

ETHICAL AND COST CONSIDERATIONS FOR ORTHOPAEDIC IMPLANTS

A considerable proportion of overall cost of care for orthopaedic patients is a result of expenditures on implants. The price of implants in total joint arthroplasty increased an estimated 130% between 1996 and 2006. Several studies have also demonstrated marked regional variation in the price of orthopaedic implants.[38] The use of generic orthopaedic implants has been advocated as an economic solution to the problem of expensive proprietary implants. In the pharmaceutical sector, an estimated $33 billion USD has been saved by Medicare in the United States through utilization of generic medications.[39] A similar reduction in healthcare expenditures through the use of generic orthopaedic implants would be consistent with the ethical principle of justice and favorable for improving healthcare value. However, given that generic implants must be manufactured, either by the same companies which produce the branded implants or by other stakeholders, there is still potential for conflict of interest.

Other strategies toward medical device cost containment include price transparency initiatives to encourage surgeon and patient selection based on implant prices. Awareness of implant prices has been shown to increase a surgeon's likelihood of selecting a lower cost implant.[40] It can be argued that a surgeon is morally bound by the principle of justice to choose a lower cost implant for a particular procedure if a more expensive alternative does not demonstrably improve quality of the surgical intervention or patient outcome.

On a systems level, the primary ethical considerations for regulation and development of orthopaedic implants are justice and nonmaleficence. The Center for Devices and Radiological Health in the Federal Drug Agency (FDA) is responsible for enforcing the regulatory framework of implant development in the United States. The approval of a given implant in the United States requires proof of the device's safety and efficacy with most orthopaedic implants classified as "class II" or "class III" devices subject to generic regulation as well as 510(k) premarket notification or approval.[41] High-profile medical device failures such as metal-on-metal hip arthroplasty have increased the pressure on surgeons to be cautious when adopting a new implant. Surgeons are also duty bound to disclose any personal conflicts of interest to patients and clinical institutions they work with. When a surgeon has a personal stake in a particular implant, there is a potential for selection bias. As many as 39% of surgeons report a conflict of interest.[42,43]

VULNERABLE POPULATIONS AND HEALTH DISPARITIES

Healthcare disparities are pervasive in the United States across medical disciplines. Numerous studies have demonstrated the increased likelihood of adverse outcomes and lower-quality care in underserved populations and racial minorities. The role of implicit racial bias in perpetuating healthcare disparities has been explored with respect to pain management and clinical decision making. Similar disparities have been reported in orthopaedic surgery with black patients having lower rates of referral for treatment, poorer outcomes tied to lower socioeconomic status, and decreased patient satisfaction after surgery.[44-47] Surgeons and the orthopaedic profession at large must make efforts to recognize these biases and propose systemic solutions to address healthcare disparities and improve access to care for all patients.

Other vulnerable populations orthopaedic surgeons encounter are underserved patients from low- and middle-income countries (LMICs) and incarcerated patients. The ethics of humanitarian surgical work are complex, but basic recommendations for orthopaedic surgeons partaking in international work include prioritizing local capacity building, using culturally appropriate care models, and ensuring proper follow-up and capability to care for complications in the host country. Obstacles of caring for incarcerated patient and recommendations for treatment are summarized in **Table 2** as adopted from an article by Dr Sraj published in 2016.[48]

A values-explicit approach to healthcare reform has been recommended as a means to systematically ensure adherence to the ethical principles society values highly in policymaking.

A summary of these values as recommended in the literature is included in[49] **Table 3**.

Such a system would need to be specific to the culture and society in which reform is taking place and the emphasized values agreed upon by principal stakeholders and community members to function properly. Most recommendations for the ethical practice of orthopaedic surgery pertaining to vulnerable populations reflect adherence to the principle of solidarity. Solidarity is embodied by a commitment beyond empathy with others and dictating willingness to act on their behalf. This principle espouses a framework for ethical decision making built on the recognition that an individual's fate is intrinsically tied to the fate of another. It is best described by Prainsack and Buyx in their 2012 paper differentiating the three tiers of solidarity along interpersonal, group, and contractual levels and emphasizing the importance of symmetry in relationships.[50]

©Copyright 2021 American Academy of Orthopaedic Surgeons

TABLE 2 Obstacles of Care of Incarcerated Patients

Situation	Obstacle	Suggestion	Risk	Ethics Principle
Timely intervention required	Delay in authorization	Contact administrator or consider direct admit	Increased use of resources, more complex treatment and complications	Duty to rescue Utilitarianism Nonmaleficence Justice
Immobilization recommended	Security (potential use for weaponry)	Avoid metal and plastic for immobilization and assist devices	Injury to others, insufficient immobilization for patient	Nonmaleficence Justice
Rehabilitation	Unavailable resources	Patient education, self-administered exercises	Inadequate rehabilitation leading to suboptimal outcomes	Justice (disparities) Beneficence
Follow-up	Unreliable Malingering	Systemization and communication with provider pool. Some recommend nondisclosure of follow-up plan with inmate		Nonmaleficence Beneficence Solidarity Professionalism Shared decision-making
Poor access to advanced imaging	Resource availability	Establish protocol for advanced imaging	Delayed treatment, practical barrier to implementation	Justice Access to care

MORAL CONSIDERATIONS FOR INNOVATION AND TECHNOLOGICAL ADVANCES IN ORTHOPAEDIC SURGERY

Advances in technology and preclinical research in orthopaedic surgery are creating new and diverse ethical quandaries for surgeons to consider. The demand for use of stem cell therapy and biologics in orthopaedic surgery has outpaced evidence supporting its efficacy. This has led to increased scrutiny of direct-to-consumer marketing for these products. Breaches of integrity, failure to disclose financial conflicts of interest, and incidents of direct patient harm from unindicated use of biologics in orthopaedic surgery have led to increased physician advocacy to create patient awareness, consistent with nonmaleficence. The advent of robotic surgery has generated difficult questions of cost, precision, and surgical autonomy for the orthopaedic community to ponder as well. As the degree of involvement from robotic tools and automated processes for surgical procedures increase, questions of liability, cost, and surgeon responsibility arise. The implementation of new technology in orthopaedic surgery should address at minimum six questions:

TABLE 3 Essential Values Framework for Healthcare Policy

Essential Value	Objective
Fair access	Access to adequate care independent of financial, geographic, and cultural barriers
Quality	Maximize likelihood of desired health outcome
Efficiency	Minimize expenditure and maximize value
Respect for patients	Facilitate informed consent and voluntary treatment, prioritize autonomy
Patient advocacy	Promotion of individual patient's rights and benefits from the physician

1. How is the safety of a new technology or technique ensured?
2. What are the process and timing by which a hospital implements a new technology?
3. How are patients informed prior to undergoing a technique using new technology?
4. What is the process for training and credentialing surgeons in a new technology or technique?
5. How are the outcomes of the new technology or technique evaluated and tracked?
6. By what means are the responsibilities to individual patients and society at large balanced?

These are basic considerations for the ethical use of new technology consistent with informed consent, justice, and beneficence. More farfetched future scenarios in which robotic surgery advances to the point that the surgeon's active technical role is diminished substantially may create other thorny moral issues. Should the technology's vendor acquire some responsibility for patient stewardship in such a scenario? Would computer code programmers bear some of the responsibility for surgical complications secondary to instrument failure or robotic technical failure independent of the operating surgeon? If technology advanced to the point that a single surgeon could oversee multiple concomitant surgeries, should

©Copyright 2021 American Academy of Orthopaedic Surgeons

it be permitted and what would be the ethical consequences of such a clinical scenario? These issues are beyond the scope of this textbook chapter but are relevant questions as technological advances continue.

SUMMARY

In this chapter, the myriad of ethical considerations that arise in the clinical practice of orthopaedic surgery were summarized and reviewed. In a surgical field that continues to rapidly change, it is incumbent on orthopaedic surgeons to familiarize themselves with a well-defined moral framework to dictate their relationships with patients and to guide their interactions with the health-care system at large. Challenges in delivering equitable, affordable care in orthopaedic surgery will continue to arise, and it is essential that measures are taken to provide the highest quality of ethically sound orthopaedic care to all patients.

REFERENCES

1. Beauchamp TL: *The "four principles" approach to health care ethics*, in *Principles of Health Care Ethics*, ed 2. 2007. doi:10.1002/9780470510544.ch1.
2. Nuremberg Military Tribunal: The Nuremberg Code. *J Am Med Assoc* 1996;276(20):1691. doi:10.1001/jama.1996.03540200077043.
3. Crawshaw R, Pennington TH, Pennington CI, Reiss H, Loudon I, Bende BC: The Hippocratic oath. *BMJ* 1994;309:952. doi:10.1136/bmj.309.6959.952.
4. Namm JP, Siegler M, Brander C, Kim TY, Lowe C, Angelos P: History and evolution of surgical ethics: John Gregory to the twenty-first century. *World J Surg* 2014;38(7):1568-1573. doi:10.1007/s00268-014-2584-1.
5. Johnson RWG: Surgical ethics. *BMJ* 2000;320(7230):320A. doi:10.1136/bmj.320.7230.320/a.
6. American Medical Association (AMA): AMA Code of Medical Ethics. *Am Med Assoc* 1980. https://ama.com.au/sites/default/files/documents/AMA%20Code%20of%20Ethics%202004.%20Editorially%20Revised%202006.%20Revised%202016_0.pdf.
7. Little M: The fivefold root of an ethics of surgery. *Bioethics* 2002;16(3):183-201. doi:10.1111/1467-8519.00281.
8. Annas GJ: HIPAA regulations — a new era of medical-record privacy? *N Engl J Med* 2003;348(15):1486-1490. doi:10.1056/NEJMlim035027.
9. Jones K: Surgeons' silence: A history of informed consent in orthopaedics. *Iowa Orthop J* 2007;27:115-120. doi:10.1016/j.ijid.2008.03.032.
10. Barry MJ, Edgman-Levitan S: Shared decision making — the pinnacle of patient-centered care. *N Engl J Med* 2012;366(9):780-781. doi:10.1056/NEJMp1109283.
11. Birkmeyer JD, Reames BN, McCulloch P, Carr AJ, Campbell WB, Wennberg JE: Understanding of regional variation in the use of surgery. *Lancet* 2013;382(9898):1121-1129. doi:10.1016/S0140-6736(13)61215-5.
12. Fisher ES, Bell J-E, Tomek IM, Esty AR, Goodman DC: Trends and regional variation in hip, knee, and shoulder replacement. The Dartmouth Atlas Project. *Dartmouth Inst Heal Policy Clin Pract* 2010. doi:10.1177/004057368303900411.
13. Elwyn G, Frosch D, Thomson R, et al: Shared decision making: A model for clinical practice. *J Gen Intern Med* 2012;27(10):1361-1367. doi:10.1007/s11606-012-2077-6.
14. Stacey D, Légaré F, Lewis K, et al: Decision aids for people facing health treatment or screening decisions. *Cochrane Database Syst Rev* 2017;4:CD001431. doi:10.1002/14651858.CD001431.pub5.
15. Arterburn D, Wellman R, Westbrook E, et al: Introducing decision aids at group health was linked to sharply lower hip and knee surgery rates and costs. *Health Aff* 2012;31(9):2094-2104. doi:10.1377/hlthaff.2011.0686.
16. Kohn LL, Corrigan JJ, Donaldson MM. *To Err Is Human: Building a Safer Health System. (Institute of Medicine)*. Washington, DC, National Academies Press, 2000. doi:10.1017/S095026880100509X.
17. Lipira LE, Gallagher TH: Disclosure of adverse events and errors in surgical care: Challenges and strategies for improvement. *World J Surg* 2014;38(7):1614-1621. doi:10.1007/s00268-014-2564-5.
18. Mello MM, Studdert DM, Kachalia A: The medical liability climate and prospects for reform. *J Am Med Assoc* 2014;312(20):2146-2155. doi:10.1001/jama.2014.10705.
19. Kachalia A, Sands K, Niel MV, et al: Effects of a communication-and-resolution program on hospitals' malpractice claims and costs. *Health Aff* 2018;37(11):1836-1844. doi:10.1377/hlthaff.2018.0720.
20. Souter KJ, Gallagher TH: The disclosure of unanticipated outcomes of care and medical errors: What does this mean for anesthesiologists? *Anesth Analg* 2012;114(3):615-621. doi:10.1213/ANE.0b013e3182228604.
21. Snyder L: American College of Physicians Ethics, Professionalism, and Human Rights Committee. American College of Physicians Ethics Manual: sixth edition. *Ann Intern Med* 2012;156(1 pt 2):73-104. doi:10.7326/0003-4819-117-11-947.
22. Berger FR: John Stuart mill on justice and fairness. *Can J Philos* 1979;9:115-136. doi:10.1080/00455091.1979.10717097.
23. Lerner JC, Fox DM, Nelson T, Reiss JB: Perspective: The consequence of secret prices: The politics of physician preference items. *Health Aff* 2008;27(6):1560-1565. doi:10.1377/hlthaff.27.6.1560.
24. Obama B: United States health care reform: Progress to date and next steps. *J Am Med Assoc* 2016;316(5):525-532. doi:10.1001/jama.2016.9797.
25. Bosco J, Iorio R, Barber T, Barron C, Caplan A: Ethics of the physician's role in health-care cost control: AOA critical issues. *J Bone Joint Surg Am* 2016;98(14):e58. doi:10.2106/JBJS.15.00889.
26. Higgins TF, Klatt JB, Beals TC: Lower Extremity Assessment Project (LEAP) – the best available evidence on limb-threatening lower extremity trauma. *Orthop Clin North Am* 2010;41(2):233-239. doi:10.1016/j.ocl.2009.12.006.
27. Humbyrd CJ, Sugarman J: Ethical considerations related to impaired driving after orthopaedic injuries. *J Bone Joint Surg Am Vol* 2016;98(14):e60. doi:10.2106/JBJS.15.00875.
28. Sciberras N, Gregori A, Holt G: Ethics in practice : The ethical and practical challenges of patient noncompliance in orthopaedic surgery. *J Bone Joint Surg Am* 2013;95(9):1-6. doi:10.2106/JBJS.L.00483.
29. Williamson S, Landeiro F, McConnell T, et al: Costs of fragility hip fractures globally: A systematic review and meta-regression analysis. *Osteoporos Int* 2017;28(10):2791-2800. doi:10.1007/s00198-017-4153-6.
30. Toson B, Harvey LA, Close JCT: The ICD-10 Charlson Comorbidity Index predicted mortality but not resource utilization following hip fracture. *J Clin Epidemiol* 2015;68(1):44-51. doi:10.1016/j.jclinepi.2014.09.017.
31. AAP Committee on Bioethics: Informed consent, parental permision, and assent in pediatric practice. *Pediatrics* 1995;95(2):314-317.
32. Mercuri JJ, Vigdorchik JM, Otsuka NY: Moral dilemmas in pediatric orthopedics. *Orthopedics* 2015;38(12):e1133-e1138. doi:10.3928/01477447-20151123-04.
33. Keehan SP, Poisal JA, Cuckler GA, et al: National health expenditure projections, 2015-25: Economy, prices, and aging expected to shape spending and enrollment. *Health Aff* 2016;35(8):1522-1531. doi:10.1377/hlthaff.2016.0459.
34. Iorio R, Bosco J, Slover J, Sayeed Y, Zuckerman JD: Single institution early experience with the bundled payments for care improvement initiative. *J Bone Joint Surg Am Vol* 2017;99(1):e2. doi:10.2106/JBJS.16.00066.
35. Wright E, Tzeng H, Ginnetti M, et al: Effect of smoking on joint replacement outcomes: Opportunities for improvement through preoperative smoking cessation. *Instr Course Lect* 2016;65:509-520.

©Copyright 2021 American Academy of Orthopaedic Surgeons

36. Bronson WH, Lindsay D, Lajam C, Iorio R, Caplan A, Bosco J: Ethics of provider risk factor modification in total joint arthroplasty. *J Bone Joint Surg Am Vol* 2014;97(19):1635-1639. doi:10.2106/JBJS.O.00564.

37. Liu JH, Zingmond DS, McGory ML, et al: Disparities in the utilization of high-volume hospitals for complex surgery. *J Am Med Assoc* 2006;296(16):1973-1980. doi:10.1001/jama.296.16.1973.

38. Haas DA, Kaplan RS: Variation in the cost of care for primary total knee arthroplasties. *Arthroplast Today* 2017;3(1):33-37. doi:10.1016/j.artd.2016.08.001.

39. Sheingold S, Nguyen N: Impacts of generic competition and benefit management practices on spending for prescription drugs: Evidence from Medicare's Part D Benefit. *Medicare Medicaid Res Rev* 2014;4(1):E1-E15. doi:10.5600/mmrr.004.01.a01.

40. Wasterlain AS, Melamed E, Karia R, et al: The Effect of price on surgeons' choice of implants: A randomized controlled survey. *J Hand Surg Am* 2017;42(8):593-601. doi:10.1016/j.jhsa.2017.05.005.

41. Maak TG, Wylie JD: Medical device regulation: A comparison of the United States and the European Union. *J Am Acad Orthop Surg* 2016;24(8):537-543. doi:10.5435/JAAOS-D-15-00403.

42. Zuckerman JD, Prasarn M, Kubiak EN, Koval KJ: Conflict of interest in orthopaedic research. *J Bone Joint Surg Am* 2004;86(2):423-428. doi:10.2106/00004623-200402000-00030.

43. Labek G, Neumann D, Agreiter M, Schuh R, Böhler N: Impact of implant developers on published outcome and reproducibility of cohort-based clinical studies in arthroplasty. *J Bone Joint Surg Am* 2011;93(suppl 3):55-61. doi:10.2106/JBJS.K.01108.

44. Driesman A, Fisher N, Konda SR, Pean CA, Leucht P, Egol KA: Racial disparities in outcomes of operatively treated lower extremity fractures. *Arch Orthop Trauma Surg* 2017;137(10):1335-1340. doi:10.1007/s00402-017-2766-z.

45. Driesman A, Mahure SA, Paoli A, Pean CA, Konda SR, Egol KA: Race and Ethnicity have a mixed effect on the treatment of tibial plateau fractures. *J Orthop Trauma* 2017;31(10):e309-e314. doi:10.1097/BOT.0000000000000917.

46. Dy CJ, Lane JM, Pan TJ, Parks ML, Lyman S: Racial and socioeconomic disparities in hip fracture care. *J Bone Joint Surg Am Vol* 2016;98(10):858-865. doi:10.2106/JBJS.15.00676.

47. Ibrahim SA, Kim H, McConnell KJ: The CMS comprehensive care model and racial disparity in joint replacement. *J Am Med Assoc* 2016;316(12):1258. doi:10.1001/jama.2016.12330.

48. Sraj SA: Providing orthopaedic care for the incarcerated. *J Am Acad Orthop Surg* 2016;24(9):607-614. doi:10.5435/jaaos-d-15-00215.

49. Priester R: A values framework for health system reform. *Health Aff* 1992;11(1):84-107. doi:10.1377/hlthaff.11.1.84.

50. Prainsack B, Buyx A: Solidarity in contemporary bioethics – towards a new approach. *Bioethics* 2012;26(7):343-350. doi:10.1111/j.1467-8519.2012.01987.x.

©Copyright 2021 American Academy of Orthopaedic Surgeons

39

Ethical Principles of Clinical Research

Roy K. Aaron, MD
Jennifer Racine-Avila, MBA
Jerry Menikoff, MD, JD

Keywords: *Ethics; Human Subjects Research; Informed Consent*

INTRODUCTION

Medical experimentation on humans is an essential part of the process of translating to the clinic basic discoveries of importance to human health. How human experimentation is accomplished has been the subject of evolving ethical and technical standards. The promulgation of standards for human experimentation has emphasized protection and safety of the research subjects, voluntary, uncoerced consent and opportunity for withdrawal, and competency and responsibilities of the research team. This chapter places contemporary standards for human biomedical experimentation into their evolutionary context and describes the ethical and regulatory environments of clinical research. In this chapter, "clinical research" is used synonymously with "human experimentation" to mean research on human subjects, materials, or data. The chapter is particularly timely since the US federal regulations governing clinical research have just undergone their first major revision since their inception 28 years ago.

HISTORICAL CONTEXT—THE EVOLUTION OF ETHICS OF RESEARCH ON HUMAN SUBJECTS

Prior to the Second World War, there were few standards governing human experimentation and the regulatory environment for clinical research was the province of individual investigators and institutions. Physicians in Nazi concentration camps performed grotesque, abusive, and sadistic medical experiments on unwilling subjects resulting in the death and mutilation of many individuals, primarily Jews, Russians, Poles, prisoners of war, and Gypsies.[1] At the conclusion of the war, the American army conducted a series of military tribunals in Nuremberg for war crimes. Tribunals 1 and 2 have become known as the Doctors' Trials. Physicians and administrators responsible for forced experimentation on concentration camp prisoners were tried, and some were subjected to capital sentences or imprisonment. The Nuremberg tribunal felt it needed to go further than the trial and sentencing and developed a document describing standards to prevent abusive medical experimentation that became known as the Nuremberg Code (**Table 1**). This became an influential statement of ethical principles governing experimentation on humans, emphasizing absolute requirements for

Dr. Aaron or an immediate family member has received research or institutional support from Orthofix, Inc. and serves as a board member, owner, officer, or committee member of the Orthopaedic Research Society. Ms. Racine-Avila or an immediate family member serves as a board member, owner, officer, or committee member of the Orthopaedic Research Society. Neither Dr. Menikoff nor any immediate family member has received anything of value from or has stock or stock options held in a commercial company or institution related directly or indirectly to the subject of this chapter.

The views expressed in this chapter are those of the authors and not necessarily those of the US Department of Health & Human Services, or its division, the Office of the Assistant Secretary for Health.

©Copyright 2021 American Academy of Orthopaedic Surgeons

TABLE 1 The Nuremberg Code: a 10-Point Statement Delimiting Permissible Medical Experimentation on Human Subjects

1. The voluntary consent of the human subject is absolutely eessential.
2. The experiment should be such as to yield fruitful results for the good society, unprocurable by other methods or means of study, and not random and unnecessary in nature.
3. Experiment should be based on animal experimentation...and natural history of the disease...anticipated results will justify the performance of the experiment.
4. The experiment should be so conducted as to avoid all unnecessary physical and mental suffering and injury.
5. No experiment should be conducted where there is a reason to believe that death or disabling injury will occur.
6. The degree of risk to be taken should never exceed...the importance of the problem to be solved by the experiment.
7. Proper preparations should be made...to protect the experimental subject against even remote possibilities of injury, disability, or death.
8. The experiment should be conducted only by scientifically qualified persons.
9. During the course of the experiment the human subject should be at liberty to bring the experiment to an end....
10. During the course of the experiment the scientist in charge must be prepared to terminate the experiment at any stage, if he has probable cause to believe...that a continuation of the experiment is likely to result in injury, disability, or death to the experimental subject.

Based on "Trials of War Criminals before the Nuremberg Military Tribunals under Control Council Law No. 10". Washington, DC: U.S. Government Printing Office, 1949, vol 2, pp. 181-182.

voluntary consent and withdrawal by the research subject, the need to protect the subject from harm, and the competency and responsibilities of the researchers.[2-4] Subsequently, in 1964, the World Medical Association (WMA) organized the Nuremberg Code into a series of ethical principles known as the Declaration of Helsinki that has influenced the conduct of clinical research for many years.[3] Written and revised over many years, it is a substantial document not easily summarized. The current version of the Declaration of Helsinki is found at this website: https://www.wma.net/policies-post/wma-declaration-of-helsinki-ethical-principles-for-medical-research-involving-human-subjects/. A resolution adopted by the World Medical Association held that, "Under no circumstances is a doctor permitted to do anything which would weaken the physical or mental resistance of a human being except from strictly therapeutic or prophylactic indications imposed by the interest of the patient."[5]

Regulations of research on human subjects in the United States have been codified by the federal government. In the mid-1950s, the Clinical Center of the National Institutes of Health (NIH) adopted guidelines taken directly from the Nuremberg Code that applied to the use of normal volunteers in research.[6] Subsequently, the NIH and the FDA developed more extensive regulations of clinical research.[7] In 1966, the NIH developed a policy of approving funding for research with human subjects only if the grantee institution provided prior review of research methods and an analysis of the risks and benefits of the research proposal.[6,7]

Despite these codifications, abusive clinical research continued, including in the United States.[5] A partial list of experiments performed without informed consent are plutonium injections by Manhattan Project physicians (1945-1947), radioactive iodine and other isotope administration experiments by the Atomic Energy Commission (1950-1970), radiation experiments in the Marshall Islands (1954), CIA studies of hallucinogens (1953) and pertussis (1955), the Willowbrook Experiments on psychiatric patients (1965), and the exposure of US service personnel to atomic radiation tests (1940-1971).[1,5] The Tuskegee Syphilis Experiment (1972) that observed the progression of untreated syphilis in poor black men despite an available treatment was a particularly notorious example of abusive clinical research.

The series of ethical abuses in human subjects research, particularly the Tuskegee Experiment, led Congress to pass the National Research Act (1974) which created the National Commission for the Protection of Human Subjects of Biomedical and Behavioral Research, whose charge it was to articulate ethical principles, and to develop guidelines, for human subjects research. After four years of discussions, the Commission published, "*Ethical Principles and Guidelines for the Protection of Human Subjects of Research*" also known as the *Belmont Report* (1979). The *Belmont Report* defined research as distinct from clinical practice. *Clinical practice* was defined as an intervention solely for the purpose of providing diagnosis, preventive treatment, or therapy to an individual whereas *research* tested hypotheses and was designed to create information generalizable to the population at large. The Report delineated three fundamental ethical principles for human subjects research: respect for persons, beneficence, and justice (**Table 2**). *Respect for persons* stipulated that individuals should be considered as autonomous agents and, in general, required informed consent for participation in research. *Beneficence*

©Copyright 2021 American Academy of Orthopaedic Surgeons

TABLE 2 The Belmont Report

Respect for Persons	Protecting the autonomy of all individuals, treating them with courtesy and respect, and requiring informed consent. Individuals with restricted autonomy are entitled to research protections.
Beneficence	Maximizing benefits for the research project while minimizing risks to the research subjects.
Justice	Ensuring that nonexploitative and well-considered procedures are administered fairly. The distribution of costs and benefits to potential research participants should be considered with fairness.

should underlie the assessment of risk/benefit considerations in research. *Justice* should inform the selection or exclusion of research participants.

In 1981, the Department of Health and Human Services revised federal regulations to be as consistent as possible with the principles articulated in the *Belmont Report*. These principles were subsequently codified in the Code of Federal Regulations (45 CFR part 46) (1991) as the "Federal Policy for the Protection of Human Research Subjects," based largely on the *Belmont Report*, and issued by 16 federal departments and agencies.[8] This became known as the Common Rule, and it applied to research that was either funded or conducted by those federal agencies (**Table 3**). The Common Rule provides the contemporary United States conceptual framework for research on human subjects and has governed the conduct of much of the research on human subjects including clinical trials. Among the concepts embodied by, or underlying, the Common Rule are informed consent and the right to voluntary withdrawal, the need for a well-articulated, testable hypothesis, an appropriate research design with consideration of risks to subjects, adequate predicate information to justify a clinical study, and an appropriately trained and responsible research team.

TABLE 3 Core Principles of the Common Rule

1. Review of research by independent committee (institutional review board)
2. Minimizing risks to subjects
3. Appropriate relationship among benefits to subjects, risks to subjects, and knowledge that might be learned from the research
4. Potential risks to subjects
5. Equitable selection of subjects
6. Obtaining and documenting informed consent of subjects or their representatives

WHERE ARE WE NOW?

Because of the complexity of contemporary clinical research, among other things, the agencies following the Common Rule have over the past several years been involved in a process to update it. Separately, some commentators have felt that the principles of the *Belmont Report* were also in need of updating.

THE BELMONT REPORT

Five themes for possible revision have been identified: (1) distinctions between clinical research and clinical practice, (2) harms to communities, (3) transparency of research activities, (4) implications of protectionism, and (5) the relationship between Belmont's ethical principles and their applications (**Table 4**).[9] "The *Belmont Report* was an impressive and inspiring response to the ethical issues of its day. Since its release, the field of research involving human subjects has developed in complex and unexpected ways, challenging the report's ethical framework to respond to not only the fears related to research abuses that it stemmed from, but also to the increasing commodification of biomedicine, the exclusion of many groups from research, the globalization of research, the desires of many to have access to experimental drugs, the lack of generalizability and reproducibility of many research findings, and the unique harms and histories that communities have experienced as a result of research."[9]

THE COMMON RULE

As mentioned above, because of advances in biomedicine and the resulting complexity of clinical research, among other things, the federal agencies which follow the Common Rule had undertaken a process to consider ways to revise it. The intent was to enhance government oversight of clinical research and to clarify and simplify the research approval process with the dual goals of improving patient protections and decreasing the regulatory burden on investigators. This has been a multi-year process that consisted, in part, of public commentary on an Advance Notice of Proposed Rulemaking (ANPRM). The ANPRM consisted of 155 questions with input from the Common Rule agencies that were designed to stimulate discussion. Questions were organized into seven categories (**Table 5**). (One of the authors [JR-A], reviewed the public commentary, assessed the comments of concern, and quantified the issues of most interest especially those concerns over increasing the regulatory burden for investigators.) Researchers were most concerned with the regulation of biospecimens, especially consent requirements for research use of biospecimens, including tissues removed incidental to surgery, the rights of research subjects to the information, products or services that were derived from

©Copyright 2021 American Academy of Orthopaedic Surgeons

TABLE 4 Reconsidering the Belmont Report

1. Research and Practice Research is designed to contribute to clinical knowledge generalizable to the population, while practice is meant to contribute to individual and communal well-being. However, in the years since the publication of the Report, the distinctions between research and practice have become vague, challenging regulatory agencies responsible for protections of individuals and research integrity.
2. Harms to Communities This concerns communal harm to groups that have been subjected to historical abuses in clinical research including racial and ethnic minorities. This critique argues that the principle of informed consent of individuals fails to take into account the unique harms that can be done to communities as cultural entities, such as violating widespread trust or taking ownership of a community's stories. The issue of cultural harm is described eloquently in the publication, *Rethinking the Belmont Report.*
3. Transparency in Research Much of biomedical research in the United States is now funded by industry, is complex in scope, and is often multi-institutional, making transparency and the management of conflicts of interest more difficult to attain. Another contemporary development that compromises transparency are new technologies including social media and digital monitoring that collect personal data and pose novel and unpredictable risks to research participant's privacy and confidentiality of personal or health information.
4. Protectionism The *Belmont Report* emphasized protection of vulnerable research subjects. While protections of individuals and groups is an essential part of an ethical construct, a negative result of the emphasis on protectionism is that some groups considered vulnerable have been excluded from the research process, and as a consequence, health data relevant to them are lacking (eg, pregnant women, children, embryos, the institutionalized, the elderly). As with the Women's Health Initiative which defined differences in physiologic performance between the genders, physiologic and pharmacologic differences of racial and ethnic groups that have been protected are now becoming apparent.
5. Relationship Between Ethical Principles and Applications The articulation of ethical principles and their practical applications are not identical and are subject to narrow or expansive interpretations. A criticism of the Belmont Report is that its interpretations are narrow. Respect for persons applies to informed consent; beneficence to risk–benefit analysis; and justice to subject selection. But more expansive interpretations of these ethical principles can be invoked and "*Rethinking the Belmont Report*" should be read for a more thorough treatment.

Data based on Friesen P, Kearns L, Redman B, Caplan AL: Rethinking the Belmont Report? *Am J Bioeth* 2017;17(7):15-21.

the research using their tissues, and the right to share in any derived profits. Because of the extent of interest in the disposition and value of human biospecimens, this subject merits special consideration.

TABLE 5 Health and Human Service Categories in the ANPRM

I.	Refining existing risk-based regulatory framework
II.	Single IRB review of multicenter studies
III.	Improving informed consent and process
IV.	Establishment of mandatory data security and information protection standards for all studies involving identifiable data
V.	Creation of a systematic approach for recording adverse events
VI.	Extension of federal regulatory protections, regardless of funding source to institutions that receive federal funding for human subjects research
VII.	Clarifying multiagency guidance rules

ANPRM = Advance Notice of Proposed Rulemaking

THE VALUE OF HUMAN TISSUES AND THE REGULATORY ENVIRONMENT

HENRIETTA LACKS AND HELA CELLS

Henrietta Lacks (1920-1951) was an African-American woman who was being treated for cervical cancer at Johns Hopkins Hospital. Consent to participate in research was not standard at that time. Her tumor cells, obtained from biopsies performed during the treatment, were taken for research without her consent and placed in tissue culture. They exhibited a property of multiple replications without dying and were termed "immortalized" and became known as "HeLa" cells. HeLa cells have been widely distributed to laboratories throughout the country and have been used for research into cancer, AIDS, toxicity studies, gene mapping, cloning, and the development of the polio vaccine. It is estimated that over 10,000 patents have been filed from research with HeLa cells. Ms Lacks's physicians did not seek her consent before using her tissues for research, nor did they receive any personal financial gain from the cell line. The cell line did, however, become extremely lucrative and, although it is difficult to precisely quantify the total revenue generated from the HeLa cell line, it is estimated to be in the hundreds of millions of dollars.

 ©Copyright 2021 American Academy of Orthopaedic Surgeons

Genetically modified versions of the cell line currently sell for as much as $10,000.[10] The Lacks family has never received any financial benefits from the HeLa cell line.

WI-38 CELLS

Another instructive case is that of the WI-38 cell line that is derived from the lung tissue of a surgically aborted fetus and has been used worldwide for the production of many human virus vaccines since the mid-1960s. Although it cannot be accurately determined, it is probable that the commercial sale of vaccines produced in WI-38 cells is in the multiple billions of dollars.[11]

Issues relating to the rights of individuals over their own tissues, the possible need for investigators to obtain consent to use biological specimens and data and behavioral information, and the potential profitability of information derived from experiments on human specimens have sparked a debate over whether the individuals who are sources of biospecimens must be informed about the fate of that material, including the potential commercial products that may be developed using their specimens, and whether they have any claim to compensation or to share in profits. One of the judicial precedents in this debate is *Moore v. Regents of the University of California*.[12]

MOORE V. REGENTS OF THE UNIVERSITY OF CALIFORNIA

In 1976, John Moore was treated at the UCLA Medical Center for leukemia, a treatment that included a splenectomy. Prior to surgery, his physician had determined that he was going to use portions of Moore's spleen in research activities he was conducting, but did not inform his patient about those intentions. Moore signed a standard surgical consent form for the therapeutic procedure, but the form did not include consent for use of the surgically removed tissue for research. In subsequent visits, blood samples were obtained, some of which may have been used for research. Cell cultures were developed with Moore's tissues, and in 1984, a patent was issued to the University of California for an "Mo cell line" that was developed from these cultures. In collaboration with Genetics Institute and Sandoz Pharmaceutical, several products were developed from the Mo cell line.[13] The case raised several issues, dealt with separately by several California courts, including, (1) whether individuals have the right to be informed about how biospecimens obtained from them will be used and (2) whether individuals from whom biospecimens are obtained have patent or financial rights to methods, services, or products subsequently developed from their tissues.

The California Supreme Court held (1) that in circumstances where a physician is pursuing research activities that might impact the physician's professional judgment, there was an explicit duty to obtain informed consent to those activities, which may include consent to use biospecimens for research. The court recognized that the dual role of the physician as healer and researcher created an inherent conflict of interest for the physician and imposed an obligation for the physician/researcher to disclose that conflict of interest, including potentially profiting from the research, if that profit existed.[13] (2) However, the court also held that Moore did not have a property interest in his removed tissues. In a penetrating analysis, "It is important to realize that patent rights are only available to the inventor who reduces his idea to practice. 'Products of nature', no matter how exceptional, cannot be the subject of patent protection. Thus, patent protection is not available for human tissue in its unaltered form, and the fact that patent protection has been granted to the inventor of a cell-line (or other genetically engineered substance) has no bearing on what rights the source of the original tissue may possess in that tissue."[13] Other legal precedents have supported the view that patients do not have a property interest in tissues used for research.

A DEBATE OVER PAYING PATIENTS FOR BIOSPECIMENS

Substantial debate has persisted in the scientific community as to whether patients should be paid for their tissues or share in moneys generated for research including salaries, funds to institutions, intellectual property, patents, products, or medical devices. Some feel that biological tissue has limited intrinsic value and that value is produced by the experiment. Others feel that biological tissues have inherent, independent value.

The Policy Forum published in *Science* in 2012 presented aspects of this debate. Financial compensation was held to be unnecessary when biospecimens were obtained incidental to needed care, but compensation was considered appropriate when biospecimen donation imposed added effort, burden, or risk.[10] In keeping with the Moore decision, payments in these cases are made for performance of a service rather than for transfer of property (biospecimens). The authors would deny patients a right to payment for research that yields profits based upon the legal norms that tissues separated from the body are not the ongoing property of the individual. Rather, it is the researchers, not the patients, whose intellectual efforts lead to the creation of "value." Other investigators have taken a different view and have expressed support for payment for biospecimens.[14] How this debate is resolved could have enormous impact on research with human tissues.

CHANGES TO THE COMMON RULE

As mentioned above, in the Fall of 2009, the federal Office of Management and Budget convened a working group to examine ways to revise the Common Rule.[15] That undertaking led to the 2011 release of an advance notice of proposed rulemaking, or ANPRM.[16] That document explained the need for

©Copyright 2021 American Academy of Orthopaedic Surgeons

updating the regulations as follows: "The current regulations governing human subjects research were developed years ago when research was predominantly conducted at universities, colleges, and medical institutions, and each study generally took place at only a single site. Although the regulations have been amended over the years, they have not kept pace with the evolving human research enterprise, the proliferation of multi-site clinical trials and observational studies, the expansion of health services research, research in the social and behavioral sciences, and research involving databases, the Internet, and biological specimen repositories, and the use of advanced technologies, such as genomics."

The next major step in the process to revise the Common Rule took place in September, 2015, when 16 federal agencies signed onto and released for public comment a Notice of Proposed Rulemaking (NPRM).[17] That document, unlike the ANPRM that preceded it, proposed a variety of specific changes to the regulations. There were two main themes behind the proposed changes: eliminating inappropriate barriers to the conduct of research that the current regulations posed (eg, administrative burdens that did little to improve the well-being of subjects), while increasing protections for subjects in circumstances where that was appropriate.

Among the most significant changes proposed in the NPRM were the following:

1. Implementing a number of changes designed to improve informed consent, so as to "better assure that subjects are appropriately informed before they decide to enroll in a research study."
2. In general, requiring that a researcher must obtain the informed consent of someone before using a stored biospecimen that had been taken from that person, even if the researcher never is given information that would allow her to know the identity of that person. This proposal would have changed the existing rule that such a use of a nonidentified biospecimen would not constitute the use of a human subject and thus would not be subject to the Common Rule (which only applies to research with human subjects). The new informed consent requirement would generally be met by obtaining a "broad" consent from the subject, in which they agreed to allow future open-ended research studies with their biospecimens. Paired with this change would be a change in the rules relating to the ability of Institutional Review Board (IRB) to waive the requirement to obtain informed consent so that such waivers would rarely be allowable with regard to research involving biospecimens (even if nonidentified).
3. "Excluding" from being subject to the Common Rule certain types of activities, either because they involve low risk or there are already other protections similar to those that are provided by the Common Rule.
4. Expanding the categories of research that are "exempt" from needing to follow the Common Rule. Related to this change was a proposal to allow researchers to determine whether their studies are exempt without needing to go through any IRB or other administrative review. Among the new categories of exempt research would be (1) certain research involving benign interventions with adult subjects; (2) survey and related types of research, including the collection of identifiable and sensitive private information, so long as appropriate data security and privacy protection policies are followed; (3) certain secondary research use of identifiable private information, where notice of such possible use had been given; and (4) storing or maintaining biospecimens or identifiable private information for future unspecified secondary research, and conducting such research, if a broad consent template is used, certain privacy safeguards are followed, and limited IRB approval of the consent process is obtained.
5. Requiring that for multi-institutional research conducted by US institutions within the United States, there must be one IRB that serves as the IRB of record for all of those institutions.
6. The requirement for annual continuing IRB review of research would be eliminated for studies that are approved by expedited review and for studies that have reached the point where all subjects have completed any study interventions and the only remaining parts of the research involve analyzing data or standard clinical care and observational follow-up.
7. Extending the scope of the Common Rule to apply to all clinical trials, regardless of whether they are federally funded, conducted at US institutions that receive at least some federal funding for nonexempt research with human subjects.

CONCERNS OVER THE USE OF BIOSPECIMENS

During the public comment period, more than 2,100 comments were received. Most of them were from people who wrote in their individual capacity. Although many aspects of the proposed changes received comments, one specific proposal was an outlier in terms of the extent of attention that it received: the proposal to require consent on most research involving the use of nonidentified biospecimens. Almost half of the people commenting on any aspect of the proposed changes also commented on this particular proposal. In terms of magnitude, that was several multiples higher than the number of people commenting on the next most commented-on proposal.

Approximately 80% of the comments on the biospecimen consent proposal were opposed to its implementation. A variety of reasons were provided, including a concern that implementing the proposal would adversely affect the ability to do research with biospecimens that were collected for clinical care purposes.

In January, 2017, a "final rule" was released, which implemented a subset of the changes that had been proposed.[8,18] As of January 2019, regulated entities are required to comply with

 ©Copyright 2021 American Academy of Orthopaedic Surgeons

most of the changes. January 2020 is when they will have to comply with one of the changes, relating to having a single IRB of record review certain multi-institutional research.

PROPOSED CHANGES THAT WERE NOT ADOPTED

One of the proposed changes that ended up not being adopted was the proposal regarding consent for the research use of nonidentified biospecimens. In announcing that proposal, the 2015 NPRM had stated: "Regardless of the scale on which harms may have occurred in the past, continuing to allow secondary research with biospecimens collected without consent for research places the publicly funded research enterprise in an increasingly untenable position because it is not consistent with the majority of the public's wishes, which reflect legitimate autonomy interests." In other words, the NPRM had based this proposal on an empirical claim about the public's views regarding when research is acceptable. The public comments on the proposal, as discussed above, appeared to contradict that claim: a large majority of the public commenters actually supported the existing policy of research without consent.

Another proposal that did not get adopted was the one relating to expanding the coverage of the Common Rule to almost all clinical trials, including those that are not federally funded. Public comments on that proposal had raised several concerns relating to its complexity. Among the issues raised was the fact that the new proposal would only apply where an institution was receiving some federal funding for nonexempt research with human subjects, and the possible difficulty of implementing that criterion. Another concern was the use of a definition of clinical trial that would encompass a variety of minimal risk research, and thus would be inconsistent with the goal of extending coverage primarily to higher-risk studies. For those and other reasons, it was decided that further deliberation would be appropriate before implementing this type of change.

The concept of "excluding" certain activities from being subject to the regulations was ultimately rejected: many commenters found that the creation of this new dividing line "added a layer of unnecessary complexity in determining what studies fall under the Common Rule." Instead, the final rule merely modified an existing concept—the definition of research—to carve out some activities from being subject to regulation.

CHANGES THAT WERE ADOPTED REGARDING INFORMED CONSENT AND BIOSPECIMENS

Considering the changes that were implemented in the final rule, perhaps the most significant is a set of changes to improve informed consent. *The goal is to better inform prospective subjects about the consequences of choosing to participate in a particular research study* (**Table 6**).

TABLE 6 Improved Informed Consent in the Revised Common Rule

1. "Reasonable person" standard
2. Information presented in sufficient detail
3. Begin with a presentation of key information
4. Information organized to facilitate comprehension
5. Research with deidentified biospecimens without additional consent
6. Potential commercial profit
7. Sharing of research results
8. Potential for genome sequencing
9. Broad consent for secondary research

1. The regulations now require that prospective subjects be given the information that "a reasonable person would want to have to make an informed decision" about whether to participate. A reasonable person standard is a standard that has long been used in the law for determining what information to provide when a doctor obtains consent for clinical care. In that context, it is viewed as the more ethical standard compared with the competing "professional" standard, which instead requires physicians and other care givers to only disclose the information that they think a patient needs to know.
2. In addition, the information provided must be "in sufficient detail relating to the research." This change was made in response to the circumstance that current consent forms may not uncommonly give only vague information about certain aspects of what might happen to someone in a particular research study, even though there is more specific information that might have been very helpful. As one example, the section of a cancer clinical trial consent form discussing the possible benefits from participating might merely say one might or might not benefit. However, if it is known that the possible benefit would be at best a reduction of the patient's pain, and not any change in how long she or he might survive, this would be important information that should be provided.
3. An important part of the new consent changes is a requirement that consent "must begin with a concise and focused presentation of the key information that is most likely to assist a prospective subject...in understanding the reasons why one might or might not want to participate in the research." This change was made in recognition that consent forms, over the years, have been getting longer and longer, and the information that might be most useful to prospective subjects would be buried in the midst of less important information. As a result of this new requirement, even if the consent form remained long, at least the first few pages would contain the information that would be most helpful to the subject in making a decision about participation.

©Copyright 2021 American Academy of Orthopaedic Surgeons

4. An additional new requirement, which applies to both the concise presentation at the beginning of the consent form, and also to the consent form as a whole, is that the information "must be organized and presented in a way that facilitates comprehension." So, for example, rather than presenting separate discussions of benefits, risks, and alternatives, a consent form might discuss the interrelationships of these elements and how those interrelationships might be relevant to a person's decision about participation.
5. In addition, a new element was added to the "basic elements" of informed consent, and three new elements were added to the "additional elements" of informed consent. The new basic element requires that in research involving the collection of identifiable private information or identifiable biospecimens, prospective subjects must be informed about the possibility that identifiers could be removed from the information or biospecimens, after which additional research could take place without consent. As an alternative to providing such a statement, the consent form could instead include a promise to not conduct such research with de-identified information or biospecimens.
6. As for the new "additional" elements, the *first* requires informing prospective subjects about the possibility of their biospecimens being used for commercial profit, if indeed that might happen. It also requires telling the subjects whether or not they would share in such profit. A *second* element requires telling subjects whether clinically relevant research results (including results specific to the subject) will be shared with them, and if so, under what circumstances. And the *third* new element, for research with biospecimens, is a disclosure about whether the research might include whole genome sequencing.
7. The final rule also adopted new provisions for a type of "broad consent"—namely, a person providing consent to unspecified future secondary research with identifiable private information or identifiable biospecimens. ("Secondary" research means research involving information or biospecimens that were initially collected for some other "primary" purpose.) While rules governing broad consent were initially proposed in the 2015 NPRM, the reason for proposing them largely related to the new requirement for obtaining informed consent before conducting research with nonidentified biospecimens. As that consent requirement was not adopted, the result is that the new broad consent rules end up instead serving as a voluntary option that supplements the existing (and largely unchanged) ways in which secondary research can take place.

As mentioned above, the proposal to "exclude" certain activities from being subject to the Common Rule was not implemented. But a similar outcome was achieved by removing some of those activities from meeting the definition of research. Three of the changes relate to activities that will generally be conducted by, or at the request of, governmental entities. The broadest of these changes is probably one that applies to public health surveillance activities that are conducted, among other possibilities, by or at the request of a "public health authority," which is a term defined in the revised regulations.

The one change to the definition that is not related to government activities is for "scholarly and journalistic activities (eg, oral history, journalism, biography, literary criticism, legal research, and historical scholarship)...that focus directly on the specific individuals about whom the information is collected."

The proposals to expand the exemption provisions, and create some new exemptions, were adopted in many respects, though with some significant changes. Similar to what was proposed, there is now a new exemption category for certain types of research that only involve "benign behavioral interventions." The category of survey and related research was indeed expanded to allow the collection of sensitive private information, though such research would need to undergo "limited" IRB review for the purpose of verifying that appropriate privacy and confidentiality provisions are in place. The two proposed exemptions for the storage and secondary research use of certain biospecimens and identifiable private information were adopted, though they only apply to identifiable biospecimens (as the proposal relating to nonidentified biospecimens was not adopted). In addition, various forms of limited IRB review are required to qualify for the exemptions. The proposed exemption relating to providing notice of certain types of secondary research was not adopted, although a different exemption relating to research use of identifiable health information that was subject to certain HIPAA protections was adopted.

The proposal that for multi-institutional research conducted by US institutions within the United States, there must be one IRB that serves as the IRB of record for all of those institutions was adopted. As mentioned above, this is the one change that has a later date by which institutions must comply with the requirement: January 20, 2020.

Finally, the proposal to eliminate the requirement of continuing annual IRB review of research was adopted.

SUMMARY

This chapter has traced the evolution of contemporary ethical and legal thinking governing experimentation with human subjects. It is recognized that research on humans, including in particular clinical research, is essential to translate basic information to the clinic and to improve human health. While preserving these needs, it has proven to be essential to perform clinical research within ethical bounds supported by a legal framework to ensure both that useful information is produced and that research subjects are protected from harm. Because clinical science is dynamic, ethical and legal frameworks need to evolve along with clinical techniques and technologies.

©Copyright 2021 American Academy of Orthopaedic Surgeons

REFERENCES

1. Annas GJ, Grodin MA: *The Nazi Doctors and the Nuremberg Code: Human Rights in Human Experimentation*. Oxford, UK, Oxford University Press, 1995.
2. Barondess JA: Medicine against society. Lessons from the Third Reich. *J Am Med Assoc* 1996;276(20):1657-1661.
3. Fuson RL, Sherman M, Van Vleet J, Wendt T: The conduct of orthopaedic clinical trials. *J Bone Joint Surg Am Vol* 1997;79(7):1089-1098.
4. Katz J: The Nuremberg code and the Nuremberg trial. A reappraisal. *J Am Med Assoc* 1996;276(20):1691.
5. Beecher HK: Ethics and clinical research. *N Engl J Med* 1966;274(24): 1354-1360.
6. Glantz L: The influence of the Nuremberg Code on U.S. Statutes and regulations, in Annas G, Grodin M, eds: *The Nazi Doctors and the Nuremberg Code*. Oxford, Oxford University Press, 1995, pp 183-200.
7. Curran WJ: Governmental regulation of the use of human subjects in medical research; the approach of two federal agencies. *Daedalus* 1969;98:542-594.
8. Menikoff J, Kaneshiro J, Pritchard I: The common rule, updated. *N Engl J Med* 2017;376(7):613-615.
9. Friesen P, Kearns L, Redman B, Caplan AL: Rethinking the Belmont report? *Am J Bioeth* 2017;17(7):15-21.
10. Truog RD, Kesselheim AS, Joffe S: Research ethics. Paying patients for their tissue: The legacy of Henrietta Lacks. *Science* 2012;337(6090):37-38.
11. Hayflick L: Paying for tissue: The case of WI-38. *Science* 2012; 337(6100):1292.
12. *Moore v. Regents of University of California*, in 793 P.2d 479, 271 Cal. Rptr. 146, 51 Cal. 3d 120,(1990), California Supreme Court.
13. Dorney M: Moore v. the Regents of the University of California: Balancing the need for biotechnology innovation against the right of informed consent. *High Technol Law J* 1990;5(2):333-369.
14. Kominers SD, Becker GS: Paying for tissue: Net benefits. *Science* 2012;337(6100):1292-1293.
15. Emanuel EJ, Menikoff J: Reforming the regulations governing research with human subjects. *N Engl J Med* 2011;365(12):1145-1150.
16. Human subjects research protections: Enhancing protections for research subjects and reducing burden, delay and ambiguity for investigators. *Fed Reg* 2011;76:44512.
17. Federal policy for the protection of human subjects. *Fed Reg* 2015;80:53933.
18. Federal policy for the protection of human subjects. *Fed Reg* 2017; 82:7149.

©Copyright 2021 American Academy of Orthopaedic Surgeons

40

Principles of Clinical Studies

Joel J. Gagnier, ND, MSc, PhD

Keywords: *bias; causation versus association; choice of study design; data types; hypotheses; outcome measurement; research questions; sample size calculations; statistical tests; validity*

OVERVIEW

This chapter outlines a selection of basic principles surrounding preparing and implementing clinical research. This includes overviews of study designs, the choice of an appropriate design for specific questions, and a review of biases, sampling, validity, and power calculations. I also cover the types of outcomes to consider in clinical trials, implementing those outcomes, as well as the details of scale metrics and psychometrics. Finally, I cover some basics of data management and data analytics in clinical research. This chapter contains some of the key concepts common across clinical research that are applicable to the topics and material covered in follow-up chapters in this text.

INTRODUCTION

PREPARATION

When preparing for clinical research, or research of any kind, careful preparation will save you a considerable amount of time and prevent many headaches. It is not advisable to dive straight into a clinical research project with significant preparatory work. First you need to define, even generally, your area of interest. Questions or areas of interest can arise from a number of sources: from clinical encounters, lectures, conversations with colleagues, and reading, of course. Once you have a broad idea of what you might do a project on, you need make a concerted effort to refine and vet your ideas. In particular, you should start by becoming familiar with the subject matter and, in particular, peer-reviewed publications, including systematic reviews and meta-analysis, in your area of interest. This means much reading and thinking.

To properly review the relevant literature in your area of interest you must search for, obtain, and read articles—many articles. To do this validly and comprehensively, I recommend following the methods of performing a systematic review. This may even turn into a publication for you. The specificity of the search depends on where you are at in terms of your question formation. If you do not really have a well-defined question yet, then you will of course start by broadly searching the literature, first reading review papers, and possibly focusing in on area specific journals. Examining citations in relevant papers will help further refine your idea. Think about your ideas in terms of an actual question. What is the sample of interest, what is the intervention or exposures of interest, and what are the outcomes of interest? We will discuss components of a refined and specific question below.

If you have a well-defined question, then searching will be much more specific. This will help you identify studies that are similar, maybe exactly as you were planning. But maybe the prior work had flaws that you can correct in a follow-up project. Or possibly the intervention is now out of date, or the sample is different. There are many ways to tweak your research idea to make it unique, or you can simply change your focus and begin with a new question. But, remember, if there are only a small number of studies on the exact question you are interested in, there is no harm in repeating it, except in the event that it was a very large study with definitive findings, which would make any additional work not needed and unethical.

Databases to consider searching include MEDLINE, PubMed, EMBASE, the Cochrane Library, CINAHL, and other topic-specific databases where relevant (eg, PsychInfo, SportDiscus, PEDro). I would highly recommend including library and information scientists in your searching effort especially for complex searches with many terms in the search

Dr. Gagnier serves as a paid consultant to or is an employee of Bartimus Frickleton Robertson Rader P.C. and Rubin Anders Scientific and serves as a board member, owner, officer, or committee member of the Orthopaedic Research Society.

©Copyright 2021 American Academy of Orthopaedic Surgeons

strategy. Furthermore, consider hand searching relevant journals that are not indexed in these electronic databases and contact experts for additional resources. The found literature can help you in refining your question and will help you with planning the methods, writing rationale, and implementing your study as well as reporting it.

QUESTION FORMATION

Following this introductory work, you should have refined and specific research question. Ideally, the question should include several components: the so-called P.I.C.O. format.

P: Participants/population
I: Intervention/exposure
C: Control/comparison group
O: Outcome

The primary question should include all of these components to be sufficiently specific. You can have multiple questions of interest but one primary question of interest, because it is this primary question from which your primary hypothesis is derived, which informs the sample size calculation. Remember, you have only one primary hypothesis, which is associated with a single outcome of interest (eg, pain), or put differently, a single statistic. Your secondary hypotheses relate to other questions of interest, maybe related to other outcomes (eg, quality of life, physical function, activities of daily living, satisfaction). You now must decide on how you are going to test your hypotheses. What study design do you need to use?

CLINICAL STUDY DESIGNS

OBSERVE VERSUS EXPERIMENT

From the preparatory work, the literature should provide some guidance on the type of study design needed to test the question. The first thing to decide is: are you experimenting or observing? An experimental design requires that you are exposing human participants to some intervention (ie, therapeutic, preventive, diagnostic, etc.). Or, are you planning an observational study; are you collecting data on patients that are self-chosen to their exposures, or, as is frequently the case, the decision of exposure is a combined decision of the patients together with their physicians. Next, you need to decide on the timing element. That is, do you need to do a prospective study or are you doing a retrospective study? Any experimental study is by its very nature prospective. But, in some cases, the data are already collected (say in their health record); therefore, the researcher has no control over the exposures or the type of outcomes collected, which becomes a retrospective study because you are collecting data that already exist. In the case where some data of interest already exist, there can also be a combination of prospective and retrospective data collection. For example, through health records but additional data/outcomes are also collected in a prospective manner. Finally, there are studies that collect new data on patients only, but collect both the exposure and outcome at the same time resulting in a cross-sectional study, one type of observational study. Other forms of observational studies include cohort studies, case-control studies, case series, and interrupted time series. Types of experimental studies include

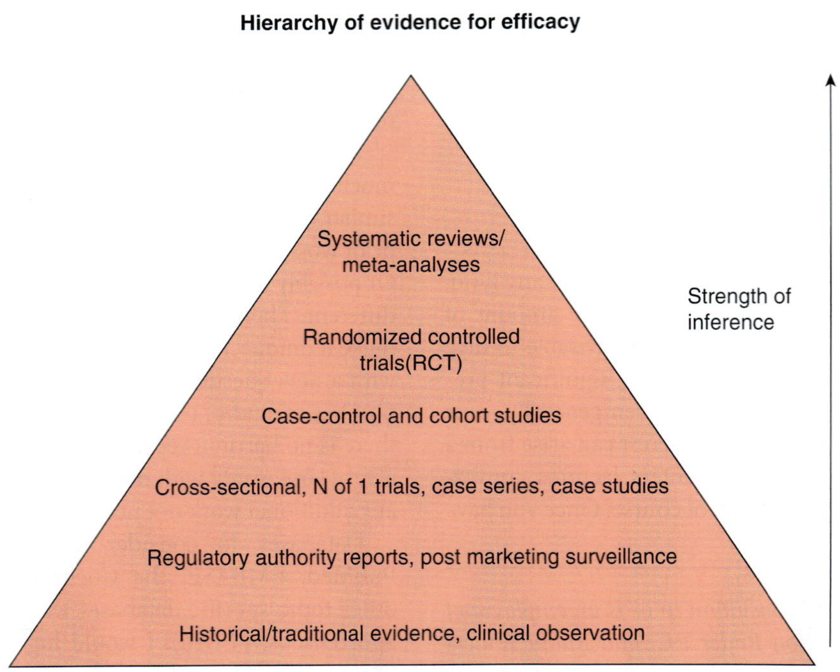

FIGURE 1 Graph showing hierarchy of evidence for efficacy.

©Copyright 2021 American Academy of Orthopaedic Surgeons

randomized trials, nonrandomized comparative studies, and before and after studies. There is a generally accepted hierarchy of evidence (**Figure 1**). All things being equal, systematic reviews and meta-analyses (well-performed on level I evidence) are the peak of the evidence pyramid, having the designs with the most powerful inferential capabilities, then comes randomized trials, and then observational studies and so on.

COHORT STUDIES

A cohort study is one of the most common clinical study designs in orthopaedics. A cohort is a group of persons with some common characteristic or set of characteristics. The groups are "self" chosen and you compare some exposure (eg, surgery) to some other exposure (eg, rehabilitation or no treatment) and then measure a subsequent outcome (**Figure 2**). The outcome always follows, or should follow, the exposure in a cohort study. Some of the advantages of cohort studies are as follows: groups of participants are self-chosen and therefore essentially any self-chosen exposure can be looked at; given this self exposure, these studies reflect the real world and real-world clinical practice and, thus, have greater generalizability. Also rare exposures (rare treatments), or rare conditions, or conditions that take a lot of time to develop can be studied but require large sample sizes and considerable resources to implement. The main disadvantage of a cohort study is that the cohorts being compared may differ at the start of the study on variables other than the differing exposure. The differences between the comparison groups may result in unequal risk of the outcome, given the exposure. That is, some effect modifier (eg, baseline disease severity or some relevant comorbidity) may influence the cohort's chances of some outcome or modify the effect of the exposure, which may be some type of treatment (eg, surgery). Therefore, every attempt must be made to explore such important variables in the participants that may modify the effect of the intervention on some outcome. This is termed effect modification.

Effect modification occurs when an exposure has varying effects among different subgroups of patients, sometimes termed heterogeneity of treatment effect. You also need to be careful to identify any confounding variables, which are variables that distort the association between the exposure and outcome, but which are not themselves causally related to the exposure outcome relationship. For example, smoking may be confounding variable for the risk of deep vein thrombosis (DVT) following total hip replacements with two comparative devices. That is, the device (exposure) group is not causally related to risk of smoking, but smoking increases the risk of DVTs. If the proportion of patients who smoke is different between the exposure groups, then the relationship between one exposure and the outcome is confounded by smoking. On the other hand, if older patients are more suited to receiving device A, and age increases the risk for DVTs, then age is an effect modifier, so should it be explored. That is, age is causally associated with the device and the outcome, and, therefore, is an effect modifier. Both types of variables should be identified if present and their effects examined. If they are not examined, any exposure outcome relationship found in the study is potentially biased.

There are a variety of ways to control for variables influencing the outcome of interest. Ideally you want to know which variables are effect modifiers and which are potential confounders up front, before participant selection and inclusion into the study. Then, particular patients, say with known confounders can be excluded, and analyses can be planned to explore the influence of known effect modifiers. That is, subgroup analyses and regression analyses can help elucidate the influence of effect modifiers. If you cannot eliminate all known confounder, then you can also use regression analyses to "adjust" for these variables.

CASE-CONTROLLED STUDIES

Next we have the case-control design, in which you gather patients who already have some outcome of interest (eg, severe osteoarthritis of the knee), who are referred to as "cases." This "case" group is compared with "controls," the latter of which does not have the outcome of interest. Ideally the controls are matched to the cases on important effect modifiers, which depend entirely on the characteristics of the outcome of interest and the causal pathway from the exposure of interest. Then you look back in time and review the history of the cases and controls for some exposure of interest (eg, participation in high-impact sports). If the exposure is causally related to outcome of interest, and the groups are otherwise equivalent,

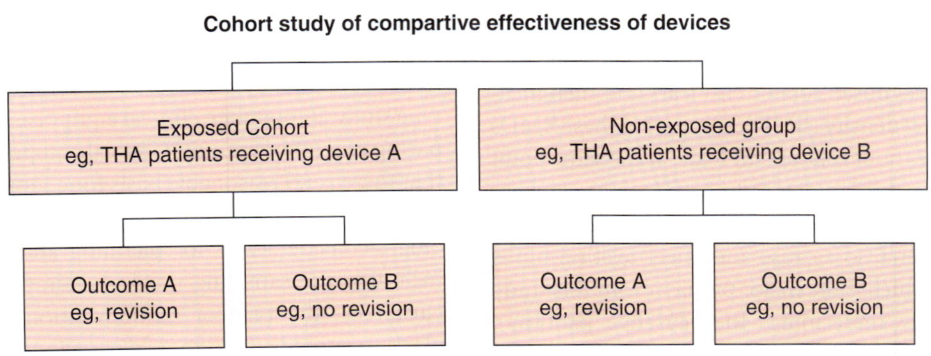

FIGURE 2 Chart demonstrating cohort study design.

©Copyright 2021 American Academy of Orthopaedic Surgeons

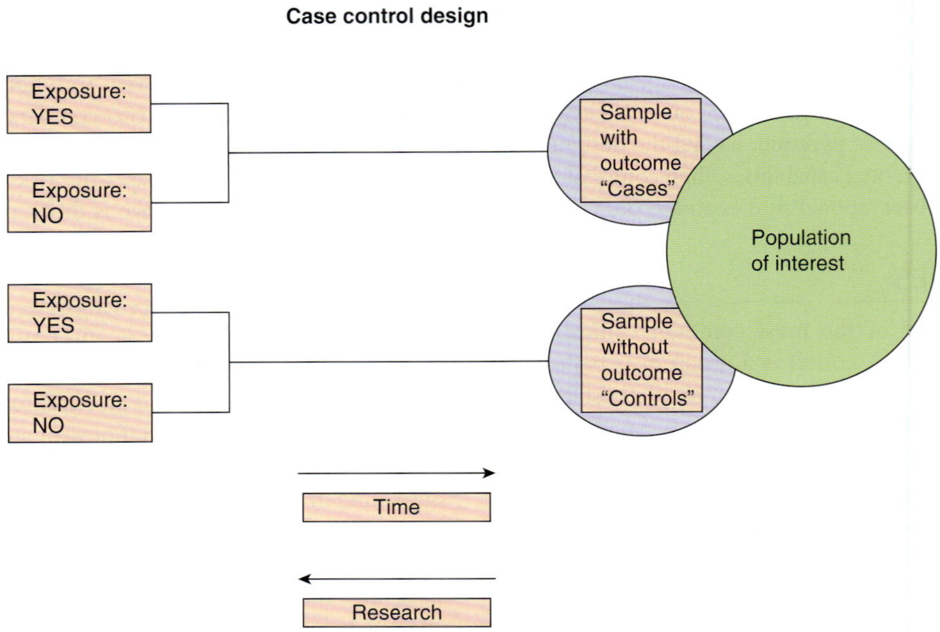

FIGURE 3 Chart demonstrating case-controlled studies.

then you would expect a greater frequency of exposure in the cases compared with the controls (**Figure 3**). The advantages of case-control studies include the fact that groups are self chosen; therefore, you can look at any outcome and related exposure, and you can easily study rare outcomes or outcomes that take a long time to develop. These latter two advantages are the major benefits of this design. Of course, case-control studies have several potential disadvantages, including the fact that the investigator must be careful to control for confounding variables and explore effect modifiers, because the cases and control may be different at the start of the study for reasons other than the exposure of interest. Also, you must be certain the exposure preceded the outcome; otherwise, this undermines causation. Also, depending on the exposure, the data source should be vetted for accuracy and completeness. For example, relying on patient recall could cause biases.

CROSS-SECTIONAL STUDIES

The next study design is the cross-sectional design. In this type of observational study, the outcome is measured at the exact same time as the exposure. For example, you might identify patients with newly diagnosed rotator cuff tears and then measure their bone mineral density (BMD), comparing these BMDs to matched patients without rotator cuff tears, at the same point in time. But, of course, this is a descriptive study only—you are not testing an exposure on some outcome, but instead looking at coexisting phenomena, so a cause-and-effect relationship is difficult to establish, which is the major problem with this study design (ie, chronology undermines the causative pathway). There are other forms of observational studies such as interrupted time series, before-and-after studies, and case series.

RANDOMIZED TRIALS

Next, we get into the experimental studies including randomized trials (**Figure 4**). The single best experimental design for establishing cause-and-effect relationships is the randomized controlled trial (RCT). RCTs have distinct features: the outcomes of interest are not present at the time of enrollment into the study (they are prospective), a concurrent control or comparison group is used, assignment to groups is random (via random number generator), and the exposure to groups is under the control of the investigator (experimental). The major advantage of the RCT is the randomization process, which theoretically should equally distribute all uncontrolled variables between the groups if the sample is large enough. There are disadvantages of this design including: random allocation is not always possible for questions where random assignment to some exposure may be unethical (eg, a harmful exposure), these studies also take a long time to complete, are expensive, and frequently require large sample sizes, and they are typically not suitable for the study of distant or rare events. RCTs can either compare an active intervention to a placebo, to no intervention or to some other active intervention, the latter of which would be a comparative effectiveness type study. Remember, clinical equipoise is needed when comparing two interventions. Clinical equipoise is the assumption that there is no reasonable basis for choosing one intervention over another in a specific patient. There are many methodologic considerations for planning and implementing RCTs including the sampling methods (simple random, stratified, clustered), the type of randomization to be used (simple, black, stratified), how to achieve allocation concealment (ie, the concept that the person allocating patients into groups

©Copyright 2021 American Academy of Orthopaedic Surgeons

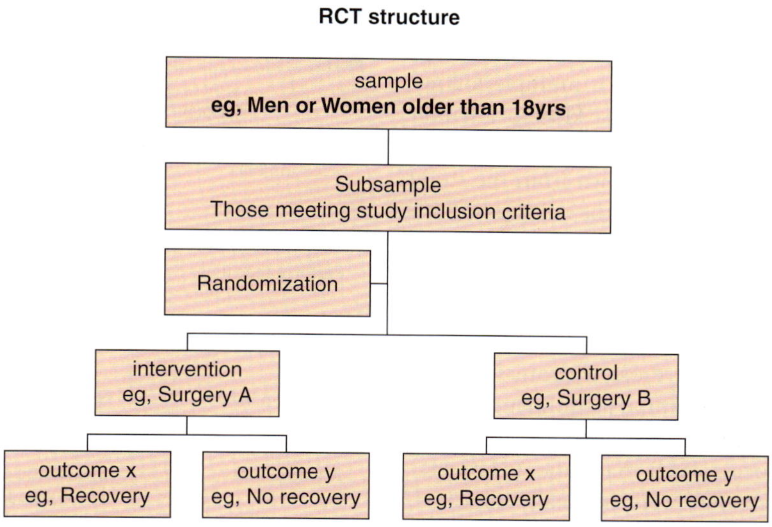

FIGURE 4 Chart demonstrating randomized trials.

has no knowledge of which intervention specific patients are getting), the blinding of specific parties involved in the study (patients, clinicians, outcome assessors, data analysts, etc.), and if crossovers are needed. All of these considerations are dictated by the question and hypothesis(ses) being tested.

CLINICAL RESEARCH CONCEPTS

CAUSATION, ASSOCIATION, AND CORRELATION

There are many ways that variables within a study may be related to each other. There can be a causative relationship, an association or a correlation, or no relationship at all. A causative relationship means by definition that some variable X is a necessary component in the existence or level of some other variable say Y. That is, X is a causative factor for Y. If there is a causal relationship, X causes Y, then X and Y are also associated. But, X and Y may be associated, for instance, when a third variable A causes both X and Y. That is, X and Y have a common cause. Association means that one variable provides some sort of information about another variable, but it does not infer causation. Remember, that spurious associations are likely when many variables are examined in complex systems. These arise simply by chance. Correlation is a type of association, where variables show some common trend, either increasing or decreasing. But correlations do not infer causation, though correlated variables can be causally related. The term "correlated" is frequently used as a catch-all term for any association, but, technically, this is incorrect because correlation does not mean causation. Generally one should avoid using the term "correlated" or "correlated with" when intending to infer causation. Also, be aware that high/strong correlations can arise in random data. Furthermore, biases can make it seem as though there is an association when in reality there is not.

BIASES IN CLINICAL RESEARCH

Bias is defined as the systematic deviation from the truth and can arise at any stage in clinical research. There are many forms of bias including these following classes: Selection bias, performance bias, detection bias, attrition bias, reporting bias, and biases due to conflicts of interest (eg, funding source, intellectual property, etc.). First, selection bias arises when participant inclusion and allocation procedures result in unequal characteristics in the groups being compared, identified by examining baseline and demographic variables in each group. In an observational study, patients are not allocated to interventions; therefore, the sampling procedure and any related matching methods dictate the similarity of the groups. In RCTs, the allocation methods, random assignment, and allocation concealment (methods to prevent foreknowledge of the forthcoming allocations) dictate group similarity. Next, performance bias refers to systematic differences between groups in the care provided or in exposures other than the interventions related to the research questions and hypotheses (ie, confounders or effect modifiers). In RCTs, blinding procedures of study participants and study personnel reduce the risk that any knowledge of the intervention received can affect the outcomes. In observational studies (eg, a cohort study), performance bias may arise due to subtle differences in the interventions received, such that in a comparative effectiveness study, group A, for example, has varying cointerventions that are distinct from those in group B. Therefore, the groups are being differentially exposed to cointerventions that could potentially influence the measured outcomes. Careful patient selection and allocation as well as the measurement of all known confounders and cointerventions can mitigate performance bias. Next, detection bias refers to systematic differences in how outcomes are being measured between the groups. In all prospective clinical research, blinding of the outcome assessors can mitigate this as can careful attention to outcomes assessments being performed

©Copyright 2021 American Academy of Orthopaedic Surgeons

in the same manner in each group. Next, attrition bias refers to systematic differences in the withdrawals from a study or from incomplete data (eg, missing data points for multiple follow-ups). Withdrawals or incomplete data arise due to attrition (where patients are lost to follow-up for a variety of reasons) and exclusions (where patients are withdrawn from the study after initial inclusion and participation in the study). In both scenarios, the loss of outcome data can systematically alter the data and bias the comparisons. There are several methods to mitigate bias due to attrition such as imputation methods for missing data (filling in the missing data) and sensitivity analyses (eg, doing separate analyses for those with missing data vs. those with no missing data, to examine the influence of this missingness). In RCTs, intention to treat analyses (ITT) preserve the randomization process, such that patients are analyzed in the groups to which they were originally allocated, even if they did not actually receive that intervention (at all or in part), controlling for attrition bias. Reporting bias refers to systematic differences between reported and unreported findings, or when outcome priority is changed from the protocol to the published report (eg, secondary outcomes are switched to primary outcomes). Generally, statistically significant differences are more likely to be reported than nonsignificant ones, and outcome priority, when changed, is changed in favor of statistically significant findings. This is also called outcome reporting bias or selective reporting bias. To mitigate reporting biases, it is important not to change outcome priority or to selectively publish particular findings. If you have a legitimate reason to do either, you must fully report this; transparency is key. Finally, depending on the question, hypotheses and study design or implementation other biases may be relevant. Some biases may specifically relate to particular study designs. For example, when performing cluster randomized studies one must be careful analytically to account for relevant grouping variables (eg, recruitment site) and when performing crossover studies carry-out effects must also be examined and considered. **Table 1** outlines the categories of bias in clinical research.

When planning clinical research you should be careful to control for these biases up front or attempt to account for or control for them in the data analysis. Of course, when you are reading and interpreting research, you should carefully and comprehensively think through the risk of bias of that research. There are several accepted risk of bias assessment tools you can use to determine the potential bias that a study is at risk of.[1]

TABLE 1 Categories of Bias in Clinical Research

Categories of Bias in Clinical Research	Definition
Selection bias	Systematic differences between baseline characteristics of the groups that are compared
Performance bias	Systematic differences between groups in the care that is provided, or in exposure to factors other than the interventions of interest
Detection bias	Systematic differences between groups in how outcomes are determined
Attrition bias	Systematic differences between groups in withdrawals from a study
Reporting bias	Systematic differences between reported and unreported findings
Other biases	Other sources of bias that are relevant only in certain circumstances

VALIDITY

When discussing risk of bias, we are referring to the internal validity of a study. Internal validity is generally defined as how "true" a study's results are for the sample of included participants. Put differently, validity is the extent to which the results for a particular outcome (dependent variable) are attributable to the exposure of interest (independent variable). Internal validity hinges squarely on the study design and implementation or, generally, the study methods. External validity, on the other hand, is the degree to which the results can be generalized or applied to participants outside of the study. External validity hinges on how similar the participants are to those you are attempting to apply the study findings to and how similar the exposure is in the study compared with the exposure in the participants outside of the study. This brings us to two related concepts: efficacy and effectiveness. Efficacy is measured in clinical research under ideal circumstances when you want to make a strong inference for cause and effect. These are also called explanatory studies. Effectiveness, on the other hand, is measured in clinical research that more so reflects clinical practice or real-world settings. Effectiveness studies are also termed pragmatic studies.

SAMPLE SIZE CALCULATIONS AND STATISTICAL ERRORS

Sample size calculations must be done for all clinical research. In some cases, pilot and feasibility clinical research can go without an a-priori sample size calculation when designed to test the feasibility of study methods (eg, recruitment, follow-up, etc.) or to collect data to be used for a sample size calculation for a larger follow-up study. In most cases, even for a pilot study, a sample size calculation can be done, but when absolutely no other data are available for the question under study, and no data for closely related questions are available, then a sample size calculation is simply not possible and any tangentially applied findings to such a calculation would be misleading. Of course, sample sizes are simply not possible or needed for case series or systematic review and meta-analyses. To calculate the sample size you will require data from related research, and the exact type of data will depend on the type

©Copyright 2021 American Academy of Orthopaedic Surgeons

of primary outcome data you are planning to collect. We will focus on dichotomous and continuous data here only, though sample size calculations are possible for any type of data (nominal, ordinal, dichotomous, ratio, continuous). For continuous data (eg, range of motion in degrees) you will require the following: alpha (α; typically set at $P = 0.05$ in biomedical research) or your risk of type I error; beta (β; typically set at 0.20), which is your risk of type II error (making your power 0.80 or 80%); some expected mean difference (delta) between your comparison groups on your primary outcome (eg, 20 degrees); and a measure of the variance for this difference, either a standard error (SE) or SD are typical.

When we have dichotomous data (eg, revision surgery within 1 year or not: Yes or No), to perform a sample size calculation you require the total number of events in the exposure group A (eg, those getting knee device A) and the total number of participants exposed in this group and the number of event events in the exposure group B (eg, knee device B) and the total number of participants exposed in the this group. So you will have two values, one for group A and one for group B. These could be risk ratios (RR) or odds ratios (OR) or some other ratio value.

Finally, it is important to account for potential drop-outs or loss-to-follow-up data, especially if you are performing prospective research. Typically you should account for 15% to 20% drop-outs. The exact amount will be dictated by the type of interventions and outcomes and can be found from pilot data or from related published research. Consult your biostatistician to help with these calculations. We must account for potential drop-outs because we do not want to be underpowered to detect a difference in outcomes if we do not have enough patients at some follow-up point. So, if our sample size yielded 50 patients total, and we expect 15% of our sample to drop out, then we need to equate the following and solve for X: $X/100\% = 50/80\%$ which results in $50/0.80 = 62.5$ patients total, which in a two-group study results in 31.25 patients per group, and we must round up to 32 patients per group, resulting in a total of 64 patients required.

The figure below highlights type I and II errors at statistical probabilities in a two-by-two table (**Figure 5**). A type I error is the probability of rejecting the null hypothesis (H_0) in favor of the alternative hypothesis (H_1) when in fact the null hypothesis is true. Conversely, a type II error is the probability of failing to reject the H_0, while the truth is that the null hypothesis should be rejected in favor of the H_1.

MEASUREMENT OF OUTCOMES

When embarking on clinical research, you must have some sort of outcome or a selection of outcomes that you are interested in and that are or can be influenced by the exposure or treatment. These can be objective (eg, laboratory test, blood values, imaging, muscle biopsies, physical examination, functional tests) or subjective (eg, self-report measures such as patient-reported outcome measures) or you can have both. But you can only have one primary outcome measure, and everything else is considered secondary. Refer back to your research question (P.I.C.O.), which should highlight your primary outcome. You cannot have a whole set of primary outcomes, because there is only one outcome, one piece of data, that dictates your required sample size and therefore is the hypothesis being tested. Everything else is secondary. Of course, it is advisable to make sure you have sufficient power to detect the differences in your secondary outcomes as well, but, technically and scientifically, this is not a requirement. You can have a whole selection of secondary outcomes, but be careful not to overburden your research team or your patients with an unreasonable number of questions or forms.

There are several ways to identify how your outcome was measured, which generally should start with the knowledge gained from your review of the literature. You should have a good idea of how your outcome has been measured. But this does not mean this is exactly what you should do. For example, you may be interested in measuring patient-reported shoulder

Statistical probabilities

Statistical decision on the basis of observation or experiment	True state	H_0	H_1
	Decide H_0	P[decide H_0 | H_0true]	P[decide H_0 | H_1true]= P[Type II error] β
	Decide H_1	P[decide H_1 | H_0true]= P[Type I error] α	P[decide H_1 | H_1true] 1-β (power)

FIGURE 5 Statistical errors.

©Copyright 2021 American Academy of Orthopaedic Surgeons

function following a type of surgical repair for a full thickness rotator cuff tear, and you may note that a particular patient-reported outcome measure (PROM) is used and reported frequently in the literature. But be very careful as you must comprehensively vet these measures and their quality before they are blindingly applied. They may not have good measurement properties, meaning they may not be reliable, valid, or responsive. That is, you must make a rational and logical decision of what to measure and how to measure it. This goes for any other measures like a laboratory measure as well (eg, a serum marker). You must be certain first that the measure squarely focuses on, or at least partly focuses on, the phenomenon you want to measure and track. Then, if it does, how good are the measurement properties of it? For example, if we find a PROM that proposes to measures the phenomena we are interested in (eg, rotator cuff physical function) then we must look for evidence of its psychometric/measurement properties.

Just like any other type of outcome, you need to make sure a PROM is valid, reliable, responsive, and interpretable. A measurement tool is considered valid when it actually measures what it proposes to measure. There are several types of validity including content, construct, and criterion validity. Reliability is the property of measuring some phenomenon in a predictable manner (repeatability). Some forms of reliability include internal consistency, test-retest or intra-rater, and inter-rater reliability. Responsiveness is the ability to detect change in the underlying construct over time, even if the changes are small. Finally, interpretability refers to the ability to derive meaning from the scores of the PROM; that is, is it clear what high or low scores mean, clinically or for the patient, or are there cutoffs or important values on the measure, etc.? The table below describes the psychometric properties you should consider (**Table 2**). Sometimes, you can find a systematic review of measurement properties to help guide you on how good a measure is, but in some cases, you need to gather the evidence yourself and make a determination if it is good or not. Simply using an outcome measure because it appears in the literature with high frequency is not justification for using it in your research. Using a poor measure severely biases your outcome measurement and can, as a result, harm patients to which such incorrect findings are applied or waste resources. Another consideration is the ease of use of a measure. That is, you should be able to actually implement the measurement tool for the types of patients you have, for the particular question of interest, for the timing needed, and, in some cases, you need to allocate funds to cover the cost of the measure. In particular, the timing or staging of an outcome measure is very important. In some cases, you make be looking at only one time point, but in many cases, you will have multiple time points—for example, when performing longitudinal research. The exact timing depends on the measure you are using, what phenomenon you are measuring, and the research participants' ability to complete the measure.

SCALE METRICS

There are a variety of scale metrics or statistics to consider when doing research with and attempting to interpret outcome measures that produce quantitative data. First, we have precision, which is defined as the property of having nearly the same value on each repeated measurement (also called

TABLE 2 Psychometric Properties of Patient-Reported Outcome Measures

Property	Description
Reliability	
Internal consistency	The extent to which items in a questionnaire (sub)scale are correlated (homogeneous), thus measuring the same concept
Reliability	The extent to which patients can be distinguished from each other, despite measurement error (relative measurement error)
Measurement error	The extent to which the scores on repeated measures are close to each other (absolute measurement error)
Validity	
Content validity	The extent to which the domain of interest is comprehensively sampled by the items in the questionnaire
Structural validity	The extent to which the scores of an instrument are an adequate reflection of the dimensionality of the construct to be measured
Hypothesis testing	The extent to which scores on a particular instrument relate to other measures in a manner that is consistent with theoretically derived hypotheses concerning the concepts that are being measured
Criterion validity	The extent to which scores on a particular instrument relate to a benchmark
Responsiveness	
Responsiveness	Responsiveness is a measure of longitudinal validity. In analogy to construct validity, longitudinal validity should be assessed by testing predefined hypotheses, eg, about expected correlations between changes in measures, or expected differences in changes between "known" groups

 ©Copyright 2021 American Academy of Orthopaedic Surgeons

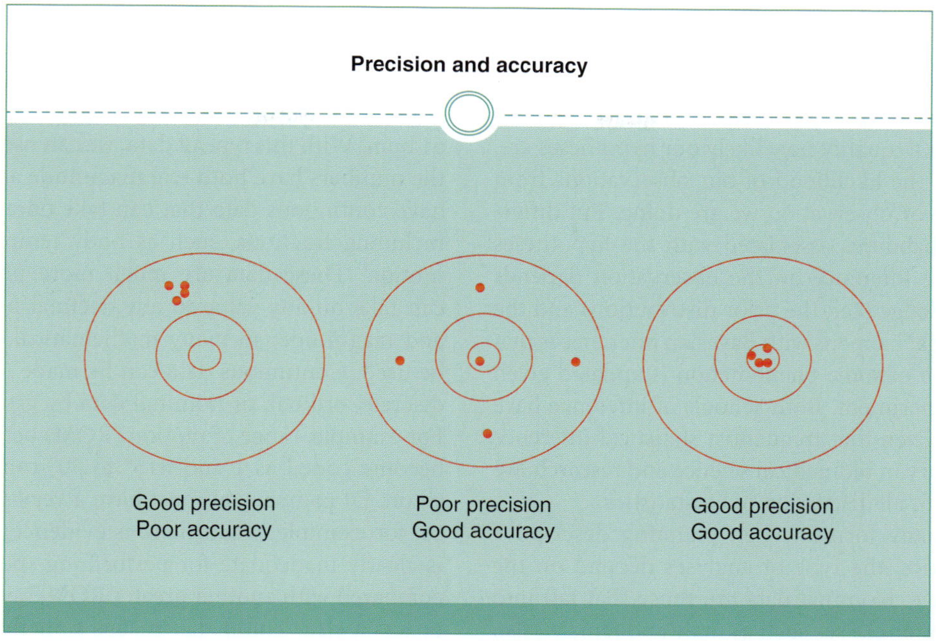

FIGURE 6 Chart demonstrating precision and accuracy.

test-retest reliability). Then we have accuracy, which is the degree to which a measurement, or an estimate based on measurements, represents the true value of the attribute that is being measured. The figure below illustrates these properties (**Figure 6**).

Furthermore, a measurement tool can be characterized in terms of sensitivity, specificity, positive predictive value (PPV), or negative predictive value (NPV). The sensitivity of an instrument is the probability that it identifies people with some phenomena or characteristic (eg, knee osteoarthritis) in those who truly have the phenomena or characteristic. Sensitive tests are very useful for screening because they are unlikely to miss patients with a disease, for example. A highly sensitive test will rule out patients without the condition with confidence (SnOut = sensitivity rules out individuals). Specificity is the probability that a test result will be negative in patients without the disease. Specific tests are useful for confirmation that a person does not have some condition or disease as they do not result in treatment of an unaffected individual. A highly specific test will rule in patients with a high degree of confidence (SpIN = Specificity rules in). A false-positive is a patient without the disease who has a positive test result. A false-negative is a patient with disease who has a negative test result. One can construct a receiver operating characteristic (ROC) curve by plotting the sensitivity of some test verses 1-specificity. The total area under the curve gives a good measure of the accuracy of a test or instrument. This ROC curve is very useful in evaluating the diagnostic ability of a test to discriminate the true state of subjects, finding the optimal cutoff values for the measure, and comparing two alternative diagnostic tests when each is performed on the same subject. Next, a positive predictive value (PPV) is the probability that a patient with a positive test result actually has the disease. Next, a negative predictive value (NPV) is the probability that a patient with a negative test actually has no disease. Remember the PPV and NPV are dependent on the prevalence of disease. Prevalence is the total number of cases of a disease present at any one point in time, whereas incidence is the number of newly reported cases of a disease during a given time period.

DATA MANAGEMENT AND INTRODUCTION TO STATISTICS FOR CLINICAL RESEARCH

In this section, we discuss some basic concepts related to biostatistical theory, summarizing data, and several other key concepts related to clinical research data. First, we must distinguish between descriptive and inferential statistics. Descriptive statistics are the set of methods for organizing and summarizing your data or observations. This might include tables, graphs, and numerical summary measures such as measures of central tendency (eg, mean, median, mode) and measures of dispersion, or spread of the data (eg, confidence intervals, standard error, SD, interquartile range). Inferential statistics take empirical data and attempts to make inferences about the world from it. That is, data from some experiment or observation are used to make judgments about phenomena in the world. There are two broad classes of inferential statistics: frequentist and Bayesian. Frequentist statistical inference draws conclusions from data from a sample by using frequency and proportion applications to the data, by performing hypothesis testing, and using confidence intervals, for example. The assumption is that the probabilities in an experiment represent long-term frequencies of repeatable random experiments. That is, frequentist statistics states that any given experiment

©Copyright 2021 American Academy of Orthopaedic Surgeons

can be considered as one of the potential results of the theoretical infinite repetitions of the same experiment. Whereas, Bayesian statistical inference suggests that because we typically have some knowledge of prior experiments, we can use this prior knowledge to qualify how likely our hypotheses are, which then changes the likelihood of our observations from the new experiment or observation we are doing. Put differently, there are probabilities associated with the hypotheses and the data, so the inference on the observation depends on both prior knowledge (call the prior distribution) and the observed data. So what happens with Bayesian inference is that the prior distribution of some phenomenon is updated given the data from an experiment. Both schools of inference have strong supporters. Given that frequentist statistical inference is the dominant theory in biomedical science and research, we will defer to it here for all discussion of biostatistics.

Data come in many forms. When planning descriptive or inferential statistics, the type of analyses depend on the type of data you have. Nominal data are those that fall into unordered categories or classes such as male and female (also dichotomous) or device types A, B, and C. With nominal data, the numbers serve as labels only (eg, the devices could be coded as device 1, 2, and 3) but the numbers themselves have no mathematical meaning. Ordinal data are those that fall into ordered categories such as severity of injury classed as mild, moderate, or severe. There is an inherent order to the classes, but the difference between classes is not necessarily equal. That is, the difference in injury severity between mild and moderate may not be quantitatively or qualitatively the same as the difference between moderate and severe. Next, discrete data are those in which both order and magnitude are important, such as the number of births (1, 2, or 3) or beats per minute of the heart (eg, 70 bpm). In these cases, the numbers represent measurable quantities and they are typically counts or integers. You cannot have 1/2 beat or 1/3 birth. It happens or it does not happen. And the difference between 1 birth and 2 births is the same as between 2 and 3 births. There is also a natural order to the data in that 60 bpm comes before 61 bpm. With this type of data, we can use arithmetic, because the numbers have both real magnitude and order. Finally, we have continuous data that can take on any numerical value, including fractions, such as body temperature or range of motion. These data are much more precise, because they can take on any value to any decimal place and have order and magnitude, so many mathematical operations can also be used. Continuous data can be made ("transformed") into discrete, ordinal, or nominal data by grouping observations. For example, range of motion (ROM) between 0° and 15° can become coded as 1 and >15° to 30° can be coded as 2 and so on. Of course, you must have a very good rationale to do so; for example, when there is evidence that a certain ROM is clearly inadequate for performing specific daily activities compared with another greater ROM, say when there is more or less a clear cutoff that means something for the patients. But doing so decreases the granularity of the data, so preciseness suffers. As we move from nominal to ordinal to discrete to continuous, the possible data values become more complex, which necessitates different statistical analyses and data representations.

PARAMETRIC AND NONPARAMETRIC DATA

When looking at summaries of the continuous data you must determine whether the data are parametric or nonparametric. That is, are the data normally distributed (**Figure 7**)? When plotted in a line graph, there should be a relatively obvious grouping of observations in the center of the figure and less as you move out from the center. The "bell-shaped" curve

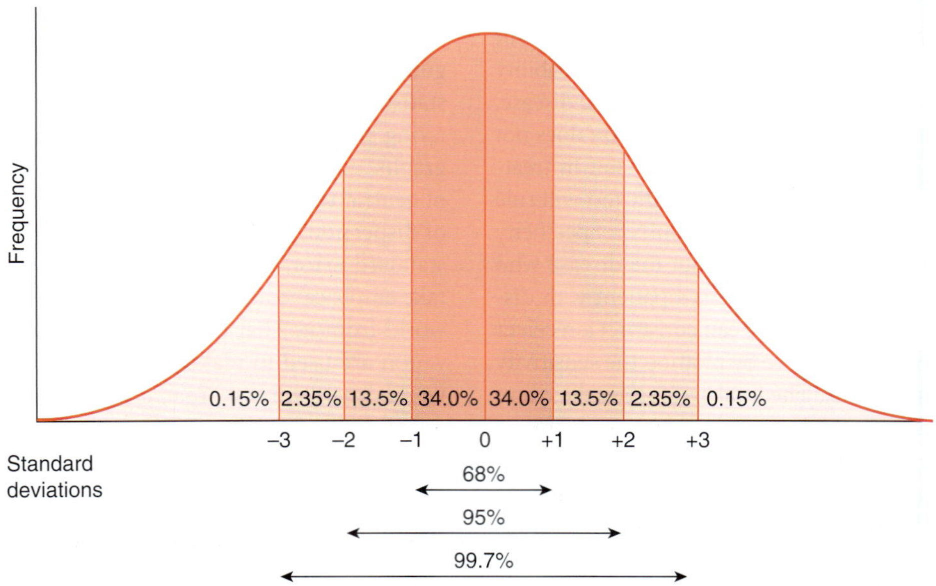

FIGURE 7 Graph demonstrating normal curve.

©Copyright 2021 American Academy of Orthopaedic Surgeons

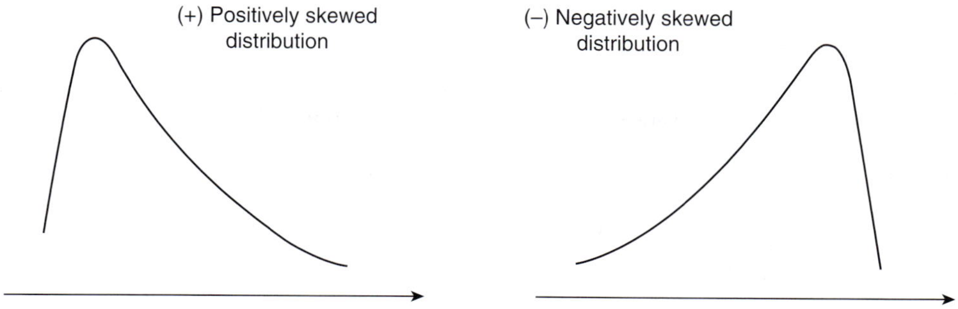

FIGURE 8 Line graph demonstrating skewed distributions.

seen below is a classic example of a parametric distribution of data or a normal distribution, though you will likely not see such a symmetric plot of real data from a sample. You can see from this plot that as you move out from the center of bell (marked with 0), the frequency of observations goes down. SDs are marked on this figure indicating the percent of the area under the curve or percent of observations in each shaded area. Within the area between −1 and +1 SD, there is approximately 68% of the sample of observations. An SD is a measure of the distance from the "center" of the sample (eg, mean). When using descriptive statistics to summarize parametric continuous data, a mean and a measure of variance (SD, or a confidence interval; CI) are sufficient. An SD is essentially the average deviation from the mean of all observations, and it is in the same units as the mean. A CI is another measure of the spread of the observations and gives some idea of the precision of an estimate. Generally, a 95% confidence interval means we are 95% confident that the values between the lower and upper limit contain the true parameter value, out there in the real world, that this data set is attempting to explain. More specifically, a 95% CI means that if we take 100 random samples from the same population and calculate 100 different confidence intervals approximately 95 would cover the true population mean and 5 would not. Thus, a 95% confidence interval is an estimate of these 100 CIs. Several parametric inferential statistical tests for continuous data include *t*-tests, repeated measures *t*-tests, ANOVAs, and repeated measures ANOVAs.

However, the distribution or curve may not be symmetric and may not approximate a normal/parametric curve. The figure below (**Figure 8**) illustrates two nonparametric curves, the one on the left positively skewed, meaning there is a long tail of observations to the right of the center of the curve, in the direction of positive values. The curve on the right is negatively skewed, with a long tail of observations to the left of the center of the curve, in the direction of negative values. In the case of nonparametric continuous data, you will need to use nonparametric statistical tests including the sign test, Wilcoxon signed rank test, Mann-Whitney test, Kolmorogov-Smirnov text, Kruskal-Wallis test, and Friedman test. The table below compares parametric and nonparametric tests for different forms of parametric and nonparametric data (**Table 3**).

To determine if your sample of data is normal or not, you can visually examine the distribution of data as we suggest above: the so-called "eyeball" test. But, in addition, there are a several formal statistical tests you can run including the Kolmogorov-Smirnov test and Shapiro-Wilk test, which are both available in most statistical packages.

P-VALUES

Finally, once you have done all of your descriptive analyses and inferential testing, you can calculate effect estimates and a *P*-value for these effect estimates. A *P*-value is the probability of obtaining a more extreme test statistic than what was observed if the null hypothesis is true. It is not the probability that the null hypothesis is true or that the result is due to chance. A *P*-value reflects the extent to which the hypothesis being tested is compatible with the observed results. The smaller the *P*-value, the less compatible the null hypothesis is with the observed results. In most applications, the hypothesis being tested is the null hypothesis of no association between the exposure or treatment of interest and the outcome. An important caveat is that the accuracy of the *P*-value is only

TABLE 3 Parametric and Nonparametric Statistical Tests

Number of Samples Being Compared	Parametric Tests	Nonparametric Tests
One	One sample *t*-test	Sign test Wilcoxon signed rank test
Two	Paired *t*-test Unpaired *t*-test (Student *t*-test)	Sign test Wilcoxon signed rank test Mann-Whitney test Kolmorogov-Smirnov test
K-samples	Analysis of variance Two-way analysis of variance	Kruskal-Wallis test Jonckheere test Friedman test

©Copyright 2021 American Academy of Orthopaedic Surgeons

as good as the underlying statistical model and the related assumptions used to arrive at it. If the model is appropriate, a small *P*-value casts doubt on the null hypothesis. In contrast to common belief, statistical findings never tell us whether there is or is not a treatment or exposure effect. Rather, statistical results—estimated associations—convey a continuum of information that we use, along with other information, to make inferences about hypothesized effects. Confidence intervals are recommended to complement the interpretation of findings because they convey information about the magnitude and direction of the association as well as the precision with which the parameter has been estimated.

MISSING DATA

In clinical research, you may have missing data, and this occurs for variety of reasons. For example, you may be performing a prospective clinical trial that involves an intervention with some serious unintended effects and patients are dropping out frequently and earlier than expected. In this case, you have data missing for particular patients from one point going forward. Missing data due to systematic drop-outs (or similar reasons) are problematic such that it changes the distribution of patients, especially if there is uneven dropout from one arm compared with another in a randomized study. In other studies, you may have frequent and many outcome measures to collect; so in some cases, you may have missing data points for particular follow-ups across an array of patients, but who have not completely dropped from the study. In other cases, you may have patients who, in an experimental study, do not comply with the allocated intervention to some extent. For example, they may not take an intended oral medication as instructed.

When you have missing data due to drop-outs or missing outcomes, then you must in some way deal with this. The first option is that you could ignore it, which would not be wise, because the findings in your study could be biased away or toward the null. You can withdraw or remove all patients with incomplete data, which can also be problematic because your remaining sample will not be representative of the sample you had at the start. If the study was randomized, then withdrawing such patients potentially undermines the original randomization performed. So, what can be done in the analysis of clinical research with missing or unavailable data?

If there is a substantial amount of missing data, then no analytic methods can rescue the study. But, if the amount of missing data is minimal or relatively small, then there is whole selection of imputation methods that can be helpful. Imputation simply means to fill in the missing data using other data that you actually do have from that study. A single imputation method is that of "last observation carried forward," also called end point analysis. It involves making the assumption that all future observations would have remained constant, which in many cases is not a valid assumption. Multiple imputation procedures are more robust than single imputation and involve the use of regression methods followed by the standard analysis for each imputation method, after which the findings are compared. In this manner, you get an array of possible outcomes depending on the exact imputation specifications, the range of which should contain the "true" findings had there not be any missing data.

When conducting an experimental study, and in particular a randomized trial, one has to consider how to deal with noncompliance with experimental interventions. Generally, if you have a selection of patients who either never take the intended intervention, do so to a lesser extent than planned (eg, a lower dose), or take some other intervention, then, to preserve the randomization process, you must do what is called an intention to treat (ITT) analysis. An ITT analysis means you analyze the outcome of the patients as if they actually got the intended intervention, even if they did not. This is done because the randomization procedure theoretically equally distributed all potential covariates or confounders between the assignment groups, and therefore, to not analyze certain individuals due to a lack of compliance may cause imbalance in the remaining group compositions, which may bias the treatment effect estimates. An alternative approach is the per protocol (PP) method, which only analyzes those patients who actually got the intended planned interventions, and everyone else is excluded from the analyses. Of course, certain patients could have been noncompliant in a systematic manner; they could all share some characteristic or set of characteristics that are confounders or effect modifiers or they could have been differentially noncompliant between the intervention groups. Either way, the patients left in the study, and those in one of the treatment groups, may be different than those originally assigned to those intervention groups. The ITT and PP analyses are only two options and can be implemented in a variety of different ways. There is also the "as treated" method, which can sometimes be used and generally refers to including all subjects and doing comparisons on the interventions they actually received, where possible.

There are a variety of methodologic implementations that can decrease the risk of missing data or withdrawals or lack of compliance. Of course, these partly depend on the exact question of the clinical study and sometimes are difficult to avoid. Generally, interventions that are easy to comply with or have substantial support for compliance are better. Also, less frequent and less invasive or obtrusive outcome measures decrease risks to data losses. Furthermore, patient incentives, monetary or otherwise, are helpful as is frequent patient contact (ie, by phone, e-mail, in person) about the research, its progress, and impact.

DATA MONITORING COMMITTEES

Two additional items for consideration in prospective clinical studies are the need to include a data monitoring committee (DMC), sometimes called a data and safety monitoring committee (DSMC), and statistical stopping rules. DMCs are

©Copyright 2021 American Academy of Orthopaedic Surgeons

typically composed of individuals who are independent of the study team with relevant expertise in the clinical field or specialty, individuals with expertise in the conduct of clinical studies, clinical epidemiologists, biostatisticians, and for particular studies bioethicists and patient advocates. This group regularly monitors the response variables or other patient outcomes (eg, adverse events) for early dramatic benefits or potential harmful effects. This involves looking at the data and the outcomes in a continual manner and suggesting relevant additional analyses to gain insight into the study progress and risk or not to patients. The primary objective of the DMC is to ensure the safety of the patients. The points at which the DMC meet should be predetermined in the study protocol but should also be responsive to the need for additional meetings in light of data and communications from the investigators. The process for making a decision to stop or continue a study can be complex and no single statistical procedure, or stopping rule, is adequate across all circumstances. But when taken together with other material, statistical stopping boundaries can assist the DMC in making decisions. There are many statistical stopping rules available and while these must always be preplanned, before patient enrollment and data collection, the exact statistical methods used are dictated by the study questions and planned outcome data. Friedman et al[2] include excellent recommendations for DMCs and give an overview of statistical stopping rule procedures.

SUMMARY

Clinical research is sometimes difficult but always rewarding. Careful consideration of methodologic aspects as you are planning your study can save considerable effort and protect your study from bias. This chapter gave an overview of a selection of principles in clinical research[3] that, if carefully considered, can strengthen planned research and improve your ability for critical interpretation of the literature. Data from clinical research can influence clinical practice, patient outcomes, and the use of healthcare resources, so every effort must be made to perform these studies with rigor in integrity.

REFERENCES

1. Centre for Evidence-Based Medicine: Critical Appraisal Tools. Available at: https://www.cebm.net/2014/06/critical-appraisal/. Accessed February 8, 2019.
2. Friedman LM, Furberg CD, DeMets DL, Reboussin DM, Granger CB: *Fundamentals of Clinical Trials*, ed 5. New York, Springer, 2015.
3. Hulley SB, Cummings SR, Browner WS, Grady DG, Newman TB: Designing Clinical Research, 4th ed. Philadelphia, Lippincott Williams & Wilkins, 2013.

©Copyright 2021 American Academy of Orthopaedic Surgeons

41

Observational Studies

William A. Cantrell, BS
Kurt P. Spindler, MD

Keywords: *case-control; cross-sectional; prospective cohort; retrospective cohort*

INTRODUCTION

Observational studies are conducted to evaluate a patient population and then to determine prognosis of outcomes of interest. The studies first report the distribution of outcomes and potential predictors (risk factors) for the outcomes of interest in the population. Then, by analyzing these distributions, the associations between predictor and outcome can be understood, and thus prediction of outcomes can be inferred.[1] To gain these insights, different types of observational studies can be employed. The most common types of observational studies are a prospective cohort and retrospective cohort. Other types include cross-sectional and case-control. This chapter will define these study types, describe the differences between them, and suggest the situations for which each study design is optimal.

Dr. Spindler or an immediate family member has received royalties from nPhase; serves as a paid consultant to or is an employee of Cytori-Scientific Advisory Board, Mitek, and NFL; has received research or institutional support from National Institutes of Health (NIAMS and NICHD); and serves as a board member, owner, officer, or committee member of the American Academy of Orthopaedic Surgeons, the American Orthopaedic Society for Sports Medicine, and the Orthopaedic Research Society. Neither Dr. Cantrell nor any immediate family member has received anything of value from or has stock or stock options held in a commercial company or institution related directly or indirectly to the subject of this chapter.

CROSS-SECTIONAL STUDIES

The cross-sectional study design provides insight into the population being studied at a single point or moment in time.[1] Thus, they are best suited for the descriptive studies, as opposed to predictive studies. When using a cross-sectional design to gain descriptive information, the investigator must recognize that only prevalence, and not incidence, can be determined. Prevalence describes the number of patients in a population who have a condition at a single point in time, whereas incidence is defined as the proportion of the population who have newly developed the condition over a set period of time.[1] Prevalence holds significant weight in the clinical environment because it informs clinicians of a patient's likelihood of having a certain condition before obtaining a thorough workup, which, in statistical language, is labeled that patient's prior probability of having the disease.[1] A good example of the cross-sectional study design and the importance of understanding prevalence is the study by Sher et al. published in *The Journal of Bone and Joint Surgery* (JBJS) in 1995, where MRI findings on 96 asymptomatic shoulders were described.[2] The study reported that 54% of patients (25/46) above 60 years of age with an asymptomatic shoulder had a rotator cuff tear visible on MRI of that shoulder, with 52% of those (13/25) being full-thickness tears.[2] The high prevalence of rotator cuff tears in patients with asymptomatic shoulders is a reminder to clinicians to be cautious when correlating rotator cuff as only cause of shoulder pain and symptoms.[2]

Although the cross-sectional design is better for a descriptive study, it can have limited use to study associations. When doing so, it is of the utmost importance to carefully draft an appropriate hypothesis, because in this case that hypothesis defines the predictors and outcomes.[1] Sometimes determining which variables serve which roles is rather straightforward, such as when using demographic factors such as age or sex,

©Copyright 2021 American Academy of Orthopaedic Surgeons

as they are never dependent and so always serve as predictors. However, teasing out which is the cause and which is the effect sometimes is unknown. For example, if an obese patient has a low Marx activity score, it is challenging at that moment in time to determine which is the predictor and which is the outcome, and so those roles are dependent on the hypothesis applied. Therefore, in general, cross-sectional studies are primarily for descriptive purposes.

STRENGTHS AND WEAKNESSES OF CROSS-SECTIONAL STUDIES

Convenience is one of the major strengths of a cross-sectional design, as these studies are quick to complete and relatively inexpensive.[1] As a result, these types of studies are often included as an initial component of randomized controlled trials or cohort studies. One common reason for this approach is to obtain information, including demographic data, about the patients at baseline. In other study types, especially cohort and randomized controlled trials, losing patients to follow-up is a major concern because of the bias it can introduce into the results; however, because follow-up is not required for cross-sectional studies, this potential problem does not affect them.[1]

Although these strengths are often useful, it is important to recognize and acknowledge the limitations of the cross-sectional study design. First and foremost, determining causal relationships is quite difficult in this approach, especially because of the lack of time-related data.[1] It can be difficult to distinguish whether a factor has a causative influence on a disease or whether it is merely associated with the disease being present. Answers to these types of questions can be explored better with the study designs discussed later in this chapter. Another area in which the cross-sectional study design does not perform particularly well is when the investigator intends on studying rare diseases or rare events; in this situation, the cross-sectional design is impractical because of the exceptionally large sample size that would be required.[1] Despite this limitation, one way that the cross-sectional study design has been applied with utility in this context is through a case series approach, where observations are reported on a sample that exclusively contains patients who have the desired condition or who have experienced the event in question.[1] The case series works well for providing information about disease characteristics, but it does not work well for answering comparative questions.[1]

PROSPECTIVE COHORT STUDIES

In a cohort study, a group of patients is selected and observed over a period of time.[1] This can be done either prospectively, where patients are identified by the investigator and then followed into the future, or retrospectively, where patients are identified and their past records are examined.[1] The objective of a prospective cohort study is to measure or record potential predictors (risk factors especially modifiable ones) of outcome and then to follow up with the patients periodically to determine patient outcomes.[1] One of the most commonly known studies of this kind is the Framingham cohort study, which has given significant insight into many areas including the heart health, hypertension, and even noncardiac diseases such as dementia.[3-5]

In orthopaedic surgery, one of the major prospective cohort studies is the Multicenter Orthopaedics Outcome Network (MOON).[6,7] Over 3,500 patients who underwent anterior cruciate ligament reconstruction (ACLR) were enrolled.[7] For these patients, numerous hypothesized predictors were recorded at the time of surgery, including body mass index (BMI), smoking status, age, preoperative physical examination, and a Marx activity score to indicate the patient's preinjury level of activity. Baseline information for a variety of patient-reported outcome measures (PROMs), namely IKDC, KOOS, WOMAC, and Marx activity rating score, were also obtained. Each surgeon documented intraoperative data, including the presence of meniscus pathology (and treatment conducted) and the location and severity of cartilage defects. For follow-up time points, PROMs were completed by patients who were contacted either passively (via a direct mail questionnaire) or actively (via phone calls to the patients) at 2, 6, and 10 years postoperatively.[7] From this cohort, numerous important insights have been gained, including the ACLR prognosis for PROMs at 10 years after ACLR and the modifiable risk factors of patient-reported outcomes (PROs) at that time.[6] PROs were initially measured at 2 years postoperatively and then stayed constant at the 6- and 10-year follow-up points.[6,7] Because of the prospective design and high rate of follow-up (greater than 80%), the risk factors for worse outcomes at 10-year follow-up were able to be identified in a level I prognostic cohort. They were lower baseline scores on the PROMs, higher BMI, smoking, having a surgery for meniscus pathology before index ACLR, undergoing lateral meniscectomy during the index ACLR, undergoing a revision ACLR, grade 3 or 4 defects in the articular cartilage of any knee compartment, and undergoing a subsequent surgical procedure on the ipsilateral knee after the index ACLR.[6] Knowledge of these predictors helps us better identify which patients are at a higher risk of worse outcome, better educate patients on modifiable risk factors, and encourage clinicians to act in ways to reduce risk of these factors developing (eg, choosing meniscectomy over meniscus repair in situations where repair success is in avascular zone because of the significant negative influence of a second surgery on outcomes).

Another example of an excellent prospective cohort study is the Multicenter ACL Revision Study (MARS).[8] Patients

©Copyright 2021 American Academy of Orthopaedic Surgeons

who underwent revision ACLR were enrolled in the study prospectively. In a similar fashion to MOON, preoperative and intraoperative data collection occurred on a variety of predictors including demographics, pathology, and surgical technique used. PROMs were also administered at baseline and then at 2 years follow-up.[8] One of the most influential studies from this cohort showed that allograft had worse PROMs as compared with autograft for revision ACLRs at 2 years and the graft re-rupture rate for allografts was significantly higher.[8]

STRENGTHS

The greatest advantage of a prospective cohort study is that the results identify both prognosis and predictors of outcomes. This is demonstrated in the MOON and MARS the studies referenced above. Cohort studies also have the significant advantage of providing appropriate information to determine incidence.[1] The causal inference can be more strongly asserted in a cohort design compared with other observational designs because the predictors are examined and recorded before the outcome.[1] An additional advantage in the case of the prospective cohort study is that the lack of knowledge of the outcome (its presence or absence, characteristics about it) reduces the potential for bias in the measurement of the predictors; thus, variable measurement in prospective studies is typically more accurate and complete than in retrospective studies.[1] Risk of recall bias, where patients with the outcome remember a predictor disproportionately to patients without the outcome, is significantly decreased in prospective studies compared with retrospective ones.[1]

WEAKNESSES

Confounding is a significant issue in cohort studies; confounders are variables that are related to both the outcome and the predictor, and they thereby can cause associations/predictions to be erroneous. These variables can be difficult to control for in all observational studies, including cohort studies.[1] However, with careful hypotheses and understanding of the disease processes, an investigator can account for confounders by including them in the model as long as the sample size is large enough to allow many variables to be tested and/or included. However, unknown confounders cannot be controlled for in modeling. This is a major statistical advantage of a randomized controlled trial. Another issue with prospective cohort studies, which is also experienced in cross-sectional studies, is that they are inefficient when the primary objective is to study rare results.[1] However, unlike the cross-sectional design, prospective cohort studies are very expensive, especially if sufficient follow-up is obtained (>70%).[1]

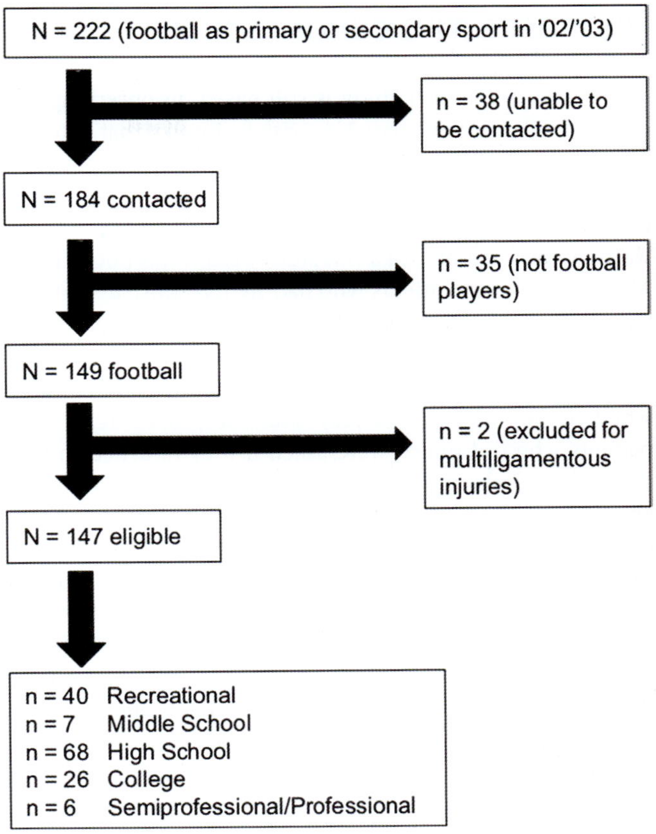

FIGURE 1 STROBE diagram representing patients screened, excluded (including exclusion reason), and enrolled in the retrospective cohort study by McCullough et al on return to high school and college football after anterior cruciate ligament reconstruction. (Data from McCullough KA, Phelps KD, Spindler KP, et al: Return to high school- and college-level football after anterior cruciate ligament reconstruction: a Multicenter Orthopaedic Outcomes Network (MOON) cohort study. *Am J Sports Med* 2012;40:2523-2529.)

KEY POINT ON ENROLLMENT

In the creation of a prospective cohort study, one of the most important elements is the definition of the cohort itself and thereby the enrolling of patients. When enrolling patients, there must be a balance between rigidity and laxity in the inclusion and exclusion criteria. If too rigid, the sample size will be too small or it will take an excessive amount of time to reach the enrollment goal. If the sample becomes too heterogeneous because of less controlled criteria, the results may not be able to be interpreted appropriately. In addition, once the study begins, there must be a system to document the number of patients screened and enrolled so that the influence of selection bias, if any, can be explicitly shown. The Strengthening the Reporting of Observational Studies in Epidemiology (STROBE) diagram (see **Figure 1**) is the optimal way to represent these enrollment data for publication.[9,10]

©Copyright 2021 American Academy of Orthopaedic Surgeons

RETROSPECTIVE COHORT STUDIES

A retrospective cohort study is still based on observing outcome and identifying predictors (risk factors) of that outcome, like the prospective cohort study. However, the retrospective study differs because it is completed by looking into the past to find the predictors, as opposed to following patients forward. A good example of a this study design was published by McCullough et al. Patients who had ACL reconstructions and who recorded football as either their primary or secondary sport on a preoperative questionnaire (obtained as a component of a different study) were contacted after ACLR to inquire whether they returned to play after the procedure.[11] Those patients who did return were asked if they returned to their prior level of play, and those who did not return were asked about their reasons for not returning. It was found that 63% of high school athletes and 69% of collegiate players returned to football. 27% of all players stated that they never returned to their preinjury performance level, while 30% never returned to play. Of those who did not return to play, fear of further damage or reinjury was reported in 50%.[11] Because of these data, clinicians were now more accurately able to inform patients of the likelihood that they would return to play and the most significant reasons why players failed to return.

STRENGTHS AND WEAKNESSES

The strengths and weaknesses of the retrospective cohort study are similar in most respects to those for the prospective variety.[1] Retrospective cohort studies allow prediction of outcome, although not with the same strength of prospective studies. When compared against the prospective version, retrospective studies have the advantage of being able to be completed much more quickly and more cheaply.[1] However, the increased efficiency comes at a cost, as the investigator has a limited ability to control follow-up time and the sampling of the population.[1] There are also concerns about the quality and accuracy of measurements obtained at baseline.[1] Confounding is still a major factor, and it is often more difficult to adjust for in retrospective studies because the data available can often be of questionable accuracy, measured in ways that are not ideal for the investigation, or even incomplete.[1]

STATISTICS OF COHORT STUDIES

The majority of cohort studies, both prospective and retrospective, require multivariate modeling, which can be quite complex and, as such, goes beyond the scope of this chapter. It is often very helpful if not necessary for a statistician to conduct the analysis to ensure an accurate and appropriate interpretation of the data.

CASE-CONTROL STUDIES

Case-control studies are conducted such that two groups of patients, one with the outcome (also known as cases) and one without (also known as the control group), are included in the study and then predictors are compared between the two groups to determine which influence the outcome. This design is optimal for studying rare outcomes or diseases.[1] In these cases, multivariable modeling cannot be performed because there is too low of an incidence for the outcome of interest.

Cohort studies can be prospective or retrospective, whereas case-control studies are mainly retrospective; they always identify a group with the disease/outcome and a group without, and then the investigator looks back in time to judge the differences between the groups with respect to potential predictors.[1]

An excellent example of a case-control study was published by Beynnon et al in AJSM in 2015.[12] The authors recruited 88 patients who had a first-time ACL tear (grade III, resulting from a noncontact injury) and 88 matched-control subjects who were uninjured.[12] Each subject enrolled underwent an MRI on either the injured knee in the cases or the corresponding knee in the matched controls, and measurements were determined for the size of the ACL and femoral intercondylar notch.[12] In addition, information on the geometry of multiple anatomic structures was recorded; the structures were meniscus, articular cartilage, subchondral bone of the tibial plateau, and the tibial spines.[12] Then, multivariate logistic modeling was completed to determine the risk of noncontact ACL injury in males and in females. The modeling showed that, for males, the highest risk of noncontact ACL injury was incurred with a decreased ACL volume and decreased wedge angle in the lateral compartment between the posterior meniscus and the subchondral bone. For females, the anatomic factors that led to the greatest increased risk of noncontact ACL injury were a decreased width of the femoral notch and an increased slope of the tibial articular cartilage when measured in a posteroinferior direction.[12]

STRENGTHS AND WEAKNESSES

Like cohort studies, case-control studies can inform the investigator both about descriptive characteristics of the disease/outcome of focus and about predictors of that outcome. The primary outcome in this study type is an odds ratio, which represents an approximate strength of the association between the outcome and the predictor variable.[1] In addition to the descriptive and predictive information, case-control studies are often useful for generating hypotheses for future studies.[1]

©Copyright 2021 American Academy of Orthopaedic Surgeons

Case-control studies do have several noteworthy weaknesses. One is that only a single disease or outcome can be examined at a time, whereas multiple outcome variables can be studied in cohort studies.[1] Another weakness of the case-control design is that they cannot give insight into prevalence or incidence, because the proportion of case to control is determined by the investigator during study design.[1] Finally, and most significantly, bias is a more severe concern in case-control studies than in cohort studies.[1] Not only is selection bias a concern, but recall bias is also a problem. Recall bias is where patients who have a condition may recall their exposure to a predictor better than the controls.[1]

NESTED CASE-CONTROL STUDY

This subtype of case-control study occurs when the cases and controls are selected from a cohort that is either as a part of a separate cohort study or defined as the first step in the study.[1] This approach is often taken to obtain both the cases and controls from a patient population that is notably at risk for the disease or outcome.[1]

One good example of a nested case-control study was published by Westermann et al; it compares the outcomes of patients who had combined ACL and medial collateral ligament (MCL) injuries based on whether they had surgical or nonsurgical management.[13] It is a nested case-control study because the patients serving as both cases and controls were selected from those enrolled in a multicenter prospective cohort study on ACL reconstruction.[13] This study reported that patients who had surgical treatment had lower PROMs at 2 years follow-up.[13] In addition, the surgical treatment group had a higher percentage of cases that required revision surgery for arthrofibrosis.[13] Marx activity scores were also lower at 2 years in the surgical group.[13] All of the data from this case-control study suggested that patients with nonsurgical management have better outcomes; however, it did clarify that there may be an unidentified subset of patients with ACL and MCL injuries who do better with surgical management but have not been identified.[13]

DECISION-MAKING

When designing an observational study, several factors contribute to the design chosen. The first decision is whether to make the study single center or multicenter. Multicenter studies are much more difficult to manage and organize, but they can be very helpful for increasing enrollment, especially in the case of rare outcomes, and for increasing generalizability. Single-center studies are easier to manage, but they can take much longer to reach the enrollment goal. The two situations where observational design decisions should be clearest are the following: when the objective is to improve an already successful treatment and identify the factors that can influence this, a single-center prospective cohort is the optimal approach; in the event where the condition or outcome is rare, a case-control design should be undertaken.

SUMMARY

Cross-sectional studies look at a population at one point in time. They are quick to complete and inexpensive to conduct. Although they can provide useful baseline information and are not subject to concerns about loss to follow-up that other studies are, the design is not well suited to make comparative statements or determine causal relationships.[1]

Prospective cohort studies follow a group of the patients into the future to determine predictors of outcomes. They allow for much better understanding of predictors of outcomes than any other study type, and bias is less of an issue because of the lack of knowledge of outcome at the start of the study. However, confounding is a major concern, and so it is important to have a well-planned design that allows the investigator to account for potential confounding variables. In addition, prospective cohort studies can be expensive and can take a long time to complete, especially for uncommon outcomes.[1]

Retrospective cohort studies also look at prediction, and they do so in a quicker and cheaper way than prospective studies. However, they have an increased risk of bias, a limited ability to control sampling, and they have an even higher risk of confounding and data issues, including missing data elements or inadequate recording of data.[1]

Case-control studies involve studying an outcome or disease in questions, especially a rare one, by identifying a group with the disease and a group without and then retrospectively studying predictors. They are generally cheaper, but they have a number of significant limitations including an increased risk for bias, the inability to comment on incidence or prevalence, and the lack of ability to examine more than one outcome.[1]

Finally, please see **Table 1** for a summary of the investigator experience and minimum level of assistance recommended for cohort and case-control trials based on the variables/outcomes of interest and the type of study.

©Copyright 2021 American Academy of Orthopaedic Surgeons

TABLE 1 Recommended Minimum Investigator Experience and Assistance for Studies

Design	PRO F/U	PE Testing F/U	Imaging	Biomarkers	Minimum PI Experience	Minimum Assistance
Single-center cohort (PRO only)	Yes	No	No	No	Limited	Research assistant (maybe)
Single-center cohort (with PE)	Yes	Yes	No	No	Limited	Research assistant
Single-center cohort (incl. imaging and/or biomarkers)	Yes	Yes	Yes	Yes	Some experience	Research coordinator
Multicenter cohort	Yes	Yes/No	Yes/No	Yes/No	Moderate to extensive	Research coordinator and methodologist (biostatistics, epidemiology)
Case-control	Yes	No	Maybe	Maybe	Limited	Biostats Preexisting database

This is a summary table for each type of observational study based on the variables/outcomes the investigator would like to include. Given the study design and elements included/collected at follow-up, the table recommends the minimum level of experience the investigator should have and the minimum assistance required to complete the study well.
PE = physical exam, PI – principal investigator, PRO = patient-reported outcome

REFERENCES

1. Hulley SB, Cummings SR, Newman TB: Designing cross-sectional and cohort studies, in *Designing Clinical Research*. Philadelphia, PA, Wolters Kluwer/Lippincott Williams & Wilkins, 2013, (Chap 7); Newman TB, Browner WS, Cummings SR, Hulley SB: Designing case-control studies, in *Designing Clinical Research*. Philadelphia, PA, Wolters Kluwer/Lippincott Williams & Wilkins, 2013, (Chap 8).
2. Sher JS, Uribe JW, Posada A, Murphy BJ, Zlatkin MB: Abnormal findings on magnetic resonance images of asymptomatic shoulders. *J Bone Joint Surg Am* 1995;77:10-15.
3. Kannel WB: Framingham study insights into hypertensive risk of cardiovascular disease. *Hypertens Res* 1995;18:181-196.
4. Parikh NI, Pencina MJ, Wang TJ, et al: A risk score for predicting near-term incidence of hypertension: the Framingham Heart Study. *Ann Intern Med* 2008;148:102-110.
5. Satizabal CL, Beiser AS, Chouraki V, et al: Incidence of dementia over three decades in the Framingham Heart Study. *N Engl J Med* 2016;374:523-532.
6. MOON Knee Group, Spindler KP, Huston LJ, Chagin KM, et al: Ten-year outcomes and risk factors after anterior cruciate ligament reconstruction: A MOON longitudinal prospective cohort study. *Am J Sports Med* 2018;46:815-825.
7. Vega JF, Spindler KP: To MOON and back. *Clin Sports Med* 2018;37:495-503.
8. Wright RW, Huston LJ, Haas AK, et al: Effect of graft choice on the outcome of revision anterior cruciate ligament reconstruction in the Multicenter ACL Revision Study (MARS) Cohort. *Am J Sports Med* 2014;42:2301-2310.
9. Vandenbroucke JP: Strengthening the reporting of observational studies in epidemiology (STROBE): Explanation and elaboration. *Ann Intern Med* 2007;147:W163-W194.
10. Egger M, Jüni P, Bartlett C, CONSORT Group (Consolidated Standards of Reporting of Trials: Value of flow diagrams in reports of randomized controlled trials. *J Am Med Assoc* 2001;285:1996-1999.
11. McCullough KA, Phelps KD, Spindler KP, et al: Return to high school- and college-level football after anterior cruciate ligament reconstruction: A Multicenter Orthopaedic Outcomes Network (MOON) cohort study. *Am J Sports Med* 2012;40:2523-2529.
12. Sturnick DR, Vacek PM, DeSarno MJ, et al: Combined anatomic factors predicting risk of anterior cruciate ligament injury for males and females. *Am J Sports Med* 2015;43:839-847.
13. Westermann RW, Spindler KP, Hettrich CM, Wolf BR: Outcomes following ACL and grade III MCL injuries. *Orthop J Sports Med* 2017;5 (3 suppl3).

 ©Copyright 2021 American Academy of Orthopaedic Surgeons

42

Randomized Controlled Trials

Heng An Lin, MBBS, MMEd(Ortho), FRCSEd
Patrick D.G. Henry, MD, FRCSC
David Wasserstein, MD, MSc, MPH, FRCSC

Keywords: *level of evidence; prostpective; randomized controlled trials; study design*

INTRODUCTION

The practice of orthopaedic surgery has evolved tremendously over the last two decades, with an emphasis on evidence-informed care. Critical appraisal of the literature is an inherent challenge in this environment, primarily due to the sheer volume and heterogeneity of published literature quality.[1-4] This necessary skill requires appropriate interpretation of the data, which may not always be concordant with the authors' conclusions. Readers must also recognize the benefits and limitations of each study, and this starts with an understanding of the study design. In the world of medical evidence, no type of study has achieved a greater reverence than a well-designed, well-executed, randomized controlled trial.

Randomized controlled trials (RCTs) are a form of prospective, analytical study that allows for the comparison of therapeutic options. When well designed and executed, the RCT minimizes bias in comparison to other study designs, and thus, the evidence it produces is considered "level 1," based on the Centre for Evidence-Based Medicine Level of Evidence Classification.[5] However, the proper design and execution of RCTs can be tedious, time consuming, and involve high cost. A study labeled as an "RCT" alone is not enough to ensure it has achieved this highest level of quality.

This chapter will outline the fundamental characteristics of the RCT, using landmark studies from the Orthopaedic literature as case examples.

UNDERSTANDING RANDOMIZED CONTROLLED TRIALS

An RCT is a prospective study design typically used to investigate the effectiveness of an intervention on a primary outcome of interest for a particular study population. For the trial, the study population is divided into at least two groups for comparison, each group receiving a different treatment. The process by which patients are distributed into the groups is called "randomization." Randomization is the allocation of included patients into groups "at random," rather than selecting patients for the groups by a particular feature or characteristic that they share. There are several different RCT designs including parallel, crossover, and factorial RCTs.

The most common type of RCT is the parallel design (**Figure 1**). In the parallel design, the study population is divided into groups (by the process of randomization), with each subject in each group exposed to only one intervention. Typically, one of these interventions is a new drug or treatment that is being tested, and the other group is considered the "control" group and is treated with either no treatment or another treatment that is considered the benchmark. The groups are then compared to determine whether one intervention is superior at achieving a particular outcome of interest. For example, Moseley JB et al (*NEJM* 2002)[6] randomized 180 patients in a parallel design to arthroscopic débridement, arthroscopic lavage, or placebo surgery, in the management of

Dr. Henry or an immediate family member is a member of a speakers' bureau or has made paid presentations on behalf of CONMED Linvatec. Neither of the following authors nor any immediate family member has received anything of value from or has stock or stock options held in a commercial company or institution related directly or indirectly to the subject of this chapter: Dr. Lin and Dr. Wasserstein.

©Copyright 2021 American Academy of Orthopaedic Surgeons

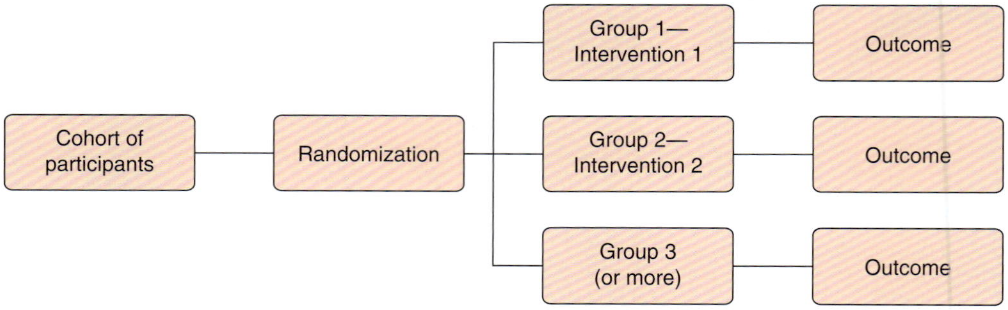

FIGURE 1 Diagram of parallel design.

knee osteoarthritis. They found no difference in knee-specific pain scores or functional improvement in walking, bending, or climbing stairs.

In a crossover design (**Figures 2** and **3**), two or more groups both receive the same intervention(s), but at different time periods. In this case, the subjects serve as their own controls. In the Denosumab Adherence Preference Satisfaction study (Freemantle et al, *Osteoporosis Int* 2012),[7] 250 postmenopausal women across 25 North American centers were given alendronate then denosumab, or denosumab then alendronate, over successive 12-month periods for each of the treatment. The similarities of the effectiveness of the drugs allowed the investigators to elucidate practical outcomes, like adherence, using the crossover design RCT.

Another major advantage of the crossover design is the avoidance of confounders (eg, age or sex) within the study and control groups, because the same people make up each group. This leads to statistical efficiency, meaning fewer patients (smaller sample size) are required. However, the disadvantages of crossover RCTs include a longer study duration, difficulty in managing dropout who had completed only a single evaluation phase, the possibility of unblinding when the participants noticed significant differences between the treatment phases, and the possibility of carryover effects between evaluation phases, especially if the "washout" phase is insufficient. Due to its nature, this design is almost impossible to carry out when testing surgical interventions and is therefore used more extensively in medical specialties.

"Crossover design" should not be confused with "treatment crossover," which is the switching from one intervention arm to another and is common to all RCT designs. For example, in the Spine Patient Outcomes Research Trial (SPORT),[8,9] 245 patients were assigned to the standard open diskectomy group and 256 to the nonsurgical group. By the end of 1 year, 41% of those assigned to the nonsurgical arm had undergone surgery and 43% of patients assigned to surgery did not receive it. Only 59% of the patients assigned to the surgical arm had surgery performed on them by the end of 4 years.

In a factorial design RCT, it is possible to study several intervention arms within the study population at the same time.[10] In a simple 2 × 2 factorial design RCT (**Figure 4**), there are two permutations to each of the two intervention arms (ie, yes/no). Hence, individual participants can be randomized to receive a single treatment, both treatments, or no treatment (control/placebo). The effect of each intervention can be compared with one another, with the control/placebo, as well as with a combination of treatments. This is the only design that allows the testing for interactions between different treatments.[11] In Fluid Lavage of Open Wounds (FLOW) study (FLOW group, *NEJM*, 2015),[12] 2,551 patients with open fractures from across 41 centers in North America, Norway, Australia, and India were centrally randomized into one of the six treatment arms, in permutations of cleansing solution (either soap or normal saline) and pressure (high pressure, low pressure or gravity)—known as a 2 × 3 factorial RCT design. The rate of revision surgery was similar regardless of pressure, although the soap solution group had a higher revision surgery rate compared with that of normal saline.

RANDOMIZATION AND ALLOCATION

Randomization is the process of allocating subjects (patients) into groups within a study, and this process aims to reduce selection bias. Selection bias is the error introduced when the criteria used in selecting the subjects do not correctly

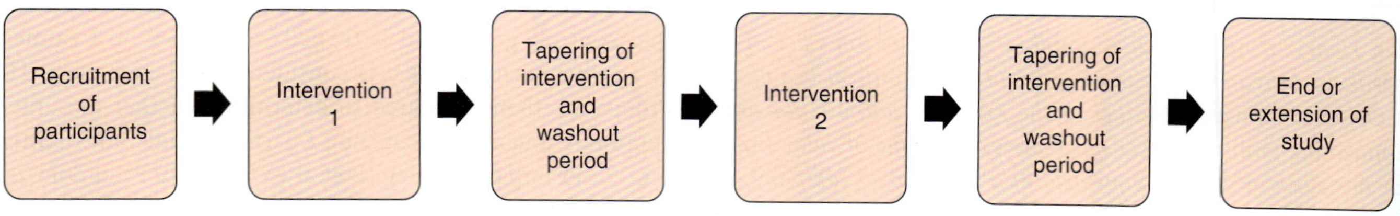

FIGURE 2 Diagram of crossover study design (single group).

©Copyright 2021 American Academy of Orthopaedic Surgeons

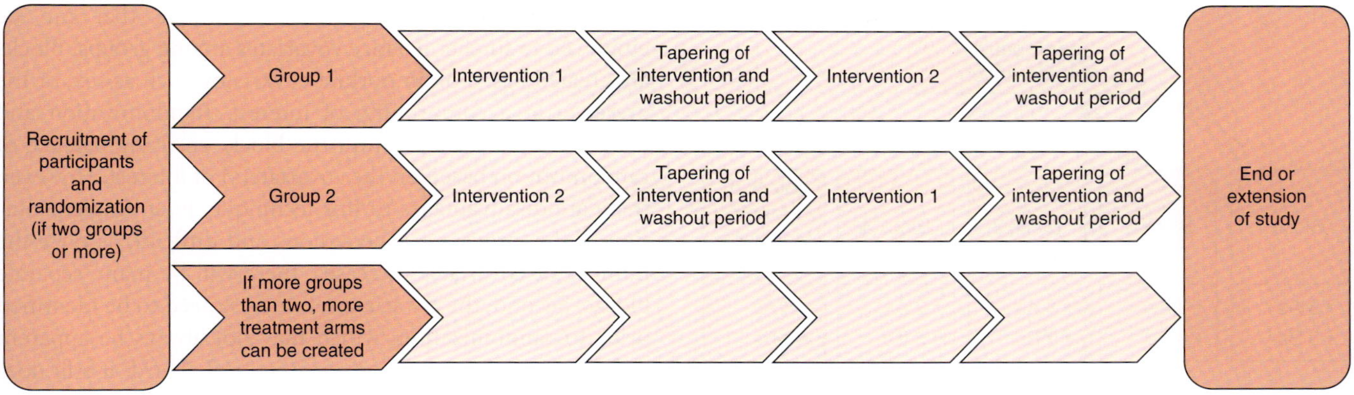

FIGURE 3 Diagram of crossover study design (two groups or more).

represent the target population of interest being evenly distributed in both (or all) groups.[13] While it might seem more reliable to take a study population and go through each patient one by one and try to "match" each person up with someone with similar characteristics and place them in opposite groups, it is impossible to find every characteristic about each patient. Randomization increases the likelihood of a balanced profile of subjects within each of the groups, including both known and unknown demographic, confounding, or prognostic factors,[14] such that the groups only differ in the interventions to be compared. The theoretical balancing of unknown confounding factors is a significant advantage of the RCT over matched, nonrandomized prospective studies where the likelihood of unknown confounders is higher—and this may bias the results.

Randomization can be achieved in several ways, including simple randomization, block randomization, stratified randomization, and covariate adaptive randomization.[14]

In simple randomization, subjects are allocated based on a single algorithm of random assignment. The classic example is a flip of the coin. Modern techniques utilize a random computer-generated number, and allocation is based on an odd or even number. Although it is easy to implement, simple randomization does not control the number of patients allocated to each group and can lead to imbalance of the group sizes.

Block randomization (**Figure 5**) is designed to prevent this problem by randomizing patients in "blocks." A block consists of a predetermined number of subjects. The number of subjects within the block is determined by the number of groups in the study. For a study with two groups, the number of subjects within the block should be in multiples of 2; multiples of 3 with 3 groups, etc. Within each block, subjects are randomized and allocated to intervention groups, which ensures balanced numbers. Block randomization is most useful when dealing with a small sized cohort (**Figure 6**).

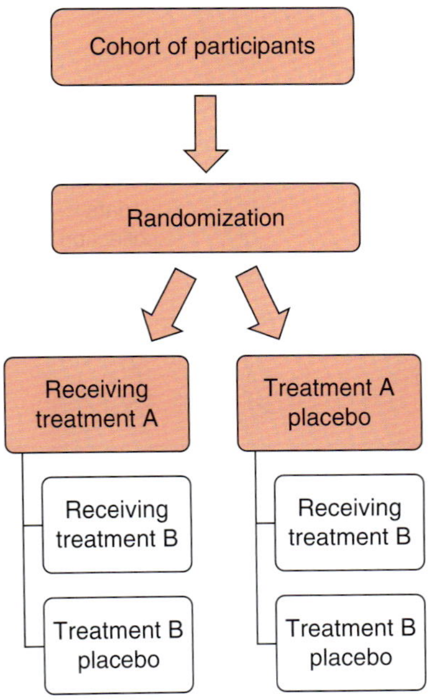

Groups	Treatment A — Yes	Treatment A — No (placebo)
Treatment B—Yes	1	2
Treatment B—No (placebo)	3	4

FIGURE 4 Diagram of factorial design (2 × 2).

©Copyright 2021 American Academy of Orthopaedic Surgeons

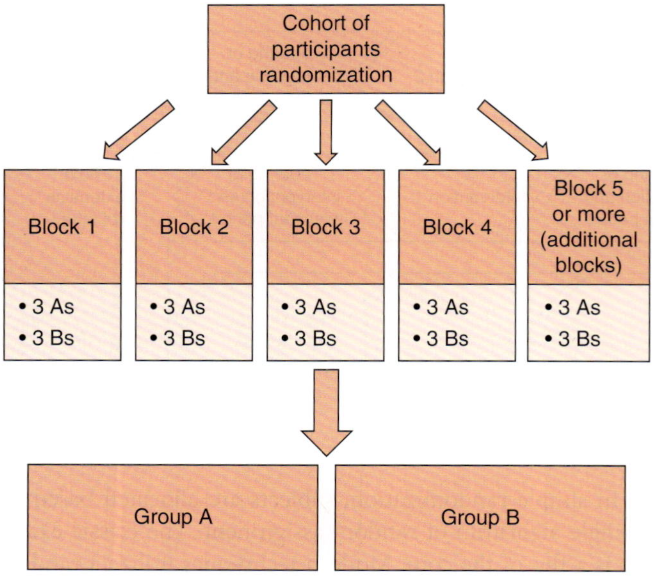

FIGURE 5 Diagram of block randomization. Each Block will consist of participants in multiples of number of groups.

As stated above, randomization helps balance confounding factors, such as underlying medical problems for example. However, simple and block randomizations may still result in groups of patients with very different baseline characteristics (also called "covariates" when these characteristics are used in part of the statistical analysis). Thus, despite randomizing, an investigator may still end up with two differing groups of patients, one relatively healthy compared with the other, or older than the other, etc. The risk of this occurring is greater with smaller samples.

Stratified randomization is a technique that can be employed to further balance covariates among groups. Blocks are created based on important covariates, such as sex, or the presence of a comorbidity of interest. Randomization and allocation then occur within the block, ensuring balance of randomization based on the covariate(s) of interest. However, there are disadvantages to this technique. First, implementation of this process can be tedious and difficult, as once the number of covariates increases, there will be many separate blocks. Second, the covariates of interest need to be identified prior to randomization, which may not always be apparent right from the start of a prospective trial. Third, it still does not account for unknown covariates.

The Moseley et al (*NEJM* 2002) trial[6] utilized a block randomization with stratification RCT design. In the randomization process of the trial, the participants were stratified according to the severity of osteoarthritis (ie, the main covariate in the study). This was followed by a stratified allocation with fixed blocks of six, wherein patients were randomized to one of three treatment arms. The goal of stratification was to allow an even distribution of mild to severe knee osteoarthritis across the various treatment arms. This was an effective design for at the time what was a landmark trial. In retrospect, separating the groups entirely based on severity of arthritis may have provided more pertinent data, as it is only the group of patients with no or very mild osteoarthritis (OA) where contention still exists as to the efficacy of this particular intervention![15]

Adaptive randomization also allows for consideration of covariates. In this method of randomization, each new subject is assigned sequentially to a group based on the specific covariates that they have, taking into consideration previous subject allocations.[16]

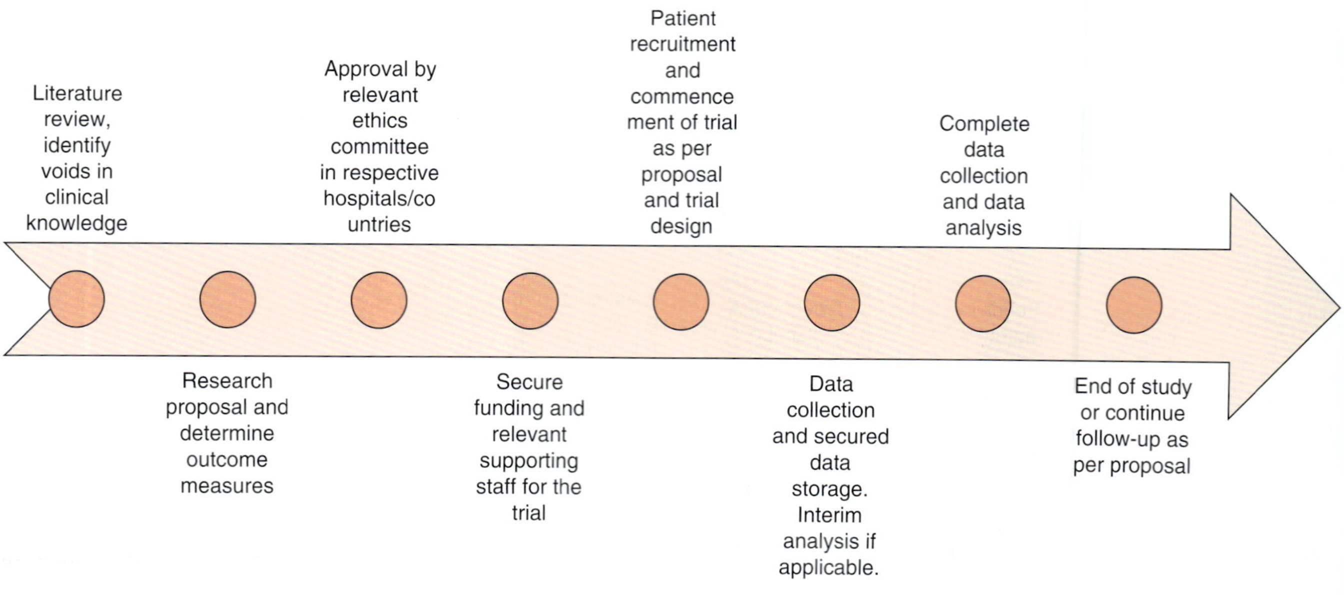

FIGURE 6 Diagram of general workflow.

©Copyright 2021 American Academy of Orthopaedic Surgeons

CONCEALMENT AND BLINDING

In addition to being "random," group allocation should also be "concealed." Allocation concealment refers to the technique where the next treatment allocation is concealed from the researcher randomizing and assigning the patient, until the moment of assignment. (Note that this is different than "blinding," which has to do with either patient or researcher being kept unaware of the treatment group even after assignment.) Concealment reduces selection bias that might otherwise be caused by the investigators, as they might influence the patient treatment assignment. For example, in a trial comparing different grafts in anterior cruciate ligament reconstruction, a surgeon who favors bone–patella tendon–bone autograft may be influenced to assign his patients into this treatment group, as opposed to other graft options. Concealment prevents this surgeon from doing this.

Ideally, participants in an RCT should also be blinded. A "blinded trial" refers to a study where treatment allocation is kept secret for the entire duration of the trial. A "blinded" person does not know what treatment was received by each patient. Patients, healthcare providers, researchers, and outcome analyzers may all potentially be blinded depending on the intervention studied. A single-blinded trial conceals the allocation from the subjects; a double-blinded trial conceals allocation from the subjects and investigators; a triple-blinded trial conceals allocation from the investigators, subjects, and outcome assessors/analysts. Blinding reduces observer bias from the investigators, placebo and nocebo effect bias from the subjects, and bias of data analysis and interpretation by eliminating the possibility of that person (patient, provider, or outcome assessor) injecting their own preconceived notions into their role in the study.

The process of blinding is not easy and, in some cases, is not possible, particularly in surgery. In a review of RCTs published in the *Journal of Bone and Joint Surgery* (American) from 1988 till 2000,[17,18] it was noted that there were more higher quality double-blinded trials on drugs as compared with surgical intervention. Though it is possible to blind the assessors and sometimes the patients in a surgical trial, surgeons cannot be blinded.

INCLUSION AND EXCLUSION CRITERIA

Ideal RCT cohort selection consists of participants from a relatively homogenous population—this will minimize confounders (ie, differences between the baseline characteristics in participants in each group that might affect the outcome). For example, the age of the target population is of importance as the physiology in a child differs greatly from that of an adult; therefore, narrowing the age criteria of a study to patients between the ages of 18 and 60 years would eliminate the chance that there would be more children in one group compared with the other. "Inclusion and exclusion criteria" help refine the target population. By adhering to strict criteria, it is possible to make the study population very homogenous, which will minimize bias and thus increase the "internal validity" of the study (ie, it increases the likelihood that the conclusions you make in your study are valid *for that specified patient population*).

However, if a population selected for inclusion is too narrow, then the study will lack external validity; meaning the results may not be applicable to many patients in real-life practice (as the typical clinical practice usually involves patients of various ages and medical profiles). Defining a narrow population can also lead to difficulty in patient recruitment and, subsequently, failure to complete a study or recruit enough patients to power the analysis. Finding the right balance in the selection criteria is challenging and depends on many factors, and this usually involves a good literature review and a seasoned team of investigators.

SETTING PRIMARY AND SECONDARY OUTCOME MEASURES

The primary outcome measure is the most important dependent variable which the study aims to evaluate. This must be identified prior to the start of the study to set a clear goal around which the study design can be developed. The remaining dependent variables that the authors are interested to look at, but are not part of the main hypothesis, are known as secondary outcome measures.

The primary outcome measure is typically used to calculate the sample size of the study. It must be set before the study which avoids a post hoc (ie, after study completion) selection of statistically significant secondary outcome. This is just one of the reasons authors are encouraged to register RCTs publicly before recruitment (eg, registration can be done on the website www.clinicaltrials.gov)—an almost mandatory step to facilitate eventual peer-review publication.

Secondary outcome measures should also be judiciously selected to minimize the probability of reporting falsely significant results. In any RCT, there are many data that can be potentially used as outcomes. However, when multiple variables are examined, the risk of false-positive findings is increased. Thus, the primary outcome is the most important, and secondary outcome findings should be interpreted with caution, especially when there are numerous secondary outcome measures.[19]

DETERMINATION OF SAMPLE SIZE

The sample size of the RCT should be determined prior to start of the study. The sample size is defined as the adequate number of participants required to detect a difference in the effect of different intervention arms on the primary outcome at a

©Copyright 2021 American Academy of Orthopaedic Surgeons

predetermined level of statistical significance.[20] Undersized or underpowered studies may not achieve significant results. On the other hand, recruiting more patients than are needed will be neither time nor cost efficient and exposes participants unnecessarily to different treatments when the most efficacious one may already be known.

Various factors are considered when calculating sample size. These include power of study, type 1 error, expected effect size of the intervention, and assumptions of variability in the control group.

If the primary outcome measure is highly variable, a general rule is that a larger sample size will be required to assess whether the observed effect is true. Conversely, if the treatment arm is very effective and can be observed frequently, chances are the sample size required to detect this effect is smaller.[21] Even in a relatively well-designed RCT, the variability in the primary outcome measure can prevent readers and investigators from drawing reasonable conclusions about their own studies. Pearce et al[22] raised this point in response to recent articles that concluded there is no role for surgery in the management of displaced intra-articular calcaneal fractures. In the multicenter, two-arm parallel group RCT UK heel fracture trial,[23] the authors concluded that surgery did not result in symptomatic or functional advantage compared with conservative management. However, Pearce et al pointed out that only 502 out of 2006 patients who presented with calcaneal fractures were deemed eligible for the trial, of which many excluded patients were ones that likely needed surgery. In addition, only 30% of the eligible patients consented to the trial, and as the trial recruitment occurred after initial clinical consultation, patient recruitment may have been influenced by surgeon opinion—contributing to selection bias. Furthermore, the authors selected only one surgical option, the extended lateral approach, which may not be the single best option to treat certain calcaneal fractures as well; for example, tongue-type fractures could be much easily fixed via percutaneous approach. This may have contributed to poorer outcomes and higher complication rates. Lastly, the follow-up period was short at two years and therefore may have missed an important long-term outcome which is posttraumatic arthritis and that may have been influenced by choice of intervention.[22]

EFFECT SIZE

The expected effect size is the expected difference between the intervention and the control arm for the primary outcome. A good RCT should consider the minimal clinically important difference (MCID). The MCID is the smallest change that is clinically relevant to patients. The process for establishing the MCID of an outcome is beyond the scope of this chapter, but it ensures that any differences seen between treatment arms is not only statistically significant but meaningful to practical patient care. Assumptions of variability in the control group is essentially the assumed "characteristics," or variation among subjects within the group, for any given outcome measure of interest and serves as the reference for the MCID. For example, in a study of the effects of quadriceps strengthening after anterior cruciate ligament reconstruction,[24] the primary outcome was the single leg hopping distance. This can be expressed in centimeters, with standard deviations reflecting the innate difference of participants within the control group. Both minimally clinically relevant difference and variability of the control group can be extrapolated from the literature or pilot studies.

The type of comparisons to be made in the trial will also affect the sample size. Clinical superiority, statistical superiority, equivalence, and noninferiority trials each have different formulae based on the above factors.

One of the common pitfalls in RCT reporting is a lack of information with regard to sample size determination. In a review article by Charles (BMJ, 2009),[20] among 215 RCT studies published in six general medical journals with high impact factors, only about a third described sample size calculations adequately. This lack of information may include innate errors in sample size calculations, of which the resulting sample size may not be ideal. As noted, small sample size risks inconclusive results, and large resource inefficiency and potentially exposing more subjects to unnecessary treatment risks.

DATA COLLECTION, FOLLOW-UP, STORAGE OF DATA, AND INTERIM ANALYSIS

Planning the type of data and its means of collection is important. The choice of assessment tools or forms should be decided prior to the start of the study and consistently applied across different treatment groups.

Many types of assessment tools and scores exist. These include scoring systems or assessments that are performed by assessors (such as measuring range of motion) and those which participants complete independently (ie, questionnaires). Physical characteristics such as height and weight are best measured rather than reported. Functional measurements performed by assessors, such as joint range of motion, muscle power, or knee stability, can suffer from interobserver variability. This can be a confounding factor and may eventually lead to inaccurate results if there are multiple assessors in a study. The prospective Multicenter Orthopaedic Outcomes Network (MOON) shoulder cohort study took a sophisticated approach to this issue by establishing interobserver reliability beforehand.[25]

With functional measures, there is also a risk of assessor bias if the assessors are not blinded. One way to reduce this potential bias is to utilize assessment tools such as isokinetic measurement machines that take away the "human factor." As

©Copyright 2021 American Academy of Orthopaedic Surgeons

far as possible, the assessors should be blinded and follow a standardized assessment plan specific to the trial and established before the study began.

The utilization of patient-reported outcome measures (PROM) will also mitigate some of the risks of using assessors. PROMs can be disease or joint specific, or general in nature. Examples include the International Knee Documentation Committee (IKDC) form or 36-Item Short Form Survey Instrument (SF-36). They are filled by participants based on their own interpretation of factors such as self-function and quality of life. Although there are no elements of external party bias involved, participants from different cultural backgrounds may interpret the questionnaire differently.

Follow-up time points are important assessment milestones that help to determine the effects of an intervention in the short, mid, or long term. The objective of each follow-up and the relevant assessments should be clearly defined. The total duration and intervals of follow-up should be based on the needs of the primary study objective. Typical postoperative follow-up periods are at one month, three months, six months, one year, two years, and/or longer, and these may or may not coincide with the ideal follow-up time-point for a study's primary outcome.

Although patients may display early enthusiasm to participate in a study, ensuring completion and follow-up can be a difficult task. Patient compliance with the follow-up schedule can be improved with mail, e-mail, or phone reminders prior to the follow-up dates, but in general, loss-to-follow-up increases with time. To reduce default rates, a follow-up action plan should be drafted and form part of the RCT protocol. The reasons for defaulting should be sought and addressed as needed. There is no standard agreement on the minimum amount of loss to follow-up that is acceptable, but most would agree that greater than 20% loss to follow-up results in the introduction of a relatively higher level of bias.

All patient information, including outcomes must be stored on a secure platform as approved by the research ethics board review committee or its equivalent. In medical research, this is especially sensitive as the data collected often involves personal health information. Physical data storage must be on encrypted devices and kept only in certified locations based on institution policy. Cloud data storage is possible but requires a high level of compliance.

Interim analysis is the analysis of data gathered midway through the trial. This is essential in prospective trials that span a long period of time or expose patients to risk and where safety must be assessed. A statistically significant superior treatment option (early superiority) or a treatment with adverse events may be identified at this stage and the trial terminated early due to ethical reasons. This function is usually performed by a Data Safety and Monitoring Board. Studies may also be terminated prior to completion due to reasons such as futility (when recruitment completion is expected to be improbable or required extensive time and cost), redundancy (when a similar study has been published which made the ongoing trial unnecessary), or funding abandonment (when the source of funding has been terminated).[26]

ANALYSIS AND INTERPRETATION OF RANDOMIZED CONTROLLED TRIAL RESULTS

Interpretation of RCT results is often complex and requires a skilled statistician to ensure the data are analyzed properly and for credible conclusions to be drawn based on the primary and secondary outcome measured. The tools and formulae used for statistical analysis are extensive and beyond the scope of this chapter—a dedicated text on statistical analysis is recommended.

CONSOLIDATED STANDARDS OF REPORTING TRIALS

Consolidated Standards of Reporting Trials (CONSORT) is a standardized, comprehensive guide on how to properly report the results of an RCT.[27] It is comprised of various recommendations, guided by evidence, to achieve a high-quality manuscript, which in turn typically reflect a high-quality study. It also serves as a template to evaluate the quality of a published RCT, and every practicing surgeon should be familiar with it.

The history of the CONSORT group goes back to 1993, where a group of medical journal editors, clinical epidemiologists, methodologists, and trialists met in Ottawa, Canada. As many published RCTs in the past were found to be written up poorly, the group focused on ways to improve the quality of RCT reports. Critical components of RCTs were identified. These are items which, if absent or poorly reported, would lead to biased or grossly inaccurate results. These were consolidated into a 32-item checklist and flow diagram. At the same time, an American group (Asilomar Working Group on Recommendation for Reporting of Clinical Trials in the Biomedical Literature, California, USA) was also working on a similar guide on RCTs. The two groups met and merged the two RCT guide proposals into the first CONSORT statement in 1996. The statement consists of a set of recommendations for the reporting of RCTs, which is considered the minimum standard required. Revisions have been published in 2001 and 2010.

The current CONSORT statement, published in 2010, consists of a 25-item checklist and a flow diagram. The checklist items guide users on how to design, interpret, and analyze the data in RCTs, while the flow diagram provides guidance on the steps to take in recruiting and following the participants through a trial (**Tables 1** and **2**).

In addition, the CONSORT group also developed extensions of the CONSORT statement, updated in 2012. These are additional guides targeted at RCTs of specific designs, such as cluster randomized trials or noninferiority and equivalence

©Copyright 2021 American Academy of Orthopaedic Surgeons

TABLE 1 CONSORT 2010 Checklist of Information to Include When Reporting a Randomized Trial[a]

Section/Topic	Item No	Checklist Item	Reported on Page No.
Title and Abstract			
	1a	Identification as a randomized trial in the title	
	1b	Structured summary of trial design, methods, results, and conclusions (for specific guidance see CONSORT for abstracts)	
Introduction			
Background and objectives	2a	Scientific background and explanation of rationale	
	2b	Specific objectives or hypotheses	
Methods			
Trial design	3a	Description of trial design (such as parallel, factorial) including allocation ratio	
	3b	Important changes to methods after trial commencement (such as eligibility criteria), with reasons	
Participants	4a	Eligibility criteria for participants	
	4b	Settings and locations where the data were collected	
Interventions	5	The interventions for each group with sufficient details to allow replication, including how and when they were actually administered	
Outcomes	6a	Completely defined prespecified primary and secondary outcome measures, including how and when they were assessed	
	6b	Any changes to trial outcomes after the trial commenced, with reasons	
Sample size	7a	How sample size was determined	
	7b	When applicable, explanation of any interim analyses and stopping guidelines	
Randomization			
Sequence generation	8a	Method used to generate the random allocation sequence	
	8b	Type of randomization; details of any restriction (such as blocking and block size)	
Allocation concealment mechanism	9	Mechanism used to implement the random allocation sequence (such as sequentially numbered containers), describing any steps taken to conceal the sequence until interventions were assigned	
Implementation	10	Who generated the random allocation sequence, who enrolled participants, and who assigned participants to interventions	
Blinding	11a	If done, who was blinded after assignment to interventions (eg, participants, care providers, those assessing outcomes) and how	
	11b	If relevant, description of the similarity of interventions	

©Copyright 2021 American Academy of Orthopaedic Surgeons

Statistical methods	12a	Statistical methods used to compare groups for primary and secondary outcomes
	12b	Methods for additional analyses, such as subgroup analyses and adjusted analyses
Results		
Participant flow (a diagram is strongly recommended)	13a	For each group, the numbers of participants who were randomly assigned, received intended treatment, and were analyzed for the primary outcome
	13b	For each group, losses and exclusions after randomization, together with reasons
Recruitment	14a	Dates defining the periods of recruitment and follow-up
	14b	Why the trial ended or was stopped
Baseline data	15	A table showing baseline demographic and clinical characteristics for each group
Numbers analyzed	16	For each group, number of participants (denominator) included in each analysis and whether the analysis was by original assigned groups
Outcomes and estimation	17a	For each primary and secondary outcome, results for each group, and the estimated effect size and its precision (such as 95% confidence interval)
	17b	For binary outcomes, presentation of both absolute and relative effect sizes is recommended
Ancillary analyses	18	Results of any other analyses performed, including subgroup analyses and adjusted analyses, distinguishing prespecified from exploratory
Harms	19	All important harms or unintended effects in each group (for specific guidance see CONSORT for harms)
Discussion		
Limitations	20	Trial limitations, addressing sources of potential bias, imprecision, and, if relevant, multiplicity of analyses
Generalizability	21	Generalizability (external validity, applicability) of the trial findings
Interpretation	22	Interpretation consistent with results, balancing benefits and harms, and considering other relevant evidence
Other Information		
Registration	23	Registration number and name of trial registry
Protocol	24	Where the full trial protocol can be accessed, if available
Funding	25	Sources of funding and other support (such as supply of drugs), role of funders

[a]We strongly recommend reading this statement in conjunction with the CONSORT 2010 Explanation and Elaboration for important clarifications on all the items. If relevant, we also recommend reading CONSORT extensions for cluster randomized trials, noninferiority and equivalence trials, nonpharmacological treatments, herbal interventions, and pragmatic trials. Additional extensions are forthcoming: for those and for up to date references relevant to this checklist, see www.consort-statement.org.

©Copyright 2021 American Academy of Orthopaedic Surgeons

TABLE 2 Effect of Crossover

Trials	Aim of Study	Study Design	Data Analysis	Patient Allocation post Randomization	Remarks
KANON trial—knee anterior cruciate ligament, nonsurgical versus surgical treatment trial (*BMJ* 2013)	To look at 5-yr outcomes in acutely ACL-ruptured individuals managed with early reconstruction (ACLR) + exercise therapy (physical therapy [PT]), PT alone, and with option of delayed ACLR in the PT group	Patients are assigned to either PT + early ACLR group, or PT + option of delayed ACLR if needed. Initial early ACLR + PT group n = 62 PT + option of delayed ACLR n = 59	Per protocol (PP)	Early ACLR with PT (n = 62) 1 lost to follow-up. 2 did not have ACLR/complete PT-excluded per PP 30/59 had PT + delayed ACLR within 5 yr, which left 20/59 with PT alone	**1.** 30/59 patients in PT group had opted for delayed ACLR, resulting in a much smaller patient number remaining compared with early ACLR + PT. Small subgroup analysis is prone to spurious results **2.** Patients with PT alone appeared to give equivalent or better result than early ACLR with PT; however, it cannot be generalized in patients with ACL rupture, as the patients who had trouble coping with PT alone would have moved on to a delayed ACLR
SPORTS trial—spine patient outcomes research trial. on surgical versus nonoperative treatment for lumbar disk herniation (*Spine* 2008)	To compare surgical (standard open diskectomy) and nonsurgical treatment (patient education, physical therapy, NSAIDs if tolerated) for patients with lumbar disk herniation	Two cohorts; one is observational cohort (n = 743) while the other is randomized cohort (n = 501) Within the randomized cohort, 245 were assigned to surgery, 256 assigned to nonsurgical treatment	Intention to treat (ITT), PP	At one year, only 139 in the surgery group had undergone surgery, whereas 106 in the nonsurgical group had undergone surgery By the end of 4 yr, only 144 in the surgery group had undergone surgery. 115 in the nonsurgical group had undergone surgery	**1.** Analysis of crossover patients showed for those who were older, less pain with higher income were more likely to cross over from surgery to nonsurgical group. Patients with less income, dissatisfied with their symptoms, less physical function, and who expressed preference for surgery were more likely to cross from nonsurgical group to surgery **2.** Although the initial analysis used ITT, as the number of cross over patients was significant; analysis subsequently was based on the actual treatment received
MeTeOR trial—meniscal tear in osteoarthritis research trial (*JBJS* 2016)	To compare arthroscopic partial meniscectomy (APM) with physical therapy (PT) versus physical therapy alone in the management of degenerative meniscal tear	Patients who are 45 yr of age or older with mild to moderate osteoarthritis and degenerative meniscal tear are randomized to APM + PT group or PT alone Allocated: APM + PT n = 174 PT only n = 177	ITT, PP	APM + PT group—10/174 did not undergo APM PT-only group—48/177 crossed over to receive APM in first 140 d; another 16 crossed over between 140 d and 2 yr	**1.** Interpretation of post APM outcome is prone to confounders, as those who crossed over to receive APM were not randomized with the initial APM + PT group **2.** Patients in PT group with higher pain score, shorter duration of presentation are more likely to cross over

©Copyright 2021 American Academy of Orthopaedic Surgeons

trials. In 2013, there were further extensions of the CONSORT statement guiding trials that report patient-reported outcomes. Known as CONSORT-PRO extension, the guide expands on five items of the initial CONSORT statement to further optimize reporting of RCTs that involve patient-reported outcomes as primary or secondary end points.

COMMON PROBLEMS IN RANDOMIZED CONTROLLED TRIAL AND HOW TO OVERCOME THEM

MANAGEMENT OF DEVIATIONS AND FOLLOW-UP LOSSES

In the course of a trial, it is inevitable that some participants will deviate from the intended protocol. This deviation and/or loss of patient follow-up can be due to various factors. Patients can deviate from the assigned treatment arm due to self-initiated use of traditional or alternative medications, crossover of treatment arms, or stopping the treatment prematurely due to cost or personal beliefs. Patients can be lost to follow-up due to death, incapacity, change in contact, logistical difficulty in attending follow-up, or social reasons such as job commitment or migration. Whatever the reason, deviation and follow-up losses do cause a data void which can potentially upset the balance in participant numbers across arms. This inevitably results in a poorer and potentially skewed interpretation of data.

Compliance to treatment arms and follow-ups should be emphasized to participants. To a certain extent, it is inevitable that a study would encounter such issues, especially when the sample size is large. When dealing with such data, common strategies to tackle these problems are the concepts of intention to treat (ITT) or per protocol (PP).

ITT refers to the principle of including all participants within the various treatment arms in the analysis of data, regardless of whether they deviated from the protocol; whereas PP is the principle of analyzing data only for participants who have complied totally with the study protocol. Any noncompliant participants (crossover) or dropouts are excluded in the analysis. In application, PP forms the subset of compliant participants within the ITT.

We will use the Knee Anterior Cruciate Ligament, Nonsurgical versus Surgical Treatment (KANON) trial[15] to illustrate some of these points. In the KANON trial, patients with anterior cruciate ligament (ACL) injury were divided into those who received exercise therapy with early ACL reconstruction, or exercise therapy alone with the option of delayed ACL reconstruction. In this trial, there were 62 patients assigned to exercise therapy with early ACL reconstruction, and 59 assigned to exercise therapy with the option of delayed ACL reconstruction. Three patients were excluded from the early ACL reconstruction group as they did not follow through with the study protocol. Within the group with the option of delayed ACL reconstruction, 30 of the 59 patients opted for delayed ACL reconstruction within 5 years. The trial did not show any better outcome in early ACL reconstruction with exercise therapy as compared with exercise therapy with option of delayed surgery.

Analysis using the ITT principle tends to give conservative outcome results on the effect of any treatment arm.[28] This is because ITT accepts the chance of noncompliance to treatment and loss to follow-up, which realistically reflects the situation in everyday practice. Also, if the participants drop out from the study even before starting the treatment, they are still included under the treatment arm. The overall effect of an intervention may be blunted due to this dilution effect. Simply put, in a treatment arm with 500 compliant and 500 noncompliant/dropout participants, if 400 compliant participants reported effective intervention at the end of the trial, the rate of effectiveness will be 400/1,000, or 40% going by the ITT principle. In contrast, this would be 400/500, or 80% if the noncompliant and dropout participants are excluded. This can be further skewed as the participants who reported effectiveness are likely to be the ones who continued with the treatment. Likewise, in the KANON trial, 30 out of 59 patients in the exercise therapy group had opted for delayed ACL reconstruction. Although this was not technically considered a crossover of treatment arm (as the exercise therapy group had the option of delayed surgery), there was a change in treatment. 23 of them had the ACL reconstruction done in the first 2 years of the trial, while seven had the surgery performed after 2 years, up to the fifth year of follow-up. These were the patients who had persistent instability despite exercise therapy. In the reported results, although the outcome of exercise therapy alone appeared to be noninferior to that of early ACL reconstruction, we can appreciate that those who stayed on in this group are the responders to exercise therapy (as the nonresponders had opted for delayed ACL reconstruction). Without the option of delayed ACL reconstruction in the exercise therapy group, the dropout rate or functional outcome scores would likely be a lot worse than reported, as 30 of them subsequently opted for delayed ACL reconstruction. Similarly, the apparent positive outcome scores of good responders who had stayed on in the exercise therapy group are not representative of the general population of patients with ACL injury.

When using the ITT principle, the reporting of deviations and dropouts is a requirement, which is in keeping with the recommendation from the CONSORT group with regard to participant accountability. It also preserves the sample size, and by doing so, preserves the power of the study. The US FDA and International Conference on Harmonisation (ICH) E9 guidelines recommend the use of ITT as a routine method of analysis, and this should be reported in the study even if it is not the author's primary method of analysis.[29]

There are downsides to using ITT alone. The dilution of noncompliant and dropout participants can reduce the estimated positive treatment results. This may mask the true effectiveness of the treatment, resulting in the treatment falsely interpreted as ineffective, or the magnitude of effect underestimate. Furthermore, many readers simply want to know which treatment was "better" for those patients who actually received the treatment.

5: Principles of Clinical Information

©Copyright 2021 American Academy of Orthopaedic Surgeons

A good secondary analysis tool adjunct to ITT is the application of the PP principle. This can be more useful when comparing the efficacy of various interventions, as the protocol violators have been excluded from the analysis. This gives a "cleaner" and better matched data as compared with ITT. However, using PP alone without the application of ITT first carries a higher degree of bias and is prone to misinterpretation of data. Adverse reportable events such as the complication rate from a surgical treatment can be falsely low in the analysis. The simplest example is if patients assigned to the surgical treatment arm have a higher mortality rate as a result of surgery, but they are excluded from the study as they have not completed the intended treatment protocol.

The Committee for Proprietary Medicinal Products (CPMP) guidelines recommends the use of both ITT and PP analysis, with ITT being the primary and PP the supportive mode of analysis for superiority trials. If both ITT and PP analyses arrived at the same results, there is a higher chance that the results will be true.

FUNDING

As a final note, no discussion of RCTs (or any research study for that matter) would be complete without some commentary regarding funding. One of the key components in RCT planning is an estimation of funds required for the trial (the budget) and then ensuring that that amount of funds is available to conduct the trial. A reality for medical research is that trials are expensive, and adequate funding is necessary to complete a trial and obtain useful information. Costs of an RCT can accumulate quickly, especially if expensive medication or testing is required (eg, MRI). However, even the cost of research administration and data collection can be substantial.

Common sources of funding include government agencies, tertiary institutions, or companies in related industries. When sourcing for funds, it is important to identify whether there is a potential conflict of interest, especially if the funds are coming from industry-related companies; if so, these should be declared

SUMMARY

The planning and logistics of carrying out an RCT can be painstaking, and the execution of that research plan is even more difficult. However, a well-planned and well-executed randomized controlled trial will yield the highest level of evidence possible. Careful consideration to the study design, outcome measures, and adherence to the study protocol are crucial components of a good RCT. Often this requires the combined effort of a well-organized team of investigators.

REFERENCES

1. Hopewell S, Dutton S, Yu L, Chan A, Altman DG: The quality of reports of randomised trials in 2000 and 2006: Comparative study of articles indexed in PubMed. *BMJ* 2010;340:c723.
2. Bhandari M, Swiontkowski MF, Einhorn TA, et al: Interobserver agreement in the application of levels of evidence to scientific papers in the American volume of the Journal of Bone and Joint Surgery. *J Bone Joint Surg Am* 2004;86-A(8):1717-1720.
3. Obremskey WT, Pappas N, Attallah-Wasif E, Tornetta P III, Bhandari M: Level of evidence in orthopaedic journals. *J Bone Joint Surg Am* 2005;87(12):2632-2638.
4. Heneghan C, Goldacre B. Mahtani KR: Why clinical trial outcomes fail to translate into benefits for patients. *Trials* 2017;18:122.
5. Oxford Centre for Evidence-based Medicine – Levels of Evidence (March 2009). Produced by Bob Phillips, Chris Ball, Dave Sackett, Doug Badenoch, Sharon Straus, Brian Haynes, Martin Dawes since November 1998. Updated by Jeremy Howick March 2009. https://www.cebm.net/2009/06/oxford-centre-evidence-based-medicine-levels-evidence-march-2009/.
6. Moseley JB, O'Malley K, Petersen NJ, et al: A controlled trial of arthroscopic surgery for osteoarthritis of the knee. *N Engl J Med* 2002;347:81-88
7. Freemantle N, Satram-Hoang S, Tang ET, et al: Final results of the DAPS (denosumab adherence preference satisfaction) study: A 24-month, randomized, crossover comparison with alendronate in postmenopausal women. *Osteoporos Int* 2012;23(1):317-326. doi:10.1007/s00198-011-1780-1.
8. Weinstein JN, Tosteson TD, Lurie JD, et al: Surgical vs nonoperative treatment for lumbar disk herniation the spine patient outcomes research trial (SPORT): A randomized trial. *J Am Med Assoc* 2006;296(20):2441-2450. doi:10.1001/jama.296.20.2441
9. Weinstein JN, Lurie JD, Tosteson TD, et al: Surgical versus non-operative treatment for lumbar disc herniation: Four-year results for the spine patient outcomes research trial (SPORT). *Spine* 2008;33(25):2789-2800.
10. Montgomery AA, Peters TJ, Little P: Design, analysis and presentation of factorial randomised controlled trials. *BMC Med Res Methodol* 2003;3:26.
11. Pandis N, Walsh T, Polychronopoulou A, Katsaros C, Eliades T: Factorial designs: An overview with applications to orthodontic clinical trials. *EJO (Eur J Orthod)* 2014;36(3):314-320.
12. FLOW study. A trial of wound irrigation in the initial management of open fracture wounds. *N Engl J Med* 2015;373:2629-2641. doi:10.1056/NEJMoa1508502.
13. Delgado-Rodríguez M, Llorca J: Bias. *J Epidemiol Community Health* 2004;58(8):635-641.
14. Suresh KP: An overview of randomization techniques: An unbiased assessment of outcome in clinical research. *J Hum Reprod Sci* 2011;4(1):8-11.
15. Brignardello-Petersen R, Guyatt GH, Buchbinder R, et al: Knee arthroscopy versus conservative management in patients with degenerative knee disease: a systematic review. *BMJ Open* 2017;7(5):e016114.
16. Kalish LA, Begg GB: Treatment allocation methods in clinical trials a review. *Stat Med* 1985;4:129-144.
17. Mundi R, Chaudhry H, Mundi S, Godin K, Bhandari M: Design and execution of clinical trials in orthopaedic surgery. *Bone Joint Res* 2014;3(5):161-168.
18. Bhandari M, Richards RR, Sprague S, Schemitsch EH: The quality of reporting of randomized trials in the Journal of Bone and Joint Surgery from 1988 through 2000. *J Bone Joint Surg [Am]* 2002;84-A:388-396.
19. Freemantle N: Interpreting the results of secondary end points and subgroup analyses in clinical trials: Should we lock the crazy aunt in the attic? *BMJ* 2001;322(7292):989-991.
20. Charles P, Giraudeau B, Dechartres A, Baron G, Ravaud P: Reporting of sample size calculation in randomised controlled trials: Review. *BMJ* 2009;338:b1732.

©Copyright 2021 American Academy of Orthopaedic Surgeons

21. Noordzij M, Tripepi G, Dekker FW, Zoccali C, Tanck MW, Jager KJ: Sample size calculations: Basic principles and common pitfalls. *Nephrol Dial Transplant* 2010;25(5):1388-1393.
22. Pearce CJ, Wong KL, Calfer JDF: Calcaneal fractures, selection bias is key. *Bone Joint J* 2015;97-B:880-882.
23. Griffin D, Parsons N, Shaw E, et al: Operative versus non-operative treatment for closed, displaced, intra-articular fractures of the calcaneus: randomized controlled trial. *BMJ* 2014;349:4483.
24. Harput G, Ulusoy B, Yildiz TI, et al: Cross-education improves quadriceps strength recovery after ACL reconstruction: A randomized controlled trial. *Knee Surg Sports Traumatol Arthrosc* 2019;27(1):68-75.
25. Kuhn JE, Dunn WR, Ma B, et al; Multicenter Orthopaedic Outcomes Network-Shoulder (MOON Shoulder Group): Interobserver agreement in the classification of rotator cuff tears. *Am J Sports Med* 2007;35(3):437-441.
26. Piuzzi N, Chughtai M, Khlopas A, et al: Early termination of randomized controlled trials in orthopaedics. *Surg Technol Int* 2017;30:290-294.
27. http://www.consort-statement.org/.
28. Heritier SR, Gebski VJ, Keech AC: Inclusion of patients in clinical trial analysis: The intention-to-treat principle. *Med J Aust* 2003;179:438-440.
29. Sandeep K: Intent to treat- a review. *Perspect Clin Res* 2011;2(3):109-112.

©Copyright 2021 American Academy of Orthopaedic Surgeons

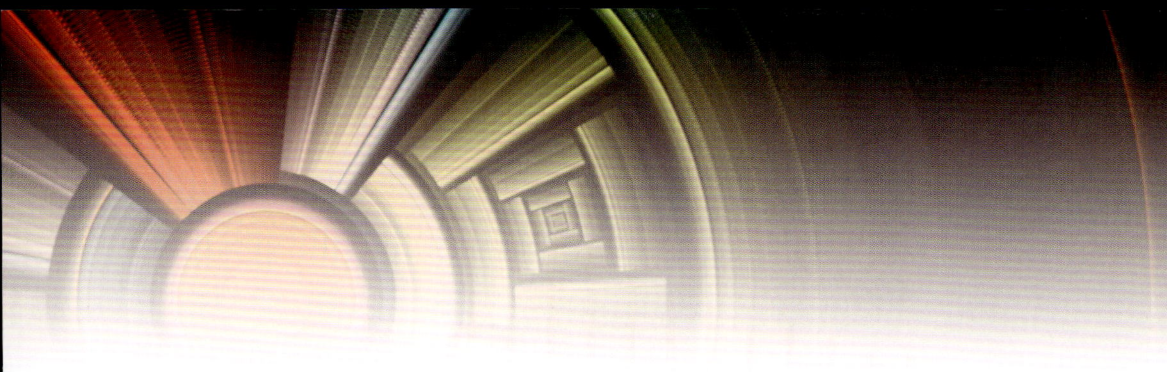

Systematic Reviews and Meta-Analysis

Joseph T. Patterson, MD
Saam Morshed, MD, PhD, MPH

Keywords: *meta-analysis; network meta-analysis; review; systematic review*

INTRODUCTION

New research relevant to practicing orthopaedic surgeons is constantly being published. A sample of articles published in the top 25 highest impact factor orthopaedic journals each year suggests that the rate of publication of new, primary orthopaedic literature increases annually (**Figure 1**), which suggests that the body of orthopaedic literature is expanding at an exponential rate. A single practicing surgeon can no longer locate, read, and synthesize all published reports relevant to most clinical questions in a reasonable amount of time.

Published reviews of the scientific literature have come to serve an important role as summaries of information from the flood of primary scientific publications. The most common types of reviews are the narrative review and the systematic review. Quantitative derivatives of the systematic review include meta-analysis of published data, pooled reanalysis, and network meta-analysis. Systematic reviews serve a central role in evidence-based medicine, or the process of integrating individual clinical expertise with the best available external clinical evidence from published research to guide decisions about patient care.[1]

Dr. Morshed or an immediate family member serves as a paid consultant to or is an employee of Synthes and serves as a board member, owner, officer, or committee member of the Orthopaedic Trauma Association. Neither Dr. Patterson nor any immediate family member has received anything of value from or has stock or stock options held in a commercial company or institution related directly or indirectly to the subject of this chapter.

The objectives of this chapter are to define the types of literature reviews, to compare the indications and limitations of each type of review within orthopaedic surgery, and to provide the practicing orthopaedic surgeon with an understanding of the methods behind each type of review as well as the skills to interpret and implement review findings.

TYPES OF REVIEWS

NARRATIVE REVIEW

A narrative review summarizes literature selected by an author or group of experts based on the author(s)' opinion of relevance to a topic of interest. The review may touch on multiple topics around one theme: for example, a narrative review on clavicle fractures might include sections on anatomy, types of clavicle fractures, forms of nonsurgical and surgical fixation, and different techniques for fixation. Narrative reviews are useful for providing a broad overview of evaluating and managing a particular condition, for offering historical context, and for characterizing "what's new?" or the "state of the art" in a particular area. A *critical analysis review* is a narrative review that attempts to consider all sides of controversial issues in an even-handed manner and use published evidence to make care recommendations in a standard format.[2]

A narrative review is inherently biased. The method of selecting studies is unlikely to be objective or systematic. Relevant data, findings, or publications may be selectively presented or omitted, while interpretation is usually qualitative and based on opinion or experience.[3] Clinical recommendations from narrative reviews may lag behind or conflict with recently published evidence: an incomplete review of recent literature may fail to identify a new treatment of proven efficacy or recommend a therapy that has

©Copyright 2021 American Academy of Orthopaedic Surgeons

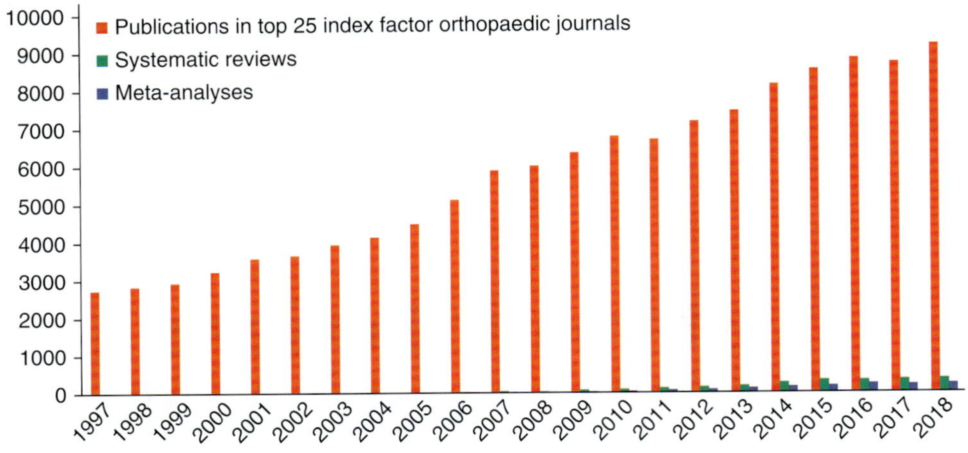

FIGURE 1 Bar graph demonstrates annual generation of orthopaedic primary scientific publications and reviews 1997-2018 published in the top 25 orthopedic journals ranked by impact factor. (NIH PubMed.)

since been proven harmful or useless.[4] For these reasons, the narrative review is no longer an appropriate means of summarizing the best or most current evidence for answering a specific question.

SYSTEMATIC REVIEW

A systematic review is a scientific investigation of published literature. Published studies are the "subjects" of this type of research. All available publications relevant to a specific question are sought, quantitatively assessed for bias, and synthesized if possible in a quantitative or qualitative manner. The full process is detailed later in the chapter.

The purpose of a systematic review is to answer a specific question using published information, favoring the highest level of available evidence. For example, the American Academy of Orthopaedic Surgeons conducts systematic reviews as the basis for developing clinical practice guidelines.[5] Major applications to clinical care also include pooling data across studies to improve statistical power or precision while comparing treatment options, diagnostic tests, or measures of outcome.[6,7]

The limitations of a systematic review include its narrow scope and sensitivity to publication bias. A systematic review cannot cover the breadth of topics possible in a narrative review. Additionally, published trials in orthopaedic surgery are more likely to describe positive treatment effects than negative or null treatment effects,[8] while negative results are less likely to be published[9]—and unpublished results are impossible to include in a systematic review. The efficacy of a treatment, or treatment effect, can therefore be overestimated by a methodologically sound systematic review which has captured publications of selectively published positive results.

META-ANALYSIS

A systematic review pools data from published information. Conventional *meta-analysis* is the quantitative synthesis of that data. *Pooled reanalysis* describes the same techniques applied to unpublished raw data provided by original investigators. These techniques can be used when the individual studies evaluate the same test, exposure, or treatment in similar populations using equivalent outcome assessments. For example, three randomized, controlled trials of single versus double bundle anterior cruciate ligament (ACL) reconstruction that used KT-1000 arthrometer measurements and pivot-shift testing as primary outcomes were sufficiently similar in study methodology to permit meta-analysis of the published data.[10] The reported outcomes in the treatment and control groups in each study were tallied. Associations between the type of ACL reconstruction and the two outcomes were then tested with the data aggregated from the three studies using the statistical techniques for meta-analysis. The authors of the meta-analysis reported a statistically significant finding that double-bundle versus single-bundle ACL reconstruction was associated smaller side-to-side differences in KT-1000 arthrometer laxity measurements that were closer to measurements from the uninjured controls knees.

Meta-analysis improves the power of the statistical analysis, increasing the precision of the result. Greater precision increases the likelihood that any association or difference may be interpreted as statistically significant. However, clinically important or functionally relevant differences may not necessarily exist even if statistically significant differences are reached with meta-analysis. As in the ACL example, that statistical difference established by the higher-powered meta-analysis did not translate to a minimal clinically important difference; there was no clinical advantage or functional benefit conferred to patients by the double-bundle ACL reconstruction over the single bundle technique.

Caution should be exercised when interpreting meta-analysis and considering translating the findings to clinical practice. Pooling similar studies to improve power may sacrifice validity if there is *heterogeneity* among the studies. Heterogeneity refers to differences between studies in selection criteria, characteristics of the sample populations, exposures

©Copyright 2021 American Academy of Orthopaedic Surgeons

or interventions, method of allocating patients to exposures or interventions, distributions of potentially confounding variables across the exposure/intervention and control groups, blinding of the study patients or outcome assessments, outcome assessment techniques, timing of outcome assessment, data collection methods, follow-up, or any other study characteristic or method that differs between studies in a way that could affect—and therefore bias—the measured outcome. Simply, heterogeneity means that a meta-analysis is not comparing apples to apples. Heterogeneity also has a quantitative statistical definition which will be discussed later in this chapter.

Meta-analysis is an additional step performed upon the product of a systematic review. Just as a systematic review does not eliminate any form of bias already present in the included studies, neither does meta-analysis reduce or eliminate bias. The quality of evidence produced from a properly conducted systematic review or meta-analysis is only as good as the quality of the studies that constitute it.

HOW TO PERFORM A SYSTEMATIC REVIEW AND META-ANALYSIS

OVERVIEW

A review begins with a clinical question. In developing a question, a useful starting point is to specifying the target ***p***opulation (condition and context), ***i***ntervention (treatment or exposure), ***c***omparator(s), and primary ***o***utcome(s) to be studied (PICO).[11] A protocol for the review and a search strategy are developed around the question, often with assistance from a research librarian. Studies are identified, screened, and selected for inclusion. The risk of bias, or the quality, of the included studies is assessed. Data are then abstracted. In a systematic review without meta-analysis, the findings from included studies are summarized and discussed qualitatively. In a quantitative systematic review, the findings are pooled and analyzed with statistical methods. The protocol and findings are reported according to accepted guidelines.

Citation manager software such as EndNote (Thomson Reuters, Carlsbad, CA), RefWorks (RefWorks, Bethesda, MD), Zotero (George Mason University, Fairfax, VA) as well as software specifically designed for systematic reviews such as Covidence (Covidence, Melbourne, Victoria) can be helpful for organizing and performing the search, citation review, study appraisal, and data abstraction portions of a systematic review.

PROTOCOL

As with any scientific investigation, a reproducible literature search strategy or protocol is planned prospectively and must be published with the review. The systematic review protocol details the research question, search strategy, methods of assessment, specific data to abstract, and planned analysis. The review protocol is the key feature that differentiates a systematic review from a narrative review. The Preferred Reporting Items for Systematic Reviews and Meta-Analyses Protocol (PRISMA-P) guidelines represent a consensus standard for the necessary elements of a systematic review and an extensive modification of the QUOROM statement from which PRISMA and PRSIMA-P were developed[12-14] (**Table 1**). For systematic reviews of observational studies and other types of research, we recommend consulting the EQUATOR (Enhancing the QUAlity and Transparency Of health Research) Network for the appropriate guideline[15] (a brief list is included in **Table 2**).

HOW TO CRITICALLY READ A SYSTEMATIC REVIEW

Understanding the process involved in generating a systematic review greatly informs the act of critically reading a systematic review.[16] The PRSIMA-P guidelines provide an excellent framework[12] (**Table 2**). Questions to consider include[17]

- Does the review address a specific question formulated with the PICO framework?
- Was the protocol registered as published?
- Is the protocol reproducible?
- Is the search strategy comprehensive, or does the strategy systematically omit a body of relevant research such as a key journal or negative outcome?
- Is there a clear flowchart of study inclusion and exclusion with explanations?
- Are the included studies sufficiently homogenous in their methods and populations to pool the data?
- Are the data extraction and synthesis appropriate?
- Do forest and inverted funnel plots support meta-analysis?
- Did the review address confidence in estimates of effect? Are there sources of funding that could introduce bias?
- Do the results apply directly to my patient?

Current practice now favors publishing the systematic review protocol *before* undertaking the review. Prospective publication of review protocols in a permanent record such as PROSPERO (an international register of systematic reviews supported by the United Kingdom National Health Service) prevents researchers from undertaking overlapping reviews and reduces the opportunity for reporting bias.[18] Before detailing a protocol, the review question should be queried using an electronic web-based search engines as well as the PROSPERO registry to see if an overlapping review has already been published or is underway.

©Copyright 2021 American Academy of Orthopaedic Surgeons

TABLE 1 PRISMA-P 2015 Checklist: Recommended Items to Include in a Systematic Review Protocol

Section/Topic	Item #	Checklist Item
Administrative Information		
Title		
Identification	1a`	Identify the report as a protocol of a systematic review
Update	1b	If the protocol is for an update of a previous systematic review, identify as such
Registration	2	If registered, provide the name of the registry (eg, PROSPERO) and registration number
Authors		
Contact	3a	Provide name, institutional affiliation, and e-mail address of all protocol authors; provide physical mailing address of corresponding author
Contributions	3b	Describe contributions of protocol authors and identify the guarantor of the review
Amendments	4	If the protocol represents an amendment of a previously completed or published protocol, identify as such and list changes; otherwise, state plan for documenting important protocol amendments
Support		
Sources	5a	Indicate sources of financial or other support for the review
Sponsor	5b	Provide name for the review funder and/or sponsor
Role of sponsor/funder	5c	Describe roles of funder(s), sponsor(s), and/or institution(s), if any, in developing the protocol
Introduction		
Rationale	6	Describe the rationale for the review in the context of what is already known
Objectives	7	Provide an explicit statement of the question(s) the review will address with reference to participants, interventions, comparators, and outcomes (PICO)
Methods		
Eligibility criteria	8	Specify the study characteristics (eg, PICO, study design, setting, time frame) and report characteristics (eg, years considered, language, publication status) to be used as criteria for eligibility for the review
Information sources	9	Describe all intended information sources (eg, electronic databases, contact with study authors, trial registers, or other grey literature sources) with planned dates of coverage
Search strategy	10	Present draft of search strategy to be used for at least one electronic database, including planned limits, such that it could be repeated
Study records		
Data management	11a	Describe the mechanism(s) that will be used to manage records and data throughout the review
Selection process	11b	State the process that will be used for selecting studies (eg, two independent reviewers) through each phase of the review (ie, screening, eligibility, and inclusion in meta-analysis)
Data collection process	11c	Describe planned method of extracting data from reports (eg, piloting forms, done independently, in duplicate), any processes for obtaining and confirming data from investigators
Data items	12	List and define all variables for which data will be sought (eg, PICO items, funding sources), any preplanned data assumptions and simplifications
Outcomes and prioritization	13	List and define all outcomes for which data will be sought, including prioritization of main and additional outcomes, with rationale
Risk of bias in individual studies	14	Describe anticipated methods for assessing risk of bias of individual studies, including whether this will be done at the outcome or study level, or both; state how this information will be used in data synthesis

©Copyright 2021 American Academy of Orthopaedic Surgeons

TABLE 1 PRISMA-P 2015 Checklist: Recommended Items to Include in a Systematic Review Protocol (Continued)

Section/Topic	Item #	Checklist Item
Data		
Synthesis	15a	Describe criteria under which study data will be quantitatively synthesized
	15b	If data are appropriate for quantitative synthesis, describe planned summary measures, methods of handling data, and methods of combining data from studies, including any planned exploration of consistency (eg, I^2, Kendall's tau)
	15c	Describe any proposed additional analyses (eg, sensitivity or subgroup analyses, meta-regression)
	15d	If quantitative synthesis is not appropriate, describe the type of summary planned
Meta-bias(es)	16	Specify any planned assessment of meta-bias(es) (eg, publication bias across studies, selective reporting within studies)
Confidence in cumulative evidence	17	Describe how the strength of the body of evidence will be assessed (eg, GRADE)

Adapted from Shamseer L, Moher D, Clarke M, et al, PRISMA-P Group: Preferred reporting items for systematic review and meta-analysis protocols (PRISMA-P) 2015: elaboration and explanation. *BMJ* 2015;349:g7647. Used under Creative Commons Attribution License 4.0, http://creativecommons.org/licenses/by/4.0/.

SEARCH STRATEGY

The search strategy begins with specifying the types of studies to include or exclude the following: randomized controlled trials, prospective nonrandomized trials, retrospective observational series, biomechanical studies, animal studies, etc. The range of publication dates and languages are specified. Search terms are then developed using the study question; modifications are made specific to the query language of each electronic web-based source to be queried (PubMed, Embase, Cochrane Controlled Trials Registry, Biosis, Google Scholar, ClinicalTrials.gov). Alternate sources are also identified (conference proceedings and abstracts) for manual reviewed. A useful starting point for developing search terms is to manually develop a list of "must-include" citations, then iteratively modify a search query for each literature source until each query captures all of the critical citations. Then all sources are searched using the final queries.

TITLE AND ABSTRACT REVIEW

Titles and abstracts are screened against the protocol inclusion and exclusion criteria. Full-text manuscripts of the included studies are then retrieved and reviewed again for final inclusion. To limit investigator bias, all reference citations should be screened for validity by at least two independent reviewers. Reviewers should be blind to identifying information such as study authors, journal, and year of publication when possible. If the reviewers disagree on inclusion or exclusion, an additional reviewer can serve in an arbitration role.[19] The PRISMA-P guidelines specify that the study selection process by reported graphically with a flow diagram[14] (**Figure 2**).

STUDY APPRAISAL AND DATA EXTRACTION

The quality of a systematic review can only be as good as the methodologic quality of the studies the review canvasses. "Quality" in this sense is perhaps best described as the risk of bias—or conversely, the probability that the reported findings are both precise and accurate. There is controversy over how a reviewer should go about appraising study quality. For example, a number of tools have been published that generate ordinal grades or numeric scores for the quality of the methods used by each study included in a systematic review, such as the Jadad/Oxford quality scoring system for clinical trials,[20] the Newcastle-Ottawa Scale for nonrandomized studies,[21] and the GRADE system for certainty in evidence and strength of clinical practice recommendations.[22] Conversely, the Cochrane Collaboration does not support the use of quality scales, recommending instead a tabular reporting of assessments of multiple forms bias across studies[23] (**Figure 3**). All of these methods attempt to identify shortcomings in study design and reporting that could bias the outcome falsely away from the true result. The Cochrane Handbook for Systematic Reviews of Interventions offers a thorough discussion of the type and detriments of bias.[23] As tools for identifying bias remain an area of active development, we recommend consulting the EQUATOR Network for up-to-date recommendations for reporting guidelines and bias assessments specific to the type of studies that are included in a systematic review[15] (**Table 2**).

Data are extracted from the included studies using a collection form. The integrity of the process is strengthened by using at least two reviewers as well as blinding of the reviewers to author, institution, journal names, and funding sources.[24] Final assessments of study quality and decisions to exclude studies are sometimes made after data extraction.

©Copyright 2021 American Academy of Orthopaedic Surgeons

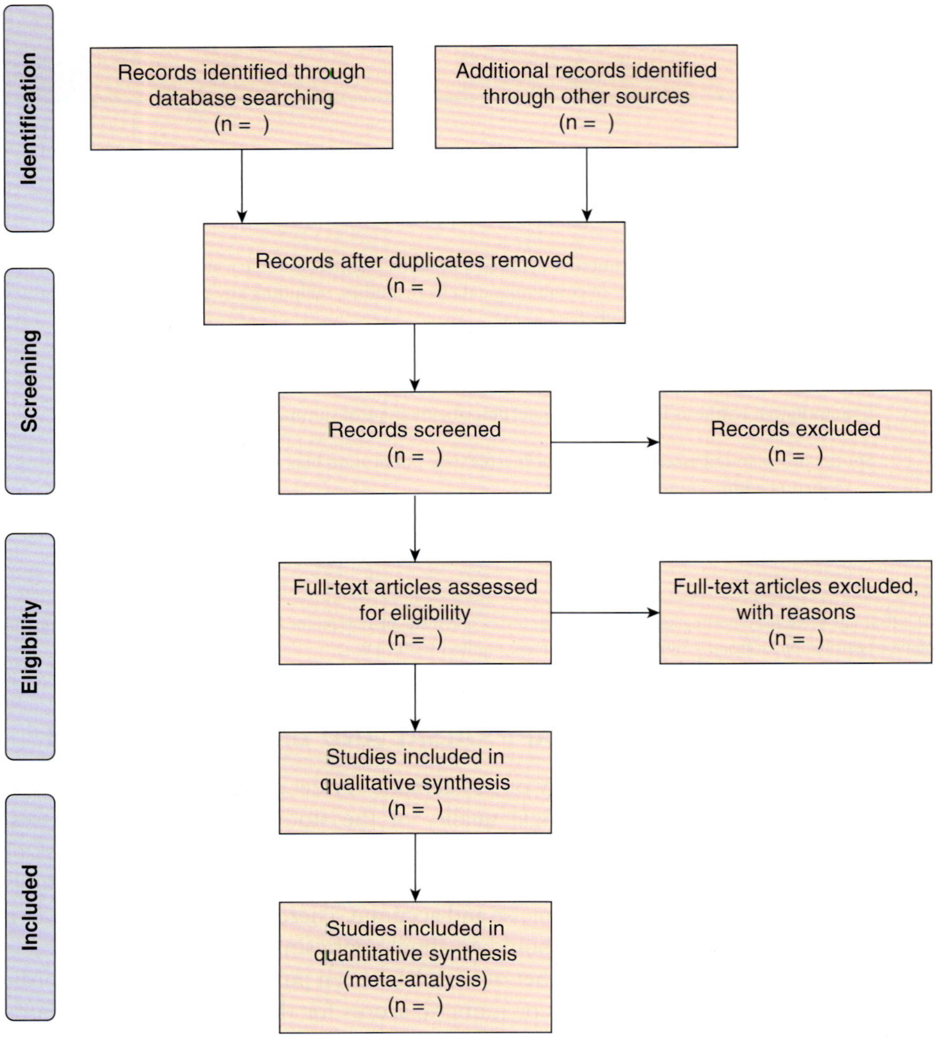

FIGURE 2 PRISMA 2009 flow diagram. (Adapted from Moher D, Liberati A, Tetzlaff J, Altman DG, The PRISMA Group: Preferred reporting items for systematic reviews and meta-analyses: The PRISMA statement. *PLOS Med* 2009;6(7):e1000097. Used under Creative Commons Attribution License 4.0, http://creativecommons.org/licenses/by/4.0/.)

META-ANALYSIS

Meta-analysis estimates a pooled treatment effect size. Pooled results are used to increase statistical power and lead to more precise estimates of treatment effect.[25] Requirements for a meta-analysis include quantitative, similar outcomes from methodologically similar studies collected via systematic review. *Heterogeneity* and *publication bias* are major concerns to the validity of a meta-analysis.

To undertake a valid analysis of pooled data from multiple studies, the studies should use similar methods to assess the effect of similar treatments in similar populations. If the studies are unbiased (or identically biased), the treatment effect will not vary across the studies. If the studies use different methods or outcomes, or are biased in different ways, the treatment effect will vary between studies. *Heterogeneity* is the magnitude of the statistical diversity of the treatment effect that exists among the included studies.[23] An explanation of commonly reported statistical measures of heterogeneity is included in **Table 3**.

A study must be published in some form to appear in a systematic review. As not all studies have an equal chance of being published, publication is a source of bias. Small studies, nonrandomized studies, and studies with negative results are less likely to be published.[25] Time-lag bias can occur if one study is published more rapidly than other, subsequently published, studies with differing results. There also may be detection bias if reviewers cannot read or write searches in a particular language. *Publication bias* can be detected by reviewing a scatter plot of sample size, standard error, or variance against the effect estimate for a collection of studies. Asymmetry, or nonrandom deviation away from zero, indicates bias. The inverted funnel plot, or Egger test, is usually skewed or otherwise asymmetric in the presence of publication bias (as in **Figure 4**). The "cone" of the plot typically represents a 95% confidence interval for the standard error expected for a given effect size.[24]

The actual meta-analysis is a calculation of the treatment effect using the pooled data from the included studies, with or without weights. The pooled treatment effect is usually

©Copyright 2021 American Academy of Orthopaedic Surgeons

	Random sequence generation	Allocation concealment	Blinding of participants and personnel	Blinding of outcome assessment	Incomplete outcome data	Selective reporting	Other bias
Study 1	+	+	+	–	+	+	–
Study 2	+	–	+	?	+	+	+
Study 3	–	+	?	–	–	?	+
Study 4	+	–	–	+	–	–	?
Study 5	+	?	+	?	+	?	–

FIGURE 3 Example of Cochrane "risk of bias" assessment tool for randomized controlled trials. Each hypothetical listed study is judged on specific criteria that constitute study quality, forgoing a summary score.

reported as an average of effect measurements (risk ratio, odds ratio, risk difference) weighted by sample size or precision of the individual study estimates, for example, inverse variance weighting. In this type of weighted pooling, each study is assigned a weight based on the precision of its results, and precise estimates of treatment effect are assigned more weight in the computation of averages.

Forest plots are routinely used to visually summarize the results of a meta-analysis in the context of the results individual reviewed studies (**Figure 5**). A forest plot typically has two main components: data that identify the individual studies and the plot itself. A vertical line is drawn through the center of the plot to represent the null hypothesis (no difference between patients in the treatment and control groups). A square and a horizontal line correspond to each study's estimate of effect (the odds ratio, risk ratio, or risk difference) and confidence interval, respectively. The size of the square reflects the weight given to the study in the analysis.[24] At the bottom of the plot is the pooled overall estimate, with its 95% confidence interval represented by a diamond. The center of the diamond on the vertical plane represents the average treatment effect, and the left and right apices represent the confidence intervals.[26]

Software packages for performing meta-analysis of studies gathered in a systematic review are available for standard statistical software such as R, SAS, SPSS, STATA, etc.[27] Many of these packages offer advanced techniques such as meta-regression and subgroup analysis that may be used to investigate causes of heterogeneity. The reader of a meta-analysis need not be familiar with these statistical procedures, but should evaluate whether pooling of study results was justified, whether heterogeneity and sources of systematic bias considered, and if found, how they were investigated and reported.

TABLE 2 Reporting Guidelines by Study Type

Study Type	Reporting Guideline
Randomized controlled trials	CONSORT
Observational studies	STROBE
Systematic reviews	PRISMA
Study protocols	SPIRIT, PRISMA-P
Diagnostic/prognostic studies	STARD, TRIPOD
Case reports	CARE
Clinical practice guidelines	AGREE, RIGHT
Qualitative research	SRQR, COREQ
Animal preclinical studies	ARRIVE
Quality improvement studies	SQUIRE
Economic evaluations	CHEERS

The EQUATOR Network: Reporting guidelines. Equator Network, 2019. Available at: https://www.equator-network.org/reporting-guidelines/. Accessed October 9, 2019.

TABLE 3 Statistical Tools for Reporting Heterogeneity in Meta-analysis

Statistic	Derivation	Limitations
Cochran's Q	Weighted sum of squared differences between individual study effects and the pooled effect across studies, with the weights being those used in the pooling method.	Underpowered to detect between-study variability when the number of studies is small, which is usually the case.[29] Overpowered if the number of studies is large.[30]
Higgins I_2	Proportion (0%-100%) of total variation in the estimates of treatment effect that is due to heterogeneity between studies, independent of the number of studies as well as the metric for treatment.[23]	Does not communicate a confidence level regarding heterogeneity, unless reported with a confidence interval.[30]
L'Abbé plot	Plot of event rate in the intervention group against the event rate in the control group	Qualitative, visual representation

©Copyright 2021 American Academy of Orthopaedic Surgeons

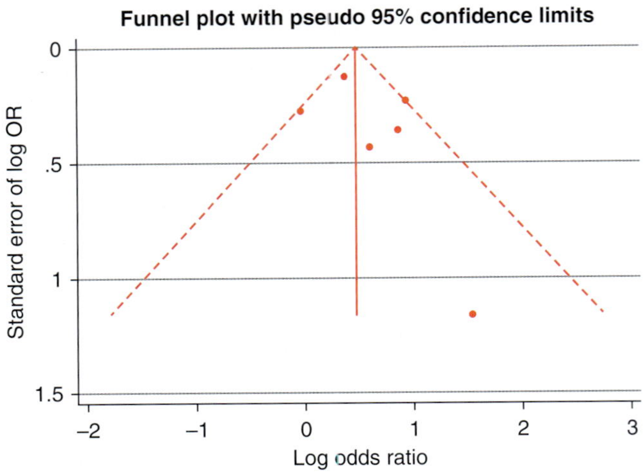

FIGURE 4 Inverted funnel (Egger) plot demonstrating asymmetry suggesting publication bias in systematic review of allogeneic transfusion versus control following primary total hip and knee arthroplasty. (Reproduced with permission from Kim JL, Park J-H, Han S-B, Cho IY, Jang K-M: Allogeneic blood transfusion is a significant risk factor for surgical-site infection following total hip and knee arthroplasty: A meta-analysis. *J Arthroplasty* 2017;32(1):320-325.)

NETWORK META-ANALYSIS

Conventional meta-analysis is applied to direct comparisons of a treatment/exposure and a comparator: does treatment A have a greater effect than treatment B? Consider a situation with more than two treatments. A group of trials show that treatment A has a greater treatment effect than treatment B. Then, a separate group of trials show that treatment B has less of an effect than treatment C. *Network meta-analysis* refers to the suite of mathematical tools an investigator can use to indirectly determine the relative effect (relative risk, risk difference, odds ratio, etc.) of treatment A versus treatment C, using the existing evidence comparing A to B and B to C and without a direct comparison of A to C. More generally, several trials each comparing two or more interventions on one common outcome each provide direct evidence. Indirect comparisons of treatment effect can be made between interventions not directly compared in an actual trial by organizing the studies into closed- and open-loop networks.[9]

A comprehensive overview of the methodological and statistical considerations required to design or report a network meta-analysis are beyond the scope of this chapter and readers

Rate of transfusion: Effect of TXA administration

Model	Study name	Odds ratio	Lower limit	Upper limit	Z-Value	p-Value
	Lee	0.275	0.104	0.729	−2.594	0.009
	Emara	0.098	0.018	0.531	−2.692	0.007
	Zuffrey	0.477	0.223	1.022	−1.904	0.057
	Sadeghi	0.450	0.169	1.199	−1.597	0.110
	Vijay	0.276	0.101	0.753	−2.514	0.012
	Mohib	0.303	0.121	0.756	−2.559	0.011
	Drakos	0.691	0.364	1.310	−1.133	0.257
	Tengberg	0.818	0.237	2.829	−0.317	0.751
	Xie	0.333	0.013	8.421	−0.667	0.505
	Watts	0.596	0.262	1.358	−1.231	0.218
	Kashyap	0.025	0.003	0.207	−3.418	0.001
	Clinical Trial Pfizer	0.787	0.220	2.819	−0.368	0.713
Fixed		0.435	0.326	0.582	−5.610	0.000
Random		0.407	0.278	0.594	−4.656	0.000

(Statistics for each study)

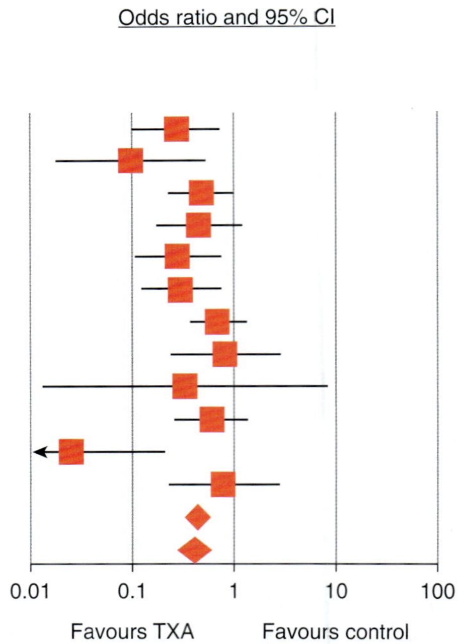

Meta-analysis

FIGURE 5 Forest plot of tranexamic acid versus control demonstrating a significant pooled reduction in blood transfusion in orthopaedic trauma surgery. (Reproduced with permission from Gausden EB, Qudsi R, Boone MD, O'Gara B, Ruzbarsky JJ, Lorich DG: Tranexamic acid in orthopaedic trauma surgery: A meta-analysis. *J Orthop Trauma* 2017;31(10):513-519.)

©Copyright 2021 American Academy of Orthopaedic Surgeons

desiring more detail are referred to these "Users' Guides" by Foote et al and Chaudhry et al.[9,28] The following principles, however, will aid in the interpretation of published analyses using these techniques. *Transitivity* is an extension of *homogeneity* that describes sufficient similarity in patients, interventions, and outcomes across the studies in the network that direct comparisons can be reasonably used to estimate indirect comparisons. *Incoherence* describes disagreement between direct and indirect estimates, which indicates that heterogeneity or bias in the published direct comparisons has propagated in the indirect comparisons. Indirect comparisons are estimates based on estimates, which implies a layer of uncertainty upon uncertainty. The more complex the network of comparisons, the more uncertain each indirect estimate. Conversely, the more studies or patients available for each direct comparison, the more certain each indirect estimate of treatment effect.

Estimated treatment effects are relative: each treatment has a certain probability of being ranked 1st or most effect, a different probability of being ranked 2nd most effective, and so on. Visual "rankograms" and surface under the cumulative ranking curve (SUCRA) scores help represent the magnitude, direction, and uncertainty in the network treatment effect comparisons. These reporting tools for network meta-analysis may not communicate bias, incoherence, or intransitivity.[28] Translating the findings of a network meta-analysis to clinical practice may be challenging without the assistance of a statistician or familiarity with the methods and their shortcomings. The utility of this type of analysis will continue to improve with publication of additional level 1 evidence comparing well-defined treatments.

SUMMARY

Reviews are a useful way for the practicing orthopaedic surgeon to stay abreast of new research. Narrative reviews are not an appropriate source for clinical practice recommendations based on the best available evidence, but are useful as broad overviews of a topic, descriptions of author-preferred surgical techniques, digests of recent publications, and developments in the field. Systematic reviews are protocol-driven investigations, narrow in focus, that represent the backbone of evidence-based medicine. Familiarity with the process of conducting a systematic review permits the reader to assess clinical utility and potential sources of bias. Meta-analysis increases confidence in the magnitude of a treatment effect, but requires a high-quality systematic review and caution with regard to heterogeneity and publication bias among the included studies when interpreting results.

PEARLS

- Reviews synthesize the findings of published literature
- A narrative review is an inherently biased discussion of arbitrarily selected studies based on expert preference
- A narrative review may provide a broad perspective or expert experience not possible with a systematic review
- A systematic review is a protocol-driven research investigation of published literature focused on a single question
- Systematic review protocols should be prospectively registered and reported according consensus guidelines
- Meta-analysis is the quantitative analysis of data pooled from multiple studies
- Meta-analysis increases confidence in the estimate of a treatment effect if constituted by sufficiently similar primary studies of high quality
- Consensus reporting guidelines offer frameworks for critically interpreting published studies and literature reviews

REFERENCES

1. Sackett DL, Rosenberg WM, Gray JM, Haynes RB, Richardson WS: Evidence based medicine. *Br Med J* 1996;313:170.
2. *JBJS Reviews*. Instructions for Authors. Available at: https://journals.lww.com/jbjsreviews/Pages/Instructions-for-Authors.aspx.
3. Montori VM, Swiontkowski MF, Cook DJ: Methodologic issues in systematic reviews and meta-analyses. *Clin Orthop Relat Res* 2003;413:43-54.
4. Antman EM, Lau J, Kupelnick B, Mosteller F, Chalmers TC: A comparison of results of meta-analyses of randomized control trials and recommendations of clinical experts: Treatments for myocardial infarction. *J Am Med Assoc* 1992;268:240-248.
5. American Academy of Orthopaedic Surgery. *Evidence-Based Clinical Practice Guidelines*. Available at: https://www.aaos.org/cpg/?ssopc=1.
6. Zlowodzki M, Zelle BA, Cole PA, Jeray K, McKee MD: Treatment of acute midshaft clavicle fractures: Systematic review of 2144 fractures. On behalf of the evidence-based orthopaedic trauma working group. *J Orthop Trauma* 2005;19:504-507.
7. Ball C, Pratt AL, Nanchahal J: Optimal functional outcome measures for assessing treatment for Dupuytren's disease: A systematic review and recommendations for future practice. *BMC Muscoskelet Disord* 2013;14:131.
8. Dijkman BG, Abouali JA, Kooistra BW, et al: Twenty years of meta-analyses in orthopaedic surgery: Has quality kept up with quantity? *J Bone Joint Surg* 2010;92:48-57.
9. Foote CJ, Chaudhry H, Bhandari M, et al: Network meta-analysis: Users' guide for surgeons: Part I – Credibility. *Clin Orthop Relat Res* 2015;473:2166-2171.
10. Meredick RB, Vance KJ, Appleby D, Lubowitz JH: Outcome of single-bundle versus double-bundle reconstruction of the anterior cruciate ligament: A meta-analysis. *Am J Sports Med* 2008;36:1414-1421.

©Copyright 2021 American Academy of Orthopaedic Surgeons

11. Richardson WS, Wilson MC, Nishikawa J, Hayward RS: The well-built clinical question: A key to evidence-based decisions. *ACP J Club* 1995;123:A12-A13.
12. Moher D, Shamseer L, Clarke M, et al: Preferred reporting items for systematic review and meta-analysis protocols (PRISMA-P) 2015 statement. *Syst Rev* 2015;4:1.
13. Moher D, Cook DJ, Eastwood S, Olkin I, Rennie D, Stroup DF: Improving the quality of reports of meta-analyses of randomised controlled trials: The QUOROM statement. *Oncol Res Treat* 2000;23:597-602.
14. Moher D, Liberati A, Tetzlaff J, Altman DG: Preferred reporting items for systematic reviews and meta-analyses: The PRISMA statement. *Int J Surg* 2010;8:336-341.
15. Enhancing the QUAlity and Transparency Of health Research (EQUATOR) Network. Reporting guidelines for main study types, 2018. Available at: https://www.equator-network.org/.
16. Murad MH, Montori VM, Ioannidis JP, et al: How to read a systematic review and meta-analysis and apply the results to patient care: Users' guides to the medical literature. *J Am Med Assoc* 2014;312:171-179.
17. Drucker AM, Fleming P, Chan AW: Research techniques made simple: Assessing risk of bias in systematic reviews. *J Invest Dermatol* 2016;136:e109-e114.
18. University of York Center for Reviews and Dissemination: About PROSPERO. Available at: https://www.crd.york.ac.uk/prospero/#aboutpage.
19. Wright RW, Brand RA, Dunn W, Spindler KP: How to write a systematic review. *Clin Orthop Relat Res* 2007;455:23-29.
20. Jadad AR, Moore RA, Carroll D, et al: Assessing the quality of reports of randomized clinical trials: Is blinding necessary? *Contr Clin Trials* 1996;17:1-12.
21. Wells GA, Shea B, O'Connell D, et al: *The Newcastle-Ottawa Scale (NOS) for Assessing the Quality of Nonrandomised Studies in Meta-Analyses*, 2018. Available at: http://www.ohri.ca/programs/clinical_epidemiology/oxford.asp.
22. GRADE Working Group: *What is GRADE?* 2018. Available at: http://www.gradeworkinggroup.org/.
23. Cochrane Collaboration: *Cochrane Handbook for Systematic Reviews of Interventions*, 2008. Cochrane Collaboration.
24. Egger M, Davey-Smith G, Altman D: *Systematic Reviews in Health Care: Meta-Analysis in Context*, 2008. John Wiley & Sons.
25. Lau J, Ioannidis JP, Schmid CH: Quantitative synthesis in systematic reviews. *Ann Intern Med* 1997;127:820-826.
26. Lewis S, Clarke M: Forest plots: Trying to see the wood and the trees. *Br Med J* 2001;322:1479.
27. Sterne JAC, Bradburn MJ, Egger M, in Egger M, Smith GD, Altman DG eds: *Systematic Reviews in Health Care.* Wiley, 2008, (Chap 18: Meta-analysis in Stata).
28. Chaudhry H, Foote CJ, Guyatt G, et al: Network meta-analysis: Users' guide for surgeons. Part II–Certainty. *Clin Orthop Relat Res* 2015;473:2172-2178.
29. Gavaghan DJ, Moore RA, McQuay HJ: An evaluation of homogeneity tests in meta-analyses in pain using simulations of individual patient data. *Pain* 2000;85:415-424.
30. Higgins JP, Thompson SG, Deeks JJ, Altman DG: Measuring inconsistency in meta-analyses. *Br Med J* 2003;327:557.

©Copyright 2021 American Academy of Orthopaedic Surgeons

44

Evidence-Based Medicine and Best-Practice Guidelines

Caroline Boyle, BA
Niv Marom, MD
Robert G. Marx, MD

Keywords: *best-practice guidelines; evidence-based medicine; level of evidence; systematic review*

INTRODUCTION

A desire to provide standardized and competent care has driven the medical field to implement evidence-based medicine. The goal of evidence-based medicine is for physicians to use the best available evidence, as well as their clinical experience, to guide their clinical decision making. In order for physicians to determine which research studies provide the best evidence, medical journals classify publications based on their level of evidence. The higher the level of evidence, the less chance there is that the results of the study might be affected by bias or confounding. Systematic reviews and meta-analyses compile available evidence to make it easier for physicians to review all of the publications on a certain topic. Once there is a sufficient amount of evidence on a given topic, healthcare organizations, such as the American Academy of Orthopaedic Surgery, develop best-practice guidelines to inform health care in their field. Best-practice guidelines have important implications both legally (malpractice litigation) and economically (healthcare insurance company coverage); thus, it is very important that people understand, and critically evaluate, how they are developed and modified when new evidence becomes available.

Dr. Marx or an immediate family member has stock or stock options held in Mend and serves as a board member, owner, officer, or committee member of the International Society of Arthroscopy, Knee Surgery, and Orthopaedic Sports Medicine. Neither of the following authors nor any immediate family member has received anything of value from or has stock or stock options held in a commercial company or institution related directly or indirectly to the subject of this chapter: Ms. Boyle and Dr. Marom.

HISTORY OF EVIDENCE-BASED MEDICINE

In 2007, *The British Journal of Medicine* published a list of the 15 most important medical milestones since the Journal originated in 1840.[1] On that list were vaccinations, the discovery of DNA, as well as the concept of evidence-based medicine (EBM). This concept was originally described by Gordon Guyatt at McMaster University in 1992.[2] Guyatt explained that with EBM, clinical decisions are made based on the best available evidence and patients' values, rather than exclusively on medical practitioners experience or intuition. A good practitioner will combine both their experiences and the best available literature to make medical decisions.[3] The challenge to handle an increased demand for healthcare services required an effective way to determine the most successful treatment plan for each patient.

Advances in orthopaedics between 1940 and 1970s were made based on case series for treatments such as total joint replacement, internal fixation of fractures, and instrumentation for the spine. However, after these major advances, it became clear different research methods (case-control studies, prospective cohort studies, and randomized controlled trials) were needed to continue to improve patient outcomes.[4] The *Journal of Bone and Joint Surgery* began to publish "*Evidence-Based Orthopaedics*" in 2000 which published randomized controlled trials (RCTs) and provided a commentary to put the evidence presented in the RCT into context. The journal did this to help orthopaedic surgeons use the best evidence available to inform their clinical practice.[5]

©Copyright 2021 American Academy of Orthopaedic Surgeons

LEVELS OF EVIDENCE

Sacket et al first broached the concept of levels of evidence in 1996 when he explained that there are not always RCTs available to inform medical decisions.[6] In these scenarios, one must be able to evaluate the evidence that is available and determine what is of the most significance. See the pyramid in **Figure 1** which depicts the quality of evidence of different research studies. RCTs are considered to be the strongest type of evidence followed by cohort studies, case series, and finally by expert opinions (**Figure 1**). Systematic reviews are considered the strongest because they combine all available evidence.

The level of evidence table is a tool that was developed to help organize the hierarchy of different types of research studies. In 2003, the *Journal of Bone and Joint Surgery* published their first level of evidence table and began to assign every article published a level of evidence. This was done in an effort to help readers classify the evidence that they were reading and to encourage authors/researchers to improve their research methodology.[5] See **Table 1** which is the updated version of the Level of Evidence table that is used by the Journal today (**Table 1**). There are four different types of studies which can then be assigned levels I to V. Therapeutic studies evaluate the effect of a treatment on patient outcomes. Prognostic studies consider the effect of patient characteristics on patient outcomes. Diagnostic studies study if the results of a test are related to the presence of a disease. Lastly, economic studies consider the cost of a certain treatment.[7]

The reason some types of studies are given higher level of evidence over others is because of their ability to limit bias and confounding. Bias is described as systematic error introduced by the design of the study.[8] This can come in the form of selection bias, in which case the selection of participants results in a group that is different than the study population. For example, if observing complication rates after a procedure, and one only surveys people who are still attending follow-up visits, this might lead to the conclusion that there is a higher complication rate because patients who continue to attend follow-up visits often have increased complaints they want to share with their surgeon. Healthy patients are less likely to attend long-term follow-up visits as they do not have anything to share with their surgeon. Thus, the population of people still attending follow-up visits may have a higher concentration of patients with bad outcomes. Additionally, information bias is defined as a systematic error in the measurement of exposures or outcomes.[8] For example, if patients are asked to report on the state of their condition, those who have had problems may be more likely to remember more details. This is known as recall bias.

Confounding is when there is another variable other than the independent or dependent variables that is associated with either the exposure or the outcome. This can lead to either masking a true correlation in the study results or to creating a correlation that is not actually present.[8] Both bias and confounding can be limited with good study design.

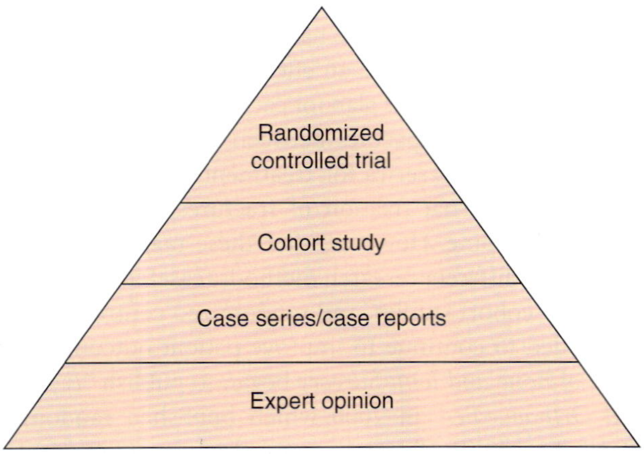

FIGURE 1 Illustration showing the hierarchy of research studies. (Adapted from Murad MH, Asi N, Alsawas M, Alahdab F: New evidence pyramid. *Br J Med* 2016;21:125-127.)

RANDOMIZED CONTROLLED TRIAL

A randomized controlled trial is given the highest level of evidence because it has the best potential to limit bias and confounding. In this type of study, patients are randomly assigned to the intervention group (receive a treatment) or the control group (receive no treatment or receive the standard treatment). As patients are randomly assigned to a treatment group, it is assumed that factors that cause confounding or bias are evenly distributed between the two groups. However, RCTs often have extremely narrow inclusion/exclusion criteria to achieve randomization. This can limit the generalizability of the results to specific patients. One thing that can limit the quality of an RCT is when randomization is not done properly. Additionally, when the outcome assessors are not blinded to the group designation there can be bias with outcome evaluation.

There are many issues specific to RCTs when randomizing to surgical or nonsurgical treatment. For example, differences in surgeon experience level may affect the uniformity of the surgery arm of the RCT. This is a limitation that is not present in drug-related RCTs. Crossover is another issue that is often found in surgical RCTs, and this can introduce patient selection bias. Crossover is when patients assigned to the nonsurgicalerative group crossover and undergo surgery. For example, Frobell et al published a RCT randomizing patients to either rehabilitation or anterior cruciate ligament reconstruction (ACLR), and by 5 years post randomization, 51% of the patients in the nonsurgical group had chosen to undergo ACLR.[9] This increases the complexity of the analysis for the comparison between groups. Overall, while RCTs are assigned the highest level of evidence, they are often very expensive and not always possible in the surgical environment due to ethical concerns and patient/surgeon preferences.[10]

©Copyright 2021 American Academy of Orthopaedic Surgeons

TABLE 1 Levels of Evidence for Primary Research Question[a,b]

Study Type	Question	Level I	Level II	Level III	Level IV	Level V
Diagnostic—Investigating a diagnostic test	Is this (early detection) test worthwhile?	• Randomized controlled trial	• Prospective[c] cohort[d] study	• Retrospective[e] cohort[d] study • Case-control[f] study	• Case series	• Mechanism-based reasoning
	Is this diagnostic or monitoring test accurate?	• Testing of previously developed diagnostic criteria (consecutive patients with consistently applied reference standard and blinding)	• Development of diagnostic criteria (consecutive patients with consistently applied reference standard and blinding)	• Nonconsecutive patients • No consistently applied reference standard	• Poor or nonindependent reference standard	• Mechanism-based reasoning
Prognostic—Investigating the effect of a patient characteristic on the outcome of a disease	What is the natural history of the condition?	• Inception[c] cohort study (all patients enrolled at an early, uniform point in the course of their disease)	• Prospective[c] cohort[d] study (patients enrolled at different points in their disease) • Control arm of randomized trial	• Retrospective[e] cohort[d] study • Case-control[f] study	• Case series	• Mechanism-based reasoning
Therapeutic—Investigating the results of a treatment	Does this treatment help? What are the harms?[g]	• Randomized controlled trial	• Prospective[c] cohort[d] study • Observational study with dramatic effect	• Retrospective[e] cohort[d] study • Case-control[f] study	• Case series • Historically controlled study	• Mechanism-based reasoning
Economic	Does the intervention offer good value for dollars spent?	Computer simulation model (Monte Carlo simulation, Markov model) with inputs derived from level-I studies, lifetime time duration, outcomes expressed in dollars per quality-adjusted life years (QALYs) and uncertainty examined using probabilistic sensitivity analyses	Computer simulation model (Monte Carlo simulation, Markov model) with inputs derived from level-II studies, lifetime time duration, outcomes expressed in dollars per QALYs and uncertainty examined using probabilistic sensitivity analyses	Computer simulation model (Markov model) with inputs derived from level-II studies, relevant time horizon, less than lifetime, outcomes expressed in dollars per QALYs and stochastic multilevel sensitivity analyses	Decision tree over the short time horizon with input data from original level-II and III studies and uncertainty is examined by univariate sensitivity analyses	Decision tree over the short time horizon with input data informed by prior economic evaluation and uncertainty is examined by univariate sensitivity analyses

[a]This chart was adapted from OCEBM Levels of Evidence Working Group, "The Oxford 2011 Levels of Evidence," Oxford Centre for Evidence-Based Medicine, http://www.cebm.net/ocebm-levels-of-evidence/. A glossary of terms can be found here: http://www.cebm.net/glossary/.

[b]Level-I through -IV studies may be graded downward on the basis of study quality, imprecision, indirectness, or inconsistency between studies or because the effect size is very small; these studies may be graded upward if there is a dramatic effect size. For example, a high-quality randomized controlled trial (RCT) should have ‡80% follow-up, blinding, and proper randomization. The level of evidence assigned to systematic reviews reflects the ranking of studies included in the review (ie, a systematic review of level-II studies is level II). A complete assessment of the quality of individual studies requires critical appraisal of all aspects of study design.

[c]Investigators formulated the study question before the first patient was enrolled.

[d]In these studies, "cohort" refers to a nonrandomized comparative study. For therapeutic studies, patients treated one way (eg, cemented hip prosthesis) are compared with those treated differently (eg, noncemented hip prosthesis).

[e]Investigators formulated the study question after the first patient was enrolled.

[f]Patients identified for the study on the basis of their outcome (eg, failed total hip arthroplasty), called "cases," are compared with those who did not have the outcome (eg, successful total hip arthroplasty), called "controls."

[g]Sufficient numbers are required to rule out a common harm (affects >20% of participants). For long-term harms, follow-up duration must be sufficient.

Reproduced with permission from Marx RG, Wilson WS, Swiontokowski MF: Updating the assignment levels of evidence. *J Bone Joint Surg Am* 2015;64(1):1-2; Table 1.

©Copyright 2021 American Academy of Orthopaedic Surgeons

COHORT STUDY

A cohort study involves two groups of patients with similar characteristics who are followed for a period of time to assess for a certain outcome. The two groups can have two different treatments or different risk factors, depending on the type of study (therapeutic or prognostic etc.). A cohort study can be either prospective or retrospective. In a prospective cohort study, the treatment is assigned and then the group is followed and assessed for a certain outcome. The only difference between a well-done prospective cohort study and an RCT is that in a prospective cohort study, the group assignment is not random and not blinded. In a retrospective cohort study, the outcomes are assessed via patient records/patient reports and then compared between two groups. Additionally, many outcomes can be assessed at once. Disadvantages of cohort studies are that they are susceptible to selection bias and as treatment groups are not randomly assigned or blinded, patients and physicians sometimes choose to change the primary assigned treatment and can further limit the quality of the study.

Case-control studies are a subset of cohort studies in which patients with a certain outcome of interest are matched to a similar patient without that outcome. The control patients are matched to the patients with the intervention on the basis of patient characteristics such as age and sex. The two groups are compared to assess for "exposure" to a specific variable to determine if that variable is associated with the outcome. Case-control studies are good for rare outcomes and are a relatively inexpensive and fast alternative to cohort studies.[11]

CASE SERIES

Case series are similar to cohort studies in that they can evaluate patient outcomes in a retrospective or prospective nature. The key difference between cohort studies and case series is that case series do not have a control or comparison group. In case series, all the patients analyzed are in the same group and thus experience the same exposure.

SYSTEMATIC REVIEWS

In the field of orthopaedics, due to the limited number of RCTs, there is not always a high level of evidence study for every research question. Additionally, it can be difficult to analyze all the evidence available for one research question when there are an unmanageable amount of publications. To solve these problems, systematic reviews and meta-analysis allow for a nonbiased review of all available evidence on a specific research question. While the terms "systematic review" and "meta-analysis" are often used interchangeably, they are actually very different. A systematic review is a comprehensive summary of all high-level evidence available to answer a specific research question. On the other hand, a meta-analysis uses statistical analysis to pool data from multiple studies and analyze it all at once.[11,12]

To avoid the introduction of bias in a systematic review/meta-analysis, one must develop a detailed review protocol and stick to it. This protocol should include a specific research question about a specific population and disease. Additionally, this should include the inclusion and exclusion criteria for the studies that will be included in the review. For example, the Preferred Reporting Items for Systematic reviews and Meta-Analysis for Protocols (PRISMA-P) is a checklist authors are encouraged to use to ensure that they are publishing a high-quality systematic review.[13] This checklist was published in 2015 and recommends that review protocols include the sources used, the search strategy, the goal of the review, the selection process, the data synthesis plan, and the plan to assess for bias of the review.[13]

BEST-PRACTICE GUIDELINES

Evidence-based medicine and systematic reviews come together to inform best-practice guidelines, which are defined by the Institute of Medicine as "statements to assist practitioner and patient decisions about appropriate health care for specific clinical circumstances."[14] The development of Best-Practice Guidelines began in the 1980s in response to rising healthcare costs, and physicians' desire to maintain their own autonomy.[15] Prior to 2018, over 2000 best-practice guidelines were available for review through the National Guideline Clearinghouse (NGC) website; however, in July 2018 the government defunded the National Guideline Clearinghouse.[16] The Emergency Care Research Institute (ECRI), an independent nonprofit patients safety organization, has since taken over the role of the NGC.[17]

In the past, best-practice guidelines were determined by the consensus of an expert panel; however, this was shown to result in a high degree of variability in the guidelines that were developed.[18] Even now, when best-practice guidelines are generally based on the best evidence available, there is variability in how experts interpret evidence. For example, in 2009 the American College of Chest Physicians (ACCP) and the American Association of Orthopaedic Surgeons (AAOS) reviewed the same body evidence regarding prevention of venous thromboembolism (VTE) after total joint arthroplasty and came to very different conclusions in their best-practice guidelines.[19] This was eventually resolved in 2012 when the ACCP endorsed aspirin as an acceptable prophylaxis; however, this is an example of how the group who reviews the evidence can greatly affect the conclusions reached and the guidelines developed.[20]

One common debate in the development of best-practice guidelines is who should be involved in reviewing the evidence and making a recommendation. Some argue that the best option is to have research methodologists write clinical guidelines as they have no stake in the medical practice and therefore are less susceptible to bias. However, others argue that clinical experts should have a role in guideline

©Copyright 2021 American Academy of Orthopaedic Surgeons

development because they have experience with the conditions being treated and are more familiar with the evidence presented.[21] Best-practice guidelines hold a lot of power as they inform healthcare providers about how to treat their patients and also have monetary effects on which treatments will be covered by health insurance companies. Therefore, the methods to generate best-practice guidelines must be rigorous and transparent to reduce the risk of bias and ensure that they are accurate.

BIAS IN BEST-PRACTICE GUIDELINES

There are two main types of bias that can potentially occur in the development of best-practice guidelines; financial or intellectual. Financial bias can come in many different forms:[22]

1. The person involved in developing the guideline has ownership or financial interest in the guideline topic. For example, if someone involved in developing a guideline relating to a certain drug has ownership in that pharmaceutical company.[22]
2. The person involved in developing a guideline for a certain treatment makes a living administering said treatment. For example, if the guideline recommends surgery for a certain condition and the person is a surgeon who would profit from performing this surgery.[22]
3. The person involved in developing the guideline has a long-term relation with a healthcare government organization or private insurer, which might make their overall goal cost rather than care. For example, someone who is a long-time government employee might be more focused on keeping costs down rather than selecting the best possible treatment.[22]

Intellectual bias can also come in a few different forms:

1. The person developing the guideline has authored/published on a topic relating to the guideline.[22]
2. The person developing the guideline has clinical experience regarding the guideline topic that overly affects their decision making.[22]

DEVELOPMENT OF BEST-PRACTICE GUIDELINES

There has been an effort to improve the development of best-practice guidelines and make the process more transparent to reduce the potential for bias. The AAOS clinical practice guideline methodology is available for review, and it follows the suggestions of the Institute of Medicine. Clinical practice guidelines developed by the AAOS combine the efforts of clinical experts who are familiar with the topic, as well as methodologists, who can evaluate the evidence being reviewed for credibility and bias.[23] Those who have a financial conflict of interest are not allowed to participate in the development group. The guideline development group uses the following steps for guideline development:[23]

1. The clinical experts develop a focused research question to direct the systematic review using the PICO method: Population (who is this guideline for), Intervention (what is the treatment), Comparison (what is the treatment being compared with), and Outcome (what is the desired outcome).
2. The methodologists then review the available evidence using the systematic review guidelines and rate the available evidence using the level of evidence distinctions discussed above.
3. After the systematic review is complete physicians meet for a recommendation meeting.
4. Methodologists and physicians then come together to review the recommendations and make a final recommendation and rationale.
5. The final recommendation is subjected to the peer review process, and any necessary changes are made.

By following these steps, the chance of introducing bias into best-practice guidelines is decreased.[23] However, even when these steps are followed, the guidelines developed are not always foolproof. This is often because the evidence available for a certain topic is not of a high level. In these situations, the strength of the guideline recommendation is decreased. The AAOS has standardized language that they use to explain the strength of a recommendation (**Table 2**). The higher the level of evidence evaluated, the stronger the recommendation. This makes sense as studies with higher levels of evidence have a lower chance of having their results be affected by bias or confounding.

UPDATING BEST-PRACTICE GUIDELINES

As of 2018, AAOS has 19 best-practice guidelines published. It is important that these guidelines are updated to stay current with new published evidence. Prior to being shut down, it was the policy of the NGC that guidelines must be updated or removed every 5 years. AAOS follows this policy, but other medical organizations update guidelines as frequently as every year. The Institute of Medicine recommends guidelines "should be updated when new evidence suggests the need for modification of clinically important recommendations."[24] However, in a systematic review of handbooks that explain the methodology of developing best-practice guidelines, less than half of the handbooks had any information on the process of updating best-practice guidelines. Even the handbooks that mention updating clinical practice guidelines offer extremely vague methodological information.[25] For example, the AAOS methodological handbook states guidelines will "be revised in accordance with new evidence" and that "they will

©Copyright 2021 American Academy of Orthopaedic Surgeons

TABLE 2 Strength of Recommendation Terminology

Strength	Overall Strength of Evidence	Description of Evidence Quality	Strength Visual
Strong	Strong	Evidence from two or more high-quality studies with consistent findings	4 stars
Moderate	Moderate	Evidence from two or more moderate-quality studies with consistent findings, or from a single high-quality study	3 stars
Limited	Low strength or conflicting evidence	Evidence from two or more low-quality studies with consistent findings, or from a single moderate-quality study, or evidence is insufficient/ conflicting	2 stars
Consensus	No evidence	No supporting evidence, recommendation based on clinical opinion	1 star

American Academy of Orthopaedic Surgeons: *AAOS Clinical Practice Guideline and Systematic Review Methodology, v2.0*. Available at: https://www.aaos.org/uploadedFiles/PreProduction/Quality/Guidelines_and_Reviews/Guideline%20and%20Systematic%20Review%20Processes_v4.0_Final.pdf. Accessed October 9, 2019.

be updated or withdrawn in 5 years"; however, there is no specific explanation of how this will be accomplished.[23] Some organizations have methods in place to detect when there has been a sufficient amount of new evidence to warrant an update for example, a new RCT is published, a new drug is released to market.[24] The process of updating best-practice guidelines in far from standardized. Policies to streamline the update process and disseminate the updates to the necessary groups are still needed.[24]

ETHICAL AND LEGAL IMPLICATIONS OF BEST-PRACTICE GUIDELINES

The need to understand and perfect the development and revision of best-practice guidelines stems from the goal of providing the most accurate and effective recommendations for patient care. Beyond the desire to provide physicians with the best advice possible, best-practice guidelines can have both ethical and legal implications. One key concern with best-practice guidelines is whether or not clinicians are actually using them. It is difficult to increase adherence to best-practice guidelines.[26-28] The legal question is whether or not a physician is considered negligent if they do not abide by best-practice guidelines. If a doctor is considered negligent for not abiding by best-practice guidelines, they could be subject to a malpractice suit. Court cases in the past few decades have used best-practice guidelines on both sides of the malpractice suit;[29] that is, physicians have used them to defend their actions and patients have used them to claim negligence on the part of the physician. For example, in *Washington v. Washington Hospital Center*, a patient sued the hospital for not using a certain monitor, and the court found the hospital liable. Later it was confirmed that the American Association of Anesthesiology's guideline, that recommends that certain monitor, was sufficient to find the doctor/hospital negligent.[30] On the contrary, in *Levine v. Rosen*, a physician was sued for failing to diagnose breast cancer. The court ruled in favor of the physician stating "a physician will not be held responsible if in the exercise of his judgment he followed a course of treatment advocated by a considerable number of recognized and respected professionals in his given area of expertise."[31] The standard definition of negligence is whether the physician met "the standard of care"; however, the standard of care is another elusive term that changes frequently.[32] The court still uses a fair degree of judgment when determining which guidelines warrant adherence and which do not. This judgment often stems from what evidence was used to develop the guidelines.[32,33] This emphasizes the importance of using strong evidence to develop best-practice guidelines, as well as the importance of transparency in the methodology of guideline development.

Another ethical/legal implication of best-practice guidelines is how they are used to inform what kind of treatments will be covered by insurance companies. Many insurance companies have policies that once a best-practice guideline is endorsed by a specialty society (such as AAOS), the coverage for that guideline must be provided. Insurance companies often have their own version of "developing practice guidelines" so that they can determine what should be covered. However, this process is greatly improved if the people developing the guidelines are experts in the field and research methodologists.[29] These are just two examples of the ethical and legal implications of best-practice guidelines, but it is clear how important it is to ensure that the guidelines developed are done so accurately and without bias.

 ©Copyright 2021 American Academy of Orthopaedic Surgeons

SUMMARY

Evidence-based medicine has had a huge impact on the medical field. The practice of making clinical decisions based on the highest level of evidence available has helped to ensure that care will lead to the best patient outcomes. The use of systematic reviews to identify relevant literature can help practitioners to be aware of the evidence available in a more timely fashion. Additionally, systematic reviews are now used to help inform best-practice guidelines, as this is perhaps the most unbiased way to evaluate the evidence available in a comprehensive and efficient manner. Best-practice guidelines have improved significantly in the last few years due to the changes in how they are developed, designed to reduce conflict of interest and bias. However, there is still a long way to go in developing a practical method to update best-practice guidelines.

REFERENCES

1. Godlee F: Milestones on the long road to knowledge. *Br J Med* 2007;334:2-3.
2. Hopppe DJ, Bhandari M: Evidence-based orthopaedics: A brief history. *Indian J Orthop* 2008;42(2):104-110.
3. Guyatt G: Evidence based medicine: Past, present and future. *McMaster Univ Med J* 2003;1(1):27-32.
4. Hayashi AC: A case for evidence-based orthopaedic clinical research. *J Orthop Res* 2011;29(6):1-III.
5. Wright JG, Swiontkowski MF, Heckman JD: Introducing levels of evidence to the journal. *J Bone Joint Surg* 2003;85:1-3.
6. Sackett DL, Rosenberg WMC, Gray JAM, Richardson SW: Evidence based medicine: What it is and what it isn't. *Br J Med* 1996;312(7023):71-72.
7. Wright JG: A practical guide to assigning levels of evidence. *J Bone Joint Surg* 2007;89:1128-1130.
8. Steinke D, Davey P: Association between antibiotic resistance and community prescribing: A critical review of bias and confounding in published studies. *Clin Infect Dis* 2001;33:S205.
9. Frobell RB, Roos HP, Roos EM, Roemer FW, Ranstam J, Lohmander SL: Treatment for acute anterior cruciate ligament tear: Five year outcome of randomised trial. *Br J Med* 2013;346:f232.
10. Burns PB, Rohrich RJ, Chung KC: The levels of evidence and their role in evidence-based medicine. *Plast Reconstr Surg* 2011;128(1):305-310.
11. Song JW, Chung KC: Observational studies: Cohort and case-control studies. *Plast Reconstr Surg* 2010;126(6):2234-2242.
12. Harris JD, Quatman CE, Manring MM, Siston RA, Flanigan DC: How to write a systematic review. *Am J Sports Med* 2014;42(11):2761-2768.
13. Moher D, Shamseer L, Clarke M, et al: Preferred reporting items for systematic review and meta-analysis protocols (PRISMA-P) 2015 statement. *Syst Rev* 2015;4:1.
14. Field MJ, Lohr KN: *Institute of Medicine Committee to Advise the Public Health Service on Clinical Practice Guidelines: Clinical Practice Guidelines: Directions for a New Program*. Washington, DC, National Academy Press, 1990.
15. Weisz G, Cambrosio A, Keating P, Knaapen L, Schlich T, Tournay VJ: The emergence of clinical practice guidelines. *Milbank Q* 2007;85(4):691-727.
16. Agency for Healthcare Research and Quality: About NGC and NQM. Available at: https://www.ahrq.gov/gam/about/index.html. Accessed January 15, 2019.
17. ECRI Institute: ECRI Institute opens Access to Clinical Practice Guidelines. Available at: https://www.ecri.org/press/ecri-institute-opens-access-to-clinical-practice-guidelines/. Accessed January 15, 2019.
18. Fretheim A, Schünemann HJ, Oxman AD: Improving the use of research evidence in guideline development: 3. Group composition and consultation process. *Health Res Policy Syst* 2006;4:15.
19. Eikelboom JW, Karthikeyan G, Fagel N, Hirsh J: American Association of Orthopedic Surgeons and American College of Chest Physicians Guidelines for venous thromboembolism prevention in hip and knee arthroplasty differ. *Chest* 2009;135(2):513-520.
20. Shah SS, Satin AM, Mullen JR, Merwin S, Goldin M, Sgaglione NA: Impact of recent guideline changes on aspirin prescribing after knee arthroplasty. *J Orthop Surg Res* 2016;11(123):1-9.
21. Hirsh J, Guyatt G: Clinical experts or methodologists to write clinical guidelines? *Lancet* 2009;374:273-275.
22. Detsky AS: Sources of bias for authors of clinical practice guidelines. *Can Med Assoc J* 2006;175(9):1033.
23. American Academy of Orthpaedic Surgeons: AAOS Clinical Practice Guideline Methodology v2.0, AAOS Clinical Practice Guideline and Systematic Review Methodology. Available at: https://www.aaos.org/uploadedFiles/PreProduction/Quality/Guidelines_and_Reviews/Guideline%20and%20Systematic%20Review%20Processes_v4.0_Final.pdf. Accessed June 24, 2018.
24. Shekelle PG: Updating practice guidelines. *J Am Med Assoc* 2014;311(20):2072-2073.
25. Vernooij RWM, Sanabria AJ, Solà I, Alonso-Coello P, Martínez García L: Guidance for updating clinical practice guidelines: A systematic review of methodological handbooks. *Implement Sci* 2014;9:3.
26. Gagliardi AR, Brouwers MC, Bhattacharyya OK: The guideline implementability research and application network (GIRAnet): An international collaborative to support knowledge exchange: Study protocol.*Implement Sci* 2012;7:26.
27. Barbour S, Beaulieu M, Gill J, Espino-Hernandez G, Reich HN, Levin A: The need for improved uptake of the KDIGO glomerulonephritis guidelines into clinical practice in Canada: A survey of nephrologists. *Clin Kidney J* 2014;7:538-545.
28. Devalia B: Adherance to protocol during the acute management of diabetic ketoacidosis: Would specialist involvement lead to better outcomes? *Int J Clin Pract* 2010;64(11):1580-1582.
29. Sanders JO, Bozic KJ, Glassman SD, Jevsevar DS, Weber KL: Clinical practice guidelines: Their use, misuse, and future directions. *J Am Acad Orthop Surg* 2014;22(3):135-144.
30. LeCraw LL: The use of clinical practice guidelines in medical malpractice litigation. *J Oncol Practice* 2007;3(5):254.
31. Justia US Law: Levine V. Rosen. Available at: https://law.justia.com/cases/pennsylvania/supreme-court/1992/532-pa-512-0.html. Accessed January 19, 2019.
32. Cooke BK, Worsham E, Reisfield GM: The elusive standard of care. *J Am Acad Psychiatry Law* 2017;45(3):358-364.
33. Mackey TK, Liang BA: The role of practice guidelines in medical malpractice litigation. *Am Med Assoc J Ethics* 2011;13(1):36-41.

©Copyright 2021 American Academy of Orthopaedic Surgeons

45

Role of Cohort Studies and Registries in Musculoskeletal Healthcare and Research

Patricia D. Franklin, MD, MBA, MPH
Jeffrey K. Lange, MD

Keywords: *orthopaedic cohort studies; orthopaedic outcomes; orthopaedic registries; real-world evidence*

INTRODUCTION: COHORTS AND REGISTRIES IN MUSCULOSKELETAL HEALTHCARE AND RESEARCH

Researchers and regulators (eg, the FDA) are prioritizing the use of real-world evidence (RWE) to generate new knowledge of best practices to treat the growing population of adults afflicted by chronic musculoskeletal conditions.[1] In addition, the FDA has called for enhanced postmarketing surveillance and safety monitoring of implantable devices using RWE.[2] Although electronic health records (EHRs) and administrative billing data are standard RWE sources, disease-specific registries and cohort studies are fundamental to evaluating outcomes of diverse treatments and longitudinal device surveillance. For example, in Sweden, both the osteoarthritis and total knee and hip replacement registries have informed clinical practice for decades.[3] For musculoskeletal outcomes, the Swedish, United Kingdom, and Australian arthroplasty registries, among others, provide data to compare outcomes across health systems, comparative effectiveness information to assess the impact of diverse treatments, and device performance and safety statistics for surgical interventions.[4,5]

Dr. Franklin or an immediate family member has received research or institutional support from Zimmer. Neither Dr. Lange nor any immediate family member has received anything of value from or has stock or stock options held in a commercial company or institution related directly or indirectly to the subject of this chapter.

A growing number of US registries and cohort studies are emerging in response to the need to evaluate both treatments and outcomes for various musculoskeletal conditions. Professional societies are taking the lead to create registries to guide clinical practice. The American Association of Orthopaedic Surgeons is developing a centralized registry infrastructure for total joint replacement, spine, foot and ankle, sports, and other procedures.[6] The American College of Rheumatology[7] and the American Physical Therapy Association[8] are developing parallel registries to capture clinical interventions, diagnoses, and outcomes. In addition, private health associations (eg, Kaiser Permanente[9]), statewide associations (eg, Michigan arthroplasty registry[10]), and national research programs (eg, the FORCE-TJR[11] and the SPORT[12] and MOON trials[13]) are being created/used to evaluate treatments for ligament pathology and to collect longitudinal outcome data for patients with a variety of musculoskeletal conditions and treatments. Longitudinal implant survivorship, postprocedure adverse events, and patient-reported health outcomes are typically measured and monitored.

In the United States today, EHRs are the primary data repository capturing the details of clinical care as well as information to support billing and administrative functions, such as visit scheduling. Thus, the EHR is the source of important RWE. In addition, EHR data are often submitted to registries or research cohorts. However, data sharing between the EHR and registries or research cohorts—including the ability to return registry data to the EHR—has the potential not only to enhance the value of EHR data but to expand the utility of registries and research to serve quality monitoring, regulatory evaluations, and research. This bidirectional sharing is often called a "learning health system (LHS)." In the LHS, electronic data collected for

©Copyright 2021 American Academy of Orthopaedic Surgeons

clinical care also serve research, and vice versa. In this way, the surgeons and health systems that participate in the registry or cohort are simultaneously contributing to research, as well as monitoring the outcomes of their own care as compared with others in the registry.

Califf and co-authors, who represent major federal research and health policy organizations (FDA, HHS, NIH, AHRQ, PCORI, CDC, etc.), have called for research to develop new methods to reliably answer questions and for new approaches to study design and conduct that will optimally collect and use RWE.[14] They list the principles of a learning health system as requiring at least two features that are often seen in well-designed cohorts and registries:

1. Operational practice networks that generate research evidence within a framework for autonomy, privacy, confidentiality, and security.
2. Common definitions, collection, and storage of digital data with informed consent, as possible, and appropriate privacy protection.

Although US public health and safety data are beginning to emerge from registries, the secondary uses of registry data for *research* and feedback to *clinicians and patients* in learning health systems are currently limited. In 2017, a National Academy of Medicine paper on engaging clinicians in the learning health system highlighted FORCE-TJR as a model for engagement. FORCE-TJR both supports federally funded research and provides real-time quality feedback to clinicians.[15] Internationally, Scandinavian arthroplasty registries have a long history of engaging in research while serving the public health reporting needs of their countries.[16]

WHAT ARE THE BENEFITS OF REGISTRIES AND COHORT STUDIES TO CLINICIANS AND PATIENTS?

Although the randomized controlled clinical trial (RCT) is the standard method for understanding the effect of a medical intervention on select groups of patients, extrapolating RCT results to clinical practice may be difficult because of the diversity of patients and healthcare factors as compared with the controlled factors of the RCT. Variation in patient and healthcare system factors will influence the intervention effects in daily practice. Cohorts and registries that include diverse patients across "real-world" clinical settings may narrow the gap between treatment intervention effects in RCTs and practice. Thus, clinicians should value the outcome analyses that emerge from cohorts and registries.

Although EHR data serve healthcare delivery *within a single* health system, EHR data elements are rarely consistently defined or structured to support aggregated use across health systems. Thus, well-designed registries and cohort studies with consistent patient, surgical, and outcome data are the keys to comparative effectiveness and outcomes research.

- Predefined measurement timing and capture across settings.

Inconsistent timing and scheduling of clinical visits is a major challenge to using EHR data for longitudinal monitoring. Thus, data-capture strategies are needed to improve the completeness of data and the consistency of timing and intervals between measures. To complement EHRs, registries can collect measures across different healthcare delivery systems and associated EHRs. Links to national death indices and administrative data are key to assessing longitudinal endpoints. Registries that integrate data submitted by patients across time and location can enhance the quality and usability of data for RWE research. Outreach to engage patients in longitudinal monitoring, especially for patients who do not return to the clinic, can improve data completeness.

- Consistent core measure sets to meet research standards.

Well-designed registries ensure consistent structure and format of data elements. For example, smoking history can be captured using a single, consistent measure (eg, pack years) or the presence or absence of relevant medical comorbid conditions may be explicitly documented rather than assuming that the absence of documentation for the condition means the absence of the condition, as can occur when using EHR data.

- Complete data automation systems to minimize bias.

Well-designed registries are programmed to prompt data collection at key intervals from all patients—both those with and without office visits. Automated data-capture protocols can be implemented through multiple capture modes (eg, web portal, phone, or in-office computers) to increase the likelihood of complete data capture. Similar automation can notify clinicians about patients who need to be reevaluated through an in-office visit based on results of certain patient-reported outcome measures.

- Integration of clinical and patient-generated data in registries.

Until recently, patient-reported outcomes (PRO) and other patient-generated data were not routinely recognized as valuable for evaluating musculoskeletal treatment outcomes. Registries can include PRO data and play a leadership role in refining relevant PRO metrics, evaluating the strengths and limitations of patient-reported data in comparative effectiveness research and public health and quality analyses. As passive data emerge from smart phones and other wearable devices, further research to define "clinically" meaningful metrics and change over time are needed.[17]

©Copyright 2021 American Academy of Orthopaedic Surgeons

WHAT ARE THE CLINICAL BENEFITS OF DATA COLLECTED FROM COHORTS AND REGISTRIES?

Although local EHRs store clinical information for patients treated within a health system, they do not house data from sites across the nation. Thus, hospital administrators and clinicians charged with managing population outcomes for quality or bundled payment initiatives must seek external data sources against which to benchmark outcomes and identify opportunities to improve. Registries designed to integrate data across health systems can readily calculate national or regional benchmarks. Such data can be valuable for comparison in individual patient care as well as at the health system or population level.

Because registries aggregate data across multiple healthcare settings, the number of patients can accumulate faster than data from a single health system. As a result, signals and trends within care patterns can be more quickly identified. Faster accumulation allows for recognition of both positive and negative outcomes, and these lessons can be readily returned to participating health systems. Furthermore, EHR software is not designed to perform sophisticated statistical analyses, whereas registry data can be easily programmed using advanced statistical techniques. As the prevalence of APIs (Application Programming Interfaces) expands, EHRs can readily submit single-site data to a registry with the expectation of real-time statistical processing and the return of risk-adjusted or other refined metrics.

Patient care and treatment decisions can be informed by real-time reports to integrate the patient's health status with national norms. APIs and other technical interfaces are available to link population analyses of real-world data with individual patient records. Collaborations between Dartmouth researchers and rheumatology registries are testing this "co-production" model.[18] A second example of translating national registry data to real-time shared-decision reports is the FORCE-TJR registry that provides real-time predictive analytics adjusted for individual patient risk factors to patients and surgeons considering total joint surgery. With PCORI funding, the impact of these shared-decision reports on decision quality and outcomes is being evaluated now in the Arthritis care through Shared Knowledge (A.S.K.) study.[19]

EXISTING COHORT AND REGISTRY RESOURCES FOR ORTHOPAEDIC SURGEONS

During the past decade, great focus has been placed on the development of high-quality data resources that can inform best practices for orthopaedic clinical care delivery. Well-designed longitudinal cohort studies help to provide answers to specific clinical questions regarding patient factors, surgical factors, and outcomes associated with particular intervention strategies. Well-established and developing registries have given us insight into orthopaedic surgical trends and basic quality and performance measures. Some of this decade's most impactful musculoskeletal cohorts and registries are summarized below. **Table 1** summarizes key resources from existing cohort studies and registries to inform best practices in high-volume orthopaedic practices.

SPINE

The Spine Patient Outcomes Research Trial (SPORT) was a multicenter randomized controlled trial with a concurrent observational cohort, studying the comparative effectiveness of surgical management and nonsurgical management of lumbar spine disease. Thirteen medical centers in 11 US states participated. With respect to the treatment of lumbar disk herniation, long-term results from the randomized cohort (501 patients) showed no statistically significant differences in bodily pain (BP), physical function (PF), or modified Oswestry Disability Index (ODI) between surgical and nonsurgical management in the intent-to-treat analysis.[12] However, improvements in secondary outcomes including sciatica bothersomeness, satisfaction with symptoms, and self-rated improvement were statistically significantly greater in the surgical group as compared with the nonsurgical group in the intent-to-treat analysis. Of note, there was significant nonadherence to treatment, and the as-treated analysis showed statistically significant and clinically meaningful greater improvements in symptoms for those patients treated surgically as compared with those treated nonsurgically in both randomized and observational cohorts (501 and 743 patients, respectively). The ultimate result of this cohort study indicated that for appropriately selected patients, surgical intervention for lumbar disk herniation can confer greater benefit than nonsurgical management at 8-year follow-up.[12] Similar midterm results were reported for surgical versus nonsurgical management of lumbar stenosis and degenerative spondylolisthesis.[20,21]

Today, the North American Spine Society (NASS) and the Michigan Spine Registry capture longitudinal outcomes for spine procedures in national (NASS) and regional (Michigan) samples. These emerging registries have the potential to guide future practice.

KNEE

The Multicenter Orthopaedic Outcomes Network (MOON) was conceived in the 1990s and began data collection in 2002.[13] MOON was established as a multicenter, prospective, longitudinal cohort study aimed at determining the factors associated with long-term success or failure of anterior cruciate ligament reconstruction (ACLR). Over 3,500 patients have been enrolled across seven centers over a 10-year period. At this point, short-, mid-, and long-term results have been published. Several key findings have influenced orthopaedic practice over the last decade, including the association between

©Copyright 2021 American Academy of Orthopaedic Surgeons

TABLE 1 Sample US Orthopaedic Cohorts and Registries[a]

Name/Date Started	Description	Enrollment	Data Collected	Other
SPORT (Spine Patient Outcomes Research Trial) (2006)	NIH-funded SPORT is a 5-year study that looked at three of the most common back conditions and compared surgical and nonsurgical treatments—intervertebral disk herniation, spinal stenosis, and degenerative spondylolisthesis.	Approximately 2,500 patients took part in the study, which was conducted at 13 US sites	Analyses of the 4-year follow-up data for three cohorts Surgical vs nonsurgical treatment outcomes; SF36 and Oswestry Disability Index at 6 wk, 3 mo, 6 mo, and 1 and 2 yr	Spine treatment calculator
The NASS Spine Registry (June 2018)	Diagnosis-based clinical data spine registry that will allow healthcare providers to collect and analyze their data on spine care and then compare it with de-identified data in the entire registry	Any spinal care provider, including physicians or allied health professionals, regardless of specialty, setting, or medical/surgical orientation	Data include demographics, diagnosis, treatment, complications, and patient-reported outcomes	Registry participants receive confidential feedback on their patients and have access to reports with benchmarking against their peers
MOON (Multicenter Orthopaedic Outcomes Network) (2001)	20+ year development and history—anterior cruciate ligament reconstruction (ACLR) multicenter cohort: 1. patient-reported outcomes and failure; 2. specialized cohort: initiation and predictors of osteoarthritis (OA)	2002-2008; N = 3,500 18 surgeons at 7 sites Two cohorts: population and nested 2-year cohort (age 12-33 injured in sports)	Risk factors of ACLR outcome: demographics, injury extent, surgical decisions, return to sports, pain, risk for additional surgery KOOS, IKDC, Marx athletic activity, SF-36, WOMAC	MOP
MOON Knee Project	Patients undergoing an ACLR	N = 3,500 patients	Follow-up at 2, 6, and 10 yr after their ACLR	
MOON Shoulder Group (2004)	Patients with surgery for shoulder injuries	16 physicians, 8 sites	Risk factors for rotator cuff disease and management of patients	
MARS (Multicenter ACLR Revision Study) (2006)	Identify modifiable predictors for revision ACLR	N = 1,205 revision patients 83 surgeons, 52 sites (US + Canada)	Data include baseline demographics, surgical technique, pathologic abnormalities, and revision rates IKDC, KOOS, WOMAC, Marx activity score Patients were followed up at 2 yr	Multivariate regression models were used to determine predictors of IKDC, KOOS, WOMAC, Marx scores, graft rerupture, and reoperation rate at 2 years after revision surgery
MeTeOR (Meniscal Tear and Osteoarthritis Research) RCT (2008)	Multicenter randomized trial comparing surgical versus nonsurgical treatment for mild to moderate OA with concomitant meniscus tears (Uses MOON or MARS sites)	2008-2011 N = 351 patients, 7 clinical centers	WOMAC, KOOS, SF-36, EQ 5D	
FORCE-TJR (2010)	Representative sample total knee and hip replacement patients; includes patients of all ages, low and high volume sites	30,000+ patients from >150 surgeons in 28 states	Complete pre-op patient risk factors, pre- and post-op K/HOOS, SF36, post-op adverse events, and annual revisions	Generates national norms for patients of all ages (Medicare and under 65 yr); CMS-certified Qualified Clinical Data Registry; Multiple federally funded ancillary research studies ongoing. www.force-tjr.org

[a]See a comprehensive list of international arthroplasty registries at http://www.isarhome.org.

©Copyright 2021 American Academy of Orthopaedic Surgeons

ACLR failure and patient age and graft type used for reconstruction. Over 40 studies have been published based on the existing data from the MOON cohort, underscoring its impact on the orthopaedic community to date.[13]

The Multicenter ACL Revision Study (MARS), inspired by the MOON cohort study, was established with the goal of identifying modifiable risk factors in the setting of revision ACLR. MARS was a multicenter prospective longitudinal cohort study, enrolling 1,205 patients over a 5-year period across 83 surgeons and 52 sites. Multiple important findings based on the results of this cohort study have been published, including the elevated risk of early revision ACLR failure with the use of allograft versus autograft, statistically significantly greater sports function outcome scores with the use of autograft versus allograft, and the identification of surgical factors associated with poorer outcomes following revision ACLR.[22-24]

The Meniscal Tear in Osteoarthritis Research (MeTeOR) trial represents another of the last decade's important orthopaedic cohorts.[25] MeTeOR was designed to explore the comparative effectiveness of physical therapy versus arthroscopic partial meniscectomy for the treatment of meniscal tear in the setting of concomitant osteoarthritis. This multicenter randomized controlled trial enrolled 351 patients across seven sites. The major finding in the intention-to-treat analysis was that there was no statistically significant difference in patient-reported outcomes (pain and function) at 6 or 12 months between groups. However, 30% crossover was noted from the nonsurgical to the surgical group. The authors placed these findings nicely in context, determining that while the ultimate role of arthroscopic partial meniscectomy remains unclear, an initial nonsurgical management strategy consisting of physical therapy with the option for later arthroscopic management in the absence of symptomatic relief is a sound approach. This trial, among others, has helped to shape current clinical management strategies for a diagnosis of meniscal tear with concomitant knee osteoarthritis.[26]

TOTAL KNEE AND HIP ARTHROPLASTY

A high volume of total hip and total knee arthroplasty surgeries are performed in the United States annually, and these procedures represent a significant expenditure for the US healthcare system.[27] There has been a great effort in the United States over the last decade to improve our understanding of total joint arthroplasty trends and to monitor for quality and safety through the establishment of new registries. Multiple new US registries have begun to emerge and have benefitted from the lessons learned by already well-established registries across the world. We summarize the major US total joint replacement registries and some of the international total joint replacement registries below.

The Function and Outcomes Research for Comparative Effectiveness in Total Joint Replacement (FORCE-TJR) registry began to enroll patients in 2010. FORCE-TJR was originally funded by the HHS Agency for Healthcare Research and Quality as an effort to create a registry based on a representative research sample of total joint replacements performed across the United States. FORCE-TJR includes over 200 surgeons in 28 states and to date has recorded over 30,000 total joint arthroplasty procedures. In addition to patient and surgical factors, FORCE-TJR records pre- and postoperative patient-reported outcome metrics. FORCE-TJR has been instrumental in developing a strong understanding of the US total joint arthroplasty experience and has generated national norms for patients of all ages, including patient-reported outcomes. Implant survivorship analyses are currently underway. This registry continues to be maintained, and its users are provided quality metrics and outcomes data in real time to assess health system performance. Multiple federally funded ancillary research studies are now ongoing.[28-32]

The Michigan Arthroplasty Registry Collaborative Quality Initiative (MARCQI) is a state-wide consortium of hospitals and surgeons dedicated to improving the quality of care for hip and knee replacement patients in Michigan. The registry includes over 250,000 cases as of February 2019. MARCQI captures 97% of the total joint replacement surgeries performed in the state of Michigan. The MARCQI annual report and associated peer-reviewed publications[10] detail the first US revision risks for specific hip and knee implants as well as trends in postoperative complications and care delivery (eg, thromboembolic events, blood transfusions, discharge disposition). The 2018 annual report captures 5 years of data and includes over 200,000 arthroplasty procedures. The registry effort is ongoing.[33]

Kaiser Permanente (KP) is a large healthcare system serving nine states, capturing over 11 million lives in the United States.[34] KP maintains registries for a variety of medical interventions, including ACLR, cardiac devices, and joint replacement surgeries. The KP total joint replacement registry has captured approximately 250,000 joint replacement procedures since 2001. Numerous studies based on the KP total joint replacement registry have been published, yielding important findings for their patient population, including implant-specific associations with increased risk of revision surgery and comparative effectiveness of postoperative DVT prophylaxis management strategies.[35,36]

The American Joint Replacement Registry (AJRR) began collecting data in 2012. As of 2017, over 650 hospitals and over 4,700 surgeons were submitting data to AJRR, representing an estimated 28% of the joint replacement volume occurring in the United States. Although membership in the AJRR is on a volunteer basis, close to 1 million procedures have been captured to date. The AJRR has recently begun to report quality metrics and to offer reporting where participants can view their own performance data benchmarked against national metrics.[37]

There are several robust total joint replacement registries that have been maintained for a decade or more across the world. In Europe alone, over 20 registries exist with combined records representing over 5 million total joint replacement surgeries.[38] Some of the most significant non-US registry efforts in the last decade have included the Swedish Hip Arthroplasty Register (SHAR), the Australian Orthopaedic Association National

©Copyright 2021 American Academy of Orthopaedic Surgeons

Joint Replacement Registry (AOANJRR), and the National Mayo Clinic Joint Replacement Database for England, Wales, Northern Ireland, and the Isle of Man (NJR). Each of these entities has recorded hundreds of thousands of joint replacement surgeries over the course of one or more decades.[3-5] Because of these sovereignties' more centralized healthcare delivery systems, they have been able to capture the vast majority of joint replacements performed over this time period. Every year, the data are analyzed and shared publicly in the form of an annual report. Some of the most important data reported include survivorship curves overall for total joint replacements, implant-specific survivorship curves, diagnosis-specific survivorship curves, patient mortality rates, and healthcare-utilization information. In addition, performance outliers can be identified in some circumstances, leading to important quality checks for poorly performing implants.[39-41]

SUMMARY

In summary, today's EHRs document individual patient care and effectively support reimbursement. However, the EHR was not designed to address consistency in data quality and data processing over time or across health systems. In contrast, well-designed cohort studies and registries can overcome these challenges: define and capture structured, consistent data, integrate real-time sophisticated analytics, provide access to comparable national or regional patient samples and norms, and link to sources of administrative and patient-reported data captured in the healthcare system. Secondarily, a registry composed of high-quality, consistent real-world data can serve research and generate new knowledge while also feeding back patient-reported data and/or external clinical events to the EHR to improve direct patient care. A high-quality registry dataset—resulting from a bidirectional relationship between EHRs and registries—supports multiple uses within clinical practice, quality and regulatory compliance, and research. The "collect once and use multiple times" principle supports efficiency.

We envision registry systems populating robust longitudinal databases that will serve both patient outcome and implant surveillance over time. US regulatory and clinical professionals need new longitudinal solutions to monitor implant survivorship, posttreatment clinical events, and PROs following surgical and nonsurgical care for musculoskeletal conditions. National registries will have sufficient sample size, as well as patient and clinician heterogeneity, to provide robust RWE for research. However, the musculoskeletal research community needs to develop best-practice standards for registry data capture, integration, and management, as well as analytic techniques.

REFERENCES

1. Sherman RE, Anderson SA, Dal Pan GJ, et al: Real-world evidence — what is it and what can it tell us? *NEJM* 2016;375(23):2293-2297.
2. Center for Devices and Radiological Health: *Strengthening Our National System for Medical Device Postmarket Surveillance: Updates and Next Steps*. U.S. Food and Drug Administration, 2013. https://www.fda.gov/media/84409/download. Accessed June 3, 2019.
3. Kärrholm J, Mohaddes M, Odin D, Vinblad J, Rogmark C, Rolfson O: *Swedish Hip Arthroplasty Register Annual Report 2017*. 2018.
4. National Joint Registry for England: *Wales, Northern Ireland and the Isle of Man. 15th Annual Report*. 2018 http://www.njrreports.org.uk/Portals/0/PDFdownloads/NJR%2015th%20Annual%20Report%202018.pdf. Accessed June 3, 2019.
5. Australian Orthopaedic Association National Joint Replacement Registry (AOANJRR): *Hip, Knee & Shoulder Arthroplasty: 2018 Annual Report*. Adelaide, AOA, 2018.
6. Glusenkamp N, Finney KM: *About the AAOS Registry Program*. July 2018. http://blog.ajrr.net/about-the-aaos-registry-program. Accessed June 3, 2019.
7. RISE (Qualified Clinical Data Registry). https://www.rheumatology.org/I-Am-A/Rheumatologist/RISE-Registry. Accessed June 3, 2019.
8. *APTA Launches Physical Therapy Outcomes Registry to Improve Patient Care*. February 2017. http://www.apta.org/uploadedFiles/APTAorg/Media/Releases/APTA/2017/APTAPressRelease_RegistryLaunch.pdf. Accessed June 3, 2019.
9. Inacio MCS, Dillon MT, Miric A, Navarro RA, Paxton EW: Mortality after total knee and total hip arthroplasty in a large integrated health care system. *Perm J* 2017;21:16-171.
10. Hughes RE, Zheng H, Igrisan RM, Cowen ME, Markel DC, Hallstrom BR: The Michigan arthroplasty registry collaborative quality initiative experience: Improving the quality of care in Michigan. *J Bone Joint Surg Am* 2018;100(22):e143.
11. Franklin PD, Allison JJ, Ayers DC: Beyond joint implant registries: A patient-centered research consortium for comparative effectiveness in total joint replacement. *J Am Med Assoc* 2012;308(12):1217-1218.
12. Lurie JD, Tosteson TD, Tosteson ANA, et al: Surgical versus non-operative treatment for lumbar disc herniation: Eight-year results for the spine patient outcomes research trial (SPORT). *Spine* 2014;39(1):3-16.
13. Lynch TS, Parker RD, Patel RM, Andrish JT, MOON Group, Spindler KP: The impact of the multicenter orthopedic outcomes network (MOON) research on anterior cruciate ligament reconstruction and orthopaedic practice. *J Am Acad Orthop Surg* 2015;23(3):154-163.
14. Califf RM, Robb MA, Bindman AB, et al: Transforming evidence generation to support health and health care decisions. *N Eng J Med* 2016;375(24):2395-2400.
15. Platt R, Blake K, Franklin P, et al: Clinician engagement for continuous learning. *NAM Perspectives*. 2017. https://nam.edu/wp-content/uploads/2017/03/Clinician-Engagement-for-Continuous-Learning.pdf. Accessed June 3, 2019.
16. Ferguson RJ, Silman AJ, Combescure C, et al: ASA class is associated with early revision and reoperation after total hip arthroplasty: An analysis of the Geneva and Swedish hip arthroplasty registries. *Acta Orthop* 2019;90(4):324-330.
17. Mobilizing mHealth Innovation for Real-World Evidence Generation: *Duke-Margolis Center for Health Policy*. 2017. https://healthpolicy.duke.edu/sites/default/files/atoms/files/duke-margolis_mhealth_action_plan.pdf. Accessed June 3, 2019.
18. Nelson EC, Dixon-Woods M, Batalden PB, et al: Patient focused registries can improve health, care, and science. *BMJ* 2016;354:i3319.
19. Franklin P, Ayers D, Berliner E: *FORCE-TJR and Patient-Centered Registries Essential Role in EHR Era*. NEJM Catalyst, 2018. https://catalyst.nejm.org/force-tjr-patient-centered-registries/. Accessed June 3, 2019.

 ©Copyright 2021 American Academy of Orthopaedic Surgeons

20. Weinstein JN, Lurie JD, Tosteson TD, et al: Surgical compared with non-operative treatment for lumbar degenerative spondylolisthesis. *JBJS Am* 2009;91:1295-1304.
21. Weinstein JN, Tosteson TD, Lurie JD, et al: Surgical versus non-operative treatment for lumbar spinal stenosis four-year results of the spine patient outcomes research trial (SPORT). *Spine* 2010;35(14):1329-1338.
22. MARS Group: Effect of graft choice on the outcome of revision anterior cruciate ligament reconstruction in the Multicenter ACL Revision Study (MARS) Cohort. *Am J Sports Med* 2014;42(10):2301-2310.
23. MARS Group: Surgical predictors of clinical outcome following revision ACL reconstruction. *Am J Sports Med* 2017;45(11):2586-2594.
24. MARS Group, Ding DY: Subsequent surgery after revision anterior cruciate ligament reconstruction: Rates and risk factors from a multicenter cohort. *Am J Sports Med* 2017;45(9):2068-2076.
25. Katz JN, Brophy RH, Chaisson CE, et al: Surgery versus physical therapy for a meniscal tear and osteoarthrits. *NEJM* 2013;368(18):1675-1684.
26. Katz JN, Brownlee SA, Jones MH: The role of arthroscopy in the management of knee osteoarthritis. *Best Pract Res Clin Rheumatol* 2014;28(1):143-156.
27. Sloan M, Premkumar A, Sheth NP: Projected volume of primary total joint arthroplasty in the U.S., 2014 to 2030. *JBJS Am* 2018;100(17):1455-1460.
28. Desai RJ, Jin Y, Franklin PD, et al: Association of geography and access to health care providers with long-term prescription opioid use in medicare patients with severe osteoarthritis: A cohort study. *Arthritis Rheumatol* 2019;71(5):712-721. doi:10.1002/art.40834. [Epub 2019 Apr 2].
29. Gandek B, Roos EM, Franklin PD, Ware JE Jr: A 12-item short form of the hip disability and osteoarthritis outcome score (HOOS-12): Tests of reliability, validity and responsiveness. *Osteoarthr Cartil* 2019;27(5):754-761.
30. Gandek B, Roos EM, Franklin PD, Ware JE Jr: Item selection for 12-item short forms of the knee injury and osteoarthritis outcome score (KOOS-12) and hip disability and osteoarthritis outcome score (HOOS-12). *Osteoarthr Cartil* 2019;27(5):746-753.
31. Gandek B, Roos EM, Franklin PD, Ware JE Jr: A 12-item short form of the knee injury and osteoarthritis outcome score (KOOS-12): Tests of reliability, validity and responsiveness. *Osteoarthr Cartil* 2019;27(5):762-770.
32. Oatis CA, Li W, DiRusso JM, et al: Variations in delivery and exercise content of physical therapy rehabilitation following total knee replacement surgery: A cross-sectional observation study. *Int J Phys Med Rehabil* 2014;suppl 5:002.
33. *Michigan Arthroplasty Registry Collaborative Quality Initiative (MARCQI) Report: 2012-2017*. Michigan Arthroplasty Registry Collaborative Quality Initiative, 2018. http://marcqi.org/dev/wp-content/uploads/2018/10/MARCQI_Six-Year_Report-2018.pdf. Accessed June 3, 2019.
34. 2017 Annual Report. Kaiser Permanente National Implant Registries https://national-implantregistries.kaiserpermanente.org/Media/Default/documents/2017 Implant Registry FINAL v2.pdf. Accessed June 3, 2019.
35. Cafri G, Paxton EW, Chen Y, et al: Comparative effectiveness and safety of drug prophylaxis for prevention of venous thromboembolism after total knee arthroplasty. *J Arthroplasty* 2017;32(11):3524-3528.
36. Cafri G, Paxton EW, Love R, Bini SA, Kurtz SM: Is there a difference in revision risk between metal and ceramic heads on highly crosslinked polyethylene liners? *Clin Orthop Relat Res* 2017;475(5):1349-1355.
37. *Fourth AJRR Annual Report on Hip and Knee Arthroplasty Data*. American Joint Replacement Registry, 2017. http://www.ajrr.net/images/annual_reports/AJRR-2017-Annual-Report--Final.pdf. Accessed June 3, 2019.
38. Lübbeke A, Silman AJ, Barea C, Prieto-Alhambra D, Carr AJ: Mapping existing hip and knee replacement registries in Europe. *Health Policy* 2018;122(5):548-557.
39. Australian Orthopaedic Association National Joint Replacement Registry (AOANJRR): *Hip, Knee & Shoulder Arthroplasty: 2007 Annual Report*. Adelaide, AOA, 2018.
40. Australian Orthopaedic Association National Joint Replacement Registry (AOANJRR): *Hip, Knee & Shoulder Arthroplasty: 2018 Annual Report*. Adelaide, AOA, 2008.
41. Australian Orthopaedic Association National Joint Replacement Registry (AOANJRR): *Hip, Knee & Shoulder Arthroplasty: 2018 Annual Report*. Adelaide, AOA, 2009.

©Copyright 2021 American Academy of Orthopaedic Surgeons

Fundamentals of Cost-Effectiveness Research

David W. Shearer, MD, MPH
Kevin J. Bozic, MD, MBA

Keywords: *cost-effectiveness; economic analysis; value-based care*

INTRODUCTION

The United States (US) health care system is in the midst of a transition from fee-for-service health care to "value-based health care" with increasing scrutiny on the high cost of orthopaedic surgical procedures.[1] Health care systems and policy makers are employing novel strategies, such as bundled payment programs, to reduce cost and improve patient outcomes. As such, research evaluating the cost-effectiveness of orthopaedic interventions has become increasingly important in both clinical and health care policy decision making. Historically, clinical decision making in orthopaedic surgery has been informed primarily by anecdotal surgeon experience, expert opinion, and small uncontrolled case series. This has evolved with greater emphasis on evidence-based medicine toward larger, multicenter clinical trials employing randomization, blinding, and patient-centered outcome measures. However, implicit in both of these approaches is the idea that the more effective intervention is always preferred, regardless of its cost. Economic analysis is an alternative approach that incorporates the cost of an intervention into the clinical and policy decision-making framework. Two underlying assumptions that are important for acceptance of this methodology are (1) resources are constrained that is, there is not an unlimited budget and (2) a more effective intervention may not always be preferred if the incremental benefit is small relative to the monetary cost.[2]

The first assumption is more widely accepted. In the United States, although health care spending is not fixed, the steady rise as a fraction of gross domestic product (GDP) over the last several decades has been labeled a health care "crisis."[3] There is no absolute threshold, but the idea that resources are not unlimited is not debated. The second assumption that certain high-cost interventions with small incremental benefit may be too expensive is more politically and ethically troublesome.[4] An attempt to factor cost into a ranking system to determine Medicaid coverage in Oregon in the 1990s led to widespread public outcry due to concerns over rationing and government control of health care.[5]

To date in the United States, the Centers for Medicaid and Medicare Services (CMS) has accepted comparative effectiveness research, but has declined to use cost-effectiveness analysis for beneficiary coverage decisions.[6,7] In other countries, economic analysis has seen greater acceptance by governments seeking to control costs of health care and maximize scarce resources. Many countries have dedicated government agencies, such as the National Institute for Clinical Excellence (NICE) in the United Kingdom, that perform economic analysis, the results of which weigh heavily in coverage decisions in the frequently nationalized healthcare systems.[8]

Dr. Bozic or an immediate family member serves as a paid consultant to or is an employee of Cardinal Analytx, Carrum Health, and Centers for Medicare and Medicaid Services; serves as an unpaid consultant to Harvard Business School; and serves as a board member, owner, officer, or committee member of the American Association of Hip and Knee Surgeons and the American Joint Replacement Registry. Neither Dr. Shearer nor any immediate family member has received anything of value from or has stock or stock options held in a commercial company or institution related directly or indirectly to the subject of this chapter.

©Copyright 2021 American Academy of Orthopaedic Surgeons

Despite the absence of an explicit use of economic analysis by CMS in the United States, there are a growing number of studies published both in the orthopaedic and other medical literature.[9,10] Review articles have been published in every orthopaedic subspecialty summarizing the existing cost-effectiveness analysis (CEA) literature.[11-16] The results are incorporated into decision making by private insurers, professional societies, and to some degree individual surgeons. It is, therefore, important for orthopaedic surgeons to have a basic understanding of the principles of economic analysis and familiarity with the interpretation of study results.

To date, the standard for CEA methodology in the United States is based on the recommendations of the Panel on Cost-effectiveness in Health and Medicine, published in 1996.[17] The panel emerged due to the lack of standardization in CEA methods and aimed to put forth a set of recommendations for each component of a CEA that would form a base case, called the reference case, that should be performed in all studies. Although the authors recognized no single method applies to all circumstances, the goal of the reference case is to allow greater comparability across economic analyses. Furthermore, it provides a framework for the reader to evaluate the methodologic quality of studies being interpreted. More recently, a second panel on Cost-effectiveness in Health and Medicine was convened to update its recommendations, which were published in *JAMA* in 2016.[18] These recommendations are incorporated throughout the chapter and summarized in an outline at its conclusions.

TYPES OF ECONOMIC ANALYSIS

Although there is variability in the nomenclature used to describe types of economic analysis, the terminology described in this chapter is generally accepted.[19,20] Each approach shares the inclusion of cost but varies in the method and degree to which other data are incorporated. **Table 1** summarizes each type of economic analysis and lists the strengths and limitations.

COST-MINIMIZATION

The first major category of economic analysis is cost-minimization, which is employed when the effectiveness of two or more interventions is considered equivalent. In this scenario, cost alone can be used to differentiate the two treatments. Cost data for both treatments are collected and the intervention with lower total cost is preferred. A simple example would be comparing the costs associated with arthroscopic versus mini-open rotator cuff repair. Collecting outcome data is unnecessary as the results have been shown to be equivalent, and therefore, an appropriate comparison can be made with cost data only. An example is a study by Adla et al[21] demonstrated equivalent outcomes but a $1850 excess cost associated with arthroscopic rotator cuff repair compared with open repair, which was attributed primarily to increased costs of instrumentation. This type of economic analysis is often simpler, and the information derived from a cost-minimization analysis can be used in future cost-effectiveness research. However, it is rare that two interventions result in an exactly equivalent outcome.

COST-EFFECTIVENESS ANALYSIS

The term cost-effectiveness analysis (CEA) is an umbrella term that seeks to identify the cost for a unit of health benefit from an intervention. It is usually expressed quantitatively in terms of the cost-effectiveness ratio. The numerator always contains cost, while the denominator can be any desired outcome of interest. Examples could include cost per life saved, cost per complication averted, or cost per unit of utility (eg,

TABLE 1 Types of Economic Analysis

	Measure of Cost	Measure of Health Effect	Output	Strengths	Limitations
Cost-minimization	$	None (assumed equal)	Cost difference	Simple to conduct	Effectiveness of two treatments usually not equal
Cost-effectiveness analysis (CEA)	$	Any measure of health benefit	Incremental cost-effectiveness ratio	Can choose health effect most relevant to intervention	Difficult to make comparisons across different diseases or interventions
Cost-utility analysis (CUA)	$	Utility (eg, QALYs)	Incremental cost-effectiveness ratio	Allows comparisons across diseases and interventions within health care	Need estimate of utility for each relevant outcome
Cost-benefit analysis (CBA)	$	$	Net monetary benefit	Policy-makers can make comparisons across health and non-health care programs	Difficult to assign monetary value to health benefits

©Copyright 2021 American Academy of Orthopaedic Surgeons

quality-adjusted life years) gained. Although using an outcome specific to an intervention may simplify an analysis, it may limit the ability to make comparisons across studies or interventions.

COST-UTILITY ANALYSIS

Cost-utility is a specific case of cost-effectiveness in which the denominator of the cost-effectiveness ratio is the preference-based measure of utility. Utility in the context of health is a measure ranging from 0 to 1 that quantifies an individual's preference for a given health state relative to perfect health (equal to 1) and death (equal to 0). The product of utility and duration of a health state yields quality-adjusted life years (QALYs), which are frequently used in the denominator of a cost-utility analysis. In the medical literature, the term cost-effectiveness analysis is often synonymous with cost-utility analysis, and the two terms may be used interchangeably, but it should be recognized that in the current taxonomy while every cost-utility analysis is a CEA, not all CEA's are a cost-utility analysis.

COST-BENEFIT ANALYSIS

In cost-benefit analysis both the cost and effect of an intervention are expressed in monetary terms. Because all terms have the same units, the result is expressed as net monetary benefit (NMB) rather than a ratio. Alolabi et al[22] used this technique to estimate the net benefit of internal fixation compared with hemiarthroplasty for displaced femoral neck fractures. The authors found a higher cost associated with internal fixation, but surveyed individuals were willing to pay more for internal fixation than hemiarthroplasty. When multiplied by the expected number of femoral neck fractures in Ontario, a total net benefit of $224,000,000 was found for internal fixation. The advantage of this approach is that it allows comparisons across broad categories of intervention that could include education, environment, criminal justice, or any other societal interest competing for scarce funds. Its use is limited in medicine, however, because assigning a monetary value to health outcomes is difficult and ethically troublesome.

Recommendations of the US Panel on Cost-effectiveness in Health and Medicine: The numerator of the cost-effectiveness ratio should contain the net cost of an intervention, while the denominator should be QALYs.

STUDY DESIGN

There are two major categories for CEA study design: clinical trial-based and model-based studies. In the former, cost data are collected in the context of a clinical trial through empiric observation. The latter relies on simulations, typically computer-generated, that make assumptions regarding the costs and effects of an intervention based on data from other sources. Each has specific advantages and disadvantages, and the two are frequently combined to achieve the best possible result.

CLINICAL TRIAL-BASED

A cost-effectiveness analysis can be conducted alongside a clinical trial by collecting economic data in addition to measuring clinical outcomes.[23] This is sometimes referred to as a CEA "piggy-backed" on a clinical trial. These studies generally require a prospective cohort design with the intention to collect data regarding every aspect of the intervention for example, procedures, hospitalization, outpatient visits, travel time, etc.

The primary advantage of a clinical trial-based CEA is that data are generated through empiric observation, which eliminates many of the assumptions necessary for modeling. However, they are often limited by the time frame of observation, which may not include important outcomes that impact health and incur cost over a longer period of time than a trial is feasible to conduct. Furthermore, all the same limitations that apply to a typical clinical trial such as a selection bias or confounding apply with the inclusion of cost. Generalizability is problematic because strict inclusion and exclusion criteria are frequently employed in trials, and efficacy observed in a trial may not reflect the effectiveness observed with more widespread use.

An example of a trial-based cost-utility analysis in orthopaedics is the Spine Patient Outcomes Research Trial (SPORT) study assessing surgical versus nonsurgical care for disk herniation, spinal stenosis, and degenerative spondylolisthesis.[24,25] In addition to reporting clinical outcomes, Tosteson et al[26] separately published the results of the cost-effectiveness of surgical decompression compared with nonsurgical care for the management of spinal stenosis with and without spondylolisthesis. The EQ-5D, a survey instrument for estimating utility, was administered to all participants and demonstrated a difference in utility of 0.17 between the surgical and nonsurgical cohorts over the 2-year follow-up period. Cost data were determined using as combination Medicare payment data for procedure and inpatient charges while remaining costs incurred, such as nonsurgical care and missed work were self-reported by the subjects in the trial. Using these data, the incremental cost-effectiveness ratio (ICER) of surgical decompression for the management of spinal stenosis was estimated to be $77,600/QALY.

MODELING

Cost-effectiveness models are typically generated after an extensive review of the available literature on the topic or in conjunction with a trial-based CEA. These models allow projection of the observed costs and benefits of an intervention over time, making lifetime estimates of the ICER more feasible.[27] Modeling is appropriate when empiric observation

5: Principles of Clinical Information

©Copyright 2021 American Academy of Orthopaedic Surgeons

is not possible, typically due to practical or ethical considerations. Practical considerations include the high-cost and time-associated with clinical trials, particularly those considered of highest quality employing randomization, blinding, and control groups. Ethical considerations include equipoise, when one treatment is known to be superior or when there is potential for harm to trial participants.

The disadvantage is that cost-effectiveness analysis models are subject to bias and often difficult to validate. Furthermore, many of the inputs required for a CEA model, including treatment costs, clinical outcome probabilities, and clinical effectiveness, may be unknown, or not previously reported in the literature. To that end, it is important that the assumptions used in formulating the model are explicitly stated. Computer-generated models can become highly complex leading to a lack of transparency, particularly to those unfamiliar with the methodology.

An example of a model-based CEA in orthopaedic surgery is a study by Slover et al[28] evaluating the cost-effectiveness of total hip arthroplasty after femoral neck fracture. The authors use a Markov model to estimate the projected cost and utility gain of total hip arthroplasty compared with hemiarthroplasty for active elderly patients over a 10-year time horizon. There were several important assumptions including an equal failure rate for both interventions and a higher postoperative utility for total hip arthroplasty. One and two-way sensitivity analysis were used to explore sensitivity in the model variables. These techniques will be discussed further in a later section. The results of the model suggest total hip arthroplasty may be highly cost-effective in this setting with an ICER of $1960/QALY.

COMBINED

It is important to recognize that modeling and clinical trial-based designs can be used in combination. This is typically done to extend the results of the trial beyond the available follow up period. There are important assumptions regarding the degree to which the effect of treatment is maintained over time, and this should be explicitly stated.

Recommendations of the US Panel on Cost-effectiveness in Health and Medicine: Researchers should use the best available data for determining the cost and effectiveness of a treatment strategy, whether from randomized controlled trials, observational studies, or descriptive series. Models should be used to supplement but not replace data directly observed in empirical study.

EXPRESSING AND INTERPRETING COST-EFFECTIVENESS

The degree of cost-effectiveness in economic studies is commonly expressed in terms of the incremental cost-effectiveness ratio (ICER), net health benefit (NHB), or net monetary benefit (NMB). These three terms are related conceptually and mathematically by the willingness-to-pay threshold (WTP or λ).

INCREMENTAL COST-EFFECTIVENESS RATIO

The ICER is a ratio of the difference in cost to the difference in effectiveness of an intervention in relation to a baseline comparator. It is expressed in the following formula:

$$\text{ICER} = \left(\text{Cost}_{\text{intervention}} - \text{Cost}_{\text{baseline}}\right) / \left(\text{Effect}_{\text{intervention}} - \text{Effect}_{\text{baseline}}\right)$$

Defining a baseline comparator is one of the most critical and frequently neglected elements of a cost-effectiveness study. There is seldom a true "do-nothing" approach that is without cost or effect on the patient. For example, a patient treated nonsurgically for a rotator cuff tear may accrue significant costs in pain medications, physical therapy, and steroid injections. They may also have significant improvement in their pain and quality of life as a result of these treatments over time. It is important that a study of the cost-effectiveness of surgical repair of the rotator cuff over a given time frame include the change in cost and utility of nonsurgical care as a comparator.

The cost-effectiveness plane is a graphical representation of the ICER that aids in its interpretation (**Figure 1**). There are four quadrants defined by whether the difference in cost and effect is positive or negative between the new intervention and the comparator. In quadrant II, the cost of the intervention is higher but the effectiveness is lower, which results in the intervention being "dominated" by the comparator. In this case, the comparator is always preferred. In quadrant IV, the intervention is more effective and less costly and therefore results in cost savings. It is therefore said to "dominate" the comparator and is always preferred. In quadrant I, the cost and effect are both higher for the intervention, which is the most common scenario. In this case, the choice is dependent upon the decision-maker's willingness to pay for a given effect. Quadrant III is the case in which the new intervention is less costly and less effective. Interpretation in this scenario

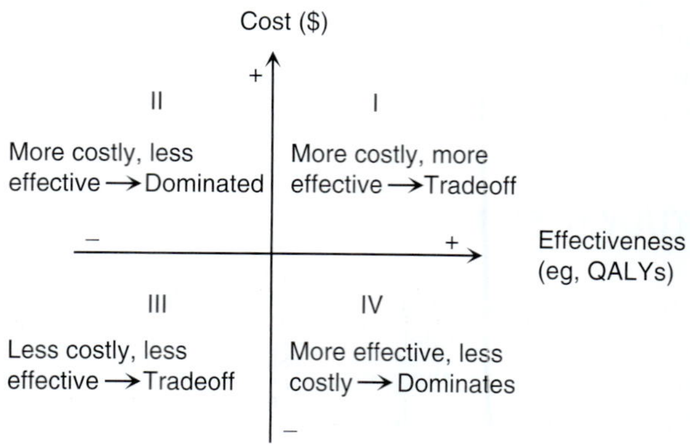

FIGURE 1 The cost-effectiveness plane.

©Copyright 2021 American Academy of Orthopaedic Surgeons

is controversial, but the concept of willingness to pay in quadrant I can again be applied, but in this case to the comparator rather than the new intervention.

Willingness-to-pay (WTP) is a concept that attempts to identify a threshold of acceptability for the incremental cost-effectiveness ratio.[29] Stated differently, it is the cost-effectiveness threshold, below which an intervention is considered to be cost-effective. Although $50,000/QALY is a frequently reported WTP threshold, it is somewhat arbitrary and is rarely used in healthcare policy decision making.

Recommendations of the US Panel on Cost-effectiveness in Health and Medicine: Economic analyses should report the total cost and effectiveness, incremental cost and effectiveness, and incremental cost-effectiveness ratios.

VALUING EFFECTIVENESS

QUALITY-ADJUSTED LIFE YEARS

The most common health outcome measure used in economic analyses is the quality-adjusted life year (QALY). The QALY is a year of life spent in a health state weighted by the utility of that health state. For example, if we assume the utility of hip osteoarthritis is 0.6, 10 years with the condition would yield 6 QALYs. An intervention that restores perfect hip function for 10 years would result in a net gain of 4 QALYs.

There are several significant assumptions underlying the QALY, not the least of which is that the preference for a health state remains constant regardless of the duration of the health state. For example, in the QALY model, 10 years with hip osteoarthritis results in exactly twice the number of QALYs as 5 years. This assumption is not supported by empirical evidence, which demonstrates that quality of life often declines over time in a chronic health state such as osteoarthritis.[30] Healthy-years equivalents (HYEs) were developed as an alternative to QALYs to avoid this assumption.[31,32] HYEs are assigned using a time-trade off approach specific to the expected duration of the disease. This is theoretically beneficial to more accurately reflect individual preference but has not been widely applied due to the time-consuming nature of collecting HYEs for all relevant health states and durations. Therefore, QALYs remain the benchmark for conducting a cost-utility analysis.

Disability-adjusted life years (DALYs) were developed and are used primarily by the World Health Organization (WHO) for estimation of global disease burden, but can also be used for economic analysis.[33] The DALY is similar to the QALY but the scale is inverse, that is, a disease with high-morbidity results in more DALY's. Unlike the QALY, the values assigned to a given disease are determined by an expert panel rather than using an empirically derived estimate of utility.

Recommendations of the US Panel on Cost-effectiveness in Health and Medicine: QALYs should be used to quantify health benefits in the denominator of the incremental cost-effectiveness ratio.

DERIVING UTILITY

There are two broad categories of methods used to estimate the utility of a health state for a CEA. The first are empiric methods, which are obtained from the general population to elicit preferences for various disease states. The standard gamble technique is the gold-standard for determining the utility of a health state.[17] It involves a choice between a given health state and a gamble between perfect health and death. The lowest probability of perfect health that is acceptable is the utility of the health state. For example, to determine the utility of hip osteoarthritis, healthy individuals could be asked to choose between having hip arthritis or taking a gamble in which there is a 99% chance of perfect health with no hip arthritis and a 1% chance of death. If this is deemed acceptable, the probability of perfect health would be lowered until reaching the threshold where the individual prefers to accept hip arthritis rather than take the gamble. If this threshold occurred when the probability of perfect health is 60% and death is 40%, the estimated utility of hip osteoarthritis would be 0.6.

An alternative method for determining utility empirically is the time trade-off (TTO) method.[34] Subjects are asked to make choice between a given time with the health state in question and a shorter duration with perfect health. The ratio of the two is an estimate of the utility of the health state. In the above example of hip osteoarthritis, an individual could be asked to trade 9 years of perfect health for 10 years with arthritis. If this were acceptable, the number of years of perfect health would be lowered until reaching the threshold where 10 years of arthritis is preferred. If the threshold of acceptability were 6 years of perfect health versus 10 years of arthritis, the estimated utility would be 0.6.

PREFERENCE-WEIGHTED GENERIC MEASURES

Because the standard gamble and TTO can be impractical to administer for all possible health states, the second method for estimating utility are survey instruments that have been developed and correlated with the empiric instruments. These surveys seek to capture relevant domains of quality of life that underlie the preference for a particular health state. Unlike the empiric instruments, most can be completed in quickly either in-person or by mail. This is much more practical in the setting of most trial-based CEAs. A few of the more common preference-weighted survey instruments are the EQ-5D and Health Utilities Index (HUI).

EQ-5D

The Euroqol group developed the EQ-5D to assess health outcomes in a practical, standardized manner. The questionnaire utilizes five distinct domains: mobility, self-care, usual activities, pain/discomfort, and anxiety/depression. There are five questions, the results of which have been correlated to results of the standardized gamble to calculate a utility value.[35]

©Copyright 2021 American Academy of Orthopaedic Surgeons

SF-6D

The SF-36 is a well-known and commonly utilized survey instrument to assess quality of life. It is not, however, designed to determine utility. The SF-6D has more recently been developed to allow calculation of utility using a subset of six SF-36 domains. It is reduced to 11-items and has been correlated with the standard gamble (SG).

Recommendations of the US Panel on Cost-effectiveness in Health and Medicine: Utilities should reflect community preferences rather than patients, providers, or investigators. Empiric measures such as the standard gamble or time-trade off and preference-weighted generic measures such as the EQ-5d are considered acceptable methods for estimating utility.

ESTIMATING COSTS

PERSPECTIVE

Determination of the relevant costs associated with a healthcare intervention is highly dependent upon the perspective of the decision-maker. Perspectives commonly considered are government or private payors, hospitals, and society. The societal perspective includes not only the direct costs of medical care, but economic effects of the intervention on employment, school, caregivers, and other societal interests.[17] These additional **effects** may be less relevant to other decision-makers with a more narrow focus. This may result in the inclusion or exclusion of certain costs from the numerator of the ICER, which could result in different conclusions. As a result, the second panel on cost-effectiveness in health and medicine recommends that investigators perform two reference cases—one from the societal perspective and the other from the health care payer perspective that does not include indirect costs.

DIRECT AND INDIRECT COSTS

Costs included in economic analyses are divided into direct and indirect sources. The direct costs of an intervention are the more readily apparent expenses stemming from medical treatment such as hospitalization, surgery, and outpatient visits. Indirect costs, which accrue from missed work, travel time, child care, and other sources of monetary loss that may be affected by an intervention are often more difficult to quantify but nevertheless important, especially when performing a CEA from a societal perspective. In modeling studies, missed time is frequently estimated by using the average time of missed work multiplied by the average wage nationally.

OBTAINING COST DATA

There are two approaches to collecting cost data: microcosting and gross-costing.[31] Microcosting is an item-by-item estimation of the costs of an intervention that could include supplies, nursing care, and other aspects of surgical care or hospitalization. This technique is more frequently used in the trial setting, where individual-level data on each resource used in the course of a treatment is recorded and tallied. In contrast, gross-costing typically uses diagnostic or procedural codes to obtain the aggregate cost of a disease or intervention from large state or national-level databases. The latter is often used in modeling studies where individual level data are unavailable. It has the benefit of being relatively generalizable and easy to obtain but has less flexibility in assessing less common diseases or subpopulations that may not have a specific code to distinguish them.

Recently, increasing emphasis has been placed on more accurately estimating health care costs using microcosting methods known as time-driven activity-based costing (TDABC), originally described by Robert Kaplan.[36] TDABC breaks down complex interventions into processes with a finite number of discrete resources each with a quantifiable cost and duration that can be measured to more accurately make cost estimates. These methods are likely to be used increasingly both in CEA and in general for programs aiming to reduce costs and improve efficiency.[37]

DISCOUNTING

Discounting is an important economic concept that stems from the principle that there is a preference for present rather than future benefits (eg, the "time-value of money"). Using a monetary example, an individual would rather receive a $10,000 reward now than in 10 years. An exact discount rate could be determined empirically by surveying individuals to determine the monetary value in 10 years that would be equivalent to a present value of $10,000. The idea of discounting medical outcomes and costs is more controversial but has been empirically studied. The US Panel on Cost-Effectiveness Analysis recommends using a 3% annual discount on both future health benefits and costs.[17] This has the effect of favoring interventions that improve health in the present rather than the future.

It is important to distinguish discounting and time preference from inflation. Inflation is the rise in prices of goods and services over time. Economic analyses should adjust all prices to present value based on the inflation rate, typically determined by the Consumer Price Index (CPI). For example, in a study of total hip arthroplasty, if costs of surgery were obtained from a database generated in the year 2000 while other costs were from 2010, the surgical costs would have to be adjusted to 2010 dollars. This is independent of the discount rate, which would remain 3%.

Recommendations of the US Panel on Cost-effectiveness in Health and Medicine: Costs should be estimated from both the societal perspective (direct and indirect costs) and the healthcare sector perspective (direct costs only). Both costs and health effects should be estimated over a lifetime time horizon, but non-health-related costs from additional years of life added by the intervention should not be included. Costs

©Copyright 2021 American Academy of Orthopaedic Surgeons

and health effects should be discounted at 3% per year, but the impact of discounting should be assessed in sensitivity analysis.

MODELING

There are a variety of modeling methods that can be used to simulate health outcomes and costs associated with an intervention ranging in complexity from a simple decision tree to dynamic models. In general, the simplest model that can effectively address the question is preferred. The vast majority of models rely on breaking a health problem and its subsequent outcomes into discrete health states. The expected progression of disease is estimated from the best available evidence whether from a trial, database, or published literature.[31]

SIMPLE DECISION TREE

There are several important considerations in selecting a model. One of the first is whether or not outcomes evolve over time or are known in a short time frame after the intervention and remain stable over time. In the latter case, a simple decision tree is well-suited, and many surgical interventions fall in this category. An example would be a patient with a tibial shaft fracture considering surgical or nonsurgical intervention. Consequences of surgery could include successful union, nonunion, or infection, while nonsurgical outcomes could be successful union, malunion, or nonunion. By one year after surgery, one could assume these outcomes are known and are unlikely to change significantly over the remainder of a patient's life. A proposed model is shown below in **Figure 2**.

The blue square represents the decision node, which is the branch point for all possible choices. The green circles are chance nodes, reflecting potential outcomes of each possible strategy. Listed below each outcome is its probability of occurring. It is important to note that at each node the sum of the probabilities is always 100%. At the far right next to the red triangles are the "rewards," which can be any outcome, cost, or both. In a CEA, cost and QALYs are the two "rewards." Through a process of "folding back," which involves a weighted sum of the rewards at each node, the expected value of each strategy can be calculated and compared or used to calculate the ICER. In the case above, the expected value of intramedullary (IM) nailing is 9.65 while the expected value of nonsurgical care is 9.5, indicating that surgical treatment is expected to result in an additional 0.15 QALYs compared with nonsurgical treatment.

MARKOV MODELING

In contrast to simple decision trees, Markov models incorporate cycling through health states over time. This facilitates a more realistic representation of the time course of diseases that progress through stages. Total joint arthroplasty procedures are commonly modeled using Markov models, as failure occurs steadily over time and is difficult to model accurately with a simple decision tree. The model output can be calculated by hand using matrix algebra but is more commonly obtained using computer-generated models. For each cycle of every health state, there is a transition probability of moving to a new health state or remaining in the same health state. The model cycles over a fixed *cycle length* (eg, 1 year) for the *time horizon* of the model, which could be a specified duration relevant to the decision-maker or the remainder of the lifetime. In a lifetime model there is usually a "dead" state referred to as an "absorbing" state because transitions can occur into but not out of the state. In a lifetime model, the Markov model cycles until the entire cohort is in the "dead" state.

A Markov model is demonstrated comparing total hip arthroplasty to nonsurgical care in **Figure 3**. With each cycle of the model, the cohort progresses through each branch of the tree. At the terminal end of each branch (red triangle) is the starting health start for the subsequent cycle. This continues until all members of the cohort are in the absorbing "dead" state. Important assumptions of the Markov model include a fixed cycle length and constant transition probabilities over time. When these assumptions are not met, there are other more complex modeling methods that can be considered.

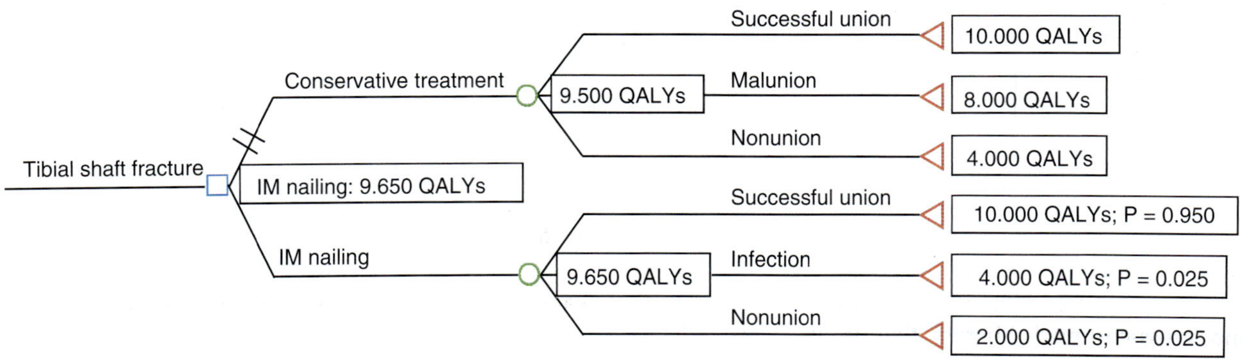

FIGURE 2 Simple decision tree comparing surgical and nonsurgical care for tibial shaft fracture.

©Copyright 2021 American Academy of Orthopaedic Surgeons

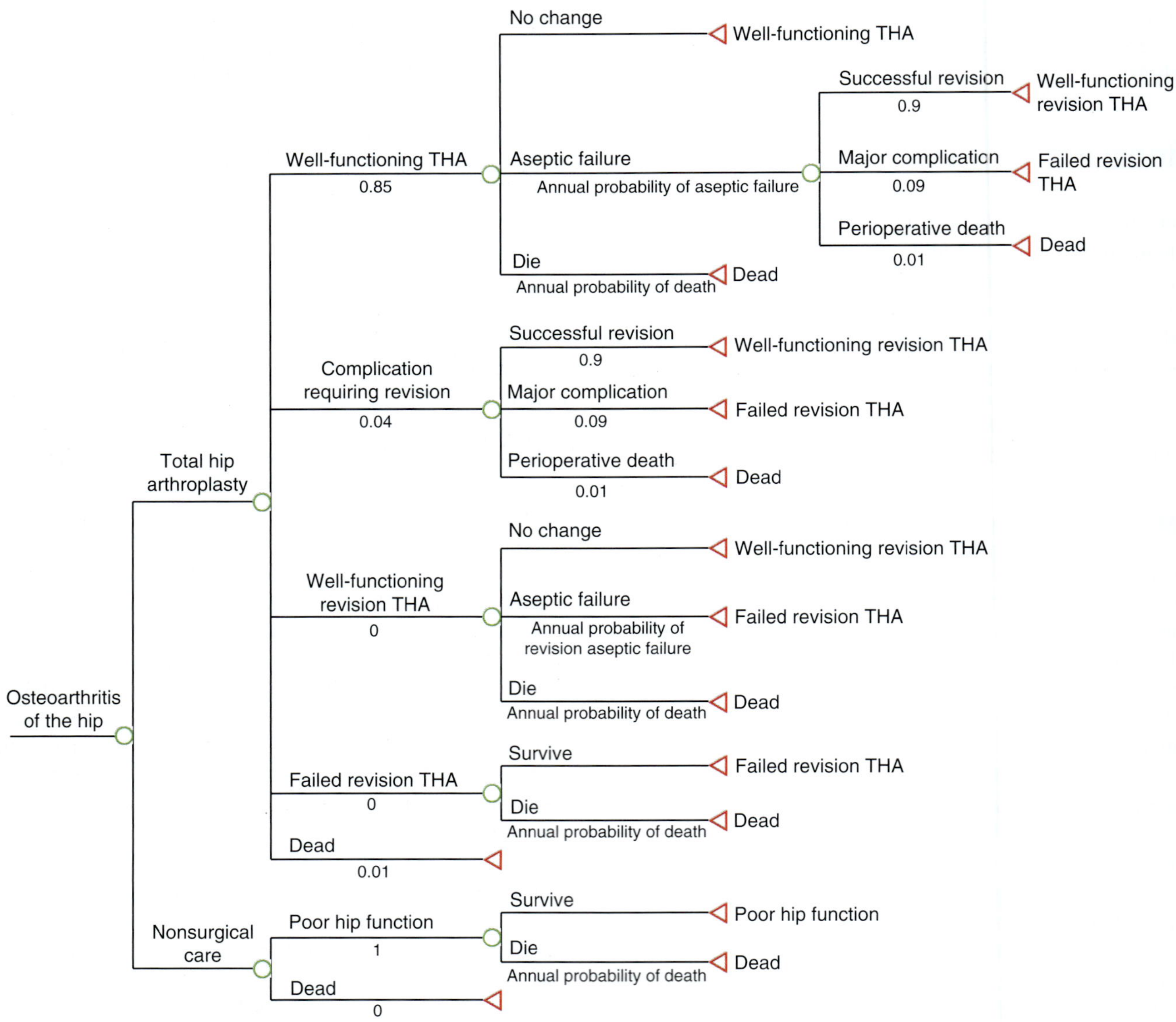

FIGURE 3 Markov model comparing total joint arthroplasty and nonsurgical care.

MANAGING UNCERTAINTY

Uncertainty exists in every aspect of a cost-effectiveness study, particularly when modeling is employed. This includes the type of model selected (model uncertainty) and the inputs to the model such as costs, utilities, and probabilities of each health state (parameter uncertainty).

PARAMETER UNCERTAINTY

Point estimates of each model variable are used, but often there are a range of plausible inputs either due to insufficient empirical data or chance error. This is referred to as parameter uncertainty. For any given model, there can be uncertainty in the estimates of cost, utilities, or the probability of events occurring within the model. The simplest method to address this is sensitivity analysis, which explores the output of the model across a range of a model input. For example, in the prior study of tibial fracture treatment, the cost-effectiveness could be calculated and plotted across a range of infection rates for surgical treatment. A sample is shown in **Figure 4** below. This figure suggests that tibial fracture treatment is cost-effective for low infection rates, but if the infection rate is above 5%, nonsurgical treatment is preferred. Identifying thresholds in an unknown variable is an important outcome of CEA's that informs clinicians and future research.

Two-way sensitivity analysis can be used to explore the impact of a plausible range of two variables. The value of each variable is plotted on each axis and the plot is coded to indicate which strategy is preferred based on the value of the two variables. A sample graph is shown below (**Figure 5**) for the tibial

©Copyright 2021 American Academy of Orthopaedic Surgeons

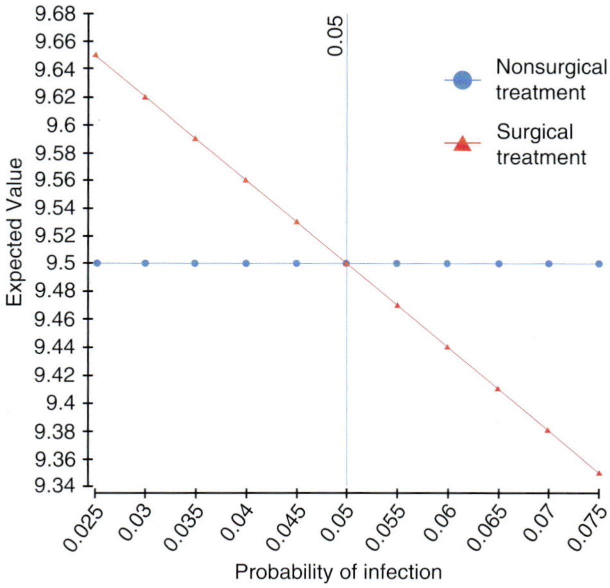

FIGURE 4 One-way sensitivity analysis.

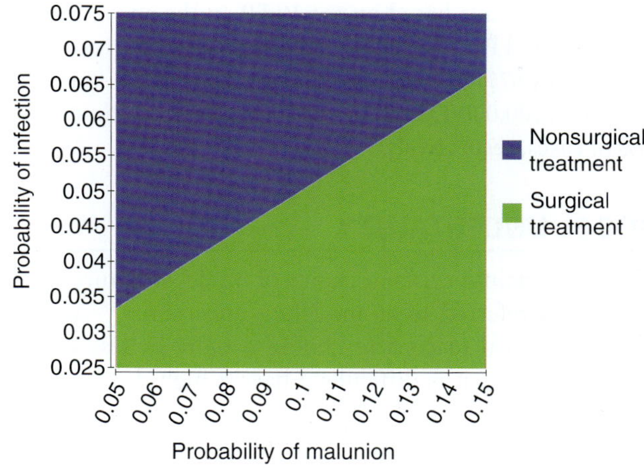

FIGURE 5 Two-way sensitivity analysis.

fracture example using the probability of infection after surgical treatment and the probability of malunion after conservative treatment. In the area denoted by a green cross-hatch, surgical treatment is preferred, while in the blue cross-hatch, nonsurgical treatment is preferred.

Sensitivity analysis becomes more difficult if there is uncertainty in more than two variables. This is not uncommon, as there is typically a degree of uncertainty in every variable included in the model. To accomplish multivariate sensitivity analysis, probabilistic sensitivity analysis (PSA) is commonly employed. This technique assigns a distribution rather than a point estimate for each variable in the model. To conduct the PSA, the model is run using computer software thousands or even millions of times in each case drawing a number for each input from the assigned distributions. The results can then be plotted and interpreted. Two common plots used are the 95% confidence ellipse and the cost-effectiveness acceptability curve, which are shown below in **Figure 6**.

The 95% confidence ellipse is a plot on the cost-effectiveness plane of all the PSA trials with an ellipse encircling the 95% of simulations nearest the point estimate. It is analogous to a 95% confidence interval and gives an idea of the upper and lower bounds of the ICER.

The cost-effectiveness acceptability curve (CEAC) can be one of the most informative methods of reporting results of a cost-effectiveness model. Along the X-axis is the willingness-to-pay (WTP) and on the Y-axis is the proportion of trials

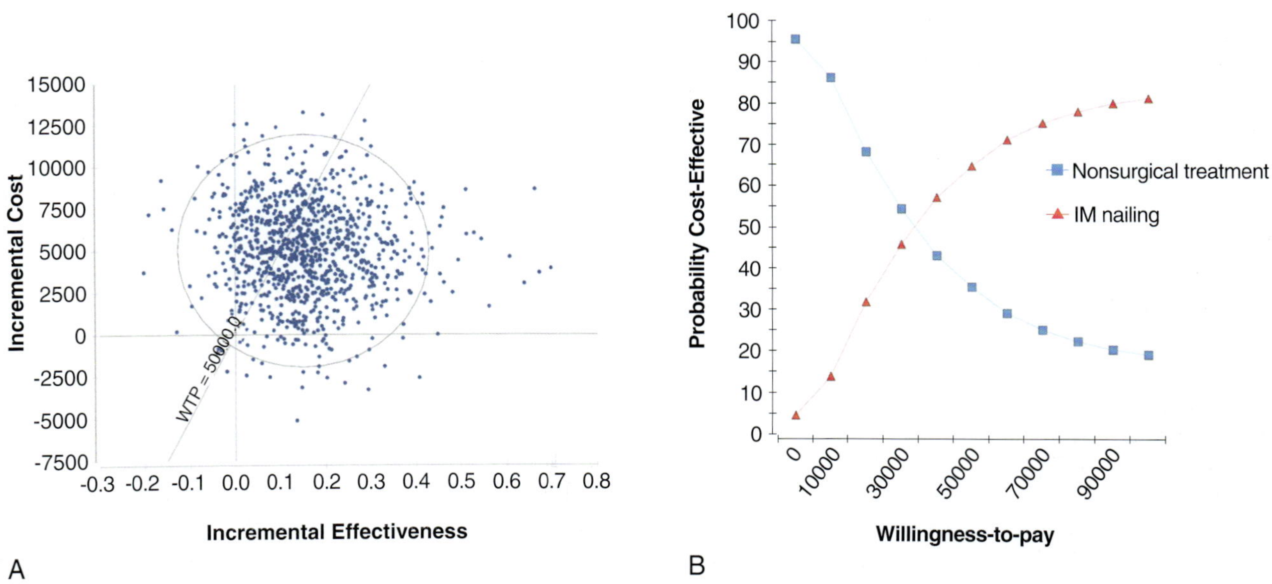

FIGURE 6 The 95% confidence ellipse (**A**) and cost-effectiveness acceptability curve (**B**).

©Copyright 2021 American Academy of Orthopaedic Surgeons

that are acceptable based on the WTP. In the above example, using low WTP of $10,000/QALY, nonsurgical treatment is preferred in 87% of cases. In contrast if the WTP is $50,000/QALY or $100,000/QALY, IM nailing is preferred in 65% and 83% of cases, respectively.

MODEL UNCERTAINTY

When uncertainty exists in choice of model structure or processes, it is referred to as modeling uncertainty.[38] Although there are logical reasons to choose a more or less complex model structure, it is difficult to have a high degree of confidence that the model ultimately chosen most accurately reflects the real-world process being modeled. This can be addressed by performing the analysis using several possible modeling methods to explore the impact of the model choice. This is limited, however, by the time and resources needed to develop one model, let alone multiple. This can therefore be addressed through validation, which is comprised of comparing model predictions to real world data or models generated by other researchers.

Recommendations of the US Panel on Cost-effectiveness in Health and Medicine: Investigators should perform both univariate and multivariate sensitivity analysis.

SUMMARY OF RECOMMENDATIONS OF THE US PANEL ON COST-EFFECTIVENESS IN HEALTH AND MEDICINE[18]

Components of numerator (costs):
- Direct costs from the health care payer perspective
- Both direct and indirect costs for the societal perspective
- Exclude costs associated with added years of life

Components of denominator (effects):
- QALYs
- Utility estimates from standard gamble/TTO or preference-weighted survey instruments (eg, EQ-5D, HUI)

Perspective: Societal and Health-care Payer Perspective (Two reference cases)
Time horizon: Lifetime
Discount: 3%, explore with sensitivity analysis
Data sources: primary or secondary, best available evidence preferred
Sensitivity analysis:
- Univariate sensitivity analysis for key assumptions at a minimum
- Multivariate sensitivity analysis recommended (eg, probabilistic sensitivity analysis)

REFERENCES

1. Porter ME, Kaplan RS: How to pay for health care bundled payments will finally unleash the competition that patients want. *Harv Bus Rev* 2016;94(7-8):88-100.
2. Weinstein MC, Stason WB: Foundations of cost-effectiveness analysis for health and medical practices. *N Engl J Med* 1977;296(13):716-721.
3. Bodenheimer T: High and rising health care costs. Part 1: Seeking an explanation. *Ann Intern Med* 2005;142(10):847-854.
4. Ubel PA, DeKay ML, Baron J, Asch DA: Cost-effectiveness analysis in a setting of budget constraints – Is it equitable? *N Engl J Med* 1996;334(18):1174-1177.
5. Firshein J: U.S. turns down Oregon plan to rank, ration Medicaid services. *J Am Health Policy* 1992;2(5):51-52.
6. Chambers JD Neumann PJ, Buxton MJ: Does medicare have an implicit cost-effectiveness threshold? *Med Decis Making* 2010;30(4):E14-E27.
7. Gold MR, Sofaer S, Siegelberg T: Medicare and cost-effectiveness analysis: Time to ask the taxpayers. *Health Aff* 2007;26(5):1399-1406.
8. Claxton K, Sculpher M, Drummond M: A rational framework for decision making by the National Institute for Clinical Excellence (NICE). *Lancet* 2002;360(9334):711-715.
9. Brauer CA, Neumann PJ, Rosen AB: Trends in cost effectiveness analyses in orthopaedic surgery. *Clin Orthop Relat Res* 2007;457:42-48.
10. Neumann PJ, Greenberg D, Olchanski NV, Stone PW, Rosen AB: Growth and quality of the cost-utility literature, 1976–2001. *Value Health* 2005;8(1):3-9.
11. Coyle S, Kinsella S, Lenehan B, Queally JM: Cost-utility analysis in orthopaedic trauma; what pays? A systematic review. *Injury* 2018;49(3):575-584.
12. Kamaruzaman H, Kinghorn P, Oppong R: Cost-effectiveness of surgical interventions for the management of osteoarthritis: A systematic review of the literature. *BMC Muscoskelet Disord* 2017;18(1):183.
13. Karhade AV, Kwon JY: Cost-utility analyses in US Orthopaedic Foot and Ankle Surgery: A systematic review. *Foot Ankle Spec* 2018:1938640018782588.
14. Lu Y, Qureshi SA: Cost-effective studies in spine surgeries: A narrative review. *Spine J* 2014;14(11):2748-2762.
15. Nwachukwu BU, Schairer WW, Bernstein JL, Dodwell ER, Marx RG, Allen AA: Cost-effectiveness analyses in orthopaedic sports medicine: A systematic review. *Am J Sports Med* 2015;43(6):1530-1537.
16. Rajan PV, Qudsi RA, Dyer GSM, Losina E: Cost-utility studies in upper limb orthopaedic surgery. *Bone Joint Lett J* 2018;100-B(11):1416-1423.
17. Gold MR: *Cost-Effectiveness in Health and Medicine.* New York, Oxford University Press, 1996, xxiii, 425 p.
18. Sanders GD, Neumann PJ, Basu A, et al: Recommendations for conduct, methodological practices, and reporting of cost-effectiveness analyses: Second panel on cost-effectiveness in health and medicine. *J Am Med Assoc* 2016;316(10):1093-1103.
19. Muennig P, EBooks Corporation: *Cost-Effectiveness Analyses in Health: A Practical Approach*, ed 2. San Francisco, Jossey-Bass, 2008, xvi, 266 p.
20. Drummond MF, McGuire A: *Economic Evaluation in Health Care: Merging Theory With Practice.* Oxford; New York, Oxford University Press, 2001, 286 p.
21. Adla DN, Rowsell M, Pandey R: Cost-effectiveness of open versus arthroscopic rotator cuff repair. *J Shoulder Elbow Surg* 2010;19(2):258-261.
22. Alolabi B, Bajammal S, Shirali J, Karanicolas PJ, Gafni A, Bhandari M: Treatment of displaced femoral neck fractures in the elderly: A cost-benefit analysis. *J Orthop Trauma* 2009;23(6):442-446.
23. Drummond M: Economic analysis alongside clinical trials: Problems and potential. *J Rheumatol* 1995;22(7):1403-1407.
24. Weinstein JN, Lurie JD, Tosteson TD, et al: Surgical versus nonoperative treatment for lumbar disc herniation: Four-year results for the Spine Patient Outcomes Research Trial (SPORT). *Spine* 2008;33(25):2789-2800.

©Copyright 2021 American Academy of Orthopaedic Surgeons

25. Weinstein JN, Lurie JD, Tosteson TD, et al: Surgical compared with nonoperative treatment for lumbar degenerative spondylolisthesis. Four-year results in the Spine Patient Outcomes Research Trial (SPORT) randomized and observational cohorts. *J Bone Joint Surg Am* 2009;91(6):1295-1304.
26. Tosteson AN, Lurie JD, Tosteson TD, et al: Surgical treatment of spinal stenosis with and without degenerative spondylolisthesis: Cost-effectiveness after 2 years. *Ann Intern Med* 2008;149(12):845-853.
27. Stahl JE: Modelling methods for pharmacoeconomics and health technology assessment: An overview and guide. *PharmacoEconomics* 2008;26(2):131-148.
28. Slover J, Hoffman MV, Malchau H, Tosteson AN, Koval KJ: A cost-effectiveness analysis of the arthroplasty options for displaced femoral neck fractures in the active, healthy, elderly population. *J Arthroplasty* 2009;24(6):854-860.
29. Olsen JA, Smith RD: Theory versus practice: A review of 'willingness-to-pay' in health and health care. *Health Econ* 2001;10(1):39-52.
30. Bala MV, Wood LL, Zarkin GA, Norton EC, Gafni A, O'Brien BJ: Are health states "timeless"? The case of the standard gamble method. *J Clin Epidemiol* 1999;52(11):1047-1053.
31. Muennig P, Khan K: *Designing and Conducting Cost-Effectiveness Analyses in Medicine and Health Care*, ed 1. San Francisco, Jossey-Bass, 2002, xxvi, 356 p.
32. Mehrez A, Gafni A: Quality-adjusted life years, utility theory, and healthy-years equivalents. *Med Decis Making* 1989;9(2):142-149.
33. Murray CJ, Acharya AK: Understanding DALYs (disability-adjusted life years). *J Health Econ* 1997;16(6):703-730.
34. Bleichrodt H, Johannesson M: Standard gamble, time trade-off and rating scale: Experimental results on the ranking properties of QALYs. *J Health Econ* 1997;16(2):155-175.
35. Shaw JW, Johnson JA, Coons SJ: US valuation of the EQ-5d health states: Development and testing of the D1 valuation model. *Med Care* 2005;43(3):203-220.
36. Kaplan RS, Anderson SR: Time-driven activity-based costing. *Harv Bus Rev* 2004;82(11):131-138.
37. Kaplan RS, Porter ME: How to solve the cost crisis in health care. *Harv Bus Rev* 2011;89(9):46-52.
38. Kim SY, Goldie SL, Salomon JA: Exploring model uncertainty in economic evaluation of health interventions: The example of rotavirus vaccination in Vietnam. *Med Decis Making* 2010;30(5):E1-E28.

©Copyright 2021 American Academy of Orthopaedic Surgeons

47

The Product Development Process From Discovery, Through the FDA, and Into the Clinic

Scott P. Bruder, MD, PhD
Kristen Allen, BS, RAC
Spencer Bailey, BS, MBA
James Petricek, MSE, MBA

Keywords: *FDA; orthobiologics; product development; regulatory strategy; reimbursement*

INTRODUCTION

To drive the discovery, development, and commercialization of therapeutic orthopaedic products into routine clinical practice with greater speed, certainty, and financial efficiency, a symbiotic relationship between academic, clinical, and industrial investigators is essential. Approaches that successfully weave the technology, tools, and clinical applications from the laboratory bench to the clinical bedside stand a greater chance of being successful in the marketplace. The purpose of this chapter is to provide practical information and insights regarding the pathways and processes required to bring innovations, particularly in the field of implantable devices, orthobiologics, and regenerative medicine, to the commercial market. The chapter will provide an overview of the product development cycle, with emphasis on recent changes to the regulatory landscape and requirements for reimbursement in the hospital and office setting. **Figure 1** illustrates the major programmatic elements and stage gates that must be navigated in the journey from product concept through scientific validation, clinical testing, FDA approval, market launch, and reimbursement. Virtually all products follow this course, though subtle differences exist depending on the nature of the product (eg, device vs biologic) and the regulatory burden necessary for market launch (eg, 510(k), PMA, or BLA). At the close of the chapter, readers will have a greater understanding of the multiyear, multistep, interactive process involving multiple government agencies, private third-party payors, industry sales planning, and the efforts required to successfully commercialize new products.

Dr. Bruder or an immediate family member serves as a paid consultant to or is an employee of AgNovos Inc., AnGes Inc., Asahi Kesai, Avanos, Collagen Matrix Inc., CreOsso, Embody, Kuros BioSciences AG, Lipogems, MTF Biologics, Myant, Novadip Biosciences, Ortho RTI, Ossio, TissueGen, and Wright Medical Technology, Inc.; and has stock or stock options held in Embody, Kuros BioSciences AG, Lipogems, MicroMedicine, Myant, Spinal Elements, and Stryker; and serves as a board member, owner, officer, or committee member of the Global Spine Outreach. Ms. Allen or an immediate family member serves as a paid consultant to or is an employee of Lipogems and TranS1. Mr. Bailey or an immediate family member serves as a paid consultant to or is an employee of Embody and Lipogems. Mr. Petricek or an immediate family member serves as a paid consultant to or is an employee of Carmell Therapeutics, Embody, Wright Medical Technology, Inc., Ossio, and CreOsso; serves as an unpaid consultant to TulangCo; and has stock or stock options held in Embody.

©Copyright 2021 American Academy of Orthopaedic Surgeons

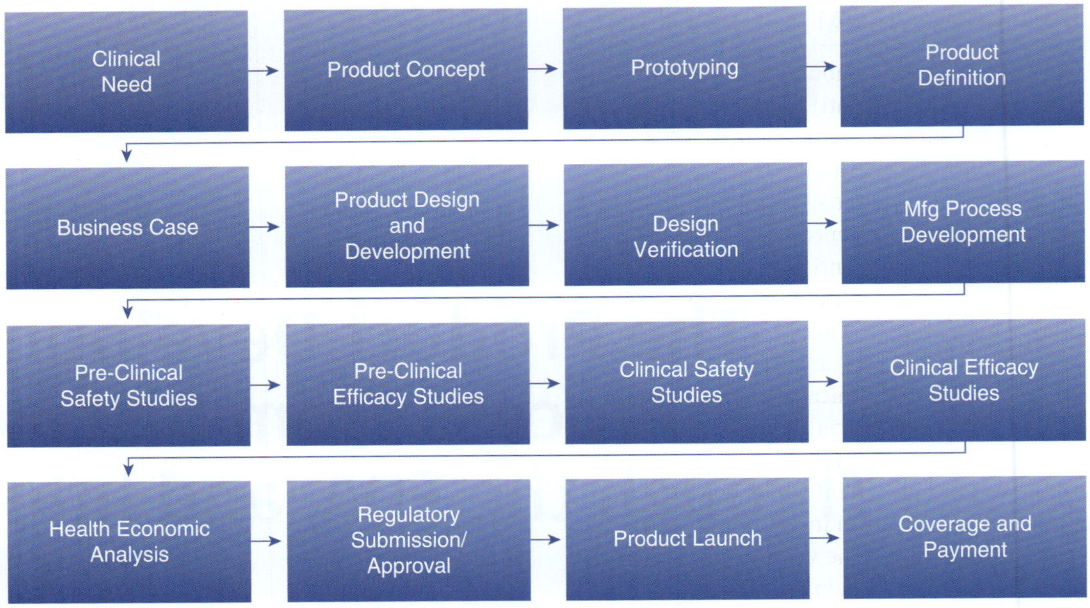

FIGURE 1 Illustration of the product development process. Any successful product development effort must navigate most, if not all, of the steps defined in this sequence. Depending on the device, drug, biologic, or combination designation, plus the Class of the product (I, II, or III), the requirements for Clinical Studies will vary from none to multiple randomized controlled clinical trials. The precise sequence of these steps may also vary depending on the nature of the product.

INNOVATING IN ORTHOPAEDICS

DEFINING AN UNMET NEED

Product development is the formalized process by which new technologies, concepts, and ideas are shaped into tangible, marketed products. Ideally, the cornerstone of any product development effort starts with the identification of a specific "unmet need" (ie, the problem). Within interventional orthopaedic care, unmet needs are abundant and may include objectives such as:

- Improving patient outcomes
- Reducing variability in patient outcomes
- Improving patient safety
- Addressing surgeon/OR staff safety
- Reducing economic cost (ie, product cost or waste)
- Improving operating room efficiencies (ie, reducing procedure time and complexity)

Once a clinical need is clearly established, an inventor or product development team can then examine possible ideas, concepts, and strategies to address the problem, through the creation of a medical device or biologic implant (for the purposes of this text), such as a surgical or diagnostic instrument or implant. In this very early stage of product development, the concept may be further fleshed out through the creation of prototypes, drawings, or models to determine if the initial design concept has merit. Prototype designs can be vetted in a variety of ways, such as through "simulated use" testing, cadaveric studies, laboratory studies, engineering testing, or "hands-on" evaluation from orthopaedic surgeons who would be likely users of the device. This process is often iterative in nature, as the creation of prototypes or drawings frequently generates feedback that spurs new creative thinking or identifies opportunities and weaknesses with the original product concept. Through this dynamic process, new design or performance requirements may begin to emerge. Consequently, this process is vital to ensuring the proposed design will adequately serve its intended purpose in the market.

Too often however, the process begins exactly backward, with an invention or a design looking for a problem to solve. This scenario is frequently encountered in the process of "technology transfer" in a university setting, whereby the creators of a technology seek practical application for an invention. This situation can be challenging to navigate (and explain to the inventor) as commonly these inventions have not fully considered the drivers and dynamics of the commercial orthopaedic market, such as the size of the market opportunity, cost of development, manufacturability, regulatory pathway and timeline, cost of goods, operating room logistics/demands, sterilization, storage, and shipping requirements, among a host of other considerations. Although no doubt there are examples of commercially successful technology transfers, the product development process is notably more "efficient" and has a higher probability of returning a greater value per invested dollar if the process starts with the clear identification of the problem, a search for potential solutions and "pressure testing" of the idea (ie, surgeon feedback) before committing significant resources to further advance development.

©Copyright 2021 American Academy of Orthopaedic Surgeons

INVENTION VERSUS INNOVATION

As part of this overall narrative, it should be noted there is a meaningful nuance between "invention" and "innovation." From a product development perspective, an *invention* refers to a novel idea, concept, or approach, whereas an *innovation* is the embodiment or implementation of an innovation into a tangible product or service. The essence of product development is the transformation of an invention into an innovation. It has been said, "good ideas are a dime a dozen, but people who implement them are priceless." This statement is no more true than in the medical technology arena, where successful innovations must not only work technically, but must address a clinical need, have sufficient commercial demand to justify the time and expense of developing the technology, be manufacturable at commercial scale, must not infringe upon third-party intellectual property, and satisfy prevailing regulatory and quality standards (which differ around the world), to name just a few critical considerations. Quite often, extraordinary scientific breakthroughs do not directly become innovative product offerings, but do so only after they have been simplified to a reproducible embodiment that addresses a specific unmet need. The notion of creating a product with elegant simplicity will have much more appeal than a technically complex solution.

PRODUCT DEFINITION

Once proof of concept has been adequately vetted through experience testing and initial customer feedback, the next step involves further defining the product in a more formalized way through the creation of a Target Product Profile (TPP). The TPP identifies and "memorializes" the desired performance elements, required features, and intended use for the proposed product. A properly constructed TPP is a tool intended to serve as roadmap to help focus and guide the R&D teams as the design matures. Creating a TPP is frequently instructive for the design team, as the process often shines a light on issues that may impact the product's future marketability. By way of example, a detailed TPP will address the following product design and business considerations:

- Clinical purpose/need and intended benefit
- Target patient population/profile
- Intended use
- Composition/configuration (including packaging)
- Product performance attributes (physical, biological, mechanical, electrical, chemical, human factors, reliability)
- Proposed labeling statements and claims
- Manufacturing considerations (anticipated unit volumes, cost of goods, identification of key manufacturing processes/quality standards)
- Storage, handling, shipping, and other environmental requirements
- Commercial objectives (markets, pricing and revenue estimates, launch dates, and targets)

In the early stages of the design process, it may not be possible to fully address all aspects within the TPP. In practice, some elements of the TPP may not be knowable without further investigation or additional research. By design, however, the TPP is intended to be a "living document" that is updated as new information is learned or uncovered. A fully complete and comprehensive TPP is a key marker of a maturing product design, as the specifications and requirements are described with sufficient specificity and clarity to provide guidance to the design team and key product stakeholders.

EVALUATING THE BUSINESS OPPORTUNITY

Once the product concept has been defined through the creation of a TPP, a medical device company will typically prepare a "business plan" before committing additional resources toward development. The purpose of the business plan is to critically analyze the merits of the concept and consider the potential challenges selling the product into the market. Chiefly, the primary purpose of the business plan is to analyze the financial opportunity for the device, that is, rationalizing if the market size, demand, and potential pricing justify the financial cost, time, and risk associated with development. The business plan provides the management team with the critical information needed to authorize resources and secure funding for the project. The individual components of a business plan will vary between companies; however, typical business plans will address all of the topics and questions provided in **Table 1**. Authorship of the business plan is the primary responsibility of the marketing team; however, by its nature, creation of a well-written business plan requires broad collaboration and input from across the organization.

PROTECTING YOUR INVENTION WITH PATENTS

The medical device industry is characterized by intense competition, both from entrenched market players and emerging startup companies. To help manage these competitive threats, inventors and companies can defend their valuable intellectual property (IP) through the use of patents and an overall "patent strategy." When managed properly, a nexus of issued patents can become a valuable asset, helping a firm maintain its competitive edge, protecting it from would-be competitors. Patents are issuable from the United States Patent Office for inventions that are novel, nonobvious, and useful, and the invention must differ from existing intellectual property or "prior art" in a meaningful way. A patent portfolio represents a collection of patents protecting a device from being copied directly, as well as variants of the design that achieve the same intended use and clinical benefit. Importantly, within the academic and clinical communities, there is often a misconception as to what benefit a patent actually provides. To be sure, securing IP (patents) does *not* give the inventor a right

©Copyright 2021 American Academy of Orthopaedic Surgeons

TABLE 1 Defining the Key Elements of a Business Plan

Topic	Key Questions
Market opportunity	Who needs this product? Where are the customers located? What is the market size? What are the market dynamics?
Competitive landscape	What are the alternatives to this product? What are their strengths and weaknesses? How are alternative products priced and promoted? How do we effectively compete?
Revenue projections	How much revenue can be generated with this product? How quickly can revenue grow? What factors will influence revenue growth? What pricing can the market accept?
Product development plan	What are the key milestones to bring the product to market? How much will it cost? How much time will it take? What are the key risks to the plan?
Regulatory pathway	Where do we want to market this product? What are the regulatory requirements? What are the risks of the proposed regulatory strategy? What is the timeline to obtain regulatory approval/clearance?
Manufacturing plan	How and where will this product be manufactured? What are the anticipated product margins? Can the supply chain satisfy the anticipated product forecast? What is required to scale manufacturing (time/cost)?
Sales/marketing plan	How will the product be distributed? How will the product be promoted? How will the product be priced? How do we maximize the revenue opportunity?

to practice the art of what is described in the patent, but only enables the owner of the IP to legally block OTHERS from practicing the art in the IP. In many cases, the owner may have to cross- or sublicense IP from another entity to actually sell what is defined by their own IP. For example, if an inventor develops an improved way (or material) to deliver a growth factor for the repair of certain tissues, such an invention cannot be sold by this inventor without also having the basic right to use the growth factor that is claimed by the original patent for that growth factor.

Within the orthopaedic medical device sector, two companies, Kyphon and KFx Medical, provide prime examples of the value of a well-constructed patent portfolio. In the early 2000s, Kyphon introduced a "balloon tamp" and instrument set for "kyphoplasty," an interventional procedure to address pain associated with osteoporotic vertebral compression fractures. At the time, several of the major spine companies sought to design similar instrument sets; however, Kyphon's vast patent estate covering the balloon technology prevented other companies from copying the Kyphon design. After Medtronic failed in its attempt to commercialize its Arcuate device to compete with the Kyphon balloon, Medtronic subsequently acquired Kyphon for $4.2 billion to enter the balloon kyphoplasty market.

Similarly, KFx Medical introduced its novel technology for soft-tissue fixation in the early 2000s. KFx's technology for double row fixation in rotator cuff repair surgery was readily adopted by orthopaedic surgeons, but was readily copied by the major orthopaedic companies servicing the sports medicine market. However, because of the strength of its patent portfolio, KFx was able to successfully defend its intellectual property rights, resulting in a legal judgment against Arthrex and leading to license agreements with industry bellwethers Smith & Nephew, Mitek/JNJ, ConMed, Wright Medical, and Zimmer Biomet. The KFx example is notable, given the company's small size relative to the other market players, and underscores the leverage a defensible patent portfolio can provide.

DESIGNING PRECLINICAL STUDIES FOR THE FDA

The foundation for establishing the safety and efficacy of any implantable device requires testing in preclinical studies or animal models. (Human clinical studies may be required in the context of a "significant-risk" experimental device, drug, or biologic; however, the foundation of any clinical trial is predicated on preclinical work.) Because of the importance of these studies in establishing "proof of concept" for a design, the FDA requires these types of nonclinical safety and efficacy studies to be performed under GLP (good laboratory practices) conditions. GLP represents a set of international standards governing the conduct and execution of preclinical studies, which have been established to ensure their uniformity, consistency, reliability, and reproducibility.[1] These standards effectively "raise the bar" for the execution of preclinical safety trials, often requiring them to be performed at organizations with the corporate structure, expertise, and business discipline to satisfy GLP requirements. It should be noted that GLP requirements generally exceed the capabilities of a typical university environment and are more costly than comparably designed non-GLP studies. Consequently, most nonclinical studies intended to support regulatory submissions are conducted at third-party contract research labs that have the necessary infrastructure and experience to navigate GLP requirements. Those aspects of study performance and underlying architecture that fulfill the primary tenets of GLP include the following:

- Utilization of properly qualified personnel to conduct studies
- Establishment of study director to oversee research and ensure quality

©Copyright 2021 American Academy of Orthopaedic Surgeons

- Appropriate facilities for the care, feeding, and housing of animals
- Provisions for equipment maintenance and calibration
- Standard operating procedures to document all procedure and test methods
- Provisions to ensure test articles are properly stored and handled
- Identification of test facilities, equipment, materials, and reagents
- Development of protocol, testing plan, and reporting methodology
- Provisions for archiving records and test data
- Test facilities are subject to FDA inspection

DESIGNING FOR MANUFACTURABILITY

Manufacturability refers to the ability of a given design to be fabricated at commercial scale at a cost that can be supported by the market. Manufacturability should be considered in the early stages of the product development cycle, as any design approach that cannot be fabricated in an economically feasible way should be abandoned. For many inventors, the challenges of manufacturability may be underappreciated, as the issues that may confound large-scale production may not be obvious. In practice, manufacturability (and the cost to manufacture) is influenced by a variety of factors, including design complexity, quality requirements, supply constraints, raw material costs, labor costs, and manufacturing environment needs. Real-world examples of manufacturability issues include sourcing constraints posed by the use of human allograft tissue (eg, need for cadaveric ligaments of a particular size) and implant designs with complex geometries requiring advanced 3D printing fabrication techniques. Collectively, manufacturability is a key input to the cost/benefit analysis of any project and can significantly affect the direction and scope of the recommended design solution. Lastly, from a practical standpoint, when preclinical GLP studies are required as part of an FDA application, the work must be performed using implants manufactured according to the final process, which also conforms to the tightly regulated clinical good manufacturing process (cGMP) standards.

DEFINING SUCCESS—ACADEMIA VERSUS INDUSTRY

In general terms, industry and academia measure "success" of product development differently, which itself can represent an additional challenge in efficiently translating inventions from the laboratory to the market. Within the academic framework, a technological discovery represents the foundation of product development (**Figure 2**, top panel), and the "Design of Therapy" practical discovery is advanced through bench testing, in vitro studies, and animal models. If the efforts lead to a "first in man" clinical trial, the academic community typically declares victory and is justifiably delighted. Within academia,

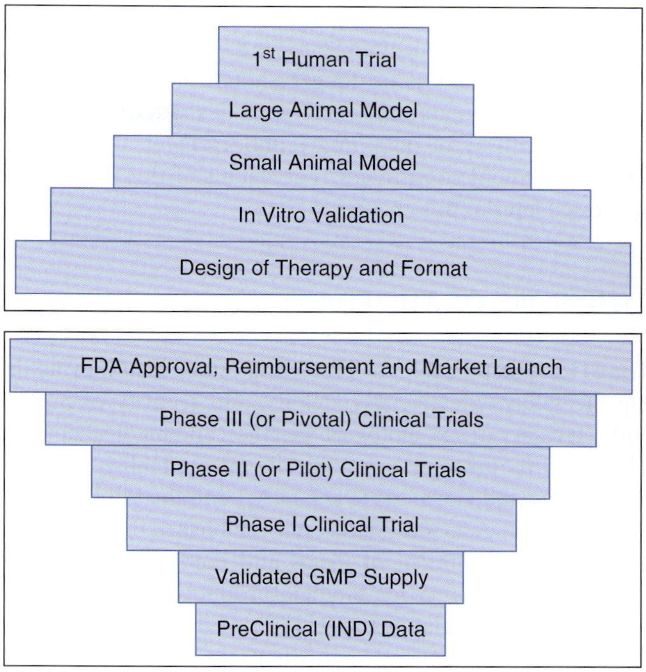

FIGURE 2 Illustration of academic and industrial foundations of product development. The top panel illustrates a typical academic hierarchy of success, which begins with the design of a therapy and ends with its first use in humans. By contrast, the lower panel turns this model upside-down, and illustrates that early human data are just the beginning of many product development efforts. Performance of a series of clinical studies, followed by FDA approval, is necessary to apply for the reimbursement required for a successful market launch.

inventions are often considered "translated" upon their first use in a human subject, and as consequence, this is often the aspirational goal of the academic researcher. However, this important academic milestone is actually just the beginning of what is required to develop and launch a meaningful product. From an industry perspective, this human use is more like the very beginning, and most professional models of product development would turn the academic pyramid upside-down (**Figure 2**, lower panel) to reflect what must be done to support the launch of a successful product.

As noted above, industry's primary objective is to develop products that achieve commercial success, a goal which often starts with human clinical use. From an industry perspective, product development planning ideally starts with commercial objectives in mind and with R&D teams "working backward" to identify the individual milestones needed to bring new technologies to market. Within the FDA's product development framework, human studies are often at the *beginning* of the product development journey. In particular, product safety is evaluated in phase I (pilot and safety) and phase II (dosing or confirmatory) human clinical trials, and if successful, phase III (pivotal) trials are used to provide evidence of safety and efficacy data to support regulatory submissions. As recently as 10 years ago, the mere approval of a product by the FDA was

©Copyright 2021 American Academy of Orthopaedic Surgeons

sufficient to begin marketing and sales efforts, but this is no longer the case in the United States and elsewhere. Nowadays, FDA approval alone is no longer enough to support meaningful revenue generation, and companies must navigate the complex pathway of obtaining reimbursement and hospital value assessment committees. The details of this process are addressed later in this chapter.

THE ROLE OF THE FDA

The FDA is responsible for protecting public health by assuring the safety, effectiveness, quality, and security of human and veterinary drugs, biologics, vaccines, and medical devices. They do this through enforcing the laws established in the Food, Drug and Cosmetic (FD&C) Act and the Public Health Service (PHS) Act. The FD&C Act establishes the basic laws governing development of drugs and medical devices, and the PHS Act does so for biologic products. These laws are translated into regulations in Title 21 of the Code of Federal Regulations (21 CFR) and are further interpreted for industry through publication of FDA Guidance Documents. The combination of these laws, regulations, and guidance documents provides the quality standards by which new medical products must be developed and marketed.

The FDA is led by the Office of the Commissioner and is divided into offices/directorates that oversee the core functions of the agency. New medical products fall under the regulatory purview of the Office of Medical Products and Tobacco, which is further divided into centers that specialize in product categories:

- *Center for Drug Evaluation and Research (CDER):* Over-the-counter and prescription drugs, including biological therapeutics and generic drugs
- *Center for Devices and Radiological Health (CDRH):* Medical devices and radiation-emitting products
- *Center for Biologics Evaluation and Research (CBER):* Biological and related products

To determine the regulations that pertain to a new orthopaedic product and which FDA center will oversee compliance, it must first be determined whether the product will be categorized as a drug, device, biologic, or some combination of these.

IS YOUR INVENTION A DRUG, DEVICE, BIOLOGIC, OR COMBINATION PRODUCT?

Determining whether the FDA will categorize a new product as a drug, device, biologic, or a combination product can often be tricky. It is critical that this is determined thoughtfully and carefully from idea conception, because the category of the product will dictate the regulations that apply to the product. This translates to the level of rigor of the quality standards and evidence required for marketing authorization. The intended use of the product is critical to this evaluation.

The appropriate product category and marketing pathway is easily determined for most implantable orthopaedic devices; for instance, a new bone plating system for fracture fixation in the feet would be considered a medical device, and therefore regulated by the CDRH. However, the framework for other medical products such as orthobiologics can be much less clear and open to interpretation. To determine the regulatory requirements for this group of products, one must carefully determine the intended use and mode of action (the means by which a product achieves its intended therapeutic effect or action). See **Table 2** for further details.

ORTHOBIOLOGICS AND THE REGULATION OF HUMAN CELLS, TISSUES, AND CELLULAR AND TISSUE-BASED PRODUCTS

Human cells, tissues, and cellular and tissue-based products (HCT/Ps) consist of human cells or tissues that are intended for implantation, transplantation, infusion, or transfer into a human recipient. Examples of such products include bone, ligament, skin, dura mater, heart valve, cornea, hematopoietic stem/progenitor cells derived from peripheral and cord blood, manipulated autologous chondrocytes, epithelial cells on a synthetic matrix, and semen or other reproductive tissue. The regulatory framework for HCT/Ps is established in sections 351 and 361 of the PHS Act, and 21 CFR 1271.[2] The FDA has been challenged with how to regulate these products and has developed comprehensive guidance documents that expand on the fundamental criteria of minimal manipulation and homologous use. An HCT/P will be regulated as a tissue (not considered a drug/biologic/device) if it meets certain criteria listed in 21 CFR 1271.10 for minimal manipulation and homologous use. These tissue products are regulated solely under section 361 of the PHS Act and, therefore, do *not* require premarket authorization from FDA. To be considered a "361 HCT/P," the product must meet *all* of the criteria as outlined in **Figure 3**. HCT/Ps that do not meet all of the criteria above are regulated as drugs, biologicals, or devices, based primarily on the mechanism of action on the body to achieve its intended purpose. These products are subject to Section 351 of the PHS Act and the applicable 21 CFR regulations, and are known as "351 HCT/Ps." These products must have premarket clearance or approval by the FDA, which typically requires a long and arduous development, qualification, and clinical trial series. Examples of such 351 HCT/Ps include culture-expanded chondrocytes for cartilage repair; ground and lyophilized amniotic membrane for modulating inflammation such as in the case of osteoarthritis; any purified stem cell preparation from fat, marrow, blood, or other tissue; and any combination of a tissue with another material. Interpreting and applying these criteria can be challenging, and therefore, it is important to communicate with the FDA early in the development process to verify there is shared understanding of the regulatory requirements.

©Copyright 2021 American Academy of Orthopaedic Surgeons

TABLE 2 Medical Product Categories and Corresponding Agency Oversight

Medical Product	Definition	Regulatory Oversight	Marketing Pathway
Drug	Articles intended for use in the diagnosis, cure, mitigation, treatment, or prevention of disease, and intended to affect the structure or any function of the body; chemically synthesized, well-defined structure, can be fully characterized	CDER	IND-NDA
Device	An instrument, apparatus, implement, machine, contrivance, implant, in vitro reagent, or other similar or related article, including a component part, or accessory which is intended for use in the diagnosis of disease or other conditions, or in the cure, mitigation, treatment, or prevention of disease, and which does not achieve its primary intended purposes through chemical action within or on the body of man or other animals and which is not dependent upon being metabolized for the achievement of its primary intended purposes	CDRH	IDE-PMA, 510(k), or exempt from premarket notification requirements
Biologic	Virus, therapeutic serum, toxin, antitoxin, vaccine, blood, blood component or derivative, allergenic product, or analogous product, applicable to the prevention, treatment, or cure of a disease or condition; derived from or made with the aid of living organisms, complex in structure, not fully characterized	CBER	IND-BLA
Combination product	Therapeutic and diagnostic products that combine drugs, medical devices, and/or biological products. Examples: monoclonal antibody combined with therapeutic drug, device coated with a drug or biologic, prefilled delivery systems such as insulin injector pens	The Office of Combination Products (assigns a "lead-center" based on the primary mode of action)	Dependent on category of product

BRINGING YOUR PRODUCT TO MARKET

There are various processes through which the FDA reviews information about products to verify they are safe and effective before they are allowed to be sold in the United States. In order for a medical product to be legally marketed in the United States, it is required to be *cleared* or *approved* by the FDA (unless it is 510(k) exempt). The term *cleared* refers to medical devices that have used the 510(k) Premarket Notification Process, and the FDA has determined them to be substantially equivalent (similar) to another legally marketed device. The term *approved* refers to medical devices and/or biologic products that the FDA has approved through the Premarket Approval (PMA) or Biologic License Application (BLA) process, that have been determined to be safe and effective for their intended use. The PMA and BLA processes also require clinical investigations that are subject to FDA preapproval through the Investigational Device Exemption (IDE) or Investigational New Drug (IND) processes, respectively. The 510(k), IDE/PMA, and IND/BLA processes are described in detail below.

"PARTNERING" WITH THE FDA—THE PRESUBMISSION PROCESS

The marketing pathway for medical products can be very complex and lengthy depending on the product category and how it is regulated. Early interaction with the FDA will likely improve the quality of subsequent submissions and facilitate the development process for new products. The presubmission process is a voluntary program through the CDRH that provides the sponsor an opportunity to obtain feedback and advice before submitting an Investigational Device Exemption (IDE) or marketing application (PMA, 510(k), BLA), and also enables the FDA to have a full understanding of the new product early in the process. Agency guidance can include, but is not limited to, product development, planned nonclinical evaluations, proposed clinical study protocols, and statistical design. Pre-Sub feedback can be obtained through an in-person meeting, teleconference, written or e-mail response. The goal for FDA's feedback is within 75 to 90 days of submission receipt.

THE PREMARKET NOTIFICATION—510(K) PATHWAY

For medical devices, the first step in determining the appropriate marketing application is to classify the device. Devices are classified using a risk-based system based on the device's intended use and indications for use, and the level of control needed to assure adequate safety. To market a Class I, II, or III device in the United States intended for human use, there are various levels of evidence required as outlined in **Table 3**. In cases where a PMA is not already required per regulation, a

©Copyright 2021 American Academy of Orthopaedic Surgeons

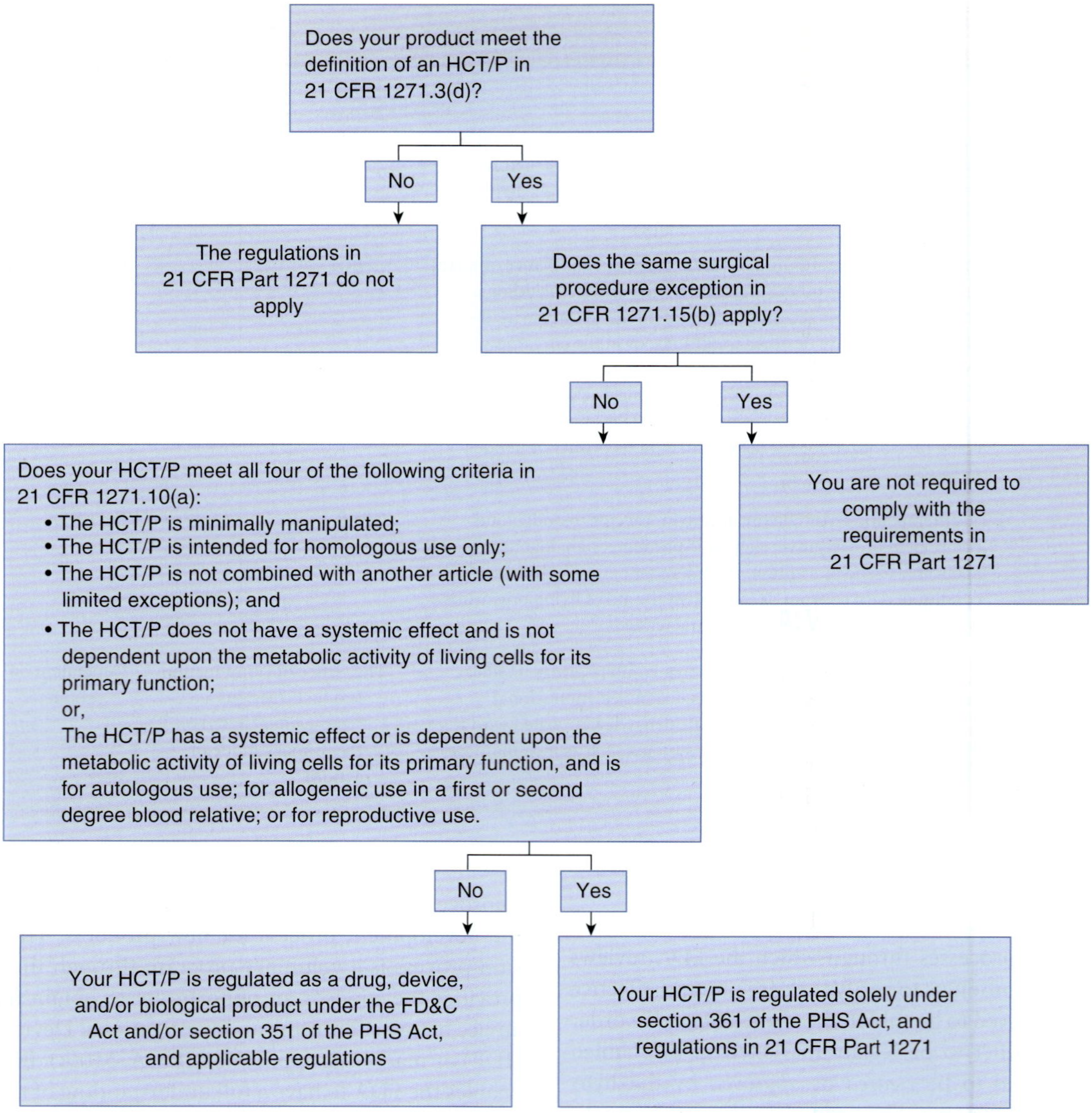

FIGURE 3 Flow chart regarding the FDA regulatory path of HCT/Ps. This diagram reflects the latest thinking from the FDA. (Reproduced from *Regulatory Considerations for Human Cells, Tissues, and Cellular and Tissue-Based Products: Minimal Manipulation and Homologous Use. Food and Drug Administration, November 2017.)*

510(k) premarket notification must be submitted to the FDA/CDRH unless the device is exempt from 510(k) requirements of the FD&C Act (such as certain HCT/Ps described above and Class I products). A 510(k) submission contains detailed technical, safety, and performance information about your device. The documentation must demonstrate the product in question is at least as safe and effective (substantially equivalent, SE) to a legally marketed device (predicate device) not subject to a Class III PMA. If the FDA determines that your device is substantially equivalent to the predicate device, they will "clear" your product for marketing in the United States. See **Figure 4** for a graphical comparison of the timeline and requirements across various regulatory pathways.

Most Class II medical devices are subject to the 510(k) program, and often a determination of SE can be supported with bench testing, logic, and animal data instead of clinical evidence. Because of this, the cost of developing a 510(k) device is much lower, and timelines are much shorter than devices subject to PMA requirements. Depending on the complexity of the submission and agency questions for the sponsor, 510(k)s are reviewed between 30 and 90 days. Although there are timeline advantages to the 510(k) pathway, such clearances to market generally lack the ability to make any meaningful clinical outcome claims. This balance must be considered as part of the overall business strategy.

©Copyright 2021 American Academy of Orthopaedic Surgeons

TABLE 3 FDA Device Classifications and Representative Orthopaedic Products

Device Classification	Risk	Market Authorization Requirement	Examples
Class I	Low risk	Exempt from premarket notification	Tongue depressors, examination gloves, plaster cast materials
Class II	Moderate risk	Most require 510(k) clearance based on substantial equivalence to a legally marketed predicate	Bone void fillers, interbody spine fusion devices, suture anchors, resorbable mesh, and most hip and knee prostheses
Class III	High risk, surgically invasive, and many are life-supporting or life-sustaining	Investigational Device Exemption (IDE) Clinical Study and Premarket Approval (PMA)	Viscosupplements, BMP (InFuse), artificial cervical and lumbar disks

De novo: If a sponsor determines their product should be Class I/Class II but there is no legally marketed predicate upon which to declare Substantial equivalence, a de novo application can be submitted to FDA to make a risk-based classification determination.

THE IDE/PMA DEVICE PATHWAY

Premarket Approval (PMA) is the FDA's process of scientific and regulatory review to evaluate Class III device safety and effectiveness. A PMA is the most stringent device marketing application required by the FDA reserved for the highest risk devices. PMA approval is based on an FDA determination that there is sufficient valid scientific evidence to assure the device is safe and effective for its intended use. To determine that there is reasonable assurance that a device is safe and effective, the type of evidence required typically includes animal studies, nonclinical in vitro studies, and well-controlled clinical investigations.

To study an unapproved device in a clinical investigation, the sponsor must obtain an Investigational Device Exemption (IDE) before the study commences. To do this, the sponsor must demonstrate that there is reason to believe that the risks to human subjects are outweighed by the anticipated benefits, the investigation is scientifically sound, and device as proposed for use will be effective. Studies of significant risk devices must also have an IDE approved by the FDA before the study commences. See **Table 4** for clinical study comparison for drugs/biologics and devices.

The PMA application includes technical information consisting of details for manufacturing the device, nonclinical laboratory studies, and clinical investigations. The FDA will perform an in-depth scientific, regulatory, and quality system

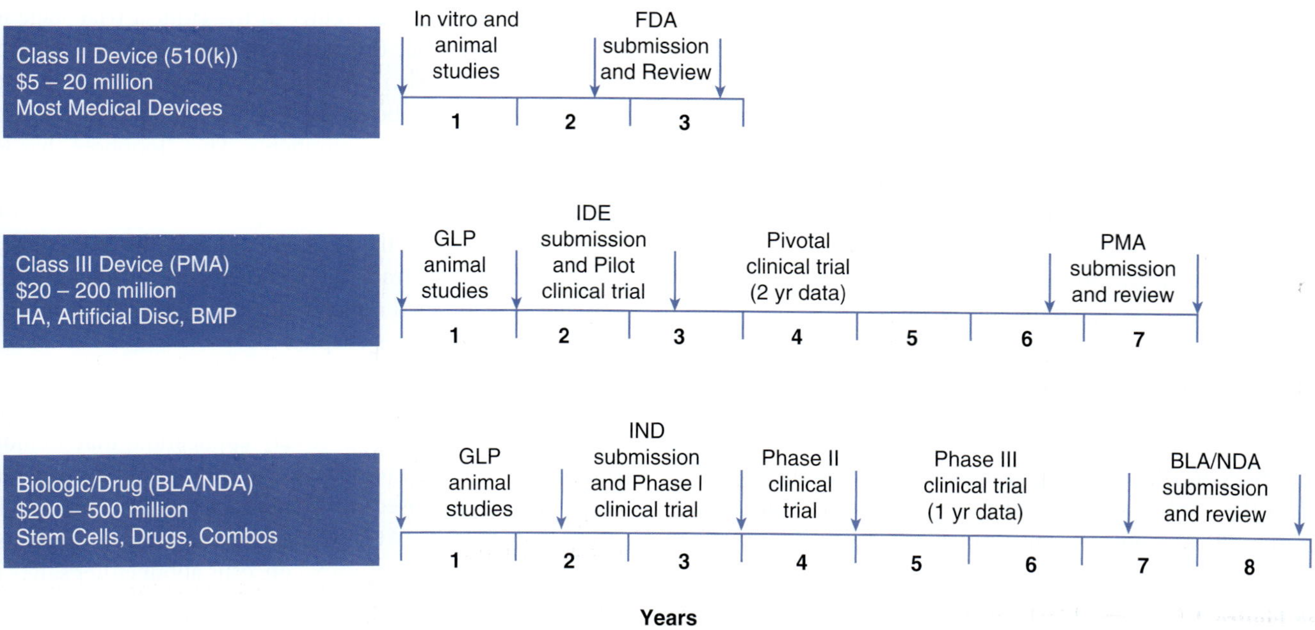

FIGURE 4 Illustration shows time/cost comparison of 510(k), PMA, and BLA/NDA premarket submissions.

©Copyright 2021 American Academy of Orthopaedic Surgeons

TABLE 4 Clinical Study Comparison for Drugs/Biologics and Devices

Drugs/Biologics	Devices
Preclinical/GLP Animal Studies: animal testing to collect efficacy, toxicology, and pharmacokinetic information	Preclinical/GLP Animal Studies: animal testing to collect efficacy, toxicology, and pharmacokinetic information
Phase 1: First-in-human study; small group of healthy subjects (10-80) Study safety Typical Duration about 1 yr	Pilot: Small study (10-30 patients with pathology for treatment) Determine preliminary safety and efficacy Typical duration about 1-2 yr
Phase 2: Larger group of subjects (100-300 with pathology for treatment) Study effectiveness and further evaluate safety Typical duration about 1 yr	Pivotal: Larger study (150-300 patients with pathology for treatment) Determine efficacy and adverse effects Typical duration 2-3 yr
Phase 3: Large group of subjects (1,000-2,000 with pathology for treatment). Phase 3 studies are randomized, multicenter trials To confirm effectiveness and monitor side effects Usually have a longer duration (several years)	PostApproval Study: Collect long-term data and adverse effects
Phase 4: Postapproval study Collect long-term data and adverse effects	

review by appropriate personnel. An advisory panel of independent experts will also review the technical evidence and provide recommendations regarding approvability of the device, suggested conditions of approval, and labeling. In some cases, the FDA may request a preapproval inspection to verify that the manufacturer is in compliance with the appropriate regulations. There are often postapproval studies required as a condition of approval. Supplemental information is required to be submitted to the FDA periodically after approval, including any changes related to manufacturing the device. Postapproval inspections are conducted within 8 to 12 months of approval, which focus on any changes made to the device design, manufacturing process, or quality systems. FDA regulations provide 180 days to review a PMA and make a determination, but after all the interactive dialogue and various meetings take place, the total the timeline often takes a year longer. As such, these timelines must be factored into the business plan.

THE IND/BLA BIOLOGIC PATHWAY

If your product is classified as a biologic, including 351 HCT/Ps, a Biologics License Application (BLA) must be submitted to the FDA and approved to legally market your product. The BLA requires a different kind of scientific review to ensure safety and effectiveness for biologic products. It is similar to the PMA process for devices, in that the application requires submission of product manufacturing and technical information, preclinical studies, and well-controlled clinical investigations. In the field of orthopaedics, the best-known examples of products approved through the BLA pathway are the culture-expanded cartilage repair products, which in some cases have taken more than 10 years of development and study to gain approval. Other cell- and tissue-based products (for bone repair and treatment of osteoarthritis or degenerative disk disease) are currently in the clinical trial stage for the BLA pathway, but this is a long, expensive, and difficult journey. Alternatively, if your product qualifies as a "361 HCT/P" as defined above, then it is exempt from the BLA marketing application requirements. This "loophole" has led some unscrupulous organizations to launch HCT/P products without proper FDA review and approval, and they have done so with the hopes that the FDA will not have the interest, ability, or bandwidth to track them and enforce regulations. The consequences for such noncompliance can be severe and will be discussed later in this chapter.

Similar to the IDE/PMA process, to study an unapproved biologic/drug product, a sponsor must submit an Investigational New Drug (IND) application that demonstrates there is reason to believe that the risks to human subjects from the proposed investigation are outweighed by the anticipated benefits. At any stage of the clinical or animal studies, if data raise significant concerns about either safety or effectiveness, the FDA may request additional information, or they may halt ongoing clinical studies.

©Copyright 2021 American Academy of Orthopaedic Surgeons

The BLA application includes technical information consisting of details for manufacturing the product, preclinical studies, and clinical investigations. To be considered, the license application must provide the multidisciplinary FDA reviewer team (medical officers, microbiologists, chemists, biostatisticians, etc) with the efficacy and safety information necessary to make a risk/benefit assessment and to recommend or oppose the approval of the product. During this time, the FDA will perform a preapproval inspection during which production as it is in progress is examined in detail. After approval of the BLA, postmarket trials are often conducted to identify and evaluate the long-term effects of the product in a greater number of patients. Supplemental information is required to be submitted to the FDA periodically after approval, including any changes related to manufacturing. The BLA application is submitted after completion of phase 3 trials, and standard review time for an original BLA filing is 12 to 14 months from receipt date.

NONCOMPLIANCE PENALTIES CAN BE SEVERE

The FDA is authorized to take action against firms and individuals found to be in violation of the laws and regulations governing human medical products. Examples of violations include issues with manufacturing processes, lack of appropriate marketing authorization, and advertising products for uses not approved by the FDA. This is often discovered during facility inspections and review of company website materials. Specific enforcement activities include actions to correct and prevent violations, removal of violative products from the market, and punishment of offenders. The type of enforcement activity the FDA uses will depend on the nature of the violation. In the extreme, the FDA can and does work with the Federal Government to write injunctions, cease, and desist orders, and they have the ability to levy financial damages on companies and individuals, as well as criminally prosecute those responsible for the noncompliance. These are serious matters and FDA's jurisdictional reach should not be taken lightly.

THE CURRENT LANDSCAPE

The rapid growth in the field of regenerative medicine and stem cells has led to the FDA's increase in oversight and enforcement in this area. The FDA issued guidance in November 2017[2] that clarifies their position on regenerative medicine and gives the agency a solid platform to take enforcement action against offenders. Several warning letters have recently been issued[3-5] to firms promoting their 361 HCT/Ps as treating degenerative conditions, and the agency put the industry on notice by issuing a press release[6] and sending letters to firms and providers of stem cell treatments reiterating their compliance and enforcement policies.[7]

GETTING PAID FOR YOUR PRODUCT

WHAT IS REIMBURSEMENT?

A fundamental question in a new product's life cycle is "Who will ultimately pay for it?", or what is commonly referred to as reimbursement. At its core, reimbursement is the payment—typically from a third-party insurer—that is made to a physician or facility provider for medical services rendered to a patient. Although the various mechanisms of reimbursement are complex, the objective is simple—a new technology that is financially attractive to users will be adopted more broadly. Reimbursement is often thought of as a single concept but is actually the interaction of three distinct variables: coding, payment and coverage.

THE IMPORTANCE OF CODING

Facilities, such as hospitals and ambulatory surgery centers (ASCs), perform medical services and submit claims to insurance providers for the services rendered. Medical procedures, devices, drugs, and even a patient's diagnosis are translated into codes for the purpose of billing. Coding is often referred to as the language of reimbursement, because the codes that are reported on a claim are what drive the payment for those services.

New technologies, procedures, and devices may be described by existing codes or may require new codes to be created by the groups that maintain them. The American Medical Association maintains physician procedure codes, often called CPT codes (or Common Procedural Terminology). The Centers for Medicare and Medicaid Services (CMS) maintains the codes that describe devices and drugs, often called HCPCS codes (or Healthcare Common Procedure Coding System). **Table 5** provides an overview of commonly used coding modalities, and they are important because of the multifactorial nature of obtaining maximal reimbursement.

The process of determining which existing codes apply to a new technology, or whether new codes should be created, needs to be validated with the appropriate governing body of each code set. The American Academy of Orthopaedic Surgeons (AAOS) Coding and Reimbursement Committee is an adjunct to AMA decision-making, which oversees the appropriate use of CPT codes. AAOS is the appropriate group to facilitate a determination on whether new orthopaedic procedures or devices are adequately described by existing codes or will require a new code. If a new procedure is not described by existing codes, then adopters will face significant challenges in seeking reimbursement from payers. The sponsor company may need to work with AAOS to seek a new code for the procedure and use of the device; however, if a new code is obtained, it can provide significant value to the sponsor.

©Copyright 2021 American Academy of Orthopaedic Surgeons

TABLE 5 Overview of Common Coding Modalities

Scope	Code-Set	Description	Governing/Oversight Body
Diagnosis coding	ICD-10-CM (International Classification of Diseases—Clinical Modification)	Describe patients' diseases and/or conditions (69,000+ codes)	CDC (Centers for Disease Control)
Physician procedure coding	CPT (Common Procedural Terminology)	Describe physician services/procedures (7,000+ codes)	AMA (American Medical Association)
Device/drug codes/miscellaneous use codes	HCPCS (Healthcare Common Procedural Coding System)	Describes drugs, devices, temporary codes (5,000+ codes)	CMS (Centers for Medicare and Medicaid Services)
Procedure coding (hospital inpatient only)	ICD-10-PCS (International Classification of Diseases—Procedure Coding System)	Describe hospital services/procedures (72,000+ codes)	CMS (Centers for Medicare and Medicaid Services)
Inpatient DRG reimbursement code	MS-DRG (Medicare Severity Diagnosis Related Group)	List of payment groups applicable to hospital inpatient encounters (1,000 codes)	CMS (Centers for Medicare and Medicaid Services)

CREATING AND ASSIGNING CPT CODES

There are two main requirements for new CPT codes to be created—a clinical evidence requirement and a substantial use requirement. Published, peer-reviewed clinical evidence must support the efficacy of a new procedure, and these clinical evidence requirements are described in **Table 6**. Depending on the utilization and technological features of the procedure and possible device, the number and nature of the publications will vary from reports of a prospective, statistically significant randomized control trial to a case series or even an "expert opinion." The AMA's definition of the various minimum levels of evidence required to secure a distinct code are provided in **Table 7**. To be clear, although none of the listed scenarios require level 1a or 1b data, it is still possible that AAOS or AMA will require that for certain situations before a new code is created. Lastly, a substantial use requirement means that practicing physicians are incorporating the new procedure into their clinical practice and are therefore able to report the time and resources necessary to perform the new procedure to the AMA. This is typically provided in what is referred to as a "clinical vignette" justification following commercial launch. The upshot of all of this is that for products cleared by the FDA through the 510(k) pathway without clinical evidence, a multiyear effort to collect postmarket clinical data is typically required before a reimbursement code is granted. For products approved through a PMA, there may be sufficient data collected before market launch to qualify for a unique CPT code.

TERMS OF PAYMENT AND SITES OF SERVICE

When a claim is submitted to an insurance provider for services rendered to a patient, that claim contains a list of billing codes that describe the services provided. The codes are tied to payment amounts that are specified in contracts with commercial

TABLE 6 AMA Level of Evidence Requirements

Category I Literature Requirements	Utilization	Typical	Typical	Limited, Specialized or Humanitarian	Limited, Specialized or Humanitarian
	Technology	New	Existing or Noncontributory	New	Existing or Noncontributory
# of peer-reviewed publications		5	5	5	3-5
Minimum # with US patient populations		1	1	1	1
Minimum # with different patient populations		2	2	1	1
Minimum level of evidence[a] for at least one article		2a	3a/3b	3b	4

[a]Level of Evidence is defined by AMA Scoring System illustrated in **Table 7**.

©Copyright 2021 American Academy of Orthopaedic Surgeons

TABLE 7 AMA Level of Evidence Scoring

Level of Evidence	Type of Study
1a	Evidence obtained from systematic review of randomized controlled trials
1b	Evidence obtained from an individual randomized controlled trial
2a	Evidence obtained from systematic review of cohort studies
2b	Evidence obtained from an individual cohort study
3a	Evidence obtained from systematic review of case-control studies
3b	Evidence obtained from a case-control study
4	Evidence obtained from case series
5	Evidence obtained from expert opinion without explicit critical appraisal

insurers or published payment rates for governmental insurers such as Medicare. Governmental payers such as Medicare and Medicaid publish fee schedules and reimbursement terms and the stated payment amounts for each code or group of codes are publicly available, albeit sometimes difficult to access or calculate. In the case of private commercial insurance plans, payment amounts are negotiated between the provider and insurer and specified in contracts. The payment amounts in commercial insurance contracts are not publicly available and may differ from one provider to the next for the same service, depending on the terms of the contract.

Payments are also impacted by variables such as the level of care a patient receives (inpatient vs outpatient) or the locale where services are rendered. Medicare payments to ASCs, for example, are much lower than corresponding payments to a hospital for the same procedure, because providing care in a hospital is more costly than in an ASC. Medicare also lists national average payment amounts for each service, and then modifies those amounts to reflect the area wage index, or relative cost factor for that geography. A Medicare payment for a procedure in San Francisco, CA, may be 30% to 40% higher than in Topeka, KS. It is important to look at payment amounts across insurers, across various venues of care, and in different geographies to develop an understanding of the payment landscape for a given product or service.

WHY DOES REIMBURSEMENT MATTER?

Facility providers such as hospitals and ASCs review the potential financial impact of a new technology before they decide to adopt it. This is a discipline often referred to as "value analysis," and is characterized by a process typically consisting of a committee of hospital stakeholders that review the business implications of adopting a new, possibly more expensive technology. If the reimbursement that the hospital or ASC will receive from insurers is sufficient to cover the cost of a new technology, they will be more likely to adopt it. Hospital and ASC buyers are reluctant to adopt new technologies that will hurt the financial performance of their institution. However, if a surgical innovation can reduce, for example, surgical time, blood loss, or infection rates, these compelling features could sway a site's decision to adopt the new technology. Developing an understanding of the "bigger picture" economic impact of a new technology on a hospital may uncover value beyond episode-of-care economics. Importantly, commercializing organizations must understand that approvals for use are often required for each individual hospital, or hospital system, and as such, resource planning and the months required to secure approval must be considered in any product launch.

WHAT DETERMINES COVERAGE FOR NEW TECHNOLOGIES?

At its core, coverage is simply whether an insurance company will pay for a therapy and under what conditions. Insurers evaluate new and existing therapies to determine whether they are medically necessary to treat a certain condition or disease. Therapies that are shown to be effective, based on the body of published clinical evidence, may be deemed medically necessary and therefore covered. Therapies that lack sufficient clinical evidence may be noncovered. In some cases, insurers have not evaluated the effectiveness of a therapy at all and are silent on coverage. That said, in the setting where payors are silent or even have policies for noncoverage, it is still possible to build a modest market for the self-paying segment of the population. This can lead to the creation of more and better clinical data, as well as a substantial use justification with health economic data, that eventually are useful in establishing a reimbursement case and code.

Truly novel technologies seldom have a body of published evidence sufficient to persuade insurers to cover a new technology. Medical innovators need to assume that clinical evidence, over and above that which is required for regulatory approval, will be necessary to obtain coverage from insurers. Evaluating the coverage landscape for a new medical technology will inform whether insurers will pay claims for the therapy and how much clinical evidence will be needed to improve the coverage profile. Because creating new procedure codes and/or payment groups can be a lengthy and complex process, evaluation of the requirements and synthesis of a thoughtful strategy is an essential aspect in the business case analysis of whether to invest the resources necessary to bring a product to market.

©Copyright 2021 American Academy of Orthopaedic Surgeons

SUMMARY

The product development process from scientific discovery, through the FDA and into the clinic requires discipline, tenacity, and perseverance. Fortunately, in the field of orthopaedics, the pathways for demonstrating preclinical, as well as clinical, safety and efficacy are very well established and governed by a variety of clearly documented guidelines promulgated by the FDA and the US Code of Federal Regulations. Navigating these development hurdles is resource intensive, and at the very least, requires several million dollars for a simple device cleared through the 510(k) pathway (eg, interference screws or fracture fixation devices), but may require hundreds of millions of dollars for a novel biologic or combination product requiring a BLA or a PMA (eg, Carticel or Infuse BMP-2). Even after successfully meeting the FDA's requirements for market launch, one must consider the reimbursement landscape and requirements for getting paid. More specifically, it is no longer enough to "simply" obtain FDA approval for one's product to be successful in the marketplace—today, there is an entirely different set of requirements to fulfill in order for a new technology or product to get reimbursed in the hospital or ambulatory care setting by Medicare or third-party payors, and in fact, each of these settings is oftentimes different from one another. Therefore, careful development planning, and the creation of a commercialization strategy early in the process, is essential to determine whether the investment will meet the revenue and profitability objectives of those underwriting the project. With that in mind, ensuring that developers have a robust understanding of the product development process, or that they engage with partners who themselves have a keen understanding of the journey from "bench to bedside," will increase the likelihood of both clinical and commercial success. When meaningful technological advancements are properly shepherded through the FDA (and other regulatory bodies), it is possible to make both important clinical contributions to the field of orthopaedics, as well as create significant value for those who invest the time and money to succeed.

REFERENCES

1. U.S. Food and Drug Administration. Good Laboratory Practice for Nonclinical Laboratory Studies. Available at: https://www.accessdata.fda.gov/scripts/cdrh/cfdocs/cfcfr/CFRSearch.cfm?CFRPart=58. Updated September 4, 2018. Accessed June 29, 2019.
2. U.S. Food and Drug Administration. Regulatory Considerations for Human Cells, Tissues, and Cellular and Tissue-Based Products: Minimal Manipulation and Homologous Use. Available at: https://www.fda.gov/regulatory-information/search-fda-guidance-documents/regulatory-considerations-human-cells-tissues-and-cellular-and-tissue-based-products-minimal. Published November, 2017. Updated December, 2017. Accessed June 29, 2019.
3. U.S. Food and Drug Administration. Warning Letter, Genetech, Inc. Available at: https://www.fda.gov/inspections-compliance-enforcement-and-criminal-investigations/warning-letters/genetech-inc-561808-11292018. November 29, 2018. Accessed June 29, 2019.
4. U.S. Food and Drug Administration. Warning Letter, Cord for Life Inc. Available at: https://www.fda.gov/inspections-compliance-enforcement-and-criminal-investigations/warning-letters/cord-life-inc-572770-03292019. March 29, 2019. Accessed June 29, 2019.
5. U.S. Food and Drug Administration. Warning Letter, US Stem Cell Clinic, LLC. Available at: https://www.fda.gov/inspections-compliance-enforcement-and-criminal-investigations/warning-letters/us-stem-cell-clinic-llc-524470-08242017. August 24, 2017. Accessed June 29, 2019.
6. U.S. Food and Drug Administration. FDA sends warning to company for marketing dangerous unapproved stem cell products that put patients at risk and puts other stem cell firms, providers on notice. Available at: https://www.fda.gov/news-events/press-announcements/fda-sends-warning-company-marketing-dangerous-unapproved-stem-cell-products-put-patients-risk-and. December 20, 2018. Accessed June 29, 2019.
7. U.S. Food and Drug Administration. Mary A. Malarkey, Director, Office of Compliance and Biologics Quality. Center for Biologics Evaluation and Research. Available at: https://www.fda.gov/media/119936/download. December 20, 2018. Accessed June 29, 2019.

©Copyright 2021 American Academy of Orthopaedic Surgeons

Index

Note: Page numbers followed by "*f*" indicate figures and "*t*" indicate tables.

©Copyright 2021 American Academy of Orthopaedic Surgeons

C

©Copyright 2021 American Academy of Orthopaedic Surgeons

©Copyright 2021 American Academy of Orthopaedic Surgeons

©Copyright 2021 American Academy of Orthopaedic Surgeons

©Copyright 2021 American Academy of Orthopaedic Surgeons

©Copyright 2021 American Academy of Orthopaedic Surgeons

N

O

©Copyright 2021 American Academy of Orthopaedic Surgeons

©Copyright 2021 American Academy of Orthopaedic Surgeons

P

©Copyright 2021 American Academy of Orthopaedic Surgeons

©Copyright 2021 American Academy of Orthopaedic Surgeons

©Copyright 2021 American Academy of Orthopaedic Surgeons

T

©Copyright 2021 American Academy of Orthopaedic Surgeons

©Copyright 2021 American Academy of Orthopaedic Surgeons